LABORATORY DIAGNOSIS OF INFECTIOUS DISEASES

Essentials of Diagnostic Microbiology

LABORATORY DIAGNOSIS OF INFECTIOUS DISEASES

Essentials of Diagnostic Microbiology

Paul G. Engelkirk, Ph.D., MT(ASCP), SM(AAM)

President, Biomed Ed
(Biomedical Educational Services)
Belton, Texas

Janet Duben-Engelkirk, Ed.D., MT(ASCP), CLS(NCA)

Chair, Biotechnology Department
Temple College and the Texas Bioscience Institute
Temple, Texas

. Wolters Kluwer | Lippincott Williams & Wilkins
Health

Acquisitions Editor: Peter Sabatini
Managing Editor: Kevin C. Dietz
Marketing Manager: Alison M. Noplock
Production Editor: Julie Montalbano
Designer: Doug Smock
Compositor: Aptara, Inc.

Library of Congress Cataloging-in-Publication Data

Engelkirk, Paul G.
     Laboratory diagnosis of infectious diseases : essentials of diagnostic microbiology /
Paul G. Engelkirk, Janet Duben-Engelkirk.
         p. ; cm.
     Includes bibliographical references.
     ISBN-13: 978-0-7817-9701-6
     1. Diagnostic microbiology.   2. Communicable Diseases—Diagnosis—Laboratory manuals.
I. Duben-Engelkirk, Janet L.   II. Title.
     [DNLM: 1. Communicable Diseases—diagnosis.   2. Microbiological Techniques—methods.
QW 25 E57L 2008]
     QR67.E54 2008
     616.9'0475—dc22
                                                            2007019766

DISCLAIMER

Care has been taken to confirm the accuracy of the information present and to describe generally accepted practices. However, the authors, editors, and publisher are not responsible for errors or omissions or for any consequences from application of the information in this book and make no warranty, expressed or implied, with respect to the currency, completeness, or accuracy of the contents of the publication. Application of this information in a particular situation remains the professional responsibility of the practitioner; the clinical treatments described and recommended may not be considered absolute and universal recommendations.

The authors, editors, and publisher have exerted every effort to ensure that drug selection and dosage set forth in this text are in accordance with the current recommendations and practice at the time of publication. However, in view of ongoing research, changes in government regulations, and the constant flow of information relating to drug therapy and drug reactions, the reader is urged to check the package insert for each drug for any change in indications and dosage and for added warnings and precautions. This is particularly important when the recommended agent is a new or infrequently employed drug.

Some drugs and medical devices presented in this publication have Food and Drug Administration (FDA) clearance for limited use in restricted research settings. It is the responsibility of the health care provider to ascertain the FDA status of each drug or device planned for use in their clinical practice.

This Book is Dedicated to . . .

Paul's sister Sue, her husband Bob, and Jan's brother Ken, in appreciation for the love and kindness that they unselfishly contributed to our mothers' care during their final days,

and

the many heroes—both the praised and the unsung—who have devoted their lives to the diagnosis and treatment of infectious diseases worldwide and to the equally important professionals who educated them.

About the Authors

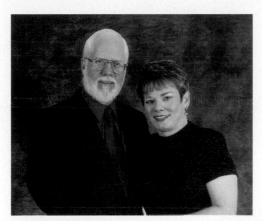

Paul G. Engelkirk, Ph.D., MT(ASCP), SM(AAM)

Dr. Engelkirk has been engaged in various aspects of clinical microbiology for more than 40 years and is a Past President of the Rocky Mountain Branch of the American Society for Microbiology. He received his bachelor's degree (in Biology) from New York University and his master's and doctoral degrees (both in Microbiology and Public Health) from Michigan State University. He received additional medical technology and tropical medicine training at Walter Reed Army Hospital in Washington, D.C., and specialized training in anaerobic bacteriology, mycobacteriology, and virology at the Centers for Disease Control and Prevention in Atlanta, Georgia.

Dr. Engelkirk served 22 years as an officer in the U.S. Army Medical Department supervising a variety of immunology, clinical pathology, and microbiology laboratories in Germany, Vietnam, and the United States. He retired with the rank of Lieutenant Colonel. Following his military service, he devoted 20 years to microbiology education, including 8 years as an Associate Professor at the University of Texas Health Science Center in Houston, Texas, teaching diagnostic microbiology to medical technology students, and 12 years as a Professor of Biological Sciences in the Science Department at Central Texas College in Killeen, Texas, teaching introductory microbiology to nursing students.

Dr. Engelkirk is the author or co-author of four microbiology textbooks, ten additional book chapters, five medical laboratory-oriented self-study courses, and many scientific articles. Over the years, he and his wife, Janet, have edited and published a variety of educational newsletters for clinical microbiology laboratory personnel on such topics as anaerobic bacteriology, clinical parasitology, medical mycology, and diagnostic microbiology. He and Janet currently provide biomedical educational services through their consulting firm (Biomed Ed), located in Belton, Texas. Dr. Engelkirk's hobbies include RVing, hiking, kayaking, nature photography, and working in his yard.

Janet Duben-Engelkirk, Ed.D., MT(ASCP), CLS(NCA)

Dr. Duben-Engelkirk has over 30 years of experience in clinical laboratory science and higher education. She received bachelor's degrees in biology and medical technology and a master's degree in technical education from the University of Akron, and her doctorate in allied health education and administration from a combined program through the University of Houston and Baylor College of Medicine in Houston, Texas.

Dr. Duben-Engelkirk began her career in clinical laboratory science education teaching students "on the bench" in a community hospital in Akron, Ohio. She then became Education Coordinator for the Clinical Laboratory Science Program at the University of Texas Health Science Center at Houston, where she taught clinical chemistry and related subjects for 12 years. In 1992, Dr. Duben-Engelkirk assumed the position of Director of Allied Health and Clinical Laboratory Science Education at Scott and White Hospital in Temple, Texas, where her responsibilities included teaching microbiology and clinical chemistry. She also served as Interim Program Director for the Medical Laboratory Technician program at Temple College. Currently, Dr. Duben-Engelkirk is the Chair of the Biotechnology Department at Temple College and the Texas Bioscience Institute in Temple, where she is responsible for the administration of the biotechnology degree and certificate programs. The Biotechnology Programs and the Texas Bioscience

Institute recently received the prestigious Bellwether Award for community colleges. Dr. Duben-Engelkirk was co-editor of a widely used clinical chemistry textbook and co-authored a clinical anaerobic bacteriology textbook with her husband, Paul. She has authored or co-authored numerous book chapters, journal articles, self-study courses, newsletters, and other educational materials.

Dr. Duben-Engelkirk has received many awards during her career, including Outstanding Young Leader in Allied Health, the American Society for Clinical Laboratory Science's Omicron Sigma Award for outstanding service, and Teaching Excellence Awards. Her professional interests include instructional technology, web-based instruction, and computer applications. Outside of the office and classroom, Dr. Duben-Engelkirk enjoys taking cruises, reading, music, yoga, movies, and hiking and RVing with Paul and their miniature schnauzer, Lacy.

Preface

Microbiology—the study of microbes—is a fascinating and extremely important subject. We are surrounded by microscopic critters that impact our daily lives in a variety of ways. In addition to the numerous beneficial aspects of microbes, many of them cause disease. In recent years, the public has been bombarded by news reports about microbe-associated medical problems such as bird flu, SARS, monkeypox, flesh-eating bacteria, mad cow disease, superbugs, black mould in buildings, West Nile virus, Ebola virus, bioterrorism, anthrax, smallpox, food recalls due to the presence of bacterial pathogens, and epidemics of meningitis, hepatitis, influenza, tuberculosis. and diarrheal diseases.

Imagine how rewarding it would be to play a major role in the diagnosis of microbial diseases. *Laboratory Diagnosis of Infectious Diseases* is intended for both teaching and learning about diagnostic microbiology. Although laboratory professionals do not actually diagnose diseases, they provide valuable assistance to clinicians by furnishing them with accurate and timely laboratory observations and test results. Throughout this book, the term "laboratory diagnosis of infectious diseases" refers to the various laboratory observations and test results, which, when received and evaluated by clinicians, assist them to correctly diagnose infectious diseases and initiate appropriate therapy.

This book, unlike some of the other books on the market, focuses on the **essentials** of diagnostic microbiology and, therefore, its entire contents can be taught in a one-semester course. The book contains many pedagogical features designed to make the text **student friendly** and its contents easily learned. Each chapter contains an outline, learning objectives, study aids, key points reemphasized in the margins, a list of new terms, a chapter review, and self-assessment exercises. Also included in the book are numerous full-color illustrations, an extensive glossary, and appendices containing detailed clinical microbiology laboratory procedures, useful conversion formulas, and answers to self-assessment exercises.

Much of the material contained in more lengthy diagnostic microbiology textbooks has been omitted in an effort to provide a **concise presentation** of the information required by those who will be performing clinical microbiology laboratory procedures. However, each chapter also contains a list of References and Suggested Reading, where students may find more in-depth information on specific topics.

The first seven chapters provide a background on pathogens, infectious diseases, host defense mechanisms, clinical specimens, and the organization and responsibilities of the clinical microbiology laboratory. Chapters 8 through 25 discuss the **most important** bacterial, fungal, parasitic, and viral pathogens as well as the infectious diseases that they cause and how clinical laboratory professionals assist in the diagnosis of these diseases. Chapter 26 contains timely information regarding the role of the clinical microbiology laboratory in healthcare epidemiology and the hospital's response to bioterrorist attacks.

A variety of pedagogical features, such as additional self-assessment exercises and answers, case studies, puzzles, and in-depth discussions of selected topics, can be found on the accompanying Student CD-ROM. Appendices on the Student CD-ROM provide useful information on topics such as microbial intoxications and choice of culture media and guidance regarding the work-up of colonies that are present on primary isolation plates. At the Lippincott Williams & Wilkins Web site (www.thePoint.com), instructors will find a comprehensive test generator and an image bank.

This book has been written in response to numerous requests for a **concise, understandable,** and **easy-to-use** text that covers only the **basics** of diagnostic microbiology. The authors welcome comments from users of the book as to how future editions might be improved.

Our sincere thanks to Robert C. Fader, Ph.D., Thomas W. Huber, Ph.D., Dale D. Dingley, M.P.H., and all others who contributed to the reviewing, editing, and production of this book. Special thanks to the authors of other Lippincott Williams & Wilkins textbooks whose illustrations appear throughout the book and to Pat Hidy, Ed.D., and the LWW artists for their excellent drawings.

—P.G.E.
—J.D.E.

Consultants

Robert C. Fader, Ph.D., D(ABMM)
Section Chief, Microbiology/Virology Laboratories
Scott and White Hospital
Temple, Texas

Assistant Professor
Department of Pathology
Texas A&M System Health Science Center, College of Medicine
Temple, Texas

Thomas W. Huber, Ph.D., D(ABMM)
Microbiologist, Pathology and Laboratory Medicine
Central Texas Veterans Health Care System, Olin E. Teague Medical Center
Temple, Texas

Associate Professor
Department of Pathology and Department of Medical Microbiology and Immunology
Texas A&M System Health Science Center, College of Medicine
Temple, Texas

Reviewers

Dale D. Dingley, M.P.H., M(ASCP)
Former Chief Parasitologist for the State of Texas
Austin, Texas

Patrick K. Hidy, RN, Ed.D.
Former Chairman, Science Department
Central Texas College
Killeen, Texas

Mary Ruth Beckham, M.Ed., MT(ASCP)
Director, Program in Clinical Laboratory Science
Scott and White Hospital
Temple, Texas

Contents

SECTION

I

Introduction to Microbes and the Diseases They Cause

CHAPTER 1

Microbes and the Science of Microbiology

Chapter Outline

LEARNING OBJECTIVES

After studying this chapter, you should be able to:

- Define the terms and abbreviations introduced in this chapter (e.g., *bacteriology, capsule, cell membrane*)
- Differentiate between microbial intoxications and infectious diseases
- Compare and contrast acellular and cellular microbes, and cite an example of each
- Given diagrams of procaryotic and eucaryotic microorganisms, label the structural components
- Cite a function for each of the following parts of a eucaryotic cell: cell membrane, nucleus, ribosomes, Golgi apparatus, lysosomes, mitochondria, plastids, cytoskeleton, cell wall, flagella, cilia
- Cite a function for each of the following parts of a bacterial cell: cell membrane, chromosome, cell wall, capsule, flagella, pili, endospores
- Identify the genus and specific epithet portions of the names of species (e.g., *Escherichia coli*)
- Compare the five-kingdom and three-domain systems of classification with regard to categories of procaryotes and eucaryotes

AIDS. Malaria. Tuberculosis. Collectively, these infectious diseases cause about 5 million deaths each year. Yet they are only three of hundreds of infectious diseases—diseases that maim, cripple, and kill; diseases that can strike anyone, at anytime, and in any part of the world; diseases that may occur naturally or may be spread by carelessness or design. To compound matters, previously unrecognized infectious diseases are constantly emerging. Imagine how exciting and rewarding it would be to play a role in diagnosing these terrible diseases.

TERMS AND DEFINITIONS

Microbiology is the study of microbes. **Microbes** consist of two major groups: (1) cellular microbes, and (2) acellular microbes (Fig. 1-1).

> Microbiology is the study of microbes. The two major categories of microbes are acellular microbes and microorganisms.

Cellular microbes are composed of cells; therefore, they are considered living organisms and are usually referred to as **microorganisms** (tiny organisms).[1] Examples of cellular microorganisms are bacteria, archaea, microscopic algae, protozoa, and microscopic fungi (yeasts and moulds).[2]

---

[1] *The cell theory states that all living organisms are composed of cells. It was first proposed in the late 1830s by Matthias Schleiden (a German botanist) and Theodor Schwann (a German zoologist).*

[2] *The term for single-celled fungi may be spelled* moulds *or* molds. *Mycologists prefer* moulds; *therefore, that spelling is used throughout the book.*

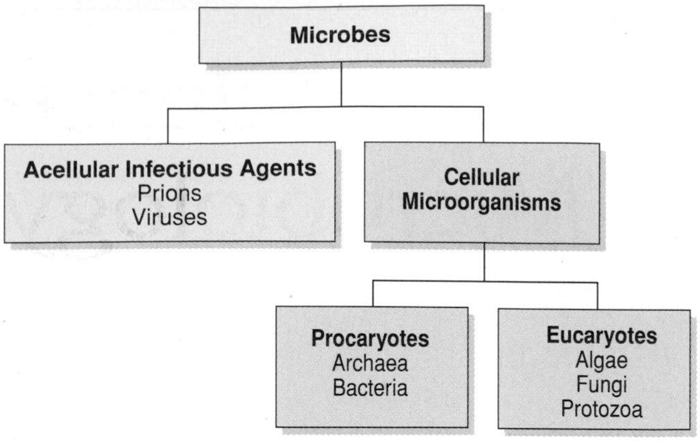

Figure 1-1. **Acellular and cellular microbes.** Acellular microbes include prions and viruses. Cellular microbes include the less complex procaryotes (archaea and bacteria) and the more complex eucaryotes (algae, protozoa, and fungi).

Acellular microbes, on the other hand, are not composed of cells. They are smaller than cells, and their structures are far less complex than those of cells. Because they are not composed of cells, the acellular microbes are considered by most scientists to be nonliving entities. They are often referred to as infectious agents or infectious particles. Viruses and prions are examples of acellular microbes. Virtually all microbes, both the cellular and acellular types, are microscopic, meaning that a microscope is required to see them.[3]

Some microbes cause disease, whereas others do not. Although sometimes referred to as "germs," the technical term for the microbes that cause disease is **pathogens**. The microbes that do not cause disease are called **nonpathogens**. For humans, some nonpathogens are beneficial and some have no effect. (Beneficial aspects of nonpathogens are briefly discussed on the CD-ROM that accompanies this book.) Other microbes, many of which live on and in the human body,[4] are called **opportunistic** pathogens (or **opportunists**). They usually do not cause any health problems, but they have the potential to cause disease if they gain access to a part of the anatomy where they do not belong. One example is the bacterium *Escherichia coli*, which lives in the human intestinal tract. This organism does not cause any harm as long as it stays in the intestinal tract, but it can cause disease if it gains

> The microbes that cause disease are called pathogens. If they only cause disease under certain conditions, they are called opportunistic pathogens.

access to the urinary bladder, the bloodstream, or a wound. Some opportunistic pathogens strike when a person becomes run down, stressed, or debilitated (weakened) as a result of some disease or condition. Opportunistic pathogens can be thought of as microbes awaiting the opportunity to cause disease.

DISEASES CAUSED BY PATHOGENS

In his discussion of Anton van Leeuwenhoek,[5] thought by many to be the father of microbiology, Paul de Kruif (see "References and Suggested Reading") described pathogens as follows:

[Leeuwenhoek] had stolen and peeped into a fantastic sub-visible world of little things, creatures that had lived, had bred, had battled, had died, completely hidden from and unknown to all men from the beginning of time. Beasts these were of a kind that ravaged and annihilated whole races of men ten million times larger than they were themselves. Beings these were, more terrible than fire-spitting dragons or hydra-headed monsters. They were silent assassins that murdered babes in warm cradles and kings in sheltered places. It was this invisible, insignificant, but implacable—and sometimes friendly—world that Leeuwenhoek had looked into for the first time of all men of all countries.

Pathogens cause two categories of diseases: infectious diseases and microbial intoxications (Fig. 1-2). An **infectious disease** results when a pathogen invades the body and subsequently causes disease. A **microbial intoxication** results when a person ingests a **toxin** (poisonous substance) that has been produced by a pathogen. Of the two categories, infectious diseases cause far more illnesses and deaths.

> Microbes cause two categories of diseases: infectious diseases and microbial intoxications.

NONLIVING, ACELLULAR INFECTIOUS AGENTS

The nonliving, acellular infectious agents discussed in this book include viruses and prions. Viruses and the diseases they cause are discussed in detail in Chapters 24 and 25.

---

[3] Helminths *(parasitic worms) are described in Chapters 21 and 23. Helminths are multicellular animals and, although they are microscopic at some stage(s) in their life cycles, they are not considered microorganisms. In fact, some adult helminths are extremely long—up to 10 meters in some cases. Helminths are included in this book because information obtained in the clinical microbiology laboratory is used in the diagnosis of helminth infections.*

[4]*Microbes that live on and in the human body are collectively referred to as the **indigenous microflora**. The older term,* normal flora, *is still in common usage. It has been estimated that the indigenous microflora of humans may number as high as 100 trillion organisms, consisting of as many as 500 to 1,000 species. Many of these microbes are beneficial. They inhibit the growth of pathogens in areas of the body where they live by occupying space, depleting the food supply, and secreting materials (waste products, toxins, antibiotics, etc.) that may prevent or reduce the growth of pathogens.*

[5]*During the mid-to-late 1600s, a Dutchman named Anton van Leeuwenhoek was the first person to observe live bacteria and protozoa, using simple microscopes he had constructed.*

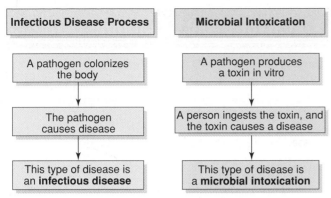

Figure 1-2. **The two categories of diseases caused by pathogens.** An infectious disease results when a pathogen colonizes (inhabits) the body and subsequently causes disease. Microbial intoxication results when a person ingests a toxin (poisonous substance) that has been produced by a microorganism in vitro (outside the body).

Prions (pronounced "pree-ons") are small infectious proteins (i.e., protein molecules capable of causing diseases).

> The two groups of acellular microbes that cause human disease are viruses and prions.

Prions cause fatal neurological diseases in animals,[6] such as scrapie (pronounced "scrape-ee") in sheep and goats; bovine spongiform encephalopathy ("mad cow disease"); and kuru, Creutzfeldt-Jakob disease, Gerstmann-Sträussler-Scheinker disease, and fatal familial insomnia in humans. Similar diseases in mink, mule deer, western whitetail deer, elk, and cats may also be caused by prions. The term *scrapie* comes from the observation that infected animals scrape themselves against fence posts and other objects in an effort to relieve the intense itching (pruritus) associated with the disease. The disease in deer and elk is called chronic wasting disease, in reference to the irreversible weight loss the animals experience. All these prion diseases are fatal spongiform encephalopathies—diseases of the brain, in which the brain becomes spongelike, filled with amyloid proteins that replace the neurons that are normally found there.

The mechanism by which prions cause disease remains a mystery, although it is thought that prions convert functional protein molecules into nonfunctional ones by causing the functional molecules to change their shape. Many scientists remain unconvinced that proteins alone can cause disease. Because the clinical microbiology laboratory currently does not play a role in the diagnosis of prion diseases, prions will not be discussed further in this book. It is possible that laboratory tests will become available in the future to diagnose prion diseases, at which time, clinical microbiology laboratory professionals may perform those procedures.

LIVING, CELLULAR MICROORGANISMS

According to the cell theory, all living organisms are composed of cells. Considerable evidence exists to indicate that between 3.5 billion and 4 billion years ago, the first bit of life to appear on the earth was a very primitive cell similar to the simple bacteria of today. Bacterial cells exhibit all the characteristics of life, although they do not have the complex system of membranes and **organelles** (tiny organlike structures) found in the more advanced organisms. These less complex cells, which include bacteria and archaea, are called **procaryotes** or procaryotic cells (Fig. 1-3). The more complex cells—those containing a true nucleus and many membrane-bound organelles—are called

> Cellular microorganisms are divided into two major categories: procaryotes and eucaryotes.

> Eucaryotic cells possess a true nucleus, whereas procaryotic cells do not.

eucaryotes or eucaryotic cells (Fig. 1-4).[7] Eucaryotes include organisms like algae, protozoa, fungi, plants, animals, and humans.

Some microbes are procaryotic, some are eucaryotic, and as previously discussed, some are not cells at all. Learning the differences in the structures of these diverse groups of microbes helps us to better

> Eucaryotic cells possess numerous membranes and membrane-bound structures. The only membrane possessed by a procaryotic cell is the cell membrane or cytoplasmic membrane.

understand pathogenic (disease-causing) mechanisms and why some drugs are effective against one group but not others. Table 1-1 summarizes key differences between procaryotic and eucaryotic cells.

Procaryotic Genome

Bacterial cells usually contain only one **chromosome**, which consists of a long, supercoiled, circular, deoxyribonucleic acid (DNA) molecule. The bacterial chromosome serves as the control center of the bacterial cell. It is capable of duplicating itself, guiding cell division, and directing cellular activities. A procaryotic cell contains neither nucleoplasm nor a nuclear membrane. The chromosome is suspended or embedded in the cytoplasm. The DNA-occupied space within a bacterial cell is sometimes referred to as the bacterial nucleoid. (The suffix *-oid* means "like" or "similar to"; *nucleoid* means "like or similar to a nucleus.")

---

[6] *Although humans are technically animals, the word* animals *is used in this book in reference to animals other than humans.*

[7] *Alternate spellings of* procaryote/procaryotic *and* eucaryote/eucaryotic *are* prokaryote/prokaryotic *and* eukaryote/eukaryotic.

TABLE 1 - 1 Key Differences Between Procaryotic and Eucaryotic Cells

Structure or Component	Procaryotic Cells	Eucaryotic Cells
Cell membrane: also known as the cellular, plasma, or cytoplasmic membrane; separates the contents of the cell from the "outer world"; its function is selective permeability, meaning that it regulates the passage of materials into and out of the cell; some materials will be able to pass through the cell membrane, whereas others will not (Fig. 1-5)	Possessed by all	Possessed by all
Cytoplasm: the semifluid, gelatinous, nutrient matrix enclosed by the cell membrane; within which are found various structures and components	Possessed by all	Possessed by all
Nucleus: a true nucleus consists of three components— a gelatinous matrix known as nucleoplasm, chromosomes, and a nuclear membrane; the nucleus serves as the "command center" of eucaryotic cells	Not found in procaryotic cells	Possessed by all (although rare, some eucaryotic cells possess more than one nucleus)
Endoplasmic reticulum (ER): a highly convoluted system of membranes running throughout the cytoplasm; ribosomes are attached to some areas of the ER, giving it a rough appearance (**rough ER**) when observed with an electron microscope; sections of ER where ribosomes are not attached are referred to as **smooth ER**	Not found in procaryotic cells	Possessed by all
Ribosomes: the sites of protein synthesis; clusters of ribosomes are referred to as polyribosomes or polysomes; ribosomes are composed of proteins and rRNA molecules	Possessed by all	Possessed by all
Golgi apparatus (also known as the Golgi complex or Golgi body): connects with the ER; where newly synthesized proteins are transformed into mature, functional proteins, which are then packaged into membrane-bound vesicles for storage within the cell or transport out of the cell; sometimes referred to as "packaging plants"	Not found in procaryotic cells	Possessed by all
Lysosomes: membrane-bound vesicles containing digestive enzymes	Not found in procaryotic cells	Possessed by all
Mitochondria (sing. *mitochondrion*): sometimes referred to as "power plants," "powerhouses," or "energy factories"; structures within which a great deal of energy is produced	Not found in procaryotic cells	Possessed by all
Plastids: the sites of photosynthesis, a process by which light energy is converted into chemical energy; a chloroplast is an example	Not found in procaryotic cells	Possessed by cells of photosynthetic eucaryotes, such as algae and plants

(continued)

TABLE 1-1   Continued

Structure or Component	Procaryotic Cells	Eucaryotic Cells
Cell wall: rigid structure lying outside of the cell membrane; provides rigidity, shape, and protection	Possessed by virtually all; notable exceptions are bacteria in the genus *Mycoplasma* (discussed later in the book)	Possessed by algal, fungal, and plant cells, but not by protozoal, animal, or human cells
Glycocalyx: slimy, gelatinous, polysaccharide material found outside of the cell wall; there are two types of glycocalyx—a **slime layer**, which consists of unorganized, loosely attached material, and a **capsule**, which consists of organized, firmly attached material	Some procaryotes possess a slime layer, others possess a capsule, and others possess neither; the capsule serves an antiphagocytic function, meaning that it protects encapsulated bacteria from being phagocytized by white blood cells	Not found in eucaryotes
Flagella (sing. *flagellum*): long appendages that enable cells to be motile; they move in a whiplike manner; the internal structure of procaryotic flagella is much different than that of eucaryotic flagella	Possessed by some; composed of threads of a protein called flagellin	Possessed by some; protozoa with flagella are referred to as flagellates; a eucaryotic flagellum contains microtubules that run the length of the flagellum
Cilia (sing. *cilium*): short, hairlike appendages that enable cells to be motile	Not found on procaryotic cells	Possessed by some; protozoa that possess cilia are referred to as ciliates; a eucaryotic cilium contains microtubules that run the length of the cilium
Pili (sing. *pilus*): long, thin appendages that enable cells to attach to surfaces; a special type of pilus known as a sex pilus is described later in the book; pili are also referred to as fimbriae	Possessed by some	Not found in eucaryotes
Spores: thick-walled structures, usually produced within cells	Possessed by some; bacterial spores are technically known as **endospores**; produced by some bacteria as a means of survival	Possessed or produced by some (e.g., moulds); their function is reproduction

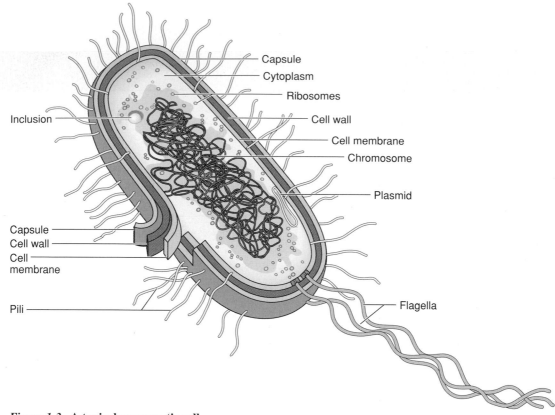

Capsule
Cytoplasm
Ribosomes
Inclusion
Cell wall
Cell membrane
Chromosome
Plasmid
Capsule
Cell wall
Cell membrane
Pili
Flagella

Figure 1-3. **A typical procaryotic cell.**

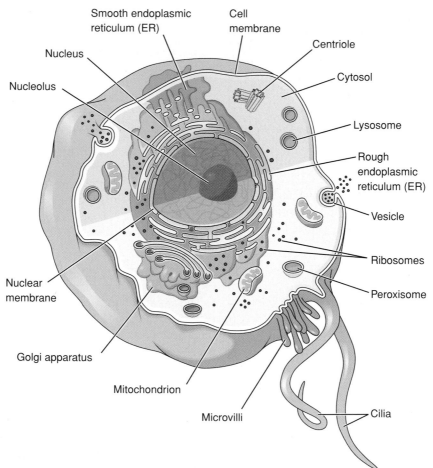

Smooth endoplasmic reticulum (ER)
Cell membrane
Nucleus
Centriole
Nucleolus
Cytosol
Lysosome
Rough endoplasmic reticulum (ER)
Vesicle
Ribosomes
Nuclear membrane
Peroxisome
Golgi apparatus
Mitochondrion
Microvilli
Cilia

Figure 1-4. **A typical eucaryotic cell.** (From Cohen BJ, Taylor JJ. Memmler's The Human Body in Health and Disease. 10th Ed. Philadelphia: Lippincott Williams & Wilkins, 2005.)

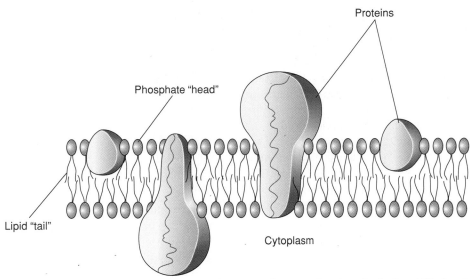

Figure 1-5. **The lipid bilayer structure of cell membranes, showing the hydrophilic heads and hydrophobic tails of phospholipid molecules.** Cell membranes also contain protein molecules, which have been described as resembling "icebergs floating in a sea of lipids."

Genes are located along the bacterial chromosome. Although genes are sometimes described as "beads on a string," each bead (gene) is actually a particular segment of the DNA molecule. Each gene contains the genetic information (or genetic code) that enables the cell to produce a **gene product**. Most gene products are proteins, but some genes code for the production of two types of ribonucleic acid (RNA): ribosomal ribonucleic acid (rRNA) and transfer ribonucleic acid (tRNA) molecules. The organism's complete collection of genes is referred to as that organism's **genotype** or **genome**.

> An organism's complete collection of genes is referred to as its genotype or genome.

Gene products influence the organism's **phenotype**, which can be thought of as all the attributes, characteristics, or properties of the organism. An organism's phenotype is a manifestation of that organism's genotype. Phenotypic characteristics of humans include such attributes as eye, hair, and skin color, and genetic tendencies to develop various hereditary diseases. Phenotypic characteristics of bacteria include the following:

> An organism's phenotype includes all the attributes, characteristics, or properties of the organism. Phenotype is determined by genotype.

- Cell shape and morphologic arrangement (grouping) of the cells

- The organism's Gram reaction (i.e., what color the cells stain in the Gram staining procedure, which is described later in the book)

- Composition of the cell wall

- Presence or absence of a capsule

- Presence or absence of flagella and, if present, their number and location on the cell

- Ability to sporulate (produce endospores)

- Presence or absence of pili (including a sex pilus)

- Presence or absence of various enzymes

The thin and tightly folded chromosome of an *E. coli* cell is about 1.5 mm (1,500 μm) long and only 2 nm wide. Because a typical *E. coli* cell is about 2 to 3 μm long, its chromosome is approximately 500 to 750 times longer than the cell itself—quite a packaging feat. Bacterial chromosomes contain between 450 and 8,000 genes, depending on the species. Thus, a bacterial chromosome contains sufficient genetic information to code for between 450 and 8,000 gene products (enzymes, other proteins, rRNA, and tRNA molecules). In comparison, the chromosomes within a human cell contain about 25,000 to 30,000 genes—enough to code for approximately 25,000 to 30,000 gene products.

Small, circular molecules of double-stranded DNA that are not part of the chromosome (referred to as extrachromosomal DNA or **plasmids**) may also be present in the cytoplasm of procaryotic cells. A plasmid may contain anywhere from fewer than 10 genes to several hundred genes. A bacterial cell may contain one plasmid, multiple copies of the same plasmid, or more than one type of plasmid (i.e., plasmids containing different genes). Thus, a bacterial cell's complete genome consists of the genes located on its chromosome *plus* the genes located on any plasmids that it possesses.

Eucaryotic Genome

As previously mentioned, the primary difference between procaryotic and eucaryotic cells is that eucaryotic cells possess a "true nucleus," whereas procaryotic cells do not. The **nucleus** unifies, controls, and integrates the functions of the entire cell and can be thought of as the "command center" of the cell. The nucleus has three components: nucleoplasm, chromosomes, and a nuclear membrane. **Nucleoplasm** is the gelatinous matrix or base material of the nucleus; like cytoplasm, nucleoplasm is a type of **protoplasm**. The chromosomes are embedded or suspended in the nucleoplasm. The membrane that serves as a "skin" around the nucleus is called the **nuclear membrane**; it contains holes (nuclear pores) through which large molecules can enter and exit the nucleus.

Eucaryotic chromosomes consist of linear DNA molecules and proteins (histones and nonhistone proteins). The number and composition of chromosomes and the number of genes on each chromosome are characteristic of the particular species of organism. Different species have different numbers and sizes of chromosomes. Human diploid cells, for example, have 46 chromosomes (23 pairs), each consisting of thousands of genes. As previously mentioned, it has been estimated that the human genome consists of about 25,000 to 30,000 genes.

When observed using a transmission electron microscope (see Chapter 6), a dark (electron-dense) area can be seen within the nucleus. This area is called the **nucleolus**; it is here that rRNA molecules are manufactured. The rRNA molecules then exit the nucleus to become part of the structure of ribosomes (ribosomes are described in Table 1-1).

TAXONOMY, MICROBIAL CLASSIFICATION, AND BINOMIAL NOMENCLATURE

Taxonomy is the science of classification of living organisms. According to *Bergey's Manual of Systematic Bacteriology* (see "References and Suggested Reading"), taxonomy consists of three separate but interrelated areas: classification, nomenclature, and identification. **Classification** is the arrangement of organisms into taxonomic groups (known as **taxa**) on the basis of similarities or relationships. Taxa include kingdoms or domains, divisions or phyla, classes, orders, families, genera, and species (see the Study Aid). Closely related organisms (i.e., organisms having similar characteristics) are placed into the same taxon. **Nomenclature** is the assignment of names to the various taxa according to international rules. **Identification** is the process of determining whether an isolate belongs to one of the established, named taxa or represents a previously unidentified species.

When attempting to learn the identity of a microorganism that has been isolated from a clinical specimen, personnel working in clinical microbiology laboratories are very much like detectives or crime scene investigators (Fig. 1-6). They gather "clues" (characteristics, attributes, properties, traits) about the organism until they have a sufficient number of clues to identify (speciate) the culprit. In most cases, the "clues" gathered will match the characteristics of an established species. (Note: Throughout this book, the phrase "to identify an organism" means to learn the organism's species name—i.e., to speciate it.) Consult the CD-ROM for more information about the connection between laboratory professionals and crime scene investigators.

The science of taxonomy is based on the binomial system developed in the 18th century by the Swedish scientist Carolus Linnaeus. In the binomial system, each organism is given two names (e.g., *Homo sapiens* for humans). The first name is the **genus (pl.** *genera*), and the second name is the **specific epithet**. The first and second names together are referred to as the **species**. Thus, *Homo* is a genus and *Homo sapiens* is a species.

> In the binomial system of nomenclature, the first name (e.g., *Escherichia*) is the genus, and the second name (e.g., *coli*) is the specific epithet. When used together, the first and second names (e.g., *Escherichia coli*) are referred to as a species.

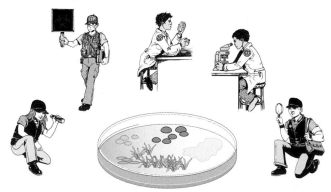

***Figure 1-6.* Clinical microbiology laboratory professionals are very much like detectives or crime scene investigators.** They gather "clues" about the organism until they have a sufficient number of clues to identify (speciate) the culprit.

TABLE 1 - 2   Examples of Bacteria Named for the Diseases They Cause[a]

Bacterium	Disease
Bacillus anthracis	Anthrax
Chlamydophila pneumoniae	Pneumonia
Chlamydophila psittaci	Psittacosis (parrot fever)
Chlamydia trachomatis	Trachoma
Clostridium botulinum	Botulism
Clostridium tetani	Tetanus
Corynebacterium diphtheriae	Diphtheria
Francisella tularensis	Tularemia (rabbit fever)
Klebsiella pneumoniae	Pneumonia
Mycobacterium leprae	Leprosy (Hansen disease)
Mycobacterium tuberculosis	Tuberculosis
Mycoplasma pneumoniae	Pneumonia
Neisseria gonorrhoeae	Gonorrhea
Neisseria meningitidis	Meningitis
Streptococcus pneumoniae	Pneumonia
Vibrio cholerae	Cholera

[a]In some cases, these bacteria cause more than one disease.

Because written reference is often made to genera and species, biologists throughout the world have adopted a standard method of expressing these names. To express the genus, the first letter of the word is capitalized and the whole word underlined or italicized—for example, *Escherichia*. To express the species, the first letter of the genus name is capitalized (the specific epithet is not capitalized) and then the entire species name is underlined or italicized—for example, *Escherichia coli*. Frequently, the genus is designated by a single-letter abbreviation, as in *E. coli*. In an essay or article about *Escherichia coli*, *Escherichia* would be spelled out the first time the organism is mentioned; thereafter, the abbreviated form, *E. coli*, could be used. The abbreviation *sp.* indicates a single species, and the abbreviation *spp.* indicates more than one species.

In addition to proper scientific names for bacteria, acceptable names like staphylococci (for *Staphylococcus* spp.), streptococci (for *Streptococcus* spp.), clostridia (for *Clostridium* spp.), pseudomonads (for *Pseudomonas* spp.), mycoplasmas (for *Mycoplasma* spp.), rickettsias (for *Rickettsia* spp.), and chlamydiae (for *Chlamydia* spp.) are com-

monly used in health care settings. Bacterial nicknames and slang frequently used within hospitals are GC and gonococci (for *Neisseria gonorrhoeae*), meningococci (for *Neisseria meningitidis*), pneumococci (for *Streptococcus pneumoniae*), staph (for *Staphylococcus* or staphylococcal), and strep (for *Streptococcus* or streptococcal). It is common to hear health care professionals using names like meningococcal meningitis, pneumococcal pneumonia, staph infection, and strep throat.

Quite often, bacteria are named for the disease that they cause (see Table 1-2 for examples). However, in a few cases, bacteria are misnamed. For example, the bacterium *Haemophilus influenzae* does not cause influenza. Influenza is a respiratory disease caused by influenza viruses.

Each organism is categorized into larger groups based on their similarities and differences. In 1969, Robert H. Whittaker proposed a five-kingdom system of classification, in which all organisms are placed into five kingdoms:

• Bacteria and archaea (which in many ways are similar to bacteria) are in the **Kingdom Procaryotae** (or Kingdom

Monera). All organisms in this kingdom are procaryotic. Nearly all are unicellular and considered microorganisms. Many bacteria cause infections in humans; bacterial infections are discussed in Chapters 8 through 18. Archaea are common in nature but are thought not to cause any type of human disease and, for that reason, are not described in this book.

- Algae and protozoa are in the **Kingdom Protista**. All organisms in this kingdom are eucaryotic; they are referred to as **protists**. Some algae are microorganisms, whereas others (e.g., certain "seaweeds") are quite large. Although algae cause various microbial intoxications, they are only rarely associated with infectious diseases. Algal infections are discussed briefly in Chapter 2. Most protozoa are unicellular, and all are considered microorganisms. Various protozoa cause human infections, which are discussed in Chapters 21 and 22.

> In the five-kingdom system of classification, procaryotic microorganisms are in the Kingdom Procaryotae. Eucaryotic microorganisms are in the Protista and Fungi kingdoms.

- Fungi are in the **Kingdom Fungi**. All organisms in this kingdom are eucaryotic. Some fungi (e.g., yeasts and moulds) are microorganisms, whereas others (e.g., mushrooms and toadstools) are not. Many yeasts and moulds are human pathogens; fungal infections are discussed in Chapters 19 and 20.

- Plants are in the **Kingdom Plantae**. All organisms in this kingdom are eucaryotic. This kingdom contains no microorganisms.

- Animals are in the **Kingdom Animalia**. All organisms in this kingdom are eucaryotic. This kingdom contains no microorganisms. As previously mentioned, although humans are in the Kingdom Animalia, in this book the word *animals* refers to animals other than humans.

Each kingdom consists of divisions or phyla, which in turn are divided into classes, orders, families, genera, and species (Table 1-3). In some cases, species are divided into subspecies, their names consisting of a genus, a specific epithet, and a subspecific epithet (abbreviated *ssp.* or *subsp.*); an example would be the bacterium *Haemophilus influenzae* ssp. *aegyptius*, the most common cause of the medical condition referred to as pink eye. Although Whittaker's five-

TABLE 1 - 3 Comparison of Human and Bacterial Classifications[a]

Classification	Human	*Escherichia coli* (a medically important Gram-negative bacillus)[b]	*Staphylococcus aureus* (a medically important Gram-positive coccus)[b]
Kingdom (Domain)	Animalia (*Eucarya*)	Procaryotae (*Bacteria*)	Procaryotae (*Bacteria*)
Phylum	Chordata	Proteobacteria	Firmicutes
Class	Mammalia	Gammaproteobacteria	Bacilli
Order	Primates	Enterobacteriales	Bacillales
Family	Hominidae	Enterobacteriaceae	Staphylococcaceae
Genus	*Homo*	*Escherichia*	*Staphylococcus*
Species (a species has 2 names; the first name is the genus; the second name is the specific epithet)	*Homo sapiens*	*Escherichia coli*	*Staphylococcus aureus*

[a]The bacteriology classification is based on Boone DR, Castenholz RW, eds. The Archaea and the Deeply Branching and Phototrophic Bacteria. New York: Springer-Verlag, 2001. Garrity GM, ed. Bergey's Manual of Systematic Bacteriology, vol 1. 2nd Ed.
[b]The terms *Gram-negative* and *Gram-positive* relate to the colors of bacteria at the end of the Gram staining procedure (see Chapter 6). If the bacteria are pink to red, they are referred to as Gram-negative bacteria. If they are blue to purple, they are referred to as Gram-positive bacteria. A bacillus is a rod-shaped bacterium, and a coccus is a round bacterium.

kingdom system of classification has been the most popular classification system for the past 30 years or so, not all scientists agree with it; other taxonomic classification schemes exist. For example, some scientists do not agree that algae and protozoa should be placed into the same kingdom, and in some classification schemes, protozoa are placed into a subkingdom of the Kingdom Animalia. Prions and viruses are not included in the five-kingdom system of classification because they are not living cells; they are acellular.

In the late 1970s, Carl R. Woese devised a three-domain system of classification that is gaining in popularity among scientists. In this system, there are two domains of procaryotes (*Archaea* and *Bacteria*) and one domain (*Eucarya* or *Eukarya*) that includes all eucaryotic organisms. The word *Archaea* comes from *archae*, meaning "ancient." Note that the domain names are italicized. Domain *Archaea* contains two phyla and Domain *Bacteria* contains 23 phyla. The three-domain system is based on differences in the structure of certain rRNA molecules among organisms in the three domains.

> In the three-domain system of classification, procaryotic microorganisms are in the *Bacteria* and *Archaea* domains.

CAREERS IN MICROBIOLOGY

Many career fields are possible within the science of microbiology. For example, a person may specialize in the study of just one category of microbe. A bacteriologist is a scientist who specializes in **bacteriology**—the study of the structure, functions, and activities of bacteria. Scientists specializing in the field of **phycology** study the various types of algae and are called phycologists. Protozoologists explore the area of **protozoology**—the study of protozoa and their activities. Those who specialize in the study of fungi, or **mycology**, are called mycologists. **Virology** encompasses the study of viruses and their effects on living cells of all types. Virologists and cell biologists may become genetic engineers who transfer genetic material (DNA) from one cell type to another. Virologists may also study prions. A parasitologist is one who specializes in **parasitology**—the study of parasites. The parasites usually studied by parasitologists include parasitic protozoa, helminths, and certain arthropods.

Other career fields in microbiology pertain more to applied microbiology—that is, how knowledge of microbiology can be applied to different aspects of society, medicine, and industry. One such career field is the exciting and rewarding field of **clinical microbiology** (also called diagnostic microbiology), which is the focus of this book. Clinical microbiology is the subdiscipline of microbiology that is associated with the diagnosis of human infectious diseases. Procedures performed in the clinical microbiology laboratory include the isolation of pathogens from human clinical specimens, tests to identify or speciate pathogens, and tests used to determine the susceptibility or resistance of pathogens to drugs. These are the laboratory procedures described in this book. The results of these tests assist clinicians in the diagnosis, treatment, and management of infectious diseases. People working in clinical microbiology must possess an extensive knowledge of pathogens and the laboratory methods required to diagnose infectious diseases. They must not only have a genuine desire to assist clinicians and patients but also enjoy detective work. Additional information about this career field can be found on the Web sites of the American Society for Microbiology (http://www.asm.org/), the American Society for Clinical Pathology (http://www.ascp.org/) and the American Society for Clinical Laboratory Science (http://www.ascls.org/).

> Clinical microbiology is the subdiscipline of microbiology associated with the diagnosis of human infectious diseases.

Information about other areas of specialization in applied microbiology can be found on the CD-ROM that accompanies this book and the Web site of the American Society for Microbiology (http://www.asm.org/). Examples of other microbiology career fields include **agricultural microbiology**, **biotechnology** (the use of microbes to make useful products), **environmental microbiology** and **bioremediation** (the use of microbes to decompose wastes, including industrial and toxic wastes), **microbial genetics** and **genetic engineering** (inserting genes into microorganisms to enable them to produce important products they previously were unable to produce), **microbial physiology, paleomicrobiology** (the study of ancient microbes), **parasitology, sanitary microbiology**, and **veterinary microbiology**. Another career field that incorporates an interest in and knowledge of microbiology is **epidemiology** (see Chapter 26). The scope of microbiology has broad, far-reaching effects on human beings and their environment.

Chapter Review

- Microbes include viruses, prions, bacteria, archaea, certain algae, protozoa, and certain fungi.

- Because viruses and prions are acellular (not composed of cells), they are often referred to as infectious agents or infectious particles, rather than microorganisms.

- Microbes that live on and in various parts of the human body are called indigenous microflora (or indigenous microbiota).

- Only a small percentage of known microbes cause disease. Those that do are called pathogens, and the diseases they cause are referred to as infectious diseases and microbial intoxications. Microbes that do not cause disease are called nonpathogens. Opportunistic pathogens do not cause disease under ordinary circumstances; however, they have the potential to cause disease if they gain access to the "wrong place" at the "wrong time."

- The cell is the fundamental unit of any living organism; it exhibits the basic characteristics of life. All living organisms are composed of one or more cells.

- Complex eucaryotic cells contain membrane-bound organelles and a true nucleus, containing DNA. Procaryotic cells (archaea and bacteria) exhibit all the characteristics of life but do not have a true nucleus or a complex system of membranes and membrane-bound organelles.

- Some eucaryotic cells have cell walls to provide rigidity, shape, and protection; these simple cell walls may contain cellulose, pectin, lignin, chitin, or mineral salts. Procaryotic bacterial cell walls are more complex, containing peptidoglycan and, in some cases, lipopolysaccharides.

- In eucaryotic cells, energy is produced within mitochondria ("energy factories"). Energy-producing reactions occur at the cell membranes of procaryotic cells.

- External to the cell wall, some bacteria have either a capsule or a slime layer. Capsules serve an antiphagocytic function and have been used in the production of certain vaccines. Determining whether a bacterium possesses a capsule or not is of value when attempting to identify the organism.

- Many bacteria have flagella that enable motility and some produce spores for survival. Determining whether a bacterium possesses flagella or not is of value when attempting to identify the organism, as are the number and location of the flagella. Likewise, the presence or absence of spores is of value when identifying bacteria.

- In the binomial system of nomenclature, the first name is the genus, the second name is the specific epithet, and the two names together represent the species.

- Taxonomic classification of organisms separates them into kingdoms, divisions, orders, classes, families, genera, and species, based on their characteristics, attributes, properties, and traits.

- In the five-kingdom system of classification, microorganisms are found in the first three kingdoms—Procaryotae (bacteria), Protista (algae and protozoa), and Fungi. In the three-domain system of classification, microorganisms are found in all three domains—*Archaea*, *Bacteria*, and *Eucarya*.

New Terms and Abbreviations

After studying Chapter 1, you should be familiar with the following terms, which are defined within the chapter and in the Glossary at the back of the book:

Acellular microbe

Bacteriology

Capsule

Cell membrane

Cell wall

Chromosome

Cilium (pl. cilia)

Cytoplasm

Endoplasmic reticulum (ER)

Endospore

Eucaryote

Flagellum (pl. flagella)

Gene

Gene product

Genotype

Genus (pl. genera)

Glycocalyx

Golgi apparatus

Indigenous microflora

Infectious disease

Lysosome

Microbial intoxication

Microbiology

Microorganism

Mitochondrion (pl. mitochondria)

Mycology

Nonpathogen

Nuclear membrane

Nucleolus

Nucleoplasm

Nucleus (pl. nuclei)

Opportunistic pathogen

Organelle

Pathogen

Parasitology

Phenotype

Phycology

Pilus (pl. pili)

Plasmid

Plastid

Prion

Procaryote

Protist

Protoplasm

Protozoology

Ribosomes

Slime layer

Species (pl. species)

Specific epithet

Spore

Taxon (pl. taxa)

Taxonomy

Toxin

Virology

References and Suggested Reading

Boone DR, Castenholz RW, eds. The Archaea and the Deeply Branching and Phototrophic Bacteria. New York: Springer-Verlag, 2001. Garrity GM, ed. Bergey's Manual of Systematic Bacteriology, vol 1. 2nd Ed.

De Kruif P. Microbe Hunters. New York: Harcourt Brace, 1926.

 ## On the CD-ROM

- How Microbes Affect Our Lives
- The CSI Connection
- Careers in Microbiology
- Additional Self-Assessment Exercises
- Puzzle

Self-Assessment Exercises

After studying Chapter 1, answer the following questions.

1. In the five-kingdom system of classification, bacteria are found in which of the following kingdoms?

   A. Animalia

   B. Plantae

   C. Procaryotae

   D. Protista

2. The microbes that usually live on or within a person are collectively referred to as

   A. germs.

   B. indigenous microflora.

   C. nonpathogens.

   D. opportunistic pathogens.

3. The field of parasitology involves the study of which of the following types of organisms?

   A. Arthropods, bacteria, fungi, protozoa, and viruses

   B. Arthropods, helminths, and certain protozoa

   C. Bacteria, fungi, and protozoa

   D. Bacteria, fungi, and viruses

4. Which of the following are even smaller than viruses?

   A. Bacteria

   B. Fungi

   C. Prions

   D. Protozoa

5. Molecules of extrachromosomal DNA are also known as

   A. the Golgi apparatus.

   B. plasmids.

   C. plastids.

   D. lysosomes.

6. Of the following, which one is *not* found in procaryotic cells?

A. Chromosome

B. Plasmid

C. Mitochondrion

D. Ribosome

7. The three-domain system of classification is based on differences in which one of the following molecules?

A. DNA

B. mRNA

C. tRNA

D. rRNA

8. Which of the following is in the correct sequence?

A. Kingdom, Division, Order, Class, Family, Genus

B. Kingdom, Order, Division, Class, Family, Genus

C. Kingdom, Division, Class, Order, Family, Genus

D. Kingdom, Class, Division, Order, Family, Genus

9. The semipermeable structure controlling the transport of materials between the cell and its external environment is the

A. cell wall.

B. cytoplasm.

C. cell membrane.

D. nuclear membrane.

10. Which one of the following statements about opportunistic pathogens is true?

A. They always cause disease.

B. They never cause disease.

C. They have the potential to cause disease but usually do not.

D. They usually cause disease but sometimes do not.

CHAPTER 2

Understanding Infectious Diseases

Chapter Outline

LEARNING OBJECTIVES

After studying this chapter, you should be able to:

☛ Define the terms and abbreviations introduced in this chapter (e.g., *acute disease, adhesin [ligand], arthropod-borne disease*)

☛ Describe a biofilm, including its biological makeup, medical significance, and susceptibility to antibiotics

☛ Identify three factors that influence the development of an infectious disease, including one pathogen factor, one host factor, and one environmental factor

☛ List the six components or "links" in the chain of infection, in the proper order

☛ Identify three examples of living reservoirs of infection and three examples of nonliving reservoirs

☛ List five principal modes of transmission of pathogens

☛ Differentiate among a communicable disease, a contagious disease, and a noncommunicable disease

☛ Differentiate among sporadic, endemic, nonendemic, epidemic, and pandemic diseases, and cite an example of each

☛ Name and discuss the four periods or phases in the course of an infectious disease

☛ Differentiate between localized and systemic infections, including the sites and severity of both types of diseases

☞ Explain the differences among acute, subacute, and chronic diseases, including speed of onset and duration of illness, and cite examples of each

☞ Define what is meant by symptoms of a disease, and cite several examples

☞ Define what is meant by signs of a disease, and cite several examples

☞ Describe latent infections, and cite one example

☞ Outline the progression from a primary infection to a secondary infection, using an example

☞ Describe six steps in the pathogenesis of an infectious disease, starting with entry of the pathogen into the body

☞ List three bacterial structures that serve as virulence factors, and describe how each functions as a virulence factor

☞ List six bacterial exoenzymes that serve as virulence factors

☞ Differentiate between endotoxins and exotoxins

☞ List six bacterial exotoxins and the diseases they cause

INFECTIOUS DISEASES VERSUS MICROBIAL INTOXICATIONS

Recall from Chapter 1 that pathogens cause two general categories of diseases: microbial intoxications and infectious diseases. A **microbial intoxication** is a disease that follows ingestion of a toxin that was produced **in vitro** (outside the body) by a pathogen.[1] Food-borne botulism is an example of a microbial intoxication. Although the clinical microbiology laboratory rarely becomes involved in the diagnosis of microbial intoxications, some information about these diseases is provided in Appendix 1 of the CD-ROM.

> Microbial intoxications are diseases that follow ingestion of toxins produced outside of the body (in vitro) by pathogens.

Infectious diseases, on the other hand, are diseases that follow colonization of the body by a pathogen.[2] Following colonization, the pathogen proceeds to

> Infectious diseases are diseases that follow colonization of the body by pathogens. Following colonization, the pathogens go on to cause disease within the body.

cause disease **in vivo** (within the body). The remainder of this chapter contains information about infectious diseases.

COLONIZATION, INFECTION, AND INFECTIOUS DISEASE

As previously noted, the term **colonization** refers to the fact that a microbe has landed on or in the human body and has taken up residence there. The person is said to be colonized with that microbe. Many microbiologists use the term *infection* to mean colonization by a pathogen. In this sense, a person colonized by a pathogen is infected with that pathogen, and the pathogen may or may not cause disease; therefore, a person may be infected without having an infectious disease. Most people, however, including most health care professionals, use the terms *infection* and *infectious disease* synonymously. To say that a child has an ear infection is the same as saying that the child has an infectious disease of the ear. Because most people use these terms synonymously, the terms *infection* and *infectious disease* are used as synonyms throughout this book.

BIOFILMS AND POLYMICROBIAL (SYNERGISTIC) INFECTIONS

It is common to hear or read about a particular microorganism being the cause of a certain disease. In reality, it is rare to find an ecological niche where only one type of microorganism is present or where only one microorganism is causing a particular effect. In nature, microorganisms are often organized into what are known as **biofilms**—complex and tenacious communities of assorted organisms. Bacterial biofilms are virtually everywhere; examples include dental plaque, the slippery coating on a rock in a stream, and the slime that accumulates on the inner walls of various types of pipes and tubing. A bacterial biofilm consists of several species of bacteria plus a gooey polysaccharide (extracellular matrix) that the bacteria secrete. The bacteria grow in tiny clusters—called microcolonies—that are separated by a network of water channels. The fluid that flows through these channels bathes the microcolonies with dissolved nutrients and carries away waste products.

Biofilms have medical significance. They form on urinary catheters and permanent medical implants, and have been implicated in diseases such as endocarditis, cystic fibrosis, middle ear infections, kidney stones, periodontal disease, and prostate infections. Microbes commonly associated with biofilms on indwelling medical devices include the yeast *Candida albicans* and bacteria such as *Staphylococcus*

---

[1] *The often-used Latin terms* in vivo *and* in vitro *literally mean "within an organism" and "outside an organism," respectively.*

[2] *When a microbe lands on or enters a person's body and establishes residence there, the person is said to be colonized with that microbe.*

aureus, coagulase-negative staphylococci, *Enterococcus* spp., *Klebsiella pneumoniae*, and *Pseudomonas aeruginosa*. In the past, scientists studied ways to control individual species of bacteria; now they are concentrating their efforts on ways to attack and control biofilms.

Biofilms are very resistant to antibiotics and disinfectants. Although an antibiotic has been shown to be effective against a pure culture of a particular organism isolated from a biofilm, that antibiotic may be ineffective against the same organism in the actual biofilm.

Example 1

In the laboratory, a particular bacterium (*Bacterium x*) has been isolated from a biofilm and has been shown to be susceptible to penicillin. However, within the biofilm, a penicillinase produced by a different bacterium will inactivate the penicillin molecule and will protect *Bacterium x* and other organisms within the biofilm from the effects of penicillin. Thus, some bacteria within the biofilm protect other species of bacteria that are also present.

Example 2

Another example of how bacteria within a biofilm cooperate with each other involves nutrients. In some biofilms, bacteria of different species cooperate to break down nutrients that any single species cannot break down by itself. In some cases, one species within a biofilm feeds on the metabolic wastes of another.

Infections caused by more than one organism are referred to as **polymicrobial (or synergistic) infections**. Examples include bacterial vaginosis and trench mouth. Consult the CD-ROM for additional information about polymicrobial infections.

> Infections caused by more than one organism (e.g., bacterial vaginosis and trench mouth) are referred to as polymicrobial or synergistic infections.

INTERACTIONS AMONG PATHOGENS, HOSTS, AND THE ENVIRONMENT

Whether or not an infectious disease occurs depends on many factors, some of which are shown in Table 2-1.

THE CHAIN OF INFECTION

There are six components of the infectious disease process (also known as links in the chain of infection). The

TABLE 2 - 1	Factors That Influence the Development of an Infectious Disease	
Factors Relating to the Pathogen	**Factors Relating to the Host**	**Factors Relating to the Environment**
Virulence of the pathogen (virulence is discussed later in this chapter; for now, think of virulence as a measure or degree of pathogenicity; some pathogens are more virulent than others)	Health status of the host (e.g., hospitalization, any underlying illnesses, invasive procedures, prosthetic devices, or catheterization)	Physical factors such as geographic location, climate, heat, cold, humidity, season of the year
Is there a way for the pathogen to enter the body (i.e., is there a portal of entry)?	Nutritional status of the host	Availability of appropriate reservoirs, intermediate hosts (see Chapter 21), and arthropod vectors
Number of organisms that enter the body (i.e., will there be a sufficient number to cause infection?)	Other factors pertaining to the susceptibility of the host (e.g., age, lifestyle [behavior], socioeconomic level, travel, hygiene, substance abuse, immune status, etc.)	Sanitary and housing conditions; adequate waste disposal
		Availability of potable (drinkable) water

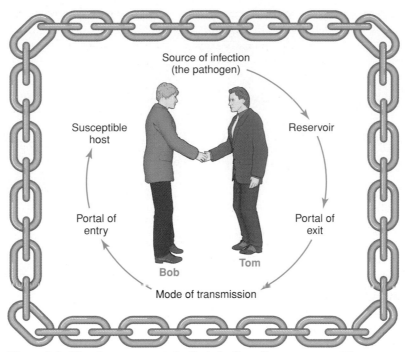

Figure 2-1. **The six components in the infectious disease process.** The process is also known as the chain of infection.

components, or links, are illustrated in Figure 2-1 and briefly described here:

1. **Pathogen.** As an example, let's assume that the pathogen is a cold virus.

2. **Reservoir** (i.e., a source of the pathogen). In Figure 2-1, the infected person on the right (Tom) is the reservoir. Tom has a cold.

3. **Portal of exit** (i.e., a way for the pathogen to escape from the reservoir). When Tom blows his nose, cold viruses get onto his hands.

4. **Mode of transmission** (i.e., a way for the pathogen to travel from Tom to another person). In Figure 2-1, the cold virus is being transferred by direct contact between Tom and his friend (Bob), by means of the handshake.

5. **Portal of entry** (i.e., a way for the pathogen to gain entry into Bob). When Bob rubs his nose, the cold virus is transferred from his hand to the mucous membranes of his nose.

6. **Susceptible host.** For example, Bob would not be a susceptible host, and therefore would not develop a cold, if he had previously been infected by that particular cold virus and had developed immunity to it.

RESERVOIRS OF INFECTION

The sources of the microbes that cause infectious diseases are many and varied. They are known as **reservoirs of** **infection** or simply **reservoirs.** A reservoir is any site where the pathogen can multiply or merely survive until it is transferred to a host. Reservoirs may be living organisms or inanimate objects or materials (Fig. 2-2).

> **Reservoirs of infection may be living organisms or nonliving objects or materials.**

Living Reservoirs

Living reservoirs include humans, household pets, farm animals, wild animals, some insects (e.g., mosquitoes and fleas), and some arachnids (e.g., ticks and mites). A human or animal reservoir may or may not actually be experiencing illness caused by the pathogen it is harboring.

Human carriers. The most important reservoirs of human infectious diseases are other humans—people with infectious diseases, as well as carriers. A **carrier** is a person who is colonized with a particular pathogen, but the pathogen is not currently causing disease in that person. The pathogen can, however, be transmitted from the carrier to others, who may then become ill. There are several types of carriers. **Passive carriers** carry the pathogen without ever having had the disease. An **incubatory carrier** is a person who is capable of transmitting a pathogen during the incubation period of a particular infectious disease. **Convalescent carriers** harbor and can transmit a particular pathogen while recovering from an infectious disease. **Active carriers** have completely recovered from the disease but continue to harbor the pathogen indefinitely. An infamous active carrier known as Typhoid Mary is described on the CD-ROM.

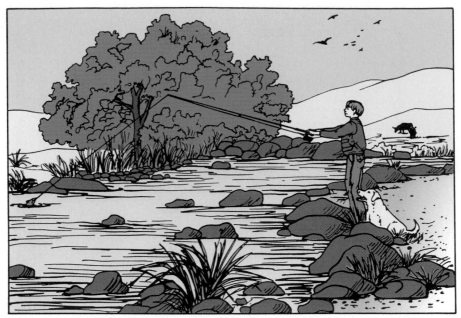

Figure 2-2. **Reservoirs of infection.** The most common reservoirs are soil, dust, contaminated water; contaminated foods; insects; and infected humans, domestic animals, and wild animals. (From Engelkirk PG, Duben-Engelkirk J, Dowell VR, eds. Principles and Practice of Clinical Anaerobic Bacteriology. Belmont, CA: Star Publishing, 1992.)

Usually, respiratory secretions or feces are the vehicles by which the pathogen is transferred, either directly from the carrier to a susceptible person or indirectly via food or water. Human carriers are very important in the spread of staphylococcal and streptococcal infections, as well as in the spread of hepatitis, diphtheria, dysentery, meningitis, and sexually transmitted diseases.

Animals. Infectious diseases that humans acquire from animal sources are called **zoonotic diseases** or **zoonoses (sing. zoonosis)**. Zoonotic diseases may be caused by viruses, bacteria, fungi, protozoa, or helminths. Many pets and other animals are important reservoirs of zoonoses. Zoonoses are acquired by direct contact with the animal, by inhalation or ingestion of the pathogen, or by injection of the pathogen by an arthropod. (Arthropods are discussed in the next paragraph.) Measures for the control of zoonotic diseases include the use of personal protective equipment when handling animals, proper use of pesticides, isolation or destruction of infected animals, and proper disposal of animal carcasses and waste products. Two of the most common zoonotic diseases in the United States are Lyme disease (discussed later in the chapter) and West Nile virus infection. Both of these diseases are **arthropod-borne diseases,** meaning they are transmitted by arthropods. Additional information about zoonoses can be found on the CD-ROM.

Arthropods. Technically, arthropods are animals, but they are being discussed separately because they are such common and important reservoirs of infection. Many types of arthropods serve as reservoirs of infection, including insects such as

mosquitoes, biting flies, lice, and fleas and arachnids such as mites and ticks. When involved in the transmission of infectious diseases, these arthropods are referred to as **vectors.** The arthropod vector first takes a blood meal from an infected person or animal and then transfers the pathogens to a healthy person. For example, consider Lyme disease, which is the most common arthropod-borne disease in the United States. First, a tick takes a blood meal from an infected deer or mouse. The tick is now infected with *Borrelia burgdorferi*, the spirochete bacterium that causes Lyme disease. Some time later, the tick takes a blood meal from a human and, in the process, injects the bacteria into the human. Ticks are especially notorious vectors. In the United States, at least 10 infectious diseases are transmitted by ticks. Lyme disease and relapsing fever are two examples; other arthropod-borne infectious diseases are shown in Table 2-2 and on the CD-ROM. Chapter 21 contains additional information about arthropods.

Nonliving Reservoirs

Nonliving or inanimate reservoirs of infection include air, soil, dust, food, milk, water, and fomites. (Fomites are described later in the chapter.) Air can become contaminated by dust or respiratory secretions of humans expelled into the air by breathing, talking, sneezing, and coughing. The most highly contagious diseases include colds and influenza, in which the respiratory viruses can be transmitted through the air on droplets of respiratory tract secretions. Air currents and air vents can transport respiratory pathogens throughout health care facilities and other buildings. Dust particles can carry

TABLE 2 - 2	Arthropods That Serve as Vectors of Human Infectious Diseases
Vectors	**Disease(s)**
Black flies (*Simulium* spp.)	Onchocerciasis (river blindness) (H)
Cyclops spp.	Fish tapeworm infection (H), guinea worm infection (H)
Fleas	Dog tapeworm infection (H), endemic typhus (B), murine typhus (B), plague (B)
Lice	Epidemic relapsing fever (B), epidemic typhus (B), trench fever (B)
Mites	Rickettsial pox (B), scrub typhus (B)
Mosquitoes	Dengue fever (V), filariasis (elephantiasis) (H), malaria (P), viral encephalitis (V), West Nile virus encephalitis (V), yellow fever (V)
Reduviid bugs	American trypanosomiasis (Chagas disease) (P)
Sand flies (*Phlebotomus* spp.)	Leishmaniasis (P)
Ticks	Babesiosis (P), Colorado tick fever (V), ehrlichiosis (B), Lyme disease (B), relapsing fever (B), Rocky Mountain spotted fever (B), tularemia (B)
Tsetse flies (*Glossina* spp.)	African trypanosomiasis (P)

B, bacterial disease; H, helminth disease; P, protozoal disease; V, viral disease.

spores of certain bacteria and dried bits of human and animal excretions containing pathogens. Bacteria cannot multiply in the air but can be transported easily via airborne particles to a warm, moist, nutrient-rich site, where they can multiply. Also, some fungal respiratory diseases (e.g., histoplasmosis) are frequently transferred via dust containing yeasts or spores. Soil contains bacterial spores of the *Clostridium* species that cause tetanus, botulism, and gas gangrene. Any of these diseases can follow the introduction of spores into an open wound.

Food and milk may be contaminated by careless handling, which allows pathogens to enter from soil, dust particles, dirty hands, hair, and respiratory secretions. If these pathogens are not destroyed by proper processing and cooking, food poisoning can develop. In the United States, foodborne diseases cause approximately 76 million illnesses; 325,000 hospitalizations; and 5,000 deaths per year. Diseases frequently transmitted via foods and water are amebiasis (caused by the ameba *Entamoeba histolytica*), botulism (caused by the bacterium *Clostridium botulinum*), cholera (caused by the bacterium *Vibrio cholerae*), *Clostridium perfringens* food poisoning, infectious hepatitis (caused by the hepatitis A virus), staphylococcal food poisoning, typhoid fever (caused by the bacterium *Salmonella typhi*), and trichinosis (a helminth disease caused by ingesting *Trichinella spiralis* larvae in pork). Other common foodborne and waterborne pathogens are shown in Table 2-3.

Human and animal fecal matter from outhouses, cesspools, or feedlots often is carried into water supplies. Improper disposal of sewage and inadequate treatment of drinking water contribute to the spread of fecal and soil pathogens. A **fomite** is an inanimate object contaminated with and capable of transmitting a pathogen. Examples of fomites found within health care facilities are patients' gowns, bedding, towels, eating and drinking utensils, doorknobs, computer keyboards, and hospital equipment like bedpans, stethoscopes, latex gloves, electronic thermometers, and ECG electrodes. These objects become contaminated with pathogens from the respiratory tract, intestinal tract, and skin of patients. Pathogens are often spread via the hands of health care workers. Health care personnel must take great care to prevent transmission of pathogens from living and nonliving reservoirs to hospitalized patients.

MODES OF TRANSMISSION

Health care professionals must be thoroughly familiar with the sources (reservoirs) of potential pathogens and pathways for their transfer. A hospital staphylococcal epidemic may begin when aseptic conditions are relaxed and a *Staphylococcus aureus* carrier transmits the bacterial pathogen to susceptible patients, such as babies, surgical patients, or debilitated persons. That type of infection could quickly spread throughout the entire hospital population.

The five principal modes by which transmission of pathogens occurs are contact (either direct or indirect),

TABLE 2 - 3   Pathogens Commonly Transmitted by Food and Water[a]

Pathogen	Vehicle	Comments
Campylobacter jejuni (bacterium)	Chickens	Most common cause of bacterial diarrhea in the United States
Cryptosporidium parvum (protozoan)	Drinking water	Highly resistant to disinfectants used to purify drinking water
Cyclospora cayetanensis (protozoan)	Drinking water, raspberries	
Escherichia coli 0157:H7 (bacterium)	Meats, produce contaminated by manure in growing fields (e.g., spinach, sprouts), drinking water	
Giardia lamblia (also called *Giardia intestinalis*) (protozoan)	Drinking water	Moderately resistant to disinfectants used to purify drinking water
Listeria monocytogenes (bacterium)	Soft cheeses and deli meats	
Salmonella enteritidis (bacterium)	Eggs	
Salmonella typhimurium DT-104 (bacterium)	Unpasteurized milk	Resistant to many antibiotics
Shigella spp. (bacteria)	Drinking water	

[a]Additional pathogens transmitted in food and water are mentioned in the text.

> The five principal modes by which infectious diseases are transmitted are contact (either direct or indirect), airborne, droplet, vehicular, and vectors.

airborne, droplet, vehicular, and vectors (Fig. 2-3 and Table 2-4). Vehicular transmission involves contaminated inanimate objects (vehicles) such as food, water, dust, and fomites. Vectors are various types of biting insects and arachnids.

COMMUNICABLE, CONTAGIOUS, AND NONCOMMUNICABLE INFECTIOUS DISEASES

As previously stated, an infectious disease is a disease that is caused by a pathogen. If the infectious disease is directly or indirectly transmissible from one human to another (i.e., person-to-person transmission), it is called a **communicable disease.** At one time, a **contagious disease** was defined as a communicable disease that is **easily transmitted** from one

> Communicable and contagious diseases are infectious diseases that are transmitted from person to person.

person to another, but today the terms are usually used synonymously. For example, both gonorrhea and influenza are communicable diseases, but influenza is considered a contagious disease because it is so easily transmitted. A **noncommunicable disease** cannot be transmitted from person to person. Examples of noncommunicable infectious diseases are tetanus, botulism, and gas gangrene.

SPORADIC, ENDEMIC, EPIDEMIC, AND PANDEMIC DISEASES

A **sporadic disease** is one that occurs only occasionally (sporadically) within the population of a particular geographic area. In the United States, sporadic diseases include botulism, cholera, gas gangrene, plague, tetanus, and typhoid fever. Quite often, particular diseases occur only sporadically because they are kept under control as a result of immunization programs and sanitary conditions. It is possible for outbreaks of these controlled diseases to occur, however, whenever vaccination programs and other public health programs are neglected.

An **endemic disease** is always present within the population of a particular geographic area. The number of cases of the disease may fluctuate over time, but the disease never dies out completely. Endemic infectious diseases of the

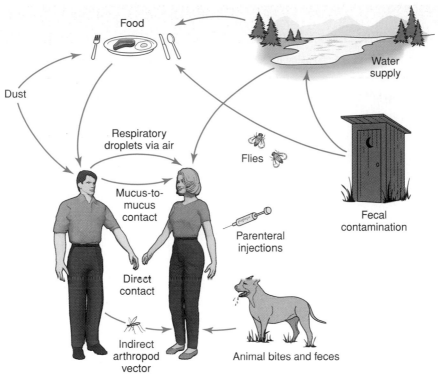

Figure 2-3. **Modes of disease transmission.**

United States include bacterial diseases like tuberculosis, staphylococcal and streptococcal infections, and the sexually transmitted diseases gonorrhea and syphilis; and viral diseases like the common cold, influenza, chickenpox, and mumps. The actual incidence of an endemic disease at any particular time depends on a balance among several factors, including the environment, the genetic susceptibility of the population, behavioral factors, the number of people who are immune, the virulence of the pathogen, and the reservoir or source of infection.[3]

Endemic diseases may on occasion become epidemic. An **epidemic disease** (or outbreak) is defined as a greater-than-usual number of cases of a disease in a particular region, usually occurring within a relatively short period. An epidemic does not necessarily involve a large number of people, although it might. If a dozen people develop staphylococcal food poisoning shortly after their return from a church picnic, that constitutes an epidemic—a small one, to be sure, but an epidemic nonetheless. Listed here are a few of the epidemics that have occurred in the United States within the past 40 years:

- **1976.** An epidemic of a respiratory disease, called Legionnaires disease or legionellosis, occurred during an American Legion convention in Philadelphia. It resulted in approximately 220 hospitalizations and 34 deaths. The bacterial pathogen (*Legionella pneumophila*, a Gram-negative bacillus) was present in the water being circu-

lated through the air-conditioning system of the hotel where the affected legionnaires were staying. Aerosols of the organism were inhaled by occupants of some of the rooms in the hotel. Subsequent epidemics of legionellosis have occurred in other hotels, hospitals, cruise ships, and supermarkets. The supermarket outbreaks were associated with the misting of vegetables. Virtually all epidemics of legionellosis have involved contaminated water and/or colonized water pipes and aerosols containing the pathogen.

- **1992–1993.** An epidemic involving hamburger meat contaminated with *Escherichia coli* 0157:H7 occurred in the Pacific Northwest, resulting in approximately 500 diarrheal cases, 45 cases of kidney failure as a result of hemolytic uremic syndrome, and the death of several young children. *E. coli* O157:H7 is a particularly virulent serotype of *E. coli*; it is also known as enterohemorrhagic *E. coli*. (The prefix *entero-* refers to the intestinal tract, and *hemorrhagic* refers to bleeding; *E. coli* O157:H7 causes intestinal bleeding.) In this epidemic, the source of the *E. coli* was cattle feces. The ground beef used to make the hamburgers had been contaminated with cattle feces during the slaughtering process. The hamburgers had not been cooked long enough, or at a high enough temperature, to kill the bacteria. There have been many epidemics associated with *E. coli* O157:H7 since the 1992–1993 epidemic.

---

[3] *The term* virulence *is a measure of pathogenicity. Some pathogens are more virulent than others. Virulence is described in more detail later in the chapter.*

TABLE 2 - 4   Common Routes of Transmission of Infectious Diseases

Route of Exit	Route of Transmission or Entry	Diseases Transmitted in This Manner
Skin	Skin discharge → air → respiratory tract	Chickenpox, common cold, influenza, measles, staphylococcal and streptococcal infections
	Skin to skin	Boils, eczema, impetigo, syphilis, warts
Respiratory	Aerosol droplet inhalation Nose or mouth → hand or inanimate object → nose	Chickenpox, common cold, influenza, mumps, measles, pneumonia, tuberculosis
Gastrointestinal	Stool → hand → mouth Stool → soil → food or water → mouth	Amebiasis, cholera, gastroenteritis, giardiasis, hepatitis, salmonellosis, shigellosis, typhoid fever
Salivary	Direct salivary transfer	Herpes labialis (cold sores/fever blisters), infectious mononucleosis, strep throat
Genital secretions	Urethral or cervical secretions	Chlamydial infection, genital herpes, gonorrhea
	Semen	AIDS, cytomegalovirus infection, syphilis, warts
Blood	Transfusion or needlestick injury	AIDS, cytomegalovirus infection, hepatitis B, malaria
	Insect bite	Malaria, relapsing fever
Zoonotic	Animal bite	Rabies
	Contact with animal carcasses	Anthrax, tularemia
	Arthropod	Lyme disease, malaria, plague, Rocky Mountain spotted fever, typhus, viral encephalitis, yellow fever

STUDY AID

Strains Versus Serotypes. Within a given species, there are usually various **strains**. For example, many strains of *E. coli* exist. If the *E. coli* that has been isolated from Patient X is producing an enzyme that is not being produced by the *E. coli* from Patient Z, the two *E. coli* isolates are considered different strains. Or if one isolate of *E. coli* is resistant to ampicillin (an antibiotic) and the other *E. coli* isolate is susceptible to ampicillin, then the two isolates are considered different strains of *E. coli*. Also, a

given species usually has various **serotypes**. Serotypes of an organism differ from each other because of differences in their surface molecules (surface antigens). Sometimes a species, like the bacteria *Chlamydia trachomatis* or *E. coli*, have different serotypes that cause different diseases.

Be careful not to confuse the terms *strains* and *serotypes*.

- **1993.** An epidemic of Hantavirus pulmonary syndrome occurred on Indian reservations in the Four Corners Region of the United States, where the borders of Colorado, New Mexico, Arizona, and Utah meet. This epidemic resulted in approximately 50 to 60 cases, including 28 deaths. The particular Hantavirus strain (now called Sin Nombre virus) was present in the urine and feces of deer mice, some of which had gained entrance to the homes of villagers. Aerosols of the virus were produced when residents swept up house dust containing the rodent droppings. The pathogen was then inhaled by people in those homes.

- **1993.** An epidemic of cryptosporidiosis, a diarrheal disease, occurred in Milwaukee, Wisconsin, as a result of drinking water contaminated with the oocysts of *Cryptosporidium parvum* (a protozoal parasite). This was the largest waterborne outbreak that has ever occurred in the United States. More than 400,000 people were affected, and more than 100 immunosuppressed patients died.

- **2002.** An epidemic of West Nile virus (WNV) infections occurred throughout the United States. More than 4,100 human cases occurred during that year, resulting in 284 deaths. In addition, more than 16,000 birds died as a result of WNV infections, and more than 14,500 horses were infected with WNV.

These and other epidemics have been identified through constant surveillance and accumulation of data by the **Centers for Disease Control and Prevention (CDC).** (Information about the CDC can be found on the CD-ROM.) Epidemics usually follow a specific pattern, in which the number of cases of a disease increases to a maximum and then decreases rapidly.

Certain infectious diseases, referred to as nationally notifiable diseases, must be reported to the CDC by all 50 states. Additional information about these diseases can be found on the CD-ROM.

The CDC prepares a weekly publication entitled *Morbidity and Mortality Weekly Report* (*MMWR*), which contains timely information about infectious disease outbreaks in the United States and other parts of the world, as well as cumulative statistics regarding the number of cases of nationally notifiable infectious diseases that have occurred in the United States during the current year. Laboratory science students are encouraged to read *MMWR*, which is accessible at the CDC Web site (http://www.cdc.gov/).

Epidemics may occur in communities that have not been previously exposed to a particular pathogen. People from populated areas who travel into isolated communities frequently introduce a new pathogen to susceptible natives of that community, and then the disease spreads like wildfire. Over the years, there have been many such examples. The syphilis epidemic in Europe in the early 1500s might have been caused by a highly virulent spirochete carried back from the West Indies by Columbus's men in 1492. Additionally, early explorers and settlers of the United States introduced Native Americans to measles, smallpox, and tuberculosis, causing epidemics that almost destroyed many tribes.

In communities where normal sanitation practices are relaxed, allowing fecal contamination of water supplies and food, epidemics of typhoid fever, cholera, giardiasis, and dysentery often occur. Visitors to these communities should be aware that they are especially susceptible to these diseases because they never developed a natural immunity by being exposed to them during childhood.

Influenza (flu) epidemics occur in many areas during certain times of the year and involve most of the population because the immunity developed in prior years is usually only temporary. Thus, the disease recurs each year among those who are not revaccinated. Epidemics of influenza cause approximately 20,000 deaths annually in the United States.

Ebola virus has caused several epidemics of hemorrhagic fever in Africa. An outbreak in Uganda in 2000 was the largest Ebola epidemic ever recorded, with 425 cases and 224 deaths. Between 50% and 90% of infected patients have died in these epidemics. The source of the virus is not yet known.

In a hospital setting, a relatively small number of infected patients can constitute an epidemic. If a higher-than-usual number of patients on a particular ward suddenly become infected by a particular pathogen, this constitutes an epidemic that must be brought to the attention of the Hospital Infection Control Committee (see Chapter 26).

A **pandemic disease** is a disease that occurs in epidemic proportions in many countries simultaneously—sometimes worldwide. The 1918 Spanish flu pandemic was the most devastating pandemic of the 20th century and is the catastrophe against which all modern pandemics are measured. That pandemic killed more than 20 million people worldwide, including 500,000 in the United States. Almost every nation on Earth was affected. Influenza pandemics are often named for the point of origin or first recognition, such as the Taiwan flu, Hong Kong flu, London flu, Port Chalmers flu, and Russian flu.

According to the **World Health Organization (WHO),** infectious diseases are responsible for approximately half the deaths that occur in developing countries, and approximately half of those are caused by three infectious diseases—HIV/AIDS, tuberculosis, and malaria—each of which is currently occurring in pandemic proportions. Together, these three diseases cause more than 300 million illnesses and 5 million deaths every year. Additional information about the WHO can be found on the CD-ROM.

THE FOUR PERIODS IN THE COURSE OF AN INFECTIOUS DISEASE

Once a pathogen has gained entrance to the body, the course of an infectious disease has four periods or phases (Fig. 2-4):

1. The **incubation period** is the time that elapses between exposure to the pathogen and the onset of

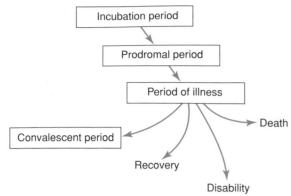

Figure 2-4. **The course of an infectious disease.**

symptoms. The length of the incubation period is influenced by many factors, including the overall health and nutritional status of the host, the immune status of the host (i.e., whether the host is immunocompetent or immunosuppressed), the virulence of the pathogen, and the number of pathogens that enter the body.

2. The **prodromal period** is the time during which the patient feels "out of sorts" but is not yet experiencing actual symptoms of the disease. Patients may feel like they are "coming down with something" but are not yet sure what it is.

3. The **period of illness** is the time during which the patient experiences the typical symptoms associated with that particular disease (e.g., sore throat, headache, sinus congestion). This period is sometimes referred to as the acute phase of the disease. Communicable diseases are most easily transmitted during this third period.

4. Assuming that the patient survives the disease, the fourth phase is the **convalescent period** (or period of convalescence)—the time during which the patient recovers. For certain infectious diseases, especially viral respiratory diseases, the convalescent period can be quite long. Although the patient may recover from the illness itself, permanent damage may be caused by destruction of tissues in the affected area. For example, brain damage may follow encephalitis or meningitis, paralysis may follow poliomyelitis, and deafness may follow ear infections. Another possible outcome of an infectious disease is death.

> The four phases or periods of an infectious disease are (1) the incubation period, (2) the prodromal period, (3) the period of illness, and (4) the convalescent period.

LOCALIZED AND SYSTEMIC INFECTIONS

Once an infectious process is initiated, the disease may remain localized to one site or it may spread. Pimples, boils, and abscesses are examples of **localized infections.** If the pathogens are not contained at the original site of infection, they may be carried to other parts of the body by way of lymph or blood, or in some cases by **phagocytes** (white blood cells capable of phagocytizing or ingesting particles). When the infection has spread throughout the body, it is referred to as either a **systemic infection** or a **generalized infection.** For example, the bacterium that causes tuberculosis, *Mycobacterium tuberculosis,* may spread to many internal organs, a condition known as miliary tuberculosis.

ACUTE, SUBACUTE, AND CHRONIC DISEASES

A disease may be described as being acute, subacute, or chronic. An **acute disease** has a rapid onset followed by a relatively rapid recovery; measles, mumps, and influenza are examples. A **chronic disease** has an insidious or slow onset and lasts a long time; examples are tuberculosis, leprosy (Hansen disease), and syphilis. Sometimes a disease having a sudden onset can develop into a long-lasting disease. Some diseases (e.g., forms of bacterial endocarditis) come on more suddenly than a chronic disease but less suddenly than an acute disease; they are referred to as **subacute diseases.** Subacute diseases usually last a longer time than acute diseases but a shorter time than chronic diseases.

SYMPTOMS AND SIGNS OF A DISEASE

A **symptom of a disease** is defined as some evidence of a disease that is experienced or perceived by the patient; it is subjective. Examples of symptoms include any type of ache or pain, a ringing in the ears (tinnitus), blurred vision, nausea, dizziness, itching, and chills. Diseases, including infectious diseases, may be either symptomatic or asymptomatic. A patient with a **symptomatic disease** (or clinical disease) experiences symptoms, whereas a patient with an **asymptomatic disease** (or subclinical disease) is unaware of the infection because he or she is not experiencing any symptoms.

In its early stages, gonorrhea is usually symptomatic in male patients (who develop a urethral discharge and experience pain while urinating) but asymptomatic in female patients. Only after several months, during which the organism has caused extensive damage to her reproductive organs, does the infected woman experience pain. In trichomoniasis (caused by the protozoan *Trichomonas vaginalis*), the situation is reversed. Infected women are usually symptomatic (experiencing vaginitis), while infected men are usually asymptomatic. These two sexually transmitted diseases are especially difficult to control because people are often unaware that they are infected and unknowingly transmit the pathogens to others during sexual activities.

A **sign of a disease** is defined as some type of objective evidence of a disease. For example, while palpating a patient, a physician might discover a lump or an enlarged liver (hepatomegaly) or spleen (splenomegaly). Other signs of disease include abnormal heart or breath sounds, blood pressure, pulse rate, or laboratory results, or abnormalities that show up on radiographs, ultrasound studies, or computed tomography scans.

LATENT INFECTIONS

An infectious disease may go from being symptomatic to asymptomatic and then some time later go back to being symptomatic. Such diseases are referred to as **latent infections.** Herpes virus infections, such as cold sores (fever blisters), genital herpes infections, and shingles are examples of latent infections. Cold sores occur intermittently, but the patient continues to harbor the herpes virus between cold sore episodes. The virus remains dormant within cells of the nervous system until some type of stress acts as a trigger. The stressful trigger may be a fever, sunburn, extreme cold, or emotional stress. A person who had chickenpox as a child may harbor the virus throughout his or her lifetime, and then later in life, as the immune system weakens, that person may develop shingles. Shingles, a painful infection of the nerves, is a latent manifestation of chickenpox.

PRIMARY AND SECONDARY INFECTIONS

One infectious disease may commonly follow another, in which case the first disease is referred to as the **primary disease** and the second disease as the **secondary disease.** For example, serious cases of bacterial pneumonia frequently follow relatively mild viral respiratory infections. During the primary infection, the virus causes damage to the ciliated epithelial cells that line the respiratory tract. The function of these cells is to move foreign materials up and out of the respiratory tract into the throat where they can be swallowed. While coughing, the patient may inhale some saliva containing an opportunistic pathogen, such as *Streptococcus pneumoniae* or *Haemophilus influenzae* bacteria. The damaged ciliated epithelial cells are unable to clear the bacteria from the lungs. The bacteria then multiply and cause pneumonia. In this example, the viral infection is the primary infection and the bacterial pneumonia is the secondary infection.

STEPS IN THE PATHOGENESIS OF INFECTIOUS DISEASES

The prefix *path-* (from the Greek *pathos*, meaning "suffering") refers to disease. Examples of words containing this prefix are **pathogen** (a microbe capable of causing disease), **pathology** (the study of the structural and functional manifestations of disease), **pathologist** (a physician who has specialized in pathology), **pathogenicity** (the ability to cause disease), and **pathogenesis** (the steps or mechanisms involved in the development of a disease).

In general, the pathogenesis of an infectious disease often follows the following sequence:

Step 1: Entry of the pathogen into the body. Portals of entry include penetration of skin or mucous membranes by the pathogen, inoculation of the pathogen into bodily tissues by an arthropod, inhalation into the respiratory tract, ingestion into the gastrointestinal tract, introduction of the pathogen into the genitourinary tract, or introduction of the pathogen directly into the blood (e.g., via blood transfusion or the use of shared needles by intravenous drug abusers).

Step 2: Attachment of the pathogen to some tissue(s) within the body.

Step 3: Multiplication of the pathogen. The pathogen may multiply in one location of the body, resulting in a localized infection (e.g., an abscess), or it may multiply throughout the body (a systemic infection).

Step 4: Invasion (or spread) of the pathogen.

Step 5: Evasion of host defenses. Host defenses are described in Chapter 3.

Step 6: Damage to host tissue(s). The damage may be so extensive as to cause death of the patient.

It is important to understand that not all infectious diseases involve *all* these steps. For example, once ingested, some exotoxin-producing intestinal pathogens are capable of causing disease without adhering to the intestinal wall or invading tissue. Exotoxins are described later in the chapter.

> The pathogenesis of many (but not all) infectious diseases follows the sequence of entry, attachment, multiplication, invasion, evasion, and damage.

MECHANISMS BY WHICH PATHOGENS CAUSE DISEASE

Virulence

Virulence is a measure or degree of pathogenicity. Although all pathogens cause disease, some are more virulent than others (i.e., they are better able to cause disease). For example, it takes fewer *Shigella* cells to cause shigellosis (a bacterial diarrheal disease) than it takes *Salmonella* cells to cause salmonellosis (another bacterial diarrheal disease). Thus, *Shigella* is considered to be more virulent than *Salmonella*. In some cases, certain strains of a particular species are more virulent than others. For example, the "flesh-eating" strains of the bacterium *Streptococcus pyogenes* are more virulent than other strains of *S. pyogenes* because they produce certain necrotizing enzymes not produced by the other strains. Similarly, only certain strains of *S. pyogenes* produce erythrogenic toxin (the cause of scarlet fever); these strains are considered more virulent than the strains of *S. pyogenes* that do *not* produce erythrogenic toxin. Strains of the bacterium *Staphylococcus aureus* that produce toxic shock syndrome toxin 1 (TSST-1) or Panton-Valentine leukocidin are considered more virulent than strains of *S. aureus* that do not produce these toxins.

Sometimes virulence is used in reference to the severity of the infectious diseases caused by the pathogens. Used in this manner, one pathogen is more virulent than another if it causes a more serious disease.

Virulent is an adjective that can be used as a synonym for *pathogenic*. For example, a particular species may have **virulent strains** and **avirulent strains** (or pathogenic and nonpathogenic strains, respectively). The virulent strains are capable of causing disease, whereas the avirulent strains are not. For example, toxigenic strains of the bacterium *Corynebacterium diphtheriae* (i.e., strains that produce diphtheria toxin) are virulent—they cause diphtheria. Nontoxigenic strains (i.e., strains that do not produce diphtheria toxin) are avirulent—they do *not* cause diphtheria. Encapsulated strains of the bacterium *Streptococcus pneumoniae* can cause disease, but nonencapsulated strains of *S. pneumoniae* cannot. As discussed in a subsequent section, piliated strains of certain pathogens are able to cause disease, whereas nonpiliated strains are not; thus, the piliated strains are virulent, but the nonpiliated strains are avirulent.

Virulence Factors

The physical attributes or properties of pathogens that enable them to attach to host cells, escape destruction by various host defense mechanisms, and/or cause disease are called **virulence factors.** Virulence factors are phenotypic characteristics that, like all phenotypic characteristics, are dictated by the organism's genotype. Toxins are obvious virulence factors, but other virulence factors are not so obvious. Some virulence factors are shown in Figure 2-5.

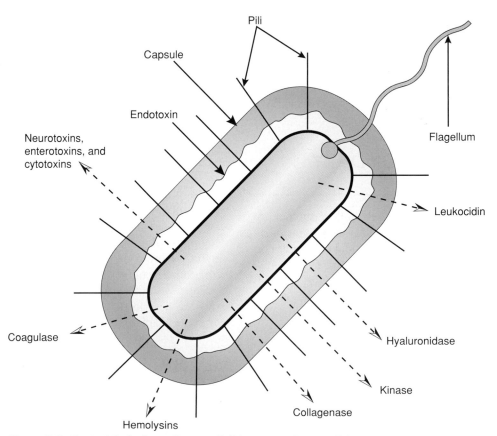

Figure 2-5. **Bacterial virulence factors.** Solid arrows point to cellular structures. Dotted arrows indicate cellular products being released from the cell.

Attachment

Perhaps you have noticed that certain pathogens infect dogs but not humans, whereas others infect humans but not dogs. Perhaps you have wondered why certain pathogens cause respiratory infections and others cause gastrointestinal infections. Part of the explanation has to do with the type or types of cells to which the pathogen is able to attach. To cause disease, some pathogens must be able to anchor themselves to cells after they have gained access to the body.

Receptors and adhesins. The general term **receptor** is used to describe the molecule on the surface of a host cell that a particular pathogen is able to recognize and to which it attaches. Glycoprotein molecules are good receptors. A particular pathogen can only attach to cells bearing its specific receptor. Thus, respiratory viruses cause respiratory infections because they are able to recognize and attach to receptors present only on cells that line the respiratory tract. Receptors are also referred to as integrins.

The general term **adhesin** is used to describe the molecule on the surface of a pathogen that is able to recognize and bind to a particular receptor. The adhesin on the envelope of HIV that recognizes and binds to the CD4 receptor is a glycoprotein molecule designated as gp120. Because possession of adhesins enables certain pathogens to attach to host cells, they are considered virulence factors. In some cases, antibodies directed against such adhesins prevent the pathogen from attaching and thus prevent infection by that pathogen. Antibodies are proteins that our immune systems produce to protect us from pathogens and infectious diseases; they are discussed in Chapter 3. Adhesins are also referred to as ligands.

Bacterial fimbriae (pili). Bacterial fimbriae (pili) are long, thin, hairlike, flexible projections composed of an array of proteins called pilin. Fimbriae are considered virulence factors because they enable bacteria to **attach** to surfaces, including various tissues within the human body. Fimbriated (piliated) strains of the bacterium *Neisseria gonorrhoeae* can anchor themselves to the inner walls of the urethra and cause urethritis (inflammation of the urethra). Should nonfimbriated (nonpiliated) strains of *N. gonorrhoeae* gain access to the urethra, they are unable to attach, are flushed out of the urethra via urination, and thus unable to cause urethritis. Therefore, with respect to urethritis, fimbriated strains of *N. gonorrhoeae* are virulent and nonfimbriated strains are avirulent.

Similarly, fimbriated strains of the bacterium *Escherichia coli* that gain access to the urinary bladder are able to anchor themselves to the inner walls of the bladder and cause cystitis (urinary bladder infection). Thus, with respect to cystitis, fimbriated strains of *E. coli* are virulent. Should nonfimbriated strains of *E. coli* gain access to the urinary bladder, they are unable to attach, are flushed out of the bladder via urination, and are unable to cause cystitis. Thus, the nonfimbriated strains are avirulent.

The fimbriae of group A β-hemolytic streptococci (*Streptococcus pyogenes*) contain molecules of M protein. M protein serves as a virulence factor in two ways: (1) it enables the bacteria to adhere to pharyngeal cells, and (2) it protects the cells from being phagocytized by white blood cells (i.e., the M protein serves an antiphagocytic function).

Other bacterial pathogens possessing fimbriae are *Vibrio cholerae*, *Salmonella* spp., *Shigella* spp., *Pseudomonas aeruginosa*, and *Neisseria meningitidis*. Because bacterial fimbriae enable bacteria to colonize surfaces, they are called colonization factors.

Capsules

Bacterial capsules are considered virulence factors because they serve an antiphagocytic function (i.e., they protect encapsulated bacteria from being phagocytized by phagocytic white blood cells). Phagocytes are unable to attach to encapsulated bacteria because they lack surface receptors for capsular polysaccharide material. If they are unable to adhere to the bacteria, they are unable to ingest them. Because encapsulated bacteria that gain access to the bloodstream or tissues are protected from phagocytosis, they are able to multiply, invade, and cause disease. Nonencapsulated bacteria, on the other hand, are phagocytized and killed. Encapsulated bacteria include *S. pneumoniae* (Fig. 2-6), *Klebsiella pneumoniae*, *Haemophilus influenzae*, and *Neisseria meningitidis*. The capsule of the yeast *Cryptococcus neoformans* is also considered to be a virulence factor.

Flagella

Recall from Chapter 1 that flagella are structures that enable bacteria to "swim." Bacterial flagella are considered virulence factors because they enable flagellated (motile) bacteria to

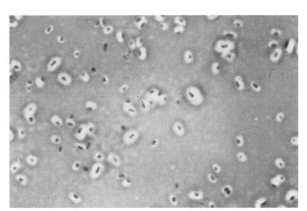

Figure 2-6. **Photomicrograph of *Streptococcus pneumoniae* type 1.** The capsules have been treated with a specific antibody to enhance their visibility; this is known as a Quellung reaction. The Quellung reaction is rarely performed in today's clinical microbiology laboratories. (From Winn WC Jr, et al. Koneman's Color Atlas and Textbook of Diagnostic Microbiology. 6th Ed. Philadelphia: Lippincott Williams & Wilkins, 2006.)

invade aqueous areas of the body that nonflagellated (nonmotile) bacteria are unable to reach. Perhaps flagella also enable bacteria to avoid phagocytosis; it is more difficult for phagocytes to catch a moving target.

> Adhesins, pili, capsules, and flagella are surface structures that serve as bacterial virulence factors.

Obligate Intracellular Pathogens

Rickettsia, Chlamydia, and *Chlamydophila* spp. (all of which are Gram-negative bacteria), *must* live within host cells to survive and multiply. They are referred to as **obligate intracellular pathogens** (or obligate intracellular parasites). Rickettsias invade and live within endothelial cells and vascular smooth muscle cells. Rickettsias are capable of synthesizing proteins, nucleic acids, and adenosine triphosphate (ATP),[4] but are thought to require an intracellular environment because they possess an unusual membrane transport system (they are said to have "leaky" membranes).

Different species and serotypes of chlamydiae invade different types of cells, such as conjunctival epithelial cells or cells of the respiratory or genital tract. Although chlamydiae are capable of synthesizing ATP, they use the ATP produced by host cells for their energy requirements. In the laboratory, obligate intracellular pathogens are propagated using cell cultures, laboratory animals, or embryonated chicken eggs.

Ehrlichia spp. and *Anaplasma phagocytophilum* are Gram-negative bacteria that are **intraleukocytic pathogens,** meaning that they live within white blood cells, or **leukocytes.**[5] *Ehrlichia* spp. live inside macrophages, causing the disease human monocytic ehrlichiosis. *Anaplasma phagocytophilum* lives within granulocytes, causing human anaplasmosis (previously known as human granulocytic ehrlichiosis). Some sporozoan protozoa, such as the *Plasmodium* spp. that cause human malaria and the *Babesia* spp. that cause human babesiosis, are **intraerythrocytic pathogens,** meaning that they live within red blood cells, or **erythrocytes.**

Facultative Intracellular Pathogens

Some pathogens, referred to as **facultative intracellular pathogens** (or facultative intracellular parasites), are capable of both an intracellular and extracellular existence. Many facultative intracellular pathogens that can be grown in the laboratory on artificial culture media are also able to survive within phagocytes. How facultative intracellular pathogens are able to survive within phagocytes is discussed next.

Phagocytes play an important role in our defenses against pathogens. The two most important categories of phagocytes in the human body (referred to as professional phagocytes) are macrophages and neutrophils. Once phagocytized, most pathogens are destroyed within the phagocytes by hydrolytic enzymes (e.g., lysozyme, proteases, lipases, DNAse, RNAse, myeloperoxidase), hydrogen peroxide, superoxide anions, and other mechanisms. However, some pathogens are able to survive and multiply within phagocytes after being ingested (Table 2-5).

Some pathogens (such as the bacterium *Mycobacterium tuberculosis*) have a cell wall composition that resists digestion. Waxes in mycobacterial cell walls protect the organisms from digestion. Other pathogens (like the protozoan *Toxoplasma gondii*) prevent the fusion of lysosomes (vesicles that contain digestive enzymes) with the phagocytic vacuole (phagosome). Other pathogens (such as the bacterium *Rickettsia rickettsii*) produce phospholipases—enzymes that destroy the phagosome membrane, thus preventing lysosome-phagosome fusion. Other pathogens (such as the bacteria *Brucella abortus, Francisella tularensis, Legionella pneumophila, Listeria monocytogenes, Salmonella* spp., and *Yersinia pestis*) can survive via mechanisms that are not yet understood.

Exoenzymes

Although adhesins, pili, capsules, and flagella are considered virulence factors, they really do not explain how bacteria and other pathogens actually *cause* disease. The major mechanisms by which pathogens cause disease are the exoenzymes and/or toxins they produce. Some pathogens (e.g., certain strains of *Streptococcus pyogenes*) produce both.

> The major mechanisms by which pathogens cause disease are the exoenzymes and/or toxins they produce.

Some pathogens release enzymes, called **exoenzymes,**[6] that enable them to evade host defense mechanisms, invade, or cause damage to body tissues. These exoenzymes include necrotizing enzymes, coagulase, kinases, hyaluronidase, collagenase, hemolysins, and lecithinase.

Necrotizing enzymes. Many pathogens produce exoenzymes that destroy tissues; these are collectively referred to as **necrotizing enzymes.** Notorious examples are the flesh-eating strains of *Streptococcus pyogenes*, which produce proteases and other enzymes that cause very rapid destruction of soft tissue, leading to a disease called necrotizing fasciitis. The various *Clostridium* species that cause gas gangrene

---

[4] *ATP is the major energy-carrying or energy-storing molecule of cells.*

[5] *The three major categories of leukocytes found in blood are monocytes (which mature to become macrophages), lymphocytes, and granulocytes. Granulocytes are named for the prominent cytoplasmic granules that they possess. The three types of granulocytes are eosinophils, basophils, and neutrophils. A neutrophil is also known as a* **PMN** *(for polymorphonuclear cell) or a poly.*

[6] *Enzymes produced within a cell that remain within the cell to catalyze reactions there are referred to as* **endoenzymes.** *Enzymes produced within the cell but subsequently released from the cell to catalyze reactions outside the cell are termed exoenzymes.*

TABLE 2 - 5	Pathogens Capable of Surviving and Multiplying Within Phagocytes	
Category of Pathogen	**Examples**	**Diseases**
Viruses	Herpes viruses	Genital herpes, herpes labialis
	HIV	AIDS
	Rubeola virus	Measles
	Poxviruses	Monkeypox, smallpox
Rickettsias	*Rickettsia rickettsii*	Rocky Mountain spotted fever
	Rickettsia prowazeki	Epidemic (louseborne) typhus
Other bacteria	*Brucella* spp.	Brucellosis
	Legionella pneumophila	Legionellosis
	Listeria monocytogenes	Listeriosis
	Mycobacterium leprae	Hansen disease (leprosy)
	Mycobacterium tuberculosis	Tuberculosis
Protozoa	*Leishmania* spp.	Leishmaniasis
	Toxoplasma gondii	Toxoplasmosis
	Trypanosoma cruzi	American trypanosomiasis (Chagas disease)
Fungi	*Cryptococcus neoformans*	Cryptococcosis

(myonecrosis) produce various necrotizing enzymes, including proteases (which break down proteins) and lipases (which break down lipids).

Coagulase. An important identifying feature of *Staphylococcus aureus* in the laboratory is its ability to produce a protein called **coagulase** (see Chapter 9). Although coagulase ends in *-ase*, like the names of many enzymes, it is technically not an enzyme. In the body, coagulase may enable *S. aureus* cells to clot plasma and thereby to form a sticky coat of fibrin around themselves for protection from phagocytes, antibodies, and other host defense mechanisms.

Kinases. Kinases (also known as **fibrinolysins**) have the opposite effect of coagulase. Sometimes the host will cause a fibrin clot to form around pathogens in an attempt to wall them off and prevent them from invading deeper into body tissues. Kinases are enzymes that lyse (dissolve) clots.

Therefore, pathogens that produce kinases are able to escape from clots. Streptokinase is the name of a kinase produced by streptococci, and staphylokinase is the name of a kinase produced by staphylococci. Streptokinase has been used to treat patients with coronary thrombosis. By producing both coagulase and staphylokinase, *Staphylococcus aureus* can not only cause the formation of clots but also dissolve them.

Hyaluronidase. The spreading factor, as the enzyme **hyaluronidase** is sometimes called, enables pathogens to spread through connective tissue by breaking down hyaluronic acid, the polysaccharide "cement" that holds tissue cells together. Hyaluronidase is secreted by several pathogenic species of *Staphylococcus*, *Streptococcus*, and *Clostridium*.

Collagenase. The enzyme **collagenase**, produced by some pathogens, breaks down collagen, the supportive protein found in tendons, cartilage, and bones. This enables the pathogens to invade tissues. *Clostridium perfringens*, the major cause of gas gangrene, spreads deeply within the body by secreting both collagenase and hyaluronidase.

Hemolysins. Hemolysins are enzymes that cause damage to the host's red blood cells (erythrocytes). The lysis of red blood cells not only harms the host but also provides the pathogens with a source of iron. In the laboratory, the effect an organism has on the red blood cells in blood agar often provides a clue to the organism's identity. Hemolysins are produced by many pathogenic bacteria, but the type of hemolysis produced by an organism is of most importance when a person is attempting to speciate a *Streptococcus* in the laboratory.

Lecithinase. *Clostridium perfringens*, the major cause of gas gangrene, can rapidly destroy extensive areas of tissue, especially muscle tissue. One of the enzymes produced by *C. perfringens* is **lecithinase,** which breaks down phospholipids collectively referred to as lecithin. This enzyme is destructive to cell membranes of red blood cells and other tissues.

> Necrotizing enzymes, coagulase, kinases, hyaluronidase, collagenase, hemolysins, and lecithinase are bacterial exoenzymes that serve as virulence factors.

Toxins

The ability of pathogens to damage host tissues and cause disease may depend on the production and release of various types of poisonous substances termed toxins. The two major categories of toxins are endotoxins and exotoxins. **Endotoxins,** which are integral parts of the cell walls of Gram-negative bacteria, can cause numerous adverse physiologic effects. **Exotoxins,** on the other hand, are toxins produced within cells and then released from the cells.

Endotoxin. Septicemia (often termed *sepsis*) is a very serious disease marked by chills, fever, prostration (extreme exhaustion), and the presence of bacteria and/or their toxins in the bloodstream. Septicemia caused by Gram-negative bacteria (e.g., *Escherichia coli, Pseudomonas aeruginosa, Haemophilus influenzae*), sometimes referred to as Gram-negative sepsis, is an especially serious type of septicemia. The cell walls of Gram-negative bacteria contain lipopolysaccharide, the lipid portion of which is called lipid A or endotoxin. Endotoxin can cause serious, adverse physiological effects, such as fever and shock. Substances that cause fever are known as pyrogens. Endotoxin is a pyrogen.

Shock is a life-threatening condition, resulting from very low blood pressure and an inadequate blood supply to body tissues and organs, especially the kidneys and brain.

The type of shock that results from Gram-negative sepsis is known as **septic shock.** Symptoms include reduced mental alertness, confusion, rapid breathing, chills, fever, and warm, flushed skin. As shock worsens, several organs begin to fail, including the kidneys, lungs, and heart. Blood clots may form within blood vessels. More than 500,000 cases of sepsis occur annually in the United States; approximately half of these are caused by Gram-negative bacteria. There is a 30% to 35% mortality rate associated with Gram-negative sepsis.

Exotoxins. Exotoxins are poisonous proteins secreted by various pathogens; they are often named for the target organs they affect. The most potent exotoxins are **neurotoxins,** which affect the central nervous system. The neurotoxins produced by the bacteria *Clostridium tetani* and *Clostridium botulinum*—tetanospasmin and botulinal toxin—cause tetanus and botulism, respectively. Tetanospasmin affects control of nerve transmission, leading to a spastic, rigid type of paralysis in which the patient's muscles are contracted. Botulinal toxin also blocks nerve impulses but by a different mechanism, leading to a generalized flaccid type of paralysis in which the patient's muscles are relaxed. Both diseases are often fatal.

Other types of exotoxins, called **enterotoxins,** affect the gastrointestinal tract, causing diarrhea and sometimes vomiting. Examples of bacterial pathogens that produce enterotoxins are *Bacillus cereus*, certain serotypes of *Escherichia coli, Clostridium difficile, Clostridium perfringens, Salmonella* spp., *Shigella* spp., *Vibrio cholerae*, and some strains of *Staphylococcus aureus*. In addition to releasing an enterotoxin (called toxin A), *C. difficile* also produces a cytotoxin (called toxin B) that damages the lining of the colon, leading to a condition known as pseudomembranous colitis.

Symptoms of toxic shock syndrome are caused by exotoxins secreted by certain strains of the bacterium *Staphylococcus aureus* and, less commonly, the bacterium *Streptococcus pyogenes*. TSST-1 primarily affects the integrity of capillary walls. The exfoliative (or epidermolytic) toxin of *S. aureus* causes the epidermal layers of skin to slough away, leading to a disease known as scalded skin syndrome. *S. aureus* also produces several toxins that destroy cell membranes.

Erythrogenic toxin, produced by some strains of *Streptococcus pyogenes*, causes scarlet fever. **Leukocidins** are toxins that destroy white blood cells (leukocytes). Thus, leukocidins (which are produced by some staphylococci and streptococci) cause destruction of the very cells that the body sends to the site of infection to ingest and destroy pathogens. Some strains of *Staphylococcus aureus* produce a leukocidin called Panton-Valentine toxin.

Diphtheria toxin, produced by toxigenic strains of the bacterium *Corynebacterium diphtheriae*, inhibits protein

TABLE 2 - 6	Examples of Infectious Diseases Caused by Bacteria[a]
Bacterial Disease	**Etiologic Agent[b]**
Anthrax	*Bacillus anthracis*
Botulism	*Clostridium botulinum*
Chlamydial genital infections	*Chlamydia trachomatis*
Cholera	*Vibrio cholerae*
Diphtheria	*Corynebacterium diphtheriae*
Gonorrhea	*Neisseria gonorrhoeae*
Hansen disease (leprosy)	*Mycobacterium leprae*
Legionellosis	*Legionella pneumophila*
Listeriosis	*Listeria monocytogenes*
Lyme disease	*Borrelia burgdorferi*
Plague	*Yersinia pestis*
Salmonellosis	*Salmonella* spp.
Shigellosis	*Shigella* spp.
Syphilis	*Treponema pallidum*
Tetanus	*Clostridium tetani*
Tuberculosis	*Mycobacterium tuberculosis*
Typhoid fever	*Salmonella typhi*
Whooping cough (pertussis)	*Bordetella pertussis*

[a]The purpose of this list is to introduce students to the names of some important pathogenic bacteria and the infectious diseases they cause. Detailed information about bacterial diseases is in Chapter 18.
[b]The term *etiologic agent* refers to the pathogen that causes the disease—in this case, a bacterium.

> Exotoxins such as neurotoxins, enterotoxins, TSST-1, exfoliative toxin, erythrogenic toxin, leukocidins, and diphtheria toxin are examples of bacterial virulence factors.

synthesis. It kills mucosal epithelial cells and neutrophils, and adversely affects the heart and nervous system. The toxin is actually coded for by a bacteriophage gene.[7] Thus, only *C. diphtheriae* cells that are "infected" with that particular bacteriophage are able to produce diphtheria toxin. Other exotoxins that inhibit protein synthesis are *Pseudomonas aeruginosa* exotoxin A, shiga toxin (produced by *Shigella* spp.), and the shigalike toxins produced by certain serotypes of *Escherichia coli*.

EXAMPLES OF INFECTIOUS DISEASES OF HUMANS

Infectious Diseases Caused by Bacteria

Examples of infectious diseases caused by bacteria are shown in Table 2-6. The table is not an all-inclusive listing of bacterial diseases of humans. For example, diseases that can be caused by more than one bacterial species, such as meningitis, pneumonia, and diarrhea, are not included.

---

[7]*Bacteriophages are viruses that infect bacteria.*

TABLE 2 - 7   Examples of Infectious Diseases Caused by Fungi[a]

Category	Name of Pathogen	Diseases
Yeasts	*Candida albicans*	Thrush, yeast vaginitis, nail infections, systemic infection
	Cryptococcus neoformans	Cryptococcosis (lung infection, meningitis, etc.)
Moulds	*Aspergillus* spp.	Aspergillosis (lung infection, systemic infection)
	Mucor spp., *Rhizopus* spp., and other species of bread moulds	Mucormycosis or zygomycosis (lung infection, systemic infection)
	Various dermatophytes	Tinea (ringworm) infections
Dimorphic fungi	*Blastomycosis dermatitidis*	Blastomycosis (primarily a disease of lungs and skin)
	Coccidioides immitis	Coccidioidomycosis (lung infection, systemic infection)
	Histoplasma capsulatum	Histoplasmosis (lung infection, systemic infection)
	Sporothrix schenckii	Sporotrichosis (a skin disease)
Other	*Pneumocystis jiroveci*[b] (previously called *Pneumocystis carinii*)	*Pneumocystis* pneumonia (PCP)

[a]The purpose of this list is to introduce students to the names of some important fungal pathogens and the infectious diseases they cause. Detailed information about fungal diseases is in Chapter 20.

[b]Although the taxonomic classification of *Pneumocystis jiroveci* is controversial, it is presently considered to be a nonfilamentous fungus.

Infectious Diseases Caused by Algae

Algal infections of humans are extremely rare. One genus of algae (*Prototheca*) has been reported to cause human infections. The disease is known as protothecosis. *Prototheca* lives in soil and on decaying organic matter. It can enter wounds, especially those located on the feet, producing a small subcutaneous lesion that can progress to a crusty, warty-looking lesion. If the organism enters the lymphatic system, it may cause a debilitating, sometimes fatal infection, especially in immunosuppressed patients. Fatal infections are extremely rare.

Prototheca spp. can be grown in the laboratory. They produce yeastlike, white to cream-colored colonies that may be dull, moist, or mucoid in appearance. Individual cells of *Prototheca* spp. are round, oval, or cylindrical and do not reproduce by budding. Some commercial miniaturized biochemical test systems (minisystems) for the identification of yeasts can be used to identify *Prototheca* spp.

Infectious Diseases Caused by Fungi

The three major categories of fungi that cause human infections—yeasts, moulds, and dimorphic fungi—are described in detail in Chapters 19 and 20. For now, think of yeasts as single-celled fungi; moulds as multicellular, filamentous fungi; and dimorphic fungi as fungi that can exist either as yeasts or moulds, depending on the temperature at which they are growing. Dimorphic fungi exist as yeasts at body temperature and as moulds at room temperature. Examples of infectious diseases caused by fungi are shown in Table 2-7. The table is not an all-inclusive listing of fungal diseases of humans.

TABLE 2 - 8 Examples of Infectious Diseases Caused by Protozoa[a]

Category of Protozoa	Name of Pathogen	Disease(s)
Amebas	*Acanthamoeba* spp.	Amebic conjunctivitis and keratoconjunctivitis (eye infections)
	Entamoeba histolytica	Amebiasis (amebic dysentery)
	Naegleria fowleri	Primary amebic meningoencephalitis (a disease of the central nervous system)
Flagellates	*Giardia lamblia*	Giardiasis (a diarrheal disease)
	Leishmania spp.	Leishmaniasis (may involve the skin, the mucosa, or internal organs)
	Trichomonas vaginalis	Trichomoniasis (a sexually transmitted disease, a cause of vaginitis)
	Subspecies of *Trypanosoma brucei*	African trypanosomiasis (a disease of the central nervous system)
	Trypanosoma cruzi	American trypanosomiasis (may lead to enlarged organs, such as the heart, esophagus, and colon)
Ciliates	*Balantidium coli*	Balantidiasis (a type of dysentery)
Sporozoa	*Babesia* spp.	Babesiosis (causes destruction of red blood cells)
	Plasmodium spp.	Malaria (causes destruction of red blood cells)
	Toxoplasma gondii	Toxoplasmosis (may involve the central nervous system, lungs, muscle, heart, and eyes)
Coccidia (a subcategory of sporozoa)	*Cryptosporidium parvum*	Cryptosporidiosis (a diarrheal disease)
	Cyclospora cayetanensis	Cyclosporiasis (a diarrheal disease)

[a]The purpose of this list is to introduce students to the names of some important parasitic protozoa and the infectious diseases they cause. Detailed information about protozoal diseases is in Chapter 22.

Infectious Diseases Caused by Protozoa
Parasitic protozoa and the diseases they cause are discussed in detail in Chapters 21 and 22. Examples of infectious protozoal diseases are shown in Table 2-8. The table does not represent an all-inclusive listing of protozoal diseases of humans.

Infectious Diseases Caused by Helminths
See Chapter 23 for a detailed discussion of helminth infections.

Infectious Diseases Caused by Viruses
Viral diseases of humans include AIDS, avian influenza (bird flu), certain types of cancer, chickenpox, cold sores (fever blisters), the common cold, dengue, diarrhea, encephalitis, genital herpes infections, German measles, Hantavirus pulmonary syndrome, hemorrhagic fevers, hepatitis, infectious mononucleosis, influenza, measles, meningitis, mumps, pneumonia, polio, rabies, severe acute respiratory syndrome, shingles, smallpox, warts, and yellow fever. Viral infections are discussed in detail in Chapter 25.

Chapter Review

- Colonization by a microbe means that the microbe has come in contact with some part of the human body, has multiplied, and has remained there.

- Microbiologists define *infection* as colonization by a pathogen. Once colonized by a pathogen, the person is said to be infected with that pathogen, whether or not the pathogen is causing disease. However, throughout this book, the terms *infection* and *infectious disease* are used synonymously.

- When people are exposed to pathogens, those microbes may or may not cause disease, depending on a number of factors, including the person's nutritional, health, and immune status and the virulence of the pathogen.

- The infectious disease process or chain of infection involves six steps: (1) a pathogen, (2) a source of the pathogen (reservoir), (3) a portal of exit, (4) a mode of transmission, (5) a portal of entry, and (6) a susceptible host.

- A reservoir is a site where the pathogen can multiply or survive until it is transferred to a host. A reservoir may be a living organism or an inanimate object.

- Examples of living reservoirs include humans, pets, farm animals, and some arthropods. Examples of nonliving reservoirs include air, soil, dust, food, and water.

- The five principal modes by which pathogens are transmitted are contact, air, droplets, vehicles, and vectors.

- An infectious disease that is directly or indirectly transmissible from one human to another is called a communicable disease. Contagious diseases are communicable diseases that are *easily* transmitted from person to person. A noncommunicable disease is one that is not transmitted by person-to-person contact (e.g., tetanus).

- A sporadic disease occurs only occasionally. An endemic disease is always present in the population of a particular geographic area. An epidemic disease affects a higher number of people than usual, often within a short period. A pandemic disease occurs in epidemic proportions in many places simultaneously, sometimes worldwide.

- Biofilms consist of various species of bacteria embedded in an extracellular polysaccharide matrix. Biofilms are medically significant and resistant to antibiotics and disinfectants.

- Pathogenicity is the ability of a microbe to cause disease, whereas pathogenesis refers to the actual steps involved in the development of a disease. Sometimes, but not always, pathogenesis follows this sequence: entry of the pathogen into the body, attachment, multiplication, invasion/spread, evasion of host defenses, and damage to host tissue(s).

- When the body loses its battle with a pathogen, clinical disease results, accompanied by characteristic signs and symptoms of the disease.

- Signs of a disease are various types of objective evidence of a disease (e.g., increased or decreased blood pressure, elevated body temperature, abnormal pulse rate, abnormalities that are discovered by palpation, and abnormal test results).

- Symptoms of a disease are various types of subjective evidence of disease that are experienced or perceived by the patient (e.g., aches or pains, chills, anorexia, nausea, itching).

- Some pathogens manifest themselves periodically, remaining dormant between episodes. The diseases caused by such pathogens are referred to as latent infections, examples being syphilis and various types of herpes infections, such as cold sores, genital herpes infection, and shingles.

- An infection may be acute, subacute, or chronic; localized or systemic; and symptomatic or asymptomatic. As the disease progresses, it may change from one stage to another.

- The four phases of an infectious disease are the incubation period, prodromal period, period of illness, and convalescent period. In some cases, the period of illness is followed by disability or death, rather than convalescence. A primary infection may set the stage for a secondary infection, which is caused by another pathogen.

- Virulence is a measure or degree of pathogenicity. Different species or even different strains of the same species vary in their ability to cause disease; thus, some are more virulent than others. Some strains of a particular species may be virulent, while other strains of the same species are avirulent.

- Virulence factors are the phenotypic characteristics of a microbe that enable it to cause disease. Some virulence factors are structural features (e.g., adhesins, pili, capsules, flagella) that enable pathogens to avoid phagocytosis and to reach and attach to various tissues within the host.

- The two major virulence factors by which bacteria cause disease are exoenzymes and toxins. Exoenzymes that are virulence factors include coagulase, kinases, hyaluronidase, collagenase, hemolysins, lecithinase, and necrotizing enzymes. These exoenzymes enable pathogens to evade host defenses, invade, and cause damage to body tissues.

- Toxins include endotoxins, which are found in the cell walls of Gram-negative bacteria, and exotoxins, which are released from the cells that produce them. Examples of exotoxins are neurotoxins, which cause paralysis; enterotoxins, which cause gastrointestinal disease; TSST-1, which causes toxic shock syndrome; exfoliative or epidermolytic toxin, which causes scalded skin syndrome; erythrogenic toxin, which causes scarlet fever; leukocidins, which destroy leukocytes; and diphtheria toxin, which causes diphtheria.

- The two most important categories of phagocytes in the human body are macrophages and PMNs. Although their primary function is to ingest and destroy pathogens, some pathogens are able to survive within phagocytes. Some pathogens prevent fusion of the phagosome with a lysosome. Others have a cell wall structure that resists the digestion process.

New Terms and Abbreviations

After studying Chapter 2, you should be familiar with the following terms, which are defined within the chapter and in the Glossary at the back of the book:

Acute disease

Adhesin

Arthropod-borne disease

Asymptomatic disease

Avirulent strain

Biofilm

Carrier

Centers for Disease Control and Prevention (CDC)

Chronic disease

Coagulase

Collagenase

Colonization

Communicable disease

Contagious disease

Convalescent period

Endemic disease

Endoenzyme

Endotoxin

Enterotoxin

Epidemic disease

Erythrocyte

Erythrogenic toxin

Exoenzyme

Exotoxin

Facultative intracellular pathogen

Fomite

Hemolysin

Hyaluronidase

Incubation period

Intraerythrocytic pathogen

Intraleukocytic pathogen

In vitro

In vivo

Kinase

Latent infection

Lecithinase

Leukocidin

Leukocyte

Localized infection

Necrotizing enzyme

Neurotoxin

Noncommunicable disease

Obligate intracellular pathogen

Pandemic disease

Pathogenesis

Pathogenicity

Pathologist

Pathology

Phagocyte

Polymicrobial infection

PMN

Primary disease

Prodromal period

Receptors

Reservoirs of infection

Secondary disease

Septic shock

Shock

Signs of a disease

Sporadic disease

Subacute disease

Symptomatic disease

Symptoms of a disease

Systemic infection

Vector

Virulence

Virulence factor

Virulent strain

World Health Organization (WHO)

Zoonosis (pl. zoonoses)

 On the CD-ROM

- A Closer Look at Polymicrobial Infections
- Typhoid Mary—an Infamous Carrier
- A Closer Look at Zoonoses
- A Closer Look at the CDC
- Nationally Notifiable Infectious Diseases in the United States
- A Closer Look at the WHO
- Additional Self-Assessment Exercises
- Puzzle

Self-Assessment Exercises

After studying Chapter 2, answer the following questions.

1. Which of the following virulence factors enable(s) bacteria to attach to tissues?

    A. Capsules

    B. Endotoxin

    C. Flagella

    D. Pili

2. Neurotoxins are produced by

    A. *Staphylococcus aureus* and *Streptococcus pyogenes*.

    B. *Clostridium difficile* and *Clostridium perfringens*.

    C. *Clostridium botulinum* and *Clostridium tetani*.

    D. *Pseudomonas aeruginosa* and *Mycobacterium tuberculosis*.

3. Which of the following pathogens produce enterotoxins?

    A. *Staphylococcus aureus* and *Vibrio cholerae*

    B. *Clostridium difficile* and *Clostridium perfringens*

    C. *Salmonella* spp. and *Shigella* spp.

    D. All the above

4. A bloodstream infection with _____ could result in the release of endotoxin into the bloodstream.

    A. *Escherichia coli*

    B. *Neisseria gonorrhoeae*

    C. *Staphylococcus aureus*

    D. both (a) and (b)

5. Communicable diseases are most easily transmitted during the

    A. incubation period.

    B. prodromal period.

    C. period of illness.

    D. latent period.

6. Enterotoxins affect cells in the

   A. respiratory tract.

   B. genitourinary tract.

   C. gastrointestinal tract.

   D. central nervous system.

7. Which bacterium produces a toxin that causes scarlet fever?

   A. *Staphylococcus aureus*

   B. *Escherichia coli*

   C. *Streptococcus pyogenes*

   D. *Clostridium tetani*

8. Which bacterium produces both a cytotoxin and an enterotoxin?

   A. *Clostridium difficile*

   B. *Clostridium tetani*

   C. *Clostridium botulinum*

   D. *Corynebacterium diphtheriae*

9. Which virulence factor enables bacteria to avoid phagocytosis by white blood cells?

   A. Cell wall

   B. Cell membrane

   C. Capsule

   D. Pili

10. Which pair of bacteria can cause toxic shock syndrome?

   A. *Clostridium difficile* and *Clostridium perfringens*

   B. *Neisseria gonorrhoeae* and *Escherichia coli*

   C. *Mycoplasma pneumoniae* and *Mycobacterium tuberculosis*

   D. *Staphylococcus aureus* and *Streptococcus pyogenes*

CHAPTER 3

Combating Pathogens and Infectious Diseases

Chapter Outline

LEARNING OBJECTIVES

After studying this chapter, you should be able to:

☛ Define the terms and abbreviations introduced in this chapter (e.g., *acquired immunity, active acquired immunity, agammaglobulinemia*)

☛ Briefly describe the three lines of defense used by the body to combat pathogens, and give one example of each

☛ Explain what is meant by *nonspecific host defense mechanisms* and how they differ from specific host defense mechanisms; include examples in your discussion

☛ Identify three ways by which the digestive system is protected from pathogens

☛ Describe how interferons function as host defense mechanisms, including specificity and mechanism of action

☛ Name three cellular and chemical responses to microbial invasion

☛ Describe the major consequences of complement activation, including its effect on inflammation, phagocytes, and foreign invaders

☛ List the four cardinal (main) signs and symptoms associated with inflammation

☛ Discuss the four primary purposes of the inflammatory response

☛ List the four steps in phagocytosis, starting with chemotaxis

☛ Identify the two major groups of phagocytes in the human body

☛ Categorize the disorders and conditions that affect the body's nonspecific host mechanisms—for example, breaks in the skin

☛ Differentiate between humoral and cell-mediated immunity, including the types of cells involved in each

☛ Distinguish between active acquired immunity and passive acquired immunity, including the source of protective antibodies in each

☛ Distinguish between natural active acquired immunity and artificial active acquired immunity, and cite an example of each

☛ Distinguish between natural passive acquired immunity and artificial passive acquired immunity, and cite an example of each

☛ Identify the two primary functions of the immune system

☛ List three types of cells that are killed by natural killer cells

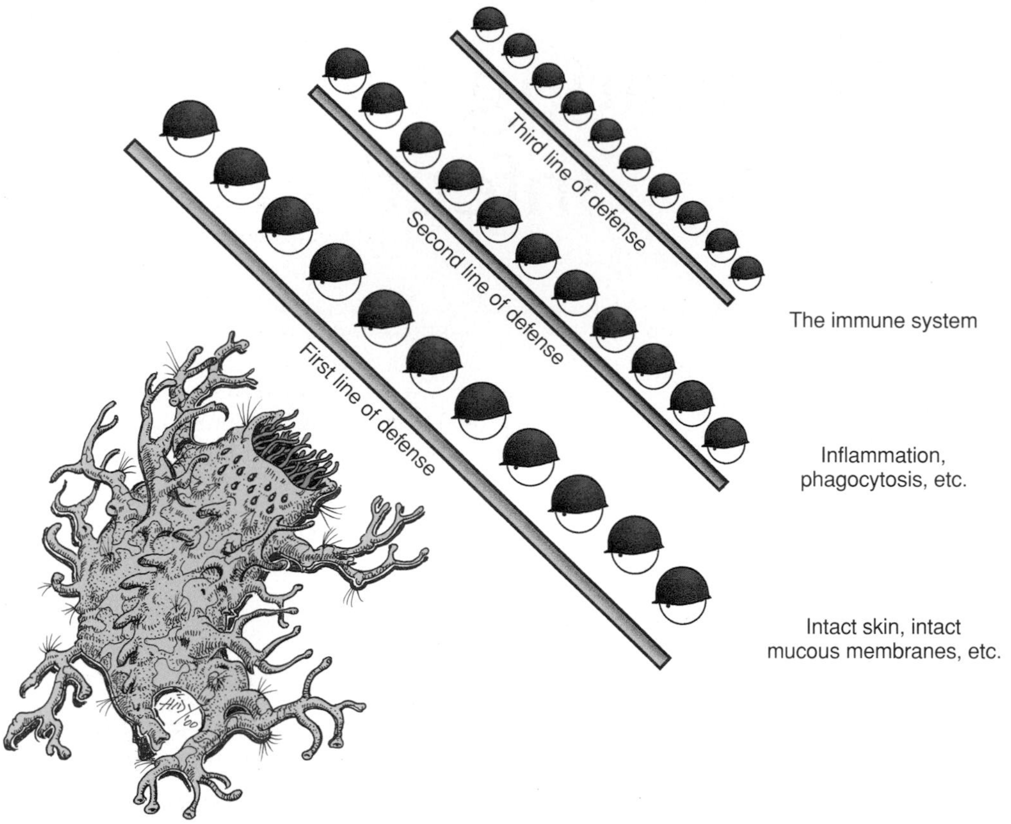

Figure 3-1. **Lines of defense.** Host defense mechanisms—ways in which the body protects itself from pathogens—can be thought of as an entrenched army consisting of three lines of defense.

Humans and animals have survived on earth for hundreds of thousands of years because they have many "built-in" or naturally occurring mechanisms of defense against pathogens and the infectious diseases they cause. The ability of humans and animals to resist these invaders and recover from disease is the result of many complex functions within the body.

Host defense mechanisms—ways in which the body protects itself from pathogens—can be thought of as an army with three lines of defense (Fig. 3-1). If the enemy (the pathogen) breaks through the first line of defense, it will encounter and, we hope, be stopped by the second line of defense. If the enemy somehow manages to evade the first two lines of defense, however, a third line of defense is ready to attack it.

The first two lines of defense are nonspecific; these are ways in which the body attempts to destroy *all* types of substances that are foreign to it, including pathogens. Some scientists refer to the first and second lines of defense as innate immunity. The third line of defense, the immune response, is very specific. It is sometimes referred to as adaptive immunity. In the third line of defense, special proteins called **antibodies** are usually produced in the body in response to the presence of foreign substances. These foreign substances are called **antigens** because they stimulate the production of specific antibodies; they are **anti**body-**gen**erating substances. The antibodies produced are very specific because they can only recognize and attach to the antigen that stimulated their production. Immune responses are discussed later in this chapter. The various categories of host defense mechanisms are summarized in Figure 3-2.

> The first two lines of defense include various nonspecific host defense mechanisms.

NONSPECIFIC HOST DEFENSE MECHANISMS

Nonspecific host defense mechanisms are general in nature and serve to protect the body against many harmful substances. One of the nonspecific host defenses is the innate, or inborn, resistance observed among some species of animals and some people who have a natural resistance to certain diseases. Innate or inherited characteristics make these

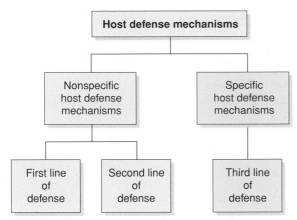

Figure 3-2. Categories of host defense mechanisms.

people and animals more resistant to some diseases than to others. The exact factors that produce this innate resistance are not well understood but are probably the result of chemical, physiological, and temperature differences between the species, as well as the general state of physical and emotional health of the person and environmental factors that affect certain races but not others.

Although we are usually unaware of it, our bodies are constantly in the process of defending us against microbial invaders. We encounter pathogens and potential pathogens many times a day, every day of our lives. Usually, our bodies successfully ward off or destroy the invading microbes. Some important nonspecific host defense mechanisms are listed in Table 3-1 (first line of defense) and Table 3-2 (second line of defense).

Complement System

Complement is not a single entity but rather a group of approximately 30 proteins (including 9 proteins designated as C1 through C9) that are found in normal blood plasma. These proteins make up what is called the complement system—so named because it "complements" the action of the immune system. Although some scientists consider the complement system part of the second line of defense, others consider it part of the immune system. The proteins of the complement system, sometimes collectively referred to as complement components, interact with each other in a stepwise manner, known as the **complement cascade.** The major consequences of complement activation are (1) initiation and amplification of inflammation, (2) attraction of phagocytes to sites where they are needed (chemotaxis, discussed later), (3) activation of leukocytes, (4) lysis of bacteria and other foreign cells, and (5) increased phagocytosis by phagocytic cells (opsonization).

Opsonization is a process by which phagocytosis is facilitated by the deposition of **opsonins** (e.g., antibodies or certain complement fragments) onto the surface of particles

or cells. In some cases, phagocytes are unable to ingest certain particles or cells (e.g., encapsulated bacteria) until opsonization occurs. One of the products formed during the complement cascade, called C3b, is an opsonin. It becomes deposited on the surface of microbes. Neutrophils and macrophages possess surface molecules (receptors) that can recognize and bind to C3b.

Complement fragments C3a, C4a, and C5a cause mast cells to degranulate and release histamine, leading to increased vascular permeability and smooth muscle contraction. C5a also acts as a chemotactic agent for neutrophils and macrophages, attracting these cells to sites where they are needed. Chemotactic agents are discussed latter in the chapter.

Inflammation

The body normally responds to any local injury, irritation, microbial invasion, or bacterial toxins by a complex series of events collectively referred to as **inflammation** or the **inflammatory response** (Fig. 3-3). Inflammation is part of the second line of defense. The three major events in acute inflammation are (1) an increase in the diameter of capillaries, a process called **vasodilation** that increases blood flow to the site; (2) increased permeability of the capillaries, allowing the escape of plasma and plasma proteins; and (3) egress (exit) of leukocytes from the capillaries and their accumulation at the site of injury. The primary purposes of the inflammatory response are to localize an infection, prevent the spread of microbial invaders, neutralize any toxins being produced at the site, and aid in the repair of damaged tissue (Fig. 3-4).

STUDY AID

The Suffix -*itis*. The suffix -*itis* is used to denote inflammation. For example, cystitis is inflammation of the urinary bladder, hepatitis is inflammation of the liver, and encephalitis is inflammation of the brain. Inflammation is often, but not always, triggered by an infection.

During the inflammatory process, many nonspecific host defense mechanisms come into play. These interrelated physiological reactions result in the four cardinal (main) signs and symptoms of inflammation: redness, heat, swelling (**edema**), and pain. (The Latin terms are *rubor, calor, tumor,* and *dolor,* respectively.) Often pus forms, and occasionally the damaged area loses some function (e.g., an inflamed elbow might prevent bending of the arm).

> The four cardinal (main) signs and symptoms of inflammation are redness, heat, swelling (edema), and pain.

A complex series of physiological events occurs immediately after the initial damage to the tissue. One of the

TABLE 3 - 1	Nonspecific Host Defense Mechanisms in the First Line of Defense
Mechanism	**Function(s)**
Intact skin and intact mucous membranes	Serve as physical or mechanical barriers. Very few pathogens are able to penetrate intact skin and intact mucous membranes.
Dryness and temperature of the skin	Many potential pathogens are unable to survive on the skin because of the dryness of certain areas and the relatively low temperature of the skin (<37°C).
Low pH of the skin (approx. pH 5.0)	Many potential pathogens are unable to survive on the skin because of its low pH (i.e., its acidity).
Sebum	The oily sebum that is produced by sebaceous glands in the skin contains fatty acids, which are toxic to some pathogens.
Perspiration	The act of perspiring flushes potential pathogens off the skin. Also, perspiration contains the enzyme lysozyme, which destroys bacterial cell walls.
Mucus	The sticky mucus produced by goblet cells within mucous membranes serves to entrap invaders. Also, mucus contains various substances (e.g., lysozyme, lactoferrin, and lactoperoxidase) that can kill bacteria or inhibit their growth. Lactoferrin is a protein that binds iron, a mineral required by all pathogens. Because they are unable to compete with lactoferrin for free iron, the pathogens are deprived of this essential nutrient. The enzyme lactoperoxidase produces superoxide radicals, highly reactive forms of oxygen, which are toxic to bacteria.
Ciliated epithelial cells that line the respiratory tract	The cilia (mucociliary covering) present on epithelial cells of the posterior nasal membranes, nasal sinuses, bronchi, and trachea sweep trapped dust and microbes upward toward the throat, where they are swallowed or expelled by sneezing and coughing. Phagocytic white blood cells in the mucous membranes may also be involved in this mucociliary clearance mechanism.
Saliva and swallowing	Lysozyme and other enzymes that lyse or destroy bacteria are present in nasal secretions, saliva, and tears. The swallowing of saliva can be thought of as a nonspecific host defense mechanism because thousands of bacteria are removed from the oral cavity with every swallow. Humans swallow about one liter of saliva a day.
Acidity of the stomach and the contents of the digestive tract	Few microbes can survive the extreme acidity of the stomach (approx. pH 1.5). The alkalinity of the intestines and the digestive enzymes they contain are capable of destroying potential pathogens. Bile, which is secreted from the liver into the small intestine, lowers the surface tension and causes chemical changes in bacterial cell walls and membranes that make bacteria easier to digest. Many invading microorganisms are trapped in the sticky mucus lining of the digestive tract, where they may be destroyed by bactericidal enzymes and phagocytes. Peristalsis and the expulsion of feces serve to remove bacteria from the intestine. Bacteria make up about 50% of feces.

(continued)

TABLE 3 - 1   Continued

Mechanism	Function(s)
The pH of the vagina	Usually, the low pH of vaginal fluid inhibits colonization of the vagina by pathogens. However, women who are taking some types of oral contraceptives are particularly susceptible to infections because the contraceptives increase the pH of the vagina.
Urination	Microorganisms are continually flushed from the urethra by frequent urination and expulsion of mucus secretions. Many urinary bladder infections result from infrequent urination, including the failure to urinate after intercourse. Conditions that obstruct urine flow (e.g., benign prostatic hyperplasia) also increase the chances of developing cystitis.
Microbial antagonism	When resident microbes of the indigenous microflora prevent colonization by new arrivals to a particular anatomical site, it is known as **microbial antagonism.** The inhibitory capability of the indigenous microflora has been attributed to (1) competition for colonization sites, (2) competition for nutrients, and (3) production of substances that kill other bacteria. Some bacteria produce antibacterial proteins (known as **bacteriocins**) that kill other bacteria. An example is **colicin**, which is produced by certain strains of *Escherichia coli*. The effectiveness of microbial antagonism is frequently decreased following prolonged administration of broad-spectrum antibiotics. The antibiotics reduce or eliminate certain members of the indigenous microflora (e.g., the vaginal and gastrointestinal flora), leading to overgrowth by bacteria and/or fungi resistant to the antibiotic(s) being administered.

initial events is vasodilation at the site of injury, mediated (caused) by vasoactive agents (e.g., histamine and prostaglandins) released from damaged cells. Vasodilation allows more blood to flow to the site, bringing redness and heat. Additional heat results from increased metabolic activities in the tissue cells at the site. Vasodilation causes the endothelial cells that line the capillaries to stretch and separate, resulting in increased permeability. Plasma escapes from the capillaries into the surrounding area, causing the site to become **edematous** (swollen). Sometimes the swelling is severe enough to interfere with the bending of a particular joint (e.g., knuckle, elbow, knee, ankle), leading to a loss of function.

Various chemotactic agents (discussed later) are produced at the site of inflammation, leading to an influx of phagocytes. The pain or tenderness that accompanies inflammation may result from actual damage of the nerve fibers because of the injury, irritation by microbial toxins or other cellular secretions (such as prostaglandins), or increased pressure on nerve endings as a result of the edema.

The accumulation of fluid, cells, and cellular debris at the inflammation site is referred to as an **inflammatory exudate.** If the exudate is thick and greenish yellow, containing many live and dead leukocytes, it is known as a **purulent exudate** or **pus.** However, in many inflammatory responses, such as arthritis or pancreatitis, there is no exudate and no invading microbes. When **pyogenic** (pus-producing) microorganisms, such as staphylococci and streptococci, are present, additional pus is produced as a result of the killing effect of the bacterial toxins on phagocytes and tissue cells. Although most pus is greenish yellow, the exudate is often bluish green in infections caused by *Pseudomonas aeruginosa*. This is a result of the bluish-green pigment (called pyocyanin) this organism produces.

When the inflammatory response is completed and the body has won the battle, the phagocytes clean up the area and help to restore order. The cells and tissues can then repair the damage and begin to function normally again in a homeostatic (equilibrated) state, although some permanent damage and scarring may result.

Phagocytosis

White blood cells that engulf or ingest foreign material are called phagocytes. The process by which they accomplish this is called **phagocytosis.** Phagocytosis is part of the second line of defense. The two most important groups of phagocytes in the human body are macrophages and

TABLE 3 - 2	Nonspecific Host Defense Mechanisms in the Second Line of Defense
Mechanism	**Function(s)**
Transferrin	Transferrin, a glycoprotein synthesized in the liver, has a high affinity for iron. Its normal function is to store and deliver iron to host cells. Like lactoferrin, transferrin serves as a nonspecific host defense mechanism by sequestering iron and depriving pathogens of this essential nutrient.
Fever	A body temperature over 37.8°C (100°F) is generally considered a fever. Fever augments the host's defenses by (1) stimulating white blood cells to deploy and destroy invaders; (2) reducing available free plasma iron, which limits the growth of pathogens that require iron for replication and synthesis of toxins; and (3) inducing the production of a cytokine called interleukin 1, which causes the proliferation, maturation, and activation of lymphocytes in the immunological response. Elevated body temperatures also slow down the rate of growth of certain pathogens, and can even kill some especially fastidious[a] pathogens. Substances that invoke fever are referred to as **pyrogens**.
Interferons	Interferons are small, antiviral proteins produced by virus-infected cells. They are called interferons because they "interfere" with viral replication. The interferons produced by a virus-infected cell are unable to save that cell from destruction, but once they are released from that cell, the interferons attach to the membranes of surrounding cells and prevent viral replication from occurring in those cells. Thus, the spread of the infection is inhibited, allowing other body defenses to fight the disease more effectively. Interferons are not virus specific, meaning they are effective against many viruses, not just the particular type of virus that stimulated their production. Interferons are species specific, however, meaning they are effective only in the species of animal that produced them. Human interferons are industrially produced by genetically engineered bacteria (bacteria into which human interferon genes have been inserted) and are used experimentally to treat certain viral infections (e.g., warts, herpes simplex, hepatitis B and C) and cancers (e.g., leukemias, lymphomas, Kaposi sarcoma in AIDS patients). Interferons also activate certain lymphocytes (NK cells) to kill virus-infected cells.
Complement and the complement cascade	See text.
Acute-phase proteins	Plasma levels of molecules collectively referred to as acute-phase proteins increase rapidly in response to infection, inflammation, and tissue injury. They serve as host defense mechanisms by enhancing resistance to infection and promoting the repair of damaged tissue. Acute-phase proteins include C-reactive protein (which is used as a laboratory marker for, or indication of, inflammation), serum amyloid A protein, protease inhibitors, and coagulation proteins.
Cytokines	Cytokines are chemical mediators released from many types of cells in the human body. They enable cells to "communicate" with each other. They act as chemical messengers both within the immune system and between the immune system and other systems of the body. A cell is able to "sense" the presence of a cytokine if it possesses appropriate surface receptors that can

(continued)

TABLE 3 - 2   Continued

Mechanism	Function(s)
	recognize the cytokine. The cytokine causes (mediates) some type of response in a cell that is able to sense its presence. Some cytokines are chemoattractants, recruiting phagocytes to locations where they are needed. Others, like interferons, have a direct role in host defense.
Inflammation	See text.
Phagocytosis	See text.

*The term *fastidious* means "fussy." Fastidious pathogens are difficult or impossible to culture in the clinical microbiology laboratory because they are nutritionally demanding or have other characteristics (e.g., sensitivity to extremes in temperature) that inhibit their growth in vitro.

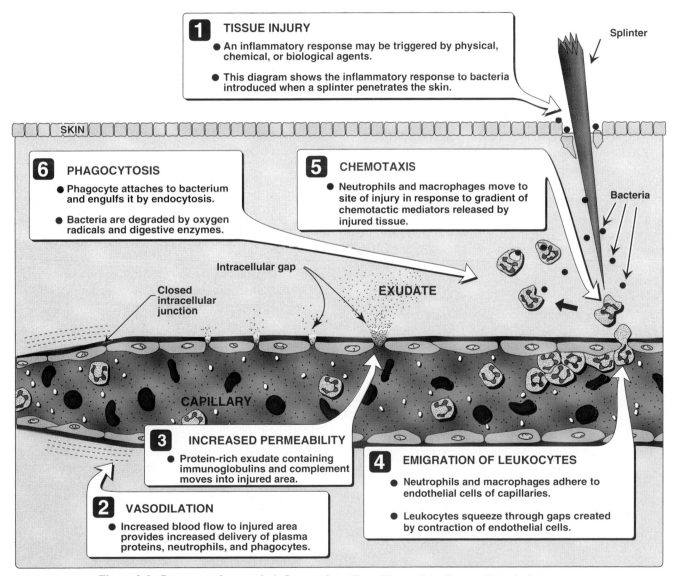

***Figure 3-3. Sequence of events in inflammation.** (From Harvey RA, Champe PA, eds. Lippincott Illustrated Reviews: Microbiology. Philadelphia: Lippincott Williams & Wilkins, 2001.)*

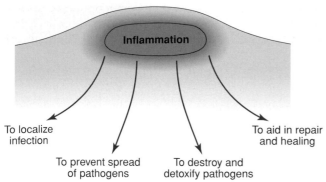

Figure 3-4. **The primary purposes of inflammation.**

Step	Brief Description
TABLE 3 - 3	**The Four Steps in Phagocytosis**
1. Chemotaxis	Phagocytes are attracted by chemotactic agents to the site where they are needed
2. Attachment	A phagocyte attaches to an object
3. Ingestion	Pseudopodia surround the object and it is taken into the cell
4. Digestion	The object is broken down and dissolved by digestive enzymes and other mechanisms

> The two most important phagocytic cells in the body are macrophages and neutrophils. They are often referred to as professional phagocytes.

neutrophils. Because phagocytosis is their major function, they are often referred to as **professional phagocytes.** Macrophages serve as a "clean-up crew" to rid the body of unwanted and often harmful substances, such as dead cells, unused cellular secretions, debris, and microbes. Neutrophils are also known as polymorphonuclear cells, PMNs, and polys.

Macrophages develop from monocytes during the inflammatory response to infections. Those that leave the bloodstream and migrate to infected areas are called **wandering macrophages. Fixed macrophages** (also known as **histocytes** or **histiocytes**) remain in tissues and organs and serve to trap foreign debris. Macrophages are extremely efficient phagocytes. They are found in tissues of the **reticuloendothelial system (RES),** which includes cells in the liver (Kupffer cells), spleen, lymph nodes, and bone marrow, as well as the lungs (alveolar or dust cells), blood vessels, intestines, and brain (microglia). The principal function of the entire RES is the engulfment and removal of foreign and useless particles, living or dead, such as excess cellular secretions; dead and dying leukocytes, erythrocytes, and tissue cells; and foreign debris and microbes that gain entrance to the body.

The four steps in phagocytosis are discussed next and are summarized in Table 3-3.

Chemotaxis. Phagocytosis begins when phagocytes move to the site where they are needed. This directed migration is called **chemotaxis,** and is the result of chemical attractants called **chemotactic agents** (also called chemotactic factors, chemotactic substances, and chemoattractants). Chemotactic agents produced by various cells of the human body are called **chemokines.**[1] Chemotactic agents are produced during the complement cascade and inflammation. When phagocytes "sense" the presence of chemotactic agents, they move along a concentration gradient; that is, they move from areas of low concentrations of chemotactic agents to

the area of highest concentration. The area of highest concentration is the site where the chemotactic agents are being produced or released (e.g., the site of inflammation). Thus, the phagocytes are attracted to where they are needed. Different types of chemotactic agents attract different types of leukocytes; some attract monocytes, others neutrophils, and still others eosinophils.

Attachment. The next step in phagocytosis is attachment of the phagocyte to the object (e.g., a yeast or bacterial cell) to be ingested. Phagocytes can only ingest objects to which they can attach. As previously mentioned, opsonization is sometimes necessary to enable phagocytes to attach to particles (e.g., encapsulated bacteria). The particle becomes coated with opsonins (either complement fragments or antibodies). Because the phagocyte possesses surface molecules (receptors) for complement fragments and antibodies, the phagocyte can now attach to the particle (see Fig. 3-5).

Ingestion. The phagocyte then surrounds the object with pseudopodia, which fuse together, and the object is ingested (phagocytized or phagocytosed; see Fig. 3-6). Phagocytosis is a type of **endocytosis** (a general term for ingestion of material from outside the cell). Within the cytoplasm of the phagocyte, the object is contained within a membrane-bound vesicle called a **phagosome.**

Digestion. The phagosome next fuses with a nearby lysosome to form a digestive vacuole (**phagolysosome**), within which killing and digestion occur (Fig. 3-7). Recall from Chapter 1 that lysosomes are membrane-bound vesicles containing digestive enzymes. Digestive enzymes found within lysosomes include

> The four steps in phagocytosis are chemotaxis, attachment, ingestion, and digestion.

---

[1] *Various types of cells within the human body, including cells of the immune system, communicate with each other. They do so via chemical "messages"— proteins known as* **cytokines.** *If the cytokines are chemotactic agents, attracting leukocytes to areas where they are needed, they are referred to as chemokines.*

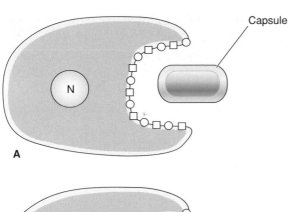

Capsule

A

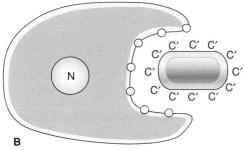

C' C' C'
C'   C'
C'   C'
C'   C'
C' C' C'

B

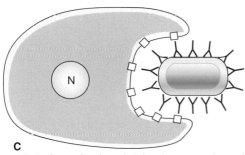

C

Figure 3-5. **Opsonization. A.** The phagocyte shown here is unable to attach to the encapsulated bacterium because there are no molecules (receptors) on the surface of the phagocyte that can recognize or attach to the polysaccharide capsule. **B.** Complement fragments (*C*) have been deposited onto the surface of the capsule. (In this example, the opsonins are complement fragments.) Now the phagocyte can attach to the bacterium because there are receptors (*circles*) on the phagocyte's surface that can recognize and bind to the complement fragments. **C.** Antibodies (*Y-shaped molecules*) have attached to the capsule. (In this example, the opsonins are antibodies.) Now the phagocyte can attach to the bacterium because there are receptors (*squares*) on the phagocyte's surface that can recognize and bind to the F$_c$ region of antibody molecules. N, nucleus.

lysozyme, β-lysin, lipases, proteases, peptidases, DNAses and RNAses, which degrade carbohydrates, lipids, proteins, and nucleic acids.

Other mechanisms participate in the destruction of phagocytized microbes. In neutrophils, for example, a membrane-bound enzyme called NADPH oxidase reduces oxygen to very destructive products such as superoxide anions, hydroxyl radicals, hydrogen peroxide, and singlet oxygen. These highly reactive reduction products assist in the destruction of the ingested microbes. Another killing mechanism involves the

enzyme myeloperoxidase. Following lysosome fusion, myeloperoxidase is released, which, in the presence of hydrogen peroxide and chloride ion, produces a potent microbicidal agent called hypochlorous acid.

Figures 3-8 and 3-9 depict various stages in the phagocytosis of *Giardia lamblia* trophozoites by rat leukocytes. *G. lamblia* (also known as *Giardia intestinalis*) is a flagellated protozoal parasite that causes the diarrheal disease giardiasis (see Chapter 22).

Mechanisms by Which Pathogens Escape Destruction by Phagocytes

During the initial phases of infection, capsules serve an antiphagocytic function, protecting encapsulated bacteria from being phagocytized. Some bacteria produce an exoenzyme (or toxin) called **leukocidin,** which kills phagocytes. Not all bacteria engulfed by phagocytes are destroyed within phagolysosomes. For example, waxes in the cell wall of *Mycobacterium tuberculosis* protect the organism from digestion. The bacteria are even able to multiply within the phagocytes and be transported by them to other parts of the body. Other pathogens capable of surviving within phagocytes are the bacteria *Rickettsia rickettsii, Legionella pneumophila, Brucella abortus, Coxiella burnetii, Listeria monocytogenes,* and *Salmonella,* and the protozoan parasites *Toxoplasma gondii, Trypanosoma cruzi,* and *Leishmania* spp. The mechanism by which each pathogen evades digestion by lysosomal enzymes differs from one pathogen to another and, in some cases, the mechanism is not yet understood. These pathogens may remain dormant within phagocytes for months or years before they escape to cause disease. Thus, these types of virulent pathogens usually win the battle with phagocytes. Unless antibodies and/or complement fragments are present to aid in the destruction of these pathogens, the infection may progress unchecked.

Ehrlichia spp., bacteria closely related to rickettsias, are obligate, intracellular, Gram-negative bacteria that live within leukocytes (i.e., they are **intraleukocytic pathogens**). The bacteria are somehow able to prevent the fusion of lysosomes with phagosomes.

SPECIFIC HOST DEFENSE MECHANISMS: A BRIEF INTRODUCTION TO IMMUNOLOGY

The terms *specific host defense mechanisms* and *third line of defense* both pertain to the immune system.[2] **Immunology** is the scientific study of the immune system and immune responses. Immune responses involve complex interactions among many types of body cells and cellular secretions.

---

[2] *Some immunologists consider both the second and third lines of defense as parts of the immune system. They refer to the second line of defense as innate immune responses and the third line of defense as acquired immune responses.*

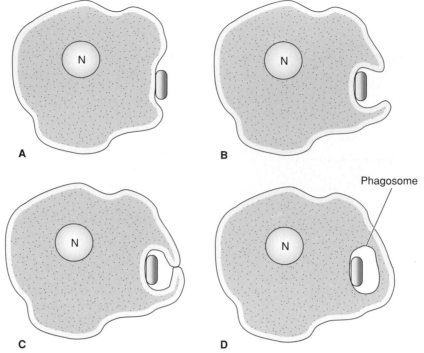

Figure 3-6. **The ingestion phase of phagocytosis. A.** A phagocyte has attached to a bacterial cell. **B.** Pseudopodia extend around the bacterial cell. **C.** The pseudopodia meet and fuse together. **D.** The bacterial cell, surrounded by a membrane, is now inside the phagocyte. The membrane-bound structure, containing the ingested bacterial cell, is called a phagosome. N, nucleus.

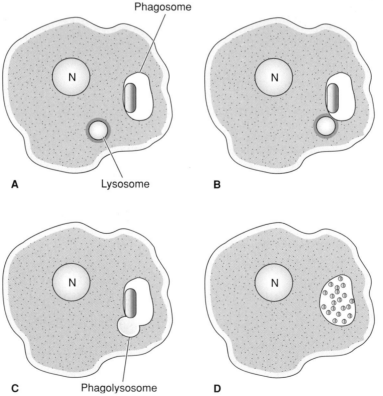

Figure 3-7. **The digestion phase of phagocytosis. A.** A lysosome, containing digestive enzymes, approaches a phagosome. **B.** The lysosome membrane fuses with the phagosome membrane. **C.** The lysosome and phagosome become a single membrane-bound vesicle, known as a phagolysosome. The phagolysosome contains the ingested bacterial cell plus digestive enzymes. **D.** The bacterial cell is digested within the phagolysosome. N, nucleus.

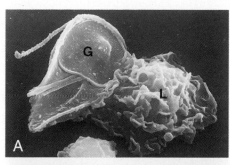

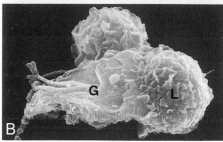

Figure 3-8. **Phagocytosis of *Giardia* trophozoites (*G*) by rat leukocytes (*L*).** Phagocytosis occurred in the laboratory under experimental conditions. (Courtesy of S. Erlandsen and P. Engelkirk.)

Only certain basic fundamentals of immunology and immune responses are presented here.

STUDY AID

The Key to Understanding Immunology. An understanding of immunology boils down to an understanding of two terms: *antigens* and *antibodies.* For the moment, think of antigens as molecules (usually proteins) that stimulate a person's immune system to produce antibodies. Think of antibodies as protein molecules that a person's immune system produces in response to antigens. Antigens and antibodies will be discussed in more detail later in the chapter. Remember, if you understand antigens and antibodies, you are well on your way to understanding immunology.

The immune system is the third line of defense. It is considered a specific host defense mechanism because it springs into action to defend against a specific pathogen that has gained entrance to the body.

According to accepted doctrine, the primary functions of the immune system are (1) to differentiate between self and nonself (foreign) and (2) to destroy that which is nonself.[3] The immune system involves very

complex interactions between many types of cells and cellular secretions. Although it encompasses the whole body, the lymphatic system is the site and source of most immune activity. The cells involved in immune responses originate in bone marrow, from which most blood cells develop. Three lines of lymphocytes—B lymphocytes (or B cells), T lymphocytes (or T cells), and natural killer (NK) cells—are derived from lymphoid stem cells of bone marrow.

There are two major types or categories of T cells: helper T cells and cytotoxic T cells. **Helper T cells** are also known as T helper cells, T_H cells, and CD4+ T cells. The term *CD4+ cells* refers to the fact that these cells possess on their surface an antigen designated as CD4. The primary function of helper T cells is secretion of cytokines. T_H1 cells and T_H2 cells are subcategories of helper T cells. Cytokines secreted by T_H1 cells (referred to as type 1 cytokines) support cell-mediated immune responses, involving macrophages, cytotoxic T cells, and natural killer (NK) cells. Cytokines secreted by T_H2 cells (referred to as type 2 cytokines) support humoral immune responses by inducing B-cell activation and differentiation of activated B cells into plasma cells.

Cytotoxic T cells are also known as T cytotoxic cells, T_C cells, and CD8+ cells. The term *CD8+ cells* refers to the fact that these cells possess on their surface an antigen designated as CD8. The primary function of cytotoxic T cells is destruction of virally infected host cells.

There are two major arms of the immune system: humoral immunity and cell-mediated immunity (Fig. 3-10). In **humoral immunity,** special glycoproteins (molecules composed of carbohydrate and protein) called **antibodies** are produced by B cells to recognize, bind with, inactivate, and destroy specific microbes. Following their production, these humoral (circulating) antibodies remain in blood plasma, lymph, and other body secretions where they protect against the specific pathogens that stimulated their production. Thus, in humoral immunity, a person is immune to a particular pathogen because of the presence of specific protective antibodies that are effective against that pathogen. Because humoral immunity is mediated by antibodies, it is sometimes referred to as **antibody-mediated immunity.**

The second major arm of the immune system—**cell-mediated immunity**—involves various cell types, with antibodies only playing a minor role, if any. These immune responses are referred to as cell-mediated immune responses; they are briefly discussed later in this chapter.

The two major arms of the immune system are humoral immunity and cell-mediated immunity.

[3]***An alternative viewpoint.*** *For more than 50 years, immunologists have relied on the self/nonself theory of immunity, which states that the immune system reacts to, or "does battle with," nonself (foreign molecules) but does not react to self (molecules that are part of the human body). However, certain immunological events are seemingly at odds with this theory. Recently, an alternative model of immunity has been proposed, called the Danger Model. This model "suggests that the immune system is more concerned with [tissue] damage than with foreignness, and is called into action by [danger or] alarm signals [emitted] from injured issues, rather than by the recognition of non-self. . . . When distressed, [the tissues] stimulate immunity, and . . . they may also determine the [specific type] of [immune] response." The immune response "is tailored to the tissue in which the response occurs, rather than being tailored by the targeted pathogen." Thus, "immunity is controlled by an internal conversation between tissues and the cells of the immune system." (From P. Matzinger. Science 2002;296:301–305.)*

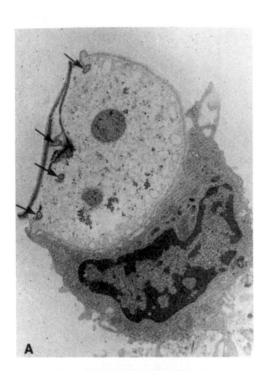
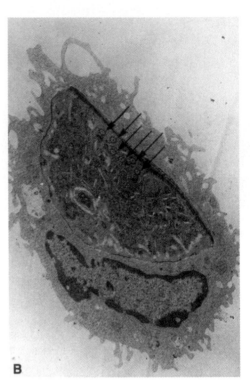
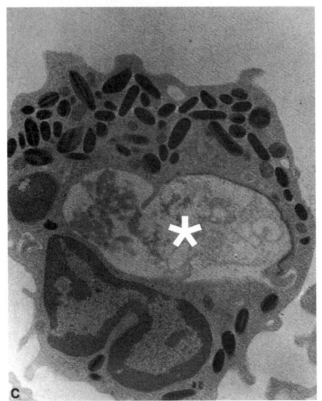

Figure 3-9. **The phagocytosis of *Giardia* trophozoites by rat leukocytes. A.** Attachment. **B.** Ingestion. **C.** Digestion. Note the cross-sections of flagella (*arrows*) in A and B, and the phagolysosome (*) and darkly stained granules in the eosinophil in C. The phagocytosis occurred in the laboratory under experimental conditions. (Courtesy of S. Koester and P. Engelkirk.)

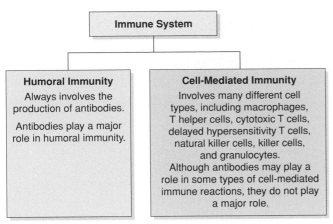

Figure 3-10. The two major arms of the immune system.

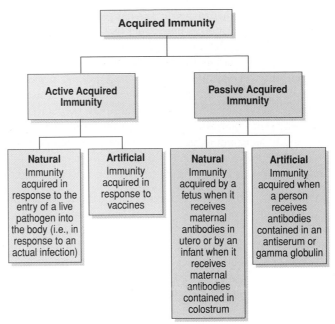

Figure 3-11. Types of acquired immunity.

Immunity

Immunity is the condition of being immune or resistant to a particular infectious disease. Humans are immune to certain infectious diseases simply because they are humans. For example, humans are not infected with some of the pathogens that infect their pets. One explanation is that human cells do not possess the appropriate cell surface receptors for some pathogens that cause diseases in pets. Other reasons for this natural or innate resistance are far more complex and, in some cases, not fully understood and will not be addressed here.

What will be discussed in this section are the various immunities that humans acquire as life progresses, from conception onward; these types of immunity are collectively referred to as acquired immunity. Such immunity is often the result of the presence of protective antibodies that are directed against various pathogens.

 CAUTION **Different Uses of the Term *Resistant*.** As discussed in Chapter 7, bacteria can become resistant to certain antibiotics, meaning that they are no longer killed by those antibiotics. Such bacteria are said to be drug resistant. Humans do not become resistant to antibiotics. Humans can become resistant (immune) to certain infectious diseases, however, in ways that are discussed in this section.

Immunity that results from the active production or receipt of antibodies during one's lifetime is called **acquired immunity.** If the antibodies are produced within the person's body, the immunity is called **active acquired immunity**; such protection is usually long lasting. In **passive acquired immunity,** the person receives antibodies produced by another person, by more than one person, or, in some cases, by an animal (e.g., antibodies in horse serum);

such protection is usually only temporary. In either case—active or passive—the immunity may result from either a natural or an artificial event. The four categories of acquired immunity are summarized in Figure 3-11.

> The four types of acquired immunity are (1) natural active acquired immunity, (2) artificial active acquired immunity, (3) natural passive acquired immunity, and (4) artificial passive acquired immunity.

Humoral Immunity

Antigens. Most **antigens** are foreign organic substances large enough to stimulate the production of antibodies; in other words, an antigen is an **anti**body-**gen**erating substance. Substances capable of stimulating the production of antibodies are said to be **antigenic.** Antigens may be proteins with molecular weight of more than 10,000 daltons,[4] polysaccharides larger than 60,000 daltons, large molecules of DNA or RNA, or any combination of biochemical molecules (e.g., glycoproteins, lipoproteins, and nucleoproteins) that are cellular components of either microbes or macroorganisms (e.g., helminths). Foreign proteins are the best antigens because of their structural complexity.

A bacterial cell has many molecules on its surface capable of stimulating the production of antibodies; these individual molecules or antigenic sites are known as **antigenic determinants** (or **epitopes**). A bacterial cell can be described as a mosaic of antigenic determinants. The

---

[4]*A dalton is a unit of mass equal to one-twelfth the mass of a carbon-12 atom. A dalton is equal to 1 in the atomic mass scale. Daltons are used to express molecular weight.*

important point is that, in most cases, antigens must be **foreign** materials that the human body does not recognize as **self** antigens. Certainly, all invading microbes fall into this category. A type of small molecule called a **hapten** may act as an antigen only when coupled with a large carrier molecule such as a protein. Then the antibodies formed against the antigenic determinant(s) of the hapten may combine with the hapten molecule when it is not coupled with the carrier protein. As an example, penicillin and other low-molecular-weight chemical molecules may act as haptens, causing some people to become allergic (or hypersensitive) to them.

Antibodies. Humoral immunity, or antibody-mediated immunity, involves the production of antibodies, as opposed to cell-mediated immunity (discussed later in this chapter), which does not involve antibody production. Antibodies are proteins produced by plasma cells in response to the presence of an antigen. (As described later, a plasma cell is derived from a type of lymphocyte called a B cell.) A bacterial cell has numerous antigenic determinants on its cell membrane, cell wall, capsule, and flagella that stimulate the production of many different antibodies. Usually, an antibody is "specific" in that it will recognize and bind only to the antigenic determinant that stimulated its production. For example, antibodies produced against molecules located on bacterial pili can only recognize and bind to those particular molecules. Occasionally, however, an antibody will bind to an antigenic determinant that is similar, but not identical, in structure to the antigenic determinant that stimulated its production; in that case, it is referred to as a cross-reacting antibody.

All antibodies are in a class of proteins called **immunoglobulins**—globular glycoproteins in the blood that participate in the immune reactions. The term *antibodies* is used to refer to immunoglobulins with particular specificity for an antigen. In addition to being found in blood, immunoglobulins are found in lymph, tears, saliva, and colostrum (Fig. 3-12). (**Colostrum** is the first milk that is secreted at the termination of pregnancy.) Antibodies found in the blood are called humoral or circulating antibodies. Those that provide protection against infectious diseases are called **protective antibodies.**

> Antibodies are secreted by plasma cells. Antibodies that provide protection against infectious diseases are known as protective antibodies.

The amount and type of antibodies produced by a given antigenic stimulation depend on the nature of the antigen, the site of antigenic stimulus, the amount of antigen, and the number of times the person is exposed to the antigen. Following the initial exposure to an antigen (such as a vaccine), there is a delayed primary response in the production of antibodies. During this lag phase, the antigen is processed by cells of the immune system.

For antibodies to be produced within the body, a complex series of events must occur, some of which are not completely

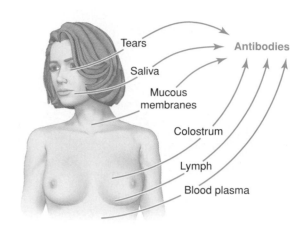

Figure 3-12. **Body fluids and sites where antibodies are found.**

understood. It is known that macrophages, T cells, and B cells often are involved in a cooperative effort. (The processing of antigens within the body is actually far more complex than the abbreviated explanation that follows.)

The majority of antigens are referred to as **T-dependent antigens,** because T cells (specifically, T_H cells) are involved in their processing; in other words, processing of these antigens is **dependent** on T cells. The processing of T-dependent antigens also involves macrophages and B cells. Other antigens are known as **T-independent antigens.** Their processing requires only B cells; in other words, the processing occurs independently of T cells (Fig. 3-13). T-independent antigens are large polymeric molecules (usually polysaccharides) containing repeating antigenic determinants; examples include the lipopolysaccharide found in the cell walls of Gram-negative bacteria, bacterial flagella, and bacterial capsules. (Table 3-4 summarizes the processing of T-independent and T-dependent antigens.) Note that the processing of either category of antigen—T independent or T dependent—results in B cells developing into **plasma cells** that are capable of secreting antibodies.

> The processing of T-dependent antigens involves T helper cells, whereas the processing of T-independent antigens does not.

The initial immune response to a particular antigen is called the **primary response.** In the primary response to an antigen, it takes about 10 to 14 days for antibodies to be produced. When the antigen is used up, the number of antibodies in the blood declines as the plasma cells die off. Other antigen-stimulated B cells become memory B cells, which are small lymphocytes that can be stimulated to rapidly produce large quantities of antibodies when later exposed to the same antigens. The increased production of antibodies following the second exposure to the antigen (e.g., a booster shot) is called the **secondary response, anamnestic response,** or **memory response.** A second booster shot of antigen many months later causes the antibody concentration to exceed the level of the secondary response. This is

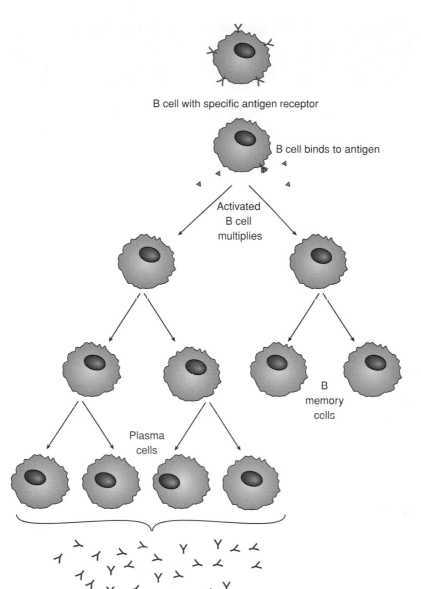

B cell with specific antigen receptor

B cell binds to antigen

Activated
B cell
multiplies

B
memory
cells

Plasma
cells

Antibodies

Figure 3-13. **Processing of T-independent antigens. See text for details.**

the reason why booster shots are given to protect against certain pathogens that a person might encounter throughout life, such as the bacterium *Clostridium tetani* (the cause of tetanus). In addition to memory B cells, memory T cells also contribute to immunological memory.

Where Do Immune Responses Occur?

Immune responses to antigens in the blood are usually initiated in the spleen, whereas responses to microbes and other antigens in tissues are generated in lymph nodes located near the area. Antigens entering the body through mucosal surfaces (e.g., following inhalation or ingestion) activate immune responses in mucosa-associated lymphoid tissues. For example, immune responses to intranasal and inhaled antigens occur in the tonsils and adenoids. Ingested antigens enter specialized epithelial cells called microfold or M cells, which then transport the antigens to Peyer patches—clusters of lymphatic nodules in the mucous membranes that line the small intestine—where the immune responses are initiated. All the various types of cells (macrophages, B cells, T cells, etc.) that collaborate to produce immune responses are present at these sites (spleen, lymph nodes, tonsils, adenoids, Peyer patches).

TABLE 3 - 4	Mechanisms by Which T-Dependent and T-Independent Antigens Are Processed by the Immune System

T-Independent Antigen	T-Dependent Antigen
Processing of T-independent antigens is initiated when an appropriate B cell makes physical contact with the free antigenic determinant (i.e., an antigenic determinant not bound to a major histocompatibility complex, or MHC, molecule[a]).	Following invasion of the body, an antigen (e.g., a bacterial cell) is ingested and digested by a macrophage.
↓	↓
The activated B cell next undergoes extensive cell division, producing a clone of identical B cells.	Within the macrophage, antigenic determinants of the bacterial cell (referred to as antigenic peptides, or APs) attach to MHC molecules.
↓	↓
Some of the members of the newly formed clone mature into antibody-producing plasma cells, whereas others become memory cells.	The combined AP-MHC molecules are then displayed on the surface of the macrophage. At this point, the macrophage is referred to as an **antigen-presenting cell.**
	↓
	A T_H cell attaches to one of the AP-MHC molecules, divides, and "sends out" (secretes) chemical signals (cytokines). Note that T_H cells assist in the production of antibodies, but do not manufacture antibodies themselves.
	↓
	When the chemical signals reach a B cell capable of recognizing that particular signal, the activated B cell divides, producing a clone of identical B cells.
	↓
	Some members of the newly formed clone mature into antibody-producing plasma cells. Antibodies are expelled rapidly for several days until the plasma cell dies. Each plasma cell makes only one type of antibody—one that will bind with the antigenic determinant that activated the B cell and stimulated production of that antibody. Members of the clone that do not become plasma cells, and some of the activated T cells, remain in the body as memory cells, able to respond very quickly should the antigen enter the body again at a later date.

[a]Major histocompatibility complex (MHC) molecules are cell membrane proteins, some of which bind antigenic determinants and serve as antigen presenting molecules. Human MHC molecules can serve as potent antigens when introduced into another person, as occurs during tissue or organ transplantation.

How Antibodies Protect Us from Pathogens and Infectious Diseases

As previously mentioned, once they are produced, antibodies are very specific. Usually, a given antibody can only recognize and bind to the antigenic determinant that stimulated its production. In the following paragraphs are several examples illustrating how antibodies protect us from pathogens and infectious diseases:

Example 1

A pathogen enters a person's body and starts producing a toxin. The person's immune system responds by producing antibodies against the toxin; these antibodies are called **antitoxins.** Once produced, the antitoxins recognize, bind to, and neutralize the toxin molecules so that they can no longer cause harm (i.e., they are no longer toxic).

Example 2

As mentioned earlier in the chapter, viruses can bind only to host cells that bear the appropriate receptor on their surfaces. The molecule on the virus that recognizes and binds to the receptor is called an adhesin. A person has received a vaccine containing an attenuated virus (a virus that is no longer infectious). The vaccine stimulates that person's immune system to produce antibodies against the adhesin molecules. At some later date, should the same virus enter the person's body, those antibodies will adhere to the adhesin molecules, making it impossible for the virus to bind to host cells. If the virus is unable to bind to the appropriate host cells, it is unable to enter the cell, and the person is protected from infection with that virus.

Example 3

A person is infected with a piliated bacterium. (Recall that pili enable bacteria to attach to host cells, which, with certain bacterial pathogens, is necessary for the bacteria to cause disease.) That person's immune system responds by producing antibodies against the pili. The antibodies bind to the pili, making it impossible for the bacterial cells to bind to tissue. If the bacteria are unable to attach to tissue, they are unable to cause disease.

Example 4

A person is infected with an encapsulated bacterium. (Recall that bacterial capsules serve an antiphagocytic function, meaning that phagocytic white blood cells are unable to phagocytize encapsulated bacteria. The reason

for this is that the phagocytes have no receptors on their surface that recognize the polysaccharide molecules. If the phagocyte is unable to attach to the encapsulated bacterium, it is unable to phagocytize it.) That person's immune system responds by producing antibodies against the capsular polysaccharide molecules. The antibodies attach to the capsule. This makes it possible for the phagocytes to bind to the encapsulated bacteria. Why? Because the phagocytes have receptors on their surfaces that can recognize and bind to antibody molecules.

Vaccines

The mere mention of the names of certain infectious diseases struck fear into the hearts of our ancestors. Today, thanks to childhood vaccines, residents of the United States rarely hear of those diseases, let alone live in fear of them. The Centers for Disease Control and Prevention (CDC) has stated, "Immunizations are one of the great public health success stories of the 20th century, having made once-common diseases such as diphtheria, measles, mumps, and pertussis diseases of the past. Vaccines are now available to protect children and adults against 21 life-threatening or debilitating diseases" (http://www.cdc.gov/programs/immun.htm). Vaccine-preventable diseases are listed on the CD-ROM.

A **vaccine** is defined as material that can artificially induce immunity to an infectious disease, usually following injection or, in some cases, ingestion of the material (e.g., oral polio vaccine). A person is deliberately exposed to a harmless version of a pathogen (or toxin), which will stimulate that person's immune system to produce protective antibodies and memory cells, but will not cause disease in that person. In this manner, the person's immune system is primed to mount a strong protective response, should the actual pathogen (or toxin) be encountered in the future. An ideal vaccine is one that

- contains enough antigenic determinants to stimulate the immune system to produce protective antibodies (i.e., antibodies that will protect people from infection by the pathogen); contains antigenic determinants from all of the strains of the pathogen that cause that disease (e.g., the three strains of virus that cause polio); such vaccines are referred to as multivalent or polyvalent vaccines;

- has few—preferably no—side effects; and

- does not cause disease in the vaccinated person.

Types of vaccines. Various materials are used in vaccines (Table 3-5). Most vaccines are made from living or dead (inactivated) pathogens or from certain toxins they produce. The use of such vaccines illustrates a very important and practical application of the principles of microbiology and immunology. In general, vaccines made from living organisms are most effective, but they must be prepared from harmless organisms

TABLE 3 - 5 Types of Available Vaccines

Type of Vaccine	Examples
Attenuated vaccines. The process of weakening pathogens is called attenuation, and the vaccines are referred to as **attenuated vaccines**. Most live vaccines are avirulent (nonpathogenic) mutant strains of pathogens that have been derived from the virulent (pathogenic) organisms; this is accomplished by growing them for many generations under various conditions or by exposing them to mutagenic chemicals or radiation. Attenuated vaccines should not be administered to immunosuppressed patients, because even weakened pathogens could cause disease in these persons.	**Attenuated viral vaccines:** adenovirus, chickenpox (varicella), measles (rubeola), mumps, German measles (rubella), polio (oral Sabin vaccine), smallpox, yellow fever **Attenuated bacterial vaccines:** bacille Calmette-Guérin (for protection against tuberculosis), cholera, tularemia, typhoid fever (oral vaccine)
Inactivated vaccines. Vaccines made from pathogens that have been killed by heat or chemicals—called **inactivated vaccines**—can be produced faster and more easily, but they are less effective than live vaccines. This is because the antigens on the dead cells are usually less effective and produce a shorter period of immunity.	**Inactivated viruses or viral antigens:** hepatitis A, influenza, Japanese encephalitis, other encephalitis vaccines, polio (subcutaneous Salk vaccine), rabies **Inactivated bacterial vaccines:** anthrax, typhoid fever (subcutaneous vaccine), Q fever
Subunit vaccines. A **subunit vaccine** (or **acellular vaccine**) is one that uses antigenic (antibody-stimulating) portions of a pathogen, rather than using the whole pathogen. For example, a vaccine containing pili of *Neisseria gonorrhoeae* could theoretically stimulate the body to produce antibodies that would attach to *N. gonorrhoeae* pili, thus preventing the bacteria from adhering to cells. If *N. gonorrhoeae* cannot adhere to cells that line the urethra, they cannot cause urethritis. The material used to protect health care workers and others from hepatitis caused by hepatitis B virus (HBV) is being produced by genetically engineered yeasts. The genes that code for hepatitis B surface protein were introduced into yeast cells, which then produced large quantities of that protein. The proteins are then injected into people. Antibodies against the protein are produced in their bodies, and these antibodies serve to protect the people from HBV.	Hepatitis B, Lyme disease, pertussis, whooping cough
Conjugate vaccines. Successful conjugated vaccines have been made by conjugating bacterial capsular antigens (which by themselves are not very antigenic) to molecules that stimulate the immune system to produce antibodies against the less antigenic capsular antigens.	Hib (for protection against *Haemophilus influenzae* type b), meningococcal meningitis (*Neisseria meningitidis* serogroup C), pneumococcal pneumonia
Toxoid vaccines. A **toxoid** is an exotoxin that has been inactivated (made nontoxic) by heat or chemicals. Toxoids can be injected safely to stimulate the production of antibodies that are capable of neutralizing the exotoxins of pathogens, such as those that cause tetanus, botulism, and diphtheria. Antibodies that neutralize toxins are called **antitoxins** and a serum containing such antitoxins is referred to as an **antiserum**.	Diphtheria, tetanus Commercial antisera containing antitoxins are used to treat diseases such as tetanus and botulism. Such antisera are also used in certain types of laboratory tests, known as immunodiagnostic procedures.

(continued)

TABLE 3 - 5   Continued

Type of Vaccine	Examples
DNA vaccines. At present, **DNA vaccines** or **gene vaccines** are only experimental. A particular gene from a pathogen is inserted into plasmids, and the plasmids are then injected into skin or muscle tissue. Inside host cells, the genes direct the synthesis of a particular microbial protein (antigen). Once the cells start churning out copies of the protein, the body then produces antibodies directed against the protein, and these antibodies protect the person from infection with the pathogen.	Laboratory animals have been successfully protected using this technique, and reports of the induction of cellular immune responses in humans to a malarial parasite antigen, using DNA vaccines, have been published.
Autogenous vaccines. An **autogenous vaccine** is one that has been prepared from bacteria isolated from a localized infection, such as a staphylococcal boil. The pathogens are killed, then injected into the same person to induce production of more antibodies.	

that are antigenically closely related to the pathogens or from weakened pathogens that have been genetically changed so that they are no longer pathogenic.

As immunologists made further studies of the characteristics of vaccines, they found that it was practical to vaccinate against several diseases by combining specific vaccines in a single injection. Thus, the diphtheria-tetanus-pertussis vaccine contains toxoids to prevent diphtheria and tetanus and portions of killed bacteria (*Bordetella pertussis*) to prevent whooping cough (pertussis). Another example is the measles-mumps-rubella vaccine.

How vaccines work. Vaccines stimulate the recipient's immune system to produce protective antibodies. The protective antibodies and/or memory cells produced in response to the vaccine then remain in the recipient's body to "do battle with" a particular pathogen should that pathogen enter the recipient's body at some time in the future.

For example, when a person receives tetanus toxoid (an altered form of the toxin tetanospasmin), protective antibodies referred to as antitoxins are produced. The antitoxins remain in the person's body. Should *C. tetani* enter the person's body at some time in the future and start to produce tetanospasmin, the antitoxins are there to attach to and neutralize the toxin.

Some vaccines stimulate the body to produce protective antibodies that are directed against surface antigens. When the pathogen enters the person's body, the antibodies attach to the surface antigens. This prevents the pathogen from adhering to host cells. In the case of viruses, if they are unable to attach, they are unable to enter the cell and are thus unable to multiply and cause cell destruction. Antibodies produced in response to molecules on the surface of bacterial pili would adhere to the pili, preventing the bacteria from attaching to tissues and thus preventing the bacteria from causing disease.

In some cases, protective antibodies attached to surface antigens act as opsonins (discussed earlier), enabling phagocytes to attach to pathogens. Once attached to a pathogen, the phagocyte can ingest and digest it. In other cases, attachment of protective antibodies to surface antigens activates the complement cascade, with the end result being lysis of the pathogen.

Cell-Mediated Immunity

Antibodies are unable to enter cells, including cells containing intracellular pathogens. Fortunately, there is an arm of the immune system capable of controlling chronic infections by intracellular pathogens (e.g., bacteria, protozoa, fungi, viruses). Cell-mediated immunity (**CMI**) is a complex system of interactions between many types of cells and the cellular secretions known as cytokines. (Only a brief overview of CMI can be provided here.) Included among the various cells that participate in CMI are macrophages, T_H cells, T_C cells, NK cells, and granulocytes. Although CMI does not involve the production of antibodies, antibodies produced during humoral immunity may play a minor role in some cell-mediated responses. A typical cell-mediated cytotoxic response would involve the following steps:

Step 1: A macrophage engulfs and partially digests a pathogen. Fragments (antigenic determinants) of the pathogen are then displayed on the surface of the macrophage (i.e., the macrophage acts as an antigen-presenting cell).

Step 2: A T_H cell binds to one of the antigenic determinants being displayed on the macrophage surface. The T_H cell produces cytokines that reach an effector cell of the immune system (e.g., a T_C cell or NK cell).

Step 3: The effector cell binds to a target cell (i.e., a pathogen-infected host cell displaying the same antigenic determinant on its surface).

Step 4: Vesicular contents of the effector cell are discharged. These include perforin and other proteins or enzymes, which literally punch holes in the target cell membrane. Other cytokines released by effector cells are tumor necrosis factor (TNF) and NK cytotoxic factor.

Step 5: Toxins produced by the effector cells enter the target cell, causing disruption of DNA and organelles. The target cell dies.

Both humoral and cell-mediated immune responses play a role in the body's defense against viral infections. In cytolytic viral infections (e.g., herpes infections), the viruses can be neutralized and destroyed by antibodies and the complement system when they move in body fluids from a lysed cell to an intact cell. When the virus is established within body cells, the cell-mediated immune response can destroy the virus-infected cells, preventing viral multiplication. If the virus is not completely destroyed, however, it may become latent in nerve ganglion cells, as in herpes infections (e.g., shingles).

T_C cells and NK cells kill infected host cells when pathogens are established inside the cells. Thus, infected liver cells are destroyed in hepatitis infections during the body's battle against the disease. The AIDS virus (HIV), which targets T_H cells, is particularly destructive because it destroys the very cells that would have helped fight the infection. The lack of T_H cells impairs both humoral and cell-mediated immunity, making AIDS patients very susceptible to many opportunistic infections and malignancies.

Natural Killer (NK) Cells

NK cells are in a subpopulation of lymphocytes called large granular lymphocytes. Although they morphologically resemble lymphocytes, NK cells lack typical T-cell or B-cell surface markers. They also differ from T and B cells in other ways. For example, they do not proliferate in response to antigen and appear not to be involved in antigen-specific recognition. As the name implies, NK cells kill target cells, including foreign cells, host cells infected with viruses or bacteria, and tumor cells. Although NK-cell activity does not depend on antibodies, NK cells have receptors on their surfaces for a portion of IgG antibodies called the F_C region. (Information about the structure of antibody molecules can be found on the CD-ROM.) These receptors enable the cells to attach to and kill antibody-coated target cells; this is known as antibody-dependent cellular cytotoxicity. Once attached to an antibody-coated target cell, the NK cell inserts a molecule called perforin into the cell membrane of the target cell, creating an opening (pore), through which cytotoxic granules called granzymes are injected. Although

firm evidence is lacking for an "immune surveillance" system within our bodies that monitors for and destroys malignant cells, NK cells may participate in such a system.

Immunosuppression

People with properly functioning immune systems are said to be **immunocompetent.** People with immune systems that do not function properly are said to be **immunosuppressed, immunodepressed,** or **immunocompromised.** The most common cause of immune deficiency worldwide is malnutrition. In addition, there are acquired and inherited immunodeficiencies.

Acquired immunodeficiencies may be caused by drugs (e.g., cancer chemotherapeutic agents, steroids, and drugs given to transplant patients), irradiation, or certain infectious diseases (e.g., HIV infection). HIV infection leads to a decrease in T_H cells, which in turn prevents the production of antibodies against T-dependent antigens and consequently results in an inability to fight off certain pathogens. These pathogens overwhelm the patient's host defenses, eventually causing death. AIDS patients usually die from various devastating infectious diseases, including viral, bacterial, fungal, and parasitic diseases. Immune responsiveness and the ability to produce antibodies also decline as the normal body ages, perhaps the result of a declining ability of T cells to regulate the immune response. This in turn results in greater susceptibility of the elderly to serious infectious diseases.

Inherited immunodeficiency diseases can be the result of deficiencies in antibody production, T-cell production, complement activity, phagocytic function, NK-cell function, or some combination of these. Examples of inherited immunodeficiency diseases include agammaglobulinemia, hypogammaglobulinemia, chronic granulomatous disease, Chediak-Higashi syndrome, severe combined immune deficiency (SCID), DiGeorge syndrome, and Wiskott-Aldrich syndrome.

Some people are born lacking the ability to produce protective antibodies. Patients with an abnormality known as **agammaglobulinemia** lack the gamma fraction of serum globulin, which is where antibodies are normally found. These people are very susceptible to infections by even the least virulent microorganisms in their environment.

Persons who produce an insufficient amount of antibodies are said to have **hypogammaglobulinemia.** Their resistance to infection is lower than normal, so they usually do not recover from infectious diseases as readily as most other persons. One type, called Bruton's hypogammaglobulinemia, is a hereditary disease in which the numbers of circulating B cells are profoundly low or totally absent.

SCID patients have deficiencies of B cells and T cells, resulting in severe recurrent infections. In DiGeorge syndrome is a congenital absence of the thymus and parathyroid glands in which patients suffer frequent infections and delayed development. Wiskott-Aldrich syndrome patients have deficiencies in B cells, T cells, monocytes, and platelets; effects on the patient include bleeding, recurrent infections, and eczema. Bone marrow transplantation and gene therapy may be of value in treating certain immunodeficiency diseases. The increased knowledge of genetics being gained from the Human Genome Project should lead to an increased understanding of these diseases and a variety of new methods by which they may be treated.

ANTIMICROBIAL AGENTS

Drugs used to treat infectious diseases are collectively called antimicrobial agents. They are only briefly mentioned here because they represent another way of combating infectious diseases. Antimicrobial agents are discussed in detail in Chapter 7.

Chapter Review

- Certain human host defense mechanisms are classified as nonspecific, whereas others are classified as specific. Nonspecific host defense mechanisms serve to protect the body from various foreign substances or pathogens. Specific host defense mechanisms are directed against a particular foreign substance or pathogen that has entered the body.

- Another way to categorize host defense mechanisms is to divide them into first, second, and third lines of defense. The first and second lines of defense are nonspecific, whereas the third line of defense (the immune system) is specific.

- The first line of defense includes innate or inborn resistance; physical barriers such as intact skin and intact mucous membranes; chemical, physiological, and temperature barriers; microbial antagonism by indigenous microflora; and overall nutritional status and state of health.

- The second line of defense includes nonspecific cellular and chemical responses such as inflammation, fever, interferon production, activation of the complement system, iron balance, cellular secretions, activation of blood proteins, chemotaxis, phagocytosis, neutralization of toxins, and the cleanup and repair of damaged tissues.

- Interferons (discussed in Table 3-2) are small, antiviral proteins that prevent viral multiplication in virus-infected cells and serve to limit viral infections.

- The complement system involves about 30 blood proteins that interact in a stepwise manner known as the complement cascade. Complement activation by immune complexes or other mechanisms aids in the initiation and amplification of inflammation, attraction and activation of leukocytes, lysis of bacteria and other foreign cells, and enhanced phagocytosis (opsonization).

- Fever is a nonspecific host defense mechanism that augments host defenses by stimulating leukocytes to deploy and destroy invaders, reducing available free plasma iron, and inducing the production of interleukin 1, which causes the proliferation, maturation, and activation of lymphocytes in the immunological response. Elevated body temperature also slows down the rate of growth of certain pathogens and kills especially fastidious ("fussy") pathogens. Substances that invoke fever are referred to as pyrogens.

- Phagocytes rid the body of unwanted or harmful substances, such as dead cells, unused cellular secretions, dust, debris, and pathogens. Following their recruitment to a particular site by chemotactic substances, they attach to, surround, ingest, and digest unwanted or harmful substances.

- The four steps in phagocytosis are chemotaxis, attachment, ingestion, and digestion.

- Indications of inflammation include redness, heat, edema, and pain. Inflammation is often accompanied by pus formation, and sometimes the inflamed part of the body loses function. The purposes of the inflammatory response are to localize an infection, prevent the spread of microbial invaders, neutralize toxins, and aid in the repair of damaged tissue.

- Lactoferrin and transferrin are host molecules that tie up iron, thereby preventing pathogens access to this essential mineral.

- Immunology is the scientific study of the immune system and immune responses, including active and passive acquired immunity to infectious agents, antibody production, cell-mediated immune responses, allergic responses, other types of hypersensitivity reactions, and autoimmune disorders.

- The immune system is the third line of defense against pathogens; it is a specific host defense mechanism. Most immune responses involve the production of antibodies that recognize, bind to, and inactivate or destroy specific pathogens or their toxins. Immune responses involving the production of antibodies are known as humoral immunity or antibody-mediated immunity.

- In protective cell-mediated immune responses, antibodies play only a minor role, if any. Cell-mediated immune responses involve several cell types, including macrophages and lymphocytes.

- Immunity to an infectious disease may be innate or acquired. If acquired, the immunity may have been acquired actively (with antibodies actively produced by the person) or passively (with the person receiving antibodies produced by others). Both active acquired and passive acquired immunity may occur naturally or artificially.

- The production of antibodies in response to a pathogen that has entered the body is an example of natural active acquired immunity. The production of antibodies in response to a vaccine is an example of artificial active acquired immunity. A fetus receiving antibodies that were produced by its mother is an example of natural passive acquired immunity. A soldier receiving antibodies contained in a shot of gamma globulin is an example of artificial passive acquired immunity.

- The various categories of vaccines include attenuated vaccines (weakened pathogens are injected), inactivated vaccines (killed pathogens are injected), subunit or acellular vaccines (only that part of the pathogen that stimulates the production of protective antibodies is injected), and toxoids (injection of toxins that have been modified as to no longer cause disease).

- Antigens can be defined as substances that stimulate the immune system to produce antibodies. Proteins make the best antigens, but large polysaccharides can also serve as antigens. Individual antigenic molecules are referred to as antigenic determinants or epitopes.

- Antigens can be classified as being either T independent or T dependent, depending on how they are processed by the immune system. Only B cells are involved in the processing of T-independent antigens. A T-dependent antigen requires the interaction of a macrophage, a T helper cell, and a B cell. The final result is the same: antibodies are secreted by plasma cells.

- The amount and type of antibodies produced by a given antigenic stimulation depend on the nature of the antigen, the site of antigenic stimulus, the amount of antigen, and the number of times the person is exposed to the antigen.

- Immune responses involve complex interactions between different types of cells and cellular secretions, occurring mostly in the lymphatic system. Cells involved in immune responses originate in bone marrow (from which most blood cells develop); they include B cells, plasma cells (antibody producers), T cells (helper T cells and cytotoxic T cells), and NK cells.

- Antibodies are glycoproteins in a class of proteins known as immunoglobulins.

- Once produced, antibodies are capable of recognizing and binding to the antigenic determinant that stimulated their production. Antibodies have several functions, including neutralizing toxins, preventing the attachment of pathogens to host cell receptors, serving as opsonins, and initiating the complement cascade.

New Terms and Abbreviations

After studying Chapter 3, you should be familiar with the following terms, which are defined within the chapter and in the Glossary at the back of the book:

Acquired immunity

Active acquired immunity

Agammaglobulinemia

Antibody

Antigen

Antigenic

Antigenic determinant

Antigen-presenting cell

Antiserum

Antitoxin

Artificial active acquired immunity

Artificial passive acquired immunity

Attenuated vaccine

Autogenous vaccine

B cell (B lymphocyte)

Cell-mediated immunity (CMI)

Chemokine

Chemotactic agent

Chemotaxis

Colostrum

Complement

Complement cascade

Conjugate vaccine

Cytotoxic T cell

DNA vaccine

Edema

Endocytosis

Erythema

Fastidious pathogen

Fixed macrophage

Granulocyte

Hapten

Helper T cell

Host defense mechanism

Humoral immunity

Hypogammaglobulinemia

Immune

Immunity

Immunocompetent

Immunoglobulin

Immunology

Immunosuppressed

Inactivated vaccine

Inflammation

Inflammatory exudate

Interferon

Macrophage

Natural active acquired immunity

Natural passive acquired immunity

Neutrophil

Nonspecific host defense mechanism

Opsonin

Opsonization

Passive acquired immunity

Phagocytosis

Phagolysosome

Phagosome

Plasma cell

Primary response

Professional phagocytes

Protective antibody

Purulent exudate

Pyogenic

Pyogenic microorganism

Reticuloendothelial system (RES)

Secondary response

Specific host defense mechanism

Subunit vaccine

T cell (T lymphocyte)

T-dependent antigen

T-independent antigen

Toxoid

Toxoid vaccine

Transferrin

Vaccine

Vasodilation

Wandering macrophage

References and Suggested Reading

Cunningham MW, Fujinami RS. Effects of Microbes on the Immune System. Philadelphia: Lippincott Williams & Wilkins, 2000.

Roitt IM, Brostoff J, Male DK. Immunology. 5th Ed. London: Mosby, 1998.

Sell S. Immunology, Immunopathology, and Immunity. Washington, DC: ASM Press, 2001.

 ## On the CD-ROM

- Vaccine-Preventable Diseases
- Vaccination—A Cautionary Note
- A Closer Look at Antibodies
- Additional Self-Assessment Exercises
- Puzzle

Self-Assessment Exercises

After studying Chapter 3, answer the following questions.

1. Of the following, which is the *least* likely to be involved in cell-mediated immunity?

   A. Macrophages

   B. Antibodies

   C. Cytokines

   D. T cells

2. Antibodies are secreted by which of the following?

   A. T_H cells

   B. Macrophages

   C. Plasma cells

   B. T_C cells

3. Humoral immunity involves all the following except

   A. T_C cells.

   B. B cells.

   C. antibodies.

   D. plasma cells.

4. Immunity that develops as a result of an actual infection is called

   A. natural passive acquired immunity.

   B. artificial active acquired immunity.

   C. natural active acquired immunity.

   D. artificial passive acquired immunity.

5. Artificial passive acquired immunity would result from

   A. receiving a gamma globulin injection.

   B. receiving an inactivated vaccine.

   C. ingestion of colostrum.

   D. having the measles.

6. The vaccines used to protect people from diphtheria and tetanus are

    A. subunit vaccines.

    B. inactivated vaccines.

    C. attenuated vaccines.

    D. toxoids.

7. Natural passive acquired immunity would result from

    A. receiving a gamma globulin injection.

    B. ingestion of colostrum.

    C. having the measles.

    D. receiving an attenuated vaccine.

8. Opsonization is best described as

    A. accumulation of cellular debris.

    B. an increase in the diameter of blood vessels.

    C. a process by which phagocytosis is facilitated.

    D. a process by which phagocytes are attracted to a site where they are needed.

9. All of the following are considered to be part of the first line of defense *except*

    A. intact skin.

    B. intact mucous membranes.

    C. ciliated epithelial cells in the respiratory tract.

    D. inflammation.

10. Antibodies are

    A. glycoproteins.

    B. secreted by plasma cells.

    C. produced by the immune system in response to antigens.

    D. all the above.

II

Introduction to the Clinical Microbiology Laboratory

CHAPTER 4

Organization and Responsibilities of the Clinical Microbiology Laboratory

LEARNING OBJECTIVES

After studying this chapter, you should be able to:

- Define the terms and abbreviations introduced in this chapter (e.g., algicidal agent, antimicrobial agents, antimicrobial susceptibility testing)

- List the steps in the diagnosis of an infectious disease

- Outline the organization of the pathology department and the clinical microbiology laboratory, including the two major divisions of pathology and the various sections (e.g., bacteriology section) of the clinical microbiology laboratory

- Name the various types of professionals that work in the clinical microbiology laboratory, and describe their educational requirements or training

- State the overall mission and responsibilities of the clinical microbiology laboratory

- Describe the general steps involved when processing a clinical specimen in the clinical microbiology laboratory

- Discuss, *in general*, how bacteria, yeasts, moulds, parasites, viruses, and mycobacteria are identified in the clinical microbiology laboratory, and describe types of specimens and most appropriate methods

- Describe the various types of safety precautions that must be followed in a clinical microbiology laboratory, including biohazard safety, biosafety levels, standard precautions, federal safety requirements, and types of biosafety cabinets

☞ Distinguish between a bactericidal and a bacteriostatic agent

☞ List three methods of sterilization that may be used in a clinical microbiology laboratory

☞ Describe an autoclave, including its purpose and proper operation (i.e., operating temperature, pressure, and time)

☞ Name three pieces of personal protective equipment that should be used in the clinical microbiology laboratory

☞ Describe the four biological or biosafety levels established by the U.S. Department of Health and Human Services; for each level, describe the types of agents that may be worked with and the appropriate safety precautions

☞ State any special safety considerations for the mycobacteriology section of the clinical microbiology laboratory

☞ Discuss the use of biosafety cabinets in the clinical microbiology laboratory, including their purpose, kinds, and type of work that may be performed in each

☞ State the purpose of a chemical fume hood and its proper operation, including positioning of the sash, ventilation, and work area

☞ Describe the purpose of material safety data sheets, including the type of information they contain

☞ Diagram a National Fire Protection Association hazard-rating sign, label it with the appropriate hazard areas and colors, and describe the numbering system

☞ Briefly discuss the proper procedures or precautions for shipping pathogens or clinical specimens to an outside or reference laboratory

☞ Discuss how quality control in the clinical microbiology laboratory relates to quality assurance

☞ List two or three of the processes that occur in the preanalytic, analytic, and postanalytic phases of quality assurance

☞ Describe the basic components of a clinical microbiology laboratory's quality control program, addressing personnel competency, policies and procedures, testing, media, reagents, equipment/instrumentation, and records or reports

☞ Explain what is meant by quality control organisms, and describe when they are used

TERMS AND DEFINITIONS

Clinical microbiology. Clinical microbiology (also called diagnostic microbiology) is the subdiscipline of microbiology associated with the diagnosis of human infectious diseases. The results of laboratory procedures performed in the clinical microbiology laboratory assist clinicians in the diagnoses of infectious diseases.[1] These laboratory procedures include the isolation of pathogens from human clinical specimens, the tests used to identify (speciate) pathogens, and antimicrobial susceptibility testing. Subsequent chapters in this book will mention these laboratory procedures, and the details of many of them can be found in Appendix A.

Diagnosis of infectious diseases. The proper diagnosis of an infectious disease requires (1) taking a complete patient history; (2) conducting a thorough physical examination of the patient; (3) carefully evaluating the patient's signs and symptoms; (4) conducting appropriate laboratory tests, as well as radiographs, ultrasound, computerized axial tomography (CAT) scans, and other types of imaging; and (5) initiating the proper selection, collection, and transport of appropriate clinical specimens. Although laboratory professionals do not actually diagnose diseases, they provide valuable assistance to clinicians by furnishing them with accurate and timely laboratory observations and test results. Most medical decisions made about patient diagnosis, treatment, and care are based on laboratory results.

Laboratory diagnosis of infectious diseases. Throughout this book, the phrase "laboratory diagnosis of infectious diseases" refers to the various laboratory observations and test results that, when received and evaluated by clinicians, assist them to correctly diagnose infectious diseases and initiate appropriate therapy.

INTRODUCTION TO THE CLINICAL MICROBIOLOGY LABORATORY

Throughout this book, the term **clinical microbiology laboratory** (hereafter referred to as the CML) refers to the laboratory within a hospital, clinic, or other health care facility where microbiological procedures are performed on human clinical specimens to assist clinicians in the diagnoses of infectious diseases. The CML is also sometimes referred to as the diagnostic microbiology laboratory.

Within a hospital setting, the CML is usually an integral part of the pathology department, which is frequently referred to simply as the lab. The pathology department is under the direction of a pathologist—a physician who has had extensive, specialized training in pathology, the study of the structural

---

[1]As used in this book, the term clinicians refers to physicians, physicians' assistants, nurse practitioners, and any other health care professionals authorized/licensed to make diagnoses, write prescriptions, and initiate appropriate therapy.

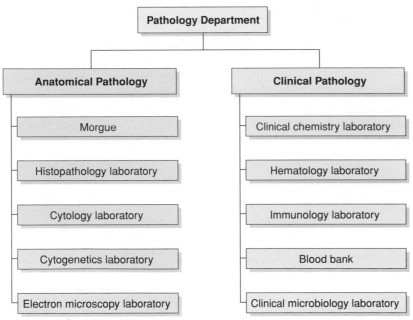

Figure 4-1. **Typical organization of a pathology department.** (Modified from Engelkirk PG. Burton's Microbiology for the Health Sciences. 8th Ed. Baltimore: Lippincott Williams & Wilkins, 2007.)

and functional manifestations of disease. As shown in Figure 4-1, the pathology department consists of two major divisions: anatomical pathology and clinical pathology. The CML is located within the clinical pathology division.

Laboratory professionals working in anatomical pathology include pathologists, cytogenetic technologists, cytotechnologists, histologic technicians, histotechnologists, and pathologists' assistants. Pathologists perform autopsies in the morgue and examine diseased organs, stained tissue sections, and cytology specimens.

Laboratory professionals working in clinical pathology include clinical pathologists; specialized scientists, such as chemists and microbiologists, who have graduate degrees in their specialty areas; **clinical laboratory scientists** (also known as CLSs, medical technologists, or MTs) who have four-year baccalaureate degrees; and **clinical laboratory technicians** (also known as CLTs, medical laboratory technicians, or MLTs) who have two-year associate degrees.

STAFFING AND ORGANIZATION OF THE CLINICAL MICROBIOLOGY LABORATORY

Depending on the size of the hospital, the CML may be under the direction of a pathologist, a microbiologist (having either a master's degree or doctorate in clinical microbiology), or, in smaller hospitals, a medical technologist who has had many years of experience working in microbiology. Most of the actual "bench work" performed in the CML is performed by CLSs and CLTs. For the remainder of this book, these people will be referred to as CML professionals.

As shown in Figure 4-2, the CML is divided into various sections that largely correspond to the various categories of microorganisms described in Chapter 1. The responsibilities of the specific sections of the CML are briefly described later in this chapter.

> Most of the procedures performed in the clinical microbiology laboratory are performed by clinical laboratory scientists and clinical laboratory technicians.

MISSION AND RESPONSIBILITIES OF THE CLINICAL MICROBIOLOGY LABORATORY

The primary mission of the CML is to assist clinicians in the diagnosis and treatment of infectious diseases. To accomplish this mission, the CML has four major responsibilities it must fulfill daily:

> The primary mission of the CML is to assist clinicians in the diagnosis and treatment of infectious diseases.

1. Process the various clinical specimens that are submitted to the CML. (Processing is described in the next paragraph. The types of clinical specimens submitted to the CML are described in Chapter 5.)

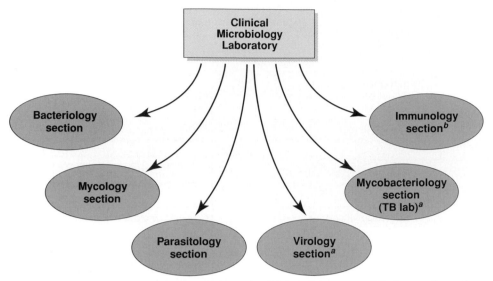

Figure 4-2. **Typical organization of a clinical microbiology laboratory.** [a]Virology and mycobacteriology sections are usually found only in larger hospitals and medical centers. Lacking these sections, most smaller hospitals would instead send virology and mycobacteriology specimens to a reference laboratory. [b]Only smaller hospitals would have immunology sections, where some immunodiagnostic procedures would be performed. Larger hospitals and medical centers would have an immunology laboratory, which would perform a much wider variety of immunological procedures and would operate independently of the clinical microbiology laboratory. (Modified from Engelkirk PG. Burton's Microbiology for the Health Sciences. 8th Ed. Baltimore: Lippincott Williams & Wilkins, 2007.)

2. Isolate pathogens from those specimens.

3. Identify the pathogens.[2]

4. Perform antimicrobial susceptibility testing when appropriate. The drugs used to treat infectious diseases are called **antimicrobial agents**. The term **antimicrobial susceptibility testing** means to test microorganisms for their susceptibility or resistance to various antimicrobial agents. Currently, in most CMLs, only bacteria are tested for their susceptibility or resistance to various antimicrobial agents. Antimicrobial agents and antimicrobial susceptibility testing are discussed in detail in Chapter 7.

> The four major daily responsibilities of the CML are to (1) process specimens, (2) isolate pathogens, (3) identify (speciate) pathogens, and (4) perform antimicrobial susceptibility testing.

The exact steps in the processing of clinical specimens vary from one specimen type to another and depend on the specific section of the CML to which the specimen is submitted. In general, processing includes the following steps (summarized in Figure 4-3):

- Examining the specimen macroscopically (i.e., with the naked eye) to confirm that it is the appropriate specimen and the container is properly labeled, and to make note of and record pertinent observations, such as cloudiness, the presence of blood or mucus, or an unusual odor

- Examining the specimen microscopically and recording pertinent observations, such as the presence of white blood cells or microorganisms

- Inoculating appropriate culture media to isolate the pathogen from the specimen and growing it in pure culture in the laboratory[3]

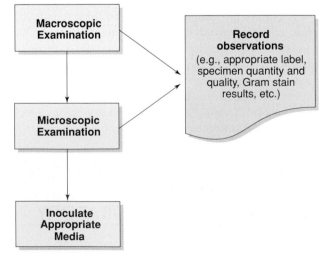

Figure 4-3. **Specimen processing in the clinical microbiology laboratory.**

---

[2]*Throughout this book, the phrases "identify a pathogen" or "identify an organism" mean to learn the pathogen's or organism's name. Although this usually involves identifying the organism to the species level (i.e., to speciate it), sometimes it is acceptable merely to identify the organism to the genus level.*

[3]*The term **pure culture** means that the organism has been isolated (separated) from other organisms and is growing alone.*

The CML is sometimes asked to assume an additional responsibility—namely, the processing of environmental samples, which are samples collected from within the hospital environment. Environmental samples are processed by the CML whenever there is an outbreak or epidemic within the hospital in an attempt to

> A fifth responsibility of the CML is to process environmental samples whenever there is an outbreak or epidemic within the hospital.

locate the source of the pathogen involved. Samples include those collected from appropriate hospital sites (e.g., floors, sink drains, shower heads, whirlpool baths, respiratory therapy equipment) and employees (e.g., nasal swabs, material from open wounds). The role of the CML in health care epidemiology is described in greater detail in Chapter 26.

ISOLATION AND IDENTIFICATION OF PATHOGENS

To isolate bacteria (including mycobacteria) and fungi (yeasts and moulds) from clinical specimens, the specimens are inoculated into liquid culture media or onto solid culture media.[4] The goal is to isolate any pathogens present in the specimen, to grow them in pure culture, and to obtain a sufficient quantity of the organism to inoculate appropriate identification and antimicrobial susceptibility testing systems. How pathogens are identified depends on which section of the CML the specimen was submitted to (e.g., the bacteriology, mycology, or parasitology section).

OVERVIEW OF CLINICAL MICROBIOLOGY LABORATORY SECTION RESPONSIBILITIES

Bacteriology Section
The major responsibility of the bacteriology section of the CML is to assist clinicians in diagnosing bacterial diseases. Chapters 8 through 18 discuss bacterial disease diagnosis in detail. In the bacteriology section, various types of clinical specimens are processed, bacterial pathogens are isolated from specimens, tests are performed to identify bacterial pathogens, and antimicrobial susceptibility testing is performed when appropriate. Once isolated from clinical specimens, bacterial pathogens are identified by gathering clues (i.e., phenotypic characteristics of the organism). Thus, the technologists and technicians working in the CML are much like detectives and crime scene

investigators, gathering clues about a pathogen until finally they can identify it.

Mycobacteriology Section
The major responsibility of the mycobacteriology section (or TB lab, as it is often called) is to assist clinicians in the diagnosis of tuberculosis and other mycobacterial infections (see Chapter 10). In the mycobacteriology section, various types of specimens (primarily sputum specimens)

> The technologists and technicians that work in the CML are much like detectives and crime scene investigators, gathering clues about a pathogen until finally they can identify it.

are processed, acid-fast staining is performed, mycobacteria are isolated and identified, and antimicrobial susceptibility testing is performed. *Mycobacterium* spp. are identified using a combination of growth characteristics—such as growth rate, colony pigmentation, photoreactivity, and morphology—and various biochemical tests. *Mycobacterium tuberculosis*, the primary cause of human tuberculosis, is a slow-growing organism. Fortunately, the acid-fast stain enables rapid presumptive diagnosis of tuberculosis, as do molecular diagnostic procedures and mycolic acid profiles (see Chapter 10).

Mycology Section
The major responsibility of the mycology section of the CML is to assist clinicians in the diagnosis of fungal infections, or mycoses. Chapters 19 and 20 discuss fungal infections in detail. In the mycology section, various types of clinical specimens are processed, fungal pathogens are isolated, and tests are performed to identify the fungal pathogens. In general, the specimens processed in the mycology section are the same types of specimens processed in the bacteriology section. However, three types of specimens are more commonly submitted to the mycology section than to the bacteriology section: hair clippings, nail clippings, and skin scrapings.

When isolated from clinical specimens, yeasts are identified by using various biochemical tests, testing their ability to catabolize (break down) carbohydrates. Moulds are usually identified using a combination of rate of growth and macroscopic and microscopic observations, *not* by performing biochemical tests. Macroscopic observations of a mould colony (mycelium) reveal characteristics like color, texture, and topography.

Susceptibility testing of fungi currently is not performed in most CMLs, although because of the ever-growing problem of drug resistance in fungi, it is likely that such testing (especially of yeasts) will become routine in the near future. Sometimes important fungal isolates are sent to reference laboratories for susceptibility testing.

---

[4]*Culture media are the nutrient-rich mixtures within or on which microorganisms are growing.*

Parasitology Section

The major responsibility of the parasitology section is to assist clinicians in the diagnosis of parasitic diseases—specifically, infections caused by endoparasites. Endoparasites are parasites that live within the body, such as parasitic protozoa and helminths (parasitic worms). Chapters 21 through 23 discuss this topic in detail. In general, parasitic infections are diagnosed by observing and recognizing various stages of the parasite life cycle (e.g., trophozoites and cysts of protozoa; microfilariae, eggs, and larvae of helminths) in clinical specimens. Parasites are identified primarily by the characteristic appearance—size, shape, internal details—of the various life cycle stages that are seen in clinical specimens. Sometimes whole worms or segments of worms are observed in fecal specimens.

Virology Section

The major responsibility of the virology section of the CML is to assist clinicians in the diagnosis of viral diseases. Chapters 24 and 25 discuss this topic in detail. Many viral diseases are diagnosed using immunodiagnostic procedures.[5] Other techniques used to identify viral pathogens include the following:

- Observation of intracytoplasmic or intranuclear viral inclusion bodies in specimens by cytologic or histologic examination

- Observation of viruses in specimens using electron microscopy

- Molecular diagnostic techniques such as nucleic acid probes and polymerase chain reaction assays (see Chapter 6)

- Virus isolation by use of cell cultures; viruses are identified primarily by the type(s) of cell lines that they are able to infect and the physical changes (called cytopathic effect, or CPE) that they cause in the infected cells

Immunology Section

The immunology laboratory in large hospitals and medical centers is where various immunological procedures are performed to diagnose infectious diseases and immune system disorders, determine tissue compatibility for organ and tissue transplants, and detect and measure various serum components. In smaller hospitals that do not have a separate immunology laboratory, some immunological procedures are performed in the microbiology, chemistry, and hematology laboratories, and some clinical specimens are sent to reference laboratories for immunological testing. In the CML of smaller hospitals, some immunodiagnostic procedures are performed in the immunology section, which is sometimes referred to as the serology section.

REPORTING AND CONFIDENTIALITY OF CLINICAL MICROBIOLOGY LABORATORY RESULTS

It is essential for CML results to be accurate and reported in a timely manner. Because of the time it takes to isolate and identify certain pathogens, the final report containing complete laboratory results may not be available for two or more days following receipt of the specimen. The **preliminary report** is furnished (often telephonically) to the physician before the final report is complete. A preliminary report often (1) is based on the initial macroscopic examination and microscopic examination of the specimen, (2) is furnished within an hour of specimen collection, (3) enables the physician to make a diagnosis and initiate appropriate therapy, and (4) saves the patient's life.

> Preliminary reports are very important. Often they enable clinicians to make diagnoses, initiate appropriate therapies, and save lives.

As with all patient information, laboratory results are confidential. Great care must be taken to prevent laboratory test results from being seen by unauthorized persons.

> All patient information, including laboratory results, are confidential.

SAFETY IN THE CLINICAL MICROBIOLOGY LABORATORY

Personnel working in the CML must be very safety conscious because of the constant danger of infection. Laboratory managers must ensure that laboratory professionals are in compliance with the regulations and standards prescribed by the **Occupational Safety and Health Administration (OSHA).** Many CML safety practices are briefly described in the following sections. Detailed safety information can be found in appropriate documents published by the Centers for Disease Control and Prevention (CDC), the Clinical and Laboratory Standards Institute (CLSI),[6] and other organizations.

Standard Precautions

CML professionals must familiarize themselves with the mandatory safety precautions universally practiced in hospital settings to prevent the transmission of pathogens. These **standard precautions,** as they are now called, prescribe proper safety practices such as hand washing; the use of gloves, masks or respirators, eye protection, and gowns; the

---

[5] *Immunodiagnostic procedures are laboratory procedures that detect either antigens or antibodies in clinical specimens. They are described in detail in Chapter 6.*

[6] ***The Clinical and Laboratory Standards Institute (CLSI)**, formerly called the National Committee for Clinical Laboratory Standards (NCCLS), is "a globally recognized, voluntary consensus standards-developing organization that enhances the value of medical testing within the health care community through the development and dissemination of standards, guidelines, and best practices" (quoted from the CLSI Web site, http://www.clsi.org/).*

handling of patient care equipment; disinfection practices; and the proper handling and disposal of "sharps" and other infectious wastes. In a CML, the term *sharps* refers to scalpel blades, pipettes, plastic loops, wooden sticks, needles, syringes, slides, and coverslips. Standard precautions include all the safety precautions previously called universal precautions. Additional information about standard precautions can be found in the section titled "Biological Safety."

Disinfection and Sterilization

Terms and Definitions

Disinfection is the destruction or removal of pathogens from nonliving objects by physical or chemical methods. Chemicals used to disinfect inanimate objects, such as laboratory countertops, floors, bedside equipment, and operating rooms, are called **disinfectants.** Most disinfectants are strong chemical substances that cannot be used on living tissue. **Antiseptics,** on the other hand, are solutions that kill or inhibit the growth of microorganisms on skin and other

living tissues. Examples of antiseptics used for preoperative preparation of skin are iodophors, alcohol-containing products, and chlorhexidine gluconate. These same antiseptics are used as hand hygiene agents, along with phenol derivatives, triclosan, and quaternary ammonium compounds.

The suffix *-cide* or *-cidal* means "killing." General terms like *germicidal agents* (*germicides*), *biocidal agents* (*biocides*), and *microbicidal agents* (*microbicides*) are disinfectants that kill microbes. **Bactericidal agents** (bactericides) are disinfectants that specifically kill bacteria but not necessarily bacterial endospores. Because spore coats are thick and resistant to the effects of many disinfectants, **sporicidal agents** are required to kill bacterial endospores. **Fungicidal agents** (fungicides) kill fungi, including fungal spores. **Algicidal agents** (algicides) are used to kill algae in swimming pools and hot tubs. **Viricidal** (or virucidal) **agents** destroy viruses. **Pseudomonicidal agents** kill bacteria in the genus *Pseudomonas,* and **tuberculocidal agents** kill the *M. tuberculosis* bacterium. Table 4-1 contains information about disinfectants used in health care settings.

TABLE 4 - 1   Examples of Disinfectants Used in Health Care Settings[a]

Disinfectant	Bactericidal	Sporicidal	Tuberculocidal	Pseudomonicidal	Fungicidal	Viricidal
Ethyl and isopropyl alcohols	Yes	No	Yes	Yes	Yes	Yes
Chlorine disinfectants	Yes	Yes	Yes	Yes	Yes	Yes
Formaldehyde	Yes	Yes	Yes	Yes	Yes	Yes
Glutaraldehyde	Yes	Yes	Yes	Yes	Yes	Yes
Hydrogen peroxide	Yes	Yes	Yes	Yes	Yes	Yes
Iodophors	Yes	Yes, with prolonged contact time	Yes	Yes	Yes	Yes
Peracetic acid	Yes	Yes	Yes	Yes	Yes	Yes
Peracetic acid/hydrogen peroxide	Yes	Perhaps, with prolonged contact time	Yes	Yes	Yes	Yes
Phenolics	Yes	No	Yes	Yes	Yes	Yes, some viruses
Quaternary ammonium compounds	Yes	No	No	Yes	Yes	Yes, some viruses

Source: Rutala WA. Selection and use of disinfectants in health care. In: Mayhall CG, ed. Hospital Epidemiology and Infection Control. 2nd Ed. Philadelphia: Lippincott Williams & Wilkins, 1999.

[a] These disinfectants are "cidal" for various groups of microbes only when used in accordance with manufacturers' directions.

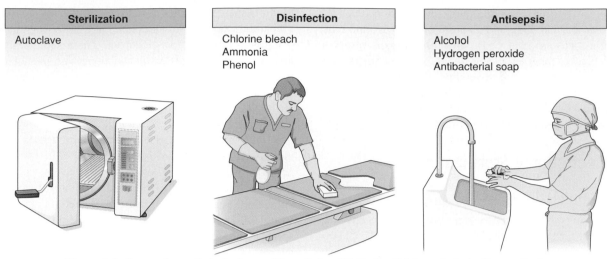

Figure 4-4. Types of aseptic techniques. (From Cohen BJ, Taylor JJ. Memmler's the Human Body in Health and Disease. 10th Ed. Philadelphia: Lippincott Williams & Wilkins, 2005.)

> Beware of similar-sounding words. If a drug or disinfectant kills bacteria, it is said to be bactericidal. If a drug or disinfectant stops bacteria from growing and multiplying, it is said to be bacteriostatic. Notice that there is an *o* in bacteriostatic but no *o* in bactericidal.

A **microbistatic agent** is a drug or chemical that inhibits growth and reproduction of microorganisms but does not kill them. Freeze drying (lyophilization) and rapid freezing using liquid nitrogen are microbistatic techniques that are used to preserve microbes for future use or study. A **bacteriostatic agent** is a drug or disinfectant that specifically inhibits the metabolism and reproduction of bacteria. Some of the drugs used to treat bacterial diseases are bacteriostatic, whereas others are bactericidal (see Chapter 7).

Sterilization is the complete destruction of all microbes, including cells, spores, and viruses. When something is **sterile,** it is devoid of microbial life. Sterilization of objects can be accomplished by dry heat, autoclaving (steam under pressure), gas (ethylene oxide), various chemicals (such as formaldehyde), and some types of radiation, such as ultraviolet light and gamma rays.

> Disinfection is the destruction or removal of pathogens, whereas sterilization is the complete destruction of all microbes.

Methods of Sterilization and Disinfection

Sepsis refers to the presence of pathogens in blood or tissues, whereas **asepsis** is the absence of pathogens. Various techniques, collectively referred to as **aseptic techniques,** are employed to eliminate and exclude pathogens. Aseptic techniques include hand washing; the use of sterile gloves, masks, and gowns; sterilization of surgical instruments and other equipment; and the use of disinfectants, including antiseptics (Fig. 4-4). **Antisepsis** is the prevention of infection. **Antiseptic technique** refers to the use of antiseptics. Antiseptic technique is a type of aseptic technique.

Sterile technique. Sterile technique is practiced when it is necessary to exclude *all* microorganisms from a particular area. It is important to use sterile technique in the CML, when inoculating culture media. Sterile technique is also employed in many other areas of the hospital, such as the operating rooms. Methods used to destroy or inhibit microbial life are either physical or chemical, and sometimes both types are used. Physical methods commonly used in hospitals, clinics, and laboratories to destroy or control pathogens include heat, a combination of heat and pressure, desiccation, radiation, sonic disruption, and filtration.

Heat. Heat is the most practical, efficient, inexpensive, and common method of sterilization of inanimate objects and materials that can withstand high temperatures. Two factors, *temperature* and *time*, determine the effectiveness of heat for sterilization. In practical applications of heat for sterilization, the type of material in which a mixture of microorganisms and/or their spores are found must be taken into consideration. Pus, feces, vomitus, mucus, and blood contain proteins that serve as a protective coating to insulate pathogens from destruction. When these substances are present on bedding, bandages, surgical instruments, and syringes, very high temperatures are required to destroy vegetative microorganisms and spores.[7] In practice, the most effective procedure is to wash away the protein debris with strong soap, hot water, and a disinfectant and then to sterilize the equipment or materials with heat.

Dry heat baking in a thermostatically controlled oven provides effective sterilization of metals, glassware, some

---

[7] *Vegetative microorganisms are microorganisms that are actively metabolizing, growing, and reproducing. Spores represent a dormant stage of the organism.*

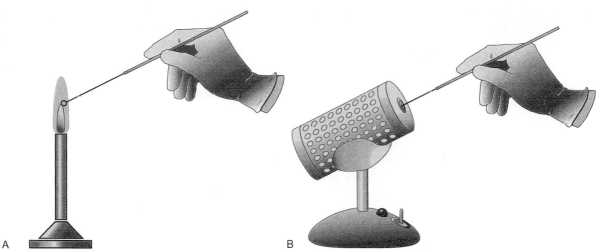

Figure 4-5. **Dry heat sterilization. A.** Flaming a wire bacteriological loop in a Bunsen burner flame. **B.** Sterilizing a bacteriological loop using an electrical heating device.

powders, oils, and waxes. These items must be baked at 160°C to 165°C for 2 hours or at 170°C to 180°C for 1 hour.[8] An ordinary oven of the type found in most homes may be used if the temperature remains constant. The effectiveness of dry heat sterilization depends on how deeply the heat penetrates throughout the material, and the items to be baked must be positioned so that the hot air circulates freely around them.

Incineration or burning is an effective means of destroying contaminated disposable materials. An incinerator must never be overloaded with moist or protein-laden materials, such as feces, vomitus, or pus, because the contaminating microorganisms within these moist substances may not be destroyed if the heat does not readily penetrate and burn them. Flaming the surface of metal forceps and wire bacteriological loops is an effective way to kill microorganisms and, for many years, was a common laboratory procedure. Flaming is accomplished by briefly holding the end of the loop or forceps in the inner blue portion of a gas flame (Fig. 4-5). Open flames are dangerous, however, and thus are rarely used in modern laboratories. Today disposable plastic inoculating loops are used most often. Whenever wire inoculating loops are employed, heat sterilization is usually accomplished using electrical heating devices.

Heat applied in the presence of moisture, as in boiling or steaming, is faster and more effective than dry heat and can be accomplished at a lower temperature. Thus, moist heat is less destructive to many materials that otherwise would be damaged at higher temperatures. Moist heat causes proteins to coagulate, as occurs when eggs are hard-boiled. Because cellular enzymes are proteins, they are inactivated by moist heat, leading to cell death.

An **autoclave** is like a large metal pressure cooker that uses steam under pressure to completely destroy all microbial life (Fig. 4-6). The increased pressure raises the temperature above the temperature of boiling water (i.e., above 100°C) and forces the steam into the materials being sterilized.

Autoclaving at a pressure of 15 pounds per square inch (psi) and a temperature of 121.5°C for 20 minutes destroys vegetative microorganisms, bacterial endospores, and viruses, as long as they are not protected by pus, feces, vomitus, blood, or other proteinaceous substances. Some types of equipment and certain materials, such as rubber, which may be damaged by high temperatures, can be autoclaved at lower temperatures for longer periods. The timing must be carefully determined based on the contents and compactness of the load. All articles must be properly packaged and arranged within the autoclave to allow steam to penetrate each package completely. Cans should remain open, bottles covered loosely with foil or cotton, and instruments wrapped in cloth. Sealed containers should not be autoclaved. Heat-sensitive autoclave tape (Fig. 4-7) and commercially

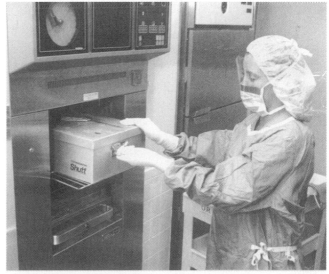

Figure 4-6. **A large, built-in autoclave.** (Courtesy of Scott & White Hospital, Temple, TX.)

---

[8] *Formulas for converting Celsius to Fahrenheit and vice versa are presented in Appendix B.*

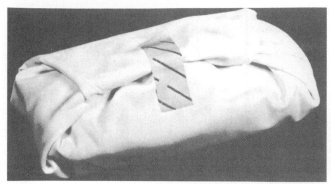

Figure 4-7. **Heat-sensitive autoclave tape showing dark stripes after sterilization.** (From Volk WA, Benjamin DC, Kadner RJ, Parson JT. Essentials of Medical Microbiology. 4th Ed. Philadelphia: JB Lippincott, 1991.)

available solutions or paper strips containing bacterial spores (Fig. 4-8) should be used as quality control measures to ensure that autoclaves are functioning properly.

Ultraviolet light. The sun is not a particularly reliable disinfecting agent because it kills only the microorganisms directly exposed to its rays. The rays of the sun include the

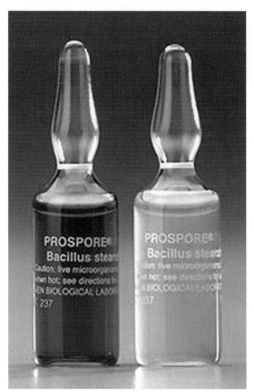

Figure 4-8. **Biological indicator used to monitor the effectiveness of steam sterilization.** Sealed ampules containing bacterial spores suspended in a growth medium are placed in the load to be sterilized. Following sterilization, the ampules are incubated at 35°C. If the spores were killed, there will be no change in the color of the medium. If the spores were not killed, acid production by the organisms will cause the medium to change from purple to yellow. (Courtesy of Fisher Scientific.)

long infrared (heat) rays, the visible light rays, and the shorter ultraviolet (UV) rays. UV rays, which do not penetrate glass and building materials, are effective only in the air and on surfaces. They can, however, penetrate a cell and cause damage to DNA. When this occurs, genes may be so severely damaged that the cell dies—especially a unicellular microorganism—or is drastically changed.

In practice, a UV lamp, often called a germicidal lamp, is useful for reducing the number of microorganisms in the air. Its main component is a low-pressure mercury vapor tube. Such lamps are found in newborn nurseries, operating rooms, elevators, entryways, cafeterias, and classrooms, where they are incorporated into louvered ceiling fixtures designed to radiate across the top of the room without striking people in the room. Sterility may also be maintained by a UV lamp placed in a hood or cabinet containing instruments, paper or cloth equipment, liquid, or other inanimate articles.

> Exercise caution when using UV lamps. Ultraviolet rays can cause serious burns, cellular damage, and eye injury.

Ultrasonic waves. In hospitals, medical clinics, and dental clinics, ultrasonic waves are a frequently used means of cleaning and sterilizing delicate equipment. Ultrasonic cleaners consist of tanks filled with liquid solvent, usually water. The short sound waves are then passed through the liquid. The sound waves mechanically dislodge organic debris on instruments and glassware. Glassware and other articles that have been cleansed in ultrasonic equipment must be washed to remove the dislodged particles and solvent and then sterilized by another method before they are used.

Filtration. Filters of various pore sizes are used to filter or separate cells, larger viruses, bacteria, and certain other microorganisms from the liquids or gases in which they are suspended. Filters with tiny pore sizes, known as cellulose-acetate filters, are used in laboratories to filter bacteria and viruses out of liquids. The variety of filters is large and includes sintered glass (in which uniform particles of glass are fused), plastic films, unglazed porcelain, asbestos, diatomaceous earth, and cellulose membrane filters. Small quantities of liquid can be filtered through a syringe, but large quantities require larger apparatuses.

A cotton plug in a test tube, flask, or pipette is a good filter for preventing the entry of microorganisms. Dry gauze or paper masks and **high-efficiency particulate air (HEPA) filters** prevent the outward passage of microbes from the mouth and nose, at the same time protecting the wearer from inhaling airborne pathogens and foreign particles that could damage the lungs. Biological safety cabinets contain HEPA filters to protect workers from contamination. HEPA filters are also located in operating rooms and patient rooms to filter the air that enters or exits the room.

> **Sterilization may be accomplished using dry heat, moist heat, UV light, or filtration.**

General Safety Precautions

Each laboratory must have an appointed laboratory safety officer—a person who has experience and/or credentials in the field of laboratory safety. A safety manual must be available within the CML, which all new employees are required to read. A laboratory security system should be in place, allowing only authorized people to have access to the laboratory. Biohazard signs must be posted at the entrance(s) to the laboratory (Fig. 4-9). Hands must be washed frequently and thoroughly in the CML, using warm water and soap. CML professionals should wash their hands after removing gloves, after working at the laboratory bench, and before leaving the laboratory. Storing of food, placing any sort of food (e.g., candy, chewing gum) into one's mouth, drinking, smoking, and applying cosmetics are strictly forbidden in the CML. The CML must also have an emergency eye wash station, a safety shower, and first aid equipment.

> **CML professionals must familiarize themselves with the various warning signs posted in the CML, such as those for biohazards and radioactivity.**

Disinfectants must be available for routine disinfection of workbenches and for cleaning biological spills. Working solutions of disinfectants must be prepared in accordance with the manufacturer's instructions, and the disinfectant must remain in contact with the surface for a sufficient time, as stated in the manufacturer's instructions. A 10% solution of household bleach is a commonly used disinfectant. Additional information about disinfectants, contact time, and preparation of solutions and dilutions can be found on the CD-ROM. Because of the inherent danger of ingesting hazardous liquids, mouth pipetting is strictly forbidden.

Because compressed gas cylinders are potentially dangerous, they should be securely fastened to a wall or lab bench, the metal valve safety cover should be in place during transport and whenever the tank is not in use, and the cylinders should be securely chained to special hand trucks or dollies when being transported.

Personal Protective Equipment (PPE)

Personal protective equipment (PPE) includes gloves, gowns, lab coats, face shields, goggles, and respirators. Gloves must always be worn while collecting or handling clinical specimens. They should also be worn when working at the laboratory bench, if the skin of the hands is chapped or broken. Even tiny breaks in the skin, such as paper cuts, represent potential portals of entry for pathogens. There are certain areas within the CML where gloves must always be worn; the TB lab is an example.

Long-sleeved, impermeable laboratory coats or gowns must be worn while working in the CML (Fig. 4-10). Coats or gowns that are worn within the laboratory must never be worn outside the laboratory. Separate coats or gowns should be

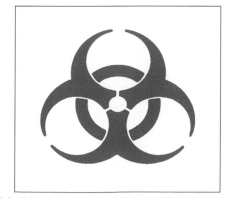

Figure 4-9. **Biohazard symbol.** (From McCall RE, Tankersley CM. Phlebotomy Essentials. 4th Ed. Baltimore: Lippincott Williams & Wilkins, 2007.)

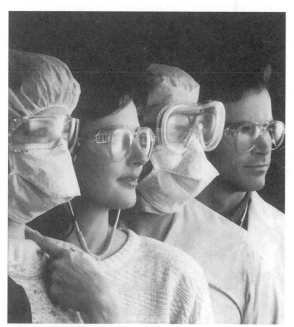

Figure 4-10. **Various pieces of personal protective equipment**, including masks, goggles, hair protection, and disposable gowns. (Courtesy of 3M Health Care.)

available for laboratory personnel who are required to draw blood from hospital patients or retrieve clinical specimens from wards and clinics. Whenever a laboratory coat or gown becomes soiled, it should be carefully removed and placed in an appropriate disposal or laundry container.

There are occasions when CML professionals should wear HEPA-filtered face masks, respirators, or face shields, or perform their work behind an acrylic splash shield. For example, a HEPA-filtered face mask or respirator is sometimes used in addition to a biological safety cabinet, when working with *M. tuberculosis*. Vortexing (high-speed mixing) or other splatter-generating practices require the use of a biosafety cabinet or acrylic splash shield.

Biological Safety

Biosafety Levels

The U.S. Department of Health and Human Services has established four levels of biosafety, based upon the degree of hazard associated with particular pathogens. The four biosafety levels (BSLs) are designated BSL-1, BSL-2, BSL-3, and BSL-4. These levels are sometimes referred to as biological levels (BLs), in which case the four levels are designated BL-1, BL-2, BL-3, and BL-4.

BSL-1 is appropriate for working with microbes thought not to cause disease in healthy adults, such as those used in high school or community college biology and microbiology laboratory settings. Although no special safety precautions are required at BSL-1, the following standard microbiological precautions are required:

- Appropriate hazard warning signs are posted on laboratory door(s)—for example, biohazard, radioactive materials, toxic chemicals—and access to the laboratory is limited or restricted whenever work with pathogens is in progress.

- A sink or sinks must be available for hand washing; hands are washed when work is finished and before leaving the laboratory.

- Eating, drinking, smoking, handling contact lenses, and applying cosmetics are forbidden.

- Sandals and open-toe shoes are inappropriate footwear in the laboratory.

- Mechanical pipetting devices are used; mouth pipetting is forbidden.

- Appropriate measures are taken to minimize aerosol and splash production; work is performed in a biosafety cabinet, whenever appropriate to do so.

- Work surfaces are decontaminated whenever a spill of viable material occurs and when the day's work is completed.

- Waste materials are segregated according to hazard type and disposed of properly; infectious wastes are decontaminated using an autoclave, chemical disinfection, or other approved method.

- Ideally, the laboratory is under negative pressure—that is, air flows into the laboratory whenever the laboratory door is opened.

- Lab coats or gowns are worn to protect street clothes; these must remain in the laboratory unless properly decontaminated.

- Gloves are worn when handling infected animals and when hands may come in contact with infectious materials and contaminated equipment or surfaces.

- Splatter shields, eye or face protection should be worn, whenever appropriate to do so.

Most CMLs are considered to be BSL-2 laboratories. BSL-2 agents (e.g., hepatitis B virus, HIV) present a low-to-moderate degree of hazard. At BSL-2, all standard microbiological practices are employed, as are the following special safety precautions:

- Some immunizations are required (e.g., hepatitis B virus).

- Extreme precautions are taken while handling needles and other sharps. Never break, bend, or recap needles. Appropriate containers must be available for disposal of needles and syringes.

- Access to the laboratory is restricted, and laboratory doors are kept closed.

- Although not required, many BSL-2 laboratories are under negative pressure.

- Although some work can be done on open benches (as at BSL-1), any work that may produce splatters or aerosols of infectious materials should be performed within a **biosafety cabinet (BSC).** A BSC must be used when processing clinical specimens. The most common type of BSC used at BSL-2 is a class II, type A BSC (described later in the chapter).

- Infectious waste must be chemically decontaminated or autoclaved.

- Work surfaces are decontaminated after working with infectious materials.

- All spills and accidents are reported, and an incident log book is maintained.

BSL-3 is suitable for work with pathogens that may cause serious or potentially lethal diseases following inhalation. BSL-3 agents include *M. tuberculosis*, *Coxiella burnetii*, and St. Louis encephalitis virus. All BSL-1 and BSL-2 safety measures must be practiced at BSL-3. In addition, work must be performed in a containment facility having self-closing double doors and negative air pressure, access to the lab must be controlled, and the lab air must be exhausted through HEPA filters to the outside. Additional PPE (e.g., respirators) is often required. All waste must be decontaminated, and lab clothing must be decontaminated before laundering. Class II, type A BSCs are suitable in BSL-3 laboratories. All work that may create aerosols or splatter is performed within the BSC. Special centrifuges and centrifugation procedures are used to prevent aerosol exposures.

BSL-4 agents present a lethal degree of hazard; examples are smallpox virus and the viruses that cause hemorrhagic fevers, such as Marburg, Lassa, and Ebola viruses. BSL-4 facilities are sometimes referred to as maximum containment laboratories or hot labs. All BSL-1, BSL-2, and BSL-3 safety measures must be practiced at BSL-4. In addition, the laboratory must be located in a separate building or isolated zone, workers must wear full-body positive-pressure suits, and they must shower on exiting the facility. All procedures must be performed in a class III BSC. Ideally, waste materials are decontaminated before their removal from the facility.

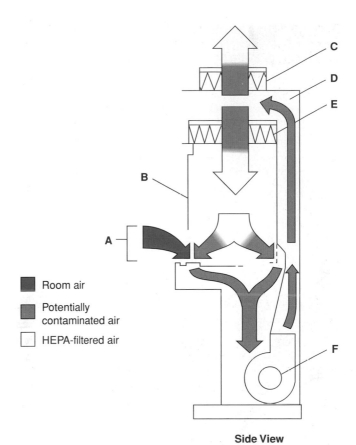

Biosafety Cabinets

BSCs are designed to protect people and the environment from pathogens and are also used to protect specimens, cultures of microorganisms, or cell cultures from contamination. In the CML, BSCs must be available for use when processing clinical specimens and when working with especially infectious pathogens (e.g., mould colonies and *M. tuberculosis*). Work should always be performed within a BSC whenever potentially infectious aerosols are produced (e.g., by grinding, mincing, vortexing, or centrifuging).

The three general types of BSCs are called class I, class II, and class III BSCs. A BSC is not required when working only with BSL-1 organisms. Class I BSCs are not recommended for biohazard work. The class II BSC is the type most commonly found in CMLs (Fig. 4-11). It is required when working with BSL-2 and BSL-3 agents. Air is drawn into the BSC by negative air pressure; it passes through a HEPA filter. Air flows in a vertical sheet in front of the person using the BSC; it serves as a barrier between the outside and inside of the BSC. The air that is exhausted from the BSC passes through HEPA filters.

Class III BSCs are required when manipulating cultures of extremely hazardous BSL-3 and BSL-4 agents (Fig. 4-12). They are used in maximum containment laboratories or BSL-4 facilities, such as those found at the CDC in Atlanta, Georgia; the U.S. Army Medical Research Institute of Infectious Diseases at Fort Detrick, Maryland; and the Maximum Containment Lab (MCL) at the National Institutes of Health in Bethesda, Maryland.

Side View

Figure 4-11. **Design of a class II type A biosafety cabinet.** A motor (*F*) draws room air into the cabinet through the front opening (*A*). The air is recirculated through a plenum (*D*). Approximately 70% of the air is recirculated into the work area through a HEPA filter (*E*). The remainder is exhausted through another HEPA filter (*C*) to the room. The work area is viewed through a glass sash (*B*). (From Winn WC Jr, et al. Koneman's Color Atlas and Textbook of Diagnostic Microbiology. 6th Ed. Philadelphia: Lippincott Williams & Wilkins, 2006.)

Processing Clinical Specimens

CML professionals must be very careful when collecting and handling *all* clinical specimens, because *any* specimen might contain highly infectious pathogens. Infectious pathogens could be present in specimens collected from patients not even suspected of having an infectious disease. Especially dangerous specimens processed in the CML are blood, amniotic fluid, cerebrospinal fluid, feces, peritoneal fluid, saliva, semen, sputum, synovial fluid, tissues, urine, vaginal secretions, and wound drainage. Gloves and gowns that are impervious to liquids must always be worn while processing clinical specimens in the CML. In general, all specimens should be processed in a class II BSC.

> Exercise caution when collecting, transporting, or processing clinical specimens. They could contain highly infectious pathogens.

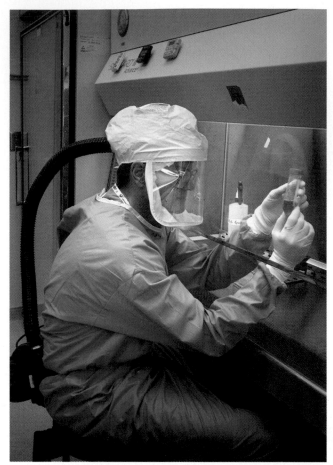

Figure 4-12. **CDC microbiologist working in a BSL-3 laboratory.** (Courtesy of James Gathany and the Centers for Disease Control and Prevention.)

Special Safety Considerations in the Mycobacteriology Section

Because of the highly infectious nature of *M. tuberculosis*, special safety precautions are necessary for the mycobacteriology section (TB lab). It should be a separate room, under negative pressure, with minimal traffic. Room air should be exhausted through HEPA filters. TB lab employees wear gowns and gloves. Personnel in BSL-3 TB labs also wear eye protection (if they wear contact lenses) and special respirators (Fig. 4-13). All bench work is performed within class II BSCs. Special centrifuges are used to prevent the formation of aerosols. Disinfectants must be tuberculocidal. The use of ultraviolet lights is recommended when no one is working in the TB lab to destroy any residual microorganisms. Employees in the TB lab should be monitored with the Mantoux PPD (purified protein derivative) skin test at least annually.

Hazardous Waste and Infectious Waste Plans

CMLs are required to have hazardous and infectious waste plans in place. The hazardous waste plan provides CML

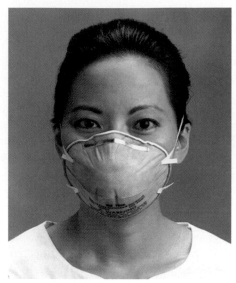

Figure 4-13. **Type N95 respirator.** (Courtesy of 3M Occupational Health and Environmental Safety Division, St. Paul, MN.)

professionals with information about any types of hazardous wastes generated within the CML. This would include corrosive, toxic, carcinogenic, flammable, extremely reactive, radioactive, and infectious wastes. The plan would contain information regarding the handling, storage, labeling, and disposal of such wastes.

The infectious waste plan identifies the various types of infectious wastes processed by or generated within the CML. The plan includes information regarding the handling, storage, labeling, treatment, and disposal of infectious wastes, as well as record keeping and mandatory infectious waste training of CML professionals. Infectious wastes generated in the CML are usually autoclaved or incinerated. Puncture-proof containers must be available for the disposal of needles, broken glass, microscope slides, and other sharps.

> New CML employees are required to familiarize themselves with the CML's hazardous and infectious waste plans.

Chemical Safety

Many hazardous chemicals are used in the CML. It is extremely important that CML professionals be aware of the hazards associated with the chemicals with which they work. In 1987, OSHA published the Hazard Communication Standard, which states that all laboratory personnel must be made aware of the hazards of the chemicals with which they work. In addition, every laboratory should have a chemical hygiene plan, manufacturer's material safety data sheets, and a written safety-training program. The chemical hygiene plan should include information about potentially hazardous chemicals, the handling and storage of such chemicals, the use of personal protective equipment, first aid measures, actions to be taken if chemical spills occur, chemical waste disposal, records to be maintained, warning signs and labels to be posted, and required personnel training.

A **material safety data sheet (MSDS)** is an OSHA-required form that contains important information about a particular chemical. An MSDS must be available for every chemical and chemical-containing product in use in the CML, and all personnel must be familiar with the location of the forms. An MSDS provides valuable information about the chemical, including the following:

> CML professionals should familiarize themselves with the MSDS for every chemical and chemical-containing product used in the CML.

- Product name and specifications

- Manufacturer's name, address, and contact information

- Physical data

- Hazardous ingredients

- Handling procedures

- Routes of entry

- Fire and explosion hazards

- Reactivity data

- Emergency and first aid procedures

- Spill and disposal procedures

- Permissible exposure levels

- Storage and transportation precautions

A sample MSDS is shown in Figure 4-14.

In addition, the laboratory door and all hazardous chemicals must be clearly labeled with the **National Fire Protection Association (NFPA)** hazard-rating label (Fig. 4-15). This diamond-shaped label, containing four individual diamond-shaped areas, is color coded to indicate health hazards (blue), flammability risk (red), reactivity/stability (yellow), and any special hazards (white). The numbers in the blue, red, and yellow diamonds indicate the severity of the hazard, with 1 being the least severe and 4 being the most severe. The white diamond is reserved for symbols that warn of any special firefighting or hazardous information (e.g., a warning not to use water, or the presence of oxidizers or radiation). The primary purpose of the NFPA symbol is to protect firefighters.

Chemical Fume Hoods

For work with potentially dangerous chemical reagents, a chemical fume hood is required to expel any noxious or hazardous fumes. Fume hoods also provide protection from potential fires or explosions. Fume hoods work by exhausting fumes and vapors to the outside of the building by means of a fan. All work should be performed at least 6 inches inside the hood with the sash—the glass window—open no more than about 12 inches. The hood should have some visual means or alarm system to indicate that it is working properly and should be inspected regularly for proper airflow and ventilation. The velocity of airflow, with the sash in the normal operating position, should be 100 to 120 feet per minute.

Fire and Electrical Safety

CMLs must post fire evacuation plans and must conduct periodic fire drills. CML professionals must be aware of the location of fire safety equipment (e.g., fire alarm boxes, fire extinguishers, and fire blankets) and receive training on their use. Categories of fire extinguishers include type A (to extinguish trash, wood, and paper fires), type B (for chemical fires), and type C (for electrical fires). Combination type ABC extinguishers can be used to extinguish any of these types of fires, but type C extinguishers are preferable for use on fires involving laboratory instruments. The appropriate phone number to call to report a fire must be posted on or near all telephones in the CML. All fire exits must be marked and remain clear of obstructions. Most institutional and laboratory safety programs include training on responding to a fire emergency. Laboratory personnel should remember the acronym RACE—**R**escue, **A**larm, **C**ontain, and **E**xtinguish.

Shipping Pathogens and Clinical Specimens

Sometimes it is necessary to send an etiologic agent or specimen to an outside or reference laboratory for identification or processing.[9] Because of the inherent danger of leakage, the shipping of potentially infectious materials is closely regulated by the International Civil Aviation Organization, the International Air Transport Association, and the U.S. Department of Transportation. Information regarding the packaging and shipment of these materials can be found in CLSI Document M29-A3 (see "References and Suggested Reading") and online at http://hazmat.dot.gov/regs/rules.htm and http://www.asm.org/. Personnel who ship infectious substances must be familiar with these regulations and must have completed an appropriate training course. CLSI Document M29-A3 states the following:

> Requirements for packaging are generally based on a three-container system, with the primary and secondary packages required to be watertight [(Fig. 4-16)]. [Absorbent material] is required between the primary and secondary packages in case of accidental breakage and spill. . . . For some packaging, for example when transporting cultures, the secondary container requires high integrity and protection against damage. For diagnostic samples, the packaging requirements

---

[9]The term **etiologic agent** means the causative agent; in other words, the pathogen that is causing the disease.

MSDS Product and Company Name

MSDS Date: 03/27/1996   MSDS: BZTYN

Submitter: F BT   LIIN: 00f048833   Tech 07/08/1996   Status C
Review: CD:

Product 17-5 METHANOL ABSOLUTE   MFN: 02
ID:

Article: N   Kit Y
Part:

Cage 21076

Responsible
Party

Name: SIGMA CHEMICAL COMPANY

Address: 3050 SPRUCE ST   Box: 14508

City: SAINT LOUIS   State: MO   Zip: 63178-5000

Country: US

Info Phone Number: 314-771-5765/800-325-3010

Emergency Phone Number: 314-771-5765/800-325-3010

Preparer's Name: N/P

Proprietary Ind: N   Review Ind: Y
Published: Y   Special Project CD:

MSDS Preparer

Cage: 21076   Assigned N
Ind:

Name: SIGMA CHEMICAL COMPANY

Address: 3050 SPRUCE ST   Box: 14508

City: SAINT LOUIS   State: MO   Zip: 63178-5000

Company Information

Cage: 21076   Name: SIGMA CHEMICAL COMPANY

Address: 3050 SPRUCE ST   Box: 14508

City: SAINT LOUIS   State: MO   Zip: 63178-5000

Country: US   Phone: 314-771-5765

Signs And Symptoms of Overexposure
IRRITATION, GI DISTURBANCES, CONVULSIONS.

Medical Cond Aggravated By Exposure
N/K

First Aid
EYES/SKIN: FLUSH W/COPIOUS AMOUNTS OF WATER FOR 15
MINS. INHALATION: REMOVE TO FRESH AIR. GIVE CPR/OXYGEN IF
NEEDED. INGESTION: WASH OUT MOUTH W/WATER PROVIDED
PERSON IS CONSCIOUS. OBTAIN MEDICAL ATTENTION IN ALL
CASES.

Spill Release Procedures
EVACUATE AREA. SHUT OFF IGNITION SOURCES. WEAR SCBA,
RUBBER BOOTS & HEAVY RUBBER GLOVES. COVER W/DRY-LIME,
SANDS/SODA ASH. PLACE IN COVERED CONTAINERS USING
NON-SPARKING TOOLS & TRANSPORT OUTDOORS. VENTILATE
AREA & WASH SITE AFTER PICKUP IS COMPLETE.

Neutralizing Agent
N/K

Waste Disposal Methods
BURN IN CHEMICAL INCINERATOR EQUIPPED W/AFTERBURNER &
SCRUBBER. USE CAUTION, MATERIAL IS HIGHLY FLAMMABLE.
DISPOSE OF IAW/FEDERAL, STATE & LOCAL REGULATIONS.

Handling And Storage Precautions
KEEP TIGHTLY CLOSED. KEEP FROM HEAT, SPARKS, & OPEN
FLAME. STORE IN A COOL DRY PLACE.

Other Precautions
DON'T BREATHE VAPORS. AVOID CONTACT W/SKIN, EYES &
CLOTHING. DON'T USE IF SKIN IS CUT/SCRATCHED. TOXIC.

Ingredients

Cas: 67-56-1   M   PC1400000   M
Code: RTECS#:   Code:

Name: METHANOL (METHYL, ALCOHOL), COLUMN SPIRITS
96-2   MFN: 02
N/K

% Text: Environmental
Wt:
200 PPM

Other REC
Limits:

OSHA PEL: 200 PPM   M
Code: OSHA STEL: Code:

ACGIH TLV: 200 PPM   M   N/P
Code: ACGIH STEL: Code:

EPA Rpt Qty: 5000 LBS   DOT Rpt Qty: 5000 LBS

Ozone Depleting Chemical: N

Health Hazards Information

LD50 LC50 Mixture ORAL LD50(RAT): 5628 MG/KG

	YES	YES	YES
Route Of Entry Inds - Inhalation:	Skin:	Ingestion:	
	NO	NO	NO
Carcinogenicity Inds - NTP:	IARC:	OSHA:	

Health Hazards Acute And Chronic
HARMFUL BY INHALATION, ABSORPTION & INGESTION. EYES/SKIN:
IRRITATION. MATERIAL IS IRRITATING TO MUCOUS MEMBRANES &
UPPER RESPIRATORY TRACT.

Explanation Of Carcinogenicity
NONE

Fire and Explosion Hazard Information

Flash Point N/P
Method:
52F

Flash Point: Flash Point Text:
N/A

Autoignition   Autoignition Temp
Temp: Text:
6   36

Lower Limits: Upper Limits:

Extinguishing Media
CO2, DRY CHEMICAL POWERDER/APPROPRIATE FOAM.

Fire Fighting Procedures
WEAR SCBA & PROTECTIVE CLOTHING.

Unusual Fire/Explosion Hazard
EXTREMELY FLAMMABLE. VAPORS MAY TRAVEL DISTANCE TO
IGNITION SOURCES & FLASH BACK. AUTOIGNITION TEMP: 725F.

Control Measures

Respiratory Protection
WEAR NIOSH/MSHA APPROVED RESPIRATOR.

Ventilation
MECHANICAL EXHAUST VENTILATION.

Protective Gloves
CHEMICAL RESISTANT

Eye Protection
SAFETY GOGGLES

Figure 4-14. **Example of a material safety data sheet (MSDS).**

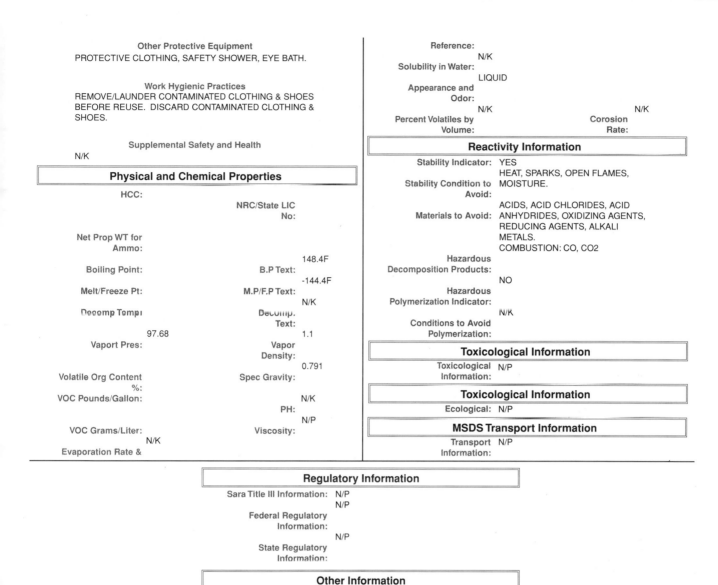

Other Protective Equipment
PROTECTIVE CLOTHING, SAFETY SHOWER, EYE BATH.

Work Hygienic Practices
REMOVE/LAUNDER CONTAMINATED CLOTHING & SHOES
BEFORE REUSE. DISCARD CONTAMINATED CLOTHING &
SHOES.

Supplemental Safety and Health
N/K

Physical and Chemical Properties

HCC:

NRC/State LIC
No:

Net Prop WT for
Ammo:

Boiling Point:	B.P Text:	148.4F
Melt/Freeze Pt:	M.P/F.P Text:	-144.4F
Decomp Temp:	Decomp. Text:	N/K
		97.68
Vapor Pres:	Vapor Density:	1.1
Volatile Org Content %:	Spec Gravity:	0.791
VOC Pounds/Gallon:	PH:	N/K
VOC Grams/Liter:	Viscosity:	N/P
		N/K
Evaporation Rate &		

Reference:
N/K
Solubility in Water:
LIQUID
Appearance and
Odor:
N/K   N/K
Percent Volatiles by   Corrosion
Volume: Rate:

Reactivity Information

Stability Indicator: YES

Stability Condition to   HEAT, SPARKS, OPEN FLAMES,
Avoid: MOISTURE.

Materials to Avoid: ACIDS, ACID CHLORIDES, ACID
                      ANHYDRIDES, OXIDIZING AGENTS,
                      REDUCING AGENTS, ALKALI
                      METALS.
                      COMBUSTION: CO, CO2

Hazardous
Decomposition Products:
                      NO
Hazardous
Polymerization Indicator:
                      N/K
Conditions to Avoid
Polymerization:

Toxicological Information

Toxicological   N/P
Information:

Toxicological Information

Ecological: N/P

MSDS Transport Information

Transport   N/P
Information:

Regulatory Information

Sara Title III Information: N/P
                            N/P
Federal Regulatory
Information:
                            N/P
State Regulatory
Information:

Other Information

Other   N/P
Information:

Figure 4-14. (continued)

are similar, but the performance test requirements are less stringent. The outer packaging usually consists of a sturdy fiberboard of sufficient size to accommodate the required labels and external markings on a single surface, without going over or around an edge.

External labels and markings include a specific United Nations number (e.g., UN 2814 is the label for an infectious substance affecting humans) and appropriate safety labels that include the international symbol for infectious substances (Fig. 4-17). If dry ice is used as a refrigerant, this information must be reported.

Safety Programs and Training

To be in compliance with OSHA and the Joint Commission on the Accreditation of Healthcare Organizations (JCAHO; http://www.jcaho.org/) regulations, a comprehensive safety-training program must be in place for training new employees and retraining experienced employees. The training program should address fire prevention, chemical safety, and infection control. Personnel should receive training regarding the proper donning, wearing, and removal of PPE. Training is required annually and should be documented for anyone identified as being at risk to occupational exposure for bloodborne pathogens.

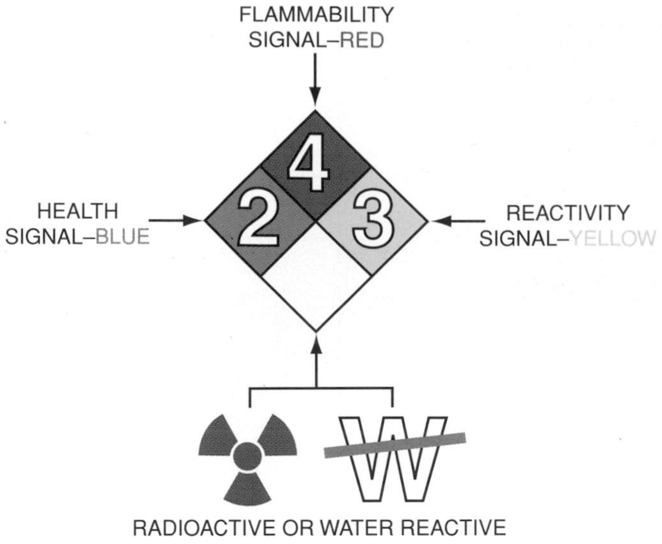

FLAMMABILITY
SIGNAL–RED

HEALTH
SIGNAL–BLUE

REACTIVITY
SIGNAL–YELLOW

RADIOACTIVE OR WATER REACTIVE

Identification of Health Hazard Color Code: **BLUE**		Identification of Flammability Color Code: **RED**		Identification of Reactivity (Stability) Color Code: **YELLOW**	
	Type of possible injury		Susceptibility of materials to burning		Susceptibility to release of energy
SIGNAL		SIGNAL		SIGNAL	
4	Materials that on very short exposure could cause death or major residual injury even though prompt medical treatment was given.	4	Materials that will rapidly or completely vaporize at atmospheric pressure and normal ambient temperature, or that are readily dispersed in air and that will burn readily.	4	Materials that in themselves are readily capable of detonation or of explosive decomposition or reaction at normal temperatures and pressures.
3	Materials that on short exposure could cause serious temporary or residual injury even though prompt medical treatment was given.	3	Liquids and solids that can be ignited under almost all ambient temperature conditions.	3	Materials that in themselves are capable of detonation or explosive reaction but require a strong initiating source or that must be heated under confinement before initiation or that react explosively with water.
2	Materials that on intense or continued exposure could cause temporary incapacitation or possible residual injury unless prompt medical treatment is given.	2	Materials that must be moderately heated or exposed to relatively high ambient temperatures before ignition can occur.	2	Materials that in themselves are normally unstable and readily undergo violent chemical change but do not detonate. Also materials that may react violently with water or that may form potentially explosive mixtures with water.
1	Materials that on exposure would cause irritation but only minor residual injury even if no treatment is given.	1	Materials that must be preheated before ignition can occur.	1	Materials that in themselves are normally stable but that can become unstable at elevated temperatures and pressures or that may react with water with some release of energy, but not violently.
0	Materials that on exposure under fire conditions would offer no hazard beyond that of ordinary combustible material.	0	Materials that will not burn.	0	Materials that in themselves are normally stable, even under fire exposure conditions, and that are not reactive with water.

Figure 4-15. **National Fire Protection Association fire hazard warning sign.** (From McCall RE, Tankersley CM. Phlebotomy Essentials. 4th Ed. Baltimore: Lippincott Williams & Wilkins, 2007.)

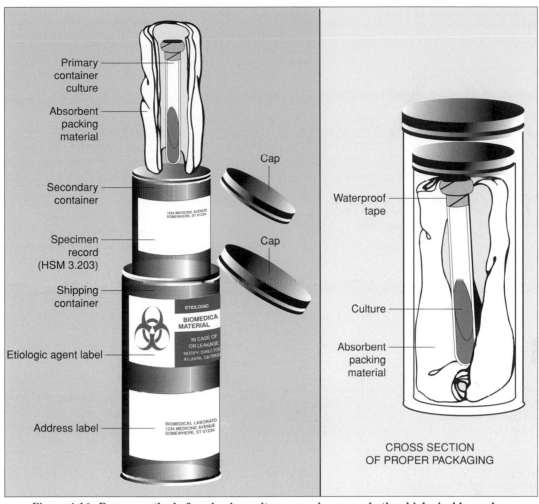

Figure 4-16. **Proper method of packaging cultures, specimens, and other biological hazardous materials.** (From Winn WC Jr, et al. Koneman's Color Atlas and Textbook of Diagnostic Microbiology. 6th Ed. Philadelphia: Lippincott Williams & Wilkins, 2006.)

QUALITY ASSURANCE AND QUALITY CONTROL IN THE CLINICAL MICROBIOLOGY LABORATORY

Quality Assurance (QA)

Quality assurance or quality assessment (QA) programs within health care facilities attempt to continuously identify, monitor, evaluate, and improve the reliability and efficiency of every aspect of patient care in the institution. Quality improvement (QI) programs, also known as continuous quality improvement (CQI) programs, are in existence to identify any problems that may exist regarding the quality of services being provided and methods to improve the quality of those services. QA and QI programs are sometimes combined under the umbrella terms of *quality management (QM)* or *total quality management (TQM)*.

The CML's quality assurance program focuses on the quality of three phases or levels of laboratory services:

- **Preanalytic processes.** Other names for this phase are pre-examination process and input phase. The processes occur *before* the performance of laboratory procedures and include the appropriateness of the tests being requested; the availability of published guidelines pertaining to proper selection, collection, and transport of clinical specimens; the quality of the clinical specimens being submitted to the CML;[10] the use of proper collection and transport devices; specimen labeling; information provided on laboratory request slips; and the times that elapse between specimen collection, arrival of the specimen at the CML, and processing of the specimen within the CML.

---

[10] *One of the most important aspects of QA, as it applies to the CML, is the quality of specimens received by the CML. Only high-quality specimens (i.e., specimens that have been properly selected, collected, and transported) are acceptable for processing in the CML. The topic of specimen quality is discussed in detail in Chapter 5.*

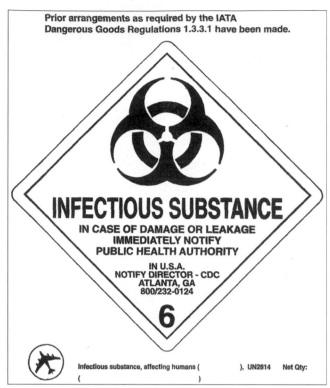

Figure 4-17. **Infectious substance label that must be affixed to the outside of any package containing potentially hazardous infectious materials.** (From Winn WC Jr, et al. Koneman's Color Atlas and Textbook of Diagnostic Microbiology. 6th Ed. Philadelphia: Lippincott Williams & Wilkins, 2006.)

- **Analytic processes.** Other names for this phase are examination process and process phase. These are events associated with the actual performance of laboratory procedures and include the quality control measures that are in effect to ensure the accuracy and precision of the tests performed in the CML (QC is discussed in the next section).[11]

- **Postanalytic processes.** Other names for this phase are postexamination process and output phase. These are events that occur following the performance of laboratory procedures and include the accuracy, clarity, and thoroughness of handwritten or computer-printed laboratory reports; the timeliness with which laboratory reports reach the patient's chart; proper interpretation of test results; how test results affect patient management; the patient's perception of the quality of laboratory services; and the ultimate benefit that the patient achieves from the laboratory services provided.

Preanalytic, analytic, and postanalytic processes are summarized in Figure 4-18.

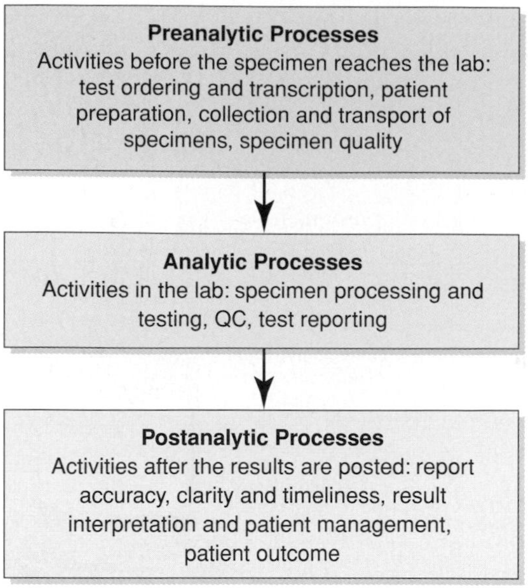

Preanalytic Processes
Activities before the specimen reaches the lab: test ordering and transcription, patient preparation, collection and transport of specimens, specimen quality

↓

Analytic Processes
Activities in the lab: specimen processing and testing, QC, test reporting

↓

Postanalytic Processes
Activities after the results are posted: report accuracy, clarity and timeliness, result interpretation and patient management, patient outcome

Figure 4-18. **Summary of preanalytic, analytic, and postanalytic QC processes.**

Quality Control (QC)

The laboratory's **quality control (QC) program**—an integral part of the hospital QA program—is designed to monitor the accuracy, reliability, and reproducibility of all tests performed within the laboratory and to identify and correct any problems that exist. The CML's QC program is based on recommendations and requirements established by the Clinical Laboratory Improvement Amendments of 1988 (**CLIA '88**),[12] the College of American Pathologists (http://www.cap.org/), JCAHO, and the CLSI. Components of a CML's QC program include the following:

- **Competency of personnel.** CLIA '88 mandates the personnel requirements for CMLs, based upon the complexity of the laboratory procedures being performed there; annual documentation of personnel competency is required; competency may be verified in various ways, including written examinations, workup of "unknowns," and performing supervised workup, interpretation, and reporting of cultures; all training and competency test results must be documented

- **Standard operating procedures manual.** The CML must maintain a policy and procedures manual that contains written proce-

> The CML must maintain a policy and procedures manual that contains written procedures for every aspect of CML work.

---

[11] Accuracy *is a measure of the truth or validity of a laboratory test result. The methods selected for use in the CML must yield valid results.* Precision *is the expression of the variability of analysis or an indication of the amount of random error that exists in an analytical process or laboratory test. An imprecise test gives completely different results each time the test is repeated, whereas a precise test gives the same result, or very similar results, each time the test is repeated.*

[12] *CLIA '88 is a federal regulation that modified the Clinical Laboratory Improvement Act of 1967. The CLIA guidelines mandate quality standards for laboratory testing, including QC, personnel, and proficiency testing standards for clinical laboratories. CLIA guidelines are based on test complexity. The more complicated the test, the more stringent the requirements. A federal agency called the Centers for Medicare and Medicaid Services oversees the enforcement of the CLIA guidelines.*

dures for *all* aspects of CML work, including preanalytic, analytic, and postanalytic phases. The original manual and any changes must be signed by the laboratory director, and the manual must be reviewed annually.

- **Test verification and validation.** CMLs must use whichever test methods provide the most accurate, repro-

> CMLs must use whichever test methods provide the most accurate, reproducible, and clinically relevant results.

ducible, and clinically relevant results; any new tests or reagents must be verified for accuracy and precision before they are used to test patient specimens. CMLs must validate existing methodologies for consistency of results.

- **Test methods and procedures.** The QC program must monitor, document, and evaluate *all* aspects of *every* test procedure performed in the CML. Positive and negative controls must be used for all qualitative tests. **QC organisms** (i.e., organisms known to give positive and negative test results) are maintained in the CML and

> The QC program must monitor, document, and evaluate *all* aspects of *every* test procedure that is performed in the CML.

used for this purpose (Appendix A contains information regarding specific QC organisms to be used for various CML procedures). QC organisms are usually obtained from the American Type Culture Collection or a commercial supplier and are stored in tryptic soy broth plus 20% glycerol (in an ultracold freezer, at least

> Manufacturers of the various kits and minisystems used for identification of microorganisms specify which particular QC organisms should be used to verify the accuracy of their products.

−50°C) or maintained in a freeze-dried (lyophilized) state until needed. The manufacturers of the various kits and minisystems used for identification of microorganisms specify which particular QC organisms should be used to verify the accuracy of their products. Two controls of different strengths or concentrations must be used for all quantitative tests. Controls and patient specimens must be tested by identical methods.

- **Media, reagents, staining solutions, antisera.** All

> Media, reagents, and stains must never be used beyond their expiration dates.

media, reagents, staining solutions, and so on are evaluated frequently for their accuracy, reliability, and reproducibility. Vials must be labeled to indicate contents, concentration, safety

hazards (if any), storage requirements, and dates of preparation and expiration. These materials must never be used beyond their expiration dates. The quality of culture media used in the CML is primarily the responsibility of commercial suppliers, but in some cases, in-house QC procedures must also be performed (appropriate QC organisms are used for this purpose). Before use, all media must be inspected for dehydration, hemolysis (if applicable), cracks, contamination, and proper fill.

- **Equipment and instruments.** All equipment should be properly maintained and monitored for performance. Maintenance and function checks are performed as specified by the manufacturers; refrigerators, freezers, incubators, and water baths should be checked daily for accuracy of temperature control. Routine preventive maintenance and all function and temperature checks must be documented.

- **Records and reports.** Not only must QC measures be performed, but also they must be documented. In addition, sufficient records must be retained by the CML to document all activities related to a specific patient specimen.

- **Proficiency testing.** The CML is expected to participate in proficiency testing programs for every type of test performed in the CML; participation is required for laboratory accreditation. There are a number of commercial sources for proficiency testing speci-

> Appropriate positive and negative controls must be used for every test procedure performed in the CML.

mens. One such source is the American Proficiency Institute (API; http://www.api-pt.com), which offers a variety of proficiency-testing services approved by the federal government, hospital/laboratory accrediting agencies, and state health departments. API offers proficiency-testing packages for bacteriology, bacterial antigens, mycobacteriology, mycology, parasitology, and virology. The API bacteriology packages include simulated specimens for culture (e.g., blood, ear, eye, genital, stool, sputum, throat, urine, and wound cultures), rapid group A strep antigen testing, Gram stain, antimicrobial susceptibility testing, and urine colony count.

By constant surveillance and frequent checking, the efficiency and reliability of the laboratory work can be maintained, so that laboratory results are accurate and of the highest quality. Additional information about QA and QC can be found in appropriate documents published by the CLSI (see "References and Suggested Reading").

Chapter Review

- In a hospital setting, the CML is generally a part of the clinical pathology division of the pathology department.

- The CML is staffed by various professionals with varying educational backgrounds and specific training in microbiology procedures and safety.

- The primary mission of the CML is to assist clinicians in the diagnosis of infectious diseases by providing accurate and timely results and information.

- The four major day-to-day responsibilities of those employed in the CML are (1) processing clinical specimens, (2) isolating pathogens from specimens, (3) identifying pathogens, and (4) performing antimicrobial susceptibility testing.

- In general, specimen processing includes (1) examining the specimen macroscopically and recording pertinent observations, (2) examining the specimen microscopically and recording pertinent observations, and (3) inoculating appropriate culture media to isolate the pathogen(s) from the specimen and to start pathogen(s) growing in pure culture in the laboratory. The actual steps in specimen processing vary from one specimen type to another and from one section of the CML to another.

- Environmental samples, collected from various sites within the hospital, are processed by the CML whenever an outbreak is suspected within the hospital.

- The CML is usually divided into various sections or benches, including bacteriology, mycobacteriology, mycology, parasitology, virology, and sometimes immunology.

- The major responsibility of the bacteriology section of the CML is to assist clinicians in the diagnosis of bacterial infections, whereas the major responsibility of the mycobacteriology section is to assist clinicians in the diagnosis of tuberculosis and other mycobacterial infections.

- The major responsibility of the mycology section is to assist clinicians in the diagnosis of fungal infections (mycoses), whereas the major responsibility of the parasitology section is to assist clinicians in the diagnosis of parasitic infections. The major responsibility of the virology section is to assist clinicians in the diagnosis of viral infections.

- To avoid becoming infected, extreme care must be taken by those involved in collecting, handling, and processing clinical specimens, particularly, blood, urine, cerebrospinal fluid, sputum, mucous membranes, and fecal specimens. CML professionals must always follow the safety precautions known as standard precautions, as well as the institution's and laboratory's safety policies.

- Disinfection is the destruction or removal of pathogens from nonliving objects by physical or chemical methods, whereas sterilization is the complete destruction of *all* microbes, including cells, spores, and viruses.

- Most CMLs operate at BSL–2.

- A BSC must be available for processing clinical specimens and when working with especially infectious pathogens. BSCs employ a HEPA filter and negative air pressure to protect the environment and laboratory personnel.

- Every laboratory should have a chemical hygiene plan, which includes MSDSs and safety training.

- A QC program is necessary to monitor the reliability and quality of the work performed in the CML. All equipment and instruments, test procedures, media, reagents, and staining solutions must be evaluated frequently to ensure that accurate test results are being obtained. A good laboratory QC program is part of the institution's overall QA program.

- Components of a CML's QC program should address personnel competency, standard operating procedures, test verification and validation, test methods and procedures, media reagents and solutions, and equipment and instruments.

- A variety of QC organisms—organisms known to give positive and negative test results—are maintained in the CML for use in its QC program.

- For safety reasons, clinical specimens and cultures of microorganisms must be shipped in accordance with regulations established by the U.S. Public Health Service.

New Terms and Abbreviations

After studying Chapter 4, you should be familiar with the following terms, which are defined within the chapter and in the Glossary at the back of the book:

Algicidal agent

Antimicrobial agent

Antimicrobial susceptibility testing

Antisepsis

Antiseptic

Antiseptic technique

Asepsis

Aseptic technique

Autoclave

Bactericidal agent

Bacteriostatic agent

Biosafety cabinet (BSC)

Biosafety level (BSL or BL)

CLIA '88

Clinical laboratory scientist (CLS)

Clinical and Laboratory Standards Institute (CLSI)

Clinical laboratory technician (CLT)

Clinical microbiology

Clinical microbiology laboratory (CML)

Clinician

Disinfectant

Etiologic agent

Final report

Fungicidal agent

High-efficiency particulate (HEPA) air filter

Material safety data sheet (MSDS)

National Fire Protection Association (NFPA)

Occupational Safety and Health Administration (OSHA)

Pathologist

Personal protective equipment (PPE)

Preliminary report

Pseudomonicidal agent

Pure culture

QC organism

Quality assurance (QA) program

Quality control (QC) program

Sepsis

Sporicidal agent

Standard precautions

Sterile

Sterile techniques

Sterilization

Tuberculocidal agent

Viricidal agent

References and Suggested Reading

Clinical Laboratory Safety: Approved Guideline. 2nd Ed. CLSI Document GP17-A2. Wayne, PA: Clinical and Laboratory Standards Institute. 2004.

Isenberg HD, ed. Essential Procedures for Clinical Microbiology. Washington, DC: ASM Press, 1998.

Protection of Laboratory Workers from Occupationally Acquired Infections: Approved Guideline. 3rd Ed. CLSI Document M29-A3. Wayne, PA: Clinical and Laboratory Standards Institute, 2005.

Rutala WA. Selection and use of disinfectants in health care. In: Mayhall CG, ed. Hospital Epidemiology and Infection Control. 2nd Ed. Philadelphia: Lippincott Williams & Wilkins, 1999.

Sewell DL, MacLowry JD. Laboratory management. In: Murray PR, Baron EJ, Jorgensen JH, Pfaller MA, Yolken RH, eds. Manual of Clinical Microbiology. 8th Ed. Washington, DC: ASM Press, 2003.

Voss A, Nulens E. Prevention and control of laboratory-acquired infections. In: Murray PR, Baron EJ, Jorgensen JH, Pfaller MA, Yolken RH, eds. Manual of Clinical Microbiology. 8th Ed. Washington, DC: ASM Press, 2003.

 On the CD-ROM

- Disinfectants and Contact Time

- Preparing Solutions and Dilutions

- Using Bleach as a Disinfectant

- Additional Self-Assessment Exercises

- Puzzle

Self-Assessment Exercises

After studying Chapter 4, answer the following questions.

1. All the following are examples of PPE *except*

   A. gloves.

   B. lab coat.

   C. fire extinguisher.

   D. respirator.

2. Which of the following is **not** one of the four major daily responsibilities of the CML?

   A. Process environmental samples

   B. Isolate pathogens from clinical specimens

   C. Identify (speciate) pathogens

   D. Perform antimicrobial susceptibility testing when appropriate to do so

3. The yellow area of the NFPA hazard rating indicates

   A. health hazard.

   B. flammability risk.

   C. reactivity or stability.

   D. any special hazard.

4. Sterilization of objects can be accomplished by all the following *except*

   A. moist heat (autoclaving).

   B. gas (ethylene oxide).

   C. antiseptics.

   D. formaldehyde.

5. Which of the following is a globally recognized, voluntary consensus organization that develops and disseminates laboratory standards, guidelines, and practices?

   A. Occupational Safety and Health Administration (OSHA)

   B. Joint Commission on the Accreditation of Healthcare Organizations (JCAHO)

   C. American Society for Clinical Laboratory Science (ASCLS)

   D. Clinical and Laboratory Standards Institute (CLSI)

6. The recommended operating parameters to achieve sterilization of most microorganisms and their spores in an autoclave are

A. 20 psi and 121° C for about 30 minutes.

B. 15 psi and 121°C for about 20 minutes.

C. 15 psi and 150.5°C for about 20 minutes.

D. none of the above.

7. In general, parasites are identified by

A. inoculating them into a series of biochemical tests.

B. their appearance when grown on various types of culture media.

C. their characteristic appearance.

D. their cytopathic effect on cells in various types of cell cultures.

8. An MSDS contains information about which of the following?

A. Storage and transportation precautions

B. Routes of entry

C. First aid procedures

D. All of the above

9. The analytic phase of quality assurance includes all the following *except*

A. specimen collection technique.

B. testing of specimens.

C. quality control measures.

D. specimen processing, including macroscopic and microscopic examination of the specimen.

10. Most clinical microbiology laboratories are considered to be operating at which biologic safety level?

A. BSL-1

B. BSL-2

C. BSL-3

D. BSL-4

CHAPTER 5

Clinical Specimens Used for the Diagnosis of Infectious Diseases

Chapter Outline

Types of Clinical Specimens Submitted to the Clinical Microbiology Laboratory

Role of Health Care Professionals in the Submission of Clinical Specimens

Importance of High-Quality Clinical Specimens

Proper Selection, Collection, and Transport of Clinical Specimens

Contamination of Clinical Specimens with Indigenous Microflora

Clinical Specimens from Various Anatomical Sites and Organ Systems
- Circulatory System
- Skin, Abscess, and Wound Specimens
- Eyes and Ears
- Respiratory System
- Central Nervous System
- Urinary Tract
- Genital Tract
- Oral Cavity
- Gastrointestinal Tract
- Body Fluids

Rejection of Clinical Specimens

LEARNING OBJECTIVES

After studying this chapter, you should be able to:

☛ Define the terms and abbreviations introduced in this chapter (e.g., *bacteremia, bacteriuria, bartholinitis*)

☛ Describe what constitutes proper selection, collection, and transport of clinical specimens

☛ Describe the proper procedures for collecting blood, urine, cerebral spinal fluid, sputum, throat, wound, gonococcal, and fecal specimens for submission to the clinical microbiology laboratory

☛ List the predominant indigenous microflora organisms at each body site discussed in the chapter

☛ State the information that must be included on specimen labels and laboratory request slips

☛ Outline the steps involved in the diagnosis of an infectious disease

☛ State at least one example of an infectious disease for each of the anatomic sites or organ systems discussed—for example, lower respiratory tract and urinary tract, among others

☛ Identify the *most* appropriate specimen for laboratory diagnoses of the following: bacteremia, septicemia, respiratory infections, urinary tract infections, meningitis, wounds, and diarrheal diseases

☛ Give four or five examples of specimens that would be considered unacceptable for workup in the clinical microbiology laboratory

☛ Use the Bartlett classification system to determine if a sputum specimen is acceptable for culture

The proper steps in the diagnosis of an infectious disease are (1) taking a complete patient history, (2) conducting a thorough physical examination of the patient, (3) carefully evaluating the patient's signs and symptoms, (4) ordering the performance of appropriate diagnostic tests, and (5) properly selecting, collecting, transporting, and processing appropriate clinical specimens. The latter topics—those involving clinical specimens—are shown in Figure 5-1 and discussed in this chapter. The other topics are beyond the scope of this book.

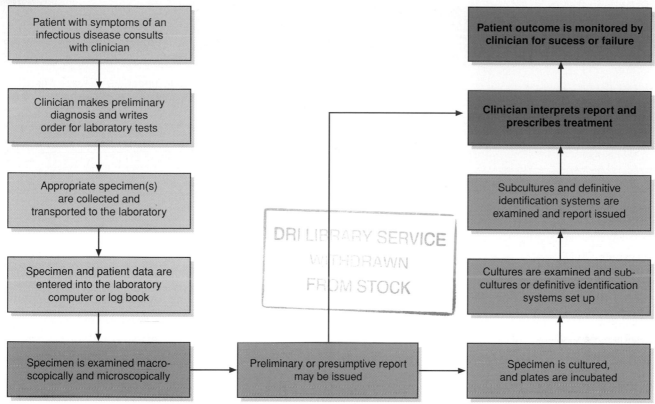

Figure 5-1. **Diagrammatic representation of the steps involved in the diagnoses of infectious diseases.** (Modified from Winn WC Jr, et al. Koneman's Color Atlas and Textbook of Diagnostic Microbiology. 6th Ed. Philadelphia: Lippincott Williams & Wilkins, 2006.)

TYPES OF CLINICAL SPECIMENS SUBMITTED TO THE CLINICAL MICROBIOLOGY LABORATORY

The various types of specimens—such as blood, urine, feces, and cerebrospinal fluid—that are collected from patients and used to diagnose or follow the progress of infectious diseases are referred to as **clinical specimens.** The most common types of clinical specimens sent to a hospital microbiology laboratory (hereafter referred to as a clinical microbiology laboratory or CML) are listed in Table 5-1. It is extremely important that a specimen is of the highest possible quality and is collected in a manner that does not jeopardize the patient's outcome or the person collecting the specimen.

ROLE OF HEALTH CARE PROFESSIONALS IN THE SUBMISSION OF CLINICAL SPECIMENS

A close working relationship among the members of the health care team is essential for the proper diagnosis of an infectious disease. When a clinician suspects that a patient has a particular infectious disease, appropriate clinical specimens must be obtained and certain diagnostic tests requested. The doctor, nurse, or other qualified health care professional must select the appropriate specimen, collect it correctly, and then properly transport it to the CML for processing. Laboratory findings must then be conveyed to the attending clinician as quickly as possible to facilitate the prompt diagnosis and treatment of the infectious disease.

Health care personnel who collect clinical specimens must adhere strictly to the safety policies known as standard precautions, which are discussed in Chapter 4. Within the laboratory, all specimens are handled carefully, following standard precautions, and ultimately disposed of as infectious waste.

IMPORTANCE OF HIGH-QUALITY CLINICAL SPECIMENS

Specimens submitted to the CML must be of the highest possible quality. High-quality clinical specimens are required to achieve accurate, **clinically relevant results**—that is, results that *truly* provide information about the patient's infectious disease. It has often been stated that the quality of the laboratory work performed in a CML can be only as good as the quality of

TABLE 5 - 1	Types of Clinical Specimens Submitted to the Clinical Microbiology Laboratory
Type of Specimen	Type(s) of Infectious Disease That the Specimen Is Used to Diagnose[a]
Blood	B, F, P, V
Bone marrow	B
Bronchial and bronchoalveolar washes	B, F, V
Cerebrospinal fluid (CSF)	B, F, P, V
Cervical and vaginal swabs	B, V
Conjunctival swab or scraping	B, V
Ear drainage	B
Feces and rectal swabs	B, P, V
Gastric and duodenal biopsy	B
Hair clippings	F
Nail (fingernail and toenail) clippings	F
Nasal swabs	B
Pus from a wound or abscess	B, F
"Scotch tape" preparations	P
Sinus washings	B
Skin scrapings	F
Skin snip	P
Sputum	B, F, P
Synovial (joint) fluid	B
Throat swabs	B, V
Tissue (biopsy and autopsy) specimens	B, F, P, V
Transtracheal aspirate	B
Tympanic membrane aspirate	B
Urethral discharge material	B
Urine (clean-catch midstream specimen, catheterized specimen, specimen collected by suprapubic bladder aspiration)	B, F, P, V
Urogenital secretions (e.g., vaginal discharge material, prostatic secretions)	B, F, P
Vesicle fluid or scraping	V
Wound aspirate or biopsy	B

[a]B, bacterial infections; F, fungal infections; P, parasitic infections; V, viral infections.

TABLE 5-2	The Three Components of Specimen Quality
Component	**Explanation**
Proper selection of the specimen	The specimen must be the appropriate type to diagnose the infectious disease suspected by the clinician.
Proper collection of the specimen	The specimen must be collected in a manner that eliminates or minimizes contamination of the specimen with indigenous microflora. Sometimes special collection devices are required.
Proper transport of the specimen	The specimen must be transported to the laboratory in a manner that ensures that the pathogen remains viable and/or preserves its morphology (e.g., rapid transport, sometimes by packing the container in ice or by using a preservative)

the specimens it receives. It is impossible for a CML to obtain and report high-quality test results if the laboratory receives poor quality specimens or the wrong types of specimens.

The three components of specimen quality are (1) proper specimen selection, (2) proper specimen collection, and (3) proper specimen transport to the laboratory (Table 5-2). The laboratory must provide written guidelines regarding specimen selection, collection, and transport, in the form of a book—often called the laboratory policies and procedures manual, or the lab P&P manual for short. Copies of the lab P&P manual must be available to every ward, floor, clinic, and department. Often it is accessible from the hospital's computer system. **The person who collects the specimen is ultimately responsible for its quality.**

> The three components of specimen quality are (1) proper specimen selection, (2) proper specimen collection, and (3) proper specimen transport to the laboratory.

> The person who collects the specimen is ultimately responsible for its quality.

When clinical specimens are improperly collected and handled, (1) the etiologic agent (causative agent) may not be found or may be destroyed, (2) overgrowth by indigenous microflora may mask the pathogen, or (3) contaminants may interfere with the identification of pathogens and the diagnosis of the patient's infectious disease. Important concepts of proper specimen selection, collection, and transport are discussed in the next section.

PROPER SELECTION, COLLECTION, AND TRANSPORT OF CLINICAL SPECIMENS

When collecting clinical specimens for microbiology, these general precautions should be taken.

The specimen must be properly selected. That is, it must be the appropriate type of specimen for diagnosis of the suspected infectious disease. For example, a blood specimen is required to diagnose malaria.

The specimen must be properly and carefully collected. Whenever possible, specimens must be collected in a manner that will eliminate or minimize contamination of the specimen with indigenous microflora. For example, diagnosis of a urinary tract infection requires either a clean-catch midstream urine specimen (described later) or a urine specimen collected from a urinary catheter. Sterile technique should be practiced during specimen collection. Other important factors in specimen collection include the following:

- The material should be collected from a site where the suspected pathogen is most likely to be found and where the least contamination is likely to occur.

- Whenever possible, specimens should be obtained before antimicrobial therapy has begun. If this is not possible, the laboratory should be informed as to which antimicrobial agent(s) the patient is receiving.

- The acute stage of the disease, when the patient is experiencing symptoms, is the appropriate time to collect most specimens. Some viruses, however, are more easily isolated during the prodromal or onset stage of disease.

- Specimen collection should be performed with care and tact to avoid harming the patient, causing discomfort, or causing undue embarrassment. If the patient is to collect the specimen, such as sputum or urine, the patient must be provided with clear and detailed collection instructions.

- A sufficient quantity of the specimen must be obtained to perform all required diagnostic tests. The amount of specimen to collect should be specified in the lab P&P manual.

- All specimens should be placed or collected into a sterile container to prevent contamination of the specimen by indigenous microflora and airborne microbes. Appropriate types of collection devices and specimen containers should be specified in the lab P&P manual.

Specimens must be properly transported to the CML. Specimens should be protected from heat and cold and promptly delivered to the laboratory to help ensure that the results of the analyses will validly represent the number and types of organisms present at the time of collection. If delivery to the laboratory is delayed, some delicate pathogens might die; therefore, certain types of specimens must be rushed to the laboratory immediately after collection. Some specimens must be placed on ice during delivery to the laboratory, whereas others should never be refrigerated or placed on ice because of the fragile and sensitive nature of the pathogens. Obligate anaerobes die when exposed to oxygen and therefore must be protected from oxygen during transport to the CML. Any indigenous microflora in the specimen may overgrow, inhibit, or kill pathogens. Specimen transport instructions should be contained in the lab P&P manual.

All specimens must be handled with great care to avoid contamination of the patients, couriers, and health care professionals. Specimens must be placed in a sealed plastic bag for immediate and careful transport to the laboratory. Whenever possible, sterile, disposable specimen containers should be used.

The specimen container must be properly labeled and accompanied by an appropriate laboratory request slip containing adequate instructions. Labels should contain the patient's name, unique hospital identification number, and hospital room number; requesting clinician's name; culture site; and date and time of collection. Laboratory request slips should contain the patient's name, age, sex, and unique hospital identification number; name of the requesting clinician; specific information about the type of specimen and the site from which it was collected; date and time of collection; initials of the person who collected the specimen; and information about any antimicrobial agents that the patient is receiving. The laboratory should always be given sufficient clinical information to aid in performing appropriate analyses. For example, the request slip that accompanies a wound specimen should not merely state "wound." Rather, it should state the specific *type* of wound (e.g., burn wound, dog bite wound, postsurgical wound infection, etc.), the anatomical site, and whether it is on the left side or right side, if applicable.

Ideally, specimens should be collected and delivered to the laboratory as early in the day as possible to give the CML professionals sufficient time to process the material,

> The laboratory request slip should always contain sufficient clinical information to enable the CML to perform appropriate analyses.

especially when the hospital or clinic does not have 24-hour laboratory service.

CONTAMINATION OF CLINICAL SPECIMENS WITH INDIGENOUS MICROFLORA

As mentioned in Chapter 1, vast numbers of microbes live on and in the human body. They are usually collectively referred to as indigenous microflora, although the older term, *normal flora*, is sometimes used. Clinical specimens must be collected in a manner that eliminates (or at least reduces) contamination of the specimens with members of the indigenous microflora. Members of our indigenous microflora are also referred to as endogenous microbes; the term *endogenous* means "within the body."[1]

> Clinical specimens must be collected in a manner that eliminates or greatly reduces contamination of the specimens with members of the indigenous microflora.

It is important for CML professionals to be aware of the various indigenous microorganisms present at various anatomical sites and to be alert to the fact that, when isolated from clinical specimens, these organisms might be contaminants. Note that they *might* be contaminants; it is also possible that these indigenous microorganisms *might* be causing an infection. Recall from Chapter 1 that many of the members of the indigenous microflora are opportunistic pathogens.

Table 5-3 presents information regarding the variety of endogenous bacteria and fungi usually present as indigenous microflora at various anatomical sites. Any of these organisms could be isolated from clinical specimens, either as contaminants or as actual causes of infectious processes.

> Indigenous microflora present in a clinical specimen might either be contaminants or the cause of the patient's infectious disease.

CLINICAL SPECIMENS FROM VARIOUS ANATOMICAL SITES AND ORGAN SYSTEMS

Specific techniques for the collection and transport of clinical specimens vary from institution to institution and are contained in the institution's lab P&P manual. Only a few of the most important considerations are mentioned here.

---

[1]*The adjectives* endogenous *and* exogenous *are used to indicate the origin of the pathogen that is causing a patient's infection.* **Endogenous microbes** *originate from within the body (e.g., members of the patient's indigenous microflora), whereas* **exogenous microbes** *originate from outside of the body (i.e., from the external environment).*

TABLE 5 - 3   Indigenous Microflora of the Human Body

Anatomical Site	Bacteria Commonly Present as Indigenous Microflora	Fungi Commonly Present as Indigenous Microflora
Skin	Coagulase-negative staphylococci, *Micrococcus* spp., diphtheroids, *Propionibacterium* spp., *Staphylococcus aureus* (less commonly)	*Malassezia*, *Candida* spp.
Ear	Essentially the same as skin	*Alternaria*, *Aspergillus*, *Candida*, *Penicillium* spp.
Eye	Similar to that of skin	
Gastrointestinal tract		
Mouth	Viridans streptococci, many anaerobes (e.g., treponemes[a]; *Actinomyces*, *Bacteroides*, *Fusobacterium*, *Peptostreptococcus*, *Prevotella*, *Propionibacterium*, *Veillonella* spp.)	*Candida*, *Geotrichum* spp.
Esophagus	Primarily transient organisms from the nares, mouth, and nasopharynx	
Stomach	Transient organisms from the nares, mouth, and nasopharynx, and acid-resistant *Helicobacter*, *Lactobacillus*, *Staphylococcus*, and *Streptococcus* spp.	Yeasts
Intestines	Many members of the family Enterobacteriaceae plus *Bacteroides*, *Bifidobacterium*, *Clostridium*, *Enterococcus*, *Eubacterium*, *Fusobacterium*, *Lactobacillus*, *Peptostreptococcus*, *Pseudomonas*, and *Streptococcus* spp.	Yeasts
Genitourinary tract		
Distal urethra	Coagulase-negative staphylococci, diphtheroids, enterococci, lactobacilli, mycoplasmas, streptococci, ureaplasmas, *Bacteroides* and *Peptostreptococcus* spp., members of the Enterobacteriaceae family	*Candida* spp.
Vagina	Coagulase-negative staphylococci, diphtheroids, enterococci, lactobacilli, micrococci, mycoplasmas, streptococci, ureaplasmas, sometimes members of the Enterobacteriaceae family	*Candida* spp.
Respiratory tract		
Nares (nose)	Similar to that of skin, *Staphylococcus aureus* (in about 30% of healthy people)	
Nasopharynx (throat)	Similar to that of the mouth; also potential pathogens such as *Haemophilus influenzae*, *Neisseria meningitidis*, *Streptococcus pneumoniae*	

[a] Spiral-shaped bacteria.

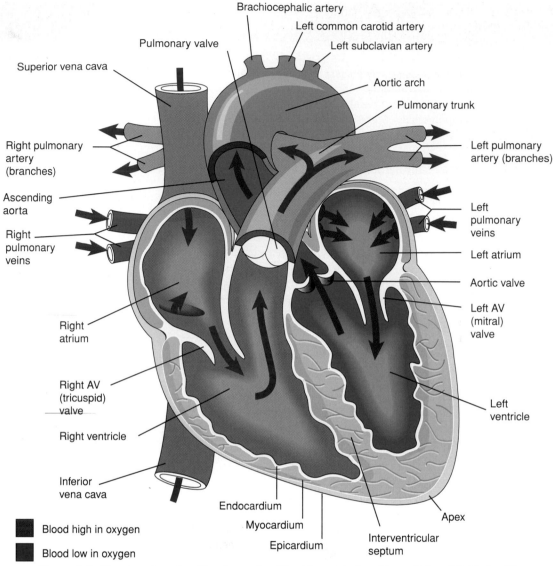

Figure 5-2. **Heart and major blood vessels.** AV, atrioventricular. (From Cohen BJ, Taylor JJ. Memmler's The Human Body in Health and Disease. 10th Ed. Philadelphia: Lippincott Williams & Wilkins, 2005.)

Circulatory System

The circulatory system consists of the cardiovascular system and the lymphatic system.

Cardiovascular System

The cardiovascular (*cardio* refers to the heart and *vascular* to the various types of blood vessels) system includes the heart, arteries, capillaries, veins, and blood (Fig. 5-2). Blood is composed of plasma, which is the liquid portion, plus the various cellular elements—red blood cells, white blood cells, and platelets.

Examples of infectious diseases of the cardiovascular system include the following:

- **Endocarditis.** Inflammation of the endocardium—the endothelial membrane that lines the cavities of the heart.

- **Myocarditis.** Inflammation of the myocardium—the muscular walls of the heart.

- **Pericarditis.** Inflammation of the pericardium—the fibrous sac surrounding the heart.

Blood and Blood Cultures

Blood is usually sterile; it contains no resident microflora. The presence of bacteria in the bloodstream—a condition known as **bacteremia**—may indicate a disease, although temporary or transient bacteremias may occur following oral surgery, tooth extraction, or even aggressive tooth brushing. However, when pathogens are capable of resisting or overwhelming the phagocytes and other body defenses, or when an person is immunosuppressed or is otherwise more susceptible than normal, a systemic disease called **septicemia** may occur. A patient with septicemia experiences chills, fever, and prostration (extreme exhaustion) and has bacteria and/or their toxins in the bloodstream. The most severe types of septicemia are caused by Gram-negative bacilli that release endotoxin from their cell walls. Endotoxin can induce fever and septic shock, which can be fatal. To diagnose either bacteremia or septicemia, two or three blood cultures or blood culture sets should be collected over a 24-hour period. Depending on the infectious disease that is suspected, specimens may be drawn from each arm, collected at least 1 hour apart, or spaced over a 24-hour period. (Specific blood culture methods are described in Chapter 6.)

STUDY AID   **"-Emias."** The suffix *-emia* refers to the bloodstream; very often, the presence of something in the bloodstream. **Toxemia** refers to the presence of toxins in the bloodstream; **bacteremia,** the presence of bacteria; **fungemia,** the presence of fungi; **viremia,** the presence of viruses; and **parasitemia,** the presence of parasites. **Septicemia,** however, is an actual disease that quite often is serious and life threatening. (See text for additional information about septicemia.) **Meningococcemia** is a specific type of septicemia, in which the bloodstream contains the bacterium *Neisseria meningitidis* (also known as **meningococci**). **Tularemia** is a bacterial disease caused by *Francisella tularensis,* a Gram-negative bacillus. **Leukemia** is a type of cancer; actually, there are several different types of leukemia. In all types, there is a proliferation of abnormal white blood cells (leukocytes) in the blood. Some types of leukemia are known to be caused by viruses.

Collecting blood for culture. To prevent contamination of the blood specimen with indigenous skin flora, health care personnel must be extremely careful to use sterile technique when collecting blood for culture. When drawing the blood, sterile gloves must be worn and changed after each patient. After locating a suitable vein, the patient's skin must be disinfected with 70% isopropyl alcohol and then with an iodophor. It should be noted that the protocol for skin disinfection varies from one medical facility to another. For example, some facilities use isopropyl alcohol alone; some use tincture of iodine alone; some use povidone-iodine alone; some use a combination of ethyl alcohol and povidone-iodine; some use chlorhexidine gluconate alone.

When disinfecting the site, a concentric swabbing motion should be used, starting at the point where the needle will be inserted and working outward (Fig. 5-3). The iodophor should

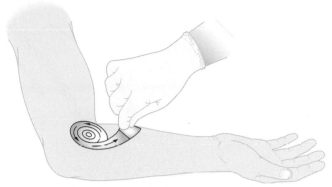

Figure 5-3. **Proper method of preparing venipuncture site when obtaining blood for culture.**

be allowed to dry. Then a tourniquet is applied and the appropriate amount of blood drawn. The site should never be touched after it has been disinfected. Under traditional methods, the blood would be injected into two blood culture bottles—one aerobic and one anaerobic. However, many different types of blood culture systems are currently available. The rubber tops of blood culture bottles must always be disinfected before the needle is inserted. The volume of blood to inject will be specified by the manufacturer of the type of blood culture used. After venipuncture, the iodophor should be removed from the skin with alcohol. Finally, the blood culture bottle(s) are transported promptly to the laboratory for incubation at 35°C. Blood culture bottles should not be refrigerated.

Lymphatic System

The lymphatic system consists of lymphatic vessels, lymphoid tissue (including lymph nodes, tonsils, thymus, and spleen), and lymph (the liquid that circulates through the lymphatic system). Lymph occasionally picks up microorganisms from the intestine, lungs, and other areas, but these transient organisms are usually quickly engulfed by phagocytic cells in the liver and lymph nodes. The lymphatic system contains many lymphocytes, which play major roles in immune responses (see Chapter 3). Diseases of the lymphatic system can be diagnosed by culturing lymph node biopsy specimens and/or by blood culture, if the pathogens have entered the bloodstream.

Following are a few examples of infectious diseases of the lymphatic system:

- **Lymphadenitis.** Inflamed and swollen lymph nodes.

- **Lymphadenopathy.** Diseased lymph nodes.

- **Lymphangitis.** Inflamed lymphatic vessels; more a sign of an infection than of disease.

Skin, Abscess, and Wound Specimens

As mentioned in Chapter 3, intact skin is a type of nonspecific host defense mechanism, serving as a physical

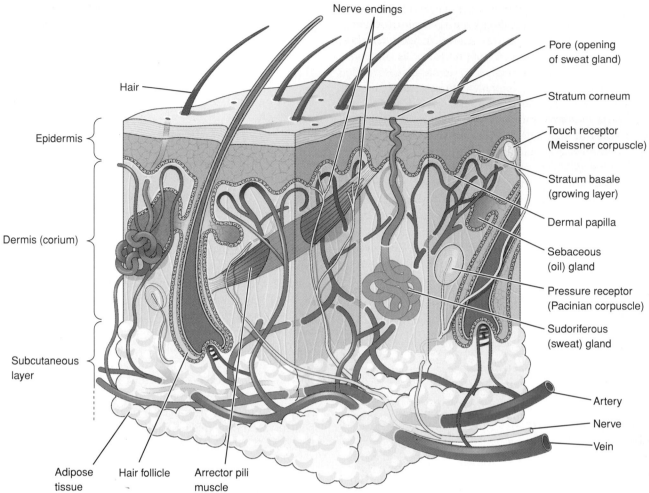

Nerve endings

Hair

Epidermis

Dermis (corium)

Subcutaneous layer

Pore (opening of sweat gland)

Stratum corneum

Touch receptor (Meissner corpuscle)

Stratum basale (growing layer)

Dermal papilla

Sebaceous (oil) gland

Pressure receptor (Pacinian corpuscle)

Sudoriferous (sweat) gland

Artery

Nerve

Vein

Adipose tissue

Hair follicle

Arrector pili muscle

Figure 5-4. **Cross section of the skin.** (From Cohen BJ, Taylor JJ. Memmler's The Human Body in Health and Disease. 10th Ed. Philadelphia: Lippincott Williams & Wilkins, 2005.)

barrier (Fig. 5-4). Very few pathogens can penetrate intact skin. The indigenous microflora of the skin, a low pH, and the presence of chemical substances like lysozyme and sebum also serve to prevent colonization of the skin by pathogens. Nonetheless, skin infections do occur. Listed here are some terms relating to skin and infectious diseases of the skin:

- **Epidermis.** The superficial epithelial portion of the skin.

- **Dermis.** The inner layer of skin, containing blood and lymphatic vessels, nerves, and nerve endings, glands, and hair follicles.

- **Dermatitis.** Inflammation of the skin.

- **Sebaceous glands.** Glands in the dermis that usually open into hair follicles and secrete an oily substance known as **sebum.**

- **Folliculitis.** Inflammation of a hair follicle, the sac that contains a hair shaft.

- **Sty (or stye).** Inflammation of a sebaceous gland that opens into a follicle of an eyelash.

- **Furuncle.** A localized pyogenic (pus-producing) infection of the skin, usually resulting from folliculitis; also known as a boil.

- **Carbuncle.** A deep-seated pyogenic infection of the skin, usually arising from a coalescence of furuncles.

Obtaining specimens from the skin. For pustules or vesicles, the overlying skin is decontaminated, the covering removed using a sterile needle, and fluid and basal cells collected from the pustule or vesicle using a small needle and syringe assembly (preferred) or a sterile swab. For petechiae, a specimen is collected by vigorously scraping the outer margin of the lesion. Skin scrapings are often sent to the mycology section of the CML to diagnose superficial mycoses, such as tinea, or ringworm, infections (see Chapter 20). Portions of skin known as skin snips are used to diagnose a helminth disease called onchocerciasis (see Chapter 23).

Pustules, Vesicles, and Petechiae. Pustules and vesicles are circumscribed, superficial, fluid-filled elevations of the skin. The fluid within vesicles is clear, whereas pustules contain purulent material (pus). Vesicles are sometimes referred to as blisters. Petechiae are pinpoint- to pinhead-sized hemorrhagic spots in the skin.

Collecting abscess specimens. After decontamination of the overlying skin, the abscess contents are aspirated using a needle and syringe. Following excision and draining of the abscess, a portion of the abscess wall should be submitted in an anaerobic transport container.

Collecting wound specimens. Whenever possible, a wound specimen should be an aspirate (i.e., pus that has been collected using a small, sterile needle and syringe assembly), or a sample taken from the advancing margin of the lesion. Specimens collected by swab are frequently contaminated with indigenous microflora and, if not submitted in some type of transport medium, often dry out before they can be processed in the CML. As previously mentioned, when collecting the specimen, the *type* of wound infection (e.g., dog bite, postsurgical, or burn wound infection) should be indicated on the laboratory request slip and the anatomic site from which the specimen was obtained. This provides valuable information that will enable CML professionals to inoculate appropriate types of media and be on the lookout for specific organisms. For example, the bacterium *Pasteurella multocida* is frequently isolated from cat and dog bite wound infections, but this Gram-negative bacillus is rarely encountered in other types of specimens. Merely stating "wound" on the request slip is not sufficient.

Eyes and Ears

Eyes

The anatomy of the eye is shown in Figure 5-5. Terms relating to the eye and infectious diseases of the eye include the following:

- **Conjunctiva.** The thin, tough lining that covers the inner wall of the eyelid and the sclera (the white of the eye).

- **Conjunctivitis.** An infection or inflammation of the conjunctiva.

- **Keratitis.** An infection or inflammation of the cornea—the domed covering over the iris and lens.

- **Keratoconjunctivitis.** An infection that involves both the cornea and conjunctiva.

The request slip that accompanies a specimen collected from the eye should specify the exact type of specimen, such as conjunctival swab, corneal scraping, or aspirate. Using separate sterile swabs, sample the conjunctiva of both eyes, even if only one eye is infected. The swab of the uninfected eye provides information about the indigenous microflora of the patient's eyes. In some medical facilities, the CML furnishes ophthalmologists with appropriate types of culture media,

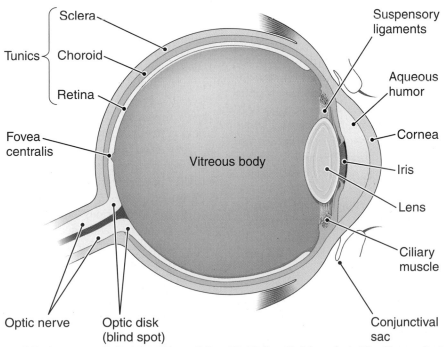

Figure 5-5. **Anatomy of the eye.** (From Cohen BJ, Taylor JJ. Memmler's The Human Body in Health and Disease. 10th Ed. Philadelphia: Lippincott Williams & Wilkins, 2005.)

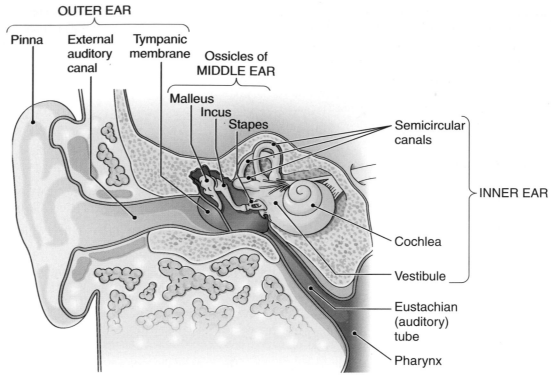

Figure 5-6. **Anatomy of the ear.** (From Cohen BJ, Taylor JJ. Memmler's The Human Body in Health and Disease. 10th Ed. Philadelphia: Lippincott Williams & Wilkins, 2005.)

allowing inoculation of the media immediately after specimen collection. Because aspirates from eye infections tend to be very small in volume, add some type of liquid culture medium (e.g., thioglycollate broth) to the aspirate to ensure that there will be a sufficient quantity of material for staining and culturing.

Ears

The anatomy of the ear is shown in Figure 5-6. There are three pathways for pathogens to enter the ear: (1) through the eustachian (auditory) tube, from the throat and nasopharynx; (2) from the external ear; and (3) via blood or lymph. Usually, bacteria are trapped in the middle ear when a bacterial infection in the throat and nasopharynx causes the eustachian tube to close. The result is an anaerobic condition in the middle ear, allowing obligate anaerobes and facultative anaerobes to grow and cause pressure on the tympanic membrane (eardrum). Swollen lymphoid (adenoid) tissues, viral infections, and allergies may also close the eustachian tube, especially in young children. Infection of the middle ear is known as **otitis media,** whereas infection of the outer ear canal is known as **otitis externa.**

The request slip that accompanies a specimen collected from the ear should specify the exact type of specimen (e.g., swab of external ear canal, fluid aspirated from the middle ear). A specimen collected by swab is not recommended for diagnosis of otitis media, unless the tympanum (eardrum) has ruptured. The ideal specimen for diagnosis of otitis

media is fluid collected by needle and syringe from behind the tympanum, a procedure known as tympanocentesis. Tympanocentesis is painful and infrequently performed, but it is the method of choice for diagnosis of otitis media.

Respiratory System

For practical purposes, the discussion of the respiratory system is divided into the upper respiratory tract (URT) and the lower respiratory tract (LRT). The URT includes the paranasal sinuses, nasopharynx, oropharynx, epiglottis, and larynx ("voice box"). The LRT includes the trachea ("windpipe"), bronchial tubes, and alveoli of the lungs. The respiratory system is depicted in Figure 5-7.

Indigenous microflora of the URT may cause opportunistic infections of the respiratory system. Infectious diseases of the URT (e.g., colds and sore throats) are more common than infectious diseases of the LRT. They may predispose the patient to more serious infections, such as sinusitis, otitis media, bronchitis, and pneumonia. LRT infections are the most common cause of death from infectious diseases.

Terms relating to infectious diseases of the respiratory system include the following:

- **Bronchitis.** Inflammation of the mucous membrane lining of the bronchial tubes; most commonly caused by respiratory viruses.

- **Bronchopneumonia.** Combination of bronchitis and pneumonia.

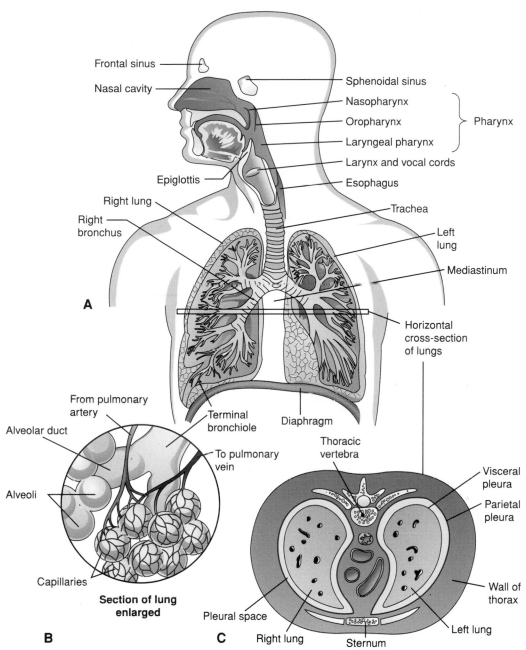

Figure 5-7. **Respiratory system. A.** Overview. **B.** Enlarged section of lung tissue showing the relationship between the alveoli (air sacs) of the lungs and the blood capillaries. **C.** A transverse section through the lungs. (From Cohen BJ, Taylor JJ. Memmler's The Human Body in Health and Disease. 10th Ed. Philadelphia: Lippincott Williams & Wilkins, 2005.)

- **Epiglottitis.** Inflammation of the epiglottis (the mouth of the windpipe); may cause respiratory obstruction, especially in children; prior to the availability of Hib vaccine, epiglottitis in children was frequently caused by the bacterium *Haemophilus influenzae* type b.

- **Laryngitis.** Inflammation of the mucous membrane of the larynx, or voice box.

- **Pharyngitis.** Inflammation of the mucous membrane and underlying tissue of the pharynx; commonly referred to as sore throat.

- **Pneumonia.** Inflammation of one or both lungs. Alveolar sacs become filled with exudate, inflammatory cells, and fibrin. Most cases of pneumonia are caused by bacteria or viruses, but pneumonia can also be caused by fungi and protozoa.

- **Sinusitis.** Inflammation of the lining of one or more of the paranasal sinuses. The most common causes are the bacteria *Streptococcus pneumoniae* and *H. influenzae*. Less common causes are the bacteria *Streptococcus pyogenes*, *Moraxella catarrhalis*, and *Staphylococcus aureus*.

Upper Respiratory Tract

Infectious diseases of the URT include pharyngitis, laryngitis, epiglottitis, and sinusitis. Examples of clinical specimens collected from the URT are throat swabs, nasal swabs, nasal washings, and nasopharyngeal swabs. By far, the most common type of URT specimen submitted to the CML is the throat swab.

Most cases of pharyngitis are caused by viruses. Routine throat swabs are collected to determine if a patient has strep throat, which is caused by the bacterium *S. pyogenes*, also known as group A strep. If any other pathogen (e.g., a bacterium such as *Neisseria gonorrhoeae* or *Corynebacterium diphtheriae*) is suspected, a specific request for culture of that pathogen must be noted on the laboratory request slip, so that the appropriate culture media will be inoculated. There is an art to the proper collection of a throat swab. Under direct observation, the swab is carefully but firmly rubbed over any areas of inflammation or exudate or over the tonsils and posterior pharynx. Routine throat swabs should be refrigerated if transport of the swab to the laboratory will be delayed beyond 1 hour.

The most common causes of laryngitis are viruses. For diagnosis, throat swabs or nasal washings should be collected and then transported in viral transport medium. Throat cultures are *not* recommended for diagnosis of epiglottitis. Touching an inflamed epiglottis could result in obstruction of the airway. The specimen of choice for diagnosis of epiglottitis is blood for culture. The only specimen of value to determine the etiologic agent of sinusitis is a needle aspirate; nasal and nasopharyngeal swabs cannot be used for this purpose.

Lower Respiratory Tract

Infections of the LRT include bronchitis, bronchopneumonia, and pneumonia. Clinical specimens submitted for diagnosis of LRT infections include bronchial washings, bronchial brushings, tracheal aspirates, transtracheal aspirates, needle biopsy, and sputum. By far the most common type of LRT specimen submitted to the CML is sputum.

Sputum specimens. Sputum is pus that accumulates deep within the lungs of a patient with pneumonia, tuberculosis, or other LRT infection. Unfortunately, many of the specimens submitted to the CML that are labeled "sputum" are actually saliva (see "Study Aid: Differentiating Between Sputum and Saliva Specimens"). A laboratory workup of a patient's saliva will not provide clinically relevant information about the patient's LRT infection, and will be a waste of time, effort, and money. This situation can be avoided if someone takes a moment to explain to the patient what is required of him/her. For example, a nurse could say, "The next time you cough up some of that thick, greenish material from your lungs, Mr. Smith, please spit it into this container." If proper mouth hygiene is maintained, the sputum will not be severely contaminated with oral flora.

STUDY AID **Differentiating Between Sputum and Saliva Specimens.** CML professionals can differentiate between a sputum specimen and a saliva specimen by examining a Gram-stained smear of the specimen. Recall that sputum is pus that accumulates deep down in the lungs of patients with LRT infections. Pus contains numerous white blood cells (WBCs). Thus, a true sputum specimen will contain numerous WBCs. If the submitted specimen contains more squamous epithelial cells than WBCs, then it is probably a saliva specimen (Fig. 5-8). Some authorities state that the best sputum specimen should contain 10 or fewer epithelial cells per ×100 field (using a ×10 ocular and ×10 objective).

> CML professionals can differentiate between a sputum specimen and a saliva specimen by examining a Gram-stained smear of the specimen.

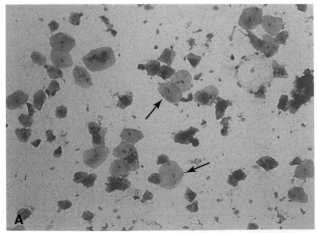

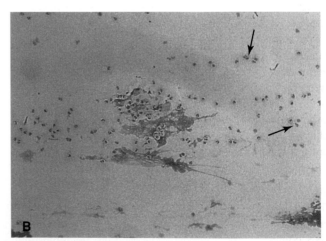

***Figure 5-8. Sputum specimens. A.** Gram stain of an unacceptable "sputum" specimen. Note the predominance of squamous epithelial cells (*arrows*). **B.** Gram stain of an acceptable sputum specimen. Note the predominance of neutrophils (*arrows*). (Courtesy of Marler LM, Siders JA, Allen SD. Direct Smear Atlas. Philadelphia: Lippincott Williams & Wilkins, 2001.)*

TABLE 5 - 4	Bartlett's Grading System for Determining the Quality of Sputum Specimens	
Number of Neutrophils per ×10 Low-Power Field[a]	Number of Epithelial Cells per ×10 Low-Power Field[a]	Grade
<10		0
10–25		+1
>25		+2
Presence of mucus		+1
	10–25	−1
	>25	−2

Source: Adapted from Winn WC Jr, et al. Koneman's Color Atlas and Textbook of Diagnostic Microbiology. 6th Ed. Philadelphia: Lippincott Williams & Wilkins, 2006.

[a]The average number of cells in about 20 to 30 separate ×10 microscopic fields.

Calculate the total. A final total of 0 or less indicates a lack of active inflammation or contamination with saliva. In such cases, a repeat specimen should be requested.

If tuberculosis is suspected, extreme care in collecting and handling the specimen should be exercised to avoid becoming infected with the pathogen. The specimen should be submitted to the CML as quickly as possible. Refrigeration of sputum specimens is not necessary, unless a delay of more than 1 or 2 hours is anticipated.

To determine which sputum specimens are suitable for culture, some CMLs use the grading system developed by Bartlett et al. (see "References and Suggested Reading") or one of several similar grading systems. Barlett's grading system is shown in Table 5-4.

Other LRT specimens. The clinician may wish to obtain a better quality specimen by bronchial aspiration through a bronchoscope or by a process known as percutaneous transtracheal aspiration. In the former procedure, a catheter is fed into the affected lung via the patient's nose, mouth, or tracheotomy site. Needle biopsy of the lungs may be necessary for diagnosis of *Pneumocystis jiroveci* pneumonia, which is common in AIDS patients, and for certain other pathogens. Although once classified as a protozoan, *P. jiroveci* is currently considered to be a fungus (see Chapter 20).

Central Nervous System

The nervous system is composed of the central nervous system (CNS) and the peripheral nervous system (Fig. 5-9). The CNS consists of the brain, the spinal cord, and the three membranes (called **meninges**) that cover the brain and spinal cord (Fig. 5-10). The CNS is well protected and remarkably resistant to infection; it is encased in bone, bathed and cush-

ioned in **cerebrospinal fluid (CSF),** and nourished by capillaries. Together with CNS tissue cells called astrocytes, these capillaries make up the blood-brain barrier, supplying nutrients but not allowing cells of the immune system, microorganisms, or larger particles—for example, macromolecules like antibodies and most antibiotics—to pass from the blood into the brain. The peripheral nervous system consists of nerves that branch from the brain and spinal cord.

There are no indigenous microflora of the nervous system. Microbes must gain access to the CNS through trauma (fracture or medical procedure), via the blood and lymph to the CSF, or along the peripheral nerves.

The following are some terms relating to infectious diseases of the CNS:

- **Encephalitis.** Inflammation of the brain. Usually caused by viruses.

- **Encephalomyelitis.** Inflammation of the brain and spinal cord.

- **Meningitis.** Inflammation of the membranes (**meninges**) that surround the brain and spinal cord.

- **Meningoencephalitis.** Inflammation of the brain and meninges.

- **Myelitis.** Inflammation of the spinal cord.

Cerebrospinal Fluid

Meningitis, encephalitis, and meningoencephalitis are rapidly fatal diseases that can be caused by various microbes,

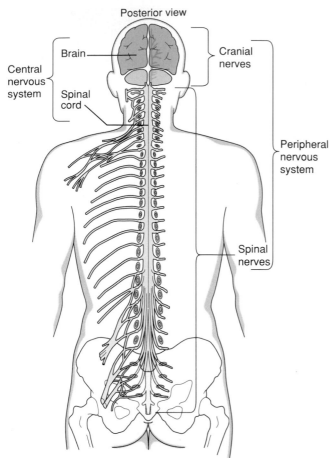

Figure 5-9. **Nervous system, consisting of the central nervous system and the peripheral nervous system.** (From Cohen BJ, Taylor JJ. Memmler's The Human Body in Health and Disease. 10th Ed. Philadelphia: Lippincott Williams & Wilkins, 2005.)

including bacteria, fungi, protozoa, and viruses. To diagnose these diseases, CSF (sometimes called spinal fluid) must be collected into a sterile tube by a lumbar puncture or spinal tap under surgically aseptic conditions (Fig. 5-11). This technically difficult procedure is performed by a physician. CSF specimens must be rushed to the laboratory. Because some of the pathogens that cause CNS infections are killed by cold temperatures, CSF specimens should never be refrigerated.

The extremely serious nature of central nervous system infections demand that CSF be treated as a "stat" specimen[2] in the CML, and a workup of the specimen must be initiated immediately. Information obtained as a result of examining a Gram-stained smear of the spinal fluid sediment will be telephonically reported to the clinician immediately. That is

> CSF specimens are treated as stat (emergency) specimens in the CML. Workup of the CSF specimen is initiated immediately upon receipt.

what is known as a preliminary report. As mentioned earlier, preliminary reports are laboratory reports that are communicated, usually by telephone, to the requesting clinician prior to the availability of the final report. Preliminary reports containing CSF Gram stain observations frequently enable clinicians to make diagnoses and initiate therapy, and often save patients' lives.

Urinary Tract

The anatomy of the urinary tract is shown in Figure 5-12. For purposes of discussion, **urinary tract infections (UTIs)** can be divided into upper and lower UTIs. Upper UTIs include infections of the kidneys and ureters. Lower UTIs include infections of the urinary bladder, the urethra, and in males, the prostate.

UTIs may be caused by any of a variety of microorganisms introduced by poor personal hygiene, sexual intercourse, the insertion of catheters, and other means. The urinary tract is usually protected from pathogens by the frequent flushing action of urination. The acidity of normal urine also discourages growth of many microorganisms. Indigenous microflora are found at and near the outer opening (meatus) of the urethra of both males and females.

Terms relating to infectious diseases of the urinary tract include the following:

- **Cystitis.** Inflammation of the urinary bladder. The most common type of UTI, cystitis is most often caused by *Escherichia coli*. Other common causes of cystitis are species of *Klebsiella*, *Proteus*, *Enterobacter*, *Pseudomonas*, and *Enterococcus*, as well as *Staphylococcus saprophyticus*, *Staphylococcus epidermidis*, and *Candida albicans*.

- **Nephritis.** General term referring to inflammation of the kidneys. **Pyelonephritis** is inflammation of the renal parenchyma, the basic cellular tissue of the kidney. *E. coli* is the most common cause of nephritis and pyelonephritis. Typically, nephritis is preceded by cystitis; the bacteria migrate up the ureters, from the urinary bladder to the kidneys. Bacteria may also gain access to the kidneys via the bloodstream.

- **Ureteritis.** Inflammation of one or both ureters. Usually caused by the spread of infection upward from the urinary bladder or downward from the kidneys.

- **Urethritis.** Inflammation of the urethra. The pathogens that cause urethritis are usually transmitted sexually. The most common causes of urethritis are *Chlamydia trachomatis*, *N. gonorrhoeae*, ureaplasmas, and mycoplasmas. Urethritis that is not caused by *N. gonorrhoeae* is often referred to as nonspecific urethritis or nongonococcal urethritis.

- **Prostatitis.** Inflammation of the prostate gland. Most often, prostatitis is not an infectious disease. If the cause

---

[2]*The term* stat *is used to indicate an emergency specimen, one that should be worked on right away.* Stat *comes from the Latin word* statim, *which means "at once" or "immediately." Unfortunately, the word has become overused, and* stat *is often written on laboratory request slips that are not truly related to emergency cases.*

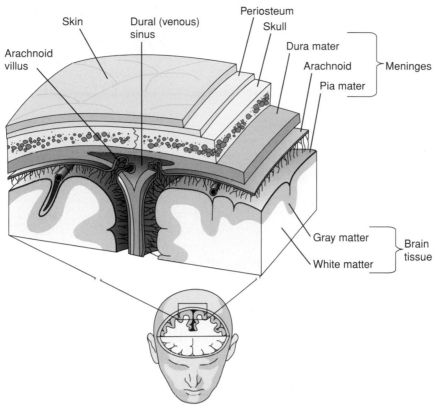

Figure 5-10. **Frontal section of the top of the head, showing the meninges and related structures.** (From Cohen BJ, Taylor JJ. Memmler's The Human Body in Health and Disease. 10th Ed. Philadelphia: Lippincott Williams & Wilkins, 2005.)

is a pathogen, it may be a bacterium, a virus, a fungus, or a protozoan.

Urine

Diagnosis of UTIs is made by culturing urine specimens. Although urine is ordinarily sterile while it is in the urinary bladder, it becomes contaminated during urination (voiding) by indigenous microflora of the distal urethra, the portion of the urethra furthest from the bladder. Thus, the mere presence of bacteria in the urine, **bacteriuria,** is not significant. Contamination can be reduced by collecting **clean-catch midstream urine.** *Clean catch* refers to the fact that the area around the external opening of the urethra is cleansed by washing with soap and rinsing with water prior to urination. This removes the indigenous microflora that live in the area. *Midstream* refers to the fact that the initial portion of the urine stream is directed into a toilet or bedpan, and then the remainder of the urine stream is directed into a sterile container. Thus, the microorganisms that live in the distal urethra are flushed out of the urethra by the initial portion of the urine stream, into the toilet or bedpan, rather than into the specimen container. In some circumstances, the clinician may prefer to collect a catheterized specimen or use the suprapubic needle aspiration technique to obtain a sterile sample of urine. In the latter technique, a needle is inserted through the abdominal wall into the urinary bladder and a syringe is used to withdraw urine from the bladder.

To prevent continued bacterial growth, all urine specimens must be processed within 30 minutes of collection, or refrigerated at 4°C until they can be analyzed. Refrigerated urine specimens should be cultured within 24 hours. Failure to refrigerate a urine specimen will cause an inflated colony count (see Chapter 18), which could lead to an incorrect diagnosis of a UTI.

> Urine specimens for culture must be collected in a manner that reduces contamination of the specimen by indigenous microflora of the distal urethra.

There are three parts to a urine culture: (1) a colony count, (2) isolation and identification of the pathogen, and (3) antimicrobial susceptibility testing. These are described in Chapter 18.

Genital Tract

As previously mentioned, indigenous microflora are found at and near the outer opening of the urethra and within the distal urethra of both males and females. Additionally, the female genital region supports the growth of many microorganisms,

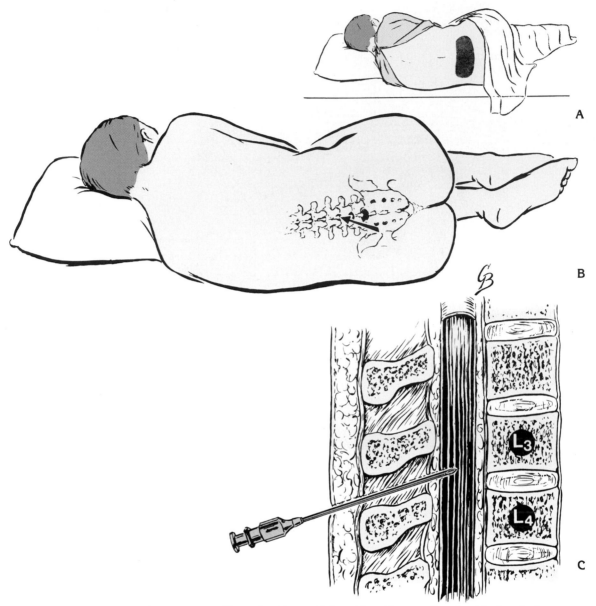

Figure 5-11. **Lumbar puncture.** The patient lies on his/her side, with knees flexed and back arched to separate the lumbar vertebrae. **A.** The patient is surgically draped, and an area overlying the lumbar spine is disinfected. **B.** The space between lumbar vertebrae L-3 and L-4 (*arrow*) is palpated with a sterilely gloved forefinger. **C.** The spinal needle is carefully directed between the spinous processes, through the intraspinous ligaments into the spinal canal. (From Winn WC Jr, et al. Koneman's Color Atlas and Textbook of Diagnostic Microbiology. 6th Ed. Philadelphia: Lippincott Williams & Wilkins, 2006.)

such as species of *Lactobacillus*, *Staphylococcus*, *Streptococcus*, *Enterococcus*, nonpathogenic *Neisseria*, *Clostridium*, *Actinomyces*, *Prevotella*, diphtheroids, enteric bacilli, and *Candida*. The relative distribution of these microbes depends on the estrogen levels and pH of the site. Should any of these or other microorganisms invade further into the genitourinary system, various infections may occur. The male and female reproductive systems are shown in Figures 5-13 and 5-14.

Following are some terms relating to infectious diseases of the female genital tract:

- **Bartholinitis.** Inflammation of the Bartholin ducts in females.

- **Cervicitis.** Inflammation of the cervix, that part of the uterus that opens into the vagina.

- **Endometritis.** Inflammation of the endometrium (the inner layer of the uterine wall).

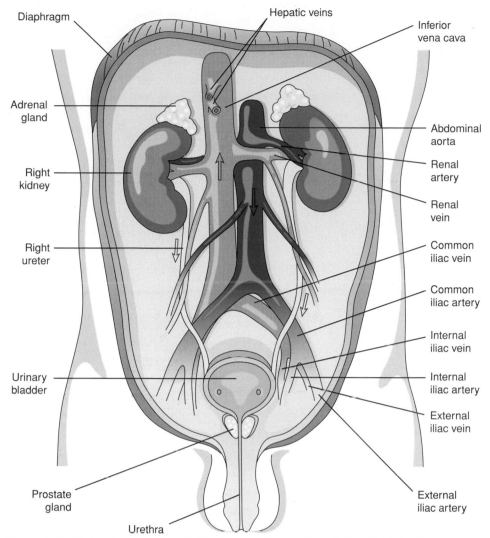

Figure 5-12. **Male urinary tract, with blood vessels shown.** (From Cohen BJ, Taylor JJ. Memmler's The Human Body in Health and Disease. 10th Ed. Philadelphia: Lippincott Williams & Wilkins, 2005.)

- **Oophoritis.** Inflammation of an ovary.

- **Pelvic inflammatory disease (PID).** Inflammation of female pelvic structures, such as the endometrium, uterine tube, and pelvic peritoneum.

- **Salpingitis.** Inflammation of the uterine tube.

- **Vaginitis.** Inflammation of the vagina. The three most common causes of vaginitis in the United States, each causing about one-third of the cases, are *C. albicans* (a yeast), *Trichomonas vaginalis* (a protozoan), and a mixture of bacteria (including bacteria in the genera *Mobiluncus* and *Gardnerella*). When caused by a mixture of bacteria, the infection is referred to as bacterial vaginosis. In general, infections that result from the actions of two or more bacteria are called synergistic or polymicrobial infections (see Chapter 2). A saline wet mount preparation

is usually used to diagnose vaginitis (see Appendix A); a Gram-stained smear is of value to diagnose bacterial vaginosis.

- **Vulvovaginitis.** Inflammation of the vulva—the external genitalia of females—and the vagina.

STUDY AID **Vaginitis Versus Vaginosis.** The similarly sounding terms *vaginitis* and *vaginosis* both refer to vaginal infections. The suffix *-itis* refers to inflammation, and inflammation usually involves the influx of white blood cells known as polymorphonuclear cells. Thus, a vaginal infection involving inflammation and the influx of polymorphonuclear cells is referred to as vaginitis. In bacterial vaginosis, there is a watery, noninflammatory discharge with few if any WBCs.

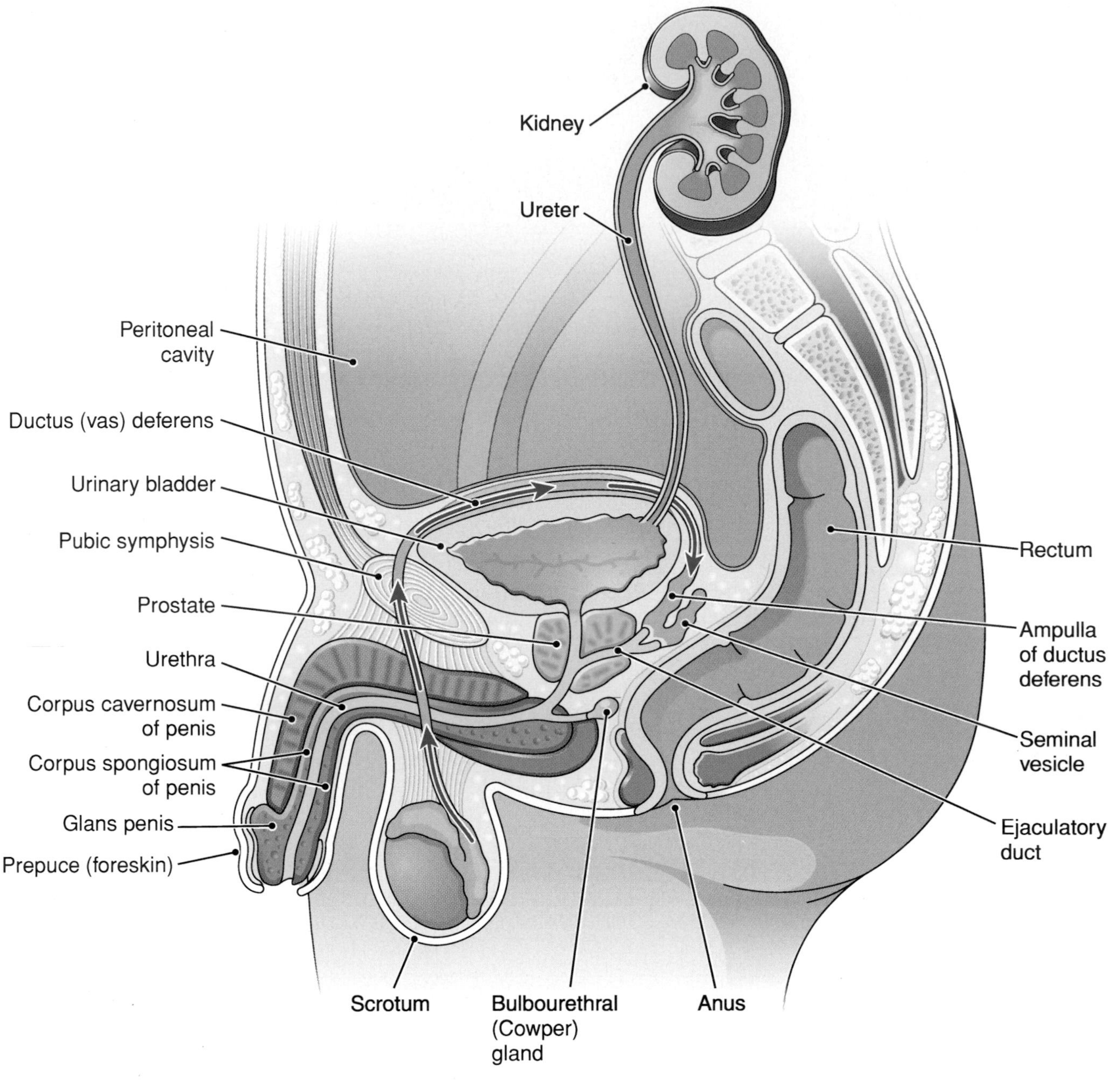

— Path of spermatozoa

Figure 5-13. **Male reproductive system.** (From Cohen BJ, Taylor JJ. Memmler's The Human Body in Health and Disease. 10th Ed. Philadelphia: Lippincott Williams & Wilkins, 2005.)

Thus, the difference between vaginitis and vaginosis boils down to the presence or absence of WBCs. Bacterial vaginosis is a synergistic infection caused by a mixture of various bacteria.

Terms relating to infectious diseases of the male genital tract include the following:

• **Epididymitis.** Inflammation of the epididymis (an elongated structure connected to the testis).

• **Orchitis.** Inflammation of the testis.

• **Prostatitis.** Inflammation of the prostate.

Genital tract specimens include vaginal and cervical swabs; pus aspirated from Bartholin gland abscesses; endometrial samples obtained by protected suction curette; culdocentesis specimens; scrapings, aspirates, and biopsy material from vulvar lesions; vaginal discharge specimens; and prostatic secretions. Genital tract specimens from

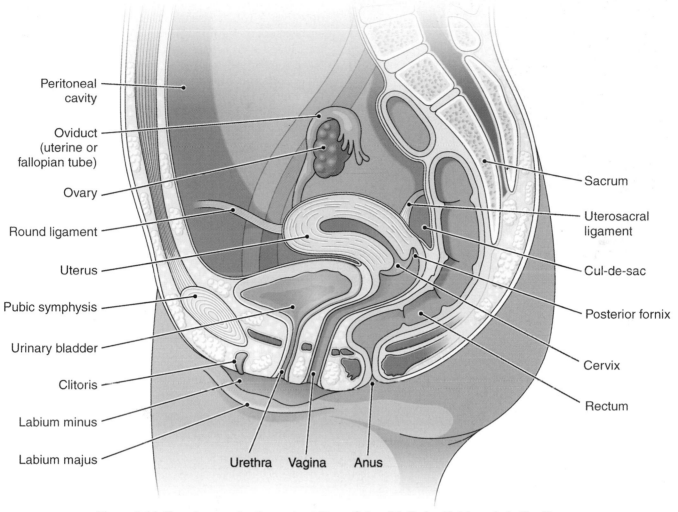

***Figure 5-14.* Female reproductive system.** (From Cohen BJ, Taylor JJ. Memmler's The Human Body in Health and Disease. 10th Ed. Philadelphia: Lippincott Williams & Wilkins, 2005.)

female patients are often contaminated with indigenous microflora.

Gonococcal (GC) Cultures

The initials *GC* stand for **gonococci or gonococcal,** terms referring to *N. gonorrhoeae. N. gonorrhoeae* is the cause of gonorrhea, a disease that can manifest itself in many ways, including urethritis and PID. *N. gonorrhoeae* is a fastidious bacterium that is capnophilic and borderline microaerophilic.[3] Only Dacron, calcium alginate, or nontoxic cotton swabs should be used to collect GC specimens. Ordinary cotton swabs contain fatty acids that can be toxic to *N. gonorrhoeae.* When attempting to diagnose gonorrhea, swabs (vaginal, cervical, urethral, throat, and rectal swabs)

should ideally be inoculated immediately onto a highly enriched and selective medium, such as Thayer-Martin or Martin-Lewis medium and incubated in a carbon dioxide (CO_2) environment. Alternatively, they should be inoculated into or onto a bottle (e.g., Transgrow) or tray (e.g., Jembec) that contains an appropriate culture medium and an atmosphere containing 5% to 10% CO_2 (Fig. 5-15). The Transgrow bottle should be held in an upright position while inoculating, to prevent loss of the CO_2. These cultures should be incubated at 37°C overnight and then shipped to a microbiology laboratory for positive identification of *N. gonorrhoeae.* If it is necessary to transport a swab specimen, the swab should be placed into an appropriate transport medium for shipment. Never refrigerate GC swabs, because the low temperature may kill the *N. gonorrhoeae.*

---

[3]*Microorganisms with especially demanding nutritional requirements are referred to as being **fastidious,** meaning "fussy." A **capnophile** is an organism that requires carbon dioxide concentrations higher than that found in room air (less than 1%) for optimum growth. A carbon dioxide concentration of between 5% and 10% is provided when attempting to culture capnophiles in the CML. A **microaerophile** is an organism that requires oxygen, but in concentrations lower than that found in the atmosphere (about 20% to 21%). An oxygen concentration of 5% (for* Campylobacter *or* Helicobacter *spp.) to 15% (for* N. gonorrhoeae*) is provided when attempting to culture microaerophiles in the CML.*

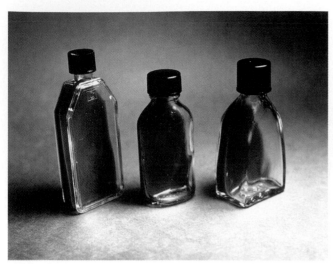

Figure 5-15. **Transgrow bottles used in gonococcal cultures.** (Courtesy of Dr. A. Schroeter and the CDC.)

Oral Cavity

The following terms relate to infectious diseases of the oral cavity:

- **Dental caries.** Tooth decay or cavities. Dental caries starts when the external surface (the enamel) of a tooth is dissolved by organic acids produced by masses of microorganisms attached to the tooth (dental plaque). This is followed by enzymatic destruction of the protein matrix, cavitation, and bacterial invasion. The most common cause of tooth decay is the bacterium *Streptococcus mutans*, which produces lactic acid as an end product in the fermentation of glucose.

- **Gingivitis.** Inflammation of the gingiva (gums).

- **Periodontitis.** Inflammation of the periodontium (tissues that surround and support the teeth, including the gingiva and supporting bone); in severe cases, teeth loosen and fall out.

The oral cavity or mouth is a complex ecosystem suitable for growth and interrelationships of many types of microorganisms. Although the actual indigenous microflora of the mouth varies greatly from one person to the next, studies have shown that it includes about 300 identified species of bacteria, both aerobes and anaerobes. Thus, it is often difficult to interpret the results of culturing oral swab specimens. When bacteria are isolated from oral swabs, it is difficult to know whether they are involved in an infectious process or are merely contaminants. Carefully collected scrapings or aspirates should be transported to the CML in some type of anaerobic transport system (see Chapter 17).

Gastrointestinal Tract

The gastrointestinal (GI) tract consists of a long tube with many expanded areas designed for digestion of food,

absorption of nutrients, and elimination of undigested materials (Fig. 5-16). Transient and resident microbes continuously enter and leave the GI tract. Most of the microorganisms ingested with food are destroyed in the stomach and duodenum by the low pH (gastric contents have a pH of approximately 1.5), and are inhibited from growing in the lower intestines by the resident microflora (microbial antagonism). They are then flushed from the colon during defecation, along with large numbers of indigenous microbes.

Following are some terms related to infectious diseases of the GI tract:

- **Colitis.** Inflammation of the colon (the large intestine)

- **Diarrhea.** An abnormally frequent discharge of semisolid or fluid fecal matter. Some CML professionals define diarrheal specimens as "stool specimens that conform to the shape of the container."

- **Dysentery.** Frequent watery stools accompanied by abdominal pain, fever, and dehydration. The stool specimens may contain blood and/or mucus.

- **Enteritis.** Inflammation of the intestines, usually the small intestine.

- **Gastritis.** Inflammation of the mucosal lining of the stomach.

- **Gastroenteritis.** Inflammation of the mucosal linings of the stomach and intestines.

- **Hepatitis.** Inflammation of the liver; usually the result of viral infection but can be caused by toxic agents.

Gastrointestinal tract specimens include duodenal contents, gastric biopsy samples, gastric aspirates, "Scotch tape" preparations, rectal and anal swabs, sigmoidoscopy specimens, and stool specimens. By far, the most common type of GI specimens submitted to the CML are stool or fecal specimens.

Fecal Specimens

Ideally, a fecal specimen (also known as feces, stool, or a stool specimen) is collected at the laboratory and processed immediately to prevent a decrease in temperature, which allows the pH to drop, causing the death of many *Shigella* and *Salmonella* species. Alternatively, the specimen may be placed in a container with a preservative that maintains a pH of 7.0.

Because the colon is anaerobic, members of the indigenous GI microflora are obligate, aerotolerant, and facultative anaerobes. However, fecal specimens are cultured anaerobically only when *Clostridium perfringens* food poisoning or *Clostridium difficile*–associated diseases are suspected. In intestinal infections, the pathogens frequently overwhelm the indigenous microflora and thus are the predominant

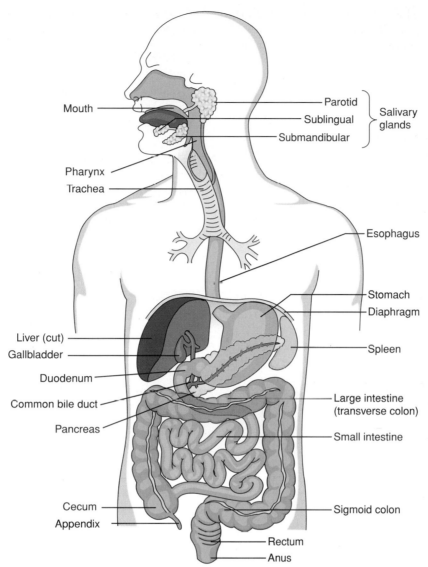

Figure 5-16. **The gastrointestinal tract.** (From Cohen BJ, Taylor JJ. Memmler's The Human Body in Health and Disease. 10th Ed. Philadelphia: Lippincott Williams & Wilkins, 2005.)

organisms seen in smears and cultures. A combination of direct microscopic examination, culture, biochemical tests, and immunological tests may be performed to identify Gram-negative and Gram-positive bacteria (e.g., enteropathogenic *E. coli*, *Salmonella* spp., *Shigella* spp., *C. perfringens*, *Vibrio cholerae*, *Campylobacter* spp., and *Staphylococcus* spp.), intestinal protozoa (*Giardia*, *Entamoeba*), and intestinal helminths. Toxin assays are used more frequently than fecal cultures to diagnose diseases associated with *C. difficile*.

Body Fluids

In addition to blood and cerebrospinal fluid (which were previously discussed), body fluid specimens include abdominal or peritoneal fluid, pleural or thoracentesis fluid, synovial (joint) fluid, and amniotic fluid. Carefully collected aspirates of amniotic and pleural fluids are usually transported to the CML in an anaerobic transport system (see Chapter 17). Peritoneal and synovial fluids should be inoculated into blood culture bottles and anaerobic transport systems for transport to the CML.

REJECTION OF CLINICAL SPECIMENS

As part of its quality assurance program, the CML maintains the right to reject any clinical specimens believed to be of poor quality. The processing of such specimens could lead to misleading and potentially dangerous laboratory results, thus jeopardizing the health of the patients. Should a poor-quality specimen be rejected by the CML, the requesting clinician would be notified and asked to submit a high-quality specimen in its place.

Example

A patient is suspected of having pneumonia. The specimen container that was received by the CML is labeled "sputum," but a Gram stain of the specimen reveals that it is actually saliva. A workup of the patient's saliva would not provide the clinician with clinically relevant information; that is, a workup of the saliva would reveal which organisms are in the patient's mouth but would not provide any information regarding the organisms, if any, present in the patient's lungs. The clinician would be informed that a saliva specimen, rather than a sputum specimen, was received by the CML, and he or she would be asked to submit a true sputum specimen.

> Poor-quality specimens are rejected as part of the CML's quality assurance program. Workup of a poor-quality specimen could generate results that are not clinically relevant and might endanger the life of the patient.

Winn et al. cite the following as reasons for rejection of specimens:

- Specimens received in formalin. Any microorganisms present would have been killed by the formalin.

- Twenty-four-hour sputum collections. Such specimens would be heavily contaminated with indigenous microflora from the oral cavity.

- Smears or secretions from the uterine cervix, vaginal canal, or anus for Gram stain detection of *N. gonorrhoeae*. Because of their similar morphology, some indigenous microflora could be mistaken for *N. gonorrhoeae*.

- A single swab submitted for multiple requests (e.g., for anaerobic culture, fungal culture, and mycobacterial culture). In all likelihood, there would be too little specimen to accomplish all that is requested.

- Specimens submitted in an improper, nonsterile, or leaking and obviously contaminated container.

- Overgrown or dried-out culture plate, unless the culture plate was obtained for one of the slower-growing pathogenic fungi.

- Specimens that are obviously contaminated, such as those containing barium, colored dyes, or oily chemicals.

- Specimens submitted for anaerobic culture that are unacceptable (see Chapter 17).

Chapter Review

- The quality of the results produced by the CML can only be as good as the quality of the clinical specimens submitted to it.

- The three components of specimen quality are proper selection, proper collection, and proper transport of the specimen.

- The CML should educate health care professionals on the proper selection, collection, and transport of clinical specimens. In addition, the laboratory is responsible for publishing a book (often called the laboratory policies and procedures manual, or lab P&P manual) that contains instructions for the proper selection, collection, and transport of clinical specimens. The information is often accessible via the hospital's computer system.

- The person who collects the clinical specimen is ultimately responsible for its quality.

- Indigenous microflora, or normal flora, are microbes usually found on and in the human body. Indigenous microflora may also be referred to as endogenous microbes.

- When collecting blood specimens for culture, the venipuncture site must be thoroughly cleansed and disinfected to prevent contamination of the specimen with indigenous skin flora.

- All clinical specimens must be properly labeled. Ideally, labels should contain the patient's name, unique hospital identification number, and room number; requesting clinician's name; culture site; and date and time of collection.

- Ideally, laboratory request slips must contain the patient's name, age, sex, and unique hospital identification number; name of the requesting clinician; specific information about the type of specimen and the site from which it was collected; date and time of collection; initials of the person who collected the specimen; and information about any antimicrobial agents that the patient is receiving. The laboratory should always be given sufficient clinical information to aid in performing appropriate analyses.

- Aspirates (i.e., pus that has been collected using a sterile needle and syringe assembly) are the preferred type of specimen for wounds. Specimens collected by swab are frequently contaminated with indigenous microflora and often dry out before they can be processed in the CML. The type of wound should always be indicated on the request slip, as well as the anatomical site and whether it is on the left or right, if applicable.

- Routine throat swabs are collected to determine if a patient has strep throat. If any other pathogen (e.g., *Neisseria gonorrhoeae* or *Corynebacterium diphtheriae*) is suspected to be causing the patient's pharyngitis, culture for that pathogen must be noted on the laboratory request slip.

- In general, sputum specimens are considered acceptable if they contain many more polymorphonuclear cells than epithelial cells.

- Because meningitis is such a serious and often rapidly fatal disease, CSF specimens are processed immediately on their receipt at the CML. Important information that is learned about the specimen is immediately reported to the requesting clinician; this is known as a preliminary report. Such reports have often saved patients' lives.

- The proper specimen to diagnose a UTI is clean-catch midstream urine. If a delay in transport is expected, urine specimens must be refrigerated until they can be transported to the laboratory.

- *N. gonorrhoeae* is a fastidious bacterium that is both capnophilic and borderline microaerophilic. Therefore, when attempting to diagnose gonorrhea, vaginal, cervical, urethral, throat, and rectal swabs should ideally be inoculated immediately onto a highly enriched and highly selective medium (such as Thayer-Martin or Martin-Lewis medium) and incubated in a CO_2 atmosphere.

- Specimens may need to be rejected because of poor quality or an improper label.

New Terms and Abbreviations

After studying Chapter 5, you should be familiar with the following terms, which are defined within the chapter and in the Glossary at the back of the book:

Bacteremia

Bacteriuria

Bartholinitis

Bronchitis

Bronchopneumonia

Capnophile

Carbuncle

Cervicitis

Clean-catch midstream urine

Clinically relevant results

Clinical specimens

Colitis

Conjunctiva

Conjunctivitis

Cerebrospinal fluid (CSF)

Cystitis

Dental caries

Dermatitis

Dermis

Diarrhea

Dysentery

Encephalitis

Encephalomyelitis

Endocarditis

Endogenous microbe

Endometritis

Enteritis

Epidermis

Epididymitis

Epiglottitis

Exogenous microbe

Folliculitis

Fungemia

Furuncle

Gastritis

Gastroenteritis

Gingivitis

Gonococci (GC)

Hepatitis

Keratitis

Keratoconjunctivitis

Laryngitis

Leukemia

Lymphadenitis

Lymphadenopathy

Lymphangitis

Meninges

Meningitis

Meningococcemia

Meningoencephalitis

Microaerophile

Myelitis

Myocarditis

Nephritis

Oophoritis

Orchitis

Otitis externa

Otitis media

Parasitemia

Pelvic inflammatory disease (PID)

Pericarditis

Periodontitis

Pharyngitis

Pneumonia

Prostatitis

Pyelonephritis

Salpingitis

Sebaceous glands

Sebum

Septicemia

Sinusitis

Sputum

Sty (stye)

Toxemia

Ureteritis

Urethritis

Urinary tract infection (UTI)

Vaginitis

Vaginosis

Vulvovaginitis

Viremia

References and Suggested Reading

Bartlett RC. A plea for clinical relevance in microbiology. Am J Clin Pathol 1974;61:867–872.

Marler LM, Siders JA, Allen SD. Direct Smear Atlas. Philadelphia: Lippincott Williams & Wilkins, 2001.

Miller JM. A guide to specimen management in clinical microbiology. 2nd Ed. Washington, DC: ASM Press, 1999.

Winn WC Jr, et al. Koneman's Color Atlas and Textbook of Diagnostic Microbiology. 6th Ed. Philadelphia: Lippincott Williams & Wilkins, 2006.

 On the CD-ROM

- Additional Self-Assessment Exercises
- Puzzle

Self-Assessment Exercises

After studying Chapter 5, answer the following questions.

1. Which of the following statements about CSF specimens is *false*?

   A. Following collection, they should be rushed to the laboratory.

   B. They are used to diagnose serious conditions such as meningitis and encephalitis.

   C. They should always be refrigerated.

   D. They are collected only by physicians.

2. All of the clinical specimens submitted to the CML must be

   A. properly and carefully collected.

   B. properly transported to the laboratory.

   C. properly labeled.

   D. all the above.

3. Who is ultimately responsible for the quality of specimens submitted to the CML?

   A. The microbiologist who is in charge of the CML

   B. The person who collects the specimen

   C. The person who transports the specimen to the CML

   D. The clinician who writes the laboratory request slip

4. Which of the following body sites or specimens is *not* considered normally sterile?

   A. CSF

   B. Blood

   C. Skin

   D. Urinary bladder

5. The proper specimen for diagnosis of a UTI is

   A. a clean-catch midstream urine sample.

   B. a routine, first-morning voided urine.

   C. a swab of the distal urethra.

   D. none of the above.

6. Which of the following statements about urine cultures is *incorrect*?

    A. The best type of specimen is a clean-catch midstream urine.

    B. There are three parts to a urine culture.

    C. The container into which the patient urinates should be sterile.

    D. A white blood cell count is part of the urine culture.

7. Regarding the proper collection of clinical specimens, which of the following statements is *incorrect*?

    A. Specimens should be collected *after* antimicrobial therapy is started.

    B. Specimens should be collected in a manner that will minimize or eliminate contamination of the specimen with indigenous microflora.

    C. A sufficient quantity of specimen should be collected to allow culture and testing.

    D. Specimens should be protected from heat and cold as much as possible.

8. If urine specimens cannot be transported immediately to the CML, they should

    A. be placed in a 35°C to 37°C incubator.

    B. be refrigerated.

    C. remain at room temperature.

    D. be discarded.

9. Keratitis is inflammation of the

    A. middle ear.

    B. cornea of the eye.

    C. kidney.

    D. meninges.

10. What is the most common cause of pharyngitis?

    A. *Neisseria gonorrhoeae*

    B. *Streptococcus pyogenes*

    C. *Corynebacterium diphtheriae*

    D. Viruses

CHAPTER 6

General Clinical Microbiology Laboratory Methods

LEARNING OBJECTIVES

After studying this chapter, you should be able to:

☞ Define the terms introduced in this chapter (e.g., *anabolism, antiserum, artificial medium*)

☞ Given one metric unit of length, convert it to another (e.g., micrometers to nanometers)

☞ State the relative sizes of viruses, bacteria, and protozoa in terms of metric units

☞ Compare and contrast various types of microscopes (e.g., simple microscopes, compound light microscopes, electron microscopes), including their applications and resolving powers

☞ Describe the functions of the various components (e.g., condenser, stage) of a compound microscope

☞ Explain how the wavelength of visible light is related to the size of objects that can be seen using the compound light microscope

☞ State the relationship between the resolving powers of the unaided human eye and the compound light microscope

☞ Differentiate among enriched, selective, and differential media, including purpose, and state at least one example of each

☞ Demonstrate the proper method for inoculating plated media to obtain well-isolated colonies

☞ Discuss the importance of practicing sterile technique, and describe types of contaminants and safety precautions

- ☞ Describe the different types of incubators used in the clinical microbiology laboratory, including the specific atmospheric environment maintained in each

- ☞ State three reasons for "fixing" smears of organisms for staining, and name two common methods of fixation

- ☞ Name the two differential staining procedures most commonly used in the bacteriology section of the clinical microbiology laboratory

- ☞ Discuss the differences between antigen detection procedures and antibody detection procedures

- ☞ Describe monoclonal antibodies, including their production and use

- ☞ Describe molecular diagnostic procedures, including their purpose, sensitivity, and specificity compared with traditional methods, examples of DNA probes commonly available, and advantages and disadvantages

- ☞ Explain the general principles of microbial growth detection in automated blood culture systems, including how growth is detected and the type of sensor used

- ☞ Explain the general principles of automated biochemical-based instruments, and describe the types of detection method used for bacteria, yeasts, and susceptibility testing

This chapter describes general clinical microbiology laboratory (CML) methods—that is, procedures that pertain to more than one category of microbes. Procedures that pertain *only* to bacteria, fungi, parasites, and viruses are discussed in Sections III, IV, V, and VI, respectively.

USING THE METRIC SYSTEM TO EXPRESS THE SIZE OF MICROBES

The metric system is used in scientific fields to express weights and measures. Units of length are based on the meter; units of weight are based on the gram; and units of volume are based on the liter. In microbiology, metric units of length, primarily micrometers and nanometers, are used to express the sizes of microorganisms. The basic unit of length in the metric system, the meter, is equivalent to approximately 39.4 inches, which is about 3.4 inches longer than a yard. A meter may be divided into 10 (10^1) equally spaced units called **decimeters**; or 100 (10^2) equally spaced units called **centimeters**; or 1,000 (10^3) equally spaced units called **millimeters**; or 1 million (10^6) equally spaced units called **micrometers**; or 1 billion (10^9) equally spaced units called **nanometers**. Interrelationships among these units are shown in Figure 6-1. Formulas that can be used to convert inches into centimeters, millimeters, and so forth are presented in Appendix B.

It should be noted that the old terms micron (μ) and millimicron (mμ) have been replaced by the terms micrometer

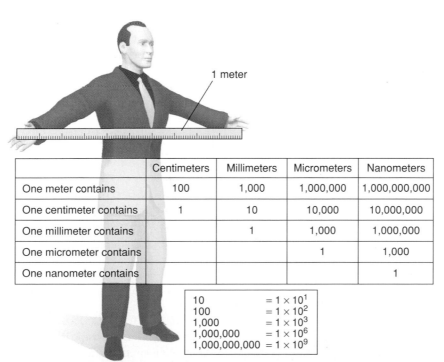

1 meter

	Centimeters	Millimeters	Micrometers	Nanometers
One meter contains	100	1,000	1,000,000	1,000,000,000
One centimeter contains	1	10	10,000	10,000,000
One millimeter contains		1	1,000	1,000,000
One micrometer contains			1	1,000
One nanometer contains				1

$$10 = 1 \times 10^1$$
$$100 = 1 \times 10^2$$
$$1,000 = 1 \times 10^3$$
$$1,000,000 = 1 \times 10^6$$
$$1,000,000,000 = 1 \times 10^9$$

Figure 6-1. **Representations of metric units of measure and exponents.**

(μm) and nanometer (nm), respectively. An **angstrom (Å)** is 0.1 nm; this unit of measure is often used in electron microscopy.

The sizes of bacteria and protozoa are usually expressed in terms of micrometers. For example, a typical spherical bacterium, or **coccus (pl. cocci)** is approximately 1 μm in diameter. Human red blood cells are about 7 μm in diameter; thus, about 7 cocci could fit side by side across a red blood cell. If the head of a pin was 1 mm (1,000 μm) in diameter, then 1,000 cocci could be placed side by side on the pinhead. The average size of a rod-shaped bacterium, or **bacillus (pl. bacilli),** is about 1 μm wide by 3 μm long, but it can be shorter, or many bacilli may form very long filaments (up to 60 μm or more). **The sizes of viruses are expressed in terms of nanometers.** Most of the viruses that cause human disease range in size from about 10 to 300 nm, although some (e.g., Ebola virus, a cause of hemorrhagic fever) can be as long as 1,000 nm (1 μm). Some very large protozoa reach a length of 2,000 μm (2 mm).

> The sizes of bacteria are expressed in micrometers, whereas the sizes of viruses are expressed in nanometers.

In the CML, the sizes of microorganisms can be measured using an ocular micrometer, a tiny ruler within the eyepiece (ocular) of the compound light microscope (Fig. 6-2). Before it can be used to measure objects, however, the ocular micrometer must first be calibrated, using a microscope stage-measuring device called a stage micrometer. Calibration (see Appendix A) must be performed for *each* of the objective lenses to determine the distance between the marks on the ocular micrometer. The ocular micrometer can then be used to measure lengths and widths of microbes and other objects on the specimen slide. The sizes of some microorganisms are shown in Figure 6-3 and Table 6-1.

> An ocular micrometer is used to measure the dimensions of objects being viewed with the microscope.

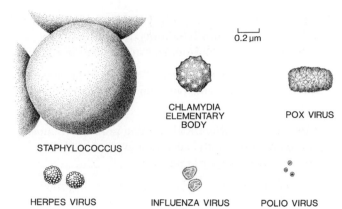

Figure 6-3. **The relative sizes of** *Staphylococcus* **and** *Chlamydia* **bacteria and several viruses.** Poliovirus is one of the smallest viruses that infect humans. (From Winn WC Jr, et al. Koneman's Color Atlas and Textbook of Diagnostic Microbiology. 6th Ed. Philadelphia: Lippincott Williams & Wilkins, 2006.)

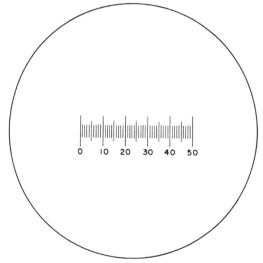

Figure 6-2. **Example of an ocular micrometer wafer, which is located within one of the eyepieces of a compound light microscope.** Ocular micrometers are discussed in detail in Appendix A. (From Winn WC Jr, et al. Koneman's Color Atlas and Textbook of Diagnostic Microbiology. 6th Ed. Philadelphia: Lippincott Williams & Wilkins, 2006.)

MICROSCOPES AND MICROSCOPY

The human eye, a telescope, a pair of binoculars, a magnifying glass, and a microscope can all be thought of as various types of optical instruments. A microscope is an optical instrument used for observing tiny objects, often objects that cannot be seen at all with the unaided human eye. Each optical instrument has a limit to what can be seen through it. This limit is referred to as the **resolving power** or **resolution** of the instrument. Resolving power will be discussed in more detail later in the chapter. Table 6-2 lists the resolving powers for various optical instruments.

Simple Microscopes

A **simple microscope** is defined as a microscope containing only one magnifying lens. Actually, a magnifying glass could be considered a simple microscope. Images seen through a magnifying glass usually appear about 3 to 20 times larger than the object's actual size.

Compound Microscopes

A **compound microscope** is a microscope that contains more than one magnifying lens. Compound light microscopes can magnify objects up to 1,000 times. Photographs taken

TABLE 6 - 1   Relative Sizes of Microbes

Microbe or Microbial Structure	Dimension(s)	Approximate Size (μm)
Viruses	Diameter	0.01–0.3
Bacteria		
Cocci (spherical bacteria)	Diameter	Average = 1
Bacilli (rod-shaped bacteria)	Width $\times$ length	Average = 1 $\times$ 3
	Filaments (width)	1
Fungi		
Yeasts	Width $\times$ length	3–5
Septate hyphae (hyphae containing cross-walls)	Width	2–15
Aseptate hyphae (hyphae without cross-walls)	Width	10–30

> A simple microscope contains only one magnifying lens, whereas a compound microscope contains more than one magnifying lens.

Because visible light, from a built-in light bulb, is used as the source of illumination, the compound microscope is also referred to as a **compound light microscope.** The wavelength of visible light (approximately 0.45 μm) limits the size of objects that can be seen using the compound light microscope. Under a compound light microscope, objects cannot be seen if they are smaller than half the wavelength of visible light. A compound light microscope is shown in Figure 6-4, and the functions of its various components are described in Table 6-3.

The compound light microscopes used in today's CMLs contain two magnifying lens systems. Within the eyepiece or ocular is a lens called the ocular lens; it usually has a magnifying power of $\times$10. The second magnifying lens system is in the objective, positioned directly above

through the lens system of compound microscopes are called **photomicrographs.**

> Total magnification of the compound light microscope is calculated by multiplying the magnifying power of the ocular by the magnifying power of the objective that is being used.

TABLE 6 - 2   Resolving Powers of Various Optical Instruments

Type of Optical Instrument	Approximate Resolving Power
The naked eye	0.2 mm
Compound light microscope	0.2 μm
Darkfield microscope	0.2 μm
Phase contrast microscope	0.2 μm
Fluorescence microscope	0.2 μm
Scanning electron microscope	20 nm
Transmission electron microscope	0.2 nm

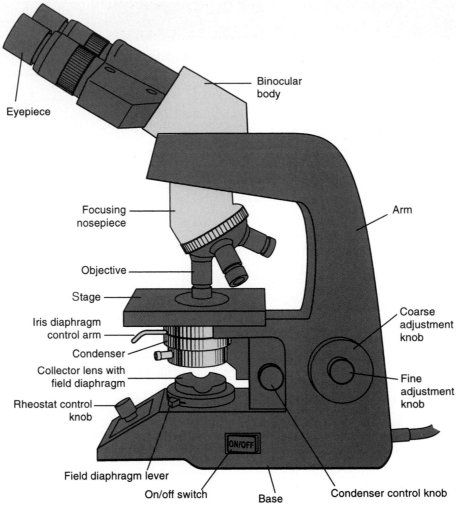

Figure 6-4. **A compound light microscope.**

the object to be viewed. The four objectives used in most lab-oratory compound light microscopes are ×4, ×10, ×40, and ×100 objectives. As shown in Table 6-4, total magnification is calculated by multiplying the magnifying power of the ocu-lar (×10) by the magnifying power of the objective that you are using.

The ×4 objective is rarely used in CMLs. Usually, specimens are first observed using the ×10 objective. Once the specimen is in focus, the high-power or "high-dry" ×40 objective is then swung into position. This lens can be used to study algae, protozoa, and other large microorganisms. However, the oil immersion objective (total magnification = ×1,000) must be used to study bac-teria because they are so tiny. To use the oil immersion objective, a drop of immersion oil must first be placed between the specimen and the objective. The immersion oil reduces the scattering of light and ensures that the light will enter the oil immersion lens.

For optimal observation of the specimen, the light must be properly adjusted and focused. The condenser,

located beneath the stage, focuses light onto the specimen, adjusts the amount of light, and shapes the cone of light entering the objective. Usually, the amount of light enter-ing the objective needs to be increased as magnification is increased.

Magnification alone is of little value unless the enlarged image pos-sesses increased detail and clarity. Image clar-ity depends on the microscope's **resolving power** (or **resolution**), which is the ability of the lens system to distinguish between two adjacent (side-by-side) objects. If two objects were to be moved closer and closer together, they eventually are so close that the lens system can no longer resolve them as two separate objects; that is, they are so close together they appear to be one object. The distance between them, where they cease to be seen as separate objects, is

> The resolving power or resolution of an optical instrument is its ability to distinguish between two adjacent objects.

TABLE 6 - 3   Components of a Compound Light Microscope

Component	Location	Function
Ocular lens; also known as an eyepiece; a binocular microscope (such as the one shown in Fig. 6-4) has two lenses		×10 magnification
Revolving nosepiece	Above the stage	Holds the objective lenses
Objective lenses	Held in place above the stage by the revolving nosepiece	Used to magnify objects placed on the stage
Stage	Directly beneath the nosepiece and objective lenses	Flat surface on which the specimen is placed
Stage adjustment knobs (not shown in Fig. 6-4)	Beneath the stage	Used to move the stage and specimen
Condenser	Directly beneath the stage	Contains a lens system that focuses light on the specimen
Condenser control knob	Beneath and to one side of the condenser	Used to adjust the height of the condenser
Iris diaphragm control arm	Attached to the condenser	Used to adjust the amount of light emitted from the condenser
Field diaphragm lever	Beneath the condenser and collector lens	Used to adjust the amount of light coming through the collector lens
Rheostat control knob	At the front of the base	Used to adjust the amount of light being emitted by the light bulb in the base
Coarse and fine adjustment knobs	On the arm of the microscope, near the base	Used to focus the lenses

referred to as the resolving power of the optical instrument. Knowing the resolving power of an optical instrument also defines the smallest object that can be seen with that instrument. For example, the resolving power of the unaided human eye is approximately 0.2 mm. Thus, the unaided human eye is unable to see objects smaller than 0.2 mm in diameter.

The resolving power of the compound light microscope is approximately 1,000 times better than the resolving power of the unaided human eye. In practical terms,

TABLE 6 - 4   Calculation of Total Magnification

Multiply the Magnifying Power of the Ocular Lens . . .	By the Magnifying Power of the Objective in Use to Achieve the . . .	Total Magnificaton
×10	×4	×40
×10	×10	×100
×10	×40	×400
×10	×100	×1,000

> The resolving power of the compound light microscope is approximately 0.2 μm, which is about one-half the wavelength of visible light.

this means that objects can be examined with the compound microscope that are as much as 1,000 times smaller than the smallest objects a person can see. Using a compound light microscope, a person can see objects down to about 0.2 μm in diameter.

Additional magnifying lenses could be added to the compound light microscope, but this would not increase the resolving power. As stated earlier, as long as visible light is used as the source of illumination, objects smaller than half the wavelength of visible light cannot be seen. Increasing magnification without increasing the resolving power is called **empty magnification.** It does no good to increase magnification without increasing resolving power.

Because objects are observed against a bright background, or "bright field," when a compound light microscope

> When using a brightfield microscope, a person can see objects against a bright background. When using a darkfield microscope, a person sees illuminated objects against a dark background.

is used, that microscope is sometimes referred to as a **brightfield microscope.** If the regularly used condenser is replaced with what is known as a darkfield condenser, illuminated objects are seen against a dark background, or "dark field," and the microscope has been converted into a **darkfield microscope.** In the CML, darkfield microscopy is routinely used to diagnose the initial stage of syphilis, known as primary syphilis. The etiologic (causative) agent of syphilis—a spiral-shaped bacterium named *Treponema pallidum*—cannot be seen with a brightfield microscope because it is thinner than 0.2 μm and therefore beneath the resolving power of the compound light microscope. *T. pallidum* can be seen using a darkfield microscope, however, much as you can "see" dust particles in a beam of sunlight. Dust particles are actually beneath the resolving power of the unaided eye and therefore cannot really be seen. What you see in the beam is sunlight being reflected off of the dust particles. With the darkfield microscope, CML professionals do not really *see* the treponemes; rather, they see the light being reflected off the bacteria, and that light is easily seen against the dark background (Fig. 6-5).

Other types of compound microscopes include phase contrast microscopes and fluorescence microscopes. **Phase contrast microscopes** can be used to observe unstained living microorganisms. Because the light refracted by living cells is different from the light refracted by the surrounding medium, contrast is increased, and the organisms are more

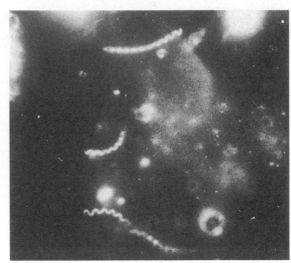

Figure 6-5. **Spiral-shaped *Treponema pallidum,* the bacterium that causes syphilis, as seen by darkfield microscopy.** (From Winn WC Jr, et al. Koneman's Color Atlas and Textbook of Diagnostic Microbiology. 6th Ed. Philadelphia: Lippincott Williams & Wilkins, 2006.)

easily seen. Phase contrast microscopy is also used in the mycology section of the CML to identify filamentous fungi (see Chapter 19). **Fluorescence microscopes** contain a built-in ultraviolet light source. When ultraviolet light strikes certain dyes and pigments, these substances emit a longer wavelength light, causing them to glow against a dark background. Fluorescence microscopy is often used in immunology laboratories to demonstrate that antibodies stained with a fluorescent dye have combined with specific antigens; this is a type of immunodiagnostic procedure. Immunodiagnostic procedures are described later in this chapter.

Electron Microscopes

Although extremely small infectious agents, such as rabies and smallpox viruses, were known to exist, they could not be seen until the electron microscope was developed. It should be noted that electron microscopes cannot be used to observe living organisms. Organisms are killed during the specimen processing procedures. Even if they were not, the organisms would be unable to survive in the vacuum that exists within the electron microscope.

Electron microscopes use an electron beam as a source of illumination instead of visible light and magnets instead of lenses to focus the beam. Because the wavelength of electrons traveling in a vacuum is much shorter than the wavelength of visible light—about 100,000 times shorter—electron microscopes have a much greater resolving power than do compound light microscopes. There are two main types of electron microscopes: transmission electron microscopes and scanning electron microscopes.

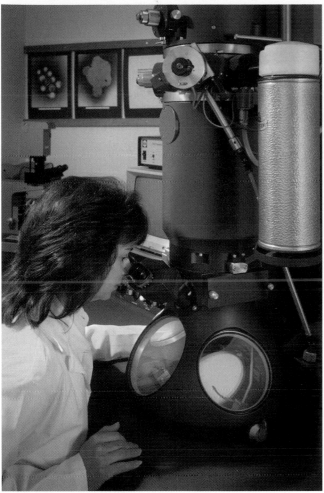

Figure 6-6. **Biologist using a transmission electron microscope.** (Courtesy of James Gathany and the Centers for Disease Control and Prevention.)

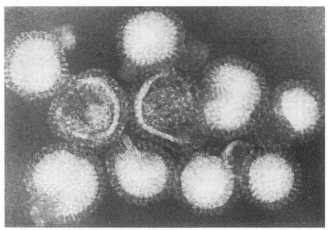

Figure 6-7. **A transmission electron micrograph of influenza virus A.** (From Winn WC Jr, et al. Koneman's Color Atlas and Textbook of Diagnostic Microbiology. 6th Ed. Philadelphia: Lippincott Williams & Wilkins, 2006.)

A **transmission electron microscope** (Fig. 6-6) has a very tall column, at the top of which an electron gun fires a beam of electrons downward. When an extremely thin specimen (less than 1 μm thick) is placed into the electron beam, some of the electrons are transmitted through the specimen, and some are blocked. An image of the specimen is produced on a phosphor-coated screen at the bottom of the microscope's column. The object can be magnified up to approximately 1 million times. Thus, using a transmission electron microscope, a magnification is achieved that is about 1,000 times greater than the maximum magnification

> The resolving power of a transmission electron microscope is approximately 0.2 nm, which is about a million times better than the resolving power of the unaided human eye and one thousand times better than the resolving power of the compound light microscope.

achieved using a compound light microscope. Even very tiny microbes (e.g., viruses) can be observed using a transmission electron microscope (Fig. 6-7). Because thin sections of cells are examined, transmission electron microscopy enables scientists to study the **internal structure** of cells. Special staining procedures are used to increase contrast between different parts of the cell. The first transmission electron microscopes were developed during the late 1920s and early 1930s, but it was not until the early 1950s that electron microscopes began to be used routinely to study cells.

A **scanning electron microscope** (Fig. 6-8) has a shorter column, and the specimen, instead of being placed into the electron beam, is placed at the bottom of the column. Electrons that bounce off the surface of the specimen are captured by detectors, and an image of the specimen appears on a monitor. Scanning electron microscopes are used to observe the outer surfaces of specimens (i.e., surface detail). Although the resolving power of scanning electron microscopes (about 20 nm) is not quite as good as the resolving power of transmission electron microscopes (about 0.2 nm), it is still possible to observe extremely small objects using a scanning electron microscope. Scanning electron microscopes became available during the late 1960s.

Both types of electron microscopes have built-in camera systems. The photographs taken using transmission and scanning electron microscopes are called **transmission electron micrographs** and **scanning electron micrographs,** respectively. They are black-and-white images. If you ever see electron micrographs in color, they have been artificially colorized. Figures 6-9, 6-10, and 6-11 show the differences in magnification and detail between light micrographs and electron micrographs. Refer to Table 6-2 for the characteristics of various types of microscopes.

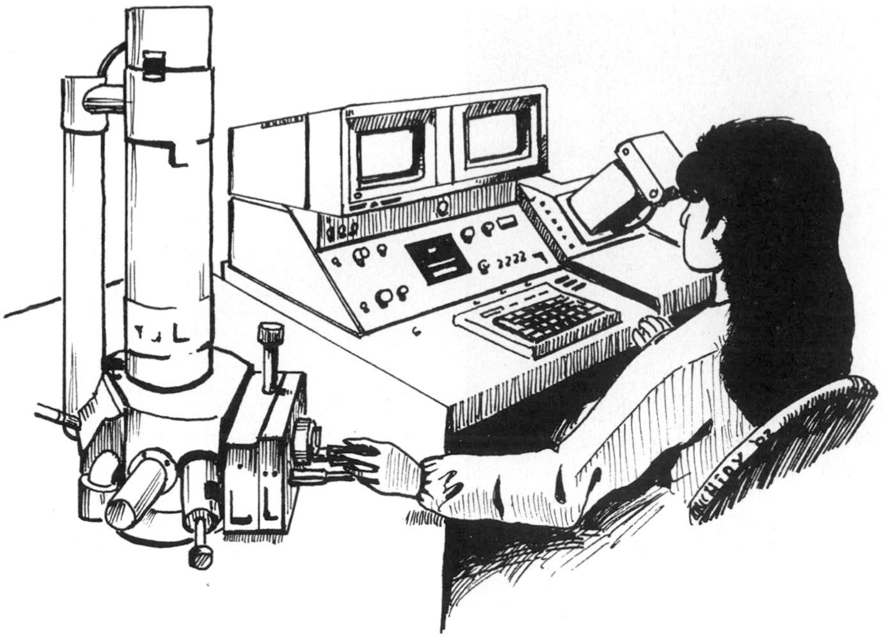

Figure 6-8. **A scanning electron microscope.**

EXAMINING CLINICAL SPECIMENS AND COLONIES USING WET MOUNTS

Unstained clinical and culture materials are sometimes examined using a very simple technique known as the **wet mount.** Wet mounts are easier and faster to perform than Gram staining or other staining procedures.

To prepare a wet mount of a liquid clinical specimen, a drop of the specimen is added to a glass microscope slide, and a glass coverslip is placed over the drop. The preparation is then examined under the microscope, using low power and high-dry objectives. The oil immersion objective is not used because the contact among the objective, immersion oil, and coverslip would cause the preparation

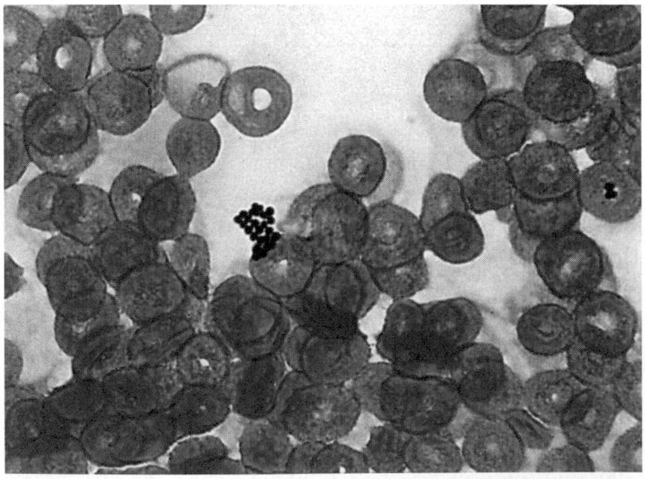

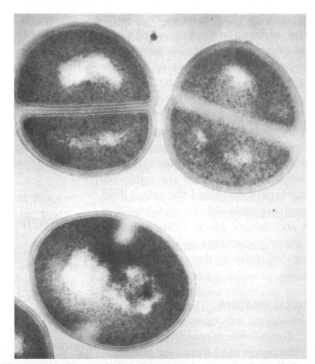

Figure 6-9. **Photomicrograph of *Staphylococcus aureus* (blue spheres) in a Gram-stained blood specimen.** (From Marler LM, Siders JA, Allen SD. Direct Smear Atlas. Philadelphia: Lippincott Williams & Wilkins, 2001.)

Figure 6-10. **Transmission electron micrograph of *Staphylococcus aureus* cells in various stages of binary fission.** (From Volk WA, Gebhardt BM, Hammarskjöld M, Kadner RJ. Essentials of Medical Microbiology. 5th Ed. Philadelphia: Lippincott-Raven, 1996.)

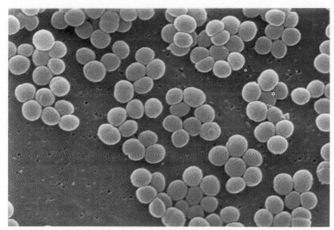

Figure 6-11. **Scanning electron micrograph of *Staphylococcus aureus*.** (Courtesy of Janice Carr, Matthew J. Arduino, and the Centers for Disease Control and Prevention.)

to move around. One of the most common uses of a wet mount is in the diagnosis of vaginitis, where vaginal discharge material is examined for the presence of yeasts (*Candida albicans*), protozoa (*Trichomonas vaginalis*), or evidence of bacterial infection. Appendix A contains details of this technique, as well as other procedures used in the CML.

A wet mount may also be used to differentiate between a bacterial colony and a yeast colony or to determine motility. To prepare a wet mount of a bacterial or yeast colony, a drop of water or saline is first added to a glass microscope slide. Using a sterile inoculating loop, a very small portion of the colony is then mixed into the drop. A glass coverslip is placed over the drop, and the preparation is then examined under the microscope. Yeast cells can be distinguished from bacterial cells by size and shape. Yeast cells are larger—up to about 10 times larger than bacteria. Also, yeast cells are usually oval shaped, and some may be observed in the process of budding. Except in extremely rare cases, bacteria do not produce buds.

Wet mounts of colonies or liquid cultures can also be used to determine if organisms are motile. If motile, they will be observed "swimming" in the wet mount. Occasionally, nonmotile objects (such as yeast cells) that have been in a wet mount and examined under a microscope for a while appear to start vibrating. This vibration, technically called **Brownian movement,** is the result of heat from the microscope bulb. The heat causes water molecules to move about rapidly, striking the objects, and causing them to vibrate.

> The movement of nonmotile objects observed under a compound light microscope is referred to as Brownian movement.

CULTURE MEDIA

The traditional method of determining the bacterial or fungal cause of a patient's infectious disease was to (1) inoculate the clinical specimen to some type of culture medium, (2) isolate the pathogen from any other microorganisms that might be present in the specimen, (3) grow the pathogen in pure culture, and (4) gather information (clues) about the pathogen's phenotype until there was sufficient information to identify or speciate the organism.

Types of Culture Media

The term *culture media* refers to the various types of nutrient-containing liquid and solid mixtures used in CMLs to culture (grow) microorganisms—primarily, bacteria and fungi. The media are referred to as **artificial media** or **synthetic media** because they do not occur naturally but are prepared in the laboratory. There are several ways to categorize culture media, as described in the paragraphs that follow.

Liquid media, also known as broths, are usually contained in tubes and are thus often referred to as tubed media. **Solid media** are prepared by adding agar to liquid media and then pouring the liquid media into tubes or circular, shallow, plastic containers called petri dishes, where the media solidifies. Petri dishes containing media are often referred to as "plates" or "plated media." Bacteria or fungi are then grown on the surface of the agar-containing solid media. Agar is a complex polysaccharide obtained from a red marine alga. It is used as a solidifying agent, much like gelatin is used as a solidifying agent in the kitchen. Examples of liquid and solid culture media are shown in Figure 6-12.

> Agar is used as a solidifying agent in the preparation of solid culture media. Solid culture media is usually contained in circular, shallow, plastic containers called petri dishes.

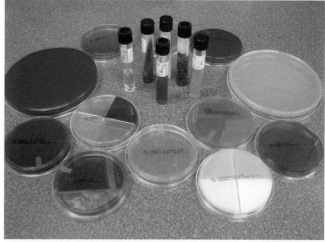

Figure 6-12. **Solid and liquid culture media.** (Courtesy of Dr. Robert Fader.)

A **chemically defined medium** is one in which all the ingredients are known, because the medium was prepared in the laboratory by adding a certain number of grams of each of the components, such as carbohydrates, amino acids, and salts. On the other hand, in a **complex medium,** the exact contents are not known. Complex media contain ground-up or digested extracts from animal organs (e.g., hearts, livers, brains), fish, yeasts, and plants, which provide the necessary nutrients, vitamins, and minerals.

An **enrichment medium** is a broth containing specific nutrients that have been added to the medium to encourage the growth of a particular organism. A clinical specimen is usually inoculated into an enrichment broth when it is suspected that only small numbers of

> An enrichment medium is used to encourage the growth of a particular organism, thereby improving the chance of isolating that organism from a clinical specimen.

the pathogen are present in the specimen. An example of an enrichment medium is Gram-negative broth, which is used to recover *Shigella* and *Salmonella* spp. from fecal specimens. Selenite broth is another example of an enrichment medium, used primarily for recovery of *Salmonella* spp.

An **enriched medium** is a broth or solid medium containing a rich supply of special nutrients that promotes the growth of fastidious ("fussy") organisms, such as most bacterial pathogens. It is usually prepared by adding extra nutrients to a medium called nutrient agar. Blood agar (nutrient agar plus 5% sheep red blood cells) and chocolate agar (nutrient agar plus powdered hemoglobin) are examples of solid enriched media routinely used in the bacteriology section of the CML. Blood and chocolate agars are described in greater detail in Chapter 8.

> An enriched medium contains sufficient nutrients to grow most bacterial pathogens.

A **selective medium** contains substances that inhibit growth of certain organisms without inhibiting growth of the organism(s) being sought. For example, MacConkey agar is used in the bacteriology section to isolate Gram-negative bacteria.

> A selective medium is used to grow an organism or organisms of interest, while inhibiting growth of unwanted organisms.

MacConkey agar contains substances that inhibit growth of Gram-positive bacteria. Thus, MacConkey agar is said to be selective for Gram-negative bacteria. Media called phenylethyl alcohol medium and colistin-nalidixic acid medium are selective for Gram-positive bacteria. (**Note:** The terms *Gram-positive* and *Gram-negative* are defined later in this chapter.) Other examples of selective media are described in Chapter 8.

A **differential medium** permits the differentiation of organisms that grow on the medium. MacConkey agar is a good example of a differential medium. It is frequently used to differentiate between various Gram-negative bacilli isolated from fecal specimens. Gram-negative bacteria that can ferment lactose (an ingredient of MacConkey agar) produce pink colonies, whereas those that cannot ferment lactose produce colorless colonies. Thus, MacConkey agar differentiates between lactose fermenting and non-lactose-fermenting Gram-negative bacteria (Fig. 6-13). Other examples of differential media are described in Chapter 8.

> A differential medium enables differentiation of various organisms that are growing on the medium.

The enriched, selective, and differential categories of media are not mutually exclusive. For example, as just described, MacConkey agar is both selective and differential.

Importance of Sterile Technique

CML professionals must practice what is known as **sterile technique,** and must understand its importance. Sterile technique is practiced when it is necessary to exclude *all* microorganisms from a particular area to make it sterile. For example, while inoculating a plated medium, it is important to keep the petri dish lid in place at all times, except for the few seconds that it takes to inoculate the specimen to the surface of the medium. Every additional second that the lid is off provides an opportunity for airborne organisms (e.g., bacterial and fungal spores) to land on the surface of the medium, where they will then grow. Such unwanted organisms are referred to as **contaminants,** and the plate is said to be **contaminated**. Of equal importance is

> Using sterile technique in the CML prevents accidental contamination of culture media.

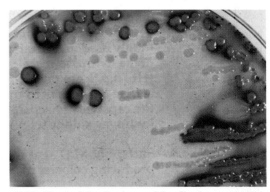

Figure 6-13. Bacterial colonies on MacConkey agar. This selective and differential medium is selective for Gram-negative bacteria, meaning that only Gram-negative bacteria will grow on MacConkey agar. Colonies of lactose fermenters (pink colonies) and non-lactose fermenters (clear colonies) can be seen. (From Winn WC Jr, et al. Koneman's Color Atlas and Textbook of Diagnostic Microbiology. 6th Ed. Philadelphia: Lippincott Williams & Wilkins, 2006.)

to maintain the sterility of the medium before inoculation and to avoid touching the agar surface with fingertips or other nonsterile objects. Inoculating media within a biological safety cabinet (BSC) minimizes the possibility of contamination and protects the laboratory worker from becoming infected with the organism(s) with which he or she is working. BSCs are discussed in Chapter 4.

Inoculation of Culture Media

Within CMLs, culture media are routinely inoculated with clinical specimens.

Inoculation of a liquid medium involves adding a portion of the specimen to the medium. Inoculation of a solid or plated medium involves the use of a sterile bacteriological loop (or inoculating loop) to apply a portion of the specimen to the surface of the medium; a process commonly referred to as streaking (Fig. 6-14). The proper method of inoculating plated media to obtain well-isolated colonies is described in Appendix A.

A different method of inoculation is used to obtain a colony count, such as that required for workup of a clean-catch midstream urine. Likewise, plates being used for antimicrobial susceptibility testing are also inoculated in a different manner. In each case, plates are inoculated in a way that will result in a **lawn of growth,** where the inoculated organism grows over the entire surface of the plate. Details of this inoculation technique can be found in Appendix A.

Inoculated plates are always labeled on the underside of the plate, not the lid. Thus, should the lid become separated from the agar-containing bottom portion of the plate, the identity of the patient and/or specimen will remain with the inoculated medium.

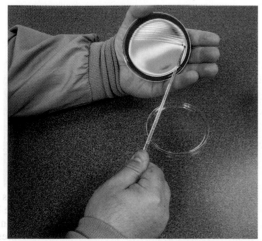

***Figure 6-14.* CML professional inoculating the surface of a plated medium.** Notice that the plate is held in the palm of one hand, and the other hand is used to lightly drag the inoculating loop over the surface of the medium. (Courtesy of Dr. Robert Fader.)

Incubation of Inoculated Culture Media

After culture media are inoculated, they must be incubated. That is, they must be placed into a chamber (called an incubator) that contains the appropriate atmosphere and moisture level. The incubator is set to maintain the appropriate temperature. To culture most human pathogens, the incubator is set at 35°C to 37°C. Three types of incubators are used in a CML:

- A **CO₂ (carbon dioxide) incubator** has a cylinder of CO_2 attached. CO_2 is periodically introduced into the incubator to maintain a concentration of about 5% to 10%. Such an incubator is used to isolate capnophiles—organisms that grow best in atmospheres containing increased CO_2. It is important to keep in mind that a CO_2 incubator contains oxygen (about 15% to 20%), in addition to CO_2. Therefore, this type of incubator is *not* anaerobic.

- A **non-CO₂ incubator** contains room air; thus, it contains about 20% to 21% O_2.

- An **anaerobic incubator** contains an atmosphere devoid of oxygen.

> An incubator provides the appropriate temperature, humidity, and atmosphere for the growth of microorganisms.

Within the incubator, plates are stacked with the underside of the plates upward. If plates were incubated with the lid side up, water vapor produced by the metabolizing organisms would accumulate on the underside of the lid and drip down onto the surface of the

> Always label the bottom of inoculated plates, and incubate the plates with the agar side up.

agar medium. This would make the agar surface too wet for some organisms to survive. Other organisms—those that are highly motile—would "swim" over the wet agar surface, preventing the formation of discrete colonies.

Some CMLs use a candle jar or candle extinction jar to obtain the proper atmosphere to isolate *Neisseria gonorrhoeae* from specimens (Fig. 6-15). Inoculated plates are stacked in a glass jar with the agar side up. A lighted candle is placed on top of the stack, and the jar is tightly sealed. The flame goes out when there is insufficient oxygen to support combustion; thus, the oxygen concentration within the jar has decreased. At the same time, the burning candle has raised the CO_2 concentration in the jar. In place of candles, many CMLs use commercial packets that produce a comparable atmosphere.

Once a particular microbial species has been isolated from a clinical specimen, it can be separated from any other organisms that were present in the specimen and can be grown as a pure culture. As mentioned in Chapter 4, the term *pure culture* refers to there being only one species present.

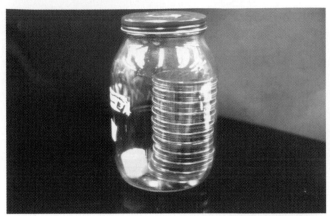

***Figure 6-15.* A candle extinction jar.** This jar is being used to culture *Neisseria gonorrhoeae.* (Courtesy of Dr. Michael Rein and the Centers for Disease Control and Prevention.)

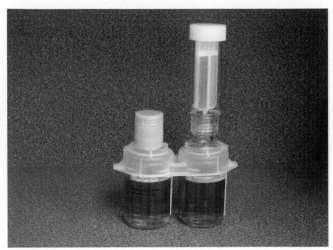

***Figure 6-16.* The Septi-Check blood culture system, manufactured by BD Biosciences.** The aerobic bottle to the right is a biphasic system, consisting of a broth-containing vial with an attached agar-coated plastic paddle. (Courtesy of Dr. Robert Fader.)

MANUAL BLOOD CULTURE METHODS

The techniques used to isolate bacteria or fungi from blood are collectively referred to as blood culture systems. Traditional blood culture techniques involve (1) inoculating a blood specimen into broth-containing culture vials, usually one aerobic vial and one anaerobic vial; (2) incubating the vials at 35°C; (3) macroscopically inspecting the vials periodically for evidence of microbial growth, such as increased turbidity, hemolysis, gas bubbles, and/or presence of colonies; (4) Gram staining the blood-broth mixture; and (5) performing subcultures. Blind subcultures (subcultures that are performed even though no visible evidence of microbial growth is observed) are usually performed at specific intervals. Traditional blood culture techniques are time consuming and labor intensive.

> The presence of increased turbidity, hemolysis, gas bubbles, and/or colonies provides evidence of microbial growth within blood culture bottles.

Newer blood culture methods include both automated and nonautomated methods. Several of the nonautomated methods are discussed here; automated methods are discussed later in the chapter. Nonautomated methods include the Septi-Chek, Oxoid Signal, and Isolator blood culture systems.

The Septi-Chek blood culture system, manufactured by BD Biosciences (http://www.bdbiosciences.com/) is shown in Figure 6-16. It consists of a broth-containing vial with an attached agar-coated plastic paddle. A culture system consisting of both a liquid medium and a solid medium is referred to as a **biphasic system.** The paddle is attached to the vial after a blood specimen is injected into the vial. Following attachment of the paddle, the vial is tipped to allow the blood-broth mixture to flood the paddle. Any microorganisms present will adhere to the agar and produce colonies. The colonies can then be used for microorganism identification and antimicrobial susceptibility testing. If no colonies are observed, the vial can be tipped again at specific intervals to reinoculate the solid medium.

Another nonautomated blood culture method is the Oxoid Signal blood culture system, manufactured by Oxoid Inc. (http://www.oxoid.ca/). Following the inoculation of blood into the broth-containing vial, a plastic signal device is attached to the vial. The device contains a long needle that extends beneath the surface of the broth. If microbial growth occurs in the broth, the gases produced as a result of metabolism rise to the headspace. The additional headspace pressure forces some of the blood-broth mixture up the needle and into the chamber of the signal device. Thus, the presence of some of the blood-broth mixture serves as a signal that microbial growth has occurred in the vial. The CML professional will then Gram stain and subculture the blood-broth mixture present in the chamber of the signal device.

The Isolator blood culture system, manufactured by Wampole Laboratories (a division of Inverness Medical; http://www.invernessmedicalpd.com/) is shown in Figure 6-17. Unlike the Septi-Chek and Oxoid Signal blood culture systems, the Isolator system is not based on growth of microorganisms in a liquid culture medium. Rather, it is based on lysis and centrifugation. A blood specimen is inoculated into the Isolator tube, which contains a solution that lyses the blood cells. Following centrifugation of the tube and removal of the liquid, the sedimented pellet is resuspended and inoculated to appropriate types of solid, plated media. Any colonies that appear on the plated media are then used for microorganism identification and antimicrobial susceptibility testing. The Isolator system is more

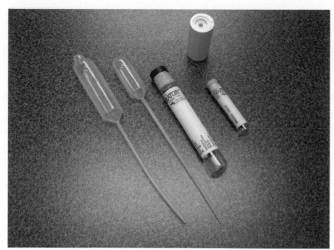

Figure 6-17. **The Isolator blood culture system, manufactured by Wampole Laboratories.** The smaller tube is used for pediatric blood specimens. (Courtesy of Dr. Robert Fader.)

labor intensive than either the Septi-Chek or Oxoid Signal blood culture systems.

STAINING TECHNIQUES

Many types of staining techniques are used in the CML, including procedures to stain bacteria, fungi, parasites, and viruses. As examples, some of the staining techniques used in the bacteriology section are briefly discussed here. Additional staining procedures will be discussed in Chapters 8, 19, and 21.

As they exist in nature, bacteria are colorless, transparent, and difficult to see. Therefore, various staining methods have been devised to enable scientists to see and examine bacteria. In preparation for staining, the bacteria are smeared onto a glass microscope slide, resulting in what is known as a smear. The smear is then air dried and fixed. Methods for preparing and fixing smears are further described in Appendix A. The two most common methods of fixation are heat fixation and methanol fixation. Heat fixation is best accomplished using a slide warmer or a heat block; overheating tends to distort the morphology of the cells. Methanol fixation, which is accomplished by flooding the smear with absolute methanol for 30 seconds, is a more satisfactory fixation technique. Fixation serves three purposes:

> The primary purpose for staining bacteria is to be able to see them.
> Simple stains enable CML professionals to determine the size, shape, and morphological arrangement of bacteria.

- It kills the organisms.
- It preserves their morphology (shape).
- It anchors the smear to the slide.

Specific stains and staining techniques are used to observe bacterial cell morphology (e.g., size, shape, morphological arrangement of cells, composition of cell wall, capsules, flagella, and endospores).

A **simple stain** is sufficient to determine bacterial size, shape, and morphological arrangement (e.g., pairs, chains, clusters). For this method, a dye, such as methylene blue, is applied to the fixed smear, rinsed, dried, and examined using the oil immersion lens of the microscope. The staining procedures used to observe bacterial capsules, spores, and flagella are collectively referred to as **structural staining procedures**.

> Structural staining procedures are used to observe bacterial structures, such as capsules, spores, and flagella.

Differential staining procedures enable CML professionals to differentiate between groups of bacteria. Two very important differential staining procedures used in the bacteriology section are the Gram staining procedure and the acid-fast staining procedure.

- The **Gram staining procedure** differentiates between bacteria that are blue to purple at the end of the staining procedure (known as Gram-positive bacteria) and those that are pink to red at the end of the procedure (known as Gram-negative bacteria). Gram-positive and Gram-negative bacteria are shown in Figure 6-18.

> Differential staining procedures enable CML professionals to differentiate between various groups of bacteria (e.g., to differentiate between Gram-positive and Gram-negative bacteria).

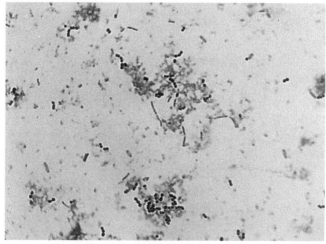

Figure 6-18. **Gram-stained material from an arm wound.** Both Gram-positive (*blue*) and Gram-negative (*red*) bacteria can be seen in this photomicrograph. (From Marler LM, Siders JA, Allen SD. Direct Smear Atlas. Philadelphia: Lippincott Williams & Wilkins, 2001.)

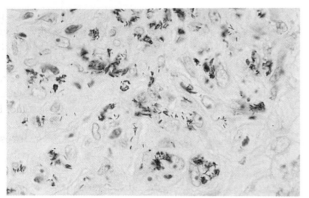

Figure 6-19. **Red acid-fast bacteria in an acid-fast stained liver biopsy specimen.** In the CML, these bacteria were later identified as members of the *Mycobacterium avium-intracellulare* complex. (From Winn WC Jr, et al. Koneman's Color Atlas and Textbook of Diagnostic Microbiology. 6th Ed. Philadelphia: Lippincott Williams & Wilkins, 2006.)

Additional information about the Gram staining procedure is in Chapter 8 and Appendix A.

- The **acid-fast staining procedure** differentiates between bacteria that are red at the end of the procedure (known as acid-fast bacteria) and bacteria that are green or blue at the end of the procedure (known as non-acid-fast bacteria). Acid-fast bacteria are shown in Figure 6-19. The acid-fast staining procedure is described in detail in Chapter 10. Chapter 10 also contains a detailed discussion of the meaning of the term *acid-fast*.

Table 6-5 summarizes the categories of staining techniques used in the bacteriology section. Table 6-6 contains examples of staining procedures used in sections of the CML other than the bacteriology section.

IDENTIFICATION OF MICROORGANISMS USING BIOCHEMICAL TESTS

Detecting the Presence or Absence of Specific Enzymes

Once a pure culture of the suspected pathogen has been obtained, it can be used to inoculate a series of biochemical tests to gather information about the organism's phenotypic characteristics. By inoculating these biochemical tests,

TABLE 6 - 5 Categories of Staining Techniques Used in the Bacteriology Section of the CML

Category	Example(s)	Purpose
Simple staining procedures	Staining with methylene blue	Merely to stain the cells so that their size, shape, and morphological arrangement can be determined
Structural staining procedures	Capsule stains	To determine whether or not the organism is encapsulated
	Flagella stains	To determine if the organism possesses flagella and, if so, their number and location on the cell
	Endospore stains	To determine if the organism is a spore former and, if so, to determine if the spores are terminal or subterminal spores
Differential staining procedures	Gram stain	To differentiate between Gram-positive and Gram-negative bacteria
	Acid-fast stain	To differentiate between acid-fast and non-acid-fast bacteria

TABLE 6 - 6	Examples of Staining Techniques Used in Sections of the CML Other Than the Bacteriology Section	
CML Section	**Staining Technique**	**Purpose**
Mycology	Calcofluor white	Can be mixed with potassium hydroxide in the KOH prep; requires the use of a fluorescence microscope; fungi (including *Pneumocystis* cysts) will fluoresce a bright bluish white or green, depending on the filter being used
	India ink wet mount (a black dye called nigrosin can be used in place of India ink)	Used in the India ink prep, a negative staining procedure for presumptive diagnosis of cryptococcal meningitis
	Lactophenol cotton blue	Used to stain fungal cultures in tease mount and cellophane tape preparations
Parasitology	Calcofluor white	Used to stain cysts of free-living amebae (e.g., *Naegleria* and *Acanthamoeba* spp.)
	Giemsa, Wright, and Wright-Giemsa stains	Used to stain peripheral blood smears to detect malaria parasites, *Babesia*, trypanomastigotes, microfilariae, etc.
	Modified Kinyoun acid-fast stain	Used to detect *Cryptosporidium*, *Isospora*, and *Cyclospora* in fecal preparations
	Trichrome stain	Used to stain intestinal parasites in fecal preparations
	Iodine	Used to stain intestinal parasites in fecal preparations

CML professionals learn what enzymes the organism does or does not possess.

Enzymes are protein molecules that serve as biological catalysts, meaning that they cause biochemical reactions to occur or speed up the rate at which they occur. Enzymes are very specific. A given enzyme can catalyze only one specific reaction. The molecule on which the enzyme acts or exerts its effect is called the **substrate** for that enzyme.

> Learning which enzymes an organism does or does not produce provides important clues about the organism's identity.

An organism's ability to produce or not produce a particular enzyme is part of that organism's phenotype. Thus, when a CML professional discovers what enzymes an organism does or does not produce, that person is gathering clues to the identity of the organism. Specific enzymes to be discussed in future chapters include catalase, coagulase, oxidase, and urease.

STUDY AID **Names of Enzymes.** An enzyme is usually named by adding the suffix *-ase* to the name of the compound or types of compounds on which the enzyme acts or exerts its effect. For example, proteases, carbohydrases, and lipases are enzymes specific for proteins, carbohydrates, and lipids, respectively. The specific molecule on which an enzyme acts is referred to as that enzyme's substrate. Each enzyme has a particular substrate on which it exerts its effect; thus, enzymes are very specific. Although most enzymes end in *-ase*, some do not, like lysozyme and hemolysins.

Determining an Organism's Ability to Catabolize Various Substrates

The term **metabolism** relates to *all* the biochemical reactions that occur within an organism—biochemical reactions collec-

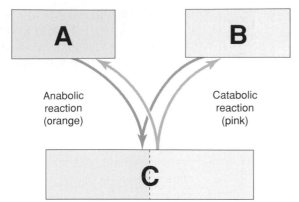

Figure 6-20. **Anabolic and catabolic reactions.** An anabolic reaction joins smaller molecules (**A, B**) together to produce a larger molecule (**C**). A catabolic reaction breaks a larger molecule (**C**) down into smaller molecules (**A, B**).

tively referred to as **metabolic reactions.** Metabolism can be divided into two parts: **catabolism** and **anabolism** (Fig. 6-20). Key facts about catabolism and anabolism are summarized in Table 6-7. Most metabolic reactions are catalyzed by enzymes.

Many of the biochemical tests performed in the CML to identify a bacterial isolate determine which substrates (e.g., carbohydrates and amino acids) the organism is able to catabolize, or break down. In the past, each biochemical test was set up in a separate test tube, which was expensive and labor intensive. In today's CMLs, many of these biochemical tests are incorporated into rapid manual (nonautomated), semiautomated, and automated identification systems. These systems are often referred to as **minisystems,** short for "miniaturized biochemical test systems." Manual systems rely on the analytical skills of CML professionals for reading and interpreting test results. In both semiautomated and automated systems, test results are read by an instrument. In semiautomated systems, preincubated cards, panels, or trays are

inserted into the instrument. In automated systems, inoculated cards, panels, or trays are inserted into the instrument, within which they are incubated. Minisystems used for identifying bacteria are discussed in Chapter 8; those used to identify yeasts are discussed in Chapter 19. Figure 6-21 illustrates one of the more popular manual minisystems.

IDENTIFICATION OF MICROORGANISMS USING GAS-LIQUID CHROMATOGRAPHY

Gas-liquid chromatography (GLC) is frequently used in reference laboratories as an adjunct to other identification methods. GLC uses the chemical and physical properties of a particular component to separate it from other components in a mixture. Two ways in which GLC can be used in the identification of bacteria and yeasts are (1) analysis of acid end products of metabolism and (2) analysis of cellular fatty acids. Fatty acids are the building blocks of lipids. In the first technique, metabolic end products or their methyl esters are first extracted from broth cultures, and then injected into the gas-liquid chromatograph. In the second technique, bacterial cells are saponified (converted into soap) to release the fatty acids from lipids within the cells. Next the fatty acids are treated with methyl alcohol, creating volatile methyl esters. The methyl esters are then extracted from the aqueous phase into an organic solvent, base washed, and injected into a gas-liquid chromatograph. Some models are equipped with computer data systems that identify peaks obtained with the "unknown" isolates by comparing them with peaks obtained with a standard solution. Gas-liquid chromatographs, columns, and standards are available from SRI Instruments (http://www.srigc.com/) and Supelco (a division

TABLE 6 - 7	Key Differences Between Catabolism and Anabolism
Catabolism	**Anabolism**
A term referring to all of the catabolic reactions that occur within an organism.	A term referring to all of the anabolic reactions that occur within an organism.
Catabolic reactions release energy.	Anabolic reactions require energy.
Catabolic reactions involve the breaking of chemical bonds. Whenever chemical bonds are broken, energy is released.	Anabolic reactions involve the creation of chemical bonds. It takes energy to create chemical bonds.
In catabolic reactions, larger molecules are broken down into smaller molecules.	In anabolic reactions, smaller molecules are bonded together to create larger molecules.
Catabolic reactions are sometimes referred to as degradative reactions.	Anabolic reactions are sometimes referred to as biosynthetic reactions.

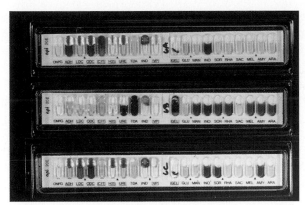

Figure 6-21. **An example of a minisystem.** These three API 20E strips were inoculated with suspensions of three different members of the Enterobacteriaceae family. After 18 to 20 hours of incubation, the colors in the compartments are interpreted as either positive or negative results. Based on the positive and negative reactions, a seven-digit biotype number is calculated. In most cases, the number is specific for a particular species. (From Winn WC Jr, et al. Koneman's Color Atlas and Textbook of Diagnostic Microbiology. 6th Ed. Philadelphia: Lippincott Williams & Wilkins, 2006.)

of Sigma-Aldrich; http://www.sigma-aldrich.com/). The MIDI Sherlock Microbial Identification System, or MIDI, is a fully automated gas chromatographic system for identification of bacteria and yeasts by cellular fatty acid analysis; it is available from MIDI Inc. (http://www.midilabs.com/).

High-pressure liquid chromatography of mycolic acids is a useful technique for identification of *Mycobacterium* spp. (see Chapter 10). Mycolic acids are high-molecular-weight fatty acids found in the cell walls of mycobacteria and related bacteria.

IMMUNODIAGNOSTIC PROCEDURES

Traditionally, the major criticism of the CML has been speed—that it takes too long to get results from the lab. This is primarily a result of it taking days, or even weeks in some cases, to isolate microbes in the laboratory—to get them growing in pure culture, in large numbers, so that sufficient inoculum is available for the tests necessary to identify them. With certain infectious diseases, it is impossible to isolate the pathogens because they will not grow on artificial media. Two approaches to diagnosing infectious diseases have greatly reduced the time it takes to obtain a diagnosis. One method is the use of immunodiagnostic procedures, which are described here, and the other is the use of molecular diagnostic procedures, which are described later in the chapter.

Immunodiagnostic procedures (IDPs) are laboratory procedures that help to diagnose infectious diseases by detecting either antigens or antibodies in clinical specimens. The results of such procedures are often available on the

same day that the clinical specimen is collected from the patient. IDPs performed on serum specimens are sometimes referred to as **serologic procedures**; for this reason, the immunology section of the CML is sometimes called the serology section. Some IDPs are designed to detect antigens, whereas others detect antibodies (Fig. 6-22).

Detection of a particular pathogen's antigens in a clinical specimen is an indication that the pathogen is present in the patient, thus providing direct evidence that the patient is infected with that pathogen. Detection of antibodies directed against a particular pathogen is indirect evidence of infection with that pathogen. However, there are three possible explanations for the presence of antibodies to a particular pathogen:

1. Present infection: the person is currently infected with the pathogen

2. Past infection: the person was infected with the pathogen in the past, and antibodies directed against that pathogen are still present in the person's body

3. Vaccination; the antibodies are the result of the person having been vaccinated against that particular pathogen at some time in the past; for example, a person's serum may contain antibodies against influenza viruses because the person received a flu shot last year

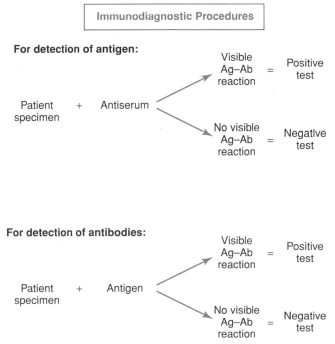

Figure 6-22. **Principles of antigen and antibody detection procedures.** Depending on the type of immunodiagnostic procedure being performed, the visible antigen-antibody (Ag-Ab) reaction might be agglutination (clumping) of cells or latex particles, formation of a precipitin line or band, fluorescence, or production of a color (as in enzyme immunoassays).

Because several explanations are possible for the presence of antibodies in a clinical specimen, the presence of **antigens** provides the best proof of current infection. Unfortunately, antigen detection procedures are not available for many infectious diseases. Another problem with antibody detection procedures is that it takes a person about 10 to 14 days to produce detectible antibodies. Thus, even if the person is infected with a particular pathogen, antibodies will not be detectible for about 2 weeks.

Two ways to increase the value of antibody detection procedures to diagnose present infection are (1) to specifically test for a particular class of antibodies called IgM antibodies and (2) to use paired sera. Because IgM antibodies are the first antibodies produced during the initial exposure to an antigen, in what is known as the primary response, and are relatively short lived, the presence of IgM antibodies directed against a particular pathogen is evidence that the pathogen is *currently* infecting the patient. To test paired sera, one serum specimen, referred to as the acute or acute-phase serum, is collected during the acute stage of the disease; another serum specimen, referred to as the convalescent or convalescent-phase serum, is collected 2 weeks later. A significant rise in antibody titer (concentration) between the acute and convalescent sera is evidence that the patient was actively producing antibodies against the pathogen during the 2-week period and therefore the pathogen is the cause of the patient's current infection. Usually, a fourfold or greater rise in antibody titer suggests a recent infection.

The reagents used to detect either antigens or antibodies are purchased from commercial companies. The reagent used to detect antigens contains antibodies and is called an **antiserum.** An antiserum is usually prepared by inoculating a laboratory animal with the pathogen—usually dead pathogens are used—and then collecting blood from the animal several weeks later. The blood is allowed to clot, and the serum is drawn off. The reagent used to detect antibodies contains antigens. This is usually a suspension of the dead pathogen.

A variety of different laboratory tests have been designed so that a visible reaction will be observed if an antigen-antibody reaction takes place. They include agglutination procedures, involving the clumping of particles such as bacterial cells, red blood cells, or latex particles; precipitin procedures, involving the production of a precipitate; immunodiffusion, immunoelectrophoresis, and immunofluorescence procedures; and enzyme-linked immunosorbent assays (ELISAs), some of which are described later in this chapter.

Antigen Detection Procedures

For detection of antigen in a clinical specimen, the specimen is mixed with a particular antiserum (see Fig. 6-22). A visible reaction is the result of the formation of antigen-antibody complexes, and indicates that the antigen is present in the clinical specimen. Thus, the test is considered positive. If the visible reaction is not observed, then the antigen is not present in the specimen and the test is considered negative.

Example

A drop of cerebrospinal fluid (CSF) from a patient with meningitis is mixed with a drop of antiserum containing antibodies against the yeast *Cryptococcus neoformans*. A visible antigen-antibody reaction is evidence that the patient's CSF contained *C. neoformans* antigens, and the patient is diagnosed as having meningitis caused by *C. neoformans*.

Purified antibodies directed against specific antigens have been produced in laboratories by an innovative technique in which a single plasma cell that produces only one type of antibody is fused with a rapidly dividing tumor cell. The new, long-lived, antibody-producing cell is called a **hybridoma.** These hybridomas are capable of producing large amounts of specific antibodies called **monoclonal antibodies.** The first monoclonal antibodies were produced in 1975, and since then many uses have been found for them. They are commonly used in IDPs. The first diagnostic kit containing monoclonal antibodies was approved for use in the United States in 1981. Many other monoclonal antibody-based IDPs have been developed over the past 25 years. Monoclonal antibodies are also being evaluated for possible use in fighting diseases, killing tumor cells, and boosting the immune system.

Antibody Detection Procedures

For detection of antibodies in a clinical specimen, the specimen is mixed with a suspension of a particular antigen (see Fig. 6-22). A visible reaction indicates that antibodies against that pathogen are present in the clinical specimen, and the test is considered positive. If the visible reaction is not observed, then antibodies against that pathogen are not present in the specimen and the test is considered negative.

Example

A drop of serum from a patient suspected of having brucellosis is mixed with a suspension of *Brucella melitensis*, the bacterium that usually causes human brucellosis. A visible antigen-antibody reaction is evidence that the patient's serum contains antibodies against *B. melitensis*, and the patient is diagnosed as having brucellosis.

Specific Types of Immunodiagnostic Procedures

Various types of laboratory tests have been designed to produce a visible reaction if an antigen-antibody reaction takes place. These tests—which include agglutination techniques, involving the clumping of particles such as bacterial cells, red blood cells, or latex beads; precipitin techniques, involving the production of a precipitate, immunofluorescence procedures; and ELISAs—are briefly described here. More-detailed descriptions are available in immunology courses. Following are some terms that relate to these tests:

- **Agglutinins** are antibodies that cause the aggregation or clumping of particulate antigens.

- **Lysins** are antibodies that dissolve cell membranes, resulting in the lysis (bursting) of cells. Hemolysins are examples of lysins; they cause the lysis of red blood cells (RBCs).

- **Precipitins** are antibodies that combine with soluble antigens to form insoluble complexes (precipitation).

Agglutination techniques. Agglutination techniques can be used to detect either antigens or antibodies. The antigens are usually located on the surface of a particle (e.g., a bacterial cell, an RBC, or a latex particle). When the antibodies (agglutinins) combine with the antigens, the particles become linked, forming visible masses or clumps. The clumping of RBCs is known as **hemagglutination.** Regardless of which type of particle is involved, the clumps provide visible evidence that an antigen-antibody reaction has occurred.

Complement and complement fixation techniques. In the presence of complement (see Chapter 3), an antigen-antibody reaction that has occurred on the surface of a cell (e.g., an RBC) will lead to lysis of the cell (**cytolysis**). If the cells are bacteria, the term **bacteriolysis** is used. If the cells are RBCs, the term **hemolysis** is used. Lysis of the cells provides visible evidence that an antigen-antibody reaction has occurred. Alternatively, the depletion of complement can be used as evidence that an antigen-antibody reaction occurred.

Precipitation techniques. In precipitation techniques, the antigen-antibody reaction results in the formation of a visible precipitate. Thus, the precipitate provides visible evidence that an antigen-antibody reaction has occurred. Examples of precipitation techniques include tube tests, gel diffusion tests (e.g., double diffusion Ouchterlony tests, immunoelectrophoresis, and counterimmunoelectrophoresis), radioimmunoassays, and enzyme-linked immunosorbent assays.

Fluorescent antibody techniques. In immunofluorescence procedures, antibodies are first conjugated with a dye that will fluoresce under ultraviolet light. **Direct immunofluorescence** procedures are used to detect antigens. The labeled antibody is added to either a clinical specimen or an unidentified organism. If an antigen-antibody reaction takes place, fluorescence will be observed when the preparation is examined under ultraviolet light. This will provide visible evidence that an antigen-antibody reaction has occurred. **Indirect immunofluorescence** is used to detect antibodies to which a labeled antibody has attached. As in direct immunofluorescence, if an antigen-antibody reaction has occurred, fluorescence will be observed when the preparation is examined under ultraviolet light.

Specificity and Sensitivity, False-Positive and False-Negative Results

When using immunodiagnostic procedures, CML professionals must take into consideration the specificity and sensitivity of the test procedure. The **specificity** of an IDP is the ability of the test to correctly identify noninfected persons. An antigen detection procedure is considered to be specific if a positive test result occurs only when the pathogen being sought is actually present. An antibody detection procedure is considered to be specific if a positive test result occurs only when antibodies directed against the pathogen being sought are actually present. For either antigen or antibody detection procedures, the test would be considered 100% specific if no false-positive results occur. If the antigen or antibody, whichever is being tested, is not actually present in the specimen but the test result is positive, the test result is considered a **false-positive result.**

The **sensitivity** of an IDP relates to the quantity of antigen or antibody that must be present for the test to be positive. For either antigen or antibody detection procedures, the test would be considered 100% sensitive if no false-negative results occur. If the antigen or antibody, whichever is being tested for, is actually present in the specimen but the test result is negative, the test result is considered a **false-negative result.**

Although the terms *specificity* and *sensitivity* are being described here, in the section on IDPs, they relate to all types of identification procedures, including biochemical tests and molecular diagnostic procedures. They also have applicability to tests performed in areas of the pathology department other than the CML.

Molecular Diagnostic Procedures

The most recently introduced types of tests for the diagnosis of infectious diseases are **molecular diagnostic procedures (MDPs)**—laboratory procedures that detect pathogen-specific DNA or RNA in clinical specimens. Because it is not necessary for the pathogens to be alive, there is less emphasis on the need for fresh specimens. Also, because of the use of what are known as amplification procedures, only small amounts of pathogen DNA or RNA need be present in the specimen.

One example of an amplification procedure is the **polymerase chain reaction (PCR),** where the enzyme DNA polymerase is used to make many additional copies of existing segments of DNA. The PCR method has revolutionized the diagnosis of certain viral infections, such as enteroviral meningitis and herpes simplex encephalitis, making it possible to diagnose these diseases in a matter of hours. The three main steps in PCR are shown in Figure 6-23.

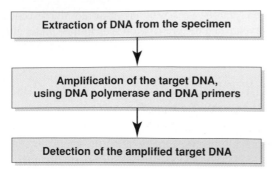

Figure 6-23.   The three main steps in polymerase chain reactions.

PCR for the detection of RNA requires that the RNA first be converted to DNA, using an enzyme called reverse transcriptase (RNA-dependent DNA polymerase). First the extracted DNA is heated to cause denaturation. Then the mixture is cooled, allowing short single-stranded segments of DNA (the DNA primers) to bind to complementary sequences of the denatured DNA. DNA polymerase then causes extension of the target or primer segments. When one cycle has been completed, the number of target molecules has doubled. Following anywhere from 30 to 50 cycles of denaturing, annealing, and extension, the quantity of target DNA will have been amplified by up to a million or a billion times.

MDPs typically provide results in as few as 4 to 6 hours after receipt of the specimen, and they tend to be more sensitive than and as specific as traditional methods of culture and identification. Various DNA probes are commercially available for the diagnosis of many infectious diseases, including bacterial, viral, fungal, and protozoal diseases.

Listed here are some additional advantages of MDPs:

- They can be used to detect slow-growing organisms or organisms that cannot be cultured in vitro.

- They can be used to detect organisms that are highly infectious and thus dangerous to work with in the CML.

- They can be used to quickly diagnose diseases that are rapidly fatal.

MDPs do have disadvantages, however, some of which are listed here:

- Usually, an MDP can test for only one organism at a time. If the test is negative, only one disease has been ruled out.

- Even if an MDP indicates that a particular organism is present, that organism may not be the cause of the patient's infectious disease. MDPs do not distinguish between colonization and disease causation. They also do not distinguish between viable and nonviable organisms.

- Even if the MDP result is a true positive, it is possible that the patient's infection is caused by more than one pathogen. Coinfection will not be detected unless labora-

tory personnel are specifically looking for multiple organisms and using multiple MDPs.

- When an MDP is positive and the specimen was not cultured, the actual organism is not available for antimicrobial susceptibility testing. However, a few MDPs can detect antimicrobial resistance genes (e.g., isoniazid resistance in *Mycobacterium tuberculosis*) and it is likely that additional MDPs for this purpose will be developed in the future.

- MDPs, especially PCRs, are so sensitive that they are prone to false-positive results because of cross-contamination of specimens and controls. As explained previously, a false-positive result means that the test result is positive even though the pathogen is not present.

- Cross-reactivity problems can arise with MDPs, meaning that the reagent may react with something other than the organism being tested for.

- An MDP may give a false-negative result—for example, because of enzyme inhibitors. As previously explained, a false-negative result means that the test result is negative even though the pathogen is present.

- MDPs tend to be more expensive than traditional methods.

Note that most of the disadvantages of MDPs also apply to IDPs.

Commercially available MDPs for direct detection of microorganisms in clinical specimens include nucleic acid probes for certain bacteria (e.g., *Chlamydia trachomatis*, *Neisseria gonorrhoeae*, and *Streptococcus pyogenes* [group A strep]) and amplification-based methods for certain bacteria (e.g., *C. trachomatis*, *M. tuberculosis*, *N. gonorrhoeae*, and methicillin-resistant *Staphylococcus aureus*) and viruses (e.g., cytomegalovirus, hepatitis C virus, HIV, and human papillomavirus). One DNA probe-based test for vaginitis can differentiate among *Candida* (a yeast), *Gardnerella* (a bacterium), and *Trichomonas* (a protozoan) from a single sample in less than 1 hour. Commercially available MDPs for identification of cultured microorganisms include nucleic acid probes for bacteria (e.g., *Campylobacter* spp., *Enterococcus* spp., *Escherichia coli*, *Haemophilus influenzae*, *Listeria monocytogenes*, *Mycobacterium* spp., *N. gonorrhoeae*, *S. aureus*, *Streptococcus agalactiae* [group B strep], *Streptococcus pneumoniae*, and *S. pyogenes*) and various fungi (e.g., *Blastomyces dermatitidis*, *Coccidioides immitis*, and *Histoplasma capsulatum*). New MDPs are constantly being developed and adopted by CMLs.

Manufacturers of MDPs include Abbott Diagnostics (http://abbottdiagnostics.com/), Siemens Medical Solutions Diagnostics (http://diagnostics.siemens.com/), BD Biosciences (http://www.bdbiosciences.com/), bioMérieux Inc. (http://www.biomerieux.com/), Digene Corporation (http://www.digene.com/), Gen-Probe Inc. (http://www.gen-probe.com/), and Roche (http://www.roche.com/).

Additional information about MDPs can be found in Winn et al. and, in other textbooks, chapters by Nolte and Caliendo, Poutanen and Tompkins, and Sandin (see "References and Suggested Reading").

AUTOMATION IN THE CLINICAL MICROBIOLOGY LABORATORY

Although automated laboratory procedures were first introduced into the chemistry and hematology sections of the pathology department, some as early as the 1960s, great strides have been made in the last three decades to automate the CML. Many CMLs now use automated methods for blood cultures, microorganism identification, antimicrobial susceptibility testing, immunodiagnostic procedures, molecular diagnostic procedures, and detection and susceptibility testing of mycobacteria.

Automated Blood Culture Techniques

Automated, or instrument-based, blood culture systems can rapidly and accurately detect positive blood cultures, and are far less time consuming and labor intensive than traditional methods. Automated blood culture systems available for use in CMLs are referred to as continuous-monitoring blood culture systems (CMBCSs). Following inoculation, the culture vials are placed within the instrument, where they are incubated and periodically monitored—usually, every 10 to 15 minutes—by the instrument for evidence of microbial growth. Thus, monitoring by instrumentation ensures that vials are checked more frequently than in the traditional system of blood culturing. This often leads to faster detection of positive cultures. When an instrument flags a vial as being positive, the CML professional removes the vial from the instrument and Gram stains and subcultures its contents. Three companies manufacture the CMBCSs used in the United States (Table 6-8).

The BacT/Alert systems employ a CO_2 sensor at the base of each vial. The sensor changes color when the CO_2 concentration increases as a result of microbial growth. A change in color alters the amount of light reflected from the sensor, and this change in reflectance is measured by the instrument (Fig. 6-24).

The BACTEC systems also employ culture vials with a CO_2 sensor at the base of the vials. An increase in CO_2 is detected by a fluorescence sensing mechanism. Increased fluorescence is evidence of microbial growth.

The ESP Culture System periodically samples headspace gases within the vials to detect either increased or decreased pressure of these gases. Headspace gases are the gases that accumulate between the vial's stopper and the surface of the broth. Changes in the pressure of these gases occur as microorganisms metabolize various substrates within the broth.

Automated Biochemical- and Enzyme-Based Methods for Microorganism Identification

One of the time-honored methods of identifying bacterial and yeast pathogens is to inoculate the organism into a series of biochemical tests that reveal what enzymes the organism does or does not possess. Each test result serves as a clue to the identity of the organism. Originally, this approach involved inoculation of a large number of test tubes, each of which contained a particular substrate—in most cases, a particular carbohydrate or amino acid. Starting in the 1970s, biochemical- and enzyme-based kits became available. These kits contained numerous biochemical tests, were relatively simple to inoculate, and often provided results in just a few hours. The results had to be read manually, however, making the process quite time consuming and subjective in some cases.

Today various automated biochemical-based methods exist for identifying bacteria and yeasts (Table 6-9). Following its inoculation, a card, tray, or panel is placed into an

TABLE 6 - 8	Continuous-Monitoring Blood Culture Systems Used in U.S. Clinical Microbiology Laboratories	
Name of System[a]	**Manufacturer**	**Method Used for Detecting Growth**[b]
BacT/Alert	bioMérieux Inc. (http://www.biomerieux.com/)	CO_2 colorimetric
BACTEC	BD Biosciences (http://www.bdbiosciences.com/)	CO_2 fluorescence
ESP Culture System	Trek Diagnostic Systems (http://www.trekds.com/)	Manometric (pressure measurement)

[a]Several models of each system are available, varying primarily in the number of vials that the instrument can accommodate.
[b]See text for details.

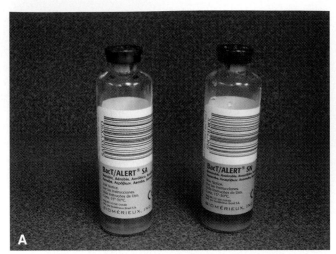
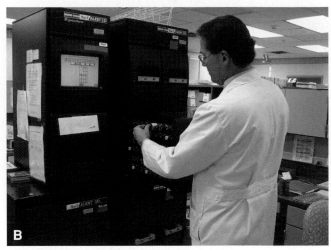

Figure 6-24. **BacT/Alert blood culture system, manufactured by bioMérieux. A.** Aerobic and anaerobic BacT/Alert blood culture bottles. **B.** Blood culture bottle being removed from the BacT/Alert instrument. (Courtesy of Dr. Robert Fader.)

TABLE 6 - 9	Examples of Biochemical-Based Automated Methods for Identifying Bacteria and Yeasts	
Name of System	**Manufacturer**	**Category of Microbe**
MicroScan Gram Pos ID Panel and MicroScan Rapid Gram Pos ID Panel	Dade Behring (http://www.dadebehring.com/)	Bacteria: Gram-positive cocci
Vitek GPI Card and Vitek ID-GPC Card	bioMérieux Inc. (http://www.biomerieux.com/)	
MIDI Sherlock System	MIDI, Inc. (http://www.midilabs.com/)	
MicroScan Rapid Neg ID Panel	Dade Behring	Bacteria: Gram-negative bacteria
Vitek GNI Card, Vitek GNI Plus Card, Vitek 2 ID-GNB Card, and Vitek NHI Card	bioMérieux Inc.	
Sensititre Gram-Negative AP80 Panel	Trek Diagnostics http://www.trekds.com/)	
Phoenix Gram-Negative Panel	BD Biosciences (http://www.bdbiosciences.com/)	
Rapid Yeast Identification Panel	Dade Behring	Yeasts
Vitek.YBC System	bioMérieux Inc.	
Biolog YT Microplate	Biolog Inc. (http://www.biolog.com/)	
Microbial Identification System (MIS)	MIDI Inc.	

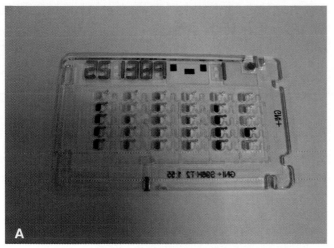
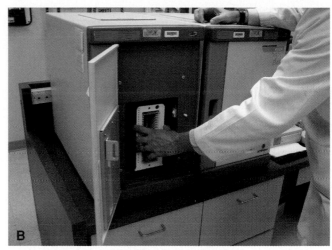

Figure 6-25. **Vitek bacterial identification system, manufactured by bioMérieux. A.** Vitek GNI Plus card, containing substrates for identification of Gram-negative bacteria. **B.** Inoculated Vitek cards being placed into the Vitek incubator/reader. (Courtesy of Dr. Robert Fader.)

instrument, within which the biochemical test results are read. The instrument then prints the test results and the name of the organism.

Instruments such as the Vitek (bioMérieux Inc.; http://www.biomerieux.com/; Fig. 6-25) and MicroScan (Dade Behring; http://www.dadebehring.com/) systems use colorimetry (color change) and/or fluorescence for microbial identification. Turbidimetry (turbidity) or nephelometry (light scattering) are used in automated antimicrobial susceptibility test systems.

Additional information about automated methods for microorganism identification can be found in Chapter 8 and, in other textbooks, chapters by Evangelista et al., O'Hara et al.,

and Wolk and Roberts (see "References and Suggested Reading").

Automated Immunodiagnostic Procedures

As stated earlier, one approach to reducing the time it takes to diagnose infectious diseases has been the development of immunodiagnostic procedures. Today the results of many IDPs are read by some type of automated instrument. Automated IDP systems are available for the detection of numerous viral, bacterial, fungal, and parasitic pathogens (Table 6-10). For additional information about automated IDPs, see chapters by Constantine and Lana and by Hodinka in other textbooks

TABLE 6 - 10	Examples of Pathogens Detected by Automated Immunodiagnostic Systems
Category of Pathogen	**Specific Pathogens**
Viruses	Adenovirus; cytomegalovirus; HIV; Epstein-Barr virus; hepatitis A, B, C, and D viruses; herpes simplex virus; influenza viruses A and B; measles virus; mumps virus; parvovirus; rubella virus
Bacteria	*Bordetella pertussis, Borrelia burgdorferi, Brucella abortus, Chlamydia trachomatis, Clostridium difficile, Escherichia coli* O157:H7, *Helicobacter pylori, Legionella pneumophila, Listeria monocytogenes, Mycoplasma pneumoniae, Salmonella* spp., *Treponema pallidum*
Fungi	*Aspergillus* spp., *Candida albicans*
Parasites	*Entamoeba histolytica, Giardia lamblia, Toxoplasma gondii, Trypanosoma cruzi*

(see "References and Suggested Reading"). Many companies manufacture automated IDP systems. Information about these companies can be found on the CD-ROM.

Automated Molecular Diagnostic Procedures

The major steps involved in amplification types of MDPs are (1) specimen processing, (2) nucleic acid amplification, and (3) product detection. The most labor-intensive step, and the one most difficult to automate, is specimen processing. Several manufacturers have developed instruments that automate the second and third steps, but few have automated all three. For additional information about automated MDPs, see chapters by Jungkind and Kessler and by Nolte and Caliendo in other textbooks (see "References and Suggested Reading").

Automated Methods for Antimicrobial Susceptibility Testing

Information about automated methods for antimicrobial susceptibility testing can be found in Chapter 7, as well as in chapters by Evangelista et al. and O'Hara et al. in other textbooks (see "References and Suggested Reading").

Automated Methods for Identification and Susceptibility Testing of Mycobacteria

Information about automated methods for identification and susceptibility testing of mycobacteria can be found in Chapter 10 and in the chapter by Roberts et al. in another textbook (see "References and Suggested Reading").

Chapter Review

- The metric system is used in scientific fields to express weights and measures. In microbiology, metric units of length, such as micrometers and nanometers, are used to express the sizes of microorganisms.

- Microscopes are optical instruments that allow observation of objects that cannot be seen with the human eye alone. Several types of microscopes are available for various application.

- The resolving power of a microscope is its ability to distinguish between two adjacent objects or points.

- Various types of liquid and solid culture media are used to grow and isolate microorganisms in the CML.

- Aseptic technique is used to avoid the introduction of unwanted contaminants when inoculating culture media.

- Three types of incubators are commonly used in the CML: CO_2, non-CO_2, and anaerobic incubators.

- The wet mount may be used to examine clinical specimens, determine motility, and differentiate a yeast colony from a bacterial colony.

- Common methods of fixation include heat and methanol fixation. The three purposes of fixation are (1) killing the organisms, (2) preserving morphology, and (3) anchoring the smear to the slide.

- Gram staining and acid-fast staining procedures are differential staining techniques. They differentiate between groups of bacteria (e.g., between Gram-positive and Gram-negative bacteria and between acid-fast and non-acid-fast bacteria).

- Microorganisms may be identified by several methods, including biochemical tests, gas-liquid chromatography, immunodiagnostic procedures, and molecular diagnostic procedures.

- Biochemical tests performed in the CML identify a microorganism by determining which substrates it is able to catabolize. This provides information about which enzymes the organism produces or does not produce.

- Gas-liquid chromatography can be used to identify a microorganism by analyzing acid end products of metabolism or the cellular fatty acids that the organism possesses.

- Immunodiagnostic procedures help diagnose infectious diseases by detecting either antigens or antibodies in clinical specimens. IDPs include agglutination, complement fixation, precipitation, and fluorescent antibody techniques.

- The specificity of an immunodiagnostic test is its ability to identify all noninfected persons correctly, whereas the sensitivity of an immunodiagnostic test relates to its ability to identify all infected persons correctly.

- Molecular diagnostic procedures detect pathogen-specific DNA or RNA.

- Automated methods are available in the CML for identifying microorganisms and performing blood cultures, antimicrobial susceptibility testing, immunodiagnostic procedures, molecular diagnostic procedures, and detection and susceptibility testing of mycobacteria.

New Terms and Abbreviations

After studying Chapter 6, you should be familiar with the following terms, which are defined within the chapter and in the Glossary at the back of the book:

Anabolic reaction

Anabolism

Antiserum

Artificial medium

Aseptic techniques

Biphasic system

Brightfield microscope

Brownian movement

Catabolic reaction

Catabolism

Chemically defined medium

Complex medium

Compound light microscope

Compound microscope

Contaminant

Culture medium

Darkfield microscope

Differential medium

Differential staining procedure

Electron micrograph

Electron microscope

Empty magnification

Enriched medium

Enrichment medium

Enzyme

Fluorescence microscope

Hemagglutination

Hybridoma

Immunodiagnostic procedure (IDP)

Incubation

Incubator

Inoculation

Lawn of growth

Metabolic reaction

Metabolism

Micrometer

Minisystem

Molecular diagnostic procedure (MDP)

Monoclonal antibody

Nanometer

Ocular micrometer

Phase contrast microscope

Photomicrograph

Polymerase chain reaction (PCR)

Resolving power

Scanning electron micrograph

Scanning electron microscope

Selective medium

Simple microscope

Simple staining procedure

Structural staining procedure

Substrate

Transmission electron micrograph

Transmission electron microscope

Wet mount

References and Suggested Reading

Constantine NT, Lana DP. Immunoassays for the diagnosis of infectious diseases. In: Murray PR, Baron EJ, Jorgensen JH, Pfaller MA, Yolken RH, eds. Manual of Clinical Microbiology. 8th Ed. Washington, DC: ASM Press, 2003.

Evangelista AT, et al. Rapid systems and instruments for antimicrobial susceptibility testing of bacteria. In: Manual of Commercial Methods in Clinical Microbiology. Washington, DC: ASM Press, 2002.

Ferraro MJ, Jorgensen JH. Susceptibility testing instrumentation and computerized expert systems for data analysis and interpretation. In: Murray PR, Baron EJ, Jorgensen JH, Pfaller MA, Yolken RH, eds. Manual of Clinical Microbiology. 8th Ed. Washington, DC: ASM Press, 2003.

Hodinka RL. Automated immunoassay analyzers. In: Manual of Commercial Methods in Clinical Microbiology. Washington, DC: ASM Press, 2002.

Jungkind D, Kessler HH. Molecular methods for diagnosis of infectious diseases. In: Manual of Commercial Methods in Clinical Microbiology. Washington, DC: ASM Press, 2002.

Menegus MA. Rapid systems and instruments for the identification of viruses. In: Manual of Commercial Methods in Clinical Microbiology. Washington, DC: ASM Press, 2002.

Nolte FS, Caliendo AM. Molecular detection and identification of microorganisms. In: Murray PR, Baron EJ, Jorgensen JH, Pfaller MA, Yolken RH, eds. Manual of Clinical Microbiology. 8th Ed. Washington, DC: ASM Press, 2003.

O'Hara CM, et al. Manual and automated systems for detection and identification of microorganisms. In: Murray PR, Baron EJ, Jorgensen JH, Pfaller MA, Yolken RH, eds. Manual of Clinical Microbiology. 8th Ed. Washington, DC: ASM Press, 2003.

Poutanen SM, Tompkins LS. Molecular epidemiology in infectious diseases. In: Gorbach SL, Bartlett JG, Blacklow NR, eds. Infectious Disease. 3rd Ed. Philadelphia: Lippincott Williams & Wilkins, 2004.

Roberts GD, et al. Mycobacteria. In: Manual of Commercial Methods in Clinical Microbiology. Washington, DC: ASM Press, 2002.

Sandin RL. Molecular biology of infectious diseases. In: McClatchey KD, ed. Clinical Laboratory Medicine. 2nd Ed. Philadelphia: Lippincott Williams & Wilkins, 2002.

Winn WC Jr, et al. Koneman's Color Atlas and Textbook of Diagnostic Microbiology. 6th Ed. Philadelphia: Lippincott Williams & Wilkins, 2006.

Wolk DM, Roberts GD. Commercial methods for identification and susceptibility testing of fungi. In: Manual of Commercial Methods in Clinical Microbiology. Washington, DC: ASM Press, 2002.

 ## On the CD-ROM

- A Closer Look at Molecular Diagnostic Procedures

- A Closer Look at PCR

- Companies That Manufacture Automated Immunodiagnostic Systems

- Additional Self-Assessment Exercises

- Puzzle

Self-Assessment Exercises

After studying Chapter 6, answer the following questions.

1. One millimeter is equivalent to how many nanometers?

   A. 1,000

   B. 10,000

   C. 100,000

   D. 1,000,000

2. What is the total magnification when using the high power (high-dry) objective of a compound light microscope equipped with a ×10 ocular lens?

   A. ×10

   B. ×40

   C. ×100

   D. ×400

3. The limiting factor of any compound light microscope (i.e., the thing that limits its resolution to 0.2 μm) is the

   A. company that made the microscope.

   B. number of condenser lenses it has.

   C. number of magnifying lenses it has.

   D. wavelength of visible light.

4. Which of the following types of microscopes has the greatest resolving power?

   A. Phase contrast microscope

   B. Darkfield microscope

   C. Electron microscope

   D. Fluorescent microscope

5. Which of the following is a good example of a *selective* medium?

   A. Blood agar

   B. Chocolate agar

   C. MacConkey agar

   D. Mueller-Hinton agar

6. The environment within a CO_2 incubator contains

    A. 5% to 10% CO_2 and 15% to 20% O_2.

    B. 10% to 15% CO_2 and 5% to 10% O_2.

    C. 20% CO_2 and 10% O_2.

    D. none of the above.

7. Fixation of a specimen to a slide accomplishes all of the following *except*

    A. killing the organism.

    B. anchoring the smear to the slide.

    C. causing the organism to change to a pink or blue color.

    D. preserving the morphology of the cells.

8. The Gram stain is an example of which of the following types of staining procedures?

    A. Simple

    B. Structural

    C. Differential

    D. Selective

9. In the CML, automated instruments like the Vitek or MicroScan identify microorganisms based on which of the following?

    A. Antigen and antibody reactions

    B. Cellular fatty acid contents

    C. DNA sequences

    D. Biochemical reactions

10. In which of the following immunodiagnostic techniques are visible masses or "clumps" of particles observed when an antigen-antibody reaction has occurred?

    A. Complement fixation technique

    B. Agglutination technique

    C. Precipitation technique

    D. None of the above

CHAPTER 7

Antimicrobial Agents and Antimicrobial Susceptibility Testing

LEARNING OBJECTIVES

After studying this chapter, you should be able to:

- ☛ Define all terms introduced in this chapter (e.g., *acquired resistance, antagonism, antibacterial agents*)
- ☛ Differentiate among chemotherapeutic agents, antimicrobial agents, and antibiotics
- ☛ List five subcategories of antimicrobial agents (e.g., antibacterial agents)
- ☛ Name two antifungal agents and two antiviral agents
- ☛ State the five most common mechanisms of action of antimicrobial agents
- ☛ Differentiate between narrow-spectrum and broad-spectrum antimicrobial agents, and describe their effectiveness against different types of bacteria and examples of each
- ☛ Identify the four most common mechanisms by which bacteria become resistant to antimicrobial agents
- ☛ Explain what is meant by empirical therapy
- ☛ List six of the factors that a clinician would take into consideration before prescribing an antimicrobial agent for a particular patient
- ☛ State three undesirable effects of antimicrobial agents
- ☛ Explain what is meant by a "superinfection," and cite three diseases that can result from superinfections
- ☛ Briefly describe the available choices for performing antimicrobial susceptibility testing of bacteria, including the "gold standard" method and the most commonly used method

☞ Given the results of a broth microdilution test, determine the minimum inhibitory concentration for each antimicrobial agent that was tested

☞ Given the results of the disk diffusion method, interpret the data as to the microorganism's susceptibility or resistance to the drugs tested

☞ Given a problem with the results of the disk diffusion method, state the most likely cause

☞ Explain how a minimum bactericidal concentration test is performed and how the results are interpreted

☞ Explain how β-lactamases function, describe their effect on the drugs' structure, and cite two examples

☞ Explain why a patient's serum specimens would be tested for their antibacterial activity

TERMS AND DEFINITIONS

Chemotherapy. Although we most often hear the term used in conjunction with cancer, **chemotherapy** actually refers to the use of any chemical or drug to treat any disease or condition. The drugs used to treat diseases are referred to as chemotherapeutic agents. By definition, a **chemotherapeutic agent** is any drug used to treat any condition or disease.

Antimicrobial agents. The chemotherapeutic agents used to treat infectious diseases are collectively referred to as antimicrobial agents. Thus, an **antimicrobial agent** is any drug used to treat an infectious disease, either by inhibiting or killing pathogens in vivo. Drugs used to treat bacterial diseases are called **antibacterial agents,** whereas those used to treat fungal diseases are **antifungal agents.** Drugs that treat protozoal diseases are called **antiprotozoal agents,** and those that treat viral diseases are **antiviral agents.** Drugs used to treat helminth infections have various names, including antihelminth drugs, anthelmintics, anthelminthics, antihelmintics, and antihelminthics.

> The chemotherapeutic agents (drugs) used to treat infectious diseases are called antimicrobial agents.

> The antimicrobial agents that treat bacterial infections are called antibacterial agents.

Antibiotics. Some antimicrobial agents are antibiotics. By definition, an **antibiotic** is a substance **produced by a microorganism** that is effective in killing or inhibiting the growth of other microorganisms. Although all antibiotics are antimicrobial agents, not all antimicrobial agents are antibiotics; therefore, the terms are not synonyms, and care should be taken to use the terms correctly. Antibiotics are primarily used to treat bacterial infections. Thus, we can think of antibiotics as antibacterial agents. Antibiotics are produced by certain moulds and bacteria, usually ones that live in soil. The antibiotics produced by soil organisms give them a selective advantage in the struggle for available nutrients in the soil. Penicillin and cephalosporin are examples of antibiotics produced by moulds, and bacitracin, chloramphenicol, erythromycin, and tetracycline are examples of antibiotics produced by bacteria.

> An antibiotic is a substance produced by a microorganism that is effective in killing or inhibiting the growth of other microorganisms.

Semisynthetic antibiotics. Although originally produced by microorganisms, many antibiotics are now synthesized or manufactured in pharmaceutical laboratories. Also, many antibiotics have been chemically modified, usually to kill a wider variety of pathogens or reduce side effects. These modified antibiotics are called **semisynthetic antibiotics.** Semisynthetic antibiotics include semisynthetic penicillins, such as ampicillin and carbenicillin.

HOW ANTIMICROBIAL AGENTS WORK

Ideally, an antimicrobial agent will inhibit or destroy the pathogen without causing damage to the person receiving the drug. To accomplish this, the agent must target a metabolic process or structure possessed by the pathogen but not possessed by the infected person.

The five most common mechanisms of action of antimicrobial agents are

- inhibition of cell wall synthesis,

- damage to cell membranes,

- inhibition of nucleic acid synthesis (either DNA or RNA synthesis),

- inhibition of protein synthesis, and

- inhibition of enzyme activity.

ANTIBACTERIAL AGENTS

Antibacterial agents work well against bacterial pathogens because the bacteria, being procaryotic, have different cellular structures and metabolic pathways that can be disrupted or destroyed by drugs that do not damage the eucaryotic host's cells. There are antibacterial agents that function by each of the five mechanisms of action listed in the previous section.

Antibacterial agents that kill bacteria are referred to as **bactericidal agents.** Those that inhibit growth of bacteria but do not kill them are referred to as **bacteriostatic agents.** Bacteriostatic agents should only be used in patients whose host defense mechanisms (see Chapter 3) are functioning properly—that is, only in patients whose bodies are capable of killing the pathogen once it has stopped multiplying. Unless absolutely necessary, bacteriostatic agents should not be administered to immunosuppressed or leukopenic patients—patients having an abnormally low number of circulating white blood cells.

> Antibacterial agents that kill bacteria are called bactericidal agents, whereas those that inhibit growth of bacteria but do not kill them are called bacteriostatic agents.

Antibiotics like vancomycin, which destroys only Gram-positive bacteria, and colistin and nalidixic acid, which destroy only Gram-negative bacteria, are referred to as **narrow-spectrum antibiotics.** Those that are destructive to both Gram-positive and Gram-negative bacteria are called **broad-spectrum antibiotics.** Examples of broad-spectrum antibiotics are ampicillin, chloramphenicol, and tetracycline. Tables 7-1 and 7-2 contain information about some of the antimicrobial drugs most frequently used to treat bacterial infections.

Multidrug Therapy

In some cases, a single antimicrobial agent is not sufficient to destroy all the pathogens that develop during the course of a disease. In such cases, two or more drugs may be used simultaneously to kill all the pathogens and to prevent resistant mutant pathogens from emerging. In tuberculosis, for example, which might involve multidrug-resistant strains of *Mycobacterium tuberculosis*, four drugs (isoniazid, rifampin, pyrazinamide, and either ethambutol or streptomycin) are routinely prescribed, and as many as 12 drugs may be required for especially resistant strains.

Synergism Versus Antagonism

Sometimes the use of two antimicrobial agents to treat an infectious disease produces a degree of pathogen inhibition or killing that is far greater than that achieved by either drug alone. This is known as **synergism** or synergy. Many urinary, respiratory, and gastrointestinal infections respond particularly well to a combination of trimethoprim and sulfamethoxazole, a combination referred to as cotrimoxazole; brand names include Bactrim and Septra.

In certain situations, however, two drugs are prescribed (perhaps by two different clinicians who are treating the patient's infection) that actually work against each other. This is known as **antagonism.** When antagonism occurs, the extent of pathogen inhibition or killing is *less* than that achieved by either drug alone. Synergism is a good thing, whereas antagonism is not.

"Superbugs"

These days, it is quite common to hear about drug-resistant microbes, or "superbugs," as they have been labeled by the press. **Superbugs** are microorganisms, primarily bacteria, that have become resistant to one or more antimicrobial agent. Infections caused by superbugs are much more difficult to treat. The worst of the superbugs are multidrug resistant, meaning that they are resistant to several different antimicrobial agents. Especially troublesome bacterial superbugs include the following:

> Superbugs are microorganisms that have become resistant to one or more antimicrobial agents. Although the term is most frequently used in discussions of multidrug-resistant bacteria, superbugs also exist within other categories of microbes, including fungi, parasites, and viruses.

- Methicillin-resistant *Staphylococcus aureus* (MRSA) and methicillin-resistant *Staphylococcus epidermidis* (MRSE). These strains are resistant to a great many antistaphylococcal drugs. Usually, MRSA and MRSE infections can be treated with vancomycin and one or two other drugs developed more recently (e.g., Synercid and Zyvox). Some strains of *S. aureus*, called vancomycin-intermediate *S. aureus* (VISA), have developed resistance to the usual dosages of vancomycin, necessitating the use of higher doses to treat infections caused by these organisms. VISA strains are sometimes referred to as glycopeptide-intermediate *S. aureus* (GISA). **Vancomycin-resistant *S. aureus* (VRSA)** strains have also been recovered from patient specimens. *S. aureus* is a very common cause of nosocomial (hospital-acquired) infections.

- Vancomycin-resistant *Enterococcus* spp. (VRE). These strains are resistant to most antienterococcal drugs, including vancomycin. *Enterococcus* spp. are common causes of nosocomial infections, especially nosocomial urinary tract infections.

- **Multidrug-resistant *M. tuberculosis* (MRTB).** Some MRTB strains are resistant to *all* antitubercular drugs and drug combinations. Patients infected with these strains may have a lung or section of lung removed—just as in the preantibiotic days—and many will die. Tuberculosis remains one of the major killers worldwide.

- **Multidrug-resistant strains of *Pseudomonas* spp., *Salmonella* spp., *Shigella* spp., and *Neisseria gonorrhoeae.***

TABLE 7 - 1   Antibacterial Agents Listed by Class or Category

Class/Category	Description/Source	Examples of Antibacterial Agents Within the Class or Category
Penicillins[a]	Naturally occurring penicillins; produced by moulds in the genus *Penicillium*	Benzylpenicillin (penicillin G), phenoxymethyl penicillin (penicillin V)
	Semisynthetic penicillins: broad-spectrum aminopenicillins	Amoxicillin, ampicillin
	Semisynthetic penicillins: broad-spectrum carboxypenicillins	Carbenicillin, ticarcillin
	Semisynthetic penicillins: broad-spectrum ureidopenicillins	Azlocillin, mezlocillin, piperacillin
	Semisynthetic penicillins: penicillinase-resistant penicillins	Cloxacillin, dicloxacillin, methicillin, nafcillin
	Penicillin + β-lactamase inhibitor	Amoxicillin-clavulanic acid (Augmentin), ampicillin-sulbactam (Unasyn), piperacillin-tazobactam (Zosyn), ticarcillin-clavulanic acid (Timentin)
Cephalosporins[a]	Derivatives of fermentation products of the mould, *Cephalosporium (Acremonium)*	Narrow-spectrum (first-generation) cephalosporins: cefazolin, cephalothin, cephapirin, cephradine; first-generation cephalosporins have good activity against Gram-positive bacteria and relatively modest activity against Gram-negative bacteria
		Expanded-spectrum (second-generation) cephalosporins: cefamandole, cefonicid, cefuroxime; second-generation cephalosporins have increased activity against Gram-negative bacteria
		Cephamycins (second-generation cephalosporins): cefmetazole, cefotetan, cefoxitin
		Broad-spectrum (third-generation) cephalosporins: cefoperazone, cefotaxime, ceftazidime, ceftizoxime, ceftriaxone; third-generation cephalosporins are less active against Gram-positive bacteria than first- and second-generation cephalosporins but are more active against members of the Enterobacteriaceae family and *Pseudomonas aeruginosa*
		Extended-spectrum (fourth-generation) cephalosporin: cefepime; fourth-generation cephalosporins have increased activity against Gram-negative bacteria
Monobactam[a]	Synthetic drug	Aztreonam
Carbapenems[a]	Imipenem is a semisynthetic derivative of thienamycin, produced by *Streptomyces* spp.	Ertapenem, imipenem, meropenem
Aminocyclitol	Produced by *Streptomyces spectabilis*	Spectinomycin, trospectinomycin
Aminoglycosides	Naturally occurring antibiotics or semi-synthetic derivatives from *Micromonospora* spp. or *Streptomyces* spp.	Amikacin, gentamicin, kanamycin, netilmicin, streptomycin, tobramycin
Ansamycin	Semisynthetic antibiotic derived from compounds produced by *Streptomyces mediterranei*	Rifampin

(continued)

TABLE 7 - 1   Continued

Class/Category	Description/Source	Examples of Antibacterial Agents Within the Class or Category
Quinolones	Synthetic drugs	Cinoxacin, garenoxacin, nalidixic acid
Fluoroquinolones	Synthetic drugs	Ciprofloxacin, clinafloxacin, enoxacin, fleroxacin, gatifloxacin, gemifloxacin, grepafloxacin, levofloxacin, lomefloxacin, moxifloxacin, norfloxacin, ofloxacin, sparfloxacin, trovafloxacin
Macrolides	Erythromycin is produced by *Streptomyces erythraeus*; the others are natural analogs of erythromycin or semisynthetic antibiotics	Azithromycin, clarithromycin, dirithromycin, erythromycin
Ketolides	Semisynthetic derivative of erythromycin	Telithromycin
Tetracyclines	Tetracycline is produced by *Streptomyces rimosus*; the others are semisynthetic antibiotics	Doxycycline, minocycline, tetracycline
Lincosamide	Clindamycin is a semisynthetic antibiotic	Clindamycin
Glycopeptide	Produced by *Streptomyces orientales*	Vancomycin
Lipopeptide	Semisynthetic antibiotic	Teicoplanin
Streptogramins	Produced by *Streptomyces* spp.	Quinupristin-dalfopristin
Oxazolidinone	Synthetic drug	Linezolid
Sulfonamides	Synthetic drugs derived from sulfanilamide	Sulfacetamide, sulfadiazine, sulfadoxine, sulfamethizole, sulfamethoxazole (SMX), sulfisoxazole, trisulfapyrimidine (triple sulfa)
Trimethoprim	Synthetic drug	Used alone or in combination with SMX (the combination is also called cotrimoxazole)
Polypeptides	Originally produced by *Bacillus polymyxa*	Polymyxins: polymyxin B, polymixin E (colistin)
	Originally produced by *Bacillus licheniformis* (formerly named *B. subtilis*)	Bacitracin
Phenicol	Originally produced by *Streptomyces venezuelae*	Chloramphenicol
Nitroimidazole	Synthetic drug	Metronidazole
Nitrofuran	Synthetic drug	Nitrofurantoin
Fosfomycin	Originally produced by *Streptomyces* spp.	

Sources: Winn WC Jr, et al. Koneman's Color Atlas and Textbook of Diagnostic Microbiology. 6th Ed. Philadelphia: Lippincott Williams & Wilkins, 2006. Yao JDC, Moellering RC Jr. Antibacterial Agents. In: Murray PR, Baron EJ, Jorgensen JH, Pfaller MA, Yolken RH, eds. Manual of Clinical Microbiology. 8th Ed. Washington, DC: ASM Press, 2003.
[a] β-lactam antibiotics (i.e., antibiotics that contain a β-lactam ring).

TABLE 7 - 2   Antibacterial Agents Listed by Mechanism of Action

Mode of Action	Agent	Spectrum of Activity	Bactericidal or Bacteriostatic
Inhibition of cell wall synthesis	Aztreonam	Gram-negative bacteria	Bactericidal
	Bacitracin (also disrupts cell membranes)	Broad spectrum[a]	Bactericidal
	Carbapenem	Broad spectrum	Bactericidal
	Cephalosporins	Broad spectrum	Bactericidal
	Daptomycin	Broad spectrum	Bactericidal
	Fosfomycin	Broad spectrum	Bactericidal
	Penicillins and semisynthetic penicillins	Broad spectrum	Bactericidal
	Vancomycin	Gram-positive bacteria	Bactericidal
Inhibition of protein synthesis	Aminoglycosides	Primarily Gram-negative bacteria and *Staphylococcus aureus*; not effective against anaerobes	Bactericidal
	Chloramphenicol	Broad spectrum	Bacteriostatic
	Clindamycin	Most Gram-positive bacteria and some Gram-negative bacteria; highly active against anaerobes	Bacteriostatic or bactericidal, depending upon drug concentration and bacterial species
	Erythromycin and other macrolides	Most Gram-positive bacteria and some Gram-negative bacteria	Bacteriostatic (usually); bactericidal at higher concentrations
	Ketolides	Broad spectrum	Bacteriostatic
	Linezolid	Gram-positive bacteria	Bacteriostatic
	Mupirocin	Broad spectrum	Bacteriostatic
	Streptogramins	Primarily Gram-positive bacteria	Bactericidal
	Tetracyclines	Broad-spectrum and some intracellular bacterial pathogens	Bacteriostatic
Inhibition of nucleic acid synthesis	Rifampin	Gram-positive and some Gram-negative bacteria (e.g., *Neisseria meningitidis*)	Bactericidal
	Quinolones and fluoroquinolones (e.g., ciprofloxacin, levofloxacin, moxifloxacin)	Broad spectrum	Bactericidal

(continued)

TABLE 7 - 2   Continued

Mode of Action	Agent	Spectrum of Activity	Bactericidal or Bacteriostatic
Destruction of DNA	Metronidazole	Effective against anaerobes	Bactericidal
Disruption of cell membranes	Polymyxin B and polymyxin E (colistin)	Gram-negative bacteria	Bactericidal
Inhibition of enzyme activity	Sulfonamides	Primarily Gram-positive bacteria and some Gram-negative bacteria	Bacteriostatic
	Trimethoprim	Gram-positive and many Gram-negative bacteria	Bacteriostatic

a Effective against both Gram-positive and Gram-negative bacteria, but spectrum may vary with the individual antimicrobial agent.

- **β-lactam-resistant strains of *Streptococcus pneumoniae* and *Haemophilus influenzae*.** Some strains of these pathogens have become multidrug resistant.

How Bacteria Become Resistant to Antimicrobial Agents

How do bacteria become resistant to antimicrobial agents? Some bacteria are naturally resistant to a particular antimicrobial agent because they lack the specific target site for that drug. For example, mycoplasmas have no cell walls and are therefore resistant to any drugs that interfere with cell wall synthesis. Other bacteria are naturally resistant for different reasons. For example, the drug may be unable to cross the organism's cell wall or cell membrane and thus is unable to reach its site of action (e.g., ribo-

somes). Such naturally occurring resistance is known as **intrinsic resistance.**

It is also possible for bacteria that were once susceptible to a particular drug to become resistant to it. This is called **acquired resistance.** Bacteria usually become resistant to antibiotics and other antimicrobial agents by one of four mechanisms, each of which is shown in Table 7-3 and briefly described here:

- Before a drug can enter a bacterial cell, molecules of the drug must first bind or attach to proteins on the surface of the cell; these protein molecules are called **drug-binding sites.** A chromosomal mutation can result in an alteration in the structure of the drug-binding site, rendering the drug unable to bind to the cell. If the drug cannot bind to the cell, it cannot enter the cell, and the organism is resistant to the drug.

TABLE 7 - 3   Mechanisms by Which Bacteria Become Resistant to Antimicrobial Agents

Mechanism	Effect
A chromosomal mutation that causes a change in the structure of a drug-binding site	The drug cannot bind to the bacterial cell
A chromosomal mutation that causes a change in cell membrane permeability	The drug cannot pass through the cell membrane and, thus, cannot enter the cell
Acquisition (by conjugation, transduction, or transformation) of a gene that enables the bacterium to produce an enzyme that destroys or inactivates the drug	The drug is destroyed or inactivated by the enzyme
Acquisition (by conjugation, transduction, or transformation) of a gene that enables the bacterium to produce a multidrug-resistance (MDR) pump (efflux pump)	The drug is pumped out of the cell before it can damage or kill the cell

- To enter a bacterial cell, a drug must be able to pass through the cell wall and cell membrane. A chromosomal mutation can result in an alteration in the structure of the cell membrane, which in turn can change the permeability of the membrane. If the drug is no longer able to pass through the cell membrane, it cannot reach its target (e.g., a ribosome or the DNA of the cell), and the organism is resistant to the drug.

- Another way in which bacteria become resistant to a particular drug is by developing the ability to produce an enzyme that destroys or inactivates the drug. Because genes code for enzymes, a bacterial cell would have to acquire a new gene to produce an enzyme that it never before produced. The primary way in which bacteria acquire new genes is by **conjugation.** In conjugation, genetic material, often in the form of a plasmid, is transferred from one cell, called the donor cell, to another cell, called the recipient cell, through a hollow sex pilus. If a plasmid containing a gene that codes for penicillinase production is transferred from a donor cell to a recipient cell, the recipient cell acquires the ability to produce penicillinase. Penicillinase, an enzyme that destroys penicillin, is described later in this chapter. A plasmid containing multiple genes for drug resistance is called a **resistance factor** or **R factor.** A recipient cell that receives an R factor becomes a multidrug-resistant super-bug. Bacteria can also acquire new genes by **transduction,** whereby bacteriophages carry bacterial DNA from one bacterial cell to another, and by **transformation,** whereby bits of "naked" DNA are taken up from the environment.

- A fourth way in which bacteria become resistant to drugs is by developing the ability to produce multidrug-resistance (MDR) pumps, also known as MDR transporters and efflux pumps. An MDR pump enables the cell to pump drugs out of the cell before the drugs can damage or kill the cell. The genes that code for these pumps are often located on plasmids that bacteria receive during conjugation. Bacteria receiving such plasmids become multidrug-resistant superbugs.

To summarize, bacteria can acquire resistance to antimicrobial agents as a result of chromosomal mutation or by the acquisition of new genes by transduction, transformation, or most commonly, conjugation.

It is important to note that bacteria are not the only microorganisms that have developed resistance to drugs. Other drug-resistant microorganisms include some viruses,

TABLE 7 - 4   Antifungal Agents

Drug[a]	Fungal Disease(s) That the Drug is Used to Treat
Amphotericin B	Aspergillosis, blastomycosis, invasive candidiasis, coccidioidomycosis, cryptococcosis, fusariosis, histoplasmosis, mucormycosis, paracoccidioidomycosis, penicilliosis, systemic sporotrichosis
Atovaquone	*Pneumocystis* pneumonia
Echinocandins	Aspergillosis, candidiasis
Fluconazole	Blastomycosis; oropharyngeal, esophageal, and invasive candidiasis; coccidioidomycosis, cryptococcosis, fusariosis, histoplasmosis, sporotrichosis
Flucytosine	Candidiasis, chromoblastomycosis, cryptococcosis,
Griseofulvin	Dermatomycosis (less toxic drugs are available, however)
Itraconazole	Aspergillosis, blastomycosis, invasive candidiasis, coccidioidomycosis, cryptococcosis, histoplasmosis, paracoccidioidomycosis, penicilliosis, pseudallescheriasis, scedosporiosis, cutaneous or systemic sporotrichosis
Ketoconazole	Blastomycosis, coccidioidomycosis, histoplasmosis, paracoccidioidomycosis
Terbinafine	Dermatomycosis
Trimethoprim-sulfamethoxazole	*Pneumocystis* pneumonia
Voriconazole	Aspergillosis, invasive candidiasis, scedosporiosis

[a]This information is provided solely to acquaint the reader with the names of some antifungal agents and should not be construed as advice regarding recommended therapy.

like HIV, herpes simplex viruses, and influenza viruses; fungi (both yeasts and moulds); parasitic protozoa; and helminths. Parasitic protozoa that have become drug resistant include strains of *Plasmodium falciparum*, *Trichomonas vaginalis*, *Leishmania* spp., and *Giardia lamblia*. For additional information on microbial drug resistance, see the section titled "Gloomy Prospects for the Future?" on the CD-ROM.

Antifungal Agents

It is much more difficult to use antimicrobial drugs against fungal and protozoal pathogens. Because fungi and protozoa are eucaryotic cells, the drugs developed to fight them can be more toxic to patients. Most antifungal agents work by

> Antimicrobial agents used to treat fungal infections are called antifungal agents.

- binding with cell membrane sterols (e.g., nystatin and amphotericin B);

- interfering with sterol synthesis (e.g., clotrimazole and miconazole);

- blocking mitosis or nucleic acid synthesis (e.g., griseofulvin and 5-flucytosine); or

- inhibiting cell wall synthesis (e.g., echinocandins).

Examples of antifungal agents are shown in Table 7-4.

ANTIPROTOZOAL AGENTS

Antiprotozoal drugs are usually quite toxic to the host and work by (1) interfering with DNA and RNA synthesis (e.g., chloroquine, pentamidine, and quinacrine) or (2) interfering with protozoal metabolism (e.g., metronidazole; brand name Flagyl). Table 7-5 lists several antiprotozoal drugs and the protozoal diseases they treat.

> Antimicrobial agents used to treat protozoal infections are called antiprotozoal agents.

ANTIVIRAL AGENTS

Antiviral agents are the newest weapons in the antimicrobial arsenal. Before the 1960s, no drugs were available for the treatment of viral diseases. Antiviral agents are particularly difficult to develop and use because viruses are produced *within* host cells. A few drugs have been found to be effective in certain viral infections. These drugs work by inhibiting viral replication within cells. Some antiviral agents are listed in Table 7-6.

> Antimicrobial agents used to treat viral infections are called antiviral agents.

The first antiviral agent effective against HIV (the etiologic agent of AIDS)—zidovudine, also known as AZT—was introduced in 1987. Various additional drugs for the treatment of HIV infection were introduced during the 1990s. Some of these antiviral agents are administered simultaneously, in combinations referred to as "cocktails." Unfortunately, these cocktails are quite expensive, and certain strains of HIV have become resistant to some or all of the drugs.

EMPIRICAL THERAPY

In some cases, a clinician must initiate therapy before laboratory results are available. This is called **empirical therapy.** In an effort to save the life of a patient, it is sometimes necessary for the clinician to "guess" the most likely pathogen and the drug most likely to be effective. It will, of course, be an "educated guess" based on the clinician's prior experiences with the patient's particular type of infectious disease. Before writing a prescription for a particular antimicrobial agent, the clinician must consider many of the factors listed in this section.

If the laboratory has reported the identity of the bacterial pathogen, the clinician can refer to a **pocket chart,** carried by clinicians in most hospitals. Published by the hospital's clinical microbiology laboratory (CML), the pocket chart contains data on antimicrobial susceptibility testing conducted over the past year. The pocket chart provides important information regarding drugs to which various bacterial pathogens were susceptible and resistant. A sample pocket chart is shown in Figure 7-1. The susceptibility and resistance patterns of bacteria are referred to as antibiograms. Antibiograms are discussed in more detail in Chapter 26. **The clinician will take many of the following factors into consideration before prescribing the drug that, according to the pocket chart, has proven to be the most successful in antimicrobial susceptibility testing in vitro:**

- **Allergies.** Is the patient allergic to any antimicrobial agents? Obviously, it would be unwise to prescribe a drug to which the patient is allergic.

- **Age.** What is the age of the patient? Some drugs are contraindicated in very young or very old patients.

- **Pregnancy.** Is the patient pregnant? Some drugs are known to be or suspected of being teratogenic (i.e., the cause of birth defects).

- **Inpatient or outpatient.** Is the patient an inpatient or outpatient? Some drugs can only be administered intravenously and therefore cannot be prescribed for outpatients.

- **Drug availability.** If the patient is an inpatient, the clinician must prescribe a drug that is available in the

TABLE 7 - 5   Antiprotozoal Agents

Drug[a]	Protozoal Disease(s) Drug Is Used to Treat
Amphotericin B	Primary amebic meningoencephalitis, mucocutaneous leishmaniasis
Artemisinin derivatives	Multidrug-resistant *Plasmodium falciparum* malaria
Benznidazole	American trypanosomiasis (Chagas disease)
Chloroquine phosphate or quinidine gluconate or quinine dihydrochloride	Malaria (except for chloroquine-resistant *P. falciparum* malaria and chloroquine-resistant *Plasmodium vivax* malaria)
Clindamycin plus quinine	Babesiosis
Diloxanide furoate	Amebiasis
Eflornithine	African trypanosomiasis (with or without CNS involvement)
Furazolidone	Giardiasis
Halofantrine	Chloroquine-resistant *P. falciparum* malaria
Iodoquinol	Amebiasis, balantidiasis, *Dientamoeba fragilis* infection
Mefloquine	Chloroquine-resistant *P. falciparum* and *P. vivax* malaria
Melarsoprol	African trypanosomiasis (with CNS involvement)
Metronidazole	Amebiasis, giardiasis, trichomoniasis
Nifurtimox	American trypanosomiasis (Chagas disease)
Nitazoxanide	Giardiasis in children and cryptosporidiosis
Paromomycin	Amebiasis, cryptosporidiosis, *D. fragilis* infection, cutaneous leishmaniasis
Pentamidine isethionate	African sleeping sickness (without CNS involvement), leishmaniasis
Primaquine phosphate	Malaria
Proguanil hydrochloride	Malaria
Pyrimethamine plus sulfadiazine	*P. falciparum* malaria, toxoplasmosis
Quinacrine hydrochloride	Giardiasis
Quinidine gluconate	*P. falciparum* malaria
Quinine	Malaria
Spiramycin	Toxoplasmosis
Stibogluconate sodium	Visceral, cutaneous, and mucocutaneous leishmaniasis
Suramin	African trypanosomiasis (with no CNS involvement)
Tetracycline hydrochloride	Balantidiasis, *Dientamoeba fragilis* infection; can be used with quinine or quinidine for *P. falciparum* malaria
Tinidazole	Amebiasis, giardiasis, trichomoniasis
Trimethoprim-sulfamethoxazole	Cyclosporiasis, isosporiasis

[a]This information is provided solely to acquaint the reader with the names of some antiprotozoal agents and should not be construed as advice regarding recommended therapy.

CNS, central nervous system.

TABLE 7 - 6 Antiviral Agents

Virus/Viral Infection(s)	Antiviral Agents[a]
Herpes simplex infections	Acyclovir, cidofovir, famciclovir, fomivirsen, foscarnet, ganciclovir, penciclovir, valacyclovir, valganciclovir, vidarabine
Respiratory viruses	Amantadine (influenza A virus), oseltamivir (influenza A and B viruses), ribavirin (respiratory syncytial virus, influenza A and B viruses, parainfluenza virus), rimantadine (influenza A virus), zanamivir (influenza A and B viruses)
HIV: nucleoside reverse transcriptase inhibitors	Abacavir, didanosine, lamivudine, stavudine, tenofovir, zalcitabine, zidovudine (AZT, ZDV)
HIV: nonnucleoside reverse transcriptase inhibitors	Delavirdine, efavirenz, nevirapine
HIV: protease inhibitors	Amprenavir, indinavir, lopinavir, nelfinavir, ritonavir, saquinavir

[a]This information is provided solely to acquaint the reader with the names of some antiviral agents and should not be construed as advice regarding recommended therapy.

hospital pharmacy (i.e., a drug that is listed in the hospital formulary).

- **Site of infection.** What is the site of the patient's infection? If the patient has cystitis (urinary bladder infection), the clinician might want to prescribe a drug that concentrates in the urine. Such a drug is rapidly removed from the blood by the kidneys, and high concentrations of the drug are achieved in the urinary bladder. To treat a brain abscess, the clinician would select a drug capable of crossing the blood-brain barrier.

- **Other medications.** What other medications does the patient take? Some antimicrobial agents will cross-react with certain other drugs, leading to a drug interaction that could be harmful to the patient.

- **Other medical problems.** What other medical problems does the patient have? Certain antimicrobial agents are known to have toxic side effects, such as nephrotoxicity, hepatotoxicity, and ototoxicity.[1] For example, a clinician would not prescribe a nephrotoxic drug to a patient who has prior kidney damage, or a hepatotoxic drug to a patient with prior liver damage.

- **Patient's immune status.** Is the patient leukopenic or immunocompromised? If so, it would be preferable to use a bactericidal agent to treat the patient's bacterial infection, rather than a bacteriostatic agent. Recall that bacteriostatic agents should only be used in patients whose host defense mechanisms are functioning properly—that is, only in patients whose bodies are capable of killing the pathogen once its multiplication has been stopped.

A leukopenic patient has too few white blood cells to kill the pathogen, and the immune system of an immunocompromised patient would be unable to kill the pathogen.

- **Cost.** The cost of the various drugs is also a major consideration. Whenever possible, clinicians should prescribe less costly, narrow spectrum drugs.

Although the patient's weight will influence the **dosage** of a particular drug, it usually is not taken into consideration when deciding which drug to prescribe.

UNDESIRABLE EFFECTS OF CHEMOTHERAPEUTIC AGENTS

Listed here are some of the many reasons why chemotherapeutic drugs should never be used indiscriminately.

- **Selecting for drug-resistant organisms.** Whenever an antimicrobial agent is administered to a patient, organisms within that patient that are susceptible to the agent will die, but resistant ones will survive. This is referred to as selecting for resistant organisms (Fig. 7-2). The resistant organisms then multiply, become dominant, and can be transmitted to other people. To prevent the overgrowth of resistant organisms, sometimes several drugs, each with a different mode of action, are administered simultaneously.

- **Development of drug allergies.** The patient may become allergic to the agent. For example, penicillin G in low doses often sensitizes those who are prone to developing

---

[1]Nephrotoxic drugs cause kidney damage, hepatotoxic drugs cause liver damage, and ototoxic drugs cause hearing problems.

	E. coli	P. aeruginosa	Klebsiella	Proteus mirabilis	Enterobacter	Proteus sp.	Serratia	Citrobacter
Total isolates	615	371	253	193	107	33	40	56
Percent Sensitive								
Ampicillin	55	1	3	58	3	15	22	7
Carbenicillin	59	88	2	59	74	91	93	24
Timentin	87	81	88	99	82	97	98	93
Piperacillin	65	91	84	68	89	94	100	96
Cefazolin	95	1	83	97	11	18	0	76
Cefotetan	100	1	100	100	77	100	100	97
Ceftriaxone	100	80	100	100	90	100	100	98
Ceftazidime	100	98	95	100	86	97	100	98
Amikacin	100	100	100	100	100	100	100	100
Gentamicin	100	88	89	93	100	92	100	97
Tobramycin	100	89	94	92	100	94	100	100
Tetracycline	84	3	78	4	97	41	41	93
Trimeth-Sulfa	84	2	75	83	96	88	100	90
Nitrofurantoin	100	1	89	21	95	92	0	100
Ciprofloxacin	100	74	80	85	100	97	100	100

Figure 7-1. **Pocket chart for aerobic Gram-negative bacteria.** Illustrated here is the type of chart that clinicians carry in their pockets for use as a quick reference whenever empirical therapy is necessary. The pocket chart, which is prepared by the medical facility's clinical microbiology laboratory, shows the percentages of organisms susceptible to the various drugs tested. **Example of pocket chart use.** A clinician is informed that *Pseudomonas aeruginosa* has been isolated from the patient's blood culture, but the antimicrobial susceptibility testing results on that isolate will not be available until tomorrow. Because therapy must be initiated immediately, the clinician refers to the pocket chart and sees that amikacin is the most appropriate drug to use. Of the 371 strains of *P. aeruginosa* tested, 100% were susceptible to amikacin. (As explained in the text, the clinician would consider other factors, such as the toxicity of the drug, *before* prescribing amikacin for this patient.) *Question:* Which drug would be the second choice, if amikacin is not available in the hospital pharmacy? *Answer:* Ceftazidime. (Note: This pocket chart is for educational purposes only and should not be used in an actual clinical setting.)

allergies. When these people receive a second dose of penicillin at some later date, they may break out in hives or have a severe reaction known as anaphylactic shock.[2]

- **Drug toxicity.** Many antimicrobial agents are toxic to humans, and some are so toxic that they are administered only for serious diseases for which no other agents are available. One such drug is chloramphenicol (Chloromycetin), which, if given in high doses for a long period, may cause a very severe type of anemia called aplastic anemia. Another is streptomycin, which can damage the auditory nerve and cause deafness. Other drugs are hepatotoxic or nephrotoxic, causing liver or

kidney damage, respectively. For more information on drug toxicity, see the section later in this chapter titled "Monitoring Serum Levels of Antimicrobial Agents."

- **Superinfections.** With prolonged use, broad-spectrum antibiotics may destroy the normal flora of the mouth, intestine, or vagina. The person no longer has the protection of the indigenous microflora and thus becomes much more susceptible to infections caused by opportunists or secondary invaders. The resultant overgrowth by such organisms is referred to as a **superinfection.** A superinfection can be thought of as a population explosion of organisms that are usually present in relatively small

---

[2] *Anaphylactic shock is a severe, often fatal form of shock characterized by smooth muscle contraction and capillary dilation (increase in diameter of blood vessels).*

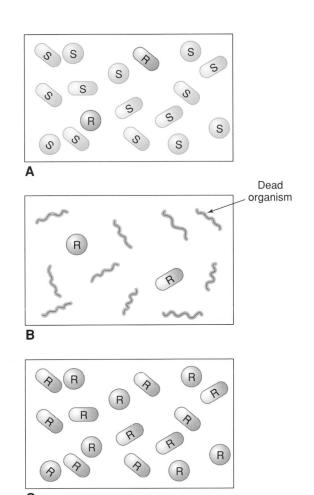

Figure 7-2. **Selecting for drug-resistant organisms. A.** Indigenous microflora of a patient before initiation of antibiotic therapy. Most members of the population are susceptible (*S*) to the antibiotic to be administered; very few are resistant (*R*). **B.** After antibiotic therapy has been initiated, the susceptible organisms are dead; only a few resistant organisms remain. **C.** As a result of decreased competition for nutrients and space, the resistant organisms multiply and become the predominant organisms in the patient's indigenous microflora.

A superinfection is an overgrowth of an organism or organisms usually present at a particular anatomical site in much lower number(s). Superinfections can lead to diseases such as antibiotic-associated diarrhea, pseudomembranous colitis, thrush, and yeast vaginitis.

numbers. For example, the prolonged use of oral antibiotics can result in a superinfection of the bacterium *Clostridium difficile* in the colon, which can lead to such diseases as antibiotic-associated diarrhea and pseudomembranous colitis. Vaginitis often follows antibacterial therapy because many bacteria of the vaginal flora were destroyed, leading to a superinfection of the indigenous yeast *Candida albicans*. This leads to the condition known as yeast vaginitis. A superinfection of *C. albicans* in the mouth can lead to a condition known as thrush.

ANTIMICROBIAL SUSCEPTIBILITY TESTING

Not only are bacterial pathogens isolated and identified in the bacteriology section of the CML, they are also tested to determine what drugs will kill them (i.e., to which drugs they are susceptible) and what drugs seem to have no effect (i.e., to which drugs they are resistant). Such testing is called **antimicrobial susceptibility testing (AST).** AST is necessary because, except in very rare cases, it is impossible to predict the drugs to which a particular bacterial isolate is susceptible or resistant. Most CMLs perform AST only on bacterial pathogens. However, with the ever-increasing number of fungi—both yeasts and moulds—becoming resistant to antifungal agents, it is likely that antifungal susceptibility testing will become a routine procedure in CMLs in the near future. The remainder of this section pertains to susceptibility testing of bacteria.

AST is performed to determine the drugs to which microorganisms are susceptible and resistant. Listed here are five methods for performing AST, the first four of which are approved by the Clinical and Laboratory Standards Institute (CLSI):

- Agar dilution method, which uses many agar plates

- Broth macrodilution or macrobroth dilution method, which uses many tubes of liquid culture media

- Broth microdilution or microbroth dilution method, which uses small plastic trays called microtiter trays

- Disk diffusion method, which uses a combination of agar plates and paper disks impregnated with antimicrobial agents

- Gradient diffusion method (the Etest)

Regardless of which method of AST is used, the testing must be performed in the exact manner prescribed by the CLSI or, when such guidelines are unavailable, in accordance with the manufacturer's instructions.

It is critical that antimicrobial susceptibility testing be performed in the exact manner prescribed by the CLSI.

Agar Dilution Method

In this method of AST, a large number of Mueller-Hinton (M-H) agar plates are used. For each antimicrobial agent being tested, several plates are needed (5 plates will be used here as an example). Thus, to test 20 agents, a total of 5 times 20 or 100 plates would be required. Although this

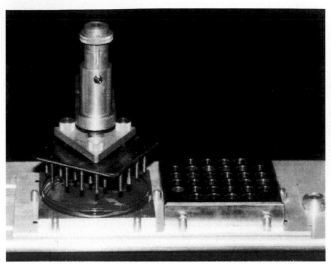

Figure 7-3. Steer's replicator. The inoculating head and prongs are fixed. On a sliding tray beneath the prongs are a metal template (to the right) and an agar plate to be inoculated (to the left). The template contains 32 wells, into each of which is added a suspension of an organism to be tested. The template is slid beneath the inoculating head and the prongs are lowered into the wells. The prongs are then lifted. The cover is removed from an agar plate and the plate is then slid into position beneath the prongs. The prongs are then lowered, thus inoculating the plate surface with each organism to be tested. (From Winn WC Jr, et al. Koneman's Color Atlas and Textbook of Diagnostic Microbiology. 6th Ed. Philadelphia: Lippincott Williams & Wilkins, 2006.)

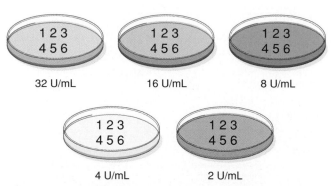

Figure 7-4. Agar dilution method of antimicrobial susceptibility testing. In this example, five Mueller-Hinton agar plates are being used to determine each organism's susceptibility to penicillin. Each plate contains a different concentration of penicillin, using doubling dilutions of penicillin from 32 U/mL to 2 U/mL. Each bacterial isolate is inoculated onto the surface of each of the five plates (a Steer's replicator can be used for this purpose). In this example, six isolates are being tested, represented by the numbers 1 through 6.

method of AST is highly accurate, it is also labor intensive and thus not practical for use in most CMLs. Even if only one isolate requires testing, someone in the CML would have to prepare a total of 100 plates. The good news is that it is possible to test more than one organism on each plate, using a multiprong inoculator called a Steer's replicator (Fig. 7-3). Because the agar dilution method is not used in many, if any, CMLs, only a brief description of the method appears here.

To test an isolate's susceptibility or resistance to penicillin, for example, a series of five plates are used, each plate containing a different concentration of penicillin (Fig. 7-4). The concentrations of penicillin shown in Figure 7-4 are for illustration purposes only. In an actual CML setting, the concentrations tested would be safe and achievable blood levels. *Safe* means that these drug levels would not be toxic to the patient. *Achievable* means that the concentrations of drug could actually be achieved in the patient's bloodstream by the usual route of administration. The concentrations of antimicrobial agents to be used in any of these methods of AST are determined by the CLSI.

The isolates to be tested are inoculated onto each of the plates. The plates are then incubated at 35°C for 16 to

20 hours in a non-CO_2 incubator.[3] At the end of the incubation period, each plate is checked for growth of the isolates. If a particular organism grew on a plate containing a particular concentration of penicillin, its growth was obviously *not* inhibited by that concentration of drug. If, on the other hand, the organism is not growing on a plate containing a particular concentration of penicillin, growth of the organism *was* inhibited by that concentration of drug (see the example in Figure 7-5).

In the example shown in Figure 7-5, isolate 1 is growing on four of the plates (the 2-U/mL, 4-U/mL, 8-U/mL, and 16-U/mL plates)[4] but is not growing on the plate containing 32 U/mL. *Question:* What result will be reported to the clinician? *Answer:* The clinician will be informed of the lowest concentration of penicillin that inhibited growth of the

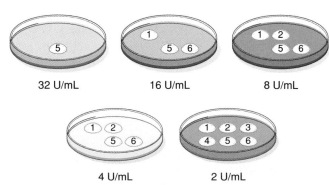

Figure 7-5. Agar dilution method of antimicrobial susceptibility testing (cont.). The same five plates as in Figure 7-4 are shown here following incubation of the plates. Small circles on the plates represent growth of the organisms being tested.

---

[3]*A CO_2 incubator must not be used routinely for AST. If plates, tubes, or trays were to be incubated in a CO_2 incubator, CO_2 could diffuse into the medium, causing the formation of carbonic acid, which would lower the pH of the medium. The lower pH could cause a change in the activity of certain antimicrobial agents. In certain situations, however, a CO_2 incubator is used—for example when testing certain fastidious bacteria, such as* Streptococcus pneumoniae, Haemophilus influenzae, *and* Neisseria gonorrhoeae, *which require CO_2 incubation for growth.*

[4]*Although drug concentrations are usually expressed in micrograms per milliliter (μg/mL), penicillin concentrations are expressed in units per milliliter (U/mL).*

> The MIC of a drug is the lowest concentration of the drug that will inhibit the growth of the organism.

organism. This is known as the **minimum inhibitory concentration (MIC).** In this example, the MIC was 32 U/mL. Thus, the laboratory report will state that the MIC for penicillin is 32 U/mL. Can you determine the MIC for the other five isolates (numbered 2 through 6)? Answers are at the end of the chapter.

The MIC for each antimicrobial agent is determined and reported to the clinician. With regard to the MIC for a given antimicrobial agent, there are really only three possibilities:

Possibility 1. The organism being tested grew on some of the plates but stopped growing at some point. The concentration of drug in the plate where it stopped growing is the MIC. In the example presented here, the MIC for penicillin was 32 U/mL.

Possibility 2. The organism being tested grew on all five plates, in which case the MIC would be greater than the highest concentration of drug that was tested. If this had been the result in the example here, the report would have stated that the MIC for penicillin was >32 U/mL.

Possibility 3. The organism being tested did not grow on any of the five plates but did grow on the growth control plate, which contained no drugs. If this had been the result in the example, the report would have stated that the MIC for penicillin was less than or equal to 2 U/mL (≤2 U/mL).

All steps in the agar dilution method are performed in accordance with the guidelines published by the CLSI. These include media preparation and storage, preparation of the inoculum, method of inoculation, time of incubation, and interpretation of results. In addition, quality control (QC) organisms are tested each time clinical isolates are tested. The QC organisms to be tested are prescribed by the CLSI.

Broth Macrodilution Method

In the broth macrodilution method of AST, sometimes referred to as the macrobroth dilution method, a large number of tubes of M-H broth are used. Several tubes are used for each antimicrobial agent being tested (5 tubes will be used here as an example). Thus, if 20 agents are to be tested, a total of 5 times 20 or 100 tubes would be required. Like the agar dilution method, the broth macrodilution method is labor intensive and impractical for use in most CMLs. Someone in the CML would have to prepare a total of 100 tubes for each isolate being tested. Because the broth

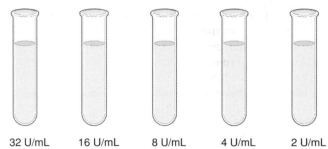

32 U/mL   16 U/mL   8 U/mL   4 U/mL   2 U/mL

Figure 7-6. **Broth macrodilution method of antimicrobial susceptibility testing.** In this example, five tubes of Mueller-Hinton broth are being used to determine the organism's susceptibility to penicillin. Each tube contains a different concentration of penicillin, using doubling dilutions of penicillin from 32 U/mL to 2 U/mL.

macrodilution method is not used in many CMLs, only a brief description of the method is presented here.

Again using penicillin as an example, to test an isolate's susceptibility or resistance to penicillin, a series of five tubes are used, and each tube contains a different concentration of penicillin (Fig. 7-6).

A standardized suspension of the isolate is inoculated into each tube. All the tubes are then incubated at 35°C for 16 to 20 hours in a non-CO_2 incubator. At the end of the incubation period, each tube is checked for growth of the isolate. If the organism grew in a tube containing a particular concentration of penicillin, it obviously was not killed by that concentration of drug. If, on the other hand, the organism is not growing in a tube containing a particular concentration of penicillin, the organism was killed by that concentration of drug. See the example shown in Figure 7-7.

In this example, the isolate is growing at 2 U/mL but not at 4, 8, 16, and 32 U/mL. *Question:* What will be reported to the clinician? *Answer:* The clinician will be informed of the lowest concentration of penicillin that inhibited growth of the organism. In this example, the MIC was 4 U/mL. Thus, the lab report will state that the MIC for penicillin is 4 U/mL.

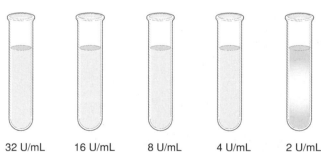

32 U/mL   16 U/mL   8 U/mL   4 U/mL   2 U/mL

Figure 7-7. **Broth macrodilution method of antimicrobial susceptibility testing (cont.).** The same five tubes as in Figure 7-6 are shown here following inoculation and incubation of the tubes. Shading represents visible growth in the tubes. As can be seen, visible growth occurred at 2 U/mL but not at 4, 8, 16, or 32 U/mL.

The MIC for each antimicrobial agent is determined and reported to the clinician. As with the agar dilution method, there are only three possibilities with regard to MICs: (1) the organism grew in some but not all of the tubes, (2) the organism grew in all the tubes, or (3) the organism did not grow in any of the tubes but did grow in the growth control tube.

As was true for the agar dilution method, all steps in the broth macrodilution method are performed in accordance with the guidelines published by the CLSI, and QC organisms are tested each time that clinical isolates are tested. The QC organisms to be tested are prescribed by the CLSI.

Broth Microdilution Method

The broth microdilution method, sometimes referred to as the microbroth dilution method, is currently the most pop-

> The broth microdilution method or microbroth dilution method is the most popular method in the U.S. for performing antimicrobial susceptibility testing.

ular method for performing AST in the United States (Fig. 7-8). There are several reasons for its popularity:

- It is an accurate method, comparing favorably with the "gold standard" agar dilution method.

- It is an appropriate method for testing any number of isolates—from just one to many.

- The microtiter trays, containing a variety of concentrations of many antimicrobial agents, are commercially available, thus saving CML professionals the time it would take to prepare the trays in the laboratory.

- The lyophilized or frozen trays can be stored until they are needed.

- The trays are very easy to inoculate.

- The results are easy to read, and with some products, results can be read by instruments.

Once a microtiter tray is inoculated with the organism being tested, the trays are incubated at 35°C for 16 to 20 hours in a non-CO_2 incubator. Determinations are then made as to whether or not the organism grew in the various concentrations of the drugs. Turbidity of the broth or a button of cells at the bottom of the well is considered evidence of growth. Results are reported in terms of MICs—the lowest concentrations of the drugs that inhibited growth of the organisms (Fig. 7-9).

What is the MIC for each of the drugs shown in Figure 7-9? Hint: The MIC for the first drug, V, is ≤2 μg/mL. It is not necessary for you to know what drugs the abbreviations stand for. Answers can be found at the end of the chapter.

As was true for the agar and broth macrodilution methods, all steps in the broth microdilution method are performed in accordance with the guidelines published by the CLSI. Whenever commercial systems are used, CML professionals must strictly follow the manufacturer's instructions regarding storage, inoculation, and incubation of the microtiter trays; interpretation of test results; and QC organisms to be used.

Some of the automated and semiautomated AST systems are listed in Table 7-7. Inoculated plastic cards, panels, or trays are incubated within the automated systems, which automatically read, record, and interpret MIC results after appropriate incubation periods. An automated system is shown in Figure 7-8B. Preincubated cards, panels, or trays are inserted into the semiautomated systems, which then

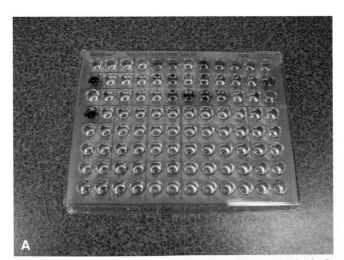
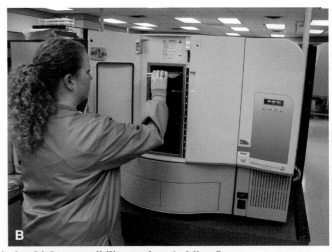

Figure 7-8. **Broth microdilution method of antimicrobial susceptibility testing. A.** MicroScan Neg/Urine Combo Panel for combined identification and antimicrobial susceptibility testing of Gram-negative bacteria isolated from urine specimens. The wells contain various substrates and multiple concentrations of antimicrobial agents. **B.** Inoculated MicroScan panel being placed into a MicroScan WalkAway instrument, manufactured by Dade Behring. (Courtesy of Dr. Robert Fader.)

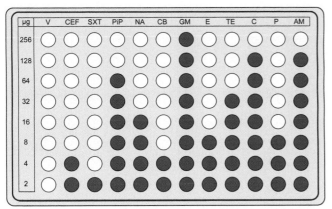

***Figure 7-9.* The broth microdilution method of antimicrobial susceptibility testing, showing test results following incubation.** Circles represent wells in the plastic microtiter tray. Shading of the wells indicates that growth of the organism being tested occurred in those wells; that is, growth occurred at those drug concentrations. Unshaded wells represent no growth; that is, growth did not occur at those drug concentrations. After reading about the broth microdilution method in the text, determine the MIC of each of the drugs that were tested. Drug concentrations are expressed in μg/mL, except for penicillin (*P*), which is expressed in Units/mL. Correct answers appear at the end of the chapter.

automatically read, record, and interpret MIC results. Depending on the system being used, cards, panels, or trays are available for testing Gram-positive bacteria, Gram-negative bacteria, Gram-negative bacteria isolated from urine specimens, and nonfermenters. In addition, some manufacturers provide cards or trays to test *Streptococcus pneumoniae* and to screen for extended-spectrum β-lactamase producers (described later in the chapter).

Disk Diffusion Method

Disk diffusion AST is also referred to as the Kirby-Bauer method, named for two microbiologists, Drs. Kirby and Bauer, who in 1966 described a standardized technique for performing disk diffusion AST. At one time, the disk diffusion method was the most popular AST method in the United States, but with the introduction of commercially prepared, antimicrobial agent–containing microtiter trays, the broth microdilution method has become the most popular method of AST in the United States. All steps in the disk diffusion method must be performed as specified in the appropriate CLSI document (see "References and Suggested Reading").

In the disk diffusion method, the organism to be tested is inoculated over the entire surface of an M-H agar plate. The inoculum may be prepared in one of two ways:

- The top portion of three to five, 18-to-24-hour-old, well-isolated, morphologically identical colonies can be transferred to a tube containing 4 to 5 mL of a suitable broth medium (e.g., tryptic soy broth). The broth culture is incubated at 35°C until the turbidity of the culture meets or exceeds the turbidity of a 0.5 McFarland turbidity standard.[5] If, after incubation, the turbidity exceeds that of the 0.5 McFarland standard, sterile saline can be added to the culture until the turbidity matches that of the standard.

- Several 18-to-24-hour-old, well-isolated, morphologically identical colonies can be transferred to a tube containing 4 to 5 mL of a suitable broth medium (e.g., tryptic soy broth) or sterile saline. The turbidity of the suspension is then adjusted (either by adding more of the organism or by adding more liquid) until it matches the turbidity of a 0.5 McFarland standard.

TABLE 7 - 7	Examples of Automated and Semiautomated Antimicrobial Susceptibility Testing Systems (ASTs)	
Type of System	**Name of System**	**Manufacturer**
Automated AST Systems	MicroScan WalkAway	Dade Behring (http://www.dedebehring.com/)
	Phoenix	BD Biosciences (http://www.bdbiosciences.com/)
	Sensititre ARIS	Trek Diagnostic Systems (http://www.trekds.com/)
	Vitek System (or Vitek 1)	bioMérieux Inc. (http://www.biomerieux.com/)
	Vitek 2	bioMérieux Inc.
Semiautomated AST Systems	MicroScan AutoScan 3 and AutoScan 4	Dade Behring
	Sensititre	Trek Diagnostic Systems

[5]*McFarland standards are a series of tubes containing various amounts of barium sulfate ($BaSO_4$). The higher the concentration of $BaSO_4$, the more turbid (cloudy) the suspension.*

Inoculation of the M-H agar plate is accomplished as described by the CLSI. In essence, it involves swabbing the entire surface of the plate three times, in three different directions, to ensure that the organism grows over the entire surface of the plate; this is known as a "lawn of growth." Note that a swab is used to inoculate the plate, rather than an inoculating loop.

Small filter paper disks, each containing a different antimicrobial agent, are then placed on the agar surface, making sure that the entire lower surface of each disk is in contact with the agar surface. The plate is then inverted and incubated for 16 to 18 hours at $35°C$ in a non-CO_2 incubator. During the incubation period, the drug diffuses into the agar (Fig. 7-10).

The selection of drugs or disks to be used depends on several factors, some of which are mentioned here:

- Is the organism being tested Gram positive or Gram negative? Certain antimicrobial agents are effective only against Gram-positive bacteria, whereas others are effective only against Gram-negative bacteria.

- If the organism being tested is a Gram-positive coccus, is it a *Staphylococcus* sp., an *Enterococcus* sp., or *S. pneumoniae*? The battery of drugs tested varies from one type of Gram-positive coccus to another.

- If the organism being tested is a Gram-negative bacillus, is it a member of the Enterobacteriaceae family, *Pseudomonas aeruginosa*, or a fastidious Gram-negative organism such as *Haemophilus influenzae* or *Neisseria*

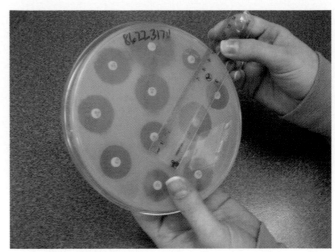

Figure 7-11. **Disk diffusion method of antimicrobial susceptibility testing (cont.).** A CML professional is measuring zone sizes, which will be recorded in millimeters. The green color is the result of pigment production by the organism that was tested—*Pseudomonas aeruginosa*. (Courtesy of Dr. Robert Fader.)

gonorrhoeae? The battery of drugs tested varies from one type of Gram-negative bacterium to another.

- What type of infection is the organism causing? For example, certain drugs are tested only if the organism is causing cystitis (urinary bladder infection). These are drugs that concentrate in the urine because they are rapidly removed from the bloodstream by the kidneys. Thus, high levels of the drug are achieved at the site of the infection, the urinary bladder.

The most recently published CLSI document describing disk diffusion AST must always be consulted when deciding which drugs to test, because recommendations change frequently.

After 16 to 18 hours of incubation, the plate is removed from the incubator, and the diameter of each **zone of no growth** is carefully measured in millimeters (Fig. 7-11). A zone of no growth around a particular disk represents an area where the growth of the organism was inhibited by the drug that diffused from that disk into the agar. In other words, the organism is not growing in that circular area because it was inhibited (perhaps killed) by the drug that diffused from the disk. A zone of no growth is also known as a **zone of inhibition** or a **zone of inhibition of growth.**

The measured zone sizes must then be compared with zone sizes listed on published charts to determine if the organism is susceptible, intermediate, or resistant to the various drugs tested.[6] The charts to be used for interpretation of zone sizes are published by the CLSI. (See examples in Table 7-8.) Even when a zone of no growth is present, the zone size might not be large enough for the organism to be considered susceptible to the drug. Also, it is not possible to

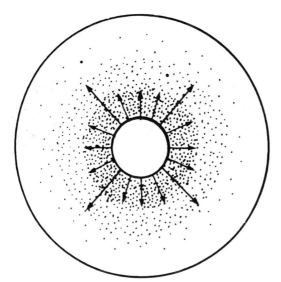

Figure 7-10. **Disk diffusion method of antimicrobial susceptibility testing.** During incubation, the drug diffuses out of the disk into the agar, creating a concentration gradient of the drug. The concentration of drug in the agar decreases as the drug diffuses further away from the disk. (From Winn WC Jr, et al. Koneman's Color Atlas and Textbook of Diagnostic Microbiology. 6th Ed. Philadelphia: Lippincott Williams & Wilkins, 2006.)

---

[6]*In the past, the "intermediate" category was called "moderately susceptible." Usually, a clinician would not prescribe a drug to which the organism is resistant or intermediate, if drugs are available to which the organism is susceptible.*

TABLE 7 - 8	Interpretation of Zone Sizes[a]		
Antimicrobial Agent	**Resistant**	**Intermediate**	**Susceptible**
Chloramphenicol, 30 µg	≤12 mm	13–17 mm	≥18 mm
Tetracycline, 30 µg	≤14 mm	15–18 mm	≥19 mm

Example 1. If the measured chloramphenicol zone size was 18 mm or greater, then the organism being tested would be considered susceptible to chloramphenicol.

Example 2. If the measured tetracycline zone size was 14 mm or less, then the organism being tested would be considered resistant to tetracycline.

[a]Shown here is a small portion of the type of interpretive criteria chart published by the Clinical and Laboratory Standards Institute. The interpretive criteria published by the CLSI are derived from a correlation between zone sizes and MICs. The symbol ≤ means "less than or equal to." The symbol ≥ means "greater than or equal to." (Note: This chart is provided for educational purposes only and should not be used in an actual CML.)

conclude that one drug is more effective than another merely because it has produced a larger zone size. The reason for this is that the disks contain different quantities of antimicrobial agents and the drugs diffuse at different rates.

Figures 7-12 and 7-13 illustrate two of the aberrant results that might be encountered when zone sizes are interpreted. Table 7-9 describes problems that can occur in the disk diffusion method when standardized steps in the procedure are not followed precisely.

Because of their fastidious nature, certain bacteria—like *H. influenzae*, *N. gonorrhoeae*, *S. pneumoniae*, and viridans group streptococci—require modified testing procedures, such as the use of chocolate agar or blood agar in place of M-H agar and incubation of the inoculated plates in a CO_2 incubator. As with all other organisms being tested,

the procedures described by the CLSI must be followed explicitly.

Predefined Gradient Method

The predefined gradient for full-range MIC determinations of antimicrobial agents (also known as the Etest) is manufactured by AB Biodisk (http://www.abbiodisk.com).

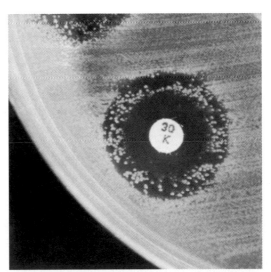

Figure 7-13. **Disk diffusion method of antimicrobial susceptibility testing (cont.).** Sometimes colonies appear within the zone of no growth. Possible explanations for this phenomenon are (1) the inoculum may not have been a pure culture, in which case the outer zone of no growth may be the result of one bacterial species, and the colonies within the zone may represent a second species; or (2) the colonies within the zone of no growth may represent colonies produced by mutants of the organism being tested—that is, colonies produced by mutants that have developed resistance to this particular drug. (From Winn WC Jr, et al. Koneman's Color Atlas and Textbook of Diagnostic Microbiology. 6th Ed. Philadelphia: Lippincott Williams & Wilkins, 2006.)

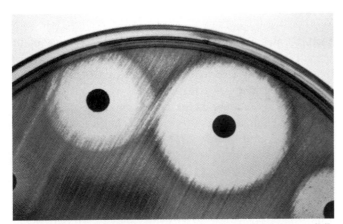

Figure 7-12. **Disk diffusion method of antimicrobial susceptibility testing (cont.).** Swarming bacteria, such as the *Proteus* species shown here, often produce zones with "fuzzy" edges. In such cases, the edge of the outermost zone of no growth should be used when measuring the zone size. (From Winn WC Jr, et al. Koneman's Color Atlas and Textbook of Diagnostic Microbiology. 6th Ed. Philadelphia: Lippincott Williams & Wilkins, 2006.)

TABLE 7 - 9	Problems That May Occur When Standardized Steps in the Disk Diffusion Method Are Not Followed Precisely[a]
Problem	**Effect**
Mueller-Hinton medium not prepared in accordance with prescribed recipe	Medium may not support the growth of the organism being tested
pH of Mueller-Hinton medium too high or too low (should be pH 7.2–7.4)	May affect the activity of some antimicrobial agents
Mueller-Hinton medium is too deep (>4 mm)	Zone sizes will be too small
Mueller-Hinton medium is too shallow (<4 mm)	Zone sizes will be too large
Inoculum too heavy	Zone sizes will be too small
Inoculum too light	Zone sizes will be too large
Disks placed too close together	Zones may overlap, making them difficult to measure
Disks not pressed flush with agar surface	May result in irregularly shaped zones
Disk strength too high	Zone sizes may be too small
Disk strength too low (incorrect or expired disk being used)	Zone sizes may be too large
Inoculated plates incubated in a CO_2 incubator	CO_2 could diffuse into the medium, causing the formation of carbonic acid, which would lower the pH of the medium

[a]A person would recognize when one or more of these problems is occurring when testing the quality control organisms.

Although the CLSI does not officially endorse any commercial products, more than 200 peer-reviewed published evaluations have demonstrated that the Etest MIC results for many antimicrobial agents and organism groups are substantially equivalent to the reference CLSI broth microdilution and agar dilution methods. Further, like other commercial AST products, Etest is regulated and cleared by the Food and Drug Administration (FDA) for clinical use in the United States. Currently, Etest is FDA-approved for testing of Gram-positive and Gram-negative aerobes, pneumococci, streptococci, *Haemophilus*, anaerobes, gonococci, and yeast.

Etest comprises a plastic strip immobilized with a preformed and predefined gradient of an antimicrobial agent on one side of the strip and the corresponding MIC reading scale on the opposite side (Fig. 7-14). The Etest concentration gradient spans across a range of 15 twofold dilutions. The ranges are optimally selected to provide on-scale MIC results for many organisms and simultaneously to cover the clinically relevant MIC interpretive breakpoints recommended for categorization of susceptibility groups.[7]

To create an even lawn of semiconfluent growth, a suspension of the test organism is inoculated onto the surface of a defined susceptibility test agar plate suitable for the organism, antibiotic, and/or resistance mechanism being detected. The Etest strips are then applied to the surface of the fully dried inoculated plate as shown in Figure 7-15, with the gradient side in contact with the agar surface (downward), and oriented so that the lowest concentration of drug is toward the center of the plate. The plate is then incubated under the appropriate conditions and for the recommended time.

When applied to an inoculated agar plate, the antimicrobial agent is immediately released from the Etest strip into the agar, creating a continuous and exponential concentration gradient of the antimicrobial agent beneath the linear axis of the carrier. After 24 to 48 hours of incubation, an elliptical zone of inhibition centered along the axis of the strip is seen if the organism is inhibited by the gradient of concentrations in that particular strip (Fig. 7-16). The zone edge intersects the strip at the concentration inhibitory to growth, and the point of intersection gives the MIC in μg/mL. MICs are read directly from the scale on the Etest strip.

---

[7]The term breakpoints *refers to MIC cutoffs used to clinically define whether an infection caused by a certain organism may respond to therapy when the MIC of the antibiotic is below the susceptible breakpoint (i.e., a susceptible organism) or may* not *respond to therapy when the MIC is above the resistant breakpoint (i.e., a resistant organism). These breakpoints are based on standard dosage regimens and routes of administration.*

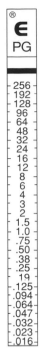

Figure 7-14. Etest. Shown here is one of the plastic carrier strips that exemplify Etest. The underside of the strip carries a preformed exponential gradient of the antimicrobial agent, and the upper-side (shown here) carries a scale for reading minimum inhibitory concentrations (MICs). One antimicrobial agent is immobilized on each plastic carrier strip. (Courtesy of AB Biodisk.)

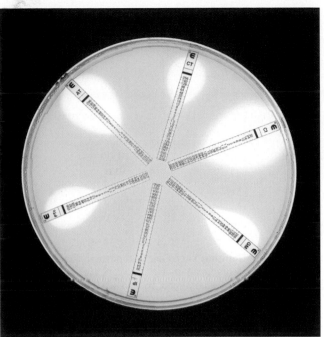

Figure 7-16. Etest (cont.). If growth of the organism was inhibited to any extent by one of the antimicrobial agents, an inhibition ellipse (such as the ones shown) is seen. Using the reading scale on the Etest strip, an MIC is determined and recorded. (Courtesy of AB Biodisk.)

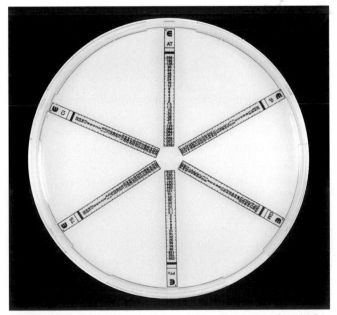

Figure 7-15. Etest (cont.). To use Etest, the agar surface is first inoculated with the test organism and dried completely. Etest strips for different antimicrobial agents are then applied to the agar surface, as shown here. Following incubation, MICs are read from the strip and recorded. (Courtesy of AB Biodisk.)

Minimum Bactericidal Concentration (MBC)

In the broth macrodilution and microdilution MIC tests described earlier, there may or may not be any live organisms in the tubes or wells showing no visible evidence of growth—that is, those that are not turbid. Too few organisms are in the tubes or wells to cause turbidity, but some live organisms *might* be present. With certain patients—usually, those who are immunosuppressed or leukopenic—clinicians might be interested in knowing the lowest concentration of drug that *kills* all the organisms.[8] That concentration of drug is known as the **minimum bactericidal concentration (MBC),** and the test used to determine that concentration is called the MBC test.

> The MBC is the lowest concentration of drug that kills 99.9% of the organisms.

The MBC test can be performed after either the broth macrodilution or microdilution procedure has been performed, following the guidelines published by the CLSI (see "References and Suggested Reading"). In the example shown in Figure 7-17, visible growth has occurred in the tubes containing 2 μg/mL and 4 μg/mL of drug, but no evidence of

---

[8]*Technically, the MBC is the concentration that resulted in a 99.9% reduction in the number of colony-forming units per milliliter (CFU/mL) compared with the organism concentration in the original inoculum.*

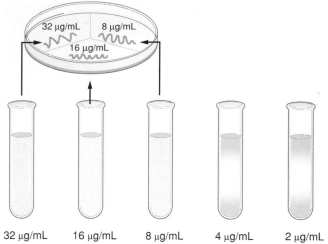

Figure 7-17. **Minimum bactericidal concentration (MBC) test.** The MIC for the organism shown here is 8 μg/mL. Aliquots of broth from the tubes containing 8, 16, and 32 μg/mL are inoculated onto a blood agar plate.

growth is visible in the other three tubes. The MIC is 8 μg/mL. The MBC test is then performed to determine if any viable (live) organisms are in the three tubes with no visible evidence of growth. An inoculating loopful of broth is aseptically removed from each of the three tubes showing no visible growth and inoculated onto a section of a blood agar (BA) plate (Fig. 7-17).

The BA plate is then incubated overnight at 35°C to 37°C in a CO_2 incubator. Following incubation, the BA plate is examined for growth (colonies). Wherever colonies are observed, it is obvious that all organisms were not killed by that concentration of drug. The MBC is the lowest concentration of drug having no colonies. In the example shown in Figure 7-18, the MBC is 16 μg/mL.

β-Lactamases and β-Lactamase Testing

At the heart of every penicillin and cephalosporin molecule is a double-ringed structure, which in penicillins resembles a

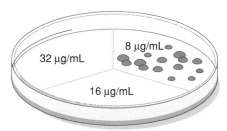

Figure 7-18. **MBC test (cont.).** Following incubation of the blood agar plate, colonies can be seen on the section of the plate labeled 8 μg/mL, but no colonies are on the sections labeled 16 and 32 μg/mL. Thus, the lowest concentration of drug that killed all the organisms is 16 μg/mL. The MBC for this drug is 16 μg/mL.

"house and garage" (Fig. 7-19). The garage is called the **β-lactam ring.** Many bacteria produce enzymes that destroy the β-lactam ring; these enzymes are known as **β-lactamases.** When the β-lactam ring is destroyed, the drug is no longer capable of killing organisms. Thus, an organism that produces a β-lactamase is resistant to antibiotics containing the β-lactam ring—drugs collectively referred to as **β-lactam antibiotics** or **β-lactams.**

There are two general categories of β-lactamases: penicillinases and cephalosporinases. **Penicillinases** destroy the β-lactam ring in penicillins; thus, an organism that produces penicillinase is resistant to penicillins. **Cephalosporinases** destroy the β-lactam ring in cephalosporins; thus, an organism that produces cephalosporinase is resistant to cephalosporins. Some bacteria produce both types of β-lactamases.

To combat the effect of β-lactamases, drug companies have developed special drugs that combine a β-lactam antibiotic with a β-lactamase inhibitor, such as clavulanic acid, sulbactam, or tazobactam. The β-lactam inhibitor irreversibly binds to and inactivates the β-lactamase, thereby enabling the companion drug to enter the bacterial cell and disrupt cell wall synthesis. Following are some of these special combination drugs:

> The two general categories of β-lactamases are penicillinases, which destroy the β-lactam ring in penicillins, and cephalosporinases, which destroy the β-lactam ring in cephalosporins.

- Clavulanic acid (clavulanate) combined with amoxicillin (Augmentin)

- Clavulanic acid (clavulanate) combined with ticarcillin (Timentin)

- Sulbactam combined with ampicillin (Unasyn)

- Tazobactam combined with piperacillin (Zosyn)

When they are isolated from clinical specimens, certain organisms, such as *H. influenzae* and *N. gonorrhoeae*, are first tested for β-lactamase production. The β-lactamase test is described in Appendix A. If the test is negative (i.e., the organism is *not* producing a β-lactamase), then AST is *not* performed. The clinician will prescribe whichever β-lactam antibiotic has traditionally been used to successfully treat infections caused by the pathogen. If, however, the test is positive (i.e., the organism *is* producing a β-lactamase), then AST must be performed to determine other drugs to which the organism may also be resistant. It is important to understand that organisms may be resistant to β-lactam antibiotics even when the β-lactamase test is negative. Such organisms are resistant to β lactams by mechanisms other than production of β-lactamases. Also, organisms producing β-lactamases may be susceptible to drugs known as extended-spectrum cephalosporin agents.

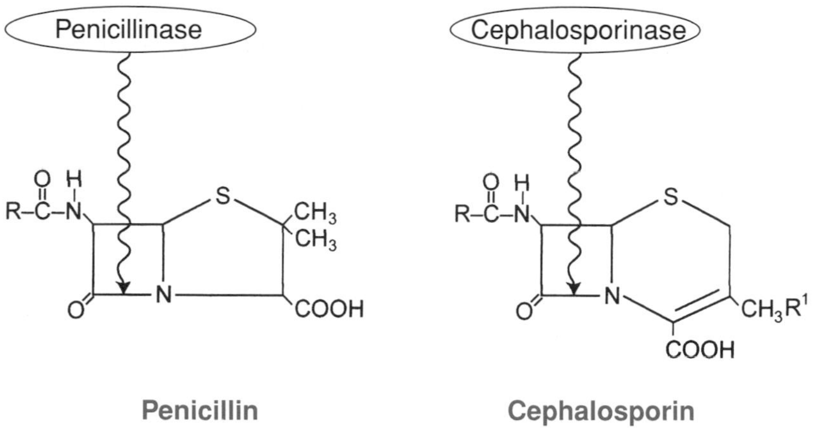

Figure 7-19. Sites of β-lactamase attack on penicillin and cephalosporin molecules.

Extended-Spectrum β-Lactamase Testing

Some Gram-negative bacilli (e.g., some isolates of *Klebsiella pneumoniae*, *K. oxytoca*, *Escherichia coli*, *Enterobacter* spp., *Citrobacter* spp., and *Proteus mirabilis*) produce enzymes known as extended-spectrum β-lactamases (ESBLs). ESBL-producing strains may be resistant to certain drugs (e.g., penicillins, cephalosporins, and aztreonam) to which most strains of these species are susceptible. The CLSI publishes methods to use in screening for these ESBL-producing strains.

MONITORING SERUM LEVELS OF ANTIMICROBIAL AGENTS

Sometimes a clinician wants to know the concentration of an antimicrobial agent in a patient's serum. The clinician may be interested in knowing if a therapeutic concentration of the drug has been achieved or, when especially toxic drugs—such as aminoglycosides, chloramphenicol, and vancomycin—are being administered, if *too much* of the drug has entered the patient's system. In some pathology departments, such testing—referred to as therapeutic drug monitoring—is performed in the chemistry laboratory, rather than the CML.

The usual times for obtaining serum specimens for testing are immediately *before* the drug is administered, called the **trough level**, and at a specific time *after* the drug is administered, called the **peak level.** The time after administration depends on whether the drug was administered intravenously, intramuscularly, or orally. The laboratory request slip that accompanies the serum specimen must state the time the drug was administered *and* the time the specimen was collected.

MEASURING THE ANTIBACTERIAL ACTIVITY OF A PATIENT'S SERUM

CML professionals are occasionally requested to test the bactericidal activity of a patient's serum against an isolate of the bacterial pathogen that is causing the patient's infectious disease. This test is referred to as the serum bactericidal test or Schlichter test. The antibacterial activity of the patient's serum is primarily a result of the presence of antimicrobial agents in the serum. Usually, peak and trough serum specimens (defined in the previous section) are collected from the patient and used in this test. Because the Schlichter test is rarely requested, details of the test will not be presented here. A standardized protocol for performing the test is available from the CLSI (see "References and Suggested Reading").

Chapter Review

- The types of chemotherapeutic agents used to treat infectious diseases are called antimicrobial agents, some of which are antibiotics. Antimicrobial agents are often referred to simply as drugs.

- Some antimicrobial agents are "cidal" agents, meaning that they kill pathogens, whereas others are "static" agents, meaning that they stop pathogens from growing and multiplying.

- An antibiotic is a substance produced by a microorganism, usually a soil organism, that is effective in killing or inhibiting the growth of other microorganisms. Some antibiotics (e.g., penicillins and cephalosporins) are produced by moulds, whereas others (e.g., tetracycline, erythromycin, chloramphenicol) are produced by bacteria.

- In some cases, a single antimicrobial agent is not sufficient to destroy all pathogens, and two or more agents may be required. When the combined effect of two antimicrobial agents is greater than that achieved by either drug alone, this is known as synergism or synergy.

- Superbugs are microbes that have become resistant to one or more antimicrobial agents. Infections caused by superbugs are difficult to treat.

- The most common ways in which bacteria become resistant to antimicrobial agents include alteration of drug-binding sites, alteration of cell membrane permeability, developing the ability to produce an enzyme that destroys or inactivates a drug, and developing multidrug-resistance (MDR) pumps or efflux pumps.

- Antifungal agents work in one of four ways: (1) they bind with cell membrane sterols, (2) they interfere with sterol synthesis, (3) they block mitosis or nucleic acid synthesis, or (4) they inhibit cell wall synthesis.

- Antiprotozoal drugs work by interfering with DNA and RNA synthesis or by interfering with protozoal metabolism.

- Antiviral agents work by inhibiting viral replication within cells.

- Empirical therapy is therapy that a clinician initiates before laboratory results are available; in other words, before the clinician knows the specific pathogen causing the patient's infectious disease and before any antibiotic susceptibility test results are available. Based on the patient's signs, symptoms, and history, the clinician must "guess" the most likely pathogen and the drug most likely to be effective. It will be an "educated guess" based on the clinician's prior experiences with similar diseases.

- Adverse effects of antimicrobial agents include selective pressure on microbial populations (i.e., selecting for drug-resistant organisms); patients becoming allergic to the agent; toxicity and damage to tissues and organs; and destruction of human indigenous microflora of the mouth, vagina, and intestine, leading to superinfections and/or increased susceptibility to infectious diseases.

- Antimicrobial susceptibility testing is performed to determine the drugs to which microorganisms are susceptible and resistant.

- Methods of susceptibility testing include agar dilution, broth macrodilution, broth microdilution, disk diffusion, and gradient diffusion. Testing must be performed in accordance with protocols established by the Clinical and Laboratory Standards Institute and/or the manufacturers of the products.

- The minimum inhibitory concentration of a drug is the lowest concentration of a drug that will inhibit the growth of the organism.

- Broth microdilution is currently the most popular method for performing antimicrobial susceptibility testing in the United States.

- The Kirby-Bauer method of antimicrobial susceptibility testing is a disk diffusion method in which all steps are standardized.

- The minimum bactericidal concentration is the lowest concentration of drug that kills all microorganisms.

- β-Lactamases are bacterial enzymes that destroy the β-lactam ring in antibiotics that contain such a structure. Such antibiotics are referred to as β-lactam antibiotics or β-lactams. Examples of β-lactamases are penicillinases and cephalosporinases, which destroy the β-lactam ring in penicillins and cephalosporins, respectively. When the β-lactam ring is destroyed, the drug no longer works. Bacteria that produce penicillinases are resistant to penicillins and those that produce cephalosporinases are resistant to cephalosporins. It is possible for an organism to produce both penicillinase and cephalosporinase.

- Some antimicrobial agents have toxic side effects. Therefore, it is sometimes necessary to monitor the serum level of the drug. Monitoring of a patient's serum for drug levels is done just before the next dose of drug is given (the trough level) or at a specific time after the drug is given (the peak level).

New Terms and Abbreviations

After studying Chapter 7, you should be familiar with the following terms, which are defined within the chapter and in the Glossary at the back of the book:

Acquired resistance

Antagonism

Antibacterial agent

Antifungal agent

Antimicrobial agent

Antiprotozoal agent

Antiviral agent

β-Lactam antibiotic

β-Lactamase

β-Lactam ring

Broad-spectrum antibiotic

Cephalosporinase

Chemotherapeutic agent

Chemotherapy

Drug-binding site

Empirical therapy

Intrinsic resistance

Minimum bactericidal concentration (MBC)

Minimum inhibitory concentration (MIC)

Methicillin-resistant Staphylococcus aureus *(MRSA)*

Methicillin-resistant Staphylococcus epidermidis *(MRSE)*

Narrow spectrum antibiotic

Penicillinase

Resistance factor (R factor)

Semisynthetic antibiotic

Superbug

Superinfection

Synergism

Vancomycin-intermediate S. aureus *(VISA)*

Vancomycin-resistant Enterococcus spp. *(VRE)*

Vancomycin-resistant S. aureus *(VRSA)*

Zone of no growth

References and Suggested Reading

Methodology for the Serum Bactericidal Test: Approved Guideline. CLSI Document M21-A. Wayne, PA: Clinical and Laboratory Standards Institute, 1999.

Methods for Antimicrobial Dilution and Disk Susceptibility Testing of Infrequently Isolated or Fastidious Bacteria: Proposed Guideline. CLSI Document M45-P. Wayne, PA: Clinical and Laboratory Standards Institute, 2005.

Methods for Antimicrobial Susceptibility Testing of Anaerobic Bacteria: Approved Standard. 6th Ed. CLSI Document M11-A6. Wayne, PA: Clinical and Laboratory Standards Institute, 2004.

Methods for Determining Bactericidal Activity of Antimicrobial Agents: Approved Guideline. CLSI Document M26-A. Wayne, PA: Clinical and Laboratory Standards Institute, 1999

Methods for Dilution Antimicrobial Susceptibility Tests for Bacteria That Grow Aerobically: Approved Standard. 6th Ed. CLSI Document M7-A6. Wayne, PA: Clinical and Laboratory Standards Institute, 2003.

Performance Standards for Antimicrobial Disk Susceptibility Tests: Approved Standard. 8th Ed. CLSI Document M2-A8. Wayne, PA: Clinical and Laboratory Standards Institute, 2003.

Performance Standards for Antimicrobial Susceptibility Testing. 15th Ed. CLSI Document NCCLS M100-S15. Wayne, PA: Clinical and Laboratory Standards Institute, 2005.

Winn WC Jr, et al. Koneman's Color Atlas and Textbook of Diagnostic Microbiology. 6th Ed. Philadelphia: Lippincott Williams & Wilkins, 2006.

Yao JDC, Moellering RC Jr. Antibacterial Agents. In: Murray PR, Baron EJ, Jorgensen JH, Pfaller MA, Yolken RH, eds. Manual of Clinical Microbiology. 8th Ed. Washington, DC: ASM Press, 2003.

Answers to the Agar Dilution MIC Question (see page 166–167)

Isolate 2:	16 U/mL
Isolate 3:	4 U/mL
Isolate 4:	4 U/mL
Isolate 5:	>32 U/mL (meaning that a concentration greater than 32 U/mL will be required to inhibit growth of this isolate)
Isolate 6:	32 U/mL

Answers to Broth Microdilution MIC Question (see caption for Figure 7-9, page 169)

V	≤2 μg/mL	GM	>256 μg/mL
CEF	8 μg/mL	E	16 μg/mL
SXT	4 μg/mL	TE	64 μg/mL
PIP	128 μg/mL	C	256 μg/mL
NA	32 μg/mL	P	16 U/mL
CB	8 μg/mL	AM	256 μg/mL

 On the CD-ROM

- Gloomy Prospects for the Future?
- Additional Self-Assessment Exercises
- Puzzle

Self-Assessment Exercises

After studying Chapter 7, answer the following questions.

1. Which of the following methods of antimicrobial susceptibility testing requires that zone sizes be measured?

    A. Agar dilution method

    B. Broth macrodilution method

    C. Broth microdilution method

    D. Disk diffusion method

2. Which of the following methods of antimicrobial susceptibility testing is the most popular method among CMLs in the United States?

    A. Agar dilution method

    B. Broth macrodilution method

    C. Broth microdilution method

    D. Disk diffusion method

3. Which of the following statements is *not* true about the disk diffusion method of antimicrobial susceptibility testing?

    A. It is also known as the Kirby-Bauer test.

    B. A pure culture of the organism is required.

    C. The plate should be incubated in a CO_2 incubator for 12 hours.

    D. The test should be performed in the exact manner described by the Clinical and Laboratory Standards Institute.

4. If the effect of two or more drugs in combination is considerably greater than that of either drug alone, this is known as

    A. synergism or synergy.

    B. antagonism.

    C. totalitarianism.

    D. metabolism.

5. An antimicrobial agent that only destroys either Gram-positive organisms or Gram-negative organisms is considered to be a

  A. bacteriostatic antibiotic.

  B. broad-spectrum antibiotic.

  C. narrow spectrum antibiotic.

  D. antagonistic antibiotic.

6. Which of the following is an antifungal agent?

  A. Clotrimazole

  B. Zidovudine

  C. Chloroquine

  D. Amoxicillin

7. A CML professional who was testing a QC organism by the disk diffusion method of susceptibility testing found that *all* the zone sizes were too small. What is the most likely cause?

  A. Inoculum was too heavy

  B. Agar depth was too shallow

  C. The pH of the medium was too low

  D. Plate was incubated in a CO_2 incubator

8. Which of the following antibiotics is produced by a mould?

  A. Penicillin

  B. Bacitracin

  C. Chloramphenicol

  D. Erythromycin

9. Bacteria become resistant to antimicrobial agents by each of the following means *except*

  A. a chromosomal mutation leads to alteration of a drug-binding site.

  B. they acquire the ability to produce an enzyme which destroys or inactivates a drug.

  C. they acquire a gene that codes for production of a capsule.

  D. they develop the ability to pump the drug out of the cell.

10. The results of a broth microdilution susceptibility test are as follows:

Tube	Concentration	Growth
1	2 µg/mL	Yes
2	4 µg/mL	Yes
3	8 µg/mL	Yes
4	16 µg/mL	No
5	32 µg/mL	No
6	64 µg/mL	No

What is the MIC for this drug?

A. 8 µg/mL

B. 16 µg/mL

C. >16 µg/mL

D. None of the above

CHAPTER 8

Introduction to Medical Bacteriology

Chapter Outline

Terms and Definitions

Classification of Medically Important Bacteria

Steps Involved in Laboratory Diagnoses of Bacterial Infections

Presumptive Versus Definitive Identifications

Laboratory Procedures Used in Diagnosing Bacterial Infections
- Culture Media
- Gathering Information About an Organism's Phenotype

LEARNING OBJECTIVES

After studying this chapter, you should be able to:

- ☛ Define the new terms introduced in this chapter (e.g., *aerotolerant anaerobe, α-hemolysis, amphitrichous*)

- ☛ List five ways in which bacteria may be classified (e.g., by atmospheric requirements)

- ☛ State eight categories of bacteria that cause human disease (e.g., Gram-positive cocci, anaerobes)

- ☛ Name four categories of culture media used in the clinical microbiology laboratory and state at least one example of each (e.g., enrichment medium, Gram-negative broth)

- ☛ Given a type of clinical specimen (e.g., wound), identify the most appropriate media to use for isolation of pathogens

- ☛ State the means by which bacteria multiply or reproduce

- ☛ Name 10 phenotypic characteristics used to identify bacteria

- ☛ State the importance of the Gram stain in the bacteriology section of the clinical microbiology laboratory

- ☛ Explain how the Gram stain differentiates between Gram-positive and Gram-negative bacteria, and the function of each Gram stain reagent

- ☛ Identify the three basic shapes of bacteria and state the name of at least one specific microorganism as an example of each

- ☛ Given the growth characteristics (i.e., growth, no growth) on various types of plated media, presumptively identify the organism as Gram positive, Gram negative, aerobic, anaerobic, fastidious, lactose fermenter, salt tolerant, or a mannitol fermenter

- ☛ Explain why some bacteria may be hemolytic, define *hemolysis*, and describe the various types of hemolysis

- ☛ Correctly describe the number and/or location of the flagella on monotrichous, amphitrichous, lophotrichous, and peritrichous bacteria

- ☛ State the purpose of spore formation (sporulation) in bacteria and the difference between terminal and subterminal spores

- ☛ Briefly explain the differences between the commercial biochemical- and enzyme-based systems used to identify bacteria (e.g., the API 20E), describe the means by which bacteria are identified, and compare automated and manual methods

- ☛ Name several examples of bacteria that can be identified using immunodiagnostic or molecular diagnostic techniques

TERMS AND DEFINITIONS

In the five-kingdom system of classification, bacteria (sing., bacterium) are in the Kingdom Procaryotae (or Monera). In the three-domain system of classification, bacteria are in a domain all by themselves, appropriately called the Domain *Bacteria*. The study of bacteria is called bacteriology, and a person who studies bacteria is called a bacteriologist. Medical bacteriology is the study of bacteria that cause human diseases. Laboratory methods described in this chapter are performed in the bacteriology section of the clinical microbiology laboratory (CML). Most bacteriology sections are organized into areas or "benches," such as the urine bench, respiratory bench, wound/miscellaneous bench, blood culture bench, and anaerobe bench (Fig. 8-1).

CLASSIFICATION OF MEDICALLY IMPORTANT BACTERIA

There are many ways to categorize bacteria, including by

• genetic similarities and differences,

• cellular morphology (shape),

• Gram reaction (whether Gram-positive or Gram-negative),

• atmospheric requirements, or

• biochemical and metabolic activities.

Bergey's Manual of Systematic Bacteriology, second edition (see "References and Suggested Readings") is considered the microbiologist's "bible" with respect to classification of procaryotes (the Domains *Bacteria* and *Archaea*).

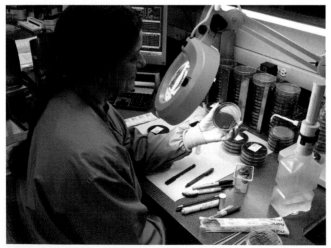

***Figure 8-1.* CML professional working at the respiratory bench in the clinical microbiology laboratory of a large hospital.** (Courtesy of Dr. Robert Fader.)

Bergey's Manual serves two major purposes: (1) to assist microbiologists in the identification (speciation) of procaryotes and (2) to indicate the relatedness that exists among the various groups of procaryotes. In *Bergey's Manual*, domains are divided into phyla, phyla into classes, classes into orders, orders into families, families into genera, and genera into species. Additional information about *Bergey's Manual* and classification of bacteria can be found on the CD-ROM.

For discussion purposes, this book divides the bacteria that cause human diseases into the following categories[1]:

• Gram-positive cocci (see Chapter 9)

• Gram-positive bacilli (see Chapter 10)

• Acid-fast bacilli (see Chapter 10)

• Gram-negative cocci (see Chapter 11)

• Gram-negative bacilli (see Chapters 12, 13, and 14)

• Curved and spiral-shaped bacilli (see Chapter 15)

• Obligate intracellular bacteria (see Chapter 16)

• Anaerobic bacteria (see Chapter 17)

STEPS INVOLVED IN LABORATORY DIAGNOSES OF BACTERIAL INFECTIONS

Traditionally, the primary way CML professionals assisted clinicians in the diagnosis of bacterial infections was to inoculate the clinical specimen to appropriate culture media, obtain a pure culture of the pathogen, and then identify or speciate the pathogen by gathering "clues" (phenotypic characteristics) to its identity. The identity of the pathogen was revealed when its phenotypic characteristics matched those of a previously characterized organism. In today's CML, many of the traditional methods of identifying bacteria have been or are in the process of being replaced by immunodiagnostic and molecular techniques (see Chapter 6). Some of the traditional methods still in use are described in this chapter. Figure 8-2 is a flowchart of the steps involved from receipt of the clinical specimen to reporting laboratory results.

PRESUMPTIVE VERSUS DEFINITIVE IDENTIFICATIONS

Presumptive identifications (IDs) of microorganisms have become more popular in recent years, primarily because of the increased emphasis on speed and cost reduction. By combining readily observable colony and Gram stain features

---

[1] *Terms not yet discussed in this book will be discussed later in this chapter and/or in the cited chapters.*

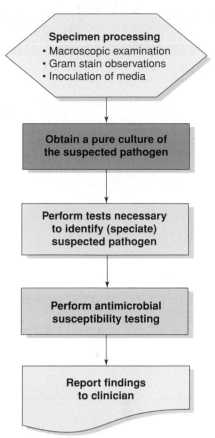

Figure 8-2. **Flowchart illustrating the sequence of events that occur within the bacteriology section of the clinical microbiology laboratory.**

with results of simple test procedures, even small CMLs are capable of making presumptive IDs of many commonly isolated and clinically important bacteria. It is important to remember, however, that some important bacterial pathogens *cannot* be identified using presumptive ID criteria. Equally important is that because they are often based solely on morphological characteristics and the results of relatively few tests, presumptive IDs may be incorrect. Nevertheless, identifications based on presumptive ID criteria are rapid, relatively inexpensive, and often correct.

Clinical and Laboratory Standards Institute (CLSI) Document M35-A, titled *Abbreviated Identification of Bacteria and Yeast: Approved Guideline* (see "References and Suggested Readings"), contains important information about presumptive IDs. Included in the document are abbreviated methods for identifying more than a dozen clinically important bacterial pathogens (Table 8-1). Some examples of CLSI abbreviated identifications are shown in Table 8-2.

When definitive IDs are required, CML professionals will find a wide variety of techniques available for their use. Examples include biochemical- and enzyme-based minisystems, gas-liquid chromatographic analysis of metabolic end products, cellular fatty acid analysis by

> Presumptive IDs of bacteria are based on readily observable colony and Gram stain features and the results of simple test procedures.

TABLE 8 - 1	Bacterial Pathogens That Can Be Identified Using Abbreviated Identification Criteria Approved by the Clinical and Laboratory Standards Institute	
Aerobic and Facultatively Anaerobic Gram-Positive Bacteria	**Aerobic and Facultatively Anaerobic Gram-Negative Bacteria**	**Anaerobic Bacteria**
Enterococcus spp.	*Escherichia coli*	*Bacteroides* spp.
Staphylococcus aureus	*Haemophilus influenzae*	*Bilophila wadsworthia*
Streptococcus agalactiae	*Moraxella catarrhalis*	Various *Clostridium* spp.
Streptococcus pneumoniae	*Proteus* spp.	*Fusobacterium nucleatum*
Streptococcus pyogenes	*Pseudomonas aeruginosa*	*Peptostreptococcus* spp.
		Porphyromonas spp.
		Various *Prevotella* spp.
		Propionibacterium acnes
		Veillonella spp.

TABLE 8 - 2   Examples of Abbreviated Identifications of Bacteria[a]

Organism	Can Be Presumptively Identified as Such If . . .
Staphylococcus aureus (Chapter 9)	Gram-positive cocci in clusters; white to yellow, creamy, opaque colonies on BA; catalase positive; slide coagulase positive or rapid 4-hour tube coagulase positive
Streptococcus pneumoniae (Chapter 9)	Gram-positive cocci in pairs and chains; α-hemolytic on BA; colonies usually transparent, slightly mucoid, or flattened, not peaked; catalase negative; bile solubility positive
Streptococcus pyogenes (Chapter 9)	Gram-positive cocci in pairs and chains; β-hemolytic on BA with a sharp periphery to the zone of hemolysis; colonies >0.5 mm in diameter after 24 hours incubation; colonies usually dry, peaked, or convex; PYR positive
Escherichia coli (Chapter 12)	Gram-negative bacilli; nonswarming on BA; LF on MAC; spot indole positive; oxidase negative
Proteus mirabilis (Chapter 12)	Gram-negative bacilli; swarming growth on BA; NLF on MAC; indole negative
Proteus vulgaris (Chapter 12)	Gram-negative bacilli; swarming growth on BA; NLF on MAC; indole positive
Pseudomonas aeruginosa (Chapter 13)	Gram-negative bacilli; oxidase positive; typical grapelike or corn tortilla–like odor; characteristic colony morphology (metallic or pearlescent, rough, blue-green pigmented, or extremely mucoid)

[a]Organisms and terms not yet discussed in this book will be discussed later in this chapter and/or in the cited chapters.

BA, blood agar; LF, lactose fermenter; NLF, non–lactose fermenter; MAC, MacConkey agar; PYR, pyrrolidonyl arylamidase.

gas-liquid chromatography, immunodiagnostic procedures, and molecular diagnostic procedures.

The decision that presumptive IDs will suffice or that definitive IDs are necessary rests with each laboratory. The choice is often based on the size of the CML and monetary restrictions. In view of the current emphasis on cost containment in clinical laboratories, presumptive IDs might suffice, especially when susceptibility test results are also furnished. Rarely isolated organisms that are difficult and/or time consuming to identify might best be sent to reference laboratories. Reference laboratories are expected to use definitive ID methods.

LABORATORY PROCEDURES USED IN DIAGNOSING BACTERIAL INFECTIONS

Culture Media

Recall from Chapter 6 that the term *culture media* refers to the various types of liquid and solid mixtures of nutrients used to culture (grow) microorganisms—primarily, bacteria and fungi—in the CML, and that there are various ways to categorize the artificial (synthetic) culture media used in the CML. These categories include the following:

- Liquid and solid culture media (see Chapter 6)
- Chemically defined and complex culture media (see Chapter 6)
- Enrichment media
- Enriched media
- Selective media
- Differential media

Enrichment Media

An example of an enrichment medium used in the bacteriology section is Gram-negative (GN) broth. GN broth contains special nutrients to support the growth of certain medically important Gram-negative bacilli (e.g., *Shigella* and *Salmonella* spp.) and ingredients that suppress the growth of Gram-positive organisms and other Gram-negative organisms. Fecal specimens are inoculated into GN broth whenever *Salmonella* or *Shigella* spp. are suspected to be present.

Examples of enrichment media are GN broth and selenite broth, both of which are used to improve the chances of recovering *Salmonella* and *Shigella* spp. from clinical specimens.

The special nutrients in the broth stimulate reproduction of these species, increasing their number and thus increasing the chances of isolating them from the specimens. Selenite broth is another example of an enrichment medium. Like GN broth, it is used to enhance the growth of *Salmonella* and *Shigella* spp. while inhibiting other bacteria present in fecal specimens.

Enriched Media

Blood agar (BA), which is nutrient agar plus 5% sheep red blood cells, and chocolate (CA) agar, which is nutrient agar plus powdered hemoglobin, are examples of solid enriched

> Blood agar and chocolate agar are examples of commonly used enriched media.

media used routinely in the bacteriology section. BA is bright red, whereas CA is brown (the color of chocolate). Although both media contain hemoglobin, CA is considered more enriched than BA because the hemoglobin is more readily accessible in CA. Also, CA contains special nutrients, like yeast extract, not found in BA. CA is used to culture important, nutritionally demanding (fastidious or "fussy") bacterial pathogens that will not grow on BA, such as *Neisseria gonorrhoeae* and *Haemophilus influenzae*.

Selective Media

Many types of selective media are used in the bacteriology section. Examples include MacConkey agar (MAC), phenylethyl alcohol agar (PEA), colistin-nalidixic acid agar (CNA), Thayer-Martin agar, and mannitol salt agar (MSA). MAC inhibits growth of Gram-positive bacteria and thus is selective for Gram-negative bacteria. PEA and CNA inhibit growth of Gram-negative bacteria and are, thus, selective for Gram-positive bacteria. PEA and CNA are blood agars to which substances have been added to inhibit growth of Gram-negative bacteria.

Thayer-Martin agar is selective for *N. gonorrhoeae* and *N. meningitidis*. It is a chocolate agar that contains extra nutrients plus several antimicrobial agents. This highly enriched medium will support the growth of even the most fastidious strains of *N. gonorrhoeae*. Specimens such as vaginal, cervical, urethral, rectal, and throat swabs all con-

> MAC, PEA, CNA, Thayer-Martin agar, and MSA are examples of commonly used selective media.

tain large numbers of indigenous microflora, which can overgrow fastidious *N. gonorrhoeae* when Thayer-Martin agar is not used. The antimicrobial agents in Thayer-Martin agar inhibit growth of any indigenous microflora that are present in the clinical specimen. Martin-Lewis agar can be used in place of Thayer-Martin agar; it contains a different formulation of nutrients and antimicrobial agents.

MSA is selective for organisms able to survive in the presence of high salt (sodium chloride or NaCl) concentrations. Organisms that "love" high salt concentrations are described as being **halophilic,** whereas those that do not "love" high salt concentrations, but can tolerate them, are described as being **haloduric.**

Differential Media

Examples of differential media used in the bacteriology section are MAC, MSA, and BA. MAC is frequently used to differentiate between various Gram-negative bacilli that are isolated from clinical specimens. One of the ingredients of MAC is lactose, a disaccharide. When lactose is fermented, acid is produced. The acid causes the pH indicator in the medium to change from a very pale pink to a rather shocking pink, resulting in bright pink colonies. Organisms capable of fermenting lactose—called lactose fermenters—produce pink colonies on MAC, whereas organisms unable to ferment lactose—called non–lactose fermenters—produce colorless colonies. Thus, MAC differentiates between lactose-fermenting and non-lactose-fermenting Gram-negative bacteria (see Fig. 6-13).

MSA contains mannitol, a sugar alcohol. When mannitol is fermented, acid is produced. The acid causes the pH indicator in the medium to turn from pink to yellow. Mannitol fermenters will cause the normally pink medium to turn yellow, whereas non–mannitol fermenters do not affect the color of the medium

> MAC, MSA, and BA are examples of commonly used differential media.

(Fig. 8-3). Thus, MSA differentiates between mannitol-fermenting and non-mannitol-fermenting organisms. MSA is often used to screen for *Staphylococcus aureus*,

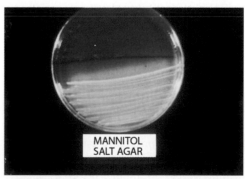

MANNITOL SALT AGAR

Figure 8-3. Mannitol salt agar. This selective and differential medium is used to screen for *Staphylococcus aureus*. Any bacteria capable of growing in a 7.5% sodium chloride concentration will grow on this medium, but *S. aureus* will turn the medium yellow because the organism can ferment the mannitol in the medium. The organism growing on the upper section of the plate is unable to ferment mannitol, but the organism growing on the lower section is a mannitol fermenter. (From Koneman EW, Allen SD, Janda WM, et al. Color Atlas and Textbook of Diagnostic Microbiology. 5th ed. Philadelphia: Lippincott Williams & Wilkins, 1997.)

TABLE 8 - 3   Plated Media Commonly Used in the Bacteriology Laboratory[a]

Name of Medium	Enriched	Selective	Differential
Blood agar (BA)	Yes. The primary purpose of BA is to isolate bacterial pathogens from clinical specimens. Most bacterial pathogens will grow on BA.	No	Yes. BA is used to differentiate between α-, β-, and γ-hemolytic organisms.
Chocolate agar (CA)	Yes. The primary purpose of CA is to isolate especially fastidious bacterial pathogens, like *Neisseria gonorrhoeae* and *Haemophilus influenzae*, that will not grow on blood agar.	No	No
MacConkey agar (MAC)	No	Yes. MAC is selective for Gram-negative bacteria.	Yes. MAC is used to differentiate between lactose fermenters and non–lactose fermenters.
Phenylethyl alcohol agar (PEA)	Yes. PEA is BA to which phenylethyl alcohol has been added.	Yes. PEA is selective for Gram-positive bacteria.	No
Colistin/nalidixic acid agar (CNA)	Yes. CNA is BA to which colistin and nalidixic acid have been added.	Yes. CNA is selective for Gram-positive bacteria.	No
Thayer-Martin agar (T-M)	Yes. T-M is chocolate agar to which additional nutrients have been added.	Yes. T-M contains several antibacterial and antifungal agents. T-M is selective for *N. gonorrhoeae* and *N. meningitidis*.	No
Mannitol salt agar (MSA)	No	Yes. MSA is selective for organisms that can tolerate high salt concentrations.	Yes. MSA is used to differentiate between mannitol fermenters and non–mannitol fermenters.

[a]Additional types of plated media are discussed in appropriate sections of subsequent chapters. In addition, CD-ROM Appendix 3 contains a recap of special media used in the bacteriology section of the clinical microbiology laboratory.

which is salt tolerant and a mannitol fermenter. Not only will *S. aureus* grow on MSA, but also it produces yellow colonies and turns the originally pink medium to yellow. The presence of yellow colonies in the absence of yellowing of the medium should not be interpreted as *S. aureus*; such organisms are most likely *Micrococcus* spp. (see Chapter 9).

BA can also be considered a differential medium because it is used to determine the type of hemolysis (alteration or destruction of red blood cells) that the bacterial isolate causes. The various types of hemolysis are described later in the chapter.

The three categories of media—enriched, selective, and differential—are not mutually exclusive. For example, as

was just described, BA is both enriched and differential. MAC and MSA are both selective and differential. PEA and CNA are both enriched and selective. Thayer-Martin agar and Martin-Lewis agar are highly enriched and highly selective. Table 8-3 further describes some of the most popular enriched, selective, and differential media used in the CML.

Primary Setup

The term **primary setup** refers to the variety of media inoculated with a particular type of clinical specimen. The primary setup varies from one type of specimen to another. For example, a routine throat swab is usually only inoculated to a BA plate. Thus, the primary setup for a routine throat swab is a BA plate. The usual primary setup for a urine specimen is a BA plate and a MAC plate. A typical primary setup for a spinal fluid or wound specimen might be a BA plate, a CA plate, a MAC plate, a PEA plate, and a tube of thioglycollate broth. Thioglycollate broth is discussed later in the chapter. CD-ROM Appendix 2 contains additional information regarding primary setups for various types of clinical specimens.

Bacterial Growth

The term *human growth* refers to an increase in size—for example, growing from a newborn to an adult. While bacteria do increase somewhat in size before cell division, the term *bacterial growth* refers to an increase in the *number* of organisms rather than an increase in their size. When each bacterial cell reaches its optimum size, it divides by **binary fission** (*bi-* meaning "two" and *fission* meaning "splitting") into two daughter cells. Each bacterium simply splits in half to become two identical cells. As shown in Figure 8-4, DNA replication must occur prior to the actual splitting (fission) of the cell, so that each daughter cell has exactly the same genetic makeup as the original or "parent" cell.[2] On solid medium, binary fission continues through many generations until a **colony** is produced

> Bacteria reproduce by binary fission. The length of time it takes for one bacterial cell to split into two cells is referred to as the organism's generation time.

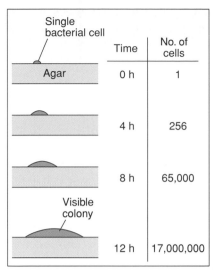

Figure 8-5. **Formation of a bacterial colony on a solid growth medium.** In this illustration, the generation time is assumed to be 30 minutes.

Time	No. of cells
0 h	1
4 h	256
8 h	65,000
12 h	17,000,000

(Fig. 8-5). A bacterial colony is a mound or pile of bacteria containing millions of cells. Binary fission continues for as long as the nutrient supply, water, and space allow and ends when essential nutrients are depleted or the concentration of cellular waste products reaches a toxic level.

The time it takes for one cell to become two cells by binary fission is called the **generation time.** The generation time varies from one bacterial species to another. In the laboratory, under ideal growth conditions, *Escherichia coli*, *Vibrio cholerae*, *Staphylococcus* spp., and *Streptococcus* spp. have a generation time of about 20 minutes, whereas some *Pseudomonas* and *Clostridium* species may divide every 10 minutes, and *Mycobacterium tuberculosis* may divide only every 18 to 24 hours. Bacteria with short generation times are referred to as rapid growers, whereas those with long generation times are referred to as slow growers.

In the laboratory, a pure culture of a single bacterial species can usually be maintained if the appropriate growth medium and environmental conditions are provided. The temperature, pH, and proper atmosphere are quite easily controlled to provide optimum conditions for growth. Appropriate nutrients must be provided in the growth medium, including appropriate energy and carbon sources. Some bacteria, described as being fastidious, have complex nutritional requirements. Think of them as being "fussy" or "picky eaters." Often special mixtures of vitamins and amino acids must be added to the medium to culture these fastidious organisms. Some organisms will not grow at all on artificial culture, including obligate intracellular pathogens, such as viruses, rickettsias, and chlamydiae. As the term implies, the only place where obligate intracellular pathogens can survive is *within* living cells. To propagate obligate intracellular pathogens in the laboratory, they must be inoculated into live animals, embryonated chicken eggs,

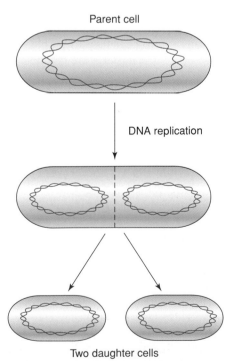

Figure 8-4. **Binary fission.** Note that DNA replication must occur prior to the actual splitting of the parent cell.

Parent cell

DNA replication

Two daughter cells

---

[2] The term DNA replication *refers to the process whereby one DNA strand is used as a template to make a duplicate DNA strand.*

or cell cultures. Other microorganisms that are unable to grow on artificial media include the bacteria *Treponema pallidum* (the etiologic agent of syphilis) and *Mycobacterium leprae* (the etiologic agent of Hansen disease or leprosy).

Gathering Information About an Organism's Phenotype

Bacterial pathogens are identified/speciated by gathering information about the organism's phenotypic characteristics, each of which can be thought of as a clue to the organism's identity. In this way, people working in the CML are like detectives and crime scene investigators, gathering clues about a pathogen until they are finally able to identify the culprit.

The various phenotypic characteristics of value in identifying bacteria include the following, each of which will be further described in this chapter:

- Gram reaction

- Cell shape (e.g., cocci, bacilli, curved, spiral-shaped, filamentous,[3] branching)

- Morphologic arrangement of cells (e.g., pairs, tetrads, chains, clusters)

- Atmospheric requirements

- Growth or no growth on various types of plated media

- Colony morphology (e.g., color, general shape, elevation, margin)

- Type of hemolysis produced

- Presence or absence of a capsule

- Motility

- Number and location of flagella

- Ability to produce spores

- Location of spores (e.g., terminal or subterminal)

- Presence or absence of various enzymes (e.g., catalase, coagulase, oxidase, urease)

- Ability to catabolize (break down) various carbohydrates and amino acids; miniaturized biochemical test systems referred to as "minisystems" are often used for this purpose

Gram Reaction

In 1883, a German physician named Hans Christian Gram developed a staining technique that bears his name—the **Gram stain** or Gram staining procedure. (Additional information about the Gram stain can be found in Table 8-4 and Appendix A.) The Gram stain has become the most important staining procedure in the bacteriology laboratory because it separates bacteria into two groups: those that are Gram positive and those that are Gram negative (terms to be explained shortly). Learning a bacterium's Gram reaction is an extremely important clue to its identity.

The color of bacteria at the end of the Gram staining procedure depends on the chemical composition of their cell walls (Table 8-5). If the bacteria were not decolorized during the decolorization step, they will be blue to purple at the conclusion of the Gram staining procedure; such bacteria are said to be Gram positive. The thick layer of peptidoglycan in the cell walls of Gram-positive bacteria makes it difficult to remove the crystal violet–iodine complex during the decolorization step.

> If a bacterium is blue to purple at the end of the Gram staining procedure, it is said to be Gram positive. If, on the other hand, it ends up being pink to red, it is said to be Gram negative.

By contrast, if the crystal violet was removed from the cells during the decolorization step and the cells were subsequently stained by safranin, they will be pink to red at the conclusion of the Gram staining procedure; pink if the cells take up only a small amount of safranin, and red if they take up a large amount. Such bacteria are said to be Gram negative. The thin layer of peptidoglycan in the cell walls of Gram-negative bacteria makes it easier to remove the crystal violet–iodine complex. In addition, the decolorizer dissolves the lipid in the cell walls of Gram-negative bacteria. This destroys the integrity of the cell wall and makes it much easier to remove the crystal violet–iodine complex. Cells with no cell walls, such as bacteria in the genus *Mycoplasma* and human cells, also stain Gram negative.

Sometimes following Gram staining of a pure culture, some of the cells will appear blue to purple, while others appear pink to red; such bacteria are referred to as being Gram variable. Gram variability may occur in the staining of older cultures that contain both live and dead cells, or when some areas of the smear are thicker than others, resulting in over- or under-decolorization of parts of the smear.

STUDY AID **A Way to Remember a Particular Bacterium's Gram Reaction.** Unfortunately, there is nothing in a bacterium's name that provides a clue to its Gram reaction. A former student used the following method to remember the Gram reaction of a particular bacterium. In her notebook, she drew two large circles. She lightly shaded in one circle, using a blue colored pencil. The other circle was lightly shaded red. Within the blue circle, she wrote the names of the Gram-positive bacteria she studied in her microbiology course. Within the red circle, she wrote the names of Gram-negative bacteria. She then studied the two circles. Later, whenever she encountered the name of a particular

---

[3] The term filamentous *refers to an organism that is long and thin, like a filament.*

TABLE 8 - 4   Steps in the Gram Staining Procedure

Step	Purpose	Color of Gram-Positive Bacteria After This Step	Color of Gram-Negative Bacteria After This Step
1. Apply the primary stain (crystal violet)	Stains all bacteria blue[a]	Blue	Blue
2. Rinse	To remove excess crystal violet	Blue	Blue
3. Apply the mordant (Gram's iodine)	Iodine forms a complex with the crystal violet, making it more difficult to remove the crystal violet from the cells	Blue	Blue
4. Rinse	To remove excess iodine	Blue	Blue
5. Decolorization step (using 95% ethanol or 50/50 mixture of acetone-ethanol)	To remove the blue color from Gram-negative bacteria	Blue	Colorless
6. Rinse	To remove the decolorizing agent and to stop the decolorizing process	Blue	Colorless
7. Apply the counterstain (safranin)	To stain the Gram-negative bacteria	Blue to purple	Pink to red
8. Rinse	To remove excess safranin	Blue to purple	Pink to red

[a] All bacteria are colorless at the start of the Gram staining procedure.

bacterium, she would remember which circle the name was in. If the name was in the blue circle, the bacterium was Gram positive. If the name was in the red circle, the bacterium was Gram negative.

Cell Shape and Morphologic Arrangement of Cells

There are three basic shapes of bacteria (Fig. 8-6): (1) round or spherical bacteria are known as **cocci (sing. coccus)**, (2) rectangular or rod-shaped bacteria are known as **bacilli**

TABLE 8 - 5   Differences Between Gram-Positive and Gram-Negative Bacteria

Characteristic	Gram-Positive Bacteria	Gram-Negative Bacteria
Color at the end of the Gram staining procedure	Blue to purple	Pink to red
Peptidoglycan in cell walls	Thick layer	Thin layer
Teichoic acids and lipoteichoic acids in cell walls	Present	Absent
Lipopolysaccharide in cell walls	Absent	Present

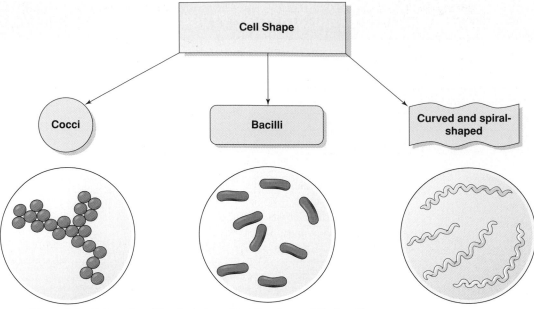

Figure 8-6. **Categories of bacteria based on the shape of their cells.**

(sing. **bacillus**), and (3) curved and spiral-shaped bacteria are sometimes referred to as spirilla. Recall that bacteria divide by binary fission—one cell splits in half to become two daughter cells. Following binary fission, the daughter cells may separate completely from each other or may remain connected, forming various morphological arrangements.

STUDY AID

Bacterial Names Sometimes Provide Clues to Their Shapes. If *-coccus* appears in the name of a bacterium, one automatically knows the shape of the organism—spherical. Examples include genera such as *Enterococcus, Peptococcus, Peptostreptococcus, Staphylococcus,* and *Streptococcus.* However, not all cocci have *-coccus* in their names (e.g., *Neisseria* spp.). If *-bacillus* appears in the name of a bacterium, one automatically knows that the organism is rod shaped or rectangular. Examples include genera such as *Actinobacillus, Bacillus, Lactobacillus,* and *Streptobacillus.* However, not all bacilli have *-bacillus* in their names (e.g., *E. coli*).

Cocci may be seen singly or in pairs (**diplococci**), chains (**streptococci**), clusters (**staphylococci**), packets of four (**tetrads**), or packets of eight (**octads**), depending on the particular species and the manner in which the cells divide (Fig. 8-7). Examples of cocci include *Enterococ-*

> Pairs of cocci are known as diplococci. Chains of cocci are known as streptococci, Clusters of cocci are known as staphylococci.

cus spp., *Neisseria* spp., *Staphylococcus* spp., and *Streptococcus* spp. A typical coccus is approximately 1 μm in diameter.

Bacilli, which are often referred to as rods, may be short or long, thick or thin, pointed or with curved or blunt ends. They may occur singly, in pairs (**diplobacilli**), in chains (**streptobacilli**), in long filaments, or branched. Some rods are quite short, resembling elongated cocci; they are called **coccobacilli** (e.g., *Haemophilus influenzae* and *Listeria monocytogenes*). Some bacilli stack up next to each other, side-by-side in a palisade arrangement, which is characteristic of *Corynebacterium diphtheriae* (the cause of diphtheria) and organisms that resemble *C. diphtheriae* in appearance (called diphtheroids). Examples of bacilli include members of the Enterobacteriaceae family (e.g., *Enterobacter, Escherichia, Klebsiella, Proteus, Salmonella,* and *Shigella* spp.), *Pseudomonas aeruginosa, Bacillus* spp., and *Clostridium* spp. A typical bacillus (e.g., *E. coli*) is approximately 1 μm in width and 3 μm in length.

CAUTION

Beware the Word *Bacillus.* Whenever the word *Bacillus* appears, capitalized and underlined or italicized, it is a particular genus of rod-shaped bacteria. However, if the word bacillus is not capitalized, underlined, or italicized, it refers to *any* rod-shaped bacterium.

Curved and spiral-shaped bacteria are placed into a third morphological grouping. For example, *Vibrio* spp., such as *V. cholerae* (the cause of cholera) and *V. parahaemolyticus* (a cause of diarrhea), are curved or comma-shaped bacilli. Spiral-shaped bacteria usually occur singly, but some species

Arrangement	Description	Appearance	Example	Disease
Diplococci	Cocci in pairs	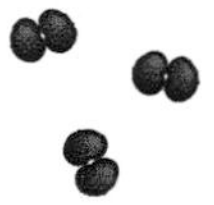	*Neisseria gonorrhoeae*	Gonorrhea
Streptococci	Cocci in chains	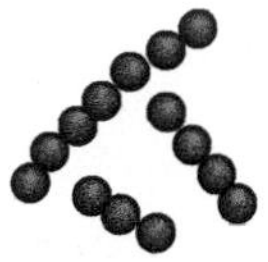	*Streptococcus pyogenes*	Strep throat
Staphylococci	Cocci in clusters	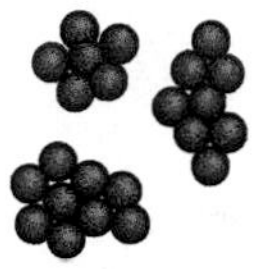	*Staphylococcus aureus*	Boils
Tetrad	Packet of 4 cocci	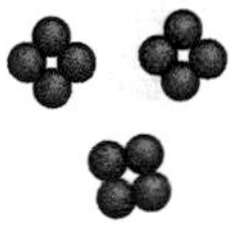	*Micrococcus luteus*	Rarely pathogenic
Octad	Packet of 8 cocci	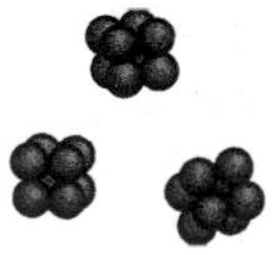	*Sarcina ventriculi*	Rarely pathogenic

Figure 8-7. **Morphological arrangements of cocci.**

> A bacterium's Gram reaction, basic cell shape, and morphological arrangement are very important clues to its identification.

may form pairs. A pair of curved bacilli resembles a bird (ᔕ), and is described as having a gull-wing morphology. *Campylobacter* spp. (a common cause of diarrhea) have a gull-wing morphology.

Spiral-shaped bacteria are referred to as spirochetes. Different species of spirochetes vary in size, length, rigidity, and the number and amplitude of their coils. Some are tightly coiled, such as *Treponema pallidum*, the cause of syphilis, with a flexible cell wall that enables them to move readily through tissues. Its morphology and characteristic motility—spinning around its long axis—make *T. pallidum* easy to recognize in clinical specimens obtained from patients with primary syphilis, when the specimens are examined by darkfield microscopy. *Borrelia* spp., the etiologic agents of Lyme disease and relapsing fever, are examples of less tightly coiled spirochetes (Fig. 8-8).

Some bacteria may lose their characteristic shape because adverse growth conditions prevent the production of

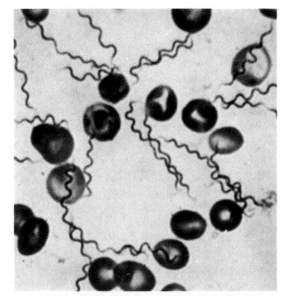

Figure 8-8. **Stained blood smear showing *Borrelia hermsii* and red blood cells.** (From Volk WA, Gebhardt BM, Hammarskjöld M, Kadner RJ. Essentials of Medical Microbiology. 5th Ed. Philadelphia: Lippincott-Raven, 1996.)

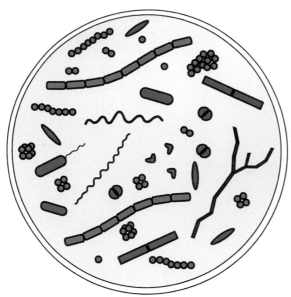

Figure 8-9. Various forms of bacteria. Illustration includes single cocci, diplococci, tetrads, octads, streptococci, staphylococci, single bacilli, diplobacilli, streptobacilli, branching bacilli, loosely coiled spirochetes, and tightly coiled spirochetes.

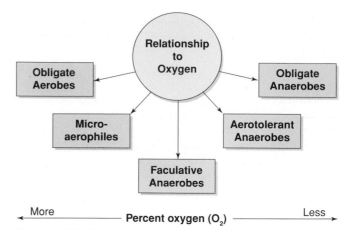

Figure 8-10. Categories of bacteria based on their relationship to oxygen.

normal cell walls. Such bacteria are referred to as cell wall–deficient bacteria. Some cell wall–deficient bacteria revert to their original shape when placed in favorable growth conditions, whereas others do not. Bacteria in the genus *Mycoplasma* do not have cell walls to define their shape and thus exist in various shapes. Bacteria that can take many shapes are described as being **pleomorphic,** and the ability to do so is known as **pleomorphism.** Because they have no cell walls, mycoplasmas are resistant to antibiotics that inhibit cell wall synthesis. Figure 8-9 illustrates the various shapes of bacteria that may be observed in a Gram-stained clinical specimen.

> Organisms that exist in various shapes are referred to as being pleomorphic.

Atmospheric Requirements

With respect to oxygen (O_2), a bacterial isolate can be classified into one of five major groups: obligate aerobes, microaerophilic aerobes (microaerophiles), facultative anaerobes, aerotolerant anaerobes, and obligate anaerobes (Fig. 8-10).

To grow and multiply, **obligate aerobes** require an atmosphere containing molecular oxygen in concentrations comparable to that found in room air (i.e., 20% to 21% O_2). Mycobacteria, *Pseudomonas* spp., and some fungi are examples of microorganisms that are obligate aerobes. **Microaerophiles,** also known as microaerophilic aerobes, also require oxygen for multiplication but in concentrations lower than that found in room air. *Campylobacter* spp., a major cause of bacterial diarrhea, are examples of microaerophilic bacteria that prefer an atmosphere containing about 5% O_2. *Neisseria gonorrhoeae*, the etiologic agent of gonorrhea, is a borderline microaerophile. It will grow in a CO_2 incubator but grows best in a microaerophilic environment. *N. gonorrhoeae* and *Campylobacter* are also capnophiles, meaning they prefer reduced concentrations of CO_2.

> Obligate aerobes and microaerophiles both require oxygen. Obligate aerobes require an atmosphere containing about 20% to 21% O_2. Microaerophiles require reduced oxygen concentrations (usually around 5% O_2).

Anaerobes can be defined as organisms that do not require oxygen for life and reproduction. However, they vary in their sensitivity to oxygen. The terms *obligate anaerobe, aerotolerant anaerobe,* and *facultative anaerobe* are used to describe the organism's relationship to molecular oxygen. An **obligate anaerobe** is an anaerobe that can only grow in an anaerobic environment—an environment containing no oxygen.

An **aerotolerant anaerobe** does not require oxygen and grows better in the absence of oxygen but can survive in atmospheres containing molecular oxygen, such as air and a CO_2 incubator. The concentration of oxygen that an aerotolerant anaerobe can tolerate varies from one species to another. **Facultative anaerobes** are capable of surviving in either the presence or absence of oxygen—anywhere from 0% to 20% or 21% O_2. Many of the bacteria routinely isolated from clinical specimens are facultative anaerobes, such as members of the Enterobacteriaceae family, most streptococci, and most staphylococci.

> Obligate anaerobes, aerotolerant anaerobes, and facultative anaerobes can thrive in atmospheres devoid of oxygen.

Thioglycollate broth (THIO) is a very popular liquid or sometimes semisolid medium for use in the bacteriology laboratory because THIO supports the growth of *all* categories of bacteria, from obligate aerobes to obligate anaerobes. How can a broth support the growth of both aerobes and anaerobes? Within the tube of THIO is a concentration gradient of dissolved oxygen. The concentration of oxygen decreases with depth: At the top of the tube, the concentration of oxygen in the broth is about 20% to 21%. At the bottom of the tube, the broth is devoid of oxygen. Organisms will grow only in that part of the broth where the oxygen concentration meets their needs (Fig. 8-11). For example, microaerophiles grow where the oxygen level is around 5%, and obligate anaerobes grow only at the very bottom of the tube, where there is no oxygen. Facultative anaerobes can grow anywhere in the tube because they can survive in the presence or absence of oxygen.

Room air contains less than 1% CO_2. Some bacteria, referred to as **capnophiles** or capnophilic organisms, grow better in the laboratory in the presence of increased concentrations of CO_2. Some anaerobes (e.g., *Bacteroides* and *Fusobacterium* spp.) are capnophiles, as are some aerobes (e.g., certain *Neisseria*, *Campylobacter*, and *Haemophilus* spp.). In the CML, CO_2 incubators are routinely calibrated to contain between 5% and 10% CO_2.

> For optimum growth in the CML, capnophiles require an atmosphere containing 5% to 10% CO_2.

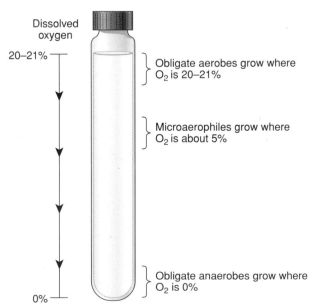

Dissolved oxygen

20–21%

Obligate aerobes grow where O_2 is 20–21%

Microaerophiles grow where O_2 is about 5%

Obligate anaerobes grow where O_2 is 0%

0%

Figure 8-11. **Culturing microorganisms in thioglycollate broth (THIO).** THIO contains a concentration gradient of dissolved oxygen, ranging from 20% to 21% O_2 at the top of the tube to 0% O_2 at the bottom of the tube. A bacterium will grow only in that part of the THIO containing the concentration of oxygen that it requires.

Growth or No Growth on Various Types of Plated Media

Recall from earlier in this chapter that the primary setup often contains a variety of enriched, selective, and differential agar plates. Clues to the identity of an isolate can be obtained by observing the plates on which the organism did and did not grow.

Example 1

A clinical specimen was inoculated onto a primary setup consisting of four plates: BA, CA, MAC, and PEA. A bacterial isolate grew only on the CA plate. *Question:* What can the CML professional conclude? *Answer:* The isolate is fastidious.

Example 2

A clinical specimen was inoculated onto a primary setup consisting of four plates: BA, CA, MAC, and PEA. A bacterial isolate grew on the BA, CA, and PEA plates but did not grow on the MAC plate. *Question:* What can the CML professional conclude? *Answer:* The isolate is Gram positive.

Example 3

A clinical specimen was inoculated onto a primary setup consisting of four plates: BA, CA, MAC, and PEA. A bacterial isolate grew on the BA, CA, and MAC plates, but did not grow on the PEA plate. The organism is producing pink colonies on the MAC plate. *Question:* What can the CML professional conclude? *Answer:* The isolate is Gram negative and a lactose fermenter.

Example 4

A clinical specimen was inoculated onto a primary setup consisting of five plates: BA, CA, MAC, PEA, and MSA. A bacterial isolate grew on the BA, CA, PEA, and MSA plates but did not grow on the MAC plate. On the MSA plate, the organism has produced yellow colonies and has caused the normally light pink agar to turn yellow. *Question:* What can the CML professional conclude? *Answer:* The isolate is Gram positive, salt tolerant, and a mannitol fermenter.

Readers who are uncertain as to the rationale leading to the conclusions in these examples should review the section in this chapter describing the functions of the various types of culture media.

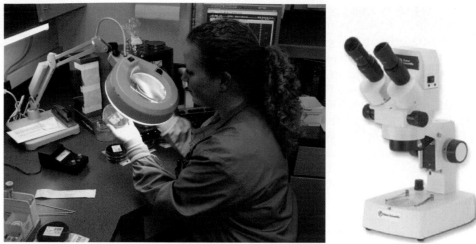

Figure 8-12. **Methods of examining colonies. A.** CML professional examining colonies using a magnifying lens with a fluorescent light attachment. **B.** Stereoscopic microscope. (Courtesy of Dr. Robert Fader [A] and Fisher Scientific [B].)

Colony Morphology

After a bacterial cell lands on the surface of a solid culture medium, it divides over and over again, ultimately producing a mound or pile of bacteria, known as a bacterial colony. A colony contains millions of organisms. The colony morphology or appearance of the colonies of bacteria varies from one species to another. As is true for cell morphology and staining characteristics, colony features serve as important clues in the identification of bacteria. Sometimes a magnifying lens with a fluorescent light attachment or a stereoscopic microscope is used to examine colonies (Fig. 8-12).

Colony morphology includes the size, color, overall shape, elevation, and the appearance of the edge or margin of the colony. The size of a colony is determined by the organism's rate of growth or generation time and is an important characteristic of a particular bacterial species. Although many bacteria produce white, gray, or cream-colored colonies, the colonies of some bacteria are quite colorful (Table 8-6). The color of bacterial colonies is influenced by various pigments produced by the organisms. Colony morphology also includes the results of enzymatic activity on various types of culture media.

SAFETY TIP

"Sniff" Warning!
It is potentially dangerous to "sniff" colonies directly to determine if they have a distinctive odor. Experienced CML professionals have developed a safe sniffing technique, whereby they hold the Petri dish beneath the nose, about six inches away from the face, and use the lid to very gently waft any aroma into the nostrils. However, a CML professional must never sniff fungal colonies (because of the presence of spores) or colonies of certain highly infectious bacteria (e.g., Mycobacterium tuberculosis or Brucella spp.)

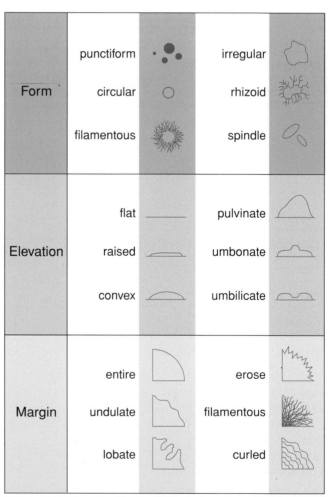

Figure 8-13. **Standardized terms used to describe the overall appearance (form), elevation, and margin of bacterial colonies.** (From Winn WC Jr, et al. Koneman's Color Atlas and Textbook of Diagnostic Microbiology. 6th Ed. Philadelphia: Lippincott Williams & Wilkins, 2006.)

TABLE 8 - 6   Examples of Bacteria That Produce Pigmented Colonies

Bacterial Species[a]	Color of Colonies
Some species of *Actinomyces* spp.	Pink to red
Brevibacterium spp.	Some strains yellow, orange, or purple
Brevundimonas vesicularis	Yellow
Burkholderia cepacia complex	Some strains chartreuse, some strains yellow
Chromobacterium violaceum	Violet
Corynebacterium nigricans	Black
Methylobacterium spp.	Pink
Micrococcus spp.	Yellow or yellowish-green
Nocardia asteroides-complex	Salmon pink to orange
Nocardia brasiliensis	Orange-tan
Nocardia otitidiscaviarum	Pale tan
Peptococcus niger	Black
Porphyromonas spp.	Brown-black
Some *Prevotella* spp.	Brown-black
Pseudomonas aeruginosa	Blue-green
Pseudomonas luteola and *P. oryzihabitans*	Dull yellow
Rhodococcus spp.	Buff, coral, orange, deep rose
Roseomonas spp.	Pink
Serratia rubidaea, some strains of *S. marcescens*	Pink-red to red
Sphingobacterium multivorum and *S. spiritivorum*	Yellow
Sphingomonas paucimobilis and *S. parapaucimobilis*	Deep yellow
Some strains of *Staphylococcus aureus*	Yellow
Stenotrophomonas maltophilia	Some strains slight yellow, some strains lavender

[a]Not all of these organisms have clinical significance, and not all of them are described in this book.

Some of the standardized terms used to describe colony morphology are listed in Table 8-7 and shown in Figure 8-13.

Although not an aspect of colony morphology, some bacteria produce a characteristic odor that may be detectable during examination for colony growth (Table 8-8). The odor is often a useful clue to identification.

Type of Hemolysis Produced

Although the word **hemolysis** usually refers to the lysis (bursting or destruction) of red blood cells, at times the term has a different meaning, as discussed later in this section. Some bacteria are **hemolytic,** meaning they cause damage or destruction to red blood cells. These bacteria are hemolytic because they produce enzymes called **hemolysins.** It is those enzymes that cause damage to or destruction of the red blood cells.

Blood agar is used to determine the type of hemolysis that an organism is producing. The following types of hemolysis may be seen on a BA plate (Fig. 8-14):

- A green zone around the bacterial colony is referred to as **α-hemolysis,** and the organism producing the green zone

TABLE 8 - 7   Terms Commonly Used to Describe Bacterial Colonies

Characteristic	Descriptive Terms
Pigmentation and color	Pigmented (state actual color), nonpigmented
Size	State size in millimeters or use terms like punctiform (pinpoint), small, medium, large
Overall shape/general appearance/form	Circular, filamentous, irregular, rhizoid (rough), spindle-like, swarming (see Fig. 8-13)
Elevation/height	Flat, raised, convex, pulvinate, umbonate (having a raised center), umbilicate (having a sunken center; see Fig. 8-13)
Edge/margin of the colony	Entire, undulate (wavelike), lobate, erose (jagged), filamentous, curled (see Fig. 8-13)
Surface	Smooth, dull, glistening (shiny, glossy), waxy, wrinkled
Consistency	Dry, moist/wet, butyrous (creamy), mucoid (sticky, viscous), brittle
Density	Transparent, translucent, opaque
Hemolysis	α-Hemolytic, β-hemolytic, nonhemolytic (γ-hemolytic)

TABLE 8 - 8   Examples of Bacteria That Produce Characteristic Odors

Organism	Description(s) of the Odor
Alcaligenes faecalis (strains previously called *Alcaligenes odorans*)	Freshly cut apples
Bartonella henselae	Caramel
Burkholderia cepacia and *B. pseudomallei*	Earthy or dirtlike
Clostridium difficile	Like a horse stable
Corynebacterium spp.	Fruity
Eikenella corrodens	Musty; like crackers, bleach, mouse cage
Nocardia and *Streptomyces*	Musty basement, earthy, root cellar, freshly plowed soil
Stenotrophomonas maltophilia	Ammonia
Pasteurella multocida	Musty
Proteus spp.	Burnt chocolate
Pseudomonas aeruginosa	Fruity; like grapes, a wine cellar, tortillas

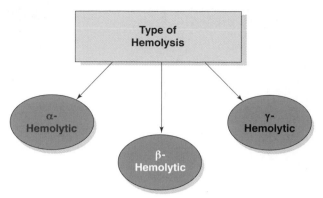

Figure 8-14. **Categories of bacteria based on the type of hemolysis they produce.**

Blood agar is considered a type of differential medium because it can be used to differentiate between the various types of hemolysis (Fig. 8-15).

Many different species of bacteria are hemolytic, but the type of hemolysis that they cause is not always an important clue when trying to identify or speciate the organism. The type of hemolysis that an organism produces is of greatest importance when attempting to identify *Streptococcus* spp. (see Chapter 9). Some species or strains of *Streptococcus* are α-hemolytic, some are α-prime hemolytic, some are β-hemolytic, and some are γ-hemolytic. The type of hemolysis that a particular *Streptococcus* isolate produces serves as a guide to what other clues are needed to identify it. For example, *S. pneumoniae* is always α-hemolytic, and *S. pyogenes* is always β-hemolytic (discussed again in Chapter 9).

> The type of hemolysis that an organism produces is of primary importance when attempting to identify a *Streptococcus* species.

is described as being **α-hemolytic.** The bacteria in the colony have caused a partial breakdown of hemoglobin in the sheep red blood cells, resulting in the green color.

CAUTION **Is It Really α-Hemolytic?** α-Hemolysis is often quite subtle. Sometimes the zone is very small, and sometimes it is difficult for the CML professional to determine if the colonies have caused a greening of the agar. Whenever determining that an organism is α-hemolytic is difficult, the CML professional can push one or more of the colonies aside, using a sterile inoculating loop. This is somewhat like sliding a hockey puck across the ice with a hockey stick. If the organism is α-hemolytic, the agar *beneath* the colony will be green.

- A clear zone around the bacterial colony is referred to as **β-hemolysis,** and the organism producing the clear zone is described as being **β-hemolytic.** The bacteria in the colony are producing a hemolysin that completely destroys the red blood cells (i.e., causes complete lysis or destruction of the red blood cells). Some bacteria (e.g., *Streptococcus agalactiae* and *Listeria monocytogenes*) produce a subtle zone of β-hemolysis. Sliding the colony aside with a sterile inoculating loop may reveal β-hemolysis beneath the colony. Alternatively, the plate can be held under or over a strong light source and viewed from the back.

- If there is neither a green zone nor a clear zone around the colony (in other words, neither α- nor β-hemolysis is seen), this is referred to as **γ-hemolysis,** and the organism is described as being **γ-hemolytic** or nonhemolytic.

- Another type of hemolysis that is rarely observed is known as α-prime or wide-zone α-hemolysis. The colony is surrounded by a narrow zone of γ-hemolysis (no hemolysis), which, in turn, is surrounded by a wider zone of β-hemolysis.

Presence or Absence of a Capsule

Recall from Chapter 1 that some bacteria produce a polysaccharide capsule that protects the organisms from phagocytosis by white blood cells. Although rarely performed in the CML, a capsule-staining procedure could enable a CML professional to determine if a bacterial isolate is producing a capsule. The capsule-staining procedure is a type of negative staining procedure. As was shown in Figure 2-6, the background stains darkly and the bacteria take up some of the stain, but the capsule remains colorless. Thus, the capsules appear as colorless halos around the bacteria.

Motility and the Number and Location of Flagella

If a bacterium is able to "swim," it is said to be motile. Bacteria unable to swim are said to be nonmotile. Bacterial motility is most often associated with the presence of flagella or axial filaments, although some bacteria exhibit a type of gliding motility on secreted slime. Most spiral-shaped bacteria and about one-half of the bacilli are motile by means of flagella, but cocci are generally nonmotile. A flagella stain can be used to demonstrate the presence, number, and location of flagella on bacterial cells, although flagella staining is not very often performed in CMLs. Various terms (e.g., **monotrichous, amphitrichous, lophotrichous, peritrichous**) are used to describe the number and location

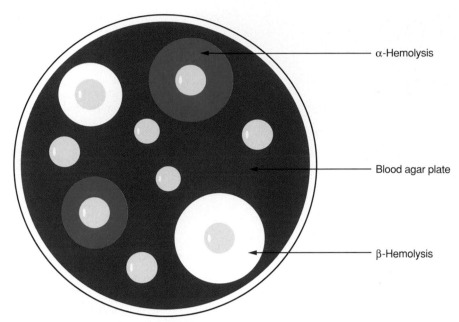

Figure 8-15. **The three types of hemolysis that can be observed on a blood agar plate.** α-Hemolysis is a green zone around the bacterial colonies. β-Hemolysis is a clear zone around the bacterial colonies. γ-Hemolysis is neither a green zone nor a clear zone around the bacterial colonies. α-Hemolytic bacteria produce an enzyme that converts red hemoglobin to green methemoglobin, thus producing the green zone. β-Hemolytic bacteria produce an enzyme that completely destroys (lyses) the red blood cells in the medium, thus producing the clear zone. γ-Hemolytic bacteria (also referred to as nonhemolytic bacteria) produce neither of these enzymes, thus causing no change in the red blood cells in the medium.

of flagella on bacterial cells (Fig. 8-16). A peritrichous bacterium is shown in Figure 8-17.

Motility can be demonstrated by stabbing the bacteria into a tube of semisolid medium or by using the hanging-drop technique. Growth or multiplication of bacteria in semisolid medium produces turbidity or cloudiness. Non-

motile organisms will grow only along the stab line; thus, turbidity will be seen only along the stab line. Motile organisms will spread away from the stab line, thereby producing turbidity throughout the medium (Fig. 8-18).

In the hanging drop method (Fig. 8-19), a drop of a bacterial suspension is placed onto a glass coverslip. The coverslip

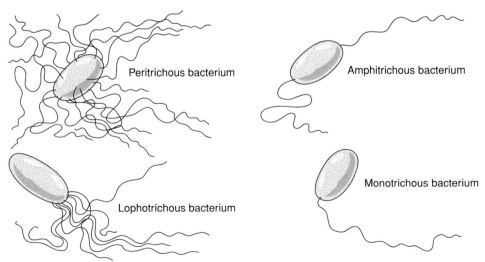

Figure 8-16. **Flagellar arrangement.** The four basic types of flagellar arrangements on bacteria are peritrichous, flagella all over the surface of the cell; lophotrichous, a tuft of flagella at one end of the cell; amphitrichous, one or more flagella at each end of the cell; and monotrichous, one flagellum.

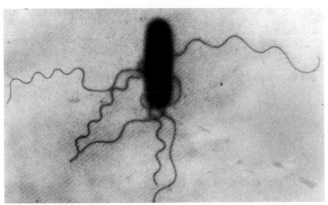

Figure 8-17. **A peritrichous *Salmonella* cell.** (From Volk WA, Gebhardt BM, Hammarskjöld M, Kadner RJ. Essentials of Medical Microbiology. 5th Ed. Philadelphia: Lippincott-Raven, 1996.)

is then inverted over a depression slide. When the preparation is examined microscopically, motile bacteria within the "hanging drop" will be seen darting about in every direction (see Appendix A for details of these procedures).

Ability to Produce Spores and Location of Spores

A few genera of bacteria (e.g., *Bacillus* and *Clostridium*) are capable of forming thick-walled spores as a means of survival when their moisture or nutrient supply is low. Bacterial spores are referred to as endospores, and the process by which they are formed is called **sporulation.** Only one spore is produced within a bacterial cell, and one vegetative bacterium emerges from the spore during germination. Although not a commonly used procedure in CMLs, endospores can be

> Associate the ability to form spores with *Bacillus* and *Clostridium* spp. Bacterial spores (technically known as endospores) serve a survival function, *not* a reproductive function.

stained using what is known as a spore stain. Once a particular bacterium's endospores are stained, CML professionals can determine whether the organism is producing terminal or subterminal spores. A terminal spore is produced at the very end of the bacterial cell, whereas a subterminal spore is produced elsewhere in the cell. Where a spore is being produced within the cell, and whether or not it causes a swelling of the cell serve as clues to the identity of the organism.

Biochemical Tests

As discussed in Chapter 6, biochemical tests are of value for learning which enzymes an organism does or does not

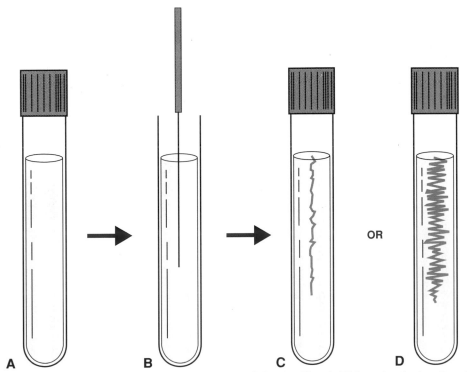

Figure 8-18. **The semisolid agar method of determining motility. A.** Uninoculated tube of semisolid agar. **B.** Same tube being inoculated by stabbing the inoculating wire into the medium. **C.** One possible result: growth occurs only along the stab line. Conclusion: the organism is nonmotile. **D.** The other possible result: Growth occurs along the stab line and in areas of the medium outward from the stab line. Conclusion: the organism is motile.

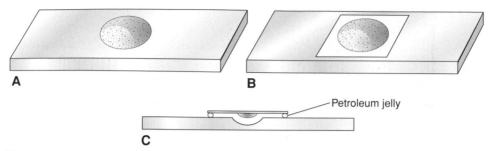

Figure 8-19. **Hanging drop preparation for study of living bacteria. A.** Depression slide. **B.** Depression slide with coverslip over the depression area. **C.** Side view of hanging drop preparation showing the drop of liquid culture medium hanging from the center of the coverslip above the depression.

possess and thus gaining information about the organism's phenotype. For many years, biochemical tests were the primary way in which bacterial isolates were identified. Isolates were inoculated into a series of test tubes, each containing a particular substrate, usually a carbohydrate or amino acid. CMLs now use various miniaturized biochemical test systems (minisystems). The more rapid minisystems test for preformed or preexisting enzymes, while others require a longer incubation period during which the organism produces enzymes in response to the presence of certain substrates. The test results (metabolic profile) achieved using these systems are compared with databases furnished by the manufacturers. Often, a code number is generated using the system, and that code number is compared with code numbers contained in a database. Some systems require manual interpretation of test results and manual comparison of code numbers. With automated systems, however, test results are read by an instrument, and organisms are identified using a built-in computer database.

Listed here are examples of substrates commonly incorporated into these identification systems:

> The term *minisystem* refers to a miniaturized biochemical test system. Most minisystems contain various substrates that enable CML professionals to learn which enzymes an organism does or does not possess.

Adonitol (an alcohol)

Arabinose (a pentose)

Dulcitol (an alcohol)

Glucose (a hexose)

Inositol (a sugar-like vitamin)

Lactose (a disaccharide)

Lysine (an amino acid)

Mannitol (a sugar alcohol)

Melibiose (a disaccharide)

Ornithine (an amino acid)

Rhamnose (a hexose)

Sorbitol (an alcohol)

Sucrose (a disaccharide)

Examples of commercial biochemical- and enzyme-based bacterial ID systems available for use in CMLs are shown in Tables 8-9 (manual systems) and 8-10 (semi-automated and automated systems). Figure 8-20 illustrates some of the more popular minisystems.

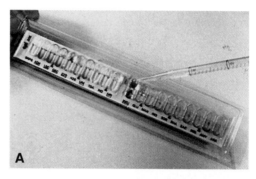

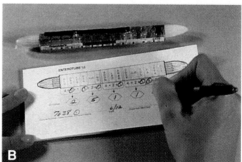

Figure 8-20. Minisystems for the identification of members of the Enterobacteriaceae family. A. A minisystem (API-20E) used to identify members of the Enterobacteriaceae family. Each of the 20 chambers contains a different substrate. If the organism is capable of breaking down a particular substrate, a change in pH will occur; this will cause the pH indicator to change color. Thus, a color change indicates a positive test result. No color change indicates a negative test result. **B.** A minisystem (Enterotube II) used to identify members of the Enterobacteriaceae family. As with the API-20E strip, color changes represent positive test results. By totaling the numerical values of the positive tests, a five-digit code number is generated. The identity of the organism is then determined by looking the number up in a codebook. (From Koneman EW, Allen SD, Janda WM, et al. Color Atlas and Textbook of Diagnostic Microbiology. 5th ed. Philadelphia: Lippincott Williams & Wilkins, 1997.)

TABLE 8 - 9	Examples of Manual Biochemical- and Enzyme-Based Bacterial ID Systems	
Name of System	**Manufacturer**	**Bacteria Identified**
ANI	bioMérieux Inc. (http://www.biomerieux.com/)	Anaerobes
API An-IDENT	bioMérieux Inc.	Anaerobes
API 20A	bioMérieux Inc.	Anaerobes
API 20E	bioMérieux Inc.	Enterobacteriaceae and nonfermenters
API 20 Strep	bioMérieux Inc.	Streptococci and enterococci
API Coryne	bioMérieux Inc.	Corynebacteria and corynebacteria-like bacteria
API 20 NE	bioMérieux Inc.	Gram-negative bacteria other than Enterobacteriaceae
API NH	bioMérieux Inc.	*Neisseria, Haemophilus,* and *Moraxella catarrhalis*
API Rapid 20E	bioMérieux Inc.	Enterobacteriaceae
API Staph	bioMérieux Inc.	Staphylococci and micrococci
Crystal Anaerobe	BD Biosciences (http://www.bdbiosciences.com/)	Anaerobes
Crystal E/NF	BD Biosciences	Enterobacteriaceae and some nonfermenters
Crystal Gram-Positive	BD Biosciences	Gram-positive cocci and bacilli
Crystal MRSA ID	BD Biosciences	Methicillin-resistant *Staphylococcus aureus*
Crystal *Neisseria/Haemophilus*	BD Biosciences	*Neisseria, Haemophilus, Moraxella, Gardnerella,* and other fastidious Gram-negative bacilli
Crystal Rapid Gram-Positive	BD Biosciences	Gram-positive cocci and bacilli
Crystal Rapid Stool/Enteric	BD Biosciences	Gram-negative stool pathogens
Enterotube II	BD Biosciences	Enterobacteriaceae
EPS (Enteric Pathogen Screen)	bioMérieux Inc.	*Edwardsiella, Salmonella, Shigella, Yersinia*
Fox Extra Gram Negative MIC/ID	Micro-Media Systems Inc.	Enteric and nonenteric Gram-negative bacteria
Fox Extra Gram Positive MIC/ID	Micro-Media Systems Inc.	Common staphylococci, micrococci, and streptococci
ID 32 Staph	bioMérieux Inc.	Staphylococci
Micro-ID	Remel (http://www.remelinc.com/)	Enterobacteriaceae
Neisseria Enzyme Test	Remel	*Neisseria* and *Moraxella*

(continued)

TABLE 8 - 9	Examples of Manual Biochemical- and Enzyme-Based Bacterial ID Systems (Continued)	
Name of System	**Manufacturer**	**Bacteria Identified**
NHI	bioMerieux	*Neisseria* and *Haemophilus*
Oxi/Ferm	BD Biosciences	Gram-negative, oxidase-positive, glucose fermenters and nonfermenters
RapID ANA II	Remel	Anaerobes
RapID CB Plus	Remel	Coryneform bacilli
RAPIDEC STAPH	bioMérieux Inc.	Staphylococci
RapID NF Plus	Remel	Nonfermenters
RapID NH	Remel	*Neisseria, Haemophilus*, and some other Gram-negative bacteria
RapID ONE	Remel	Enterobacteriaceae and other oxidase-negative bacilli
RapID SS/u	Remel	Common urinary tract pathogens
RapID STR	Remel	Streptococci
r/b Enteric Differential System	Remel	Enterobacteriaceae
Uni-N/F-Tek	Remel	Fermenting and nonfermenting Gram-negative bacilli

Source: O'Hara CM, et al. Manual and automated systems for detection and identification of microorganisms. In: Murray PR, et al., eds. Manual of Clinical Microbiology. 8th Ed. Washington, DC: ASM Press, 2003.

Analysis of Fatty Acids

As mentioned in Chapter 6, gas-liquid chromatography can be used to identify bacteria and yeasts, either by analyzing fatty acid end products of metabolism or by analyzing cellular fatty acids. Following appropriate chemical extraction procedures, a solution containing the isolate's fatty acids is injected into a gas-liquid chromatograph, and a chromatograph is produced (Fig. 8-21). Depending on the system being used, the chromatograph is then interpreted manually or by computer. Peaks obtained with the isolate are compared with peaks obtained with a standard solution containing a mixture of known fatty acids.

Immunodiagnostic Procedures

The general principles of immunodiagnostic procedures (IDPs) are presented in Chapter 6. Many commercial IDPs are available for diagnosing bacterial infections and for identifying bacterial isolates. Examples of bacteria detected by these assays are *Bordetella pertussis, Borrelia burgdorferi, Chlamydia trachomatis, Clostridium difficile* toxins, *E. coli* O157:H7, *Haemophilus influenzae, Helicobacter pylori, Legionella pneumophila, Listeria monocytogenes, Mycoplasma pneumoniae, Neisseria meningitidis, Salmonella* spp., *Streptococcus pneumoniae, Streptococcus pyogenes*, and *Treponema pallidum*. Additional information about IDPs can be found in Chapter 6.

Molecular Diagnostic Procedures

The general principles of molecular diagnostic procedures (MDPs) are presented in Chapter 6. Many commercial MDPs are available for diagnosing bacterial infections

TABLE 8 - 10	Examples of Semiautomated and Automated Biochemical- and Enzyme-Based Bacterial ID Systems		
ID System	**Semiautomated or Automated**[a]	**Manufacturer**	**Bacteria Identified**
AN Microplate	Semiautomated	Biolog Inc. (http://www.biolog.com/)	Anaerobes
GN Microplate	Semiautomated	Biolog Inc.	Aerobic Gram-negative bacteria
GNI	Automated	bioMérieux Inc. (http://www.biomerieux.com/)	Enterobacteriaceae and nonfermenters
GN and GNI+	Automated	bioMérieux Inc.	Enterobacteriaceae and nonfermenters
GP Microplate	Semiautomated	Biolog Inc.	Aerobic Gram-positive bacteria
GP and GPI	Automated	bioMérieux Inc.	Gram-positive cocci and bacilli
HNID	Automated	Dade Behring (http://www.dadebehring.com/)	*Neisseria, Haemophilus, Moraxella catarrhalis,* and *Gardnerella vaginalis*
ID-GNB	Automated	bioMérieux Inc.	Gram-negative fermenting and nonfermenting bacilli
ID-GPC	Automated	bioMérieux Inc.	Gram-positive cocci
ID Tri-Panel	Semi-automated	BD Biosciences (http://www.bdbiosciences.com/)	Gram-negative and Gram-positive bacteria
NEG ID Type 2	Automated	Dade Behring	Enterobacteriaceae and other fermenting and nonfermenting bacteria
Pos ID-2	Automated	Dade Behring	Gram-positive cocci and *Listeria*
Rapid Anaerobe	Automated	Dade Behring	Anaerobes
Rapid NEG ID Type 3	Automated	Dade Behring	Enterobacteriaceae and other fermenting and nonfermenting bacteria
Rapid POS ID	Automated	Dade Behring	Gram-positive cocci and *Listeria*
Sensititre AP 80	Automated	Trek Diagnostic Systems Inc. (http://www.trekds.com/)	Enterobacteriaceae and nonfermenters
Sensititre AP 90	Automated	Trek Diagnostic Systems Inc.	Gram-positive bacteria
UID/UID-3	Automated	bioMérieux Inc.	Urinary tract pathogens directly from urine

Source: O'Hara CM, et al. Manual and automated systems for detection and identification of microorganisms. In: Murray PR, et al., eds. Manual of Clinical Microbiology. 8th Ed. Washington, DC: ASM Press, 2003.

[a] Semiautomated systems are read-only systems.

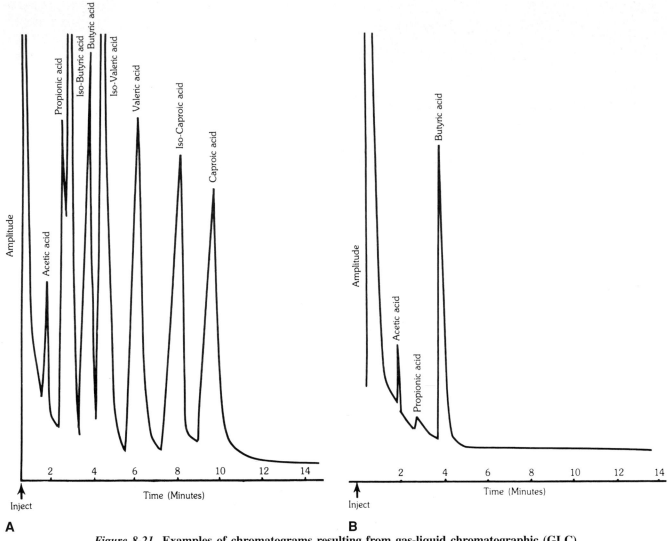

Figure 8-21. **Examples of chromatograms resulting from gas-liquid chromatographic (GLC) analysis of volatile fatty acids. A.** Chromatogram produced by GLC analysis of a standard mixture of volatile fatty acids. **B.** Chromatogram produced by GLC analysis of volatile fatty acids contained in a broth culture of *Fusobacterium mortiferum*. (From Winn WC Jr, et al. Koneman's Color Atlas and Textbook of Diagnostic Microbiology. 6th Ed. Philadelphia: Lippincott Williams & Wilkins, 2006.)

and for identifying bacterial isolates. Examples of bacteria detected by these MDPs are *Borrelia burgdorferi*, *Campylobacter* spp., *Chlamydia trachomatis*, *Enterococcus* spp., *Gardnerella vaginalis*, *Haemophilus influenzae*, *Listeria monocytogenes*, *Mycobacterium* spp., *Mycoplasma pneu-* *moniae*, *Neisseria gonorrhoeae*, *Staphylococcus aureus*, methicillin-resistant *S. aureus*, *Streptococcus agalactiae*, *Streptococcus pneumoniae*, and *Streptococcus pyogenes*. Additional information about MDPs can be found in Chapter 6.

Chapter Review

- Bacteria are in the Kingdom Procaryotae. Bacteriology is the study of bacteria, and a bacteriologist is a scientist who studies bacteria.

- Bacteria may be categorized based on genetics, cellular morphology, Gram reaction, atmospheric requirements, or biochemical and metabolic activities.

- Most bacteria may be categorized by Gram reaction into the following four categories: Gram-positive cocci, Gram-positive bacilli, Gram-negative cocci, and Gram-negative bacilli.

- Various types of culture media are used to grow bacteria in the laboratory. Categories of culture media include enrichment media, enriched media, selective media, and differential media.

- The specific type of medium used to culture a specimen depends on the source of the specimen and/or the types of organisms suspected. For example, highly enriched and highly selective Thayer-Martin medium is used to isolate and grow *N. gonorrhoeae*.

- The pattern of growth on various kinds of plated media is a good indication of the types of organisms present in the specimen. For example, Gram-negative organisms will grow on MAC, but not on PEA or CNA. Gram-positive organisms will grow on PEA and CNA, but not on MAC.

- The primary setup refers to the various types of media inoculated with a particular type of clinical specimen.

- Bacterial growth is an increase in the number of organisms and is accomplished by binary fission (i.e., one bacterial cell divides into two). The time it takes one cell to become two is called the generation time, which varies by bacterial species.

- Various phenotypic characteristics—such as Gram reaction, motility, atmospheric requirements, cell shape, and morphologic arrangement—are used in identifying bacteria.

- The Gram stain is a very important bacteriological procedure that differentiates between Gram-positive and Gram-negative bacteria based on the chemical composition of their cell walls.

- A bacterial colony is a "mound" of bacteria that takes on specific characteristics depending on the bacterial species. Colony morphology includes size, color, shape, elevation, and the appearance of the edge or margin of the colony.

- Some bacteria produce enzymes called hemolysins that damage or destroy red blood cells. Blood agar can be used to determine what type of hemolysis an organism produces. Types of hemolysis include α-hemolysis (greening of the agar), β-hemolysis (clearing of the agar), and γ-hemolysis (no hemolysis).

- Some bacteria may produce a capsule, flagella, and/or spores. These structures can help to identify the organism.

- Biochemical tests are used to determine which enzymes an organism does or does not possess. Various biochemical reactions can aid in the identification of a bacterial isolate.

- Additional means of identifying bacteria include cellular fatty acid analysis, immunodiagnostic procedures, and molecular diagnostic procedures.

New Terms and Abbreviations

After studying Chapter 8, you should be familiar with the following terms, which are defined within the chapter and in the Glossary at the back of the book:

Aerotolerant anaerobe

α-Hemolysis

Amphitrichous bacterium

Anabolism

Anaerobe

Bacillus (pl. bacilli)

β-Hemolysis

Binary fission

Capnophile

Catabolism

Coccobacillus (pl. coccobacilli)

Coccus (pl. cocci)

Colony

Diplobacilli

Diplococci

Facultative anaerobe

γ-Hemolysis

Generation time

Hemolysin

Hemolysis

Lophotrichous bacterium

Microaerophile

Monotrichous bacterium

Obligate aerobe

Obligate anaerobe

Obligate intracellular pathogen

Octad

Peritrichous bacterium

Pleomorphism

Primary setup

Sporulation

Staphylococci

Streptobacilli

Streptococci

Tetrad

References and Suggested Reading

Abbreviated Identification of Bacteria and Yeast: Approved Guideline. CLSI Document M35-A. Wayne, PA: Clinical and Laboratory Standards Institute, 2002.

Boone DR, Castenholz RW, eds. The Archaea and the Deeply Branching and Phototrophic Bacteria. New York: Springer-Verlag, 2001. Garrity GM, ed. Bergey's Manual of Systematic Bacteriology, vol 1. 2nd Ed.

Constantine NT, Lana DP. Immunoassays for the diagnosis of infectious diseases. In: Murray PR, Baron EJ, Jorgensen JH, Pfaller MA, Yolken RH, eds. Manual of Clinical Microbiology. 8th Ed. Washington, DC: ASM Press, 2003.

Hodinka RL. Automated Immunoassay Analyzers. In: Manual of Commercial Methods in Clinical Microbiology. Washington, DC: ASM Press, 2002.

Holt JG, Krieg NR, Sneath PHA, Staley JT, Williams ST, eds. Bergey's Manual of Determinative Bacteriology. 9th Ed. Baltimore: Williams & Wilkins, 1994.

Jungkind D, Kessler HH. Molecular methods for diagnosis of infectious diseases. In: Manual of Commercial Methods in Clinical Microbiology. Washington, DC: ASM Press, 2002.

Nolte FS, and Caliendo AM. Molecular detection and identification of microorganisms. In: Murray PR, Baron EJ, Jorgensen JH, Pfaller MA, Yolken RH, eds. Manual of Clinical Microbiology. 8th Ed. Washington, DC: ASM Press, 2003.

O'Hara CM, et al. Manual and automated systems for detection and identification of microorganisms. In: Murray PR, Baron EJ, Jorgensen JH, Pfaller MA, Yolken RH, eds. Manual of Clinical Microbiology. 8th Ed. Washington, DC: ASM Press, 2003.

 # *On the CD-ROM*

- Classification of Bacteria
- Additional Self-Assessment Exercises
- Puzzle

Self-Assessment Exercises

After studying Chapter 8, answer the following questions.

1. Complete hemolysis (a clear zone) surrounding a colony on blood agar is known as

   A. α-hemolysis.

   B. β-hemolysis.

   C. γ-hemolysis.

   D. ζ-hemolysis.

2. Gram-positive bacteria stain blue to purple because

   A. they possess a thick layer of peptidoglycan, making it difficult to remove the crystal violet–iodine complex during the decolorization step.

   B. they possess a thick layer of cellulose, making it difficult to remove the crystal violet–iodine complex during the decolorization step.

   C. they are unable to take up the safranin stain.

   D. none of the above.

3. Which of the following is an example of a selective and differential medium?

   A. MacConkey agar

   B. Blood agar

   C. Chocolate agar

   D. Thioglycollate broth

4. Bacterial endospores are a

   A. means of reproduction.

   B. survival mechanism.

   C. means to inactivate antimicrobial agents.

   D. means of locomotion.

5. A bacterial isolate was found to be motile by means of a single flagellum extending from one end of the cell. This organism can be described as

   A. amphitrichous.

   B. lophotrichous.

   C. monotrichous.

   D. peritrichous.

6. To isolate capnophilic organisms, the concentration of CO_2 should be maintained at

A. 1% to 5%.

B. 5% to 10%.

C. 10% to 15%

D. 15% to 20%.

7. Which bacterium is described as a Gram-positive coccus in a chain?

A. *Staphylococcus aureus*

B. *Streptococcus pyogenes*

C. *Escherichia coli*

D. *Treponema pallidum*

8. A definitive identification of a bacterial isolate may be accomplished using all of the following methods *except*

A. immunodiagnostic procedures.

B. molecular diagnostic procedures.

C. an automated biochemical-based identification system.

D. growth on specific types of culture media.

9. What can you conclude about a bacterial isolate that grows on BA, CA, and PEA but not on MAC, and is β-hemolytic on BA?

A. It is a β-hemolytic Gram-positive organism.

B. It is a β-hemolytic Gram-negative organism.

C. It is a fastidious, β-hemolytic Gram-positive organism.

D. It is a fastidious, β-hemolytic Gram-negative organism.

10. What can you conclude about a bacterial isolate that grows on BA, CA, and MAC but not on PEA, and is producing pink colonies on MAC?

A. It is a mannitol-fermenting Gram-positive organism.

B. It is a mannitol-fermenting Gram-negative organism.

C. It is a lactose-fermenting Gram-positive organism.

D. It is a lactose-fermenting Gram-negative organism.

CHAPTER 9

Gram-Positive Cocci

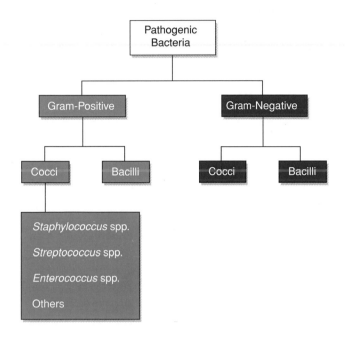

Chapter Outline

Genus *Staphylococcus*
- *Staphylococcus* Versus *Micrococcus*
- *Staphylococcus aureus*
- Coagulase-Negative Staphylococci

Other Catalase-Positive, Gram-Positive Cocci

Genus *Streptococcus*
- *Streptococcus pyogenes*
- *Streptococcus agalactiae*
- *Streptococcus pneumoniae*
- Other *Streptococcus* Species

Genus *Enterococcus*

Other Catalase-Negative, Gram-Positive Cocci

Identification of an Unknown Gram-Positive Coccus

LEARNING OBJECTIVES

After studying this chapter, you should be able to:

☛ Define the terms introduced in this chapter (e.g., *catalase, clumping factor, coagulase*)

☛ List three genera of Gram-positive cocci that contain clinically significant species

☛ Name four clinically significant species in the genus *Staphylococcus*

☛ Compare and contrast the colonial and microscopic characteristics of *Staphylococcus* spp., *Streptococcus* spp., and *Enterococcus* spp.

☛ Describe virulence factors associated with staphylococci

☛ Name some media that may be used to isolate *Staphylococcus* spp. and *Streptococcus* spp.

☞ Describe the general characteristics of *Staphylococcus* spp., including colonial and microscopic morphology, motility, atmospheric requirements, and major biochemical reactions (e.g., catalase test, coagulase test)

☞ Describe the general characteristics of *Streptococcus* spp., including colonial and microscopic morphology, motility, atmospheric requirements, and major biochemical reactions (e.g., catalase test, pyrrolidonyl arylamidase test)

☞ Explain the principles of the following tests: catalase test, modified oxidase test, pyrrolidonyl arylamidase test, A-disk test, P-disk test, ornithine decarboxylase test; describe the purpose of each test, reagent(s) used, and any products or reactions produced

☞ Given a series of cellular and colonial features and laboratory test results, presumptively identify various Gram-positive cocci

☞ Select an appropriate test to differentiate between a *Micrococcus* sp. and a *Staphylococcus* sp.

☞ Given the name of a specific infectious disease (e.g., necrotizing fasciitis), state the name of the Gram-positive coccus that causes it

☞ Discuss drug resistance in *Staphylococcus aureus*, including methicillin-resistant *S. aureus*, vancomycin-intermediate *S. aureus*, and vancomycin-resistant *S. aureus*

☞ Discuss the principles and procedures for the slide and tube coagulase tests, and explain why a tube coagulase test may be necessary after a slide coagulase test is performed

☞ Discuss the clinical significance of coagulase-negative staphylococci, including the various species most often involved in human infections and tests used to identify them

☞ Cite ways in which streptococci may be grouped (e.g., by cell wall carbohydrates and type of hemolysis)

☞ Identify two types of β-hemolysins produced by *Streptococcus pyogenes*

☞ Describe the viridans group streptococci, and cite some examples of specific species, where they are found in the body, and any associated diseases

☞ Identify the two most commonly isolated *Enterococcus* spp.

☞ Describe the common characteristics and clinical significance of *Enterococcus* spp.

Flesh-eating bacteria. Methicillin-resistant *Staphylococcus aureus*. Pneumococcal pneumonia. Scalded skin syndrome. Scarlet fever. Staph infections. Strep throat. Toxic shock syndrome. What do these organisms and diseases have in common? They all relate to bacteria discussed in this chapter.

Recall from Chapter 8 that cocci are spherical bacteria. Medically important cocci can be divided into those that are Gram positive and those that are Gram negative. Pathogenic, facultatively anaerobic Gram-positive cocci are described in this chapter. Pathogenic, aerobic and facultatively anaerobic Gram-negative cocci are described in Chapter 11. Anaerobic Gram-positive cocci are described in Chapter 17.

Of the many genera of Gram-positive cocci (GPC) that can be isolated from clinical specimens, the following three contain the most clinically significant species:

- *Staphylococcus*

- *Streptococcus*

- *Enterococcus*

> The most clinically significant Gram-positive cocci are in the genera *Staphylococcus*, *Streptococcus*, and *Enterococcus*.

According to *Bergey's Manual of Systematic Bacteriology* (see "References and Suggested Reading"), these three genera are all contained in the same phylum, same class, and same order. However, each of the three genera is in a different family. Staphylococci are in the family Staphylococcaceae, streptococci in the family Streptococcaceae, and enterococci in the family Enterococcaceae.

Although the three genera contain the most clinically significant GPC, it is sometimes necessary to distinguish members of these genera from other GPC isolated from clinical specimens. For this reason, some information is provided in this chapter and on the CD-ROM about other, less clinically significant GPC.

GENUS *STAPHYLOCOCCUS*

There are approximately 35 to 40 species in the genus *Staphylococcus*, not all of which are encountered in clinical specimens. Even when isolated from clinical specimens, many of these species are considered indigenous microflora contaminants and not clinically significant. The discussion of the genus *Staphylococcus* will be limited to the following five species:

- *S. aureus*

- *S. epidermidis*

- *S. haemolyticus*

- *S. lugdunensis*

- *S. saprophyticus*

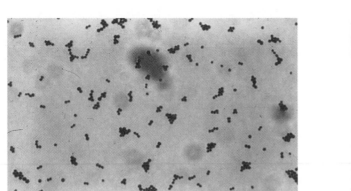

Figure 9-1. **Gram-stained broth culture of** *Staphylococcus aureus,* **showing typical grapelike clusters of cocci.** (From Winn WC Jr, et al. Koneman's Color Atlas and Textbook of Diagnostic Microbiology. 6th Ed. Philadelphia: Lippincott Williams & Wilkins, 2006.)

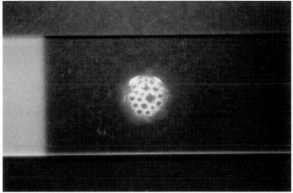

Figure 9-2. **Positive slide catalase test result.** Oxygen bubbles formed as a result of the breakdown of hydrogen peroxide. *Staphylococcus* and *Micrococcus* spp. are catalase positive. (From Winn WC Jr, et al. Koneman's Color Atlas and Textbook of Diagnostic Microbiology. 6th Ed. Philadelphia: Lippincott Williams & Wilkins, 2006.)

> Associate GPC in clusters with the genus *Staphylococcus*. The word *Staphylococcus* is derived from the Greek word *staphyle*, meaning "grapelike cluster."

Microscopically, *Staphylococcus* spp. (staphylococci) are GPC that may occur singly or in pairs (diplococci), packets of four (tetrads), short chains, or irregular or grapelike clusters (Fig. 9-1). The grapelike cluster is the morphologic arrangement most often associated with staphylococci. *Staphylococcus* spp. have the following additional characteristics:

- Facultative anaerobes, except for *S. saccharolyticus* and *S. aureus* subsp. *aureus*, which are anaerobic

- Nonmotile

- Non–spore forming

- Nonencapsulated (usually)

- Catalase positive, meaning that they produce the enzyme catalase (catalase and the catalase test are described later, and in more detail in Appendix A); anaerobic *Staphylococcus* spp. are catalase negative

- Modified oxidase negative, except for *S. lentus*, *S. scuiri*, and *S. vitulus*

Hydrogen peroxide (H_2O_2) molecules accumulate whenever oxygen (O_2) participates in various metabolic reactions. Considered a reduction product of oxygen, H_2O_2 is a highly reactive, potentially damaging molecule. To avoid damage, cells need ways to remove hydrogen peroxide from their environment. **Catalase** is an enzyme that effectively removes H_2O_2 by catalyzing the breakdown (hydrolysis) of the molecules into water and oxygen:

$$H_2O_2 \rightarrow H_2O + O_2\uparrow$$

Some bacteria produce catalase, whereas others do not. Determining whether or not a particular bacterium produces catalase is often a useful clue to the identity of an organism and is especially useful when attempting to identify GPC.

> The catalase test is especially useful when attempting to identify Gram-positive cocci.

(Note: Many laboratory tests are briefly discussed in this and subsequent chapters. Detailed information about these tests is contained in Appendix A.)

Slide catalase test. The slide catalase test is simple to perform. A colony of the organism to be tested is smeared onto a glass microscope slide, and a drop of 3% aqueous H_2O_2 is added to the smear. The immediate formation of oxygen bubbles is evidence that the organism is producing catalase (Fig. 9-2). Thus, the formation of bubbles is interpreted as a positive test result. Few or no bubbles produced after 20 seconds is interpreted as a negative test result.

CAUTION ⚠ **Blood-Containing Media Are Not Appropriate for Catalase Testing.** Red blood cells contain catalase. False-positive catalase reactions can occur when colonies are taken from blood-containing media. This is especially true if any of the medium is removed along with the colony. Whenever possible, colonies for catalase testing should be taken from media that do not contain blood.

The catalase test can be used to differentiate between *Staphylococcus* spp. and *Streptococcus* spp. **It is important for you to remember that**

> Virtually all *Staphylococcus* spp. are catalase positive, whereas all *Streptococcus* spp. are catalase negative.

virtually all *Staphylococcus* spp. are catalase positive (i.e., they produce catalase), whereas all *Streptococcus* spp. are catalase negative (i.e., they do not produce catalase).

Staphylococcus Versus *Micrococcus*

Not all catalase-positive, Gram-positive cocci isolated from clinical specimens are *Staphylococcus* spp. *Micrococcus* spp.

> When isolated from clinical specimens, *Micrococcus* spp. are usually contaminants.

are also catalase positive, and their cell shape and morphological appearance resemble those of staphylococci. Micrococci occur in pairs, tetrads, and irregular clusters. Micrococci are common members of the indigenous microflora of the skin, mucosa, and oropharynx and, when isolated from clinical specimens, are usually contaminants. However, they can cause infections in immunocompromised patients. On rare occasions, *Micrococcus luteus* has been associated with endocarditis, meningitis, pneumonia, and septic arthritis. Colonies of *Micrococcus luteus* are shown in Figure 9-3. The most common methods used to differentiate staphylococci from micrococci are shown in Table 9-1.

Susceptibility to bacitracin. Bacitracin is an antibiotic produced by *Bacillus subtilis*. Susceptibility to bacitracin can be determined by using a filter paper disk impregnated with 0.04 units (U) of bacitracin. The disk is gently pressed to the surface of an inoculated blood agar plate; the plate is incubated overnight. Then the

> *Staphylococcus* spp. are resistant to bacitracin, whereas *Micrococcus* spp. are susceptible to this antibiotic.

plate is examined for a zone of inhibition around the bacitracin disk. Staphylococci are resistant to bacitracin and will grow to the edge of the disk. Micrococci are susceptible to and killed by bacitracin, producing zone diameters that are ≥10 mm. This same type of disk can also be used to differentiate *Streptococcus pyogenes* from other β-hemolytic streptococci (discussed later in the chapter).

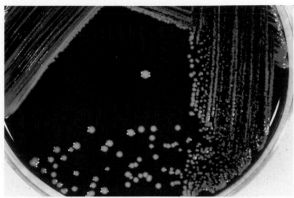

Figure 9-3. **Yellow-pigmented colonies of *Micrococcus luteus* on sheep blood agar.** (From Winn WC Jr, et al. Koneman's Color Atlas and Textbook of Diagnostic Microbiology. 6th Ed. Philadelphia: Lippincott Williams & Wilkins, 2006.)

Susceptibility to furazolidone. Furazolidone is an antimicrobial agent. Susceptibility to furazolidone can be determined using a filter paper disk impregnated with 100 μg of furazolidone. Staphylococci are susceptible to furazolidone, producing zone diameters that are ≥15 mm (Fig. 9-4). Micrococci are resistant to furazolidone, but small zone diameters (up to 9 mm) may be seen (Fig. 9-5).

> *Staphylococcus* spp. are susceptible to furazolidone, whereas *Micrococcus* spp. are resistant.

Modified oxidase test. Oxidase is an abbreviated name for cytochrome oxidase, an enzyme that participates in the electron transport chain. The modified oxidase test, using filter paper disks impregnated with tetramethyl-para-phenylene-diamine dihydrochloride (the oxidase reagent) in dimethyl sulfoxide (DMSO) can be used to differentiate between staphylococci and micrococci. (Microdase Test Disks are available from Remel; http://www.remelinc.com/.) The DMSO enables the reagent to penetrate the cell wall. When a *Micrococcus* colony is rubbed onto the disk, a blue-purple color develops within 30 seconds; this is a positive test result

TABLE 9 - 1	Methods Used to Differentiate Staphylococci from Micrococci	
Method	**Staphylococci**	**Micrococci**
Bacitracin sensitivity	Resistant	Susceptible
Furazolidone sensitivity	Susceptible	Resistant
Oxidase production	Negative, with rare exceptions	Positive
Lysostaphin	Susceptible	Resistant

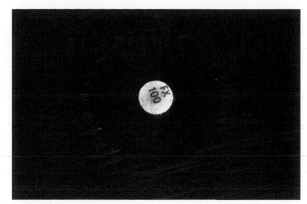

Figure 9-4. **Furazolidone disk test.** Staphylococci, such as the species that was tested here, are susceptible to furazolidone. Susceptibility to furazolidone is indicated by the zone of no growth surrounding the disk. (From Winn WC Jr, et al. Koneman's Color Atlas and Textbook of Diagnostic Microbiology. 6th Ed. Philadelphia: Lippincott Williams & Wilkins, 2006.)

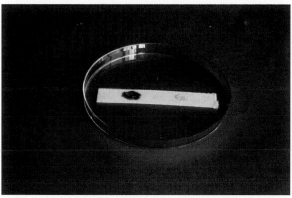

Figure 9-6. **Modified oxidase test.** A positive test result (the blue-purple color) is shown to the left, and a negative test result is shown to the right. (From Winn WC Jr, et al. Koneman's Color Atlas and Textbook of Diagnostic Microbiology. 6th Ed. Philadelphia: Lippincott Williams & Wilkins, 2006.)

(Fig. 9-6). The purple color is caused by indophenol, formed by oxidation of the oxidase reagent. When a *Staphylococcus* colony is rubbed onto the disk, no blue-purple color develops within 30 seconds; this is a negative test result. It should be noted that some of the less commonly isolated *Staphylococcus* spp. are modified oxidase test positive. A different type of oxidase test, one that does not require DMSO, is used when testing Gram-negative bacilli; it is described in Chapter 12.

> Commonly isolated *Staphylococcus* spp. are modified oxidase test negative, whereas *Micrococcus* spp. are modified oxidase test positive.

Lysostaphin susceptibility tube test. Lysostaphin is an enzyme that destroys the integrity of staphylococcal cell walls, resulting in lysis of staphylococcal cells. (A lysostaphin susceptibility tube test is available from Remel; http://www.rcmclinc.com/.) A heavy suspension of the organism to be tested is prepared in sterile saline, to which a lysostaphin solution is added. The tube is then incubated. Clearing of the suspension indicates susceptibility to lysostaphin. Organisms can also be tested using a disk diffusion method. Micrococci are resistant to lysostaphin, whereas staphylococci are susceptible. However, some staphylococci (e.g., *S. aureus* and some coagulase-negative staphylococci) are more susceptible to lysostaphin than others (e.g., *S. haemolyticus*, *S. saprophyticus*).

> *Micrococcus* spp. are resistant to lysostaphin, whereas *Staphylococcus* spp. are susceptible.

The most commonly isolated *Micrococcus* sp. is *M. luteus*, most strains of which produce bright lemon-yellow colonies (see Fig. 9-3). Micrococci are aerobic, whereas most staphylococci are facultative anaerobes.

Staphylococcus aureus

Clinical significance. *Staphylococcus aureus* is a very important human pathogen and certainly the most important of the staphylococci. It is often found in low numbers as indigenous microflora of the skin. About 20% to 30% of the general population are "staph carriers"—people whose nasal passages are colonized with *S. aureus*. As long as *S. aureus* remains localized in their nasal passages, it causes the carriers no harm. However, the organisms can be transmitted to others.

> *Staphylococcus aureus* is a *very* important human pathogen, and many strains have become multidrug resistant.

S. aureus is the most virulent *Staphylococcus* sp. It causes a wide variety of diseases, which are often referred to as staph infections. *S. aureus* is a major cause of skin, soft tissue, respiratory, bone, joint, endovascular, and wound infections. Most pimples, boils, carbuncles, and styes

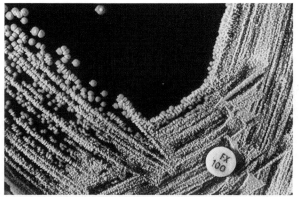

Figure 9-5. **Furazolidone disk test.** Micrococci, such as the species that was tested here, are resistant to furazolidone. (From Winn WC Jr, et al. Koneman's Color Atlas and Textbook of Diagnostic Microbiology. 6th Ed. Philadelphia: Lippincott Williams & Wilkins, 2006.)

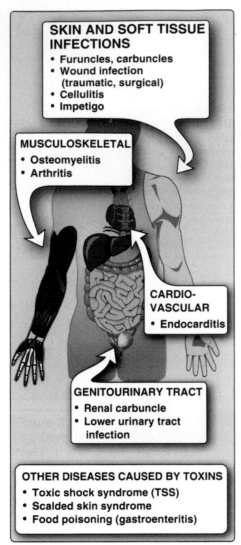

SKIN AND SOFT TISSUE INFECTIONS
- Furuncles, carbuncles
- Wound infection (traumatic, surgical)
- Cellulitis
- Impetigo

MUSCULOSKELETAL
- Osteomyelitis
- Arthritis

CARDIO-VASCULAR
- Endocarditis

GENITOURINARY TRACT
- Renal carbuncle
- Lower urinary tract infection

OTHER DISEASES CAUSED BY TOXINS
- Toxic shock syndrome (TSS)
- Scalded skin syndrome
- Food poisoning (gastroenteritis)

Figure 9-7. **Some of the diseases caused by *Staphylococcus aureus*.** (From Strohl WA, et al. Lippincott's Illustrated Reviews: Microbiology. Philadelphia: Lippincott Williams & Wilkins, 2001.)

involve *S. aureus*. It is a less common cause of pneumonia and urinary tract infections. *S. aureus* is one of the four most common causes of nosocomial infections, often causing postsurgical wound infections. **Nosocomial infections,** or hospital-acquired infections, are infections that patients develop as a result of being hospitalized; they are discussed in detail in Chapter 26. Diseases caused by *S. aureus* are summarized in Figure 9-7.

Virulence factors. Protein A is a major component of *S. aureus* cell walls. It is considered to be a virulence factor. Protein A binds to the Fc region of IgG molecules, preventing opsonization from occurring. In this manner, protein A has an antiphagocytic effect. Strains of *S. aureus* produce various exotoxins, including cytotoxins, exfoliative toxin (exfoliatin), and leukocidin. **Exfoliatin** causes a serious skin condition known as staphylococcal scalded skin syndrome.

Some strains of *S. aureus* produce Panton-Valentine toxin, which destroys leukocytes. Other strains produce toxic shock syndrome 1 (TSST-1) toxin, the cause of toxic shock syndrome (TSS). Although not the only cause of TSS, *S. aureus* is by far the most common. Some strains of *S. aureus* (those that produce an enterotoxin) are the cause of staphylococcal food poisoning, one of the most common types of food poisoning. Strains of *S. aureus* produce several exoenzymes, including protease, lipase, and hyaluronidase, which destroy tissues; hemolysins, which destroy red blood cells; coagulase, which causes clot formation; and **staphylokinase,** which dissolves clots. Figure 9-8 illustrates various virulence factors—toxins and exoenzymes—that are produced by *S. aureus*. A given strain of *S. aureus* would not be expected to produce all of these virulence factors.

Drug resistance. Virtually all strains of *S. aureus* produce penicillinase and are therefore penicillin resistant. Many strains are multidrug resistant. Strains known as methicillin-resistant *S. aureus* (MRSA) are resistant to most antibacterial agents. Drugs useful for treating most MRSA strains are vancomycin, linezolid (Zyvox), and quinupristin-dalfopristin (Synercid). Strains known as vancomycin-intermediate *S. aureus* or glycopeptide-intermediate *S. aureus* are resistant to commonly used dosages of vancomycin and other glycopeptide antibiotics but are killed by higher-than-usual doses. Strains of *S. aureus* that are completely resistant to vancomycin have been reported. They are called vancomycin-resistant *S. aureus*.

Clues to *S. aureus* Identification

Colonial morphology. All *Staphylococcus* spp. grow well on blood agar, producing abundant growth within 18 to 24 hours. *S. aureus* colonies are usually large (6 to 8 mm in diameter), smooth, entire, slightly raised, translucent, and pigmented (Fig. 9-9). Although *aureus* is from the Latin word for "golden," *S. aureus* colonies may be off-white, gray, cream-yellow, yellow, yellow-orange, or orange. As a result of several types of hemolysins produced by some strains of *S. aureus*, their colonies are often surrounded by multiple zones of hemolysis, resembling targets. Multiple zones of hemolysis serve as a clue that the organism is *S. aureus*. Small colony variants are pinpoint, nonhemolytic, and nonpigmented. As mentioned in Chapter 8, mannitol salt agar (MSA) plates are sometimes used to screen for *S. aureus* carriers—people whose nasal passages are colonized with *S. aureus*. As a result of mannitol fermentation, colonies of *S. aureus* growing on MSA will be yellow, and the normally pink medium will turn yellow.

Laboratory tests. *S. aureus* is a catalase-positive, Gram-positive coccus, usually arranged in clusters. The most common methods of identifying *S. aureus* are shown in Table 9-2.

Traditionally, the primary method used to identify *S. aureus* was the coagulase test. **Coagulase** is an enzyme that

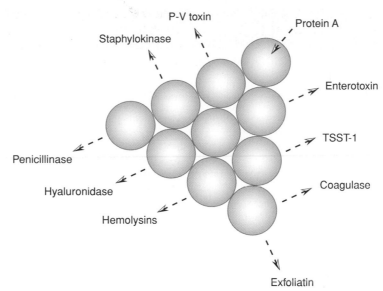

Figure 9-8. **Virulence factors of *Staphylococcus aureus*.** P-V, Panton-Valentine; TSST-1, toxic shock syndrome toxin 1.

causes the formation of clots. Specifically, coagulase catalyzes the conversion of a plasma protein called fibrinogen into a sticky substance called fibrin. *S. aureus* produces coagulase, whereas most other staphylococci isolated from clinical specimens do not. *Staphylococcus* spp. that do not produce coagulase are referred to as **coagulase-negative staphylococci (coagNS).** For reasons discussed later in the chapter, some clinical microbiology laboratories (CMLs) only speciate coagNS isolated from normally sterile body sites, such as blood, joint fluid, or cerebrospinal fluid.

> *S. aureus* is a catalase-positive, coagulase-positive, Gram-positive coccus, usually arranged in clusters.

Slide coagulase test. This rapid and easy-to-perform test detects what has been referred to as bound coagulase but is more correctly called clumping factor. Clumping factor is a protein located on the surface of *S. aureus* cells. It is capable of binding to fibrinogen but does not convert fibrinogen to fibrin. The reagent used in the slide test is rabbit plasma. Rabbit serum cannot be used in this test because serum lacks the clotting factors found in plasma, including fibrinogen.

To perform the slide coagulase test, a drop of sterile water is first placed on a microscope slide. Using a sterile inoculating loop, a colony of the organism to be tested is mixed into the drop of water, making a homogeneous suspension of the bacteria. Colonies should be obtained from media that do not contain high concentrations of salt. Salt

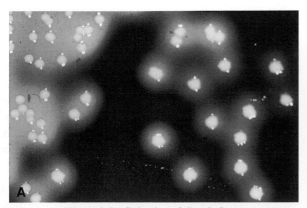
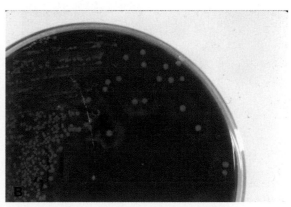

Figure 9-9. **Colonies of *Staphylococcus aureus*. A.** On sheep blood agar. **B.** Surrounded by multiple zone hemolysis. ([A] From Winn WC Jr, et al. Koneman's Color Atlas and Textbook of Diagnostic Microbiology. 6th Ed. Philadelphia: Lippincott Williams & Wilkins, 2006. [B] Courtesy of Dr. Thomas Huber.)

TABLE 9 - 2 Common Methods of Identifying *Staphylococcus aureus*

Method	Description/Example(s)[a]
Traditional slide coagulase test	Detects clumping factor (bound coagulase)
Traditional tube coagulase test	Detects staphylocoagulase (free coagulase)
Commercial hemagglutination assay that detects clumping factor	Example: BBL Staphyloslide (BD Biosciences; http://www.bdbiosciences.com/)
Commercial latex agglutination assays that detect both clumping factor and protein A	Examples: BACTiStaph (Remel; http://www.remelinc.com/); Pastorex Staph (Bio-Rad Laboratories; www.bio-rad.com); Prolex Staph Latex (Pro-Lab Diagnostics; http://www.pro-lab.com/); Staphaurex (Remel); Staphytect (Oxoid Inc.; http://www.oxoid.ca/)
Commercial latex agglutination assays that detect clumping factor, protein A, and *S. aureus* capsular antigens	Examples: Dryspot Staphytect Plus (Oxoid Inc.); Pastorex Staph-Plus (Bio-Rad Laboratories; www.bio-rad.com); Slidex Staph-Plus (bioMérieux Inc.; http://www.biomerieux.com/); Staphaurex Plus (Remel); Staphytect Plus (Oxoid Inc.)

[a]No attempt has been made to list all commercially available systems.
Source: Evangelista AT, et al. Rapid systems and instruments for the identification of bacteria. In: Manual of Commercial Methods in Clinical Microbiology. Washington, DC: ASM Press, 2002.

can cause false-positive reactions. A drop of rabbit plasma is then stirred into the bacterial suspension. The immediate formation of clumps of bacteria during the stirring process indicates a positive test result (Fig. 9-10). Clumping must occur within 10 seconds for the test result to be considered positive. A positive slide test result usually identifies the organism as *S. aureus*, but three other slide test-positive *Staphylococcus* spp.—*S. lugdunensis*, *S. schleiferi*, and some strains of *S. intermedius*—can be isolated from human clinical specimens. However, these three species are isolated less frequently than *S. aureus*. Although the absence of clumps represents a negative test result, 10% to 15% of

S. aureus strains do not produce clumping factor and are thus slide test negative. If *S. aureus* is suspected (e.g., when multiple zone hemolysis is observed) and the slide test is negative, the tube coagulase test may be performed.

Tube coagulase test. The tube coagulase test detects **staphylocoagulase,** which has also been referred to as free coagulase, meaning that the enzyme is *not* bound to the surface of the cells. The reagent used in the tube test is rabbit plasma. The tube test is more time consuming than the slide test.

To perform the tube test, a small amount of sterile rabbit plasma is first placed into a small test tube. Two drops of a broth culture of the organism to be tested are added to the rabbit plasma. The tube is then placed into a water bath at 35°C to 37°C. The tube is checked every 30 minutes for up to 4 hours to see if a clot has formed. Formation of a clot represents a positive test result (Fig. 9-11), and the organism has been identified as *S. aureus*. Some strains of staphylococci of animal origin—*S. intermedius* and *S. hyicus*—can also be tube test positive, but clot formation by these species may require 12 to 24 hours of incubation. If no clot has formed by the end of 4 hours, the test is considered negative, although a small number of strains require more than 4 hours for clot formation. For this reason, some CMLs routinely hold the tubes overnight and check them the next day. If no clot is produced, the report would state "coagulase-negative *Staphylococcus.*"

Question: Why check the tube every 30 minutes? Why not just come back after 4 hours to see if a clot has formed? *Answer:* In addition to producing staphylocoagulase, some

Figure 9-10. **Slide coagulase test.** A negative test result (no clumping of bacterial cells) is shown to the left, and a positive test result (clumping) is shown to the right. (From Winn WC Jr, et al. Koneman's Color Atlas and Textbook of Diagnostic Microbiology. 6th Ed. Philadelphia: Lippincott Williams & Wilkins, 2006.)

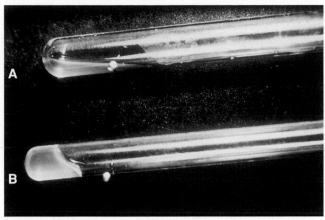

Figure 9-11. **Tube coagulase test. A.** Negative test result (no clot produced). **B.** Positive test result (a clot). (From Winn WC Jr, et al. Koneman's Color Atlas and Textbook of Diagnostic Microbiology. 6th Ed. Philadelphia: Lippincott Williams & Wilkins, 2006.)

strains of *S. aureus* produce **staphylokinase**—an enzyme that dissolves clots. If a CML professional were to wait 4 hours before checking for a clot and saw none, the test result would be called negative. However, a clot may have been produced earlier but dissolved. If that were the case, calling the test negative would represent a false-negative test result.

In most CMLs, *S. aureus* is identified by using one of the commercially available hemagglutination or latex agglutination assays (Table 9-2 and Fig. 9-12). Some hemagglutination products detect clumping factor, using sheep red blood cells that have been sensitized (coated) with fibrinogen. Some latex agglutination products detect both clumping factor and protein A, using latex particles sensitized with fibrinogen and IgG. Other latex agglutination products detect clumping factor, protein A, and *S. aureus* capsular

antigens, using latex particles sensitized with fibrinogen, IgG, and antibodies specific for *S. aureus* capsular antigens. These latter products are of value in identifying MRSA, some strains of which can mask clumping factor and protein A with their capsular antigens. With all these tests, clumping of the sheep red blood cell and bacteria mixture, or the latex particle and bacteria mixture, represents a positive test result. The technical term for clumping that results from the combination of either red blood cells plus bacteria or latex particles plus bacteria is **coagglutination.**

Clinical and Laboratory Standards (CLSI) Document M35-A (see "References and Suggested Reading") states that an isolate can be identified as *S. aureus* (with more than 95% likelihood) if it meets the following criteria:

• White to yellow, creamy, opaque colonies on blood agar

• GPC in clusters

• Catalase positive

• Conventional slide coagulase (clumping factor) test positive (two other staphylococci—*S. schleiferi* and *S. lugdunensis*—also yield positive slide coagulase test results, but such strains are expected to comprise fewer than 5% of all coagulase-positive clinical isolates) or tube coagulase test positive (neither *S. schleiferi* nor *S. lugdunensis* are tube test positive)

A large number of commercial biochemical- and enzyme-based systems are also available to identify *Staphylococcus* spp. and to differentiate *S. aureus* from other staphylococci (Table 9-3). Additionally, identification systems based on cellular fatty acid analysis are available, and molecular diagnostic procedures are being developed.

Essentials

Staphylococcus aureus

• Gram-positive cocci, usually arranged in grapelike clusters

• Catalase positive

• Coagulase positive

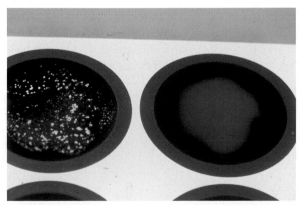

Figure 9-12. **Commercial latex agglutination test for identification of *Staphylococcus aureus*.** A positive test result (agglutination of the latex beads) is shown to the left and a negative test result (no agglutination) is shown to the right. The organism producing a positive test result would be identified as *S. aureus*. (From Winn WC Jr, et al. Koneman's Color Atlas and Textbook of Diagnostic Microbiology. 6th Ed. Philadelphia: Lippincott Williams & Wilkins, 2006.)

Coagulase-Negative Staphylococci

Coagulase-negative staphylococci are very commonly isolated from clinical specimens. **However, because many species of coagNS are members of the indigenous microflora, their isolation often represents contamination.** Some CMLs speciate coagNS only when there is good evidence that they are actually involved in an infectious process—for example, when they have been isolated from normally sterile sites (e.g., blood, joint fluid, cerebrospinal

TABLE 9 - 3   Commercial Systems for Identification of *Staphylococcus* spp.

Product[a]	Manufacturer	Also Useful for Identification of Gram-Positive Cocci Other Than Staphylococci
API RAPID Staph	bioMérieux Inc. (http://www.biomerieux.com/)	No
API Staph	bioMérieux Inc.	Yes
BBL Crystal Gram-Pos ID System	BD Biosciences (http://www.bdbiosciences.com/)	Yes
BBL Crystal Rapid Gram-Pos ID System	BD Biosciences	Yes
Biolog GP MicroPlate *Streptococcus* ID panels	Biolog Inc. (http://www.biolog.com/)	Yes
MicroScan Gram Pos ID panels	Dade Behring (http://www.dadebehring.com/)	Yes
MicroScan Rapid Gram Pos ID panels	Dade Behring	Yes
MIDI Sherlock	MIDI Inc. (http://www.midilabs.com/)	Yes
Phoenix Gram-Pos panel	BD Biosciences	Yes
Vitek GPI (Vitek 1)	bioMérieux Inc.	Yes
Vitek ID-GPC (Vitek 2)	bioMérieux Inc.	Yes

[a]No attempt has been made to list all commercially available systems.
Source: Evangelista AT, et al. Rapid systems and instruments for the identification of bacteria. In: Manual of Commercial Methods in Clinical Microbiology. Washington, DC: ASM Press, 2002.

fluid) or when they have been isolated repeatedly from a particular specimen type or site of infection. Some CMLs do not speciate coagNS at all. Four species of coagNS are described in this chapter. The names of additional species of coagNS can be found on the CD-ROM.

Staphylococcus epidermidis

Clinical significance. ***Staphylococcus epidermidis* is an opportunistic pathogen, as are the other coagNS that colonize the human body.** Virtually everyone has *S. epidermidis* as part of the indigenous microflora of their skin—thus, the specific epithet *epidermidis*, derived from *epidermis*. *S. epidermidis* is the most commonly isolated coagNS, and the coagNS most often involved in human infectious processes. *S. epidermidis* is the coagNS

> Coagulase-negative staphylococci, such as *Staphylococcus epidermidis*, are opportunistic pathogens.

most commonly associated with nosocomial infections and has been associated with bacteremia, endocarditis, postsurgical infections, urinary tract infections, infections associated with various types of prosthetic devices (e.g., artificial heart valves and joints), and intravascular catheter-associated infections. Some strains of *S. epidermidis* produce an exopolysaccharide slime layer that may enable these strains to adhere to the surface of plastics used in various prosthetic devices.

Drug resistance. Many strains of *S. epidermidis* are drug resistant. Strains called methicillin-resistant *S. epidermidis* are resistant to many antibiotics, including the penicillinase-resistant penicillins.

Clues to *S. epidermidis* Identification

Colonial morphology. Colonial morphology is of little value in identifying coagNS because their colonies usually cannot be distinguished from one another and quite often cannot be distinguished from colonies of *S. aureus*. At 24 hours, the typical coagNS colony is nonpigmented,

TABLE 9 - 4 Tests of Value in Differentiating *Staphylococcus lugdunensis* from *S. epidermidis*

Test	Results	
	S. lugdunensis	*S. epidermidis*
Ornithine decarboxylase test	Positive, usually within 8 hours of incubation	Negative after 8 hours of incubation; some strains give a delayed positive result
Pyrrolidonyl arylamidase (PYR) test	Positive	Negative

smooth, entire, glistening, slightly raised to convex, and opaque. *S. epidermidis* colonies are relatively small, ranging from 2.5 to 6 mm in diameter. Some strains produce delayed β-hemolysis, while other strains are nonhemolytic.

Laboratory tests. Like *S. aureus*, *S. epidermidis* is a catalase-positive, Gram-positive coccus, usually arranged in clusters. Unlike *S. aureus*, *S. epidermidis* is coagulase negative. It produces neither clumping factor nor staphylocoagulase. Commercial systems that can be used to identify *S. epidermidis* are listed in Table 9-3.

Staphylococcus haemolyticus

Clinical significance. *Staphylococcus haemolyticus* is the second most frequently encountered coagNS. It has been associated with opportunistic infections, including endocarditis, septicemia, peritonitis, and infections of the urinary tract, wounds, bones, and joints. Many strains of *S. haemolyticus* are multidrug resistant.

Clues to *S. haemolyticus* Identification

Colonial morphology. Colonies of *S. haemolyticus* are smooth, butyrous (butterlike), opaque, and 5 to 9 mm in diameter (larger than *S. epidermidis* colonies). Colonies may be nonpigmented or cream to yellow-orange.

Laboratory tests. Commercial systems that can be used to identify *S. haemolyticus* are listed in Table 9-3.

Staphylococcus lugdunensis

Clinical significance. *Staphylococcus lugdunensis* can cause endocarditis and has also been associated with arthritis, septicemia, and infections of the urinary tract, catheters, and prosthetic joints.

Clues to *S. lugdunensis* Identification

Colonial morphology. Colonies of *S. lugdunensis* are smooth, glossy, and 4 to 7 mm in diameter. Like colonies of

S. haemolyticus, they may be nonpigmented or cream to yellow-orange. Colonies have a flat edge and a slightly domed center.

Laboratory tests. Commercial systems that can be used to identify *S. lugdunensis* are listed in Table 9-3. Although *S. lugdunensis* is slide coagulase positive, the reaction is often delayed and is more likely to be observed when human plasma is used in place of rabbit plasma. *S. lugdunensis* can be differentiated from *S. aureus* by the tube coagulase test (*S. aureus* is positive; *S. lugdunensis* is negative). Tests of some value in differentiating *S. lugdunensis* from *S. epidermidis* are the ornithine decarboxylase test and the pyrrolidonyl arylamidase (PYR) test (Table 9-4).

> *Staphylococcus lugdunensis* can be differentiated from *S. aureus* using the tube coagulase test and from *S. epidermidis* using either the ornithine decarboxylase test or the PYR test.

Ornithine decarboxylase test. Ornithine is an amino acid. Ornithine decarboxylase is an enzyme that removes the carboxyl (acid) end of the ornithine molecule. (Decarboxylation is described in more detail in Chapter 12.) To perform the ornithine decarboxylase test, several colonies are inoculated into a tube of broth containing L-ornithine dihydrochloride. The tube contents are overlaid with sterile mineral oil, and the tube is incubated overnight at 35°C to 37°C. A change in the color of the broth, from a grayish or slightly yellowish color to violet, represents a positive test result. *S. lugdunensis* gives a positive result, often within 8 hours of incubation. A yellow color after 24 hours represents a negative test result. *S. epidermidis* gives a negative result. Yellowing of the broth is caused by glucose fermentation, whereas the violet color is a result of decarboxylation of ornithine.

PYR test. PYR stands for pyroglutamyl-β-naphthylamide. The PYR test detects the enzyme pyrrolidonyl arylamide (pyrrolidonase), which hydrolyzes PYR into L-pyrrolidone and β-naphthylamine. When β-naphthylamine combines with the PYR reagent, a red color is produced.

Several colonies are inoculated into a tube containing PYR broth, and the tube is incubated for 2 hours at 35°C. Following incubation, PYR reagent is added to the tube. Development of a red color within 2 minutes is a positive test result. *S. lugdunensis* gives a positive result. A yellow, orange, or pink color represents a negative test result. *S. epidermidis* gives a negative result. A 2-minute PYR disk test is also available.

Staphylococcus saprophyticus

Clinical significance. *Staphylococcus saprophyticus* is a common cause of urinary tract infections, sometimes progressing to septicemia, especially in young, sexually active female patients. Other infections with which *S. saprophyticus* has been associated are urethritis, prostatitis, and wound infections.

Clues to *S. saprophyticus* Identification

Colonial morphology. Colonies of *S. saprophyticus* are entire, very glossy, opaque, smooth, butyrous, and more convex than colonies of the previously described coagNS. Colonies are large (5 to 8 mm in diameter). About 50% of strains have pigmented colonies, ranging from cream to yellow-orange.

Laboratory tests. The **novobiocin resistance test** can be used to differentiate *S. saprophyticus* from most other *Staphylococcus* spp. A blood agar or Mueller-Hinton plate is inoculated with the unknown staphylococcus, in the manner described for disk diffusion antimicrobial susceptibility testing (see Chapter 7). A 5-μg novobiocin disk is gently pressed to the surface of the inoculated plate, and the plate is incubated overnight at 35°C to 37°C. A zone of no growth that is 16 mm or more in diameter indicates that the isolate is susceptible to novobiocin (Fig. 9-13). *S. saprophyticus* is resistant

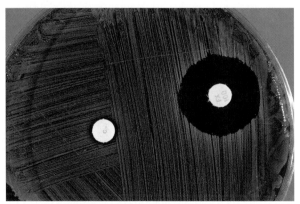

***Figure 9-13. Staphylococcus saprophyticus* on sheep blood agar.** The disk on the left contains novobiocin, to which *S. saprophyticus* is resistant. The yellow disk on the right contains furazolidone, to which *S. saprophyticus* (like other *Staphylococcus* spp.) is susceptible. (From Winn WC Jr, et al. Koneman's Color Atlas and Textbook of Diagnostic Microbiology. 6th Ed. Philadelphia: Lippincott Williams & Wilkins, 2006.)

to novobiocin, whereas *S. aureus*, *S. epidermidis*, *S. haemolyticus*, *S. lugdunensis*, and many (but not all) other coagNS are susceptible to novobiocin. Commercial systems that incorporate novobiocin and biochemical tests can be used to identify *S. saprophyticus*; some are listed in Table 9-3.

> The novobiocin resistance test can be used to differentiate *Staphylococcus saprophyticus* from most other *Staphylococcus* spp.

OTHER CATALASE-POSITIVE, GRAM-POSITIVE COCCI

In addition to *Staphylococcus* and *Micrococcus* spp., several other catalase-positive GPC may be recovered from clinical specimens. These include *Alloiococcus*, *Kocuria*, *Kytococcus*, and *Rothia* spp. These organisms are members of the indigenous microflora of the skin, mucosa, and oropharynx but can be opportunistic pathogens in immunocompromised patients. They are rare causes of septicemia, endocarditis, otitis media, endophthalmitis, central nervous system infections, pneumonia, and peritonitis. Some commercial minisystems are of value in identifying these organisms.

GENUS *STREPTOCOCCUS*

All *Streptococcus* spp. (streptococci) possess the following characteristics:

- GPC that are spherical or ovoid in shape, <2 μm in diameter, and arranged in chains (usually) and pairs

- Facultative anaerobes

- Nonmotile

- Non–spore forming

- Catalase negative (i.e., they do not produce the enzyme catalase)

Streptococcus spp. can be classified according to the type of hemolysis they produce. Recall from Chapter 8 that the type of hemolysis that an organism produces is determined by observing the

> Think of *Streptococcus* spp. as catalase-negative, Gram-positive cocci in pairs and chains.

zone(s) that surround colonies of the organism on a blood agar plate. Some species or strains of *Streptococcus* are α-hemolytic; their colonies are surrounded by a green zone. Some species or strains are α-prime hemolytic; their colonies are surrounded by two zones: an inner zone of no hemolysis and a wider outer zone of β-hemolysis. Some species or strains are β-hemolytic; their colonies are surrounded by a clear zone. Some species or strains are γ-hemolytic, causing neither α- nor β-hemolysis. The type of hemolysis that a particular *Streptococcus* isolate produces serves as a guide as to what other clues are needed to identify it.[1]

> The type of hemolysis that a *Streptococcus* sp. produces is a major clue to its identification.

Another method of classifying streptococci, primarily β-hemolytic streptococci, is based on research performed in the 1930s by Rebecca Lancefield. Streptococci can be placed into groups, referred to as Lancefield groups, based on the major cell wall carbohydrates they possess. Commercial agglutination kits are available for streptococcal grouping. At least 18 groups are recognized, designated groups A through H and K through T. Some groups (e.g., groups A and B) contain only one *Streptococcus* sp.; other groups contain more than one species; and some species of *Streptococcus* (e.g., *S. pneumoniae*) are not assigned to any group. Streptococci in groups A, B, C, and G are important pathogens, as are some small-colony streptococci and viridans group streptococci (described later in the chapter). Medically important streptococci once designated group D enterococci were reassigned to the genus *Enterococcus* (as discussed later in the chapter).

β-Hemolytic streptococci. Medically important β-hemolytic streptococci include isolates in groups A, B, C, and G. Within these four groups are strains known as large-colony (>0.5-mm diameter) formers and strains known as small-colony (<0.5-mm diameter) formers. The large-colony formers are known as **pyogenic** (pus-forming) streptococci. Although the term *group A streptococcus* has for many years been used synonymously with *Streptococcus pyogenes*, some strains of other β-hemolytic streptococci can also produce a positive reaction with group A–typing serum. Large-colony-forming, β-hemolytic group C and G streptococci are collectively referred to as *S. dysgalactiae* subsp. *equisimlis*. These organisms can cause many of the same types of infections as *S. pyogenes*, including pharyngitis. **Thus, it is important to remember that a large-colony-forming, β-hemolytic streptococcus isolated from a throat culture will not always turn out to be *S. pyogenes*.** In addition to pharyngitis, large-colony-forming, β-hemolytic streptococci in groups C and G can cause septicemia, endocarditis, meningitis, septic arthritis, and skin infections. β-Hemolytic group B streptococcus (*S. agalactiae*) is discussed later in this chapter.

Small-colony-forming, β-hemolytic group A, C, and G streptococci are members of the *Streptococcus milleri* or *Streptococcus anginosus* group, which consists of *S. anginosus*, *S. constellatus*, and *S. intermedius*. These organisms can be isolated from throat swabs as indigenous microflora

of the pharynx, but some small-colony-forming, β-hemolytic streptococci in group C (e.g., *S. constellatus* subsp. *pharyngitis*) can cause pharyngitis.

α-Hemolytic streptococci. The most clinically significant α-hemolytic streptococcus is *Streptococcus pneumoniae*. α-Hemolytic streptococci other than *S. pneumoniae* are called viridans group streptococci (VGS). VGS or oral streptococci are members of the indigenous microflora, which are occasionally involved in serious infections. *S. pneumoniae* and VGS are described later in the chapter.

> *Streptococcus pyogenes* is also known as group A strep, GAS, and strep A.

Streptococcus pyogenes

Streptococcus pyogenes is also known as group A strep, GAS, or strep A. It is the only *Streptococcus* sp. in group A, although, as mentioned previously, some strains of other β-hemolytic streptococci can also produce a positive reaction with group A–typing serum. *S. pyogenes* is a β-hemolytic, catalase-negative, Gram-positive coccus, usually arranged in chains (Fig. 9-14).

> *S. pyogenes* is a β-hemolytic, catalase-negative, Gram-positive coccus, usually arranged in chains.

STUDY AID **What's in a Name?** Let's examine the name *Streptococcus pyogenes*. Recall from Chapter 8 that the term *Streptococcus* refers to cocci in chains. *Pyo*- is from *pyon*, the Greek word for "pus." If an organism is pyogenic, it causes the formation of pus. Thus, *Streptococcus pyogenes* is a pyogenic bacterium that forms chains of cocci. *Pyogenes* is pronounced "pie-aah-gen-knees."

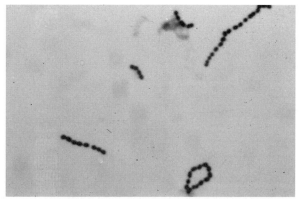

Figure 9-14. **Gram-stained *Streptococcus* sp. from a broth culture, showing typical chain formations.** (From Winn WC Jr, et al. Koneman's Color Atlas and Textbook of Diagnostic Microbiology. 6th Ed. Philadelphia: Lippincott Williams & Wilkins, 2006.)

---

[1]*Some authorities reserve the term β-hemolysis for descriptions of streptococci. Even though some bacteria other than streptococci are β-hemolytic, these authorities simply refer to the organisms as being hemolytic and/or refer to the hemolysis as complete hemolysis. If an organism is described merely as being hemolytic in subsequent chapters, assume that the organism is producing β-hemolysis. Also remember that the terms β-hemolysis and complete hemolysis are synonyms.*

Clinical significance. *S. pyogenes* is an important human pathogen, but it can also be found in low numbers as indigenous microflora of the upper respiratory tract. It is the primary cause of streptococcal pharyngitis (strep throat), and a common cause of skin infections (e.g., impetigo and erysipelas; see Chapter 18), cellulitis, and wound infections. Untreated strep throat or other *S. pyogenes* infections can lead to **sequelae** (complications) that include scarlet fever, toxic shock syndrome (TSS), rheumatic fever, rheumatoid arthritis, and glomerulonephritis (a kidney disease). Rheumatic fever is sometimes referred to as rheumatic heart disease because it induces myocarditis. Scarlet fever is caused by strains that produce erythrogenic toxin. Although some strains of *S. pyogenes* produce a toxin that causes a type of TSS, most cases of TSS are caused by *Staphylococcus aureus*. Some strains of *S. pyogenes*, referred to as flesh-eating bacteria, produce necrotizing enzymes that cause rapid and extensive destruction of tissue—a condition known as necrotizing fasciitis. Necrotizing fasciitis has a mortality rate of about 20% to 30%.

> *S. pyogenes* is a *very* important human pathogen. It is the major cause of strep throat, and some strains are the infamous flesh-eating bacteria.

> Scarlet fever is caused by *S. pyogenes* strains that produce erythrogenic toxin.

Virulence factors. *S. pyogenes* cells possess fibrillar structures on their surface that give them a "fuzzy" appearance in transmission electron micrographs. The fibrils are composed of lipoteichoic acid and M protein. M protein is thought to serve as a virulence factor in two ways: (1) by enabling *S. pyogenes* cells to adhere to surfaces and (2) by functioning as an antiphagocytic. *S. pyogenes* produces two types of β-hemolysins: streptolysin O (which is inactivated by oxygen) and streptolysin S (which is oxygen stable). The toxic shock disease caused by *S. pyogenes* is technically called toxic shock–like syndrome (TSLS) and is caused by a toxin that is similar to the TSST-1 produced by *S. aureus*. However, the TSLS toxin is different. It is called streptoccocal pyrogenic toxin (Spe). Some scientists think that the erythrogenic toxin that causes scarlet fever is a type of Spe.

S. pyogenes also produces hyaluronidase (spreading factor), two types of streptokinases, DNases, proteinases, peptidases, phosphatases, and a variety of other exoenzymes. Figure 9-15 illustrates various virulence factors (toxins and exoenzymes) that *S. pyogenes* produces. A given strain of *S. pyogenes* would not be expected to produce all these virulence factors.

> Although *Staphylococcus aureus* is the major cause of toxic shock syndrome, more than 100 new U.S. cases of TSLS were reported to the Centers for Disease Control and Prevention in 2004.

STUDY AID   What's in a Name? *Erythro-* means "red" and *-genic* means "to generate or produce." Thus, erythrogenic toxin is a toxin that produces redness, or more specifically, the red rash associated with scarlet fever. A way to remember the association between the toxin and the disease is that *erythro-* means "red," and scarlet is a shade of red.

Drug resistance. *S. pyogenes* has not developed resistance to penicillin, so penicillin remains the drug of choice to treat strep throat and most other *S. pyogenes* infections. Some strains have developed resistance to erythromycin and many strains are resistant to tetracycline.

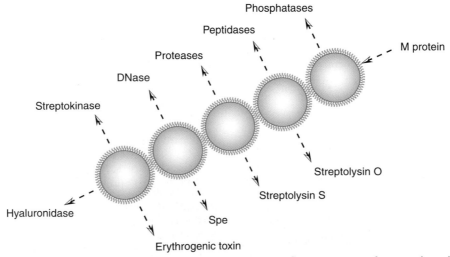

Figure 9-15. **Virulence factors of *Streptococcus pyogenes*.** Spe, streptoccocal pyrogenic toxin.

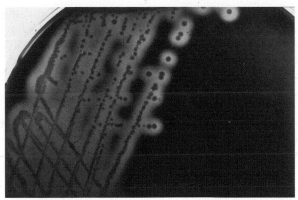

*Figure 9-16. **Streptococcus pyogenes** colonies on sheep blood agar.* (From Winn WC Jr, et al. Koneman's Color Atlas and Textbook of Diagnostic Microbiology. 6th Ed. Philadelphia: Lippincott Williams & Wilkins, 2006.)

Clues to *S. pyogenes* Identification

Colonial morphology. *S. pyogenes* is β-hemolytic. It produces a zone of β-hemolysis that is relatively wide compared with the size of the colonies (Fig. 9-16). Colonies of nonencapsulated or slightly encapsulated strains have an opaque, pearly gray appearance. Large, mucoid colonies of well-encapsulated strains of *S. pyogenes* are infrequently observed; on fresh isolation they resemble drops of oil on the surface of the blood agar plate. The colonies become dehydrated and roughened with age.

CML professionals should suspect *S. pyogenes* whenever a β-hemolytic *Streptococcus* sp. is isolated from a clinical specimen. However, some type of test must be performed to differentiate *S. pyogenes* from other β-hemolytic streptococci. Streptococcal typing sera are available for this purpose. Other tests are described next.

> *S. pyogenes* is β-hemolytic.

Laboratory tests. Various rapid group A antigen detection tests are available for the diagnosis of strep throat (Fig. 9-17). Usually, test results take only a few minutes. Although the specificity of these antigen detection tests is quite high, the sensitivity can be much lower; in other words, false-negative results occur. A throat culture should be performed whenever the antigen detection test result is negative.

The traditional method of differentiating *S. pyogenes* from other β-hemolytic *Streptococcus* spp. of human origin was the A-disk or bacitracin sensitivity test. A 0.04-U bacitracin disk is used, and any zone of inhibition of growth is considered a positive test result; that is, the organism is susceptible to bacitracin. *S. pyogenes* is bacitracin sensitive, meaning that it is killed by bacitracin. (The A in A-disk refers to group A strep.) Positive and negative A-disk test results are shown in Figure 9-18. Unfortunately, some β-hemolytic and groups B, C, and G streptococci are also bacitracin sensitive; they cause false-positive test results. Thus, the A-disk test has been largely replaced by other methods.

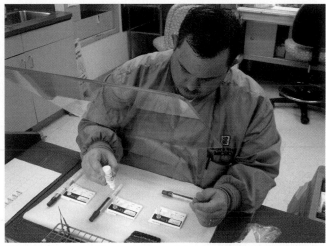

*Figure 9-17. **CML professional inoculating a rapid strep test.*** Shown here is the QuickVue Strep A test manufactured by Quidel, which provides results within 5 minutes. (Courtesy of Dr. Robert Fader.)

A better method of identifying *S. pyogenes* is the PYR test (previously described). *S. pyogenes* is PYR positive, as are most strains of *Enterococcus*. *Enterococcus* spp. (described later in this chapter) may be α- or β-hemolytic or nonhemolytic.

CLSI Document M35-A (see "References and Suggested Reading") states that an isolate can be identified as *S. pyogenes* (with more than 95% likelihood) if it meets the following criteria:

- GPC in chains (primarily) and pairs
- Catalase negative
- β-Hemolytic colonies; the zone of hemolysis has a clear-cut outer margin

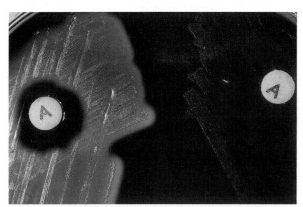

*Figure 9-18. **Bacitracin sensitivity test (also known as the A-disk test).*** *Streptococcus pyogenes*, to the left, is susceptible to bacitracin, whereas *Streptococcus agalactiae*, to the right, is resistant. (From Winn WC Jr, et al. Koneman's Color Atlas and Textbook of Diagnostic Microbiology. 6th Ed. Philadelphia: Lippincott Williams & Wilkins, 2006.)

- Colonies are usually dry, peaked, or convex, and >0.5 mm in diameter on sheep blood agar after 24 hours of incubation

- Positive PYR test result (β-hemolytic enterococci are also PYR positive, but colonies are large [>1.0 mm] and moist, and the zone of hemolysis has a softer, less clear-cut outer margin than *S. pyogenes*)

Definitive identification of *S. pyogenes* is usually made using commercially available streptococcal typing sera,

> *S. pyogenes* is PYR positive.

demonstrating that the organism is group A. Several commercial minisystems are also able to identify *S. pyogenes*, including API 20 Strep (bioMérieux Inc.; http://www.biomerieux.com/), Rapid ID 32 Strep (bioMérieux Inc.), and IDS RapID STR (Remel; http://www.remelinc.com/). In addition, nucleic acid probes are available from Gen-Probe Inc. (http://www.gen-probe.com/).

Essentials

Streptococcus pyogenes

- Also known as group A strep
- Gram-positive cocci, usually arranged in chains
- Catalase negative
- β-Hemolytic
- Bacitracin sensitive
- Identity is confirmed by using group A strep antiserum

Streptococcus agalactiae

Streptococcus agalactiae is also known as group B strep (GBS). It is the only *Streptococcus* sp. in group B. It is a catalase-negative, Gram-positive coccus, arranged in pairs and chains.

Clinical significance. *S. agalactiae* is one of the major causes of meningitis and septicemia among newborns. Neonates become infected during delivery through maternal genital tracts colonized by GBS. Adult *S. agalactiae* infections, such as septicemia, endocarditis, pneumonia, osteomyelitis, and skin and soft tissue infections, can also occur. Conditions that predispose adults to *S. agalactiae* infection are diabetes, cancer, and HIV infection.

> Another name for *Streptococcus agalactiae* is group B strep.

> *S. agalactiae* (group B strep) is a major cause of neonatal meningitis.

Virulence factors. Encapsulated strains of GBS are resistant to phagocytosis by white blood cells. Other potential virulence factors include hemolysin, CAMP factor, peptidase, and hyaluronidase.

Clues to *S. agalactiae* Identification

Colonial morphology. On blood agar, *S. agalactiae* produces gray-white colonies that are larger than colonies of other β-hemolytic streptococci. The zones of β-hemolysis surrounding *S. agalactiae* colonies have a soft outer margin and are narrower and less pronounced than the zones that surround other β-hemolytic streptococci. Some group B strains are nonhemolytic, or appear nonhemolytic until the colony is pushed aside using an inoculating loop.

Laboratory tests. Tests of value for presumptive identification of *S. agalactiae* include hippurate hydrolysis, bile-esculin hydrolysis, bacitracin sensitivity, and production of CAMP factor (Table 9-5). Specific group B antiserum is available for definitive identification of *S. agalactiae*.

Rapid hippurate hydrolysis test. This is a test to determine if the isolate produces the enzyme hippurate hydrolase

TABLE 9 - 5	Tests of Value for Identification of *Streptococcus agalactiae*	
Test	**Results**
Hydrolysis of sodium hippurate	99% of *S. agalactiae* strains are positive
Bile-esculin hydrolysis	99% to 100% of *S. agalactiae* strains are negative
Bacitracin sensitivity	>90% of *S. agalactiae* strains are resistant
Production of CAMP factor	>98% of *S. agalactiae* strains are positive

Source: Wessels MR, Kasper DL. Group B Streptococcus. In: Gorbach SL, Bartlett JG, Blacklow NR, eds. Infectious Disease. 3rd Ed. Philadelphia: Lippincott Williams & Wilkins, 2004.

(hippuricase). A turbid suspension of cells is prepared in 1% aqueous sodium hippurate and incubated for 2 hours at 35°C. Benzoic acid and glycine are produced if hippurate hydrolysis occurs. Glycine is detected by adding ninhydrin reagent and incubating for 10 minutes. Development of a deep bluish purple color, similar to the color of crystal violet, within 5 minutes is a positive reaction. *S. agalactiae* produces a positive test result. If the broth is colorless or contains only a faint tinge of purple, the test is considered negative.

Bile-esculin hydrolysis. Either a slant or a plate of bile-esculin medium is inoculated with several colonies and incubated for up to 48 hours at 35°C. Blackening of the medium, a result of esculin hydrolysis, is considered a positive test. *S. agalactiae* produces a negative test result.

> *S. agalactiae* is hippurate hydrolysis positive and bile-esculin hydrolysis negative.

Production of CAMP factor. The initials CAMP are taken from the last names of each of the three people who developed the original CAMP test: *C*hristie, *A*tkins, and *M*unch-*P*eterson. The CAMP factor is a diffusable extracellular protein that acts synergistically with staphylococcal β-lysin to cause enhanced lysis of red blood cells. A blood agar plate is inoculated by making perpendicular streaks of a β-lysin-producing strain of *Staphylococcus aureus* and the organism to be tested (Fig. 9-19). The streaks do not touch each other but are about 3 to 4 mm apart. Incubation is done overnight at 35°C. An arrowhead-shaped zone of enhanced hemolysis in the area into which both the β-lysin and the CAMP factor have diffused represents a positive test result (see Fig. 9-19).

> *S. agalactiae* is CAMP test positive.

S. agalactiae gives a positive test result. The term *enhanced hemolysis* refers to an area of more complete β-hemolysis than is produced by either the β-lysin or CAMP factor alone.

Rapid spot CAMP test. An alternative to the CAMP test just described is the rapid spot CAMP test. This test uses a spot CAMP reagent containing staphylococcal β-lysin. One drop of the reagent is placed beside a suspected GBS colony; the liquid may touch or cover the colony. The plate is incubated right-side-up in air for 20 minutes at 35°C. Using transmitted light, the plate is examined for an area of enhanced hemolysis next to the colony—that is, a zone of β-hemolysis more complete than zones of β-hemolysis surrounding untested colonies. A zone of enhanced hemolysis represents a positive test result. The plate can be reincubated for up to 30 minutes if the reaction is initially negative.

CLSI Document M35-A (see "References and Suggested Reading") states that an isolate can be identified as *S. agalactiae* (with more than 95% likelihood) if it meets the following criteria:

- GPC in pairs and chains
- Catalase negative

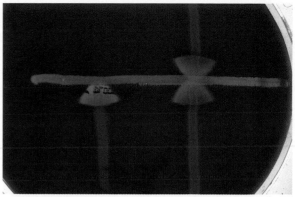

Figure 9-19. **Three positive CAMP test results.** The horizontal line is growth of a β-hemolytic *Staphylococcus aureus* strain. The three vertical lines represent growth of three isolates that were suspected of being *Streptococcus agalactiae*. The arrowhead-shaped zones of enhanced hemolysis at the junctures of the horizontal and vertical streaks are considered positive test results. Thus, all three isolates were identified as *S. agalactiae*. (From Winn WC Jr, et al. Koneman's Color Atlas and Textbook of Diagnostic Microbiology. 6th Ed. Philadelphia: Lippincott Williams & Wilkins, 2006.)

- Usually produces a narrow zone of β-hemolysis with a soft outer margin
- Either a positive rapid (2-to-4-hour) hippurate hydrolysis test result or a positive rapid (30-minute) spot test for CAMP factor (β-hemolytic enterococci may be hippurate positive, but they would be PYR positive; *S. agalactiae* is PYR negative); *S. agalactiae* also produces a positive result with group B strep typing serum

Essentials

Streptococcus agalactiae

- Also known as group B strep
- Gram-positive cocci, usually arranged in chains
- Catalase negative
- Usually produces a narrow zone of β-hemolysis with a soft outer margin
- Hippurate hydrolysis positive
- CAMP test positive
- Identity confirmed by using group B strep antiserum

Streptococcus pneumoniae

Streptococcus pneumoniae is also known as **pneumococcus (pl. *pneumococci*).** It is an encapsulated, α-hemolytic, catalase-negative, Gram-positive coccus that is usually arranged in pairs (diplococci; Fig. 9-20). **Note that this is an exception to the**

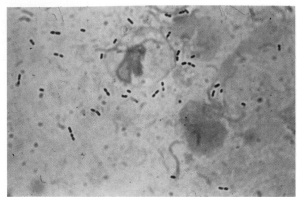

Figure 9-20. **Gram-stained smear of *Streptococcus pneumoniae* from a broth culture, showing the typical diplococcus arrangement.** A suggestion of a capsule (colorless halo) can be seen around some of the cells. (From Winn WC Jr, et al. Koneman's Color Atlas and Textbook of Diagnostic Microbiology. 6th Ed. Philadelphia: Lippincott Williams & Wilkins, 2006.)

> *Streptococcus pneumoniae* is a catalase-negative, α-hemolytic, encapsulated Gram-positive diplococcus.

general rule that streptococci are cocci arranged in chains. *S. pneumoniae* is a facultative anaerobe.

STUDY AID **What's in a Name?** Not surprisingly, bacteria having the specific epithet *pneumoniae* cause pneumonia. Examples are *Streptococcus pneumoniae*, *Klebsiella pneumoniae* (see Chapter 12), *Mycoplasma pneumoniae* (see Chapter 14), and *Chlamydophila pneumoniae* (see Chapter 16). It is important to keep in mind that these bacteria can cause other types of diseases as well.

Clinical significance. *S. pneumoniae* is an important human pathogen, but it can be found in low numbers as indigenous microflora of the upper respiratory tract. It is the most common cause of bacterial pneumonia in the world.[2]

> *Streptococcus pneumoniae* is a major cause of pneumonia, meningitis, and ear and sinus infections.

Virulence factors. *S. pneumoniae* possesses a thick polysaccharide capsule that serves an antiphagocytic function. Phagocytes are unable to attach to the capsule because they lack surface receptors that recognize the capsular polysaccharide material. Other proven or potential *S. pneumoniae* virulence factors are a cytotoxin called pneumolysin, which causes damage to cell membranes; a surface adhesin that enables *S. pneumoniae* cells to attach to tissue; a protease that may enable pneumococcal cells to escape being trapped by mucus; and production of hydrogen peroxide, which may damage tissue.

Drug resistance. The number of drug-resistant strains of *S. pneumoniae* has been steadily increasing, making it more difficult to treat pneumococcal infections. Many strains of *S. pneumoniae* are penicillin resistant. Some strains are also resistant to extended-spectrum cephalosporins, macrolides, clindamycin, fluoroquinolones, tetracyclines, chloramphenicol, trimethoprim-sulfamethoxazole, and aminoglycosides. An increasing number of strains are multidrug resistant. Because of the growth and resistance characteristics of *S. pneumoniae*, the disk diffusion method of antimicrobial susceptibility testing is not recommended. Commercial broth microdilution and Etest methods appear to be satisfactory for antimicrobial susceptibility testing of *S. pneumoniae*.

Clues to *S. pneumoniae* Identification

Colonial morphology. *S. pneumoniae* is α-hemolytic. Colonies may have depressed centers, giving them the appearance of a red blood cell,

> *S. pneumoniae* is α-hemolytic.

doughnut, nailhead, or life preserver (Fig. 9-21). Highly encapsulated strains often produce mucoid colonies.

Laboratory tests. The traditional method of differentiating *S. pneumoniae* from other α-hemolytic *Streptococcus* spp. of human origin is the P-disk (Optochin sensitivity) test. The *P* in *P-disk* stands for *pneumoniae*. In this test, an Optochin-impregnated paper disk is placed onto the surface of a blood agar plate that has previously been heavily inoculated with

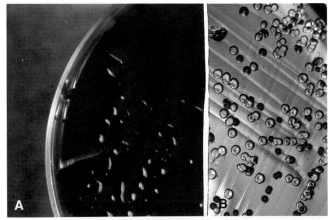

Figure 9-21. **Varied appearance of *S. pneumoniae* colonies. A.** Mucoid colonies. **B.** Colonies with collapsed centers. (From Winn WC Jr, et al. Koneman's Color Atlas and Textbook of Diagnostic Microbiology. 6th Ed. Philadelphia: Lippincott Williams & Wilkins, 2006.)

---

[2]*The pneumonia it causes is often referred to as* **pneumococcal pneumonia**. S. pneumoniae *is also a common cause of meningitis (especially in the elderly) and sinusitis and causes about one-third of the cases of otitis media (middle ear infection) in the United States.* S. pneumoniae *is a rare cause of endocarditis. Vaccines are available to prevent pneumococcal infections in children and the elderly. Although* S. pneumoniae *causes some cases of nosocomial pneumonia, it is not the major cause; members of the family Enterobacteriaceae,* Pseudomonas aeruginosa, *and* Staphylococcus aureus *are more frequent causes.*

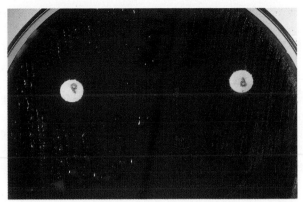

Figure 9-22. **Optochin sensitivity test (also known as the P-disk test).** *Streptococcus pneumoniae*, to the left, is susceptible to Optochin, whereas a different α-hemolytic *Streptococcus* species, to the right, is resistant. (From Winn WC Jr, et al. Koneman's Color Atlas and Textbook of Diagnostic Microbiology. 6th Ed. Philadelphia: Lippincott Williams & Wilkins, 2006.)

the isolate. Optochin is a chemical (ethyl hydrocupreine hydrochloride) that kills *S. pneumoniae* but does not kill other α-hemolytic streptococci. Following overnight incubation of the inoculated plate at 35°C in a CO_2 incubator, the plate is examined for a zone of no growth around the Optochin disk. If the zone of no growth is >14 mm (using a 6-mm-diameter disk) or >16 mm (using a 10-mm-diameter disk), the organism can be identified as *S. pneumoniae* (Fig. 9-22). If the isolate produces a smaller zone of no growth, then the isolate should be tested for bile solubility.

Bile solubility. Bile solubility can be tested using either a plate or tube method. In the plate method, a drop of either 2% or 10% bile reagent is placed onto a colony suspected of being *S. pneumoniae*. Bile will enhance an autocatalytic enzyme produced by *S. pneumoniae*, causing the colony to flatten. Flattening of the colony is considered a positive test result. In the tube method, a sufficient amount of suspect *S. pneumoniae* growth is transferred to a small tube containing 0.5 mL of the bile reagent, until the mixture becomes turbid. A decrease in turbidity after 5 to 15 minutes is considered a positive reaction.

Quellung test. Although rarely used in CMLs, the quellung test can also be used to identify *S. pneumoniae*. *Quellung* is German for "swelling." A drop of specimen or a loopful of broth culture is mixed with a loopful of omnivalent capsular antiserum containing antibodies directed against all *S. pneumoniae* capsular types. A loopful of methylene blue is then added to the mixture. After 10 minutes, a coverslip is added, and the preparation is examined microscopically. The antiserum visually enhances the capsule, making it appear larger, especially when the preparation is examined by phase contrast microscopy. Thus, encapsulated pneumococcal cells appear to be surrounded by a halo (see Fig. 2-6). The quellung test is used primarily for epidemiological purposes to determine if different *S. pneumoniae* isolates are the

same capsular type. Various antisera are available to determine specific capsular types.

A commercial latex agglutination test (Pneumoslide from BD Biosciences; http://www.bdbiosciences.com/) is also available for identification of *S. pneumoniae*. The Pneumoslide reagent is a suspension of latex beads coated (sensitized) with antipneumococcal antibodies. If agglutination occurs when an isolate suspected of being *S. pneumoniae* is mixed with a drop of the reagent, the organism has been identified as *S. pneumoniae*.

CLSI Document M35-A (see "References and Suggested Reading") states that an isolate can be presumptively identified as *S. pneumoniae* (with more than 95% likelihood) if it meets the following criteria:

- GPC, primarily in pairs, but also in short chains

- Catalase negative

- α-Hemolytic on blood agar

- Colonies are usually transparent, slightly mucoid, or flattened (resembling a checkers playing piece), not peaked

- Positive 2% or 10% bile solubility on the plate (some strains of *S. pneumoniae* may not be bile-soluble); although the CLSI document does not mention the Optochin test, Optochin susceptibility could be used in place of bile solubility, providing the organism satisfies the other criteria

> *S. pneumoniae* is bile soluble.

Essentials

Streptococcus pneumoniae

- Also known as pneumococcus

- Gram-positive cocci, usually arranged in pairs (diplococci)

- Catalase negative

- α-Hemolytic

- Optochin sensitive

Other *Streptococcus* Species

The term **viridans group streptococci (VGS)** refers to numerous α-hemolytic streptococci, including *S. anginosus*, *S. gordonii*, *S. intermedius*, *S. mitis*, *S. mutans*, *S. oralis*, *S. salivarius*, and *S. sobrinus*. Many taxonomic and nomenclature changes have occurred within this group in recent years.

VGS are common members of the indigenous microflora of the oral cavity, gastrointestinal tract, and female genital tract. Their presence in blood cultures often represents contamination, but they are the most common cause of subacute bacterial endocarditis, especially in patients with prosthetic heart valves or heart valves damaged by rheumatic heart disease. In addition to endocarditis, VGS have been associated with deep-seated liver and brain abscesses, and oral abscesses. *S. mutans* and *S. sobrinus* are often associated with dental caries and dental plaque.

VGS colonies are α-hemolytic and have a domed appearance, which differs significantly from colonies of *S. pneumoniae*. VGS are P-disk negative and are not bile soluble. Caution should be exercised when attempting to identify VGS using commercial minisystems because of the many name changes that have occurred in recent years and the large number of organisms in this category. Many CMLs identify VGS only when they are isolated from sterile sites, leukopenic patients, or patients with serious, life-threatening illnesses (e.g., endocarditis). Reference laboratories may use any of the following methods to identify members of the VGS: whole-cell-derived protein patterns by sodium dodecyl sulfate-polyacrylamide gel electrophoresis, pyrolysis mass spectrometry, monoclonal antibodies, and DNA-based methods.

Organisms previously known as *nutritionally variant streptococci* (NVS) have been reclassified as *Abiotrophia* and *Granulicatella* spp. They are members of the indigenous microflora of the oral cavity but have been associated with endocarditis, otitis media, and eye infections. Members of these two genera are Gram-positive coccobacilli. They are usually arranged in pairs and chains but may become pleomorphic and Gram variable when grown under less-than-optimal nutritional conditions. NVS will not grow on blood agar unless colonies of other bacteria or yeasts are present, in which case they form small satelliting colonies (colonies that surround colonies of other organisms; Fig. 9-23). NVS grow on or in chocolate agar, brucella agar containing 5% horse blood, thioglycolate broth, and routine blood agar that has

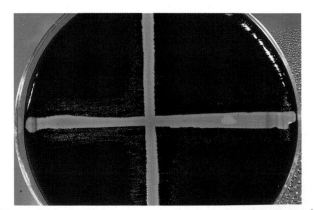

Figure 9-23. **Satelliting streptococci (also referred to as nutritionally variant streptococci).** Extremely small, shiny *Streptococcus* colonies can be seen growing in close proximity to the two grey *Staphylococcus* streaks on this sheep blood agar plate. Satelliting streptococci are currently classified in the genera *Abiotrophia* and *Granulicatella*.

been appropriately supplemented with nutrients that will support their growth. For example, if a pyridoxal disk is placed on a blood agar plate, NVS will grow around the disk.

GENUS *ENTEROCOCCUS*

Members of the genus *Enterococcus* are widespread in nature, including soil, water, and the bodies of animals. (Recall that the prefix *entero-* refers to the gastrointestinal tract.) Enterococci share the following common characteristics:

- Elongated or ovoid GPC, arranged in pairs or short chains
- Facultative anaerobes
- Optimum growth temperature is 35°C, but they can grow at 45°C
- Catalase negative
- Modified oxidase negative
- Can grow in a solution of 6.5% sodium chloride
- Bile-esculin positive
- PYR positive
- Cell walls of most strains possess Lancefield group D antigen

Their ability to grow in 6.5% sodium chloride, which is seven times the concentration found in normal tissue fluids, and their ability to grow in bile, make enterococci "mighty tough bugs."

Although more than a dozen *Enterococcus* spp. can be isolated from clinical specimens, two species—*E. faecalis* and *E. faecium*—are the most commonly isolated species. Of these two species, *E. faecalis* is isolated more frequently than *E. faecium*. Other *Enterococcus* spp. that may cause human infections and may be recovered from clinical specimens are *E. casseliflavus*, *E. raffinosus*, *E. avium*, *E. cecorum*, *E. dispar*, *E. durans*, *E. gallinarum*, *E. gilvus*, *E. hirae*, *E. mundtii*, and *E. pallens*.

Clinical significance. In humans, enterococci are opportunistic pathogens that commonly inhabit the gastrointestinal tract and, less commonly, the genitourinary tract and oral cavity. They are common causes of nosocomial infections, primarily causing disease in elderly debilitated patients, immunocompromised patients, and patients who have been hospitalized for extended periods, have implanted prosthetic devices, and/or have received prolonged antimicrobial therapy. The most common types of nosocomial infections that enterococci cause are urinary tract infections, postsurgical wound infections, endocarditis, and septicemia.

Drug resistance. Enterococci are resistant to many commonly used antimicrobial agents and some strains are multidrug resistant. All enterococci are naturally resistant to aminoglycoside and cephalosporin antibiotics; this is referred to as intrinsic resistance. Many enterococcal strains have also acquired resistance to other drugs—in some cases, to many other drugs. Antimicrobial susceptibility testing is very important for enterococci. So too is species identification, because certain *Enterococcus* spp. are more likely to be multidrug resistant than others. For example, ampicillin and vancomycin resistance is more common in *E. faecium* than in *E. faecalis* and other enterococci. Especially troublesome enterococcal strains are the vancomycin-resistant enterococci, which are resistant not only to vancomycin but also to a wide range of other antimicrobial agents. The CLSI publishes standards for performing antimicrobial susceptibility testing on enterococci and for interpreting test results.

> Infections with multidrug-resistant *Enterococcus* strains, known as vancomycin-resistant enterococci, are especially difficult to treat.

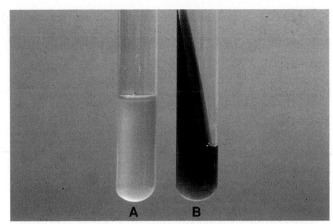

Figure 9-24. **Tests of value in identifying *Enterococcus* spp. A.** Growth in a broth containing 6.5% sodium chloride. Enterococci will grow in this concentration of sodium chloride, but group D streptococci will not. **B.** Positive bile-esculin reaction. Blackening of the inoculated slant indicates that esculin has been hydrolyzed to esculetin. Enterococci and group D streptococci are bile-esculin positive. (From Winn WC Jr, et al. Koneman's Color Atlas and Textbook of Diagnostic Microbiology. 6th Ed. Philadelphia: Lippincott Williams & Wilkins, 2006.)

Clues to *Enterococcus* spp. Identification

Colonial morphology. Most blood-containing media will support growth of enterococci, which form small, gray colonies after 24 hours of incubation at 35°C. Although some strains of *E. faecalis* and *E. durans* are β-hemolytic on certain types of blood-containing solid media, most enterococci are α-hemolytic or nonhemolytic. Various selective media are available for isolation of enterococci, including vancomycin-resistant strains. Although enterococci do not require CO_2 for growth in the laboratory, their growth is stimulated by increased concentrations of CO_2.

Laboratory tests. CLSI Document M35-A (see "References and Suggested Reading") states that an isolate can be presumptively identified as an *Enterococcus* sp. (with more than 95% likelihood) if it meets the following criteria:

> *Enterococcus* spp. are PYR positive and bile-esculin positive, and grow in a broth containing 6.5% NaCl.

- GPC or coccobacilli in pairs and chains
- Non-β-hemolytic colonies that are >1 mm in diameter
- Catalase negative
- PYR positive (enterococci are also bile-esculin positive and will grow in a broth containing 6.5% NaCl; Fig. 9-24)

Several commercial systems are available for identifying and differentiating *Enterococcus* spp.; some are listed in Table 9-6. Most enterococcal strains can be identified as an *Enterococcus* using the AccuProbe *Enterococcus* genetic probe (Gen-Probe Inc.; http://www.gen-probe.com/). Various molecular methods are available for typing *Enterococcus* strains for epidemiological purposes—for example, when tracking down the source of an *Enterococcus* outbreak within the hospital. These methods include pulsed-field gel electrophoresis, multilocus enzyme electrophoresis, and PCR-based typing methods.

Essentials

Enterococcus spp.

- Gram-positive cocci or coccobacilli in pairs and chains
- Catalase negative
- Usually α-hemolytic or nonhemolytic
- PYR positive
- Bile-esculin positive
- Will grow in 6.5% NaCl

OTHER CATALASE-NEGATIVE, GRAM-POSITIVE COCCI

Numerous less commonly isolated catalase-negative GPC can be mistaken for streptococci or enterococci. They represent a taxonomically diverse group, and the nomenclature of these organisms changes frequently. Most often, they are opportunistic agents of infections in compromised hosts. Infections with these organisms tend to occur primarily in patients with previously damaged tissues (e.g., heart valves),

TABLE 9 - 6   Commercial Systems for Identification of *Enterococcus* spp.

System	Manufacturer
API 20S system	bioMérieux Inc. (http://www.biomerieux.com/)
API Rapid ID32 STREP system	bioMérieux Inc.
Crystal Gram-Positive system	BD Biosciences (http://www.bdbiosciences.com/)
Crystal Rapid Gram-Positive system	BD Biosciences
Vitek Gram-Positive Identification Card	bioMérieux Inc.
Microscan Walk/Away Gram-Positive Identification Panel	Dade Behring (http://www.dedebehring.com/)

prolonged hospitalization, antibiotic treatment, invasive procedures, and the presence of foreign bodies. Some of the organisms within this group and diseases associated with these organisms are shown in Table 9-7.

IDENTIFICATION OF AN UNKNOWN GRAM-POSITIVE COCCUS

The first steps in identifying an unknown Gram-positive coccus are to determine its Gram-stained appearance and its catalase reaction. GPC fall into two categories, based on their catalase reaction and the morphologic arrange-

ment of their cells. GPC in category 1 are catalase negative, and their cells are arranged either in pairs or chains. GPC in category 2 are either catalase positive or catalase negative, and their cells are arranged either in clusters or irregular groups. As shown in Table 9-8, category 1 organisms include *Streptococcus* and *Enterococcus* spp., and category 2 organisms include *Staphylococcus* and *Micrococcus* spp.

The LAP test. The LAP test detects the presence of the enzyme leucine aminopeptidase (LAP). Rapid LAP disk tests are available from several manufacturers. In the presence of LAP, leucine-α-naphthylamide is hydrolyzed to leucine and free α-naphthylamine. Adding para-dimethylaminocinnamaldehyde (DMACA) reagent produces a red color. Thus, a red color represents a positive test result

TABLE 9 - 7   Infrequently Isolated Catalase-Negative, Gram-Positive Cocci

Genus/Genera	Possible Types of Infections Caused by Members of the Genus/Genera
Abiotrophia and *Granulicatella*	Endocarditis, ophthalmic infections, otitis media, brain abscess, meningitis
Aerococcus	Endocarditis, septicemia, UTI
Gemella	Endocarditis, meningitis, empyema, lung abscess, osteomyelitis, wound infections
Globicatella	Septicemia, UTI, meningitis
Helococcus	Wound infections, sebaceous cyst, breast abscess
Lactococcus	Endocarditis, septicemia, osteomyelitis
Leuconostoc	Neonatal septicemia, wound infections
Vagococcus	Wound infections

UTI, urinary tract infection.

Source: Ruoff KL. *Aerococcus, Abiotrophia,* and other infrequently isolated aerobic catalase-negative, Gram-positive cocci. In: Murray PR, Baron EJ, Jorgensen JH, Pfaller MA, Yolken RH, eds. Manual of Clinical Microbiology. 8th Ed. Washington, DC: ASM Press, 2003.

TABLE 9 - 8   Tests of Value for Identification of an Unknown Gram-Positive Coccus

GPC Category	Genus/Genera	Test Results
1	Streptococcus	Catalase negative, PYR negative (except for S. pyogenes), LAP positive, no growth in 6.5% NaCl, no growth at 10°C
	Enterococcus	Catalase negative, PYR positive, LAP positive, growth in 6.5% NaCl, BE positive, motility-variable, growth at 45°C
	Abiotrophia and Granulicatella	Catalase negative, PYR positive, LAP positive, no growth in 6.5% NaCl, BE negative, will produce a zone of growth around a pyridoxal disk placed on a blood agar plate
	Gemella	Catalase negative, PYR positive, LAP positive, no growth in 6.5% NaCl, BE negative
	Globicatella	Catalase negative, PYR positive, LAP negative, growth in 6.5% NaCl
	Lactococcus	Catalase negative, PYR-variable, LAP positive, 6.5% NaCl-variable, BE positive, motility negative, growth at 10°C
	Leuconostoc	Catalase negative, PYR negative, LAP negative
	Vagococcus	Catalase negative, PYR positive, LAP positive, 6.5% NaCl-variable, BE positive, motile, no growth at 45°C
2	Staphylococcus	Catalase positive, oxidase negative, resistant to bacitracin (0.04-U disk), susceptible to furazolidone, growth in 5% NaCl
	Micrococcus	Catalase positive, obligate aerobe, oxidase positive, susceptible to bacitracin (0.04-U disk), resistant to furazolidone, growth in 5% NaCl
	Aerococcus	Catalase negative, PYR-variable, LAP-variable
	Alloiococcus	Catalase positive, obligate aerobe, oxidase negative, growth in 6.5% NaCl
	Helococcus	Catalase negative, PYR positive, LAP negative, gamma hemolytic
	Rothia mucilaginosa	Catalase-variable, oxidase negative, PYR positive, LAP positive, no growth in 5% NaCl, ESC positive

BE, bile-esculin test; ESC, esculin hydrolysis; LAP, leucine aminopeptidase test; NaCl, sodium chloride; PYR, pyrrolidonyl arylamidase test.

(LAP positive). A pink color is a weakly positive test result, and a yellow color is a negative test result. All *Streptococcus* and *Enterococcus* spp. are LAP positive. Some less frequently isolated streptococcus-like Gram-positive cocci are LAP positive (e.g., *Lactococcus, Pediococcus, Alloiococcus, Vagococcus* spp.), whereas others (e.g., *Globicatella, Dolosicoccus, Helococcus, Aerococcus, Leuconostoc* spp.) are LAP negative. *S. pyogenes* is PYR positive and LAP positive.

In addition to the tests listed in Table 9-8, several commercial systems are available for identifying both category 1 and category 2 GPC.

Figures 9-25 through 9-27 are flowcharts that can be used in a teaching laboratory to identify commonly isolated GPC unknowns.

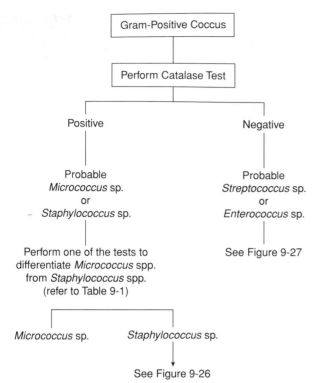

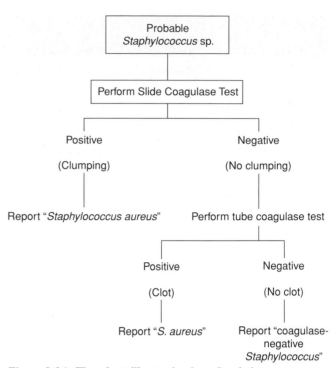

Figure 9-25. **Flowchart illustrating how *Micrococcus*, *Staphylococcus*, *Streptococcus*, and *Enterococcus* may be differentiated.** This oversimplified flowchart does not take into consideration the many other catalase-positive and catalase-negative cocci that can be isolated from clinical specimens. Thus, while useful for teaching, this flowchart should not be used in an actual clinical microbiology laboratory.

Figure 9-26. **Flowchart illustrating how *Staphylococcus aureus* can be differentiated from coagulase-negative staphylococci.** This oversimplified flowchart is for teaching purposes only and should not be used in an actual clinical microbiology laboratory.

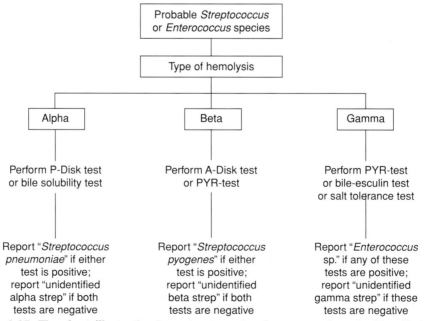

Figure 9-27. **Flowchart illustrating how streptococci and enterococci can be identified.** This oversimplified flowchart is for teaching purposes only and should not be used in an actual clinical microbiology laboratory.

Chapter Review

- The three most clinically significant genera of facultatively anaerobic Gram-positive cocci are *Staphylococcus*, *Streptococcus*, and *Enterococcus*.

- Morphologically, *Staphylococcus* spp. are Gram-positive cocci found singly, in pairs, or in grapelike clusters. Staphylococci are facultative anaerobes, nonmotile, non–spore forming, nonencapsulated (usually), and catalase positive.

- Catalase is an enzyme that removes potentially harmful hydrogen peroxide from the environment by catalyzing its breakdown into water and oxygen. Some bacteria are capable of producing catalase, whereas others are not. As a general rule, *Staphylococcus* and *Micrococcus* spp. are catalase positive, whereas *Streptococcus* and *Enterococcus* spp. are catalase negative.

- Staphylococci are resistant to bacitracin, whereas micrococci are susceptible to bacitracin.

- Oxidase is an abbreviated name for cytochrome oxidase, an enzyme that participates in the electron transport chain.

- *Micrococcus* spp. are aerobic and modified oxidase positive, whereas *Staphylococcus* spp. are facultative anaerobes and modified oxidase negative.

- *Staphylococcus aureus* is a very important pathogen. It causes many infections, including skin, soft tissue, respiratory, bone, joint, and wound infections. It also causes pimples, boils, carbuncles, styes, and toxic shock syndrome.

- *S. aureus* produces various virulence factors, including toxins and exoenzymes.

- Virtually all strains of *S. aureus* produce penicillinase and therefore are penicillin resistant. There are also methicillin-resistant strains of *S. aureus*, vancomycin-resistant strains, and vancomycin-intermediate strains.

- All *Staphylococcus* spp. grow well on blood agar. *S. aureus* usually produces large, slightly raised, translucent, β-hemolytic, cream-colored colonies.

- Of the five most commonly isolated *Staphylococcus* spp., only *S. aureus* produces the enzyme coagulase.

- Coagulase is an enzyme that causes the formation of clots. It catalyzes the conversion of fibrinogen to fibrin.

- The slide coagulase test detects clumping factor, or cell-bound coagulase, and the tube coagulase test detects staphylocoagulase, or free coagulase.

- Coagulase-negative staphylococci are members of the indigenous microflora. They include *S. epider-*midis, *S. haemolyticus, S. lugdunensis,* and *S. saprophyticus.*

- Streptococci are Gram-positive cocci, either spherical or ovoid in shape. They are facultative anaerobes, nonmotile, and non–spore forming. They do not produce the enzyme catalase; *i.e.*, they are catalase negative.

- Streptococci may be grouped according to their major cell wall carbohydrates or the type of hemolysis they produce. Streptococcal groups based on cell wall carbohydrates range from A to T. Hemolysis categories are α-, β-, or γ-hemolysis.

- *Streptococcus pyogenes* is a clinically significant β-hemolytic group A streptococcus. Microscopically, *S. pyogenes* usually appears in chains.

- The A-disk test or bacitracin sensitivity test can be used to distinguish *S. pyogenes* from most other β-hemolytic *Streptococcus* spp. *S. pyogenes* is bacitracin-sensitive.

- CAMP factor is a diffusable, extracellular protein that acts in concert with staphylococcal β-lysin to cause enhanced lysis of red blood cells. *S. agalactiae* gives a positive CAMP test result.

- *S. pneumoniae* is an opportunistic pathogen and a frequent cause of bacterial pneumonia, meningitis, sinusitis, and middle ear infections (otitis media). It possesses a polysaccharide capsule that serves an antiphagocytic function.

- The P-disk or Optochin sensitivity test may be used to distinguish *S. pneumoniae* from other α-hemolytic *Streptococcus* spp.

- Viridans group streptococci are α-hemolytic streptococci that are common members of the indigenous microflora of the oral cavity, gastrointestinal tract, and female genital tract.

- *Enterococcus* spp. are Gram-positive cocci or coccobacilli in pairs and chains. They are usually α- or γ-hemolytic, catalase negative, and PYR positive. They are opportunistic pathogens that commonly inhabit the gastrointestinal tract, and are common causes of nosocomial infections.

New Terms and Abbreviations

After studying Chapter 9, you should be familiar with the following terms, which are defined within the chapter and in the Glossary at the back of the book:

Catalase

Clumping factor

Coagglutination

Coagulase

Coagulase-negative staphylococci (coagNS)

Exfoliatin

Nosocomial infection

Oxidase

Pneumococcal pneumonia

Pneumococcus (pl. pneumococci)

Pyogenic

Sequela (pl. sequelae)

Staphylocoagulase

Staphylokinase

Viridans group streptococci (VGS)

References and Suggested Reading

Abbreviated Identification of Bacteria and Yeast: Approved Guideline. CLSI Document M35-A. Wayne, PA: Clinical and Laboratory Standards Institute, 2002.

Austrian R. *Streptococcus pneumoniae*. In: Gorbach SL, Bartlett JG, Blacklow NR, eds. Infectious Disease. 3rd Ed. Philadelphia: Lippincott Williams & Wilkins, 2004.

Bannerman TL. *Staphylococcus, Micrococcus*, and other catalase-positive cocci that grow aerobically. In: Murray PR, Baron EJ, Jorgensen JH, Pfaller MA, Yolken RH, eds. Manual of Clinical Microbiology. 8th Ed. Washington, DC: ASM Press, 2003.

Boone DR, Castenholz RW, eds. The Archaea and the Deeply Branching and Phototrophic Bacteria. New York: Springer-Verlag, 2001. Garrity GM, ed. Bergey's Manual of Systematic Bacteriology, vol 1. 2nd Ed.

Evangelista AT, et al. Rapid systems and instruments for the identification of bacteria. In: Manual of Commercial Methods in Clinical Microbiology. Washington, DC: ASM Press, 2002.

Murray BE, Bartlett JG. Enterococci. In: Gorbach SL, Bartlett JG, Blacklow NR, eds. Infectious Disease. 3rd Ed. Philadelphia: Lippincott Williams & Wilkins, 2004.

Ruoff KL. *Aerococcus, Abiotrophia*, and other infrequently isolated aerobic catalase-negative, Gram-positive cocci. In: Murray PR, Baron EJ, Jorgensen JH, Pfaller MA, Yolken RH, eds. Manual of Clinical Microbiology. 8th Ed. Washington, DC: ASM Press, 2003.

Ruoff KL. Algorithm for identification of aerobic Gram-positive cocci. In: Murray PR, Baron EJ, Jorgensen JH, Pfaller MA, Yolken RH, eds. Manual of Clinical Microbiology. 8th Ed. Washington, DC: ASM Press, 2003.

Ruoff KL, Whiley RA, Beighton D. *Streptococcus*. In: Manual of Commercial Methods in Clinical Microbiology. Washington, DC: ASM Press, 2002.

Sheagren JN, Schaberg DR. Staphylococci. In: Gorbach SL, Bartlett JG, Blacklow NR, eds. Infectious Disease. 3rd Ed. Philadelphia: Lippincott Williams & Wilkins, 2004.

Stollerman GH. *Streptococcus pyogenes* (group A streptococci). In: Gorbach SL, Bartlett JG, Blacklow NR, eds. Infectious Disease. 3rd Ed. Philadelphia: Lippincott Williams & Wilkins, 2004.

Teixeira LM, Facklam RR. *Enterococcus*. In: Murray PR, Baron EJ, Jorgensen JH, Pfaller MA, Yolken RH, eds. Manual of Clinical Microbiology. 8th Ed. Washington, DC: ASM Press, 2003.

Wessels MR, Kasper DL. Group B *Streptococcus*. In: Gorbach SL, Bartlett JG, Blacklow NR, eds. Infectious Disease. 3rd Ed. Philadelphia: Lippincott Williams & Wilkins, 2004.

 # On the CD-ROM

- A Closer Look at Coagulase-Negative Staphylococci
- A Closer Look at Streptococci
- Additional Self-Assessment Exercises
- Case Study
- Puzzle

Self-Assessment Exercises

Match the disease with the most appropriate pathogenic organism(s).

1. _____ Endocarditis

2. _____ Otitis media

3. _____ Scalded skin syndrome

4. _____ Neonatal meningitis

5. _____ Strep throat

A. Group B streptococci

B. *Staphylococcus aureus*

C. *Streptococcus pneumoniae*

D. *Streptococcus pyogenes*

E. Viridans group streptococci

6. To which Lancefield group does *Streptococcus pyogenes* belong?

    A. Group A

    B. Group B

    C. Group C

    D. None of the above

7. Which of the following organisms is catalase negative?

    A. *Staphylococcus epidermidis*

    B. *Streptococcus pyogenes*

    C. *Micrococcus luteus*

    D. *Staphylococcus aureus*

8. True or false: The tube coagulase test detects free coagulase.

9. True or false: All *Staphylococcus* spp. are coagulase positive.

10. True or false: A catalase-negative, β-hemolytic, Gram-positive coccus that is sensitive to bacitracin may be presumptively identified as group A streptococcus.

CHAPTER 10

Gram-Positive and Acid-Fast Bacilli

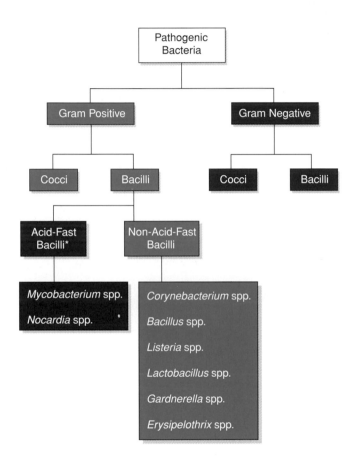

 Pathogenic Bacteria → Gram Positive / Gram Negative; Gram Positive → Cocci / Bacilli; Gram Negative → Cocci / Bacilli; Bacilli → Acid-Fast Bacilli* / Non-Acid-Fast Bacilli; Acid-Fast Bacilli*: *Mycobacterium* spp., *Nocardia* spp.; Non-Acid-Fast Bacilli: *Corynebacterium* spp., *Bacillus* spp., *Listeria* spp., *Lactobacillus* spp., *Gardnerella* spp., *Erysipelothrix* spp.

LEARNING OBJECTIVES

After studying this chapter, you should be able to:

☛ Define the terms introduced in this chapter (e.g., *acid-fast bacteria, bacteriophage, coryneform bacteria*)

☛ Identify three clinically significant species of mycolic acid-containing actinomycetes

☛ Compare and contrast the Gram-stain reaction and microscopic appearance of the aerobic actinomycetes, *Corynebacterium* spp., *Mycobacterium* spp., *Bacillus* spp., *Listeria* spp., *Lactobacillus* spp., and *Erysipelothrix* spp.

☛ Describe the pathogenesis of the following diseases: diphtheria, tuberculosis, anthrax, listeriosis, erysipeloid; describe the causative organism, mode of entry, type of illness (i.e., respiratory, cutaneous, systemic), and clinical manifestations of each

☛ Discuss the three types/forms of anthrax; describe the mode of entry and clinical signs and symptoms

☛ Describe what is meant by the terms *coryneform* and *diphtheroids*

☛ Explain why all strains of *Corynebacteria diphtheriae* do not produce the diphtheria toxin; address the topic of bacteriophages

☛ Describe the colonial and cellular morphology of the following: *Nocardia* spp., *Corynebacteria diphtheriae*, *Mycobacterium tuberculosis, M. leprae, Bacillus anthracis, B. cereus, Listeria monocytogenes,* and *Erysipelothrix rhusiopathiae*

☛ Identify the types of specimens and media routinely used to isolate the following organisms: *Nocardia* spp., *Corynebacterium diphtheriae, Mycobacterium tuberculosis, Bacillus anthracis, B. cereus, Listeria monocytogenes,* and *Erysipelothrix rhusiopathiae*

☛ List the observations and primary tests used to presumptively or definitively identify the following organisms: *Mycobacterium tuberculosis, M. leprae, Bacillus anthracis, B. cereus, Listeria monocytogenes,* and *Erysipelothrix rhusiopathiae*

☛ Given the pigmentation characteristics of a *Mycobacterium* species, classify it as a photochromogen, scotochromogen, or nonphotochromogen

☛ Identify the five species in the *Mycobacterium tuberculosis* complex

☛ Briefly outline the steps in the Ziehl-Neelsen and Kinyoun acid-fast staining procedures; describe the purpose of each step and/or reagent

☛ Discuss the clinical significance of tuberculosis, including the public health threat, specific species involved, modes of entry, and clinical signs and symptoms

☛ Given a Kinyoun- or Ziehl-Neelsen-stained slide, interpret the results

☛ Describe each of the following, including the name of the appropriate organism(s): funguslike bacteria, weakly acid-fast and partially acid-fast bacteria, "tumbling" motility, "umbrella" growth pattern, "pipe cleaner" growth pattern, serpentine cording, and cold enrichment

☛ Given the name of a specific infectious disease (e.g., diphtheria), state the name of the Gram-positive bacillus or acid-fast bacillus that causes the disease

☛ Given a series of test results from the clinical microbiology laboratory, identify the most likely Gram-positive bacillus

Anthrax. Diphtheria. Leprosy. Listeria food poisoning. Tuberculosis. These are some of the diseases that are caused by the Gram-positive and acid-fast bacilli described in this chapter.

Many Gram-positive bacilli can be involved in human infections, some of which are aerobes, some of which are facultative anaerobes, and some of which are obligate anaerobes. Several clinically significant aerobic Gram-positive bacilli are discussed in this chapter; others are discussed on the CD-ROM. Also defined and discussed in this chapter are acid-fast bacilli. Anaerobic Gram-positive bacilli are described in Chapter 17. *Actinomyces* spp., which may be microaerophilic, facultatively anaerobic, or obligately anaerobic, are also described in Chapter 17.

Collectively, the bacteria described in this chapter represent a very heterogeneous group of organisms. Each of the genera described is classified in a different family (Table 10-1). This can be quite confusing. The key to an understanding of these organisms is to memorize the key features of each.

AEROBIC ACTINOMYCETES

Actinomycetes are referred to as funguslike bacteria because they are bacteria that exhibit fungal characteristics (Fig. 10-1). Their cells are branched, filamentous hyphae that reproduce either by producing spores (conidia) or by fragmentation of the hyphae.[1] Some actinomycetes are aerobes; some are facultative anaerobes; and some are obligate anaerobes. Several of the aerobic actinomycetes— *Corynebacterium, Nocardia,* and *Mycobacterium* spp.—are discussed in this chapter. The anaerobic actinomycetes are discussed in Chapter 17.

Aerobic actinomycetes are Gram-positive to Gram-variable bacilli. Although they possess certain fungal characteristics, they are considered bacteria because their cell

---

[1] *The terms* conidia *(sing.* conidium) *and* hyphae *(sing.* hypha) *are most often used in discussions of fungi (see Chapter 19). A conidium is a spore that is produced asexually; that is, a conidium is an asexual spore. Many fungi reproduce by forming conidia. Fungal hyphae are long, thin, cytoplasmic filaments.*

TABLE 10 - 1 Classification of Gram-Positive Bacilli

Family	Genus
Corynebacteriaceae	*Corynebacterium*
Nocardiaceae	*Nocardia*
Mycobacteriaceae	*Mycobacterium*
Bacillaceae	*Bacillus*
Listeriaceae	*Listeria*
Lactobacillaceae	*Lactobacillus*
Erysipelotrichaceae	*Erysipelothrix*

Source: Boone DR, Castenholz RW, eds. The Archaea and the Deeply Branching and Phototrophic Bacteria. New York: Springer-Verlag, 2001. *Bergey's Manual of Systematic Bacteriology*, vol 1. 2nd Ed.

walls contain peptidoglycan, which is not found in fungal cell walls, and do *not* contain either chitin or cellulose, which are found in fungal cell walls. Aerobic actinomycetes are found almost everywhere in the environment, including in soil, freshwater and saltwater, and organic plant matter. Of the more than 40 genera of aerobic actinomycetes, about 16 have medical or veterinary significance.

Aerobic actinomycetes with mycolic acids (waxy substances) in their cell walls are referred to as mycolic acid–containing actinomycetes. Medically important mycolic acid–containing actinomycetes include bacteria in the genera *Corynebacterium*, *Nocardia*, and *Mycobacterium*, which are described in this chapter. Other medically important mycolic acid–containing actinomycetes, not described in this chapter, include *Dietzia*, *Gordonia*, *Rhodococcus*, *Skermania*, *Tsukamurella*, and *Williamsia* spp.

Medically important aerobic actinomycetes *lacking* mycolic acid in their cell walls include *Actinomadura*, *Amycolatopsis*, *Dermatophilus*, *Micromonospora*, *Nocardiopsis*, *Saccharomonospora*, *Saccharopolyspora*, *Streptomyces*, and *Thermoactinomyces*. These bacteria are not described in this book.

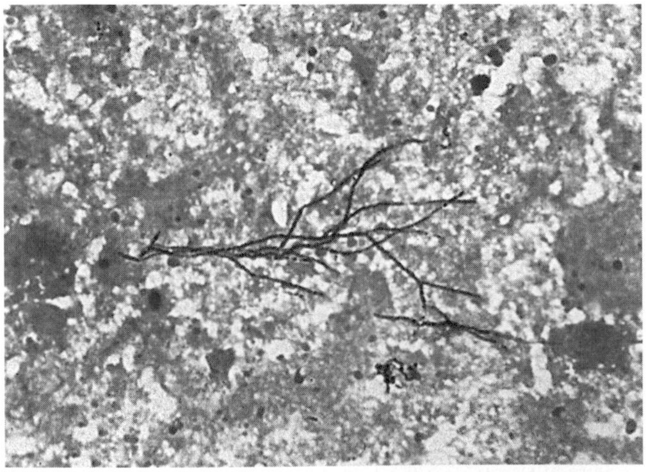

Figure 10-1. **Appearance of a typical actinomycete in a Gram-stained facial drainage specimen**. The cells are filamentous, branched, beaded, and narrow (less than 1 μm wide). Although these bacteria resemble fungi, fungal hyphae are much wider, ranging from 2 to 30 μm in width. (From Marler LM, Siders JA, Allen SD. Direct Smear Atlas. Philadelphia: Lippincott Williams & Wilkins, 2001.)

Genus *Corynebacterium* and Other Coryneform Bacteria

One group of aerobic actinomycetes is often referred to as **coryneforms** or **coryneform bacteria.** Although *coryne* is Greek for "club," there is really only one genus within the group—genus *Corynebacterium*—with club-shaped cells. The most clinically significant *Corynebacterium* species is *C. diphtheriae*, the cause of the disease diphtheria. The term **diphtheroids** refers to coryneform bacteria that resemble *C. diphtheriae* in appearance. Diphtheroids can cause disease in immunosuppressed patients and endocarditis and infections associated with catheters and prosthetic devices. The coryneform bacteria are quite diverse. Many coryneform bacteria are isolated from clinical specimens as indigenous microflora contaminants.

The genus *Corynebacterium* contains approximately 60 species. Of these, about 40 have some clinical significance. Although it is the most important *Corynebacterium* species, *C. diphtheriae* is rarely isolated in clinical microbiology laboratories (CMLs), thanks to widespread use of an effective childhood vaccine that prevents diphtheria. *C. urealyticum* is one of the most commonly isolated *Corynebacterium* species. It is a cause of urinary tract infections (UTIs) and is usually multidrug-resistant. *C. jeikeium* is also frequently isolated and often multidrug-resistant. It can cause endocarditis, septicemia, foreign body infections, and wound infections. *C. pseudodiphtheriticum* is a member of the oropharyngeal flora but can cause pneumonia and endocarditis. When they are considered clinically significant, isolates of corynebacteria other than *C. diphtheriae* are usually sent to a reference laboratory for identification.

Corynebacterium diphtheriae

Clinical significance. *C. diphtheriae* is named for the disease that it causes: diphtheria. Diphtheria is primarily an upper respiratory tract illness. Manifestations include pharyngitis (sore throat), **dysphagia** (difficulty swallowing), lymphadenitis, low-grade fever, **malaise** (extreme fatigue), and headache. A membrane sometimes forms in the throat, which can lead to obstruction of the airway. Severe systemic effects of diphtheria are myocarditis,

> Diphtheria is caused by a Gram-positive bacillus named *Corynebacterium diphtheriae.* Diphtheria is a vaccine-preventable disease.

neuritis (inflammation of a nerve), and kidney damage. *C. diphtheriae* may also cause cutaneous diphtheria. An effective vaccine has limited the number of cases of diphtheria in the United States to only a few per year. Horse serum containing antitoxins is used to treat respiratory diphtheria but is of limited value in treating cutaneous diphtheria. Serum sickness—allergic reactions to horse serum proteins—can occur in patients treated with the antitoxin.

Virulence factors. Diphtheria is caused by a toxin, appropriately named diphtheria toxin. Not all strains of *C. diphtheriae* produce diphtheria toxin. Only *C. diphtheriae*

> Only toxigenic strains of *C. diphtheriae* cause diphtheria.

cells that are infected with a particular **bacteriophage** (bacterial virus) produce diphtheria toxin, because the gene that codes for the toxin is actually a bacteriophage gene, called the "tox gene." Strains of *C. diphtheriae* that produce diphtheria toxin are called toxigenic strains; they are virulent, meaning that they cause disease. Strains of *C. diphtheriae* that do not produce diphtheria toxin are called nontoxigenic strains; they are avirulent, meaning that they do not cause disease.

Clues to *Corynebacterium* spp. Identification

Cellular morphology. The cells of most corynebacteria, including *C. diphtheriae*, are slightly curved Gram-positive bacilli with nonparallel sides. Sometimes the cells have slightly wider ends, giving them a club or dumbbell shape

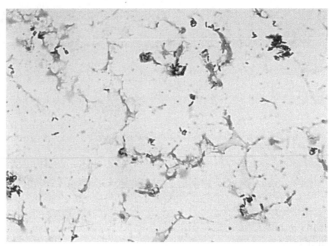

Figure 10-2. Corynebacterium **sp. in a Gram-stained blood specimen.** Occasional V, short picket fence, and Chinese letter formations can be seen. (From Marler LM, Siders JA, Allen SD. Direct Smear Atlas. Philadelphia: Lippincott Williams & Wilkins, 2001.)

(Fig. 10-2), and sometimes the cells stain unevenly. Cells from liquid media may be arranged singly, in pairs, in V forms, in **"palisades"** or **"picket fences"** (lined up side by side), or in clusters (referred to as

> Bacteria in the genus *Corynebacterium* have Gram-positive, club-shaped cells that may be observed in V forms or have the appearance of palisades, picket fences (lined up side by side), or clusters called Chinese letters.

a **"Chinese letter" arrangement**). *C. diphtheriae* cells are nonmotile and nonencapsulated.

When grown on Loeffler serum medium, *C. diphtheriae* cells contain purple-red metachromatic granules after staining with methylene blue (Fig. 10-3). The term *metachromasia*

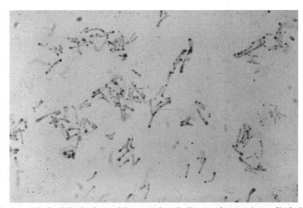

Figure 10-3. **Methylene blue-stained** *Corynebacterium diphtheriae* **cells from growth on Loeffler serum medium.** Note the beaded appearance caused by metachromatic granules within the cells. (From Winn WC Jr, et al. Koneman's Color Atlas and Textbook of Diagnostic Microbiology. 6th Ed. Philadelphia: Lippincott Williams & Wilkins, 2006.)

> Following growth on Loeffler serum medium, metachromatic granules can be seen in *C. diphtheriae* cells that have been stained with methylene blue.

refers to a change in the color of a dye that has attached to a particular substance. In this case, the blue dye becomes purple-red following attachment to granules within the *C. diphtheriae* cells. Loeffler serum medium contains beef serum and eggs.

Colonial morphology. Coryneform bacteria, including *C. diphtheriae*, grow well on blood agar. Colonial morphology differs among the four *C. diphtheriae* biotypes. Colonies of *C. diphtheriae* biotype *intermedius* are small, gray, or translucent. Colonies of the other biotypes (*belfanti*, *gravis*, and *mitis*) are white or opaque and larger—up to 2 mm in diameter after 24 hours incubation (Fig. 10-4).

Fosfomycin can be added to the blood agar to make the medium selective for corynebacteria, because most coryneform bacteria are resistant to this antimicrobial agent. Alternatively, disks containing 50 μg of fosfomycin can be added to inoculated blood agar plates; colonies showing resistance can be examined for coryneform bacteria. Most clinically relevant coryneform bacteria grow within 48 hours.

In addition to blood agar, a selective medium such as cystine-telluride blood agar (CTBA) or freshly prepared modified Tinsdale medium (preferably) should be inoculated if *C. diphtheriae* is suspected. If neither medium is available, colistin-nalidixic acid agar can be used. *C. diphtheriae* and other coryneform bacteria will grow on colistin-nalidixic acid agar, as will all other Gram-positive bacteria.

Cystine-telluride blood agar (CTBA). *C. diphtheriae* and many other Gram-positive bacteria will grow on CTBA. On CTBA, *C. diphtheriae* colonies will be black because of telluride reduction, but some other Gram-positive bacteria (e.g., other coryneform bacteria, staphylococci, streptococci) can also produce black colonies.

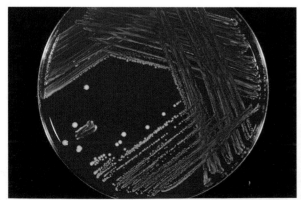

Figure 10-4. **White, creamy *Corynebacterium diphtheriae* colonies on sheep blood agar.** (From Winn WC Jr, et al. Koneman's Color Atlas and Textbook of Diagnostic Microbiology. 6th Ed. Philadelphia: Lippincott Williams & Wilkins, 2006.)

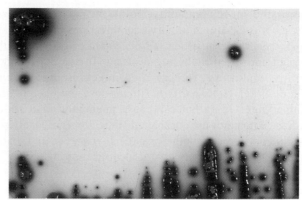

Figure 10-5. C. diphtheriae **colonies on modified Tinsdale medium.** The black *C. diphtheriae* colonies are surrounded by brown halos. (From Winn WC Jr, et al. Koneman's Color Atlas and Textbook of Diagnostic Microbiology. 6th Ed. Philadelphia: Lippincott Williams & Wilkins, 2006.)

Modified Tinsdale medium. On modified Tinsdale medium, *C. diphtheriae* colonies will be black (because of telluride reduction), surrounded by

> Associate cystine-telluride blood agar and Tinsdale medium with *C. diphtheriae.*

a brown halo caused by cystinase activity (Fig. 10-5). Other organisms can grow on modified Tinsdale medium, but the presence of the brown halos is presumptive evidence of *C. diphtheriae*. Nontoxigenic strains of *C. diphtheriae* often do not produce halos.

Many laboratory tests are briefly discussed in this and other chapters. Appendix A contains detailed information about these tests.

Laboratory tests. Presumptive identification of *C. diphtheriae* can be made by testing coryneform bacteria for the presence of cystinase, using Tinsdale medium or diagnostic tablets, and the absence of pyrazinamidase, using diagnostic tablets. Diagnostic tablets are available from Key Scientific Products (http://www.keyscientific.com/). The pyrazinamidase test is described later in the chapter. A variety of commercial minisystems are also available for identification of *C. diphtheriae* (Table 10-2). Reference laboratories can identify *C. diphtheriae* by mycolic acid profiles, using thin-layer chromatography, gas chromatography, mass spectrometry, or high-performance liquid chromatography. *C. diphtheriae* can also be identified by cellular fatty acid analysis using the Sherlock system from MIDI Inc. (http://www.midilabs.com/). An immunofluorescence procedure is also available. An organism identified as *C. diphtheriae* may or may not be toxigenic. If the isolate is nontoxigenic, it cannot be causing diphtheria.

Demonstration of toxin production is the single most important characteristic used to identify *C. diphtheriae*. Various methods are available to determine if a *C. diphtheriae* strain is producing diphtheria toxin; these include the modified Elek method, which is an immunodiffusion test

TABLE 10 - 2	Commercial Systems Available for Identification of *Corynebacterium diphtheriae*
Identification System	**Manufacturer**
API Coryne system	bioMérieux Inc. (http://www.biomerieux.com/)
BBL Crystal Gram-Pos ID System	BD Biosciences (http://www.biosciences.com/)
BBL Crystal Rapid Gram-Pos ID System	BD Biosciences
Biolog GP MicroPlate	Biolog Inc. (http://www.biolog.com/)
IDS RapID CB Plus system	Remel (http://www.remelinc.com/)
Micronaut-RPO (NAUT)	Merlin Diagnostics (http://www.merlin-diagnostika.de/engl)
MicroScan Pos ID panels	Dade Behring (http://www.dadebehring.com/)
MicroScan Rapid Gram Pos ID panels	Dade Behring
MIDI Sherlock	MIDI Inc. (http://www.midilabs.com/)
Vitek GPI card (Vitek 1)	bioMérieux Inc.
Vitek GP card (Vitek 2)	bioMérieux Inc.

Source: Evangelista AT, et al. Rapid systems and instruments for antimicrobial susceptibility testing of bacteria. In: Manual of Commercial Methods in Clinical Microbiology. Washington, DC: ASM Press, 2002.

(described on the CD-ROM), guinea pig lethality test, polymerase chain reaction, Vero cell cytotoxicity, and reversed passive latex agglutination. Such tests are performed in reference laboratories staffed with professionals possessing skill in performing the tests and interpreting the results.

Essentials

Corynebacterium diphtheriae

- Toxigenic strains cause diphtheria

- Gram-positive bacilli, often in V, picket fence, or Chinese letter arrangements

- Catalase positive

- On modified Tinsdale medium, produces black colonies surrounded by brown halos

- Cells from growth on Loeffler serum medium will contain metachromatic granules after staining them with methylene blue

Genus *Nocardia*

Clinical significance. The genus *Nocardia* comprises more than 20 species, about 13 of which have medical significance.

Nocardial infection, or nocardiosis, is rare in humans, most frequently occurring in severely immunocompromised patients. Infection is acquired by inhalation of *Nocardia* organisms in dust or by direct skin inoculation. The most common manifestations of nocardiosis are cutaneous, pulmonary, central nervous system, and systemic infections. Cutaneous nocardiosis is referred to as mycetoma or actinomycetoma, although other organisms can also cause these lesions (see Chapter 20). Pulmonary nocardiosis can mimic tuberculosis. Medically important *Nocardia* spp. include the *N. asteroides* complex, *N. brasiliensis*, and less frequently, *N. otitidiscaviarum*. The *N. asteroides* complex, which includes *N. asteroides*, *N. abscessus*, *N. farcinica*, and *N. nova*, causes most of the serious invasive *Nocardia* infections. Infections caused by the *N. asteroides* complex are widespread, whereas those caused by *N. brasiliensis* occur primarily in tropical countries and the southeastern and southwestern United States.

Direct examination of the clinical specimen, such as sputum, bronchial lavage fluid, exudate, or cerebrospinal fluid (CSF), is extremely important. The specimen should be spread out in a sterile petri dish, and clumps of microorganisms—referred to as granules, or sulfur granules if yellow—should be sought. If present, a granule should be crushed between two microscope slides and examined microscopically. Smears of the specimen should also be Gram stained and stained using the modified Kinyoun acid-fast stain (discussed later in the chapter).

Clues to *Nocardia* spp. Identification

Cellular morphology. *Nocardia* spp. form extensively branched hyphae that fragment into rod-shaped to coccoid nonmotile cells. In Gram-stained smears of specimens or cultures, *Nocardia* cells may be short or long (sometimes up to 20 μm in length), thin (0.5 to 1.0 μm in diameter), branching, often beaded Gram-positive bacilli. Clubbing of the cells may be observed. The hyphae branch at right angles and usually have secondary branches (Fig. 10-6).

> *Nocardia* spp. are filamentous, branched, and beaded Gram-positive bacilli.

Nocardia **spp. are described as being weakly acid fast.** That description refers to *Nocardia* cells becoming decolorized (i.e., they lose the red color) when the Ziehl-Neelson acid-fast staining method is used but remaining colorized (red) when the less harsh, modified Kinyoun acid-fast stain is used (Fig. 10-7). Details of both these acid-fast staining procedures are presented in Appendix A. **It is important to remember that** *Nocardia* **spp. are described as being weakly acid fast, whereas** *Mycobacterium* **spp., are described as being acid fast.** Being weakly acid fast also helps to distinguish *Nocardia* spp. from *Actinomyces* spp. (see Chapter 17), which are not acid fast.

> *Nocardia* spp. are weakly acid fast.

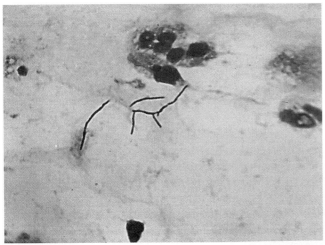

Figure 10-6. Filamentous, branched, beaded *Nocardia*-like **cells in a Gram-stained fine-needle aspirate of lung.** *Actinomyces* spp. also have this appearance (see Chapter 17). (From Marler LM, Siders JA, Allen SD. Direct Smear Atlas. Philadelphia: Lippincott Williams & Wilkins, 2001.)

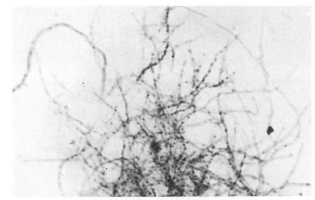

Figure 10-7. Delicate, branching, beaded *Nocardia asteroides* **cells in a Kinyoun acid-fast-stained exudate.** (From Winn WC Jr, et al. Koneman's Color Atlas and Textbook of Diagnostic Microbiology. 6th Ed. Philadelphia: Lippincott Williams & Wilkins, 2006.)

Colonial morphology. *Nocardia* spp. are aerobic, although incubation in a CO_2 incubator stimulates their growth. They will grow on simple media, but they are slow growers; it often takes 4 to 5 days before visible colonies appear. Culture plates should be held for 7 to 10 days. When aerial hyphae are absent, *Nocardia* colonies are smooth and raised. When aerial hyphae are present, colonies may appear chalky, crumbly, or may have a cotton ball appearance. In early stages of growth, aerial hyphae (when present) can only be seen microscopically (e.g., when using a stereoscopic microscope with ×10 to ×50 magnification). *Nocardia* colonies vary in color from white to pink to orange to tan, depending on the species and the type of medium on which they are growing. When growing on

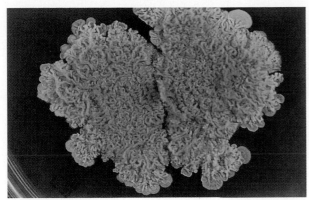

Figure 10-8. **Orange, waxy, rough colonies of *N. asteroides* on Middlebrook 7H11 medium after 7 days incubation at 30°C.** (From Winn WC Jr, et al. Koneman's Color Atlas and Textbook of Diagnostic Microbiology. 6th Ed. Philadelphia: Lippincott Williams & Wilkins, 2006.)

Sabouraud dextrose agar or brain-heart infusion agar, colonies of *N. asteroides* complex vary from salmon pink to orange (Fig. 10-8). *N. brasiliensis* colonies are usually orange-tan, and *N. otitidiscaviarum* colonies are usually pale tan. *Nocardia* colonies have a characteristic odor, which has been described as earthy, musty, or resembling a root cellar or freshly plowed soil.

Slide cultures (see Chapter 19) are useful for examination of *Nocardia* spp. When examined microscopically, branched substrate hyphae, aerial hyphae, and conidia can be observed.[2] The presence of aerial hyphae differentiates *Nocardia* from *Corynebacterium* and *Mycobacterium*, as well as other related genera.

Laboratory tests. Tests of value for identification of *Nocardia* spp. include decomposition of substrates, such as adenine, casein, hypoxanthine, tyrosine, and xanthine; growth in lysozyme; and arylsulfatase production.

Growth in lysozyme. Lysozyme (see Chapter 3) is an enzyme that destroys bacterial cell walls. The organism to be tested is inoculated into a tube containing a lysozyme solution and a control tube containing no lysozyme. The test is considered positive if good growth of the organism occurs in both tubes. A negative test result is good growth in the control tube but poor or no growth in the tube containing lysozyme. Most *Nocardia* spp. will grow in the presence of lysozyme.

Arylsulfatase production. Arylsulfatase activity is detected by the formation of a deep pink color when sodium carbonate is added to a suspension of the test organism in phenolphthalein disulfate solution. Most *Nocardia* species are arylsulfatase negative, but *N. africana* and *N. nova* are exceptions. Rapidly growing *Mycobacterium* strains, which do not posses aerial hyphae, and *N. africana*, which possesses aerial hyphae, are usually arylsulfatase positive within 3 days. Most strains of *N. nova*, which possess aerial hyphae, are positive within 14 days.

A variety of commercial biochemical test systems are available for identifying *Nocardia* spp. and other aerobic actinomycetes. Other methods of identification include antimicrobial resistance patterns, analysis of cell wall components, mycolic acid and fatty acid analysis by gas-liquid chromatography and mass spectrometry, and molecular diagnostic procedures.

Genus *Mycobacterium*

More than 100 *Mycobacterium* spp., or mycobacteria, have been described. Medically important mycobacteria include (1) those that cause tuberculosis, referred to as the *Mycobacterium tuberculosis* complex, consisting of *M. tuberculosis*, *M. bovis*, *M. africanum*, *M. microti* (very rarely isolated from humans), and *M. canettii*; (2) *M. leprae*, which causes leprosy or Hansen disease; and (3) a very large number of *Mycobacterium* spp. called **nontuberculous mycobacteria (NTM)** or **mycobacteria other than tuberculosis (MOTT)**. Organisms in the latter group live in soil and water. Diseases caused by NTM/MOTT are referred to as mycobacterioses.

Recall from Chapter 4 that special safety precautions must be practiced when working with mycobacteria. These include a negative-pressure room with air exiting through HEPA filters; a biosafety cabinet; special centrifuges to contain aerosol production; and protective clothing, such as masks, disposable gowns, gloves, caps, shoe protection, and sometimes, respirators. Personnel should be monitored annually with the Mantoux tuberculin test, in which a mycobacterial antigen is injected into the skin. People who convert from a previous negative skin test to a current positive skin test most likely have been infected with *M. tuberculosis*.

Mycobacterial cells are 0.2 to 0.6 μm wide by 1.0 to 10 μm long, straight to slightly curved, and sometimes branched. The presence of an abundance of cell wall lipids, which include waxes, makes it difficult to stain mycobacterial cells and to destain the cells once stained. **Mycobacteria are strongly acid fast. They do not stain well with the Gram staining technique because of the high and complex lipid content of their cell walls.** Although sometimes described as being Gram-positive to Gram-variable bacilli, **the Gram stain is unreliable for staining mycobacteria.** In Gram-stained specimens, they may be unstained (appearing as clear zones or "ghosts") or appear as beaded Gram-positive bacilli. Mycobacteria are nonmotile and non-spore forming. Most species are aerobic, but some can grow in a reduced-oxygen atmosphere.

> *Mycobacterium* spp. are strongly acid fast because of the presence of waxes and other lipids in their cell walls. These lipids also make it difficult to Gram stain *Mycobacterium* spp.

---

[2]*Substrate hyphae, also called vegetative hyphae, are hyphae that lie within the medium. Aerial hyphae are hyphae that project upward into the air. Fungal aerial hyphae are also called reproductive hyphae because spores are produced on these hyphae.*

CAUTION

Beware of Similar-Sounding Names. Do not confuse *Mycobacterium* spp. (mycobacteria) with *Mycoplasma* spp. (mycoplasmas). Unique features of mycobacteria are that they are acid-fast bacteria with waxes in their cell walls. The unique feature of mycoplasmas, discussed in Chapter 14, is that they have no cell walls.

Some *Mycobacterium* spp. grow on simple culture media, some are fastidious, and some (e.g., *M. leprae*) do not grow at all. Most species are slow growers, having generation times ranging from 2 to more than 20 hours. These species require more than 7 days to produce colonies large enough to work with in the CML; some species require 6 weeks or more. Other species, called rapid growers, produce colonies in less than 7 days. Optimal growth temperatures range from less than 30°C to 45°C.

Some *Mycobacterium* spp., called **photochromogens**), produce pigmented colonies only in the presence of light, whereas other species, called **scotochromogens,** produce pigment either in the presence or absence of light. Still other species, called **nonphotochromogens,** produce nonpigmented colonies whether grown in the presence or absence of light (Table 10-3). Pigmentation testing should be performed using isolated colonies from young cultures.

STUDY AID

A Way to Remember Terms Related to Mycobacterial Pigmentation. *Photo-* refers to light. **Photochromogens** produce pigment *only* in the presence of light. *Scoto-* is from the Greek word for darkness. **Scotochromogens** produce pigment in the dark *and* in the light. Associate *non*pigmented colonies with **nonphotochromogens,** which do not produce pigment at all, whether grown in the dark or in the light.

Runyon Classification Scheme

In 1965, Ernest H. Runyon devised a scheme for classification of the NTM/MOTT. These organisms were assigned to one of the following four groups:

Group I: Photochromogens

Group II: Scotochromogens

Group III: Nonphotochromogens

Group IV: Rapid growers

Although Runyon's classification scheme is still of some value, genetic and phenotypic information about these organisms that has been gained since 1965 has demonstrated

TABLE 10 - 3	Classification of Mycobacteria by Pigmentation and Photoreactivity	
Category	**Description**	**Examples**
Photochromogens	*Mycobacterium* spp. that produce slightly or nonpigmented colonies when grown in the dark but produce yellow-orange pigmented colonies after exposure to light and reincubation.	*M. marinum, M. kansasii, M. simiae, M. asiaticum*
Scotochromogens	*Mycobacterium* spp. that produce deep yellow to orange colonies when grown in either the light or the dark. Pigment production increases in some strains on continuous exposure to light.	*M. scrofulaceum, M. szulgai, M. gordonae*
Nonphotochromogens	*Mycobacterium* spp. that are nonpigmented in the light and dark or have only a pale yellow, buff, or light tan pigment that does not intensify after light exposure.	Members of the *M. tuberculosis* complex (*M. tuberculosis, M. bovis, M. africanum*), *M. avium* complex (*M. avium*, M. *intracellulare*, *M. paratuberculosis*, *M. lepraemurium*), *M. malmoense, M. ulcerans, M. xenopi, M. genavense, M. gastri, M. haemophilum, M. shimoide, M. flavescens, M. terrae* complex

that not all NTM/MOTT fit neatly into one or the other of these categories.

Acid-Fast Staining Techniques

Ziehl-Neelsen acid-fast stain. After a fixed smear is flooded with carbolfuchsin, the slide is heated until steam rises from the bright red dye. Heating enables the dye to penetrate the cell walls. After the slide cools and is washed with water, an acid-alcohol decolorizing agent is applied. After washing, the smear is counterstained using methylene blue or malachite green. The slide is then washed, blotted dry, and examined at ×400 and ×1000. Acid-fast organisms are pink to red, whereas non-acid-fast organisms are blue or green, depending on which counterstain was used (see Fig. 6-19).

Kinyoun (cold) acid-fast stain. In this acid-fast staining method, the primary stain contains higher concentrations of basic fuchsin and phenol than are used in the Ziehl-Neelsen method. The higher concentration of phenol dissolves cell wall lipids, enabling the dye to penetrate the cell walls. Heat is not used in the Kinyoun method (Fig. 10-9).

Modified Kinyoun acid-fast stain. In a modification of the Kinyoun stain, a weaker decolorizing agent (0.5% to 1% sulfuric acid) is used in place of the 3% acid-alcohol mixture.

Auramine-rhodamine fluorescent acid-fast stain. Mycobacteria fluoresce a bright yellow when stained with auramine-rhodamine (Fig. 10-10). Fluorescent acid-fast staining kits are available from several commercial sources. Kits and reagents for performing the previously mentioned acid-fast staining procedures are also commercially available. Appendix A contains detailed information about all the acid-fast staining procedures discussed here.

Mycobacterium tuberculosis Complex

The primary responsibility of the CML's mycobacteriology section (or TB lab, as it is often called) is to assist clinicians in the diagnosis of tuberculosis. Because of the expense involved in the operation of a mycobacteriology section and

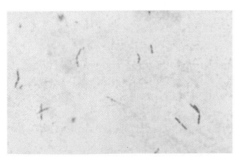

Figure 10-9. **Mycobacteria stained with the Kinyoun acid-fast staining technique.** (From Winn WC Jr, et al. Koneman's Color Atlas and Textbook of Diagnostic Microbiology. 6th Ed. Philadelphia: Lippincott Williams & Wilkins, 2006.)

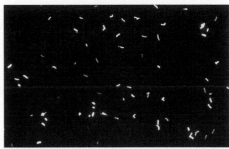

Figure 10-10. **Mycobacterial cells fluorescing a bright yellow after being stained with the auramine-rhodamine acid-fast staining procedure.** (From Winn WC Jr, et al. Koneman's Color Atlas and Textbook of Diagnostic Microbiology. 6th Ed. Philadelphia: Lippincott Williams & Wilkins, 2006.)

the stringent safety requirements required, usually only large hospitals and medical centers provide complete mycobacteriology services, including identification and susceptibility testing of *Mycobacterium* spp. Mycobacteriology services in smaller hospitals are often limited to acid-fast staining of clinical specimens, predominantly sputum, which can rapidly provide a presumptive or tentative diagnosis of tuberculosis. Positive specimens are then sent to a reference laboratory for additional mycobacteriology services.

As previously mentioned, the *M. tuberculosis* complex consists of five species: *M. tuberculosis*, *M. bovis*, *M. africanum*, *M. microti*, and *M. canettii*. Some taxonomists consider the five members of the *M. tuberculosis* complex to be so closely related that they should be thought of as subspecies of *M. tuberculosis* rather than as separate species.

Clinical significance. Tuberculosis (TB) is a serious worldwide public health concern, causing about 2 million deaths every year. *M. tuberculosis* and *M. bovis* cause most cases of TB. *M. africanum* is a common cause of TB in tropical Africa, as its name would suggest. *M. canettii* has caused generalized lymphadenitis and tuberculosis in AIDS patients in Africa.

> The primary cause of tuberculosis is *M. tuberculosis.*

M. tuberculosis is usually inhaled; thus, the lungs are the predominant portal of entry and the major target organ for *M. tuberculosis*. Patients with primary pulmonary TB may be asymptomatic or may have a fever, nonproductive (no sputum) cough, and shortness of breath. Patients with chronic pulmonary TB may have fever, night sweats, chills, fatigue, **anorexia** (loss of appetite), weight loss, cough, chest pain, and sputum production. In advanced cases, **hemoptysis** (spitting of blood) may occur. Systemic TB, referred to as miliary TB, results from **hematogenous dissemination** (via the bloodstream) of *M. tuberculosis*, and may involve the spleen, liver, lungs, bone marrow, kidneys, adrenal glands, and eyes. Central nervous system, gastrointestinal, and pericardial TB may also occur.

Clinical specimens. *Mycobacterium* spp. may infect almost any tissue or organ in the body. Although sputum and other types of pulmonary specimens, such as bronchoalveolar lavage fluids and bronchial washings, are the most common specimens submitted to the mycobacteriology section of the CML, other specimens include gastric lavage specimens, blood, urine, body fluids, tissue, wound specimens, aspirates, and material from skin lesions. Fecal specimens are acceptable when infection with the *M. avium* complex is suspected in AIDS patients.

Prior to inoculating culture media, sputum specimens are digested, decontaminated, and concentrated. Digestion procedures are used to release any mycobacteria that may be trapped in mucin and cells. The purpose of decontamination procedures is to reduce or eliminate contaminating bacteria. Sputum digestion, decontamination, and concentration procedures are discussed further in Appendix A.

Specimens are then inoculated onto selective and nonselective solid media, such as Löwenstein-Jensen medium (an egg-based medium) or Middlebrook medium (an agar-based medium), and liquid media (e.g., Middlebrook 7H9 and Dubos Tween albumin broths).

> Associate Löwenstein-Jensen and Middlebrook media with the genus *Mycobacterium*.

Additional information about these media is contained in Chapter 18.

Various alternative procedures have been developed for detecting *M. tuberculosis* in clinical specimens. These include molecular diagnostic procedures; radiometric techniques; automated, continuously monitored systems; and others.

Molecular diagnostic procedures. Commercial molecular diagnostic procedures (MDPs) are available for detection of *M. tuberculosis* in clinical specimens. These include polymerase chain reaction (PCR) and ribosomal RNA amplification procedures. The obvious advantage of MDPs is that they enable a much faster diagnosis of tuberculosis compared with conventional culture techniques. An obvious disadvantage is that no isolated organism will be available for susceptibility testing. Negative MDP results should be confirmed using conventional culture techniques. Listed here are some of the MDPs for detection of *M. tuberculosis* in clinical specimens:

- Amplified *Mycobacterium tuberculosis* Direct (MTD2) Test (Gen-Probe Inc.; http://www.gen-probe.com/)

- AMPLICOR *Mycobacterium tuberculosis* (MTB) Test (Roche; http://www.roche.com/)

- Lcx MTB Assay, Abbott Lcx Probe System (Abbott Laboratories; http://www.abbott.com/)

- BD Probe Tec ET System (BD Biosciences; http://www.bdbiosciences.com/)

Other nontraditional identification and diagnostic procedures. Other procedures that hasten the laboratory diagnosis of tuberculosis include the following:

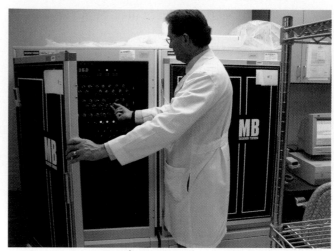

***Figure 10-11.* MB BacT System, manufactured by bioMérieux.** A liquid medium, automated, continuously monitored system for recovery of mycobacteria from clinical specimens. (Courtesy of Dr. Robert Fader.)

- BACTEC 460 TB system (BD Biosciences): a liquid medium, semiautomated, radiometric system based on $^{14}CO_2$ production. A similar, radiometric BACTEC system can be used for susceptibility testing of *M. tuberculosis*

- BACTEC 9000 MB system (BD Biosciences): a liquid medium, automated, continuously monitored, nonradiometric system based on oxygen consumption and fluorescence (Fig. 10-11)

- BACTEC MGIT 960 (BD Biosciences): a liquid medium, automated, continuously monitored, nonradiometric system based on oxygen consumption and fluorescence

- ESP-Culture System II (Trek International Inc.; http://www.trekds.com/): a liquid medium, automated, continuously monitored, nonradiometric system based on manometric measurement of gas production or consumption

- MB/BacT System (bioMérieux; http://www.biomerieux.com/): a liquid medium, automated, continuously monitored, nonradiometric system based on CO_2 production

- MB Redox (Biotest Diagnostics Corp.; http://www.biotest.com/): a liquid medium, nonautomated, nonradiometric, colorimetric system

- Septi-Chek AFB (BD Biosciences): a biphasic system (one containing both liquid and solid media), consisting of Middlebrook 7H9 broth and a paddle containing three types of solid media (modified Löwenstein-Jensen medium, Middlebrook 7H11, and chocolate agar, the latter for detection of bacterial contaminants)

Virulence factors. *M. tuberculosis* is capable of surviving within monocytes and macrophages; it is considered a facultative intracellular pathogen.[3] There are a number of

> M. tuberculosis is a facultative intracellular pathogen.

theories to explain how *M. tuberculosis* survives within host cells, but all are controversial. A mycolic acid in the cell walls of *M. tuberculosis*, called cord factor, is associated with several biologic activities, including host cell membrane cytotoxicity and inhibition of white blood cell migration.

Drug resistance. The most commonly used antitubercular drugs are isoniazid, ethambutol, pyrazinamide, and rifampin. Many strains of *M. tuberculosis* are drug resistant, many strains are multidrug-resistant, and some strains are resistant to *all* antitubercular drugs. Until the results of antimicrobial susceptibility testing are available, it is recommended that tuberculosis patients be treated with all four of the previously mentioned antitubercular drugs. Once the susceptibility results are available, they can be used to determine a specific drug regimen. Antimicrobial susceptibility testing of mycobacteria is discussed later in the chapter.

Clues to *M. tuberculosis* Identification

Colonial morphology. On complex solid culture media, *M. tuberculosis* has a generation time of 12 to 18 hours;

> Because *M. tuberculosis* is a very slow grower, it takes weeks before colonies are available to work with in the laboratory.

colonies are visible in 3 to 6 weeks. Fortunately, acid-fast staining of clinical specimens, primarily sputum, permits rapid presumptive diagnosis of tuberculosis, enabling therapy to be initiated long before culture results are available. *M. tuberculosis* colonies are off-white (buff colored) and rough on solid media (Fig. 10-12), although on moist media, colonies tend to be smoother. On solid and in liquid media,

> Associate cording or serpentine cording with *M. tuberculosis*.

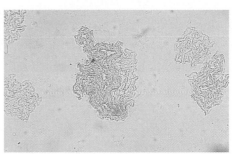

Figure 10-13. **A very young colony of *M. tuberculosis*, observed microscopically, using a low-power objective.** The pattern of the colony indicates the production of cording factor. (From Winn WC Jr, et al. Koneman's Color Atlas and Textbook of Diagnostic Microbiology. 6th Ed. Philadelphia: Lippincott Williams & Wilkins, 2006.)

virulent strains form strands or cords, referred to as cording or serpentine cording (Figs. 10-13 and 10-14). The cording is caused by a mycolic acid in *M. tuberculosis* cell walls, designated cord factor, mentioned earlier.

Colonies of *M. bovis* are small and flat on agar media, but on egg-based media, they are small and rounded, with irregular edges and a granular surface. *M. africanum* colonies are rough. *M. canettii* produces heterogenous colonies; on agar media, some colonies are flat and smooth, but most are smooth, round, and glossy, looking more like NTM/MOTT colonies than colonies produced by other members of the *M. tuberculosis* complex. *M. microti* cannot be grown on artificial media.

Laboratory tests. The first test to perform on bacteria suspected of being mycobacteria is one of the acid-fast staining procedures discussed earlier. As previously mentioned, bacteria that retain the red carbolfuchsin dye following the decolorization step of the staining procedure are called acid-fast organisms, whereas those that do not retain the red dye are called non-acid-fast organisms. **All mycobacteria are acid fast;** thus, they will be red following the acid-fast staining procedure. Acid fastness can be partially or completely lost at some stage of growth, however, which is especially true for rapidly growing mycobacteria.

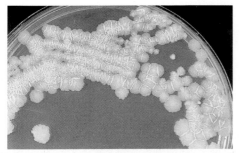

Figure 10-12. **Colonies of *Mycobacterium tuberculosis* on Middlebrook 7H10 agar after 25 days of incubation at 35°C in a CO₂ incubator.** (From Winn WC Jr, et al. Koneman's Color Atlas and Textbook of Diagnostic Microbiology. 6th Ed. Philadelphia: Lippincott Williams & Wilkins, 2006.)

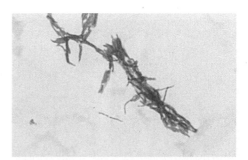

Figure 10-14. **Cording of *M. tuberculosis* cells apparent in a Kinyoun acid-fast-stained blood culture broth.** (From Winn WC Jr, et al. Koneman's Color Atlas and Textbook of Diagnostic Microbiology. 6th Ed. Philadelphia: Lippincott Williams & Wilkins, 2006.)

---

[3]*Recall from Chapter 2 that facultative intracellular pathogens are capable of living either outside of or within host cells. Obligate intracellular pathogens, on the other hand, can only survive within host cells.*

TABLE 10 - 4	Biochemical Comparison Between *Mycobacterium tuberculosis* and Other Members of the *M. tuberculosis* Complex			
	Niacin Accumulation	Nitrate Reduction	Growth on TCH	Pyrazinamidase (4-day)
M. tuberculosis	+	+	+	+
M. africanum	V	V	V	–
M. bovis	–	–	–	–
M. canettii	+	+	+	+

TCH, thiophene-2-carboxylic acid hydrazide (also known as T2H); V, variable

Members of the *M. tuberculosis* complex are slow-growing nonphotochromogens, and their optimal growth temperature is 37°C. A preliminary identification of *M. tuberculosis* can be made if the organism also produces buff-colored rough colonies and is niacin positive. Other key identifying characteristics for *M. tuberculosis* are that it is nitrate reduction positive and 68°C catalase test negative. Table 10-4 contains a biochemical comparison between *M. tuberculosis* and other members of the *M. tuberculosis* complex. Although *M. canettii* produces the same biochemical test results as *M. tuberculosis*, colonies of *M. canettii* (smooth, round, glossy) are quite different than those of *M. tuberculosis*. Although colonies of *M. africanum* resemble those of *M. tuberculosis*, keep in mind that *M. africanum* causes tuberculosis in tropical Africa. Thus, it would rarely be encountered in the United States.

> *M. tuberculosis* is niacin positive, nitrate reduction positive, and 68°C catalase test negative.

Niacin accumulation test. All mycobacteria produce niacin ribonucleotide, but some species, like *M. tuberculosis*, are unable to convert it into nicotinamide adenine dinucleotide. The niacin produced by these species is excreted and accumulates in Löwenstein-Jensen culture medium. In the niacin accumulation test, the niacin is extracted from the culture medium and transferred to a small test tube containing sterile water or saline. A cyanogen bromide–impregnated paper strip is added to the tube. Development of a yellow color indicates that niacin is present in the tube and represents a positive test result (Fig. 10-15). No yellow color represents a negative test result.

Nitrate reduction test. A few *Mycobacterium* spp. (including *M. tuberculosis*) produce the enzyme nitroreductase, which catalyzes the reduction of nitrate (NO_3) to nitrite (NO_2). Colonies removed from Löwenstein-Jensen medium are suspended in the liquid nitrate test substrate, which is then incubated. Development of a pink-to-red color when two different reagents are added to the tube indicates the presence of nitrite and that nitrate was reduced. Thus, development of a pink-to-red color represents a positive test result (Fig. 10-16). No color change represents a negative test result. A negative test result can be confirmed by adding a small amount of zinc dust to the tube. Development of a pink-to-red color at that point indicates that nitrate is still

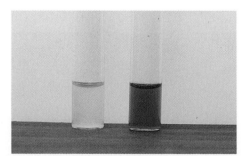

Figure 10-16. Nitrate reduction test. The tube to the left is a control tube. The tube to the right had been inoculated with an unknown *Mycobacterium* species. Appearance of red following the addition of two reagents (sulfonamide and α-naphthylethylenediamine) represents a positive test result: that nitrate had been reduced to nitrite. (From Winn WC Jr, et al. Koneman's Color Atlas and Textbook of Diagnostic Microbiology. 6th Ed. Philadelphia: Lippincott Williams & Wilkins, 2006.)

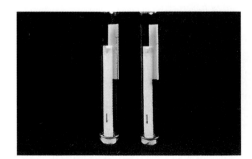

Figure 10-15. Niacin accumulation test. The yellow color of the fluid in the tube to the right indicates that niacin was present in the fluid; this is a positive test result. (From Winn WC Jr, et al. Koneman's Color Atlas and Textbook of Diagnostic Microbiology. 6th Ed. Philadelphia: Lippincott Williams & Wilkins, 2006.)

present in the tube and therefore was not reduced to nitrite. Thus, development of a pink-to-red color *after* addition of zinc dust confirms a negative nitrate reduction test result. No color change following addition of zinc dust confirms a positive test result.

68°C catalase test. The enzyme catalase was discussed in Chapter 9. The 68°C catalase test is essentially a heat tolerance test to determine if catalase can be detected following heating of the organism at 68°C for 20 minutes. All members of the *M. tuberculosis* complex are 68°C catalase test negative. Note that this is *not* the same catalase test that was described in Chapter 9.

Growth on thiophene-2-carboxylic acid hydrazide (TCH or T2H). Growth of some *Mycobacterium* spp. is inhibited by TCH that has been incorporated into Middlebrook 7H11 medium. The test is useful for differentiating *M. tuberculosis*, which grows on TCH medium, from *M. bovis*, which does not grow on TCH medium (Fig. 10-17).

Pyrazinamidase (PZA) test. The enzyme pyrazinamidase deaminates pyrazinamide to ammonia and pyrazinoic acid. The liquid test medium containing pyrazinamide is first heavily inoculated with the organism to be tested and then incubated. Ferrous ammonium sulfate is added to the tube, and the tube is observed for up to 4 hours. Development of a pink-red band in the medium indicates the presence of pyrazinoic acid; thus, presence of a pink-red band constitutes a positive test result (Fig. 10-18). *M. tuberculosis* is PZA positive, whereas *M. bovis* is PZA negative.

Culture media and reagents necessary for the tests mentioned here and for additional biochemical tests are available from several commercial sources, including BD Biosciences (http://www.bdbiosciences.com/) and Remel (http://www.remelinc.com/).

Additional techniques for the identification of *Mycobacterium* spp. include analysis of mycobacterial cell

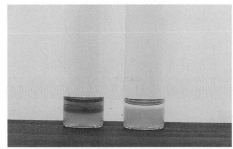

Figure 10-18. PZA test. Two tubes of Dubos broth, the one to the left containing pyrazinamide (PZA), and the one to the right serving as a control. Both tubes were inoculated with the same *Mycobacterium* species. Then ferrous ammonium sulfate was added to both tubes. The presence of a pink-red band in the tube containing PZA represents a positive test result—that PZA was deaminated. (From Winn WC Jr, et al. Koneman's Color Atlas and Textbook of Diagnostic Microbiology. 6th Ed. Philadelphia: Lippincott Williams & Wilkins, 2006.)

wall fatty acid composition by gas-liquid chromatography or high-performance liquid chromatography, and molecular techniques such as nucleic acid probes, nucleic acid sequencing, nucleic acid amplification (PCR assays), and hybridization. Nucleic acid probes (Accuprobe culture identification tests by Gen-Probe Inc.; http://www.gen-probe.com/) are available for rapid identification of the *M. tuberculosis* complex, *M. avium* complex, *M. kansasii*, and *M. gordonae*.

Mycolic acid analysis by high-performance liquid chromatography (HPLC; sometimes referred to as high-pressure liquid chromatography). Mycolic acids are high-molecular weight β-hydroxy fatty acids containing from 20 to 90 carbon atoms. They are found in the cell walls of many medically important actinomycetes, including *Corynebacterium*, *Nocardia*, *Mycobacterium*, *Dietzia*, *Gordonia*, *Rhodococcus*, *Skermania*, *Tsukamurella*, and *Williamsia* spp. HPLC of mycolic acid esters is used in reference laboratories to identify many *Mycobacterium* spp. The HPLC pattern of the test organism is compared with reference strain patterns in an atlas. A fully integrated automated fluorescence detection HPLC system, called the Sherlock Mycobacteria Identification System (SMIS), is available from MIDI Inc. (http://www.midilabs.com/).

Essentials

Mycobacterium tuberculosis

- The major cause of tuberculosis
- Slow-growing, strongly acid-fast bacillus
- Nonphotochromogen
- Optimum growth temperature is 37°C
- Buff-colored rough colonies
- Niacin accumulation positive

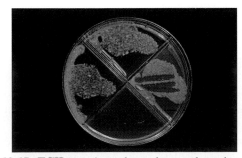

Figure 10-17. TCH test. A quadrant plate, each section of which contains thiophene-2-carboxylic acid hydrazide (TCH) in Middlebrook 7H10 agar. The plate was inoculated with three different strains of *M. tuberculosis* and one strain of *M. bovis*. The three strains of *M. tuberculosis* are growing on the plate, but *M. bovis* (bottom quadrant) is not. Hence, growth of *M. bovis* was inhibited by TCH. (From Winn WC Jr, et al. Koneman's Color Atlas and Textbook of Diagnostic Microbiology. 6th Ed. Philadelphia: Lippincott Williams & Wilkins, 2006.)

- Nitrate reduction positive
- 68°C catalase negative

SAFETY TIP

CLSI-Recommended Safety Precautions. The Clinical and Laboratory Standards Institute (CLSI) Document M29-A3 (see "References and Suggested Reading") recommends biosafety level 2 (BSL-2) practices and procedures, containment equipment, and facilities for nonaerosol-producing manipulations of clinical specimens. Aerosol-producing activities must be conducted in an annually certified biosafety cabinet. BSL-3 practices and procedures, containment equipment, and facilities are required for propagating and manipulating cultures for M. tuberculosis *in the laboratory. Every person working in a laboratory where clinical specimens that might contain* M. tuberculosis *are manipulated should be skin tested at least annually for* M. tuberculosis *infection.*

Nontuberculous Mycobacteria

Nontuberculous mycobacteria (NTM/MOTT) are usually acquired from the environment—for example, from soil, water, biofilms on home plumbing, and aquariums. NTM/MOTT can cause infections of the lungs, skin, soft tissue, bones, and lymph nodes, or infections throughout the body. Some of the most clinically important NTM/MOTT are listed in Table 10-5.

In general, members of the *M. tuberculosis* complex are considered nonphotochromogens. Pigmented mycobacteria may be preliminarily reported as NTM/MOTT and may be identified to species using biochemical tests (some of which were described earlier in the chapter), HPLC of mycolic acid esters, and molecular procedures.

Mycobacterium leprae

M. leprae is the etiologic agent of leprosy or Hansen disease. Estimates of the number of people with leprosy worldwide range from 4 million to 11 million. Most cases occur in South Asia, Southeast Asia, Africa, and Latin America. Although leprosy can be acquired in the United States, most U.S. cases are acquired elsewhere.

> *M. leprae* is the cause of leprosy or Hansen disease.

Clinical significance. Leprosy is a chronic disease with a long incubation period. Peripheral nerves and skin are principally affected. There are tuberculoid and lepromatous forms of the disease (see Chapter 18). Transmission occurs primarily by shedding of bacteria from the nose, rather than from skin lesions, and usually as a result of prolonged, intimate contact with infected persons. Leprosy occurs naturally in nine-banded armadillos, but it is unlikely that armadillos serve as important reservoirs of infection.

Clues to *M. leprae* Identification

Cellular morphology. *M. leprae* is a Gram-positive, acid-fast bacillus with rounded ends; it is 0.3 mm wide by 1.0 to 8.0 μm long.

Propagation in the laboratory. *M. leprae* will not grow in or on artificial media. When large numbers of *M. leprae* cells are required for research purposes (e.g., for development of new drugs or vaccines) they can be propagated in mouse footpads and nine-banded armadillos. Interestingly, *M. leprae* has the longest generation time of all known bacteria (about 12 days), in stark contrast to the 20-minute generation time of *E. coli*. In vivo, it is an obligate intracellular pathogen, with a special affinity for skin macrophages and peripheral nerve cells. Diagnosis of leprosy is made clinically, supported by the finding of acid-fast bacilli in slit-skin smears and/or histological examination of skin or nerve biopsy specimens. PCR methods have been developed but are not as yet commercially available.

> *M. leprae* will not grow in the laboratory on artificial media.

Antimicrobial Susceptibility Testing of Mycobacteria

Antimicrobial susceptibility testing of mycobacteria is usually only performed in large hospitals, medical centers, and reference laboratories. In the United States, the most popular methods for antimicrobial susceptibility testing of mycobacteria are the agar proportion method and a commercial method known as the BACTEC MGIT 960 method. The agar proportion method is considered to be the "gold standard" method. It uses plated media (usually Middlebrook 7H10 agar), containing antimycobacterial drugs. If a *Mycobacterium* isolate fails to grow on a particular plate, it was killed by the concentration of drug in the medium. Media for performing the agar proportion method is available from several commercial sources.

The BACTEC MGIT 960 method (BD Biosciences) employs liquid culture media, containing antimycobacterial drugs and dissolved oxygen, and an instrument equipped with a fluorescence sensor. The original amount of oxygen in the medium suppresses fluorescence. If the *Mycobacterium* isolate being tested is not killed by the drug, the organisms use the oxygen. As oxygen is depleted, fluorescence is produced, which is detected by the BACTEC MGIT 960 instrument. Thus, fluorescence indicates that the organisms were not killed by the drug. Other available susceptibility-testing methods are available, and additional methods are currently being developed and evaluated.

TABLE 10 - 5 Clinically Significant Nontuberculous Mycobacteria (NTM)

Rate of Growth	Species[a]	Clinical Significance	Pigment Production	Other Characteristics
Slow growers	M. avium complex, composed of M. avium and M. intracellulare	The most common NTM associated with human disease; a common cause of pulmonary and disseminated infection in AIDS patients	Nonphotochromogenic, but may develop a yellow pigment with age	Heterogeneous colony morphology; some colonies glossy and whitish; some smaller and translucent; some dry and flat
	M. genavense	Causes enteritis and genital and soft tissue infections in immunocompromised patients	Nonphotochromogenic	Will not grow on the media most commonly used in the TB lab
	M. haemophilum	Causes skin nodules, abscesses, cellulitis, and osteomyelitis in immunocompromised patients	Nonphotochromogenic	Prefers 30°C; requires ferric ammonium citrate or hemin for growth
	M. kansasii	Second only to M. avium complex as a cause of NTM lung disease; chronic pneumonia; less often, can cause cervical lymphadenitis, cutaneous abscesses, cellulitis, arthritis, fasciitis, osteomyelitis	Photochromogenic; the only Mycobacterium species that produces a bright yellow pigment on exposure to light	Long, beaded bacilli on acid-fast stain
	M. malmoense	Occasional cause of cervical lymphadenitis in children and chronic pulmonary infection in adults	Nonphotochromogenic	Very slow growing
	M. marinum	Causes epidemic or chronic skin lesions (swimming pool granulomas) and sporotrichoid mycobacteriosis	Photochromogenic	Often requires incubation at 30°C to 32°C for reliable recovery in vitro
	M. simiae	Causes chronic pulmonary disease	Photochromogenic	
	M. szulgai	Causes pulmonary, soft tissue, and joint infections	Scotochromogenic at 37°C; photochromogenic at 24°C	

(continued)

TABLE 10 - 5	Clinically Significant Nontuberculous Mycobacteria (NTM) (Continued)			
Rate of Growth	**Species**[a]	**Clinical Significance**	**Pigment Production**	**Other Characteristics**
Slow growers, cont.	M. ulcerans	Causes a chronic and deforming skin ulcer (Buruli ulcer) in Africa	Nonphotochromogenic	Difficult to culture in vitro
	M. xenopi	Causes chronic pulmonary disease and occasional disseminated infections	Nonphotochromogenic; some strains possess pale pigment that may intensify with age	Thermophilic; grows best at 42°C to 45°C; has been recovered from hot-water systems
Rapid growers	M. fortuitum group	Causes osteomyelitis, cellulitis, surgical wound and posttraumatic wound infections, central catheter–related infections, and rarely, chronic pulmonary disease	Nonphotochromogenic	
	M. abscessus	Causes chronic lung disease, posttraumatic wound infections, otitis media, cutaneous infections, catheter-associated bacteremia	Nonphotochromogenic	
	M. chelonae	Causes serious, disseminated nodular skin disease in immunosuppressed patients; also causes posttraumatic skin infections and catheter infections	Nonphotochromogenic	
	M. mucogenicum	An occasional cause of soft tissue infection, catheter-associated septicemia, and pulmonary infection	Nonphotochromogenic	

[a] An additional 40 or more species of NTM can be isolated from clinical specimens.

GENUS *BACILLUS*

The key feature of *Bacillus* spp. is that they produce endospores. Some people harbor the misconception that *Bacillus* spp. are the only aerobic endospore-forming bacteria, but in fact, there are approximately 10 genera of aerobic bacteria that can produce spores. Of these, the genus *Bacillus* contains the most clinically significant organisms. Thus, the following discussion will be limited to the genus *Bacillus*. The CD-ROM contains the names of other aerobic spore formers.

Although approximately 70 species are

Bacillus spp. produce spores, but they are not the only bacteria that do so. Some other aerobic bacteria also produce spores, as do anaerobes in the genus *Clostridium*.

in the genus *Bacillus*, relatively few species are of clinical significance. Of greatest medical importance is *B. anthracis*, the cause of anthrax, which has received a considerable amount of publicity in recent years as a potential bioterrorism and biological warfare agent (see Chapter 26). Next in importance is *B. cereus*, which can cause food poisoning and is an occasional cause of opportunistic infections, including eye, wound, burn, and urinary tract infections; septicemia; meningitis; endocarditis; pneumonia; and lung and brain abscesses. *B. licheniformis* and *B. subtilis* are examples of other, less clinically significant *Bacillus* spp.

> *B. anthracis*, the cause of anthrax, is a potential bioterrorism and biological warfare agent.

Although *Bacillus* spp. are Gram-positive bacilli, cells from older cultures will sometimes appear Gram variable or even Gram negative. Cells range in size from 0.4 to 2.0 μm in width by 3.0 to 9.0 μm in length. Virtually all *Bacillus* spp. are aerobes or facultative anaerobes. *Bacillus* spp. are spore formers. They produce endospores only under aerobic conditions. The spores are very resistant to heat, radiation, disinfectants, and desiccation. Most species are catalase positive. Most species are motile by means of peritrichous flagella; however, *B. anthracis* is nonmotile.

> *Bacillus* spp. are large spore-forming, Gram-positive bacilli. They produce spores only under aerobic conditions.

STUDY AID

Bacillus* versus *Clostridium. *Bacillus* spp. and *Clostridium* spp. (discussed in Chapter 17) are commonly isolated spore-forming, Gram-positive bacilli that resemble each other in Gram-stained preparations. Important distinctions between these genera are (1) their relationship to oxygen (*Bacillus* spp. are aerobic whereas *Clostridium* spp. are obligate or aerotolerant anaerobes); (2) conditions necessary for spore formation (*Bacillus* spp. sporulate only under aerobic conditions, whereas *Clostridium* spp. sporulate only under anaerobic conditions); and (3) their catalase reaction (*Bacillus* spp. are catalase positive, whereas *Clostridium* spp. are catalase negative).

Bacillus anthracis

Bacillus anthracis—the most important of the *Bacillus* spp.—is a member of the *B. cereus* group, which also contains *B. cereus*, *B. thuringiensis*, and *B. mycoides*.

Clinical significance. *B. anthracis* is the etiologic agent of anthrax, which is primarily a disease of animals such as cattle, sheep, goats, and horses. Vaccines are available to prevent anthrax in humans and animals. *B. anthracis* spores remain viable in soil for many years. Human anthrax may manifest itself in various ways, depending on the pathogen's portal of entry into the body. The most common form of anthrax—cutaneous anthrax—follows entry of *B. anthracis* spores through breaks in the skin. Cutaneous anthrax accounts for about 99% of all naturally occurring human anthrax cases. Inhalational or pulmonary anthrax follows inhalation of spores, and intestinal anthrax follows ingestion of spores.

> There are cutaneous, inhalational, and intestinal forms of anthrax.

The inhalational and intestinal forms of the disease are much more serious than cutaneous anthrax. Anthrax is sometimes referred to as woolsorter's disease because the spores may be present in wool, and people who handle unprocessed wool can become infected.

Virulence factors. Although virulent strains of *B. anthracis* produce a capsule, the capsule does not appear to protect the organisms from phagocytosis. An exotoxin is responsible for many of the clinical symptoms of anthrax. The exotoxin contains three components: protective antigen, edema factor, and lethal factor. Protective antigen binds to a host cell surface receptor, enabling edema factor and lethal factor to move into the cell. As the name implies, edema factor is responsible for the edema, or swelling, that occurs at the site of infection, but it also causes impaired neutrophil function. Lethal factor contributes to the death of host cells.

Clues to *B. anthracis* Identification

Cellular morphology. *B. anthracis* should be suspected whenever large Gram-positive bacilli are observed in blood, CSF, or material swabbed from cutaneous lesions. As stated by Logan and Turnbull (see "References and Suggested Reading"), "In a well-developed country such as the United States, it is unlikely that large numbers of Gram-positive bacteria in the blood at death are anything but *B. anthracis*."

> *B. anthracis* should be suspected whenever large Gram-positive bacilli are observed in blood, CSF, or material swabbed from cutaneous lesions.

B. anthracis cells are large (1 to 1.5 μm wide by 3 to 10 μm long), Gram-positive bacilli, with square or concave ends. They produce central-to-terminal ellipsoidal endospores, which do not cause swelling of the cells. Although spores may be seen in clinical materials, they are best observed in smears prepared from colonies. The spores do not stain with the Gram stain technique, but unstained areas within Gram-stained cells are suggestive of spores (Fig. 10-19).

Spores can be stained by flooding a fixed smear with 5% to 10% aqueous malachite green for up to 45 minutes. Heating is not required, but steaming for 3 to 6 minutes does enhance uptake of the stain into the spores and speeds the staining process. After washing, the smear is counterstained with 0.5% aqueous safranin for 30 seconds. Spores will appear green, within pink-to-red cells (Fig. 10-20). Spores

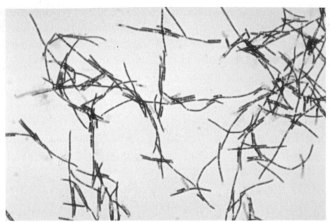

Figure 10-19. **Gram-stained** *Bacillus anthracis.* The unstained areas within the cells are spores. (Courtesy of Dr. William A. Clark and the Centers for Disease Control.)

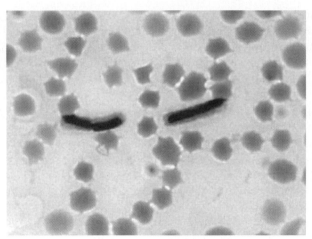

Figure 10-21. **B. anthracis stained with M'Fadyean capsule stain.** Pink-stained capsules can be seen on these *B. anthracis* cells grown in defibrinated horse blood. (Courtesy of Larry Stauffer, Oregon State Public Health Laboratory, and the Centers for Disease Control.)

can also be observed using phase-contrast microscopy. Some strains do not produce spores.

Although *B. anthracis* is encapsulated, the capsules are not observed in Gram-stained preparations. Various other stains, such as Giemsa, polychrome methylene blue, and India ink, can be used to demonstrate capsules, which are always present in tissue specimens. Using the M'Fadyean methylene blue stain, virulent *B. anthracis* strains appear as black-blue rectangular cells in very short chains (two or three cells) surrounded by a pink zone (the capsule). This appearance is known as the M'Fadyean reaction (Fig. 10-21).

Colonial morphology. On blood agar, *B. anthracis* produces large (4 to 5 mm in diameter), flat, irregular, creamy white or gray colonies, having a ground-glass texture (Fig. 10-22). Most strains are nonhemolytic. In fact, **CML professionals should suspect B. anthracis whenever a nonhemolytic, catalase-positive, aerobic Gram-positive bacillus is isolated.** Weak hemolysis is only rarely produced. *B. anthracis* grows in extended chains on solid medium, giving rise to fingerlike projections from the edge and surface of the colonies; this is

> It is important to remember that *B. anthracis* is a nonmotile and nonhemolytic *Bacillus* species.

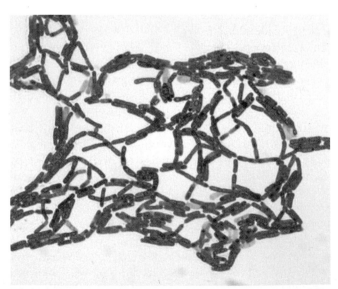

Figure 10-20. **A Bacillus species stained with malachite green/safranin spore stain.** The spores are stained green. (Courtesy of Larry Stauffer, Oregon State Public Health Laboratory, and the Centers for Disease Control.)

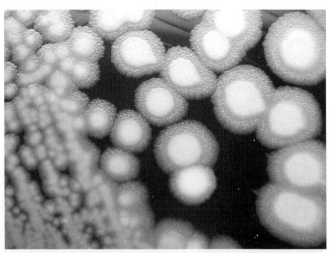

Figure 10-22. **Nonhemolytic, ground-glass colonies of B. anthracis on sheep blood agar, some in the lower-right corner with "Medusa head" projections.** (Courtesy of Larry Stauffer, Oregon State Public Health Laboratory, and the Centers for Disease Control.)

> CML professionals should suspect *B. anthracis* whenever a nonhemolytic, catalase-positive, aerobic Gram-positive bacillus is isolated.

referred to as a "Medusa head" appearance. Note that the Medusa head appearance is not unique to *B. anthracis*; other *Bacillus* spp. and *Clostridium sporogenes* also have this appearance.

Capsules will be produced if the medium contains 0.7% sodium bicarbonate and the plates are incubated overnight. This results in smooth mucoid colonies (Fig. 10-23). In the absence of bicarbonate and increased CO_2, colonies are rough. *B. anthracis* colonies are quite tenacious; they can be pulled into standing peaks, resembling beaten egg whites, with an inoculating loop. In liquid medium containing bicarbonate, *B. anthracis* produces an aromatic acid that changes the color of the broth to red. *B. anthracis* will not grow on MacConkey agar.

Polymyxin B-lysozyme-EDTA-thallous acetate (PLET) agar is selective for *B. anthracis*. On PLET agar, *B. anthracis* colonies are creamy white with a ground-glass texture and are smaller and smoother than colonies on plain heart infusion agar. Growth of most other *Bacillus* spp. is inhibited on PLET agar. *B. anthracis* is lecithinase positive on egg yolk agar, but so too are other members of the *B. cereus* group. Lecithinase will be discussed again in Chapter 17.

Laboratory tests. The catalase test can be used to differentiate *Bacillus* spp. from aerotolerant *Clostridium* spp. Bacillus spp. are catalase positive, whereas *Clostridium* spp. are catalase negative. Minisystems are available for the identification of *B. anthracis* and other *Bacillus* spp., including the API 20E/API 50CHB systems and Vitek card (bioMérieux Inc.;

www.biomerieux.com). Immunodiagnostic and molecular diagnostic procedures are also available. The MIDI system can also be used for fatty acid methyl ester analysis.

Essentials

Bacillus anthracis

- The cause of anthrax

- Large (1.0 to 1.5 wide by 3.0 to 5.0 μm long), nonmotile, aerobic Gram-positive bacilli, often in short or long chains

- Produces oval central-to-terminal spores that do not cause significant swelling of the cells

- Produces capsules in vivo, which can be demonstrated using various stains

- Produces tenacious nonhemolytic colonies on sheep blood agar, which are 2 to 5 mm in diameter

- Colonies are flat or slightly convex, irregularly round, with an irregular or wavy border and a ground-glass appearance

- Catalase positive

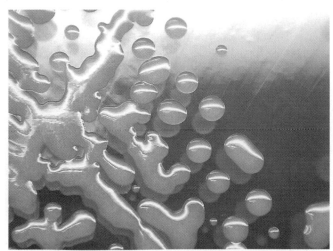

Figure 10-23. Mucoid B. anthracis colonies on 0.8% sodium bicarbonate medium. (Courtesy of Larry Stauffer, Oregon State Public Health Laboratory, and the Centers for Disease Control.)

Other *Bacillus* Species

Clinical significance. Infections caused by *Bacillus* spp. other than *B. anthracis* are extremely rare. Isolation of non-anthracis *Bacillus* spp. in the CML usually indicates contamination of the clinical specimen or the culture medium. *Bacillus cereus* can cause food poisoning and, like some other non-*anthracis Bacillus* spp. (e.g., *B. thuringiensis*, *B. licheniformis*, *B. subtilis*), is a very rare cause of opportunistic infections. *B. cereus* spores can survive normal cooking procedures. Ingestion of contaminated food can result in either of two types of food poisoning, apparently caused by different toxins. One type, characterized by diarrhea and abdominal pain, occurs 8 to 16 hours following ingestion. The other type, which occurs 1 to 5 hours after ingestion, is characterized by nausea and vomiting. Unlike *B. anthracis*, *B. cereus* is β-hemolytic and motile. Yes, it's true! *B. cereus* is pronounced "be serious." Perhaps somebody's idea of a joke?

Antibiotics produced by *Bacillus* spp. include bacitracin (produced by *B. subtilis*) and polymyxin (produced by *B. polymyxa*). *Bacillus* spp. are also used in the production

TABLE 10-6	Key Characteristics Used to Differentiate Between *Bacillus anthracis* and Other *Bacillus* spp.[a]	
Characteristic	***B. anthracis***	***B. cereus* and Other *Bacillus* spp.**
Hemolysis	Negative (usually)	Positive
Motility	Negative	Positive (usually)
Gelatin hydrolysis (7 days)	Negative	Positive
Salicin fermentation	Negative	Positive
Growth on phenylethyl alcohol (PEA) agar	Negative	Positive

Source: Koneman EW, Allen SD, Janda WM, et al. Color Atlas and Textbook of Diagnostic Microbiology. 5th ed. Philadelphia: Lippincott Williams & Wilkins, 1997.

of vitamins (B_{12}, B_2, biotin, riboflavin), antibiotic assays, monitoring of heat and gas sterilization (see Chapter 6), and the validation of disinfectants. *B. thuringiensis*, an insect pathogen, is used as an insecticide.

Laboratory tests. Key characteristics used to differentiate *B. anthracis* from other *Bacillus* spp. are shown in Table 10-6.

GENUS *LISTERIA*

There are six species in the genus *Listeria*, only one of which (*Listeria monocytogenes*) is considered a common human pathogen. *Listeria* spp. are widespread in nature. They are primarily found in soil and decaying vegetable matter but have also been isolated from silage, sewage, water, animal feed, food (e.g., fresh and frozen poultry, meats, and seafood; cheese made from unpasteurized milk), slaughterhouse waste, and in asymptomatic human and animal carriers. *L. monocytogenes* has been the cause of many foodborne (i.e., food poisoning) epidemics. The following features are common to all members of the genus:

- Short Gram-positive bacilli, 0.5 to 2 μm in length, occurring singly or in short chains; branching does not occur; filaments up to 20 mm long may be seen in older cultures, and older cultures may lose the ability to stain Gram-positive

- Motile, with one to five peritrichous flagella

- Non–spore forming

- Aerobic to facultatively anaerobic

- Optimum growth at 30°C to 37°C, but can grow at 4°C

- Catalase positive

- Oxidase negative

Listeria monocytogenes

Clinical significance. *L. monocytogenes* can grow at refrigerator temperature (4°C). **The most common portal of entry is ingestion of contaminated foods.** *L. monocytogenes* causes two general categories of infection: (1) gastrointestinal listeriosis, which has a short incubation period, usually 18 to 24 hours; and (2) invasive listeriosis, which has a longer incubation period, usually several weeks. In pregnant women, *L. monocytogenes* can cause influenza-like symptoms, followed by placentitis (infection of the placenta), amnionitis (infection of the amniotic sac), infection of the fetus, abortion, stillbirth, or premature birth. ***L. monocytogenes* is one of the major causes of neonatal meningitis.** (The other major causes of neonatal meningitis are *Streptococcus agalactiae* [group B strep], *E. coli*, and other members of the Enterobacteriaceae family.) The mortality rate is high in neonatal infections and central nervous system infections of immunocompromised patients. The organism may cause meningitis, encephalitis, and septicemia in nonpregnant adults. Less common manifestations of listeriosis include endocarditis, arthritis, osteomyelitis, intra-abdominal abscesses, endophthalmitis (inflammation of tissues within the eyeball), and pleuropulmonary infections. Observing Gram-positive bacilli in CSF, blood, amniotic fluid, respiratory secretions, placental or cutaneous swabs, gastric aspirate, or the meconium (first intestinal discharges) of a neonate could be of value for early diagnosis of listeriosis.

> *L. monocytogenes* is a cause of food poisoning and a major cause of neonatal meningitis.

Routine stool cultures to detect *L. monocytogenes* are not necessary when diagnosing gastroenteritis. However, gastrointestinal listeriosis should be suspected when routine enteric pathogens have been ruled out.

Virulence factors. *L. monocytogenes* is a facultative intracellular pathogen. It possesses carbohydrate molecules on its surface that enable it to attach to protein molecules, or receptors, on the surface of host cells. The organism then enters host cells by inducing phagocytosis. *L. monocytogenes*

> *L. monocytogenes* is a facultative intracellular pathogen.

produces at least three hemolysins, including one called listeriolysin O. The other two hemolysins are phospholipases, one of which is referred to as lecithinase. All three hemolysins destroy cell membranes. It is thought that listeriolysin O plays a role in dissolution of phagosome membranes, enabling the organisms to escape from phagosomes. By dissolving cell membranes, the hemolysins enable the organisms to move from cell to cell.

Drug resistance. Cephalosporins appear to be ineffective against *L. monocytogenes* in vivo and should not be administered when listeriosis is suspected. Some strains have shown resistance to chloramphenicol, macrolides, and tetracycline but widespread drug resistance is currently not a problem. Ampicillin is the drug of choice for treating listeriosis.

Clues to *L. monocytogenes* Identification

Cellular morphology. *Listeria* cells are short (0.4 to 0.5 μm wide by 0.5 to 2 μm long), regular, nonbranching, non-spore-forming Gram-positive bacilli that occur singly or in short chains (Fig. 10-24). Morphologically, they can be mistaken for streptococci. Older or rough colonies may contain filaments up to 20 μm long. Cells are motile at 28°C but much less so at 37°C.

Colonial morphology. *Listeria* spp. are facultative anaerobes. Colonies are small (1 to 2 mm in diameter after 1 to 2 days of incubation), smooth, and have a characteristic blue, blue-gray, or blue-green sheen on certain types of media (discussed in the following paragraphs). Although the optimum growth temperature for *Listeria* spp. is between 30°C and 37°C, growth occurs at 4°C within a few days. On blood agar, *L. monocytogenes* shows subdued narrow-zone hemolysis (Fig. 10-25). The most frequently isolated nonpathogenic *Listeria* species—*L. innocuae*—is nonhemolytic.

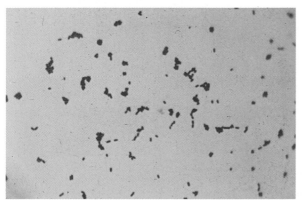

Figure 10-24. **Gram-stained smear of *Listeria monocytogenes*.** (From Winn WC Jr, et al. Koneman's Color Atlas and Textbook of Diagnostic Microbiology. 6th Ed. Philadelphia: Lippincott Williams & Wilkins, 2006.)

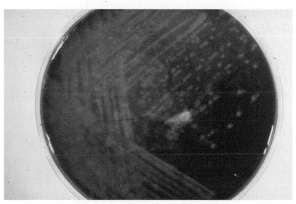

Figure 10-25. **Small, β-hemolytic colonies of *L. monocytogenes* on sheep blood agar after 72 hours incubation at 35°C to 37°C.** (From Winn WC Jr, et al. Koneman's Color Atlas and Textbook of Diagnostic Microbiology. 6th Ed. Philadelphia: Lippincott Williams & Wilkins, 2006.)

 STUDY AID **Use of the Term *Facultative*.** Throughout this book, the term *facultative* means "having a choice." For example, facultative anaerobes have a choice: they can grow either in the presence or absence of oxygen. Facultative intracellular pathogens have a choice: they can grow outside of or within host cells. The term *facultative* pops up again in Chapter 21. Facultative parasites have a choice. Although they can be parasitic, they do not have to be. They are capable of a free-living existence.

Cold enrichment. *L. monocytogenes* will grow at 4°C, whereas many other pathogens will not. A technique known as cold enrichment is sometimes used to improve recovery of *L. monocytogenes*, which is sometimes difficult to isolate from clinical specimens, especially biopsy and autopsy tissue specimens. One part of specimen is mixed with 9 parts of trypticase-soy broth, and the mixture is held at 4°C for several days or longer. The mixture is frequently subcultured onto solid media, such as blood agar and colistin-nalidixic acid agar.

Several different types of media are used to isolate and identify *L. monocytogenes*, including lithium chloride-phenylethanol-moxalactam, Oxford, modified Oxford, and polymyxin-acriflavin-lithium chloride-ceftazidime esculin-mannitol agars, and CHROMagar *Listeria*, all of which are described in the following paragraphs.

Lithium chloride-phenylethanol-moxalactam (LPM) agar. LPM is a highly selective medium for *Listeria* spp. Colonies suspected of being *L. monocytogenes* should be examined using a stereoscopic microscope at ×15 to ×25. When using obliquely transmitted light (i.e., by positioning the microscope mirror at a 45-degree angle to the light beam), *Listeria* colonies on LPM are blue. Colonies of other bacteria are yellowish or orange.

Oxford and modified Oxford agars. These media are enriched and selective. After 24 hours of incubation at 37°C, *Listeria* colonies are black, 1 to 3 mm in diameter, and surrounded by a black halo. Blackening is the result of esculin hydrolysis and the formation of black iron-phenol compounds in the medium.

Polymyxin-acriflavin-lithium chloride-ceftazidime esculin-mannitol (PALCAM) agar. On PALCAM agar, *Listeria* colonies are gray-green, about 2 mm in diameter, with black sunken centers.

A commercial product called CHROMagar *Listeria* can be used to differentiate *L. monocytogenes* from other *Listeria* spp. On this medium, *L. monocytogenes* colonies are blue with a white halo. The white halo is caused by a phospholipase produced specifically by *L. monocytogenes*. Growth of other bacteria will be inhibited, or colonies will appear blue with no halo or colorless.

Laboratory tests. Invasive listeriosis should be suspected whenever Gram-positive bacilli are observed in or isolated from blood specimens from pregnant women, as well as neonatal CSF, blood, and other types of specimens from newborns. When grown at 20°C to 25°C, *L. monocytogenes* exhibits a characteristic "tumbling" motility, which can be observed in a wet mount.

> Invasive listeriosis should be suspected whenever Gram-positive bacilli are observed in or isolated from blood specimens from pregnant women, as well as from CSF, blood, and other types of specimens from neonates.

When grown in tubes of liquid media or semisolid agar, *L. monocytogenes* exhibits a characteristic "umbrella" growth pattern near the surface of the medium (Fig. 10-26).

> Associate the terms *tumbling motility* and *umbrella growth pattern* with *L. monocytogenes*.

Presumptive identification of *L. monocytogenes* can be made based on the following observations and test results:

- Short, nonbranching Gram-positive bacilli, occurring singly or in short chains
- Observation of tumbling motility in a wet mount and/or umbrella-shaped growth in a liquid or semisolid agar medium
- Catalase positive
- Esculin hydrolysis positive (Fig. 10-27)

Additional observations of value in identification of *L. monocytogenes* are (1) growth at 4°C, (2) optimal motility at 25°C, and (3) a narrow zone of hemolysis.

CAUTION

Distinguishing Between Common Causes of Neonatal Meningitis. Both *Streptococcus agalactiae* (group B strep) and *L. monocytogenes* are common causes of neonatal meningitis. When examining Gram-stained CSF sediment, it is difficult to impossible to

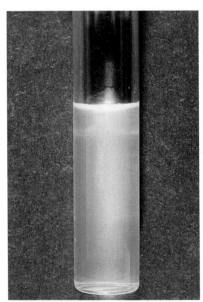

Figure 10-26. **Umbrella-shaped growth of *L. monocytogenes* after 24 hours of growth in a semisolid motility medium incubated at 25°C.** (From Winn WC Jr, et al. Koneman's Color Atlas and Textbook of Diagnostic Microbiology. 6th Ed. Philadelphia: Lippincott Williams & Wilkins, 2006.)

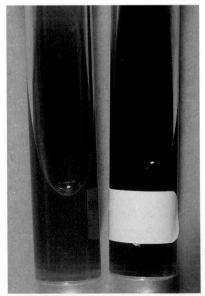

Figure 10-27. **Bile-esculin test.** To the left is an uninoculated bile-esculin agar slant. To the right is a bile-esculin agar slant that was inoculated with *L. monocytogenes*. Blackening of the medium in the inoculated slant is a result of hydrolysis of esculin. (From Winn WC Jr, et al. Koneman's Color Atlas and Textbook of Diagnostic Microbiology. 6th Ed. Philadelphia: Lippincott Williams & Wilkins, 2006.)

TABLE 10 - 7   Ways to Differentiate *Listeria* spp. from Other Gram-Positive Bacteria

	Cellular Morphology	Motility	Catalase Reaction	Ability to Grow at 4°C
Listeria spp. vs. streptococci	*Listeria* spp. are bacilli; streptococci are cocci	*Listeria* spp. are motile; streptococci are nonmotile	*Listeria* spp. are catalase positive; streptococci are catalase negative	
Listeria spp. vs. *Erysipelothrix* spp.[a]		*Listeria* spp. are motile; *Erysipelothrix* spp. are nonmotile	*Listeria* spp. are catalase positive; *Erysipelothrix* spp. are catalase negative	*Listeria* spp. grow at 4°C; *Erysipelothrix* spp. do not
Listeria spp. vs. *Lactobacillus* spp.		*Listeria* spp. are motile; *Lactobacillus* spp. are usually nonmotile	*Listeria* spp. are catalase positive; *Lactobacillus* spp. are catalase negative	

[a] Also helpful is the fact that *L. monocytogenes* is β-hemolytic, whereas *E. rhusiopathiae* produces a greenish discoloration beneath colonies on blood agar after 48 hours of incubation.

distinguish the elongated Gram-positive cocci of *S. agalactiae* from the short Gram-positive bacilli of *L. monocytogenes*. Both produce weak β-hemolysis. Both are CAMP test positive (the CAMP test is described in Chapter 9). The motility of *L. monocytogenes* may not be observed in cultures grown at 35°C. *Question:* What is the quickest way to tell the bacteria apart? *Answer:* The catalase test. *S. agalactiae* is catalase negative (as are all *Streptococcus* spp.), whereas *L. monocytogenes* is catalase positive.

Table 10-7 shows how *L. monocytogenes* can be differentiated from some other Gram-positive bacteria with which it is sometimes confused. Several minisystems are available for identification of *L. monocytogenes*, including the API-Listeria test (bioMérieux Inc.; http://www.biomerieux.com/) and Micro-ID Listeria (Remel; http://www.remelinc.com/). The API Coryne System (bioMérieux Inc.) can be used to identify *Listeria* to the genus level. A DNA probe assay, available from Gen-Probe Inc. (http://www.gen-probe.com/), can be used for rapid identification of *L. monocytogenes* from colonies on primary isolation plates.

Essentials

Listeria monocytogenes

- A cause of food poisoning and a major cause of neonatal meningitis

- Cold enrichment can be used to increase recovery from clinical specimens

- Short, nonbranching Gram-positive bacilli, occurring singly or in short chains

- Characteristic tumbling motility in a wet mount and umbrella-shaped growth in a liquid or semisolid agar medium

- Catalase positive

- Esculin hydrolysis positive

GENUS *LACTOBACILLUS*

The genus *Lactobacillus* comprises more than 50 species, some named and some unnamed. The few clinically significant species are rare causes of endocarditis, neonatal meningitis, chorioamnionitis, pleuropulmonary infections, and septicemia.

Lactobacilli are common members of the indigenous microflora of various body sites, such as the oral cavity, gastrointestinal tract, and vagina. *Lactobacillus* spp. are the predominant members of the indigenous microflora of the vagina, where they are considered "good guys" (Fig. 10-28). They produce hydrogen peroxide (H_2O_2), which keeps potentially pathogenic bacteria in check. Should something cause a decline in the vaginal *Lactobacillus* population—for instance, prolonged use of antibacterial agents—superinfections with other bacteria or yeasts may occur in the vagina. These

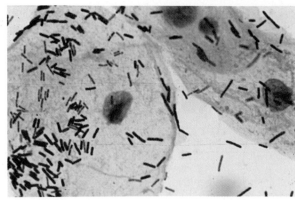

Figure 10-28. Gram-positive, *Lactobacillus* morphotype bacteria and large, pink-stained epithelial cells in a normal vaginal specimen. (From Winn WC Jr, et al. Koneman's Color Atlas and Textbook of Diagnostic Microbiology. 6th Ed. Philadelphia: Lippincott Williams & Wilkins, 2006.)

superinfections can lead to conditions such as yeast vaginitis and bacterial vaginosis. *Lactobacillus* preparations are sometimes prescribed for treatment of bacterial vaginosis and diarrheal diseases to reestablish the presence of lactobacilli in the vagina and gastrointestinal tract, respectively. The use of live microorganisms in this manner is known as **probiotics.**

Although lactobacilli are only rare causes of human infection, they are often isolated from clinical specimens as indigenous microflora contaminants. Thus, they must be differentiated from other Gram-positive bacilli. The following are the key features of *Lactobacillus* spp.:

- Slender Gram-positive bacilli that may be long or short; often have squared-off ends; may appear slightly bent, as coryneform bacilli, or sometimes as coccobacilli; occur singly, in pairs, or in short chains (Fig. 10-29)

- Most lactobacilli are microaerophiles, but some species are obligate anaerobes

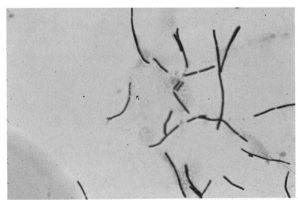

Figure 10-29. *Lactobacillus* sp. in a Gram-stained blood culture. (From Winn WC Jr, et al. Koneman's Color Atlas and Textbook of Diagnostic Microbiology. 6th Ed. Philadelphia: Lippincott Williams & Wilkins, 2006.)

- Non–spore forming (unlike *Bacillus* spp.)
- Nonmotile
- Colonies usually less than 0.5 mm in diameter
- Usually α-hemolytic
- Catalase negative (unlike *Bacillus* spp.)
- Oxidase negative
- Nitrate negative
- Do not produce hydrogen sulfide in triple-sugar iron agar (see Chapter 12)
- Many are vancomycin resistant

GARDNERELLA VAGINALIS

Clinical significance. *Gardnerella vaginalis* is the only species in the genus. It is found as part of the indigenous microflora of the vagina and the anorectal area of both males and females. *G. vaginalis* has long been thought to play a role in bacterial vaginosis, which is a synergistic infection involving several types of bacteria. Bacterial vaginosis can progress to serious complications, such as premature rupture of membranes, preterm delivery, chorioamnionitis, postpartum fever, and neonatal infections.

Gram-stained smears of vaginal discharge material from patients with bacterial vaginosis reveal the presence of large numbers of Gram-negative and Gram-variable bacilli and coccobacilli and the absence of Gram-positive lactobacilli (Fig. 10-30). Bacterial vaginosis is usually diagnosed

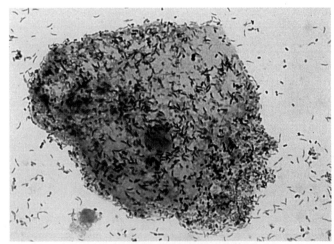

Figure 10-30. Gram-stained squamous epithelial cell in a vaginal secretion. The cell, which is covered with various Gram-positive and Gram-negative bacteria, but an absence of *Lactobacillus* morphotype bacteria, is referred to as a clue cell because the presence of these bacteria-covered cells provides evidence that the patient has bacterial vaginosis. (From Marler LM, Siders JA, Allen SD. Direct Smear Atlas. Philadelphia: Lippincott Williams & Wilkins, 2001.)

using either the Amsel criteria or the Nugent criteria (see Chapter 18).

Clues to *G. vaginalis* Identification

Cellular morphology. *G. vaginalis* cells are thin, Gram-variable bacilli and coccobacilli. Gram variability is caused by the thin layer of peptidoglycan in its cell walls. *G. vaginalis* is nonmotile.

Colonial morphology. Culture techniques are not necessary for the diagnosis of bacterial vaginosis, and *G. vaginalis* can be isolated from healthy women. If culture for *G. vaginalis* is desired, vaginal swabs should be inoculated to Vaginalis agar, and the plates should be incubated at 35°C to 37°C in a 5% CO_2 atmosphere. Colonies of *G. vaginalis* are β-hemolytic on media containing human or rabbit blood but are nonhemolytic on sheep blood agar. Usually, only a narrow band of diffuse hemolysis is present at 24 hours.

Laboratory tests. *G. vaginalis* is catalase negative and has a slow fermentative metabolism. Commercial biochemical-based identification procedures (e.g., the API Coryne system and Vitek NHI card manufactured by bio-Mérieux Inc.) and molecular diagnostic procedures are available for identification of *G. vaginalis*. Antimicrobial disks are also of some value in identification. *G. vaginalis* is inhibited by 50 μg of metronidazole and 5 μg of trimethoprim but is not inhibited by 1 mg of sulfonamide. Metronidazole is the drug of choice for treatment of bacterial vaginosis.

GENUS *ERYSIPELOTHRIX*

There are two species in the genus *Erysipelothrix*, only one of which (*E. rhusiopathiae*) is known to cause human disease. *E. rhusiopathiae* is very common in nature and is associated with many types of animals. It commonly causes a disease called swine erysipelas in pigs. Disease in humans is a zoonosis.

Erysipelothrix rhusiopathiae

Clinical significance. In humans, *E. rhusiopathiae* causes a cutaneous infection called **erysipeloid,** characterized by purplish red bumps, usually located on the hands and fingers. Less commonly, *E. rhusiopathiae* causes septicemia, endocarditis, and arthritis. The most common route of entry is through a break in the skin following an animal bite or direct contact with contaminated animals, animal products, fish, or soil. Diagnosis is usually based on clinical presentation, a history of exposure, and Gram stain and culture of skin biopsy specimens. Blood is the appropriate specimen for diagnosis of disseminated disease.

CAUTION **Beware of Similar Terms.** *Erysipelas* Versus *Erysipeloid*. Erysipelas and erysipeloid are specific types of **cellulitis** (inflammation of subcutaneous, loose connective tissue). **Erysipelas** is caused by *Streptococcus pyogenes* and is characterized by hot, red, edematous, cutaneous eruptions, usually accompanied by severe constitutional symptoms (see Chapter 9). **Erysipeloid** is typically a self-limiting cellulitis of the hand caused by *E. rhusiopathiae*. Erysipeloid appears as a dusky or shadowy erythema with a diamondlike configuration, usually at the site of a wound obtained while handling fish or meat. Erysipeloid may become generalized, with plaques of erythema and blisters and occasionally, severe toxemia.

Clues to *E. rhusiopathiae* Identification

Cellular morphology. *E. rhusiopathiae* cells are usually short (0.8 to 2.5 μm in length), nonmotile, non-spore-forming Gram-positive organisms with rounded ends (Fig. 10-31). They occur singly, in short chains or long nonbranching filaments. The presence of long, slender, Gram-positive rods in biopsy specimens from skin lesions is suggestive of *E. rhusiopathiae*. Although *E. rhusiopathiae* is Gram positive, cells can decolorize easily and, often with a beaded appearance, may look like Gram-negative bacilli with Gram-positive granules.

Colonial morphology. *E. rhusiopathiae* is a facultative anaerobe. It produces pinpoint colonies on blood agar plates after 24 hours of incubation (Fig. 10-32). After incubating for 48 hours, greenish discoloration frequently develops beneath colonies. Two distinct colony types are observed:

- Small, smooth colonies, 0.3 to 1.5 mm in diameter; transparent; convex; circular; entire edges; cells from small

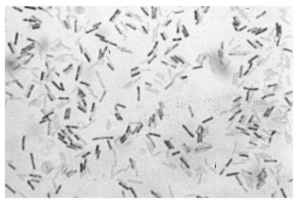

***Figure 10-31.* Gram-stained smear of *Erysipelothrix rhusiopathiae*.** (From Winn WC Jr, et al. Koneman's Color Atlas and Textbook of Diagnostic Microbiology. 6th Ed. Philadelphia: Lippincott Williams & Wilkins, 2006.)

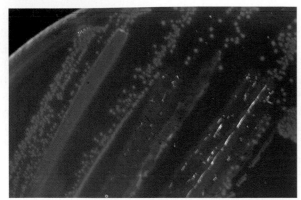

Figure 10-32. **Colonies of *E. rhusiopathiae* on sheep blood agar after 24 hours of incubation at 35°C.** (From Winn WC Jr, et al. Koneman's Color Atlas and Textbook of Diagnostic Microbiology. 6th Ed. Philadelphia: Lippincott Williams & Wilkins, 2006.)

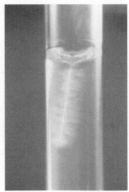

Figure 10-33. **"Test tube brush" growth of *E. rhusiopathiae* in soft gelatin agar.** (From Koneman EW, Allen SD, Janda WM, et al. Color Atlas and Textbook of Diagnostic Microbiology. 5th ed. Philadelphia: Lippincott Williams & Wilkins, 1997.)

colonies are bacilli or coccobacilli, sometimes in short chains

- Larger, rough colonies; flatter; more opaque; matt surface; irregular, fimbriated edge; cells from large colonies are long filaments, often more than 60 μm long

Laboratory tests. *E. rhusiopathiae* is catalase-, oxidase-, and urease-negative. It produces hydrogen sulfide (H_2S) in triple-sugar iron (TSI) medium. Thus, **production of H_2S in TSI medium by a Gram-positive bacillus is highly suggestive of *E. rhusiopathiae*.** (TSI and urease tests are described in Chapter 12.) Another highly characteristic trait of *E. rhusiopathiae* is its "pipe cleaner" or "test tube brush" pattern of growth in gelatin stab cultures incubated at 22°C (Fig. 10-33). *E. rhusiopathiae* can grow at temperatures from 5°C to 42°C and in high salt concentrations (up to 8.5% NaCl). This bacillus can be identified using Vitek automated systems (bioMérieux Inc.; www.biomerieux-vitek.com) or the API Coryne System (bioMérieux Inc.).

> Production of H_2S in a TSI medium by a Gram-positive bacillus is highly suggestive of *E. rhusiopathiae*.

> Associate the terms *pipe cleaner* or *test tube brush* growth with *E. rhusiopathiae*.

TABLE 10 - 8	Observations and Tests of Value for Preliminary Identification of an Unknown Gram-Positive Bacillus	
Category of Gram-Positive Bacilli	**Genus**	**Observations and Test Results**
1	*Bacillus*	Spore former
	Listeria	Non–spore former, catalase positive
	Lactobacillus	Non–spore former, catalase negative, does not produce H_2S in TSI medium
	Erysipelothrix	Non–spore former, catalase negative, produces H_2S in TSI medium
2	*Corynebacterium*	Catalase positive, club-shaped cells
	Nocardia	Produces vegetative substrate filaments/hyphae, weakly acid fast, produces aerial filaments/hyphae
	Mycobacterium	Produces vegetative substrate filaments/hyphae, strongly acid fast

H_2S, hydrogen sulfide; TSI, triple-sugar iron.

IDENTIFICATION OF AN UNKNOWN GRAM-POSITIVE BACILLUS

The first step in the identification of an unknown Gram-positive bacillus is to examine its cellular and colonial morphologies. Based on cellular morphology, Gram-positive bacilli can be divided into two categories. Category 1 Gram-positive bacilli are regular bacilli, with long edges that are parallel but not curved. Category 2 Gram-positive bacilli are irregular bacilli, with long edges that are curved but not parallel. Information in Table 10-8 pertains only to presumptive identifications of Gram-positive bacilli mentioned in this chapter. Identification of species of an unknown Gram-positive bacilli often requires chromatographic methods. Readers should bear in mind that many additional Gram-positive bacilli can be isolated from clinical specimens. Anaerobic Gram-positive bacilli are described in Chapter 17.

Chapter Review

- The aerobic actinomycetes are Gram-positive to Gram-variable bacilli. Medically important mycolic acid-containing actinomycetes are contained in the genera *Corynebacterium*, *Nocardia*, and *Mycobacterium*.

- Diphtheria is primarily an upper respiratory tract disease caused by diphtheria toxin-producing strains of *Corynebacterium diphtheriae*.

- Not all strains of *C. diphtheriae* cause disease. Only toxigenic strains (those capable of producing diphtheria toxin) are virulent. Nontoxigenic strains are avirulent.

- *C. diphtheriae* is a Gram-positive, club-shaped bacterium that grows well on blood agar or the selective media CTBA agar and Tinsdale agar.

- Medically important *Nocardia* spp. include the *N. asteroides* complex and *N. brasiliensis*. They are weakly acid fast or partially acid fast with the modified Kinyoun acid-fast stain.

- *Mycobacterium* spp. are aerobic acid-fast organisms. Medically important mycobacteria include *M. tuberculosis* complex organisms, *M. leprae*, and NTM/MOTT.

- Acid-fast staining procedures include Ziehl-Neelsen, Kinyoun (cold), modified Kinyoun, and auramine-rhodamine fluorescent techniques.

- Tuberculosis is a major health concern worldwide, with many strains of *M. tuberculosis* being multidrug resistant.

- *M. tuberculosis* is acid fast and niacin and nitrate positive.

- *M. leprae* is the etiologic agent of leprosy or Hansen disease.

- Clinically significant *Bacillus* species include *B. anthracis*, the cause of anthrax, and *B. cereus*, a cause of food poisoning. All *Bacillus* species form spores.

- There are three forms of anthrax: cutaneous anthrax (the most common type), inhalational or pulmonary anthrax, and intestinal anthrax. *B. anthracis* is a potential bioterrorism agent.

- Although *Listeria* spp. are widely distributed in nature, there is only one medically important species: *Listeria monocytogenes*, the causative agent of listeriosis.

- *L. monocytogenes* exhibits a characteristic tumbling motility in a wet mount and an umbrella growth pattern near the surface of liquid or semisolid media.

- *Lactobacillus* spp. are common members of the indigenous microflora of various body sites, including the vagina.

- *Erysipelothrix rhusiopathiae* is the cause of erysipeloid in humans. *E. rhusiopathiae* growth exhibits characteristic pipe cleaner or test tube brush patterns in gelatin stab cultures.

New Terms and Abbreviations

After studying Chapter 10, you should be familiar with the following terms, which are defined within the chapter and in the Glossary at the back of the book:

Acid-fast bacteria

Anorexia

Bacteriophage

Cellulitis

"Chinese letter" arrangement

Coryneform bacteria

Diphtheria toxin

Diphtheroid

Dysphagia

Erysipelas

Erysipeloid

Hematogenous dissemination

Hemoptysis

Malaise

Neuritis

Non-acid-fast bacteria

Nonphotochromogen

Nontuberculous mycobacteria (NTM)

Palisade arrangement

Photochromogen

Probiotics

Scotochromogen

References and Suggested Reading

Bartlett JG. Agents of actinomycosis. In: Gorbach SL, Bartlett JG, Blacklow NR, eds. Infectious Disease. 3rd Ed. Philadelphia: Lippincott Williams & Wilkins, 2004.

Bille J, et al. *Listeria* and *Erysipelothrix*. In: Murray PR, Baron EJ, Jorgensen JH, Pfaller MA, Yolken RH, eds. Manual of Clinical Microbiology. 8th Ed. Washington, DC: ASM Press, 2003.

Boone DR, Castenholz RW, eds. The Archaea and the Deeply Branching and Phototrophic Bacteria. New York: Springer-

Verlag, 2001. *Bergey's Manual of Systematic Bacteriology*, vol 1. 2nd Ed.

Broome C, et al. *Listeria monocytogenes*. In: Gorbach SL, Bartlett JG, Blacklow NR, eds. Infectious Disease. 3rd Ed. Philadelphia: Lippincott Williams & Wilkins, 2004.

Brown JM, McNeil MM. *Nocardia, Rhodococcus, Gordonia, Actinomadura, Streptomyces*, and other aerobic actinomycetes. In: Murray PR, Baron EJ, Jorgensen JH, Pfaller MA, Yolken RH, eds. Manual of Clinical Microbiology. 8th Ed. Washington, DC: ASM Press, 2003.

Evangelista AT, et al. Rapid systems and instruments for antimicrobial susceptibility testing of bacteria. In: Manual of Commercial Methods in Clinical Microbiology. Washington, DC: ASM Press, 2002.

Fennelly KP, Ellner JJ. *Mycobacterium tuberculosis* and other mycobacteria. In: Gorbach SL, Bartlett JG. Blacklow NR, eds. Infectious Disease. 3rd Ed. Philadelphia: Lippincott Williams & Wilkins, 2004.

Funke G. Algorithm for identification of aerobic Gram-positive rods. In: Murray PR, Baron EJ, Jorgensen JH, Pfaller MA, Yolken RH, eds. Manual of Clinical Microbiology. 8th Ed. Washington, DC: ASM Press, 2003.

Funke G, Bernard KA. Coryneform Gram-positive rods. In: Murray PR, Baron EJ, Jorgensen JH, Pfaller MA, Yolken RH, eds. Manual of Clinical Microbiology. 8th Ed. Washington, DC: ASM Press, 2003.

Halsey N, Bartlett JG. Corynebacteria. In: Gorbach SL, Bartlett JG, Blacklow NR, eds. Infectious Disease. 3rd Ed. Philadelphia: Lippincott Williams & Wilkins, 2004.

Koneman EW, Allen SD, Janda WM, et al. Color Atlas and Textbook of Diagnostic Microbiology. 5th ed. Philadelphia: Lippincott Williams & Wilkins, 1997.

Lockwood DNJ, McAdam KPWJ. Leprosy. In: Gorbach SL, Bartlett JG, Blacklow NR, eds. Infectious Disease. 3rd Ed. Philadelphia: Lippincott Williams & Wilkins, 2004.

Logan NA, Turnbull PCB. *Bacillus* and other aerobic endospore-forming bacteria. In: Murray PR, Baron EJ, Jorgensen JH, Pfaller MA, Yolken RH, eds. Manual of Clinical Microbiology. 8th Ed. Washington, DC: ASM Press, 2003.

Nerad JL. *Erysipelothrix rhusiopathiae*. In: Gorbach SL, Bartlett JG, Blacklow NR, eds. Infectious Disease. 3rd Ed. Philadelphia: Lippincott Williams & Wilkins, 2004.

Penn CC, Klotz SA. *Bacillus anthracis* and other aerobic Gram-positive spore-forming bacilli. In: Gorbach SL, Bartlett JG, Blacklow NR, eds. Infectious Disease. 3rd Ed. Philadelphia: Lippincott Williams & Wilkins, 2004.

Penn CC, Klotz SA. *Bacillus* species infections. In: Gorbach SL, Bartlett JG, Blacklow NR, eds. Infectious Disease. 3rd Ed. Philadelphia: Lippincott Williams & Wilkins, 2004.

Pfyffer GE, et al. *Mycobacterium*: general characteristics, isolation, and staining procedures. In: Murray PR, Baron EJ, Jorgensen JH, Pfaller MA, Yolken RH, eds. Manual of Clinical Microbiology. 8th Ed. Washington, DC: ASM Press, 2003.

Protection of Laboratory Workers from Occupationally Acquired Infections: Approved Guideline. 3rd Ed. CLSI Document M29-A3. Wayne, PA: Clinical and Laboratory Standards Institute, 2005.

Roberts GD, et al. Mycobacteria. In: Truant AL, ed. Manual of Commercial Methods in Clinical Microbiology. Washington, DC: ASM Press, 2002.

Salyers AA, Whitt DD. Bacterial Pathogenesis: A Molecular Approach. Washington, DC: ASM Press, 1994.

Vincent V, et al. *Mycobacterium*: phenotypic and genotypic identification. In: Murray PR, Baron EJ, Jorgensen JH, Pfaller MA, Yolken RH, eds. Manual of Clinical Microbiology. 8th Ed. Washington, DC: ASM Press, 2003.

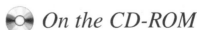 *On the CD-ROM*

- Aerobic Endospore-Forming Bacteria
- The Elek Test
- Additional Self-Assessment Exercises
- Case Study
- Puzzle

Self-Assessment Exercises

After studying Chapter 10, answer the following questions.

1. Name three medically important mycolic acid–containing actinomycetes.

   A._____

   B._____

   C._____

2. The predominant portals of entry and major target organs for *Mycobacterium tuberculosis* are

   _____.

3. On which medium will *Corynebacterium diphtheriae* colonies be black, surrounded by a brown halo?

   A. Löwenstein-Jensen

   B. MacConkey agar

   C. Tinsdale medium

   D. Sheep blood agar

4. Which of the following characteristics differentiate *Bacillus anthracis* from *Bacillus cereus*?

   A. *B. cereus* is hemolytic on blood agar and motile; *B. anthracis* is nonhemolytic on blood agar and nonmotile.

   B. *B. cereus* is nonhemolytic on blood agar and is motile; *B. anthracis* is hemolytic on blood agar and nonmotile.

   C. *B. cereus* is nonhemolytic on blood agar and is nonmotile; *B. anthracis* is hemolytic on blood agar and is motile.

   D. *B. cereus* is lipase positive and *B. anthracis* is lipase negative.

5. Which of the following genera contains aerobic spore-forming bacteria?

   A. *Listeria*

   B. *Lactobacillus*

   C. *Corynebacteria*

   D. *Bacillus*

Match the organism in the left column to the best description or appropriate disease in the right column.

6. _____ *M. marinum*   A. partially acid fast

7. _____ *E. rhusiopathiae*   B. food poisoning

8. _____ *Nocardia* spp.   C. photochromogen

9. _____ *B. cereus*   D. "pipe cleaner" or "test tube brush" growth

10. Digestion and decontamination of sputum samples for mycobacteria workup are performed to

A. reduce or eliminate contaminating bacteria.

B. concentrate any organisms for further identification.

C. release any mycobacteria that are trapped in the mucin and cells.

D. all of the above.

Gram-Negative Cocci and Related Bacteria

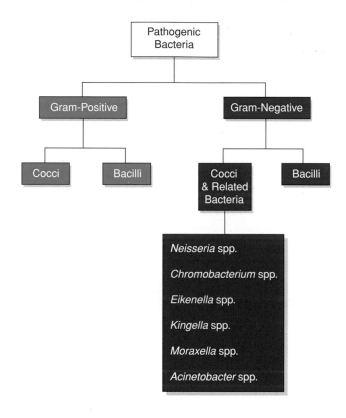

LEARNING OBJECTIVES

After studying this chapter, you should be able to:

☞ Define the terms introduced in this chapter (e.g., *autolysis, gonococcemia, gonococcus*)

☞ Identify the clinically significant Gram-negative cocci and related Gram-negative coccobacilli

☞ State the major characteristics of the genera: *Neisseria, Moraxella,* and *Acinetobacter,* including optimal growth requirements, best media for growth, major differentiating biochemical reactions, cellular and colonial morphology

☞ Relate the virulence factors for *Neisseria gonorrhoeae* and *N. meningitidis*

☞ Explain the principles of and reagents utilized in the oxidase test, superoxol test, and penicillin disk test, and identify a positive test result or reaction

☞ Given sugar oxidation reactions for *Neisseria* spp., distinguish *N. gonorrhoeae* and *N. meningitidis* from other *Neisseria* spp.

☞ Explain the pathogenesis of *N. gonorrhoeae* and *N. meningitidis* infections, including route of infection, clinical manifestations, and severity of disease

☞ Outline the proper collection procedures, specimens, and media used for isolation of *N. gonorrhoeae* and *N. meningitidis*

☞ Name and compare the different types of selective media used to isolate *N. gonorrhoeae* and *N. meningitidis*

☞ Describe the appropriate collection process and specimens for diagnosis of gonorrhea in men and women

☞ Identify the microorganisms that are members of the HACEK group

☞ Given an infectious disease, correlate it with the most probable pathogenic Gram-negative coccus, diplococcus, or coccobacillus

Gonorrhea. Meningococcal meningitis. Endocarditis. These are some of the diseases caused by the Gram-negative cocci and related bacteria that are described in this chapter.

Recall that pathogenic cocci can be divided into those that are Gram positive and those that are Gram negative. Gram-positive cocci were discussed in Chapter 9. Gram-negative cocci are discussed in this chapter, together with some closely related Gram-negative coccobacilli and Gram-negative bacilli. Of the bacteria discussed in this chapter, four genera (*Neisseria*, *Chromobacterium*, *Eikenella*, and *Kingella*) are in the Neisseriaceae family, and two genera (*Moraxella* and *Acinetobacter*) are in the Moraxellaceae family (Table 11-1).[1]

GENUS *NEISSERIA*

Most *Neisseria* spp. are Gram-negative cocci that frequently occur in pairs (diplococci), tetrads, or short chains. The diplococci have adjacent sides that are flattened, frequently giving them the appearance of side-by-side coffee beans or kidneys (Fig. 11-1). *N. elongata* and *N. weaveri* are medium-to-large plump bacilli that may occur in pairs or short chains. All *Neisseria* spp. share the following characteristics:

> *Neisseria* spp. are oxidase-positive, Gram-negative diplococci.

• Inhabit mucous membrane surfaces of warm-blooded hosts

• Aerobic

• Nonmotile

TABLE 11 - 1	Gram-Negative Bacteria Discussed in This Chapter
Genus	**Cellular Morphology**[a]
Neisseria	Predominantly GNC and GND; a few species are GNB
Chromobacterium	GNB
Eikenella	Pleomorphic GNCB
Kingella	GNCB
Moraxella	Some species are GNC; some are GND; some are GNCB
Acinetobacter	GNCB

[a]GNB, Gram-negative bacilli; GNC, Gram-negative cocci; GNCB, Gram-negative coccobacilli; GND, Gram-negative diplococci

---

[1]*The organisms discussed in this chapter are sometimes described in different sections of other textbooks. For example,* Acinetobacter, Moraxella, *and* Neisseria *spp. are sometimes discussed with nonfermenters, which in this book are described in Chapter 13.* Eikenella *and* Kingella *spp. are sometimes discussed with fastidious Gram-negative bacilli, which in this book are described in Chapter 14.* Chromobacterium *spp. are sometimes discussed with* Aeromonas *and* Vibrio *spp., because some strains are oxidase-positive fermenters; but in this book,* Aeromonas *and* Vibrio *spp. are described in Chapters 14 and 15, respectively.*

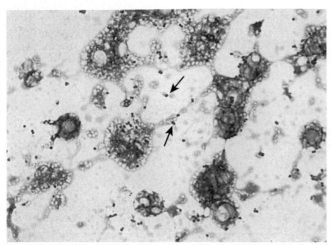

Figure 11-1. **Gram-stained blood specimen, containing numerous degenerated white blood cells, and Gram-negative diplococci resembling *Neisseria* spp.** (From Marler LM, Siders JA, Allen SD. Direct Smear Atlas. Philadelphia: Lippincott Williams & Wilkins, 2001.)

- Non–spore formers

- Optimal growth temperature for most species is 35°C to 37°C

- Produce acid from carbohydrates oxidatively, as opposed to fermentatively[2]

- Oxidase positive

- Most species are catalase positive

Pathogenic species tend to be more fastidious than nonpathogenic species. They are more nutritionally demanding, and their growth is stimulated by CO_2 and humidity.

The following *Neisseria* spp. may be isolated from human clinical specimens:

- *N. gonorrhoeae*: the cause of gonorrhea; always considered a pathogen, regardless of the anatomical site from which it is isolated

> *Neisseria gonorrhoeae* and *N. meningitidis* are *very* important human pathogens.

- *N. meningitidis*: a significant pathogen, but can also colonize the human nasopharynx without causing disease

- *N. cinerea*

- *N. elonga* subspecies *elongata, glycolytica,* and *nitroreducens*

- *N. flavescens*

- *N. kochii*

- *N. lactamica*

- *N. mucosa*

- *N. polysaccharea*

- *N. sicca*

- *N. subflava* (biovars *subflava, flava,* and *perflava*)

With the exception of *N. gonorrhoeae* and *N. meningitidis*, most human *Neisseria* spp. are members of the indigenous flora of the upper respiratory tract and are considered nonpathogenic. Only rarely have the nonpathogenic *Neisseria* spp. reportedly been associated with human infections. Nonetheless, when isolated from human clinical specimens, nonpathogenic species must be differentiated from pathogenic species. Methods used to differentiate *Neisseria* spp. include carbohydrate utilization, colorimetry involving chromogenic substrates, immunodiagnostic procedures using monoclonal antibodies, isoenzyme electrophoresis, and DNA probes. Several commercial kits are available for identification of *Neisseria* spp.

Neisseria gonorrhoeae

Clinical significance. *Neisseria gonorrhoeae* is often referred to as the **gonococcus (GC, pl. gonococci).** It is always considered a pathogen, regardless of the anatomic site from which it is isolated. The disease caused by *N. gonorrhoeae* is called gonorrhea, but

> *Neisseria gonorrhoeae* is always considered a pathogen, regardless of the anatomic site from which it is isolated.

infections by the bacteria have many clinical manifestations. Localized infections include urethritis, cervicitis, **proctitis** (inflammation of the mucous lining of the rectum), conjunctivitis, and **oropharyngitis** (inflammation of the oral portion of the throat). Neonates can be infected during their passage through the birth canal, leading to

> Although gonorrhea is often thought of as a genital infection, there are many clinical manifestations of *N. gonorrhoeae* infection.

a serious eye infection known as **ophthalmia neonatorum** or gonococcal conjunctivitis. To prevent this disease, silver nitrate or povidone-iodine drops, or tetracycline or erythromycin ointment, are instilled into the neonate's eyes within 1 hour of birth. Genital infections include pelvic inflammatory disease and epididymitis. Additional manifestations of gonorrhea include gonococcemia, septicemia, skin and joint infection, endocarditis, and pericarditis. The term **gonococcemia** refers to the presence of *N. gonorrhoeae* in the bloodstream.

---

[2] *Oxidative reactions involve oxygen, whereas fermentative reactions do not.*

What's in a Name? It should not be difficult to remember that **gonorrhea** is caused by *N. gonorrhoeae*, but note the differences in the spelling of the disease and the specific epithet. The disease ends in *-hea*, whereas the specific epithet ends in *-hoeae*. Gonorrhea, named in the second century AD, is derived from two Greek words: *gonor*, meaning "seed," and *rhoia*, meaning "flow." Apparently, it was thought that the disease was related to the flow of semen. It is not.

Virulence factors. *N. gonorrhoeae* possesses pili, but the ability to produce pili can be lost in older cultures and on subculture. Pili enable attachment of the bacterial cells to host epithelial cells. Outer membrane proteins apparently play a role in the phagocytic uptake of *N. gonorrhoeae* by host epithelial cells. *N. gonorrhoeae* may be able to survive within phagocytes. Like all Gram-negative bacteria, *N. gonorrhoeae* has cell walls that contains endotoxin. The presence of endotoxin in the bloodstream can lead to septic shock. Although some investigators have reported that *N. gonorrhoeae* possesses a capsule, its role in pathogenesis, if any, is unknown.

Drug resistance. Drug resistant and multidrug-resistant strains of *N. gonorrhoeae* are common. β-Lactamase production can be tested using the nitrocefin test. Antimicrobial susceptibility testing may be accomplished using the agar dilution method, Etest, or a modified disk diffusion method. Susceptibility testing of *N. gonorrhoeae* must be performed in accordance with Clinical and Laboratory Standards Institute (CLSI) Document M45-P (see "References and Suggested Reading"). Neither β-lactamase testing nor antimicrobial susceptibility testing are deemed necessary, because all strains of *N. gonorrhoeae* are susceptible to ceftriaxone—even penicillinase-producing strains and strains that are resistant to penicillin by mechanisms other than penicillinase production. This policy could change, however, should ceftriaxone-resistant strains emerge.

Clues to *N. gonorrhoeae* Identification

Cellular morphology. *N. gonorrhoeae* is a Gram-negative diplococcus. Each diplococcus resembles two side-by-side kidneys (Fig. 11-2). A Gram-stained smear of a urethral discharge specimen is a highly sensitive and highly specific

> A Gram-stained urethral discharge specimen is useful for diagnosis of gonorrhea in *male* patients but, because of the possible presence of "look alike" bacteria, a Gram-stained vaginal or cervical swab *cannot* be used to diagnose gonorrhea in female patients.

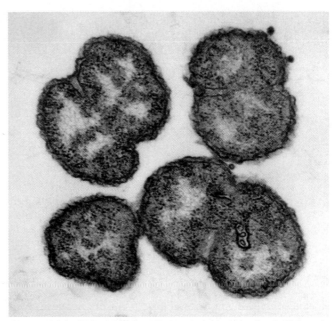

Figure 11-2. **Transmission electron micrograph of *Neisseria gonorrhoeae* diplococci, which frequently resemble two side-by-side coffee beans or kidneys.** (Courtesy of Centers for Disease Control and Prevention [CDC], VD/SCSD.)

way to diagnose genital gonorrhea in symptomatic *male* patients. The Gram-stained smear will typically reveal numerous polymorphonuclear white blood cells (PMNs)[3] and numerous intracellular and extracellular Gram-negative diplococci (Fig. 11-3). The intracellular diplococci are present within the cytoplasm of the PMNs because they were phagocytized by these white blood cells. Gram-stained

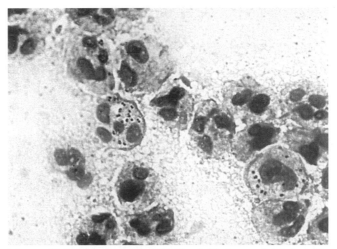

Figure 11-3. **Gram-stained urethral discharge from a male patient.** Of the numerous polymorphonuclear leukocytes (PMNs) in the specimen, some contain phagocytized Gram-negative diplococci, which most likely are *N. gonorrhoeae*. (From Marler LM, Siders JA, Allen SD. Direct Smear Atlas. Philadelphia: Lippincott Williams & Wilkins, 2001.)

---

[3] *The basis of the term* polymorphonuclear leukocyte *is that these white blood cells have various-shaped nuclei. PMNs are also called neutrophils and polys. They are important phagocytes that play a major role in the body's defenses against pathogens and infectious diseases.*

TABLE 11 - 2	Selective Media for Recovery of *Neisseria gonorrhoeae* from Clinical Specimens

Medium	Description
Modified Thayer-Martin medium	Chocolate agar supplemented with growth factors and antimicrobial agents[a]
Martin-Lewis medium	Chocolate agar supplemented with growth factors and antimicrobial agents
GC-Lect medium	Chocolate agar supplemented with growth factors and antimicrobial agents (manufactured by BD Biosciences; http://www.bdbiosciences.com/)

[a] Antimicrobial agents contained in these media include colistin (to inhibit other Gram-negative bacteria); vancomycin (to inhibit Gram-positive bacteria); trimethoprim (to inhibit swarming of *Proteus* spp.); and nystatin, amphotericin B, or anisomycin (to inhibit yeasts and moulds). The quantities of these antimicrobial agents vary from one type of selective medium to another. Some *N. gonorrhoeae* strains are susceptible to vancomycin.

smears of *female* genital tract specimens are *not* performed because of the possible presence of other morphologically similar Gram-negative cocci, coccobacilli, and bipolar-staining Gram-positive bacilli in the indigenous microflora of those sites. A bacillus that takes up greater quantities of stain at its ends or poles resembles, and can be mistaken for, a diplococcus. Gram-stained smears of colonies show uniform characteristic Gram-negative diplococci.

Colonial morphology. *N. gonorrhoeae* is fastidious, borderline microaerophilic,[4] and capnophilic. It requires enriched media, a 3% to 5% CO_2 atmosphere, and 35°C to 37°C incubation temperature. *N. gonorrhoeae* grows well on chocolate agar and will grow on blood agar *if* the inoculated plates are incubated in either a CO_2 incubator or candle extinction jar. Incubators should contain a pan of water to provide humidity and keep the media from drying out. Plates should be inspected at 24, 48, and 72 hours, before a report of no growth is issued. Neither *N. gonorrhoeae* nor *N. meningitidis* will grow on nutrient agar at room temperature without CO_2, whereas other *Neisseria* spp. will grow under those conditions. Several types of selective media (e.g., Thayer-Martin and Martin-Lewis media) are available for recovery of *N. gonorrhoeae* from specimens collected from sites that harbor various indigenous microflora organisms (Table 11-2). Anatomical sites that harbor indigenous microflora are referred to as **nonsterile sites,** as opposed to **sterile sites** (e.g., blood, cerebrospinal fluid), which do not harbor indigenous microflora. In addition to *N. gonorrhoeae*, these selective media support growth of *N. meningitidis* and *N. lactamica*. Organisms in other genera also occasionally grow on these selective media, but they can be differentiated

> *N. gonorrhoeae* is fastidious, borderline microaerophilic, and capnophilic.

from *N. gonorrhoeae* by Gram stain and/or oxidase reaction. Neither *N. gonorrhoeae* nor *N. meningitidis* will grow on MacConkey agar.[5]

Candle extinction jar (see Fig. 6-15). Candle extinction jars, or candle jars, as they are often called, are used in laboratories not equipped with a CO_2 incubator. Inoculated plates are placed medium-side up in the bottom of the jar. A lighted candle is placed on top of the plates. Candles should be made of white wax or beeswax. Scented or colored candles should not be used because they release volatile products that may inhibit growth of the organisms. The jar is then sealed and placed in an incubator at 35°C to 37°C. The major problem with candle jars is their limited capacity: they may not have sufficient room for all the inoculated plates.

N. gonorrhoeae colonies on chocolate agar are beige to gray-brown, translucent, and smooth (Fig. 11-4). Colonial appearance varies, however, depending on the degree of piliation of the organisms within the colony. Piliated organisms produce small (about 0.5 mm in diameter), glistening, raised colonies, whereas nonpiliated organisms produce larger (about 1 mm in diameter), nonglistening, flatter colonies. The colonies from nonpiliated strains may become gummy as a result of autolysis and release of cellular DNA. **Autolysis,** meaning "self-destruction," refers to the digestion or lysis of cells caused by enzymes produced within the cells. Multiple colony types on the plate may give the appearance of a mixed culture.

> Colonies of *Neisseria gonorrhoeae* vary in appearance, depending on the extent of piliation of the cells within the colony.

Laboratory tests. The oxidase test. Recall from Chapter 9 that oxidase is an abbreviated name for cytochrome oxidase, an enzyme that participates in the electron transport

---

[4] *The term* borderline microaerophilic *means that, although* N. gonorrhoeae *will grow in 15% to 21% oxygen, it grows better in reduced oxygen concentrations.*

[5] *Although MacConkey agar is selective for Gram-negative bacteria, it does* not *support the growth of* all *Gram-negative bacteria. MacConkey agar is not an enriched medium and thus will not support the growth of fastidious Gram-negative bacteria.*

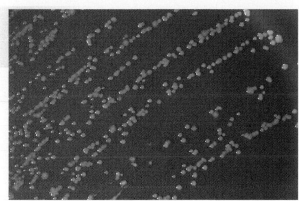

Figure 11-4. **Colonies of *N. gonorrhoeae* on modified Thayer-Martin agar after 24 hours of incubation at 35°C to 37°C in 5% to 7% CO$_2$.** (From Winn WC Jr, et al. Koneman's Color Atlas and Textbook of Diagnostic Microbiology. 6th Ed. Philadelphia: Lippincott Williams & Wilkins, 2006.)

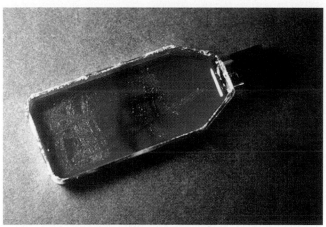

Figure 11-6. **Positive oxidase reaction.** Shown here are colonies of *N. gonorrhoeae* on modified Martin-Lewis medium within a Transgrow bottle. Some of the colonies have turned purple following the addition of oxidase reagent, indicating that *N. gonorrhoeae* is oxidase positive. (Courtesy of Dr. A. Schroeter and the CDC.)

chain.[6] The oxidase test is of value in identifying and differentiating Gram-negative bacteria, including those described in this chapter. *Neisseria*, *Eikenella*, *Kingella*, and *Moraxella* spp. are oxidase positive. *Acinetobacter* spp. are oxidase negative. *Chromobacter* spp. are oxidase variable, meaning that some strains produce oxidase while others do not.

The oxidase test is performed as follows: After saturating a portion of filter paper with one drop of dimethyl or tetramethyl oxidase reagent, a portion of a colony is rubbed onto the saturated area of the filter paper. A dark purple color appearing in 10 seconds constitutes a positive test result (Fig. 11-5). *N. gonorrhoeae*, like all *Neisseria* spp., is oxidase positive. Alternatively, growth on the agar surface can be flooded with the oxidase reagent, providing that the culture is not mixed with contaminants. Darkening (first

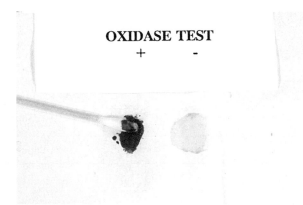

OXIDASE TEST

+   -

Figure 11-5. **Oxidase test.** A positive oxidase test result is shown to the left, and a negative test result is shown to the right. (From Winn WC Jr, et al. Koneman's Color Atlas and Textbook of Diagnostic Microbiology. 6th Ed. Philadelphia: Lippincott Williams & Wilkins, 2006.)

pink, then maroon, then black) of the colonies represents a positive oxidase test result (Fig. 11-6). If subculturing of the isolate is desired, it must be accomplished as soon as the darkening starts to occur, because the oxidase reagent kills the organisms by the time the colonies become maroon to black. The superoxol test (described next) can also be used for rapid presumptive identification of *N. gonorrhoeae* isolated from urogenital sites.

> *Neisseria gonorrhoeae* is strongly oxidase positive.

Superoxol test. To perform the superoxol test, a drop of superoxol (30% hydrogen peroxide [H$_2$O$_2$]) is placed onto a glass microscope slide. A colony of the test organism is emulsified into the drop. *N. gonorrhoeae* will produce immediate, very brisk bubbling. *Question:* Bubbles of what? (Recall from Chapter 9 why bubbles are produced when bacteria are mixed with H$_2$O$_2$.) *Answer:* The catalase enzyme causes the breakdown of H$_2$O$_2$ into water and oxygen. The bubbles are bubbles of oxygen. Some strains of *Moraxella catarrhalis* and *N. meningitidis* may also produce immediate, brisk bubbling, but *N. meningitidis* and *N. lactamica* usually produce weak, delayed bubbling. *Kingella denitrificans* produces a negative test result. It is important to exercise caution when using 30% H$_2$O$_2$ because it can burn skin.

Penicillin disk test. The penicillin disk test can be used to differentiate *Neisseria* spp. from "look alike" organisms, such as *Moraxella* and *Acinetobacter* spp. The organism to be tested is heavily streaked onto a Trypticase-soy blood agar plate to obtain confluent growth. A 10 U penicillin disk is then placed onto the inoculated area. After overnight incubation in a CO$_2$ incubator, a Gram-stained smear is prepared from growth obtained from the outer edge of the zone of inhibition (Fig. 11-7). The shape of the cells is then observed (Fig. 11-8).

---

[6] *The electron transport chain is an energy-producing biochemical pathway that is part of a larger biochemical pathway known as aerobic respiration. Aerobic respiration is a process by which aerobes, microaerophiles, and facultative anaerobes obtain energy from glucose and other substrates.*

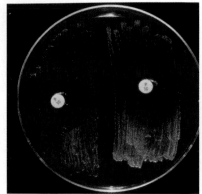

Figure 11-7. **Penicillin disk test used to distinguish between** *Neisseria* **and coccobacillary** *Moraxella* **spp.** One side of this blood agar plate was inoculated with a *Neisseria* sp. and the other side with a coccobacillary *Moraxella* sp. A penicillin disk was added to each side. After overnight incubation, there is a zone of no growth around each disk, indicating that each organism is susceptible to penicillin. Gram stains were performed on colonies removed from the edges of the zones of no growth. Results are shown in Figure 11-8. (From Winn WC Jr, et al. Koneman's Color Atlas and Textbook of Diagnostic Microbiology. 6th Ed. Philadelphia: Lippincott Williams & Wilkins, 2006.)

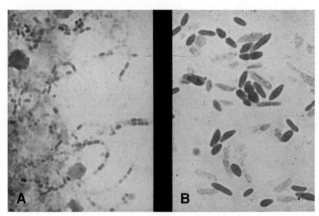

Figure 11-8. **Results of the penicillin disk test described in Figure 11-7. A.** Gram-stained *Neisseria* sp. retains its diplococcal morphology. **B.** Gram-stained *Moraxella* sp. has produced bizarre rod-shaped cells. (From Winn WC Jr, et al. Koneman's Color Atlas and Textbook of Diagnostic Microbiology. 6th Ed. Philadelphia: Lippincott Williams & Wilkins, 2006.)

TABLE 11 - 3	Differentiation of *N. gonorrhoeae* from Some Other Gram-Negative Cocci					
Bacteria	**Oxidase**	**Catalase**	**Glucose**	**Maltose**	**Lactose**	**Sucrose**
N. gonorrhoeae	+	+	+	−	−	−
N. meningitidis	+	+	+	+[a]	−	−
N. cinerea	+	+	−	−	−	−
N. elongata (rod shaped)	+	+	−	−	−	−
N. flavescens	+	+	−	−	−	−
N. kochii	+	+	+	−	−	−
N. lactamica	+	+	+	+	+	−
N. mucosa	+	+	+	+	−	+
N. polysaccharea	+	+	+	+	−	Variable
N. sicca	+	+	+	+	−	+
N. subflava	+	+	+	+	−	Variable
Kingella denitrificans	+	−	+	−	−	−
Moraxella catarrhalis	+	+	−	−	−	−

[a] Some *N. meningitidis* strains are maltose negative.

Neisseria spp., being true diplococci, will retain their diplococcal morphology in the presence of subinhibitory concentrations of penicillin (see Fig. 11-8A). Coccobacillary *Moraxella* spp. will form bizarre rod-shaped cells in the presence of subinhibitory concentrations of penicillin (see Fig. 11-8B).

Other possible penicillin disk test results include the following:

- Like *Neisseria* spp., *Moraxella catarrhalis* will retain its diplococcal morphology, although the cells may appear swollen.

- Coccobacillary *Moraxella* spp. and *K. denitrificans* form long filaments or spindle-shaped cells. Spindle-shaped cells are cells that are pointed at both ends.

- *Acinetobacter* spp., which are oxidase negative and can exhibit diplococcal morphology, form long filaments.

- *Capnocytophaga* spp. appear as pale-staining, slightly curved, spindle-shaped Gram-negative cells. *Capnocytophaga* spp. are oxidase negative and catalase negative; they are described in Chapter 14.

Sugar oxidation patterns are often used to definitively distinguish *N. gonorrhoeae* from other *Neisseria* spp. and from Gram-negative bacteria often mistaken for *N. gonorrhoeae*, such as *Kingella denitrificans* and *Moraxella catarrhalis* (Table 11-3). Traditionally, CTA sugars were used; CTA stands for cystine-tryptic digest semisolid agar-based media, which contain 1% carbohydrate and phenol red pH indicator. Glucose, maltose, lactose, and sucrose were the sugars usually tested. Heavily inoculated tubes were incubated at 35°C in a non-CO$_2$ incubator. Production of a yellow color after 4 to 72 hours of incubation constituted a positive test result.

> *Neisseria gonorrhoeae* will oxidize glucose but not maltose, lactose, sucrose, or fructose.

Many commercial systems are available for identifying *N. gonorrhoeae* and other *Neisseria* species (Table 11-4), including carbohydrate utilization, chromogenic enzyme, immunologic, and molecular diagnostic systems. Immunodiagnostic procedures and molecular diagnostic procedures are also available.

Essentials

Neisseria gonorrhoeae

- Also known as gonococcus or GC
- Gram-negative diplococci
- Fastidious

- Capnophilic and borderline microaerophilic
- Oxidase positive
- Produces acid from glucose but not from other sugars

Neisseria meningitidis

Clinical significance. Like *Neisseria gonorrhoeae*, *N. meningitidis* is strictly a human pathogen. *N. meningitidis* colonizes the nasopharyngeal mucosa of some people, who are referred to as *N. meningitidis* carriers. The bacteria may be transmitted from person to person via transfer of respiratory secretions or aerosolized droplets. *N. meningitidis* may also colonize the genital tract and conjunctiva. *N. meningitidis* is often referred to as **meningococcus (pl. meningococci)**. The usual manifestations of *N. meningitidis* disease are **meningococcemia** (*N. meningitidis* in the bloodstream), petechiae (tiny red spots on the skin), and meningitis. Meningitis caused by *N. meningitidis* is referred to as **meningococcal meningitis.** Epidemics of meningococcal meningitis are often associated with

> *Neisseria meningitidis* is often referred to as meningococcus, and meningitis caused by *N. meningitidis* is referred to as meningococcal meningitis. *N. meningitidis* is one of the major causes of meningitis.

crowded, stressful settings, such as military basic training centers, schools, and colleges. Meningococcal meningitis is a serious, rapidly progressing disease. Rarer types of *N. meningitidis* diseases are genital tract infection, proctitis, and conjunctivitis.

STUDY AID **What's in a Name?** It should not be difficult to remember that *Neisseria meningitidis* causes meningitis, because the specific epithet *meningitides* contains most of the word *meningitis*.

STUDY AID **A Closer Look at Meningitis.** Meningitis is a serious, often fatal disease. The most common symptoms of meningitis are headache, fever, chills, nausea, vomiting, photophobia, and stiffness of the neck. In addition to *N. meningitidis*, the major bacterial causes of meningitis in patients between the ages of 2 and 18 are *Streptococcus pneumoniae* and *Haemophilus influenzae*. Frequent causes of neonatal meningitis are *Streptococcus agalactiae* (group B strep), *Listeria monocytogenes*, *Escherichia coli*, and other members of the Enterobacteriaceae family. Viral meningitis is usually caused by enteroviruses, although herpes simplex viruses can also cause meningitis.

TABLE 11 - 4   Commercial Systems for Identification of *Neisseria* spp.

Commercial System	Speed	Manufacturer
AccuProbe *Neisseria gonorrhoeae* test	Rapid nucleic acid probe	Gen-Probe, Inc. (http://www.gen-probe.com/)
API-NH	Overnight multitest system	bioMérieux Inc. (http://www.biomerieux.com/)
API Quad-Ferm+	Rapid (2-hour) carbohydrate utilization test	bioMérieux Inc.
Amplicore PCR	Rapid (5-hour) PCR assay	Roche (http://www.roche.com/)
BactiCard *Neisseria*	Rapid (4-hour) enzyme substrate test	Remel (http://www.remelinc.com/)
BBL Crystal *Neisseria/Haemophilus* panel	Rapid (4 hours)	BD Biosciences (http://www.bdbiosciences.com/)
FA Test *Neisseria gonorrhoeae* Culture Confirmation Test	Rapid immunologic test	Dade Behring (http://www.dadebehring.com/)
Gonochek II	Rapid (30-minute) enzyme substrate test	E-Y Laboratories Inc. (http://www.eylabs.com/)
GonoGen I and II	Rapid immunologic tests	New Horizons Diagnostics (http://www.nhdiag.com/)
Gonostat II	Overnight	Sierra Diagnostics Inc. (http://www.sierramolecular.com/)
Gonozyme	Rapid enzyme immunoassay	Abbott Laboratories (http://www.abbott.com/)
Lcx *N. gonorrhoeae*	Rapid (5-hour) nucleic acid amplification test	Abbott Laboratories
Meritec GC	Rapid immunologic test	Meridian Bioscience Inc. (http://www.meridianbioscience.com/)
MicroScan HNID	Rapid (4-hour) multitest system	Dade Behring (http://www.dadebehring.com/)
Neisseria-Kwik	Rapid (4-hour) carbohydrate utilization test	MicroBioLogics Inc. (http://www.microbiologics.com/)
Neisstrip	Rapid enzyme substrate test	Lab M Ltd. (http://www.labm.com/)
Pace II DNA Probe	Rapid nucleic acid probe	Gen-Probe Inc.
Phadebact GC Omni Test	Rapid immunologic test	Bactus AB (http://www.bactus.se/)
RapID NH Test	Rapid multitest system	Remel
Vitek NHI Card	Rapid multitest system	bioMérieux Inc.

Source: Evangelista AT, et al. Rapid systems and instruments for the identification of bacteria. In: Manual of Commercial Methods in Clinical Microbiology. Washington, DC: ASM Press, 2002.

Virulence factors. Virulence factors of *N. meningitidis* include capsules, pili, and endotoxin.

Clues to *N. gonorrhoeae* Identification

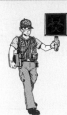

SAFETY TIP

CLSI-Recommended Safety Precautions.
When working with N. meningitidis, *CLSI Document M29-A3 (see "References and Suggested Reading") recommends biosafety level 2 (BSL-2) practices, containment equipment, and facilities for all activities using known or potentially infectious body fluids, tissues, and cultures. Additional primary containment and personnel precautions, such as those described for BSL-3, may be indicated for activities highly likely to produce droplets or aerosols and for activities involving the production of quantities or concentrations of infectious materials.*

Cellular morphology. *N. meningitidis* is an encapsulated Gram-negative diplococcus, virtually identical in appearance to *N. gonorrhoeae*. A rapid presumptive diagnosis of meningococcal meningitis can be made when PMNs and intracellular and extracellular Gram-negative diplococci are observed in Gram-stained smears of sediment obtained from centrifuged or cytocentrifuged cerebrospinal fluid specimens (Fig. 11-9). *N.*

> In Gram-stained smears, *N. meningitidis* is virtually identical to *N. gonorrhoeae* in appearance.

meningitidis cells vary in size and may resist decolorization; a pink halo may be seen around the cells of encapsulated strains.

Colonial morphology. *N. meningitidis* grows best at 35°C to 37°C in a moist 5% to 7% CO_2 environment. On blood agar, chocolate agar, or chocolate agar–based media (e.g., Thayer-Martin medium), *N. meningitidis* colonies are gray, low, convex, and glistening, with a smooth, moist entire edge (Fig. 11-10). Heavily encapsulated strains may be mucoid. *N. meningitidis* colonies are larger than those of *N. gonorrhoeae*, usually about 1 mm or more in diameter after 18 to 24 hours of incubation. Although young colonies have a smooth consistency, older colonies become gummy as a result of autolysis and release of cellular DNA. On blood agar, the medium beneath and adjacent to the colonies may be grayish green, especially in areas of confluent growth.

> *N. meningitidis* will grow on blood agar incubated in a non-CO_2 incubator, whereas *N. gonorrhoeae* will not.

Laboratory tests. Once they are isolated in the clinical microbiology laboratory, *N. meningitidis* may be identified using carbohydrate utilization or chromogenic enzyme substrate tests. Many of the commercial systems mentioned earlier for identification of *N. gonorrhoeae* can be used to identify *N. meningitidis*. Carbohydrate utilization (oxidation) by *N. meningitidis* will acidify media containing glucose and maltose but not those containing lactose, sucrose, or fructose. Recall that, of these sugars, *N. gonorrhoeae* will cause acid production only in media containing glucose.

> *N. meningitidis* will oxidize glucose and maltose but not lactose, sucrose, or fructose.

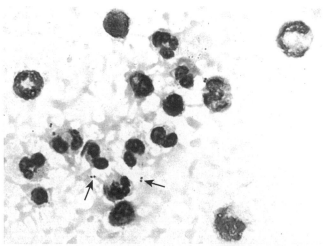

Figure 11-9. **Gram-negative diplococci (*arrows*), suggestive of *Neisseria meningitidis*, in a Gram-stained cerebrospinal fluid sediment.** (From Marler LM, Siders JA, Allen SD. Direct Smear Atlas. Philadelphia: Lippincott Williams & Wilkins, 2001.)

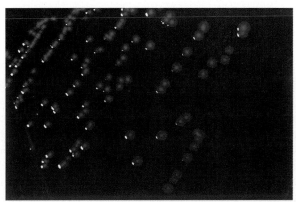

Figure 11-10. **N. meningitidis colonies on sheep blood agar after incubation for 24 hours at 35°C to 37°C in a 5% to 7% CO_2 atmosphere.** (From Winn WC Jr, et al. Koneman's Color Atlas and Textbook of Diagnostic Microbiology. 6th Ed. Philadelphia: Lippincott Williams & Wilkins, 2006.)

A Method for Remembering Carbohydrate Utilization Patterns of *Neisseria* spp. Of the usually tested sugars, *N. gonorrhoeae* will produce acid only in a medium containing glucose. Remember *G* for glucose and *gonorrhoeae*. *N. meningitidis*, on the other hand, will produce acid in both glucose- and maltose-containing media but not in media containing the other sugars. Remember *M* for maltose and *meningitidis*. *N. lactamica* will produce acid in glucose-, maltose-, and lactose-containing media. Remember *L* for lactose and *lactamica*.

Immunodiagnostic procedures (e.g., countercurrent immunoelectrophoresis, latex particle agglutination, coagglutination) are available for detection of *N. meningitidis* antigen in specimens, but they are not used as often as they were in the past. The procedures are of some use in partially treated meningococcal meningitis cases, where neither cerebrospinal fluid Gram stain nor culture is positive.

Essentials

Neisseria meningitidis

- Also known as meningococcus
- Gram-negative diplococci
- Not as fastidious as *N. gonorrhoeae*
- Oxidase positive
- Produces acid from glucose and maltose but not from other sugars

CHROMOBACTERIUM VIOLACEUM

Clinical significance. *Chromobacterium violaceum* is the only pathogenic species in the genus. It is a rare cause of human infection, primarily in tropical and semitropical areas. Most U.S. cases have occurred in Florida and Louisiana. *C. violaceum* lives in soil and water. The primarily portals of entry are through breaks in skin and oral ingestion. Entry through skin can lead to a wound infection. Other types of *C. violaceum*–associated infections that have been reported include liver, lung, spleen, and skin abscesses and septicemia (especially in leukopenic patients). *C. violaceum* produces an endotoxin and a β-lactamase. It is generally resistant to β-lactam antibiotics.

Clues to *C. violaceum* Identification

Cellular morphology. *C. violaceum* cells are motile, straight to slightly curved Gram-negative bacilli or coccobacilli that are 0.8 to 1.2 μm wide by 2.5 to 6.0 μm long. Its cells often exhibit bipolar staining.

Colonial morphology. *C. violaceum* is a facultative anaerobe. It produces round, smooth colonies, 1 to 2 mm in diameter after 24 hours at 30°C to 35°C. **The most striking characteristics of *C. violaceum* colonies are their violet color (hence, the specific epithet *violaceum*) and their hydrogen cyanide odor** (Fig. 11-11.) The violet-colored pigment is called violacein; it is ethanol soluble but not water soluble. For pigment production, the culture medium must contain the amino acid tryptophan, and the inoculated medium must be incubated in the presence of oxygen. Nonpigmented strains occur. Colonies may be β-hemolytic. *C. violaceum* will grow on MacConkey agar. Violacein has antimicrobial properties, primarily against protozoa such as soil amebae and trypanosomes. The bacterium also produces antibacterial agents.

> Associate violet-colored colonies with *C. violaceum*, although other, less commonly isolated bacteria can also produce purple colonies.

 What's in a Name? It should be easy to remember that *C. violaceum* produces violet-colored colonies: *chromo* means "color" and *violaceum* refers to violet. *C. violaceum* produces colonies having a metallic, violet sheen.

Laboratory tests. *C. violaceum* is catalase positive, generally indole negative, and nitrate reduction positive. Most strains are oxidase positive.

***Figure 11-11.* Colonies of *Chromobacterium violaceum* on blood agar.** (Courtesy of Dr. W. A. Clark and the CDC.)

EIKENELLA CORRODENS

Eikenella corrodens is sometimes grouped with similar fastidious Gram-negative bacteria into what is known as the **HACEK group:**

H *for Haemophilus aphrophilus and H. paraphrophilus*

A *for Actinobacillus actinomycetemcomitans*

C *for Cardiobacterium hominis*

E *for Eikenella corrodens*

K *for Kingella*

All members of the HACEK group are members of the oropharyngeal and/or urogenital indigenous microflora, which share other characteristics (see Chapter 14). Of the bacteria in the HACEK group, only *Eikenella* and *Kingella* are discussed in this chapter. The others are discussed in Chapter 14.

Clinical significance. *E. corrodens* is found as part of the oral, gastrointestinal, and genitourinary indigenous microflora. It is an opportunistic pathogen associated with human bites, dental extractions, or oral trauma. The most common types of *E. corrodens*–associated infections are face and hand abscesses, septic arthritis, osteomyelitis, cellulitis, abscesses of internal organs, and head and neck infections.

Virulence factors. Virulence factors of *E. corrodens* include a surface protein capable of binding to epithelial cells, pili, endotoxin, an hemolysin, and β-lactamase.

Drug resistance. *E. corrodens* strains are susceptible to penicillin (the drug of choice) but are resistant to clindamycin, lincomycin, metronidazole, aminoglycosides, erythromycin, vancomycin, first-generation cephalosporins, and penicillinase-resistant penicillins. *E. corrodens* must be tested by the agar dilution method of antimicrobial susceptibility testing; other methods are unreliable.

Clues to *E. corrodens* Identification

Cellular morphology. *E. corrodens* cells are slender, straight, nonmotile Gram-negative bacilli with rounded ends (Fig. 11-12). They are 0.3 to 0.4 μm wide by 1.5 to 4.0 μm long.

Colonial morphology. *E. corrodens* is a facultative anaerobe. Aerobic, but not anaerobic, growth requires hemin,

> Associate pitting colonies with *Eikenella corrodens*, although other bacteria can also cause pitting of the agar surface.

which is present in both blood agar and chocolate agar. CO_2 incubation enhances growth. After 48 hours at 37°C, colonies are 0.5 to 2 mm in diameter with clear

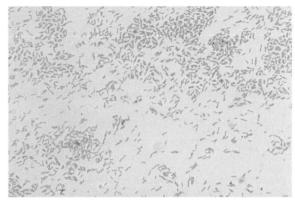

Figure 11-12. **Gram-stained *Eikenella corrodens* cells are more uniform in appearance than other HACEK group organisms, which can be coccobacillary or pleomorphic.** (From Winn WC Jr, et al. Koneman's Color Atlas and Textbook of Diagnostic Microbiology. 6th Ed. Philadelphia: Lippincott Williams & Wilkins, 2006.)

centers. They are often surrounded by spreading growth. The colonies have a characteristic pitting or corroding appearance (hence, the specific epithet *corrodens*), although not all strains corrode the agar (Fig. 11-13). Observation of pitting is facilitated by removal of the colonies with a swab, which reveals holes where the colonies were located. Pitting and nonpitting variants can occur in the same culture. Bacteria other than *E. corrodens* can cause pitting of the agar surface—for example, anaerobes in the *Bacteroides ureolyticus* group (see Chapter 17).

E. corrodens colonies may assume a slightly yellow hue after several days, which is best observed by dragging a white swab through some colonies; the yellow pigment will adhere to the swab. Although *E. corrodens* is nonmotile, strains

> *E. corrodens* is associated with a twitching motility, but so too are *Kingella* and *Acinetobacter* spp.

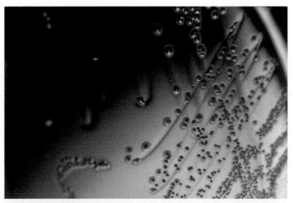

Figure 11-13. **Pitting colonies of *E. corrodens* on sheep blood agar after 72 hours of incubation at 35°C to 37°C in 5% to 7% CO_2.** (From Winn WC Jr, et al. Koneman's Color Atlas and Textbook of Diagnostic Microbiology. 6th Ed. Philadelphia: Lippincott Williams & Wilkins, 2006.)

> *Eikenella corrodens* colonies have a distinctive odor, described as smelling musty or resembling the smell of crackers, hypochlorite bleach, or mouse cages.

that corrode the agar produce a **"twitching" motility.**[7] Colonies have a characteristic odor, described as smelling musty or resembling the smell of crackers, hypochlorite bleach, or mouse cages. *E. corrodens* does not grow on MacConkey agar.

Laboratory tests. *E. corrodens* is oxidase positive and nitrate positive. It is catalase negative, indole negative, and urease negative. *E. corrodens* is resistant to clindamycin; selective media containing clindamycin or clindamycin disks have proven useful for isolating *E. corrodens*.

Essentials

Eikenella corrodens

- A member of the HACEK group
- Gram-negative bacilli (primarily) or coccobacilli
- Fastidious
- Produces colonies that pit the agar surface
- Has a twitching motility
- Has a characteristic bleachlike or musty odor
- Oxidase positive

GENUS *KINGELLA*

The genus *Kingella* consists of three species—*K. kingae*, *K. denitrificans*, and *K. oralis*—each of which can cause human infections. *Kingella* spp. are facultatively anaerobic and nutritionally fastidious.

Clinical significance. *Kingella* spp. are part of the indigenous microflora of the oral cavity and upper respiratory tract. *K. kingae* can cause bone and joint infections in children and septicemia, keratitis, endocarditis, and central nervous system infections in adults. *K. denitrificans* has caused endocarditis and granulomatous disease in AIDS patients. *K. oralis* may be associated with periodontitis.

Clues to *Kingella* spp. Identification

Cellular morphology. *Kingella* spp. are short (0.4 μm wide by 2.0 to 3.0 μm long) Gram-negative bacilli with square

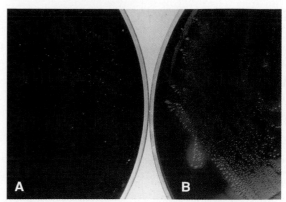

Figure 11-14. Kingella kingae colonies on sheep blood agar. **A.** After 24 hours of incubation at 35°C to 37°C in 5% to 7% CO_2, hemolysis may only be apparent beneath or immediately adjacent to the colonies. **B.** After 48 hours of incubation, however, the hemolysis is more obvious. (From Winn WC Jr, et al. Koneman's Color Atlas and Textbook of Diagnostic Microbiology. 6th Ed. Philadelphia: Lippincott Williams & Wilkins, 2006.)

ends and tend to decolorize unevenly when Gram-stained. They form pairs and short chains. Although they have no flagella, they may show twitching motility.

Colonial morphology. *K. kingae* produces 1- to-2-mm-diameter colonies on blood agar in 48 hours. Some colonies are smooth with a central nipplelike elevation, whereas others have spreading edges and pit the agar. CO_2 incubation enhances growth. *K. kingae* produces a narrow, but distinct zone of complete hemolysis (Fig. 11-14). On chocolate agar, *K. denitrificans* colonies resemble *N. gonorrhoeae* colonies (Fig. 11-15). Recovery from clinical specimens may be difficult, and viability on culture media is low. Selective media

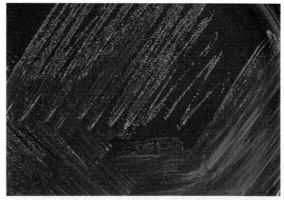

Figure 11-15. Kingella denitrificans colonies on chocolate agar. After 24 hours of incubation at 35°C to 37°C in 5% to 7% CO_2, the colonies resemble small *Neisseria gonorrhoeae* colonies. (From Winn WC Jr, et al. Koneman's Color Atlas and Textbook of Diagnostic Microbiology. 6th Ed. Philadelphia: Lippincott Williams & Wilkins, 2006.)

---

[7] The term twitching motility *refers to the ability of some nonflagellated bacteria to "crawl" over a solid surface, such as the surface of an agar medium or a glass cover slip. The bacteria possess pili/fimbriae that apparently act like grappling hooks. The pili are extended or projected forward, they bind to a surface, and then are retracted, thus pulling the cell forward. Twitching motility can be observed by examining a wet mount of the organism. Some piliated cells within colonies move in a coordinated manner, forming rafts of cells moving away from the colony edge. This can be seen by observing the edge of a colony using a dissecting or stereoscopic microscope. An Internet search for* twitching motility *will provide additional information, including videos depicting this interesting phenomenon.*

containing clindamycin or vancomycin may be helpful for isolation. Inoculation of joint fluid into blood culture bottles increases the yield in recovery of K. *kingae* from joint fluid. *K. kingae* does not grow on MacConkey agar.

Laboratory tests. *Kingella* spp. are oxidase positive and catalase negative. *K. kingae* and *K. oralis* are nitrate negative. *K. denitrificans* is nitrate positive, with production of gas.

GENUS *MORAXELLA*

Some *Moraxella* spp. are cocci, referred to as the coccal moraxellae, and some are coccobacilli, referred to as rod-shaped moraxellae. The coccal moraxellae include *M. catarrhalis*, *M. cuniculi*, and *M. caviae*. The latter two species are animal species: *M. cuniculi* is isolated from rabbits and *M. caviae* is isolated from guinea pigs. Of the coccal moraxcellae, only *M. catarrhalis* is discussed here.

Moraxella catarrhalis

Previous names for *Moraxella catarrhalis* include *Neisseria catarrhalis* and *Branhamella catarrhalis*. *Catarrh* refers to inflammation of a mucous membrane with increased flow of mucus or exudate.

Clinical significance. *M. catarrhalis* causes otitis media in children, sinusitis in children and adults, and lower respiratory tract infections (bronchitis, pneumonia) in adults. Infections in adults occur primarily in elderly and immunocompromised patients. Other infections that can be caused by *M. catarrhalis* include septicemia, endocarditis, meningitis, septic arthritis, and eye, urogenital tract, and wound infections. *M. catarrhalis* can be recovered from male and female genital tracts where, because of its diplococcal morphology, it can be confused with N. *gonorrhoeae*.

> Because of its diplococcal morphology, *M. catarrhalis* can be confused with N. *gonorrhoeae*.

Virulence factors. *M. catarrhalis* possesses endotoxin and pili, and most strains produce a β-lactamase, which is best detected using the chromogenic cephalosporin or nitrocefin test.

Clues to *M. catarrhalis* Identification

Cellular morphology. In Gram-stained clinical specimens, *M. catarrhalis* appears as extracellular, kidney-shaped Gram-negative diplococci, measuring about 0.5 to 1.5 μm in diameter.

Colonial morphology. *M. catarrhalis* grows well on blood agar and chocolate agar but not on MacConkey agar. On blood agar, colonies are gray to white, opaque, smooth, dry, and 1 to 3 mm in diameter after 24 hours of incubation. With an inoculating loop, colonies can easily be slid across the agar surface, like hockey pucks, and can be stacked like disks. Colonies on chocolate agar are pinkish brown, resembling N. *gonorrhoeae* colonies.

Tests used to identify *Moraxella catarrhalis*. Pneumonia caused by *M. catarrhalis* can be presumptively diagnosed by observing intracellular and extracellular Gram-negative diplococci in Gram-stained sputum specimens. *M. catarrhalis* is strongly oxidase positive, catalase positive, nitrate positive (most strains), and DNase positive. Many of the commercial kits used to identify N. *gonorrhoeae* and N. *meningitidis* can be used to identify *M. catarrhalis*.

DNase activity. DNase is an enzyme that breaks down DNA. DNase activity can be detected by heavily inoculating a dime-size area of DNase test agar. After overnight incubation, hydrolysis of DNA is detected by a change in color of the medium from blue to pink around and under the area of inoculation. *Neisseria* spp. are DNase negative. *M. catarrhalis* does not produce acid from glucose or other carbohydrates.

M. catarrhalis can also be distinguished from N. *gonorrhoeae* and other *Neisseria* species using the tributyrin hydrolysis test, which is a test for the enzyme butyrate esterase. *M. catarrhalis* is tributyrin hydrolysis positive, whereas *Neisseria* spp. are tributyrin hydrolysis negative. Rapid disk and spot tests to detect butyrate esterase are available commercially, and this test is incorporated into several of the rapid methods for identification of *Neisseria* and *Moraxella* spp.

CLSI Document M35-A (see "References and Suggested Reading") states that an isolate can be presumptively identified as *M. catarrhalis* if it meets the following criteria:

- Gram-negative diplococcus
- Oxidase positive
- Growth on both blood agar and chocolate agar
- Either rapid butyrate esterase positive or tributyrin hydrolysis positive; most other *Moraxella* spp. are rapid butyrate esterase positive, but they are coccobacilli rather than diplococci; although not mentioned in the CLSI document, DNase positivity could be substituted for positive reactions with either of these tests

Rod-Shaped Moraxellae

Clinical significance. The rod-shaped moraxellae include *Moraxella osloensis*, *M. nonliquefaciens*, *M. lincolnii*, *M. lacunata*, *M. atlantae*, and *M. canis*. *M. nonliquefaciens* and *M. lincolnii* are part of the indigenous microflora of the human respiratory tract. These organisms are rare causes of infections, such as conjunctivitis (pink eye), keratitis, meningitis, septicemia, endocarditis, and arthritis. The most commonly isolated species is *M. nonliquefaciens*. *M. lacunata* can cause conjunctivitis. *M. canis* is part of the upper respiratory tract flora of dogs and cats.

Clues to Identification of Rod-Shaped Moraxellae

Cellular morphology. Although referred to as rod-shaped moraxellae, these Gram-negative bacteria are often plump coccobacilli that occur predominantly in pairs and sometimes in short chains. They have a tendency to resist decolorization in the Gram-stain procedure, thus appearing Gram positive.

Colonial morphology. On blood agar, *M. nonliquefaciens* colonies are smooth, translucent to semiopaque; they are 0.1 to 0.5 mm in diameter after 24 hours and 1 mm in diameter after 48 hours. The colonies will occasionally spread and pit the agar. Colonies of *M. lincolnii* and *M. osloensis* are similar in appearance, but pitting is rare. *M. lacunata* colonies are smaller, form dark haloes on chocolate agar, and pitting is common. Colonies of *M. atlantae* are usually 0.5 mm in diameter and show spreading and pitting. Most strains of *M. canis* produce colonies that are large and smooth, resembling Enterobacteriaceae colonies (see Chapter 12). Some *M. canis* strains produce very mucoid colonies, resembling those of *Klebsiella pneumoniae* (see Chapter 12).

Laboratory tests. The rod-shaped moraxellae are non-motile and nonfermenters. They are oxidase positive, indole negative, urease negative, and nitrate variable. Except for *M. canis*, they are DNase negative. The gelatin hydrolysis test can be used to differentiate *M. lacunata* (most strains positive) from *M. nonliquefaciens* (negative).

Gelatin hydrolysis. The gelatin hydrolysis test is used to determine if an organism possesses the proteolytic enzyme(s) necessary to break down or liquify gelatin. A gelatin tube is inoculated with the test organism and incubated for up to 14 days. The tube is removed daily from the incubator and placed at 4°C, along with an uninoculated control tube. Partial or total liquefaction of the inoculated tube and complete solidification of the control tube represent a positive test result. Complete solidification of the inoculated tube following 4°C represents a negative test result.

GENUS *ACINETOBACTER*

Clinical significance. *Acinetobacter* spp. are widely distributed in nature and able to survive on most environmental surfaces, moist or dry. They are present in soil, food, water, and sewage and on animal and human skin. They are part of the indigenous microflora of the oral cavity and of the upper respiratory, genitourinary, and lower gastrointestinal tracts, as well as of skin. *Acinetobacter* spp. are opportunistic pathogens, primarily causing

> *Acinetobacter* spp. are the second most common nonfermenters isolated from clinical specimens.

infections in hospitalized, debilitated, catheterized, or immunocompromised patients. Common in the hospital environment, they cause various types of nosocomial infections, including respiratory and urinary tract infections, wound infections, and septicemia. Other *Acinetobacter*-associated infections include peritonitis, endocarditis, meningitis, osteomyelitis, arthritis, and corneal infections. The species most commonly isolated from clinical specimens are *A. baumannii*, *A. lwoffii*, *A. haemolyticus*, and *A. johnsonii*. **Acinetobacter spp. are the second-most common nonfermenters[8] isolated from clinical specimens. *Pseudomonas aeruginosa* is the most common.**

CAUTION

Beware of Similar-Sounding Names. Do not confuse the genera *Acinetobacter*, *Actinobacillus*, and *Actinomyces*. ***Acinetobacter*** spp. are Gram-negative coccobacilli; they are discussed in this chapter. ***Actinobacillus*** spp. are also Gram-negative coccobacilli; they are described in Chapter 14. ***Actinomyces*** spp. are Gram-positive bacilli; because some species are anaerobes, they are discussed in Chapter 17.

Drug resistance. Many strains are multidrug-resistant. They are generally resistant to penicillin, ampicillin, most first- and second-generation cephalosporins, gentamicin, chloramphenicol, and nalidixic acid. Resistance is more common in *A. baumannii* strains than in strains of other *Acinetobacter* spp. Multidrug-resistant *A. baumannii* strains were associated with infected war wounds in soldiers fighting in Iraq. Agents effective against most *Acinetobacter* strains include combination drugs consisting of a β-lactam agent plus a β-lactamase inhibitor, doxycycline, imipenem, quinolones, and trimethoprim-sulfamethoxazole.

Clues to *Acinetobacter* spp. Identification

Cellular morphology. *Acinetobacter* spp. are aerobic, non-motile Gram-negative coccobacilli (1.0 to 1.5 μm in width by 1.5 to 2.5 μm in length) that may appear in pairs (Fig. 11-16). They are sometimes difficult to decolorize, thus appearing Gram positive. They often resemble Gram-negative cocci in direct smears from positive blood culture bottles. Coccobacillary forms predominate on solid culture media, but bacillary forms predominate in liquid media. Although they are nonmotile, their polar fimbriae (pili) may cause a twitching motility. Some strains are encapsulated.

Colonial morphology. *Acinetobacter* spp. produce smooth, opaque, gray-white colonies that are 2 to 3 mm in diameter. Many strains grow on MacConkey agar, producing

---

[8]*The term* nonfermenters *refers to glucose nonfermentative Gram-negative bacilli, meaning Gram-negative bacilli that do not ferment glucose.* Acinetobacter spp. *are discussed in this chapter because they are members of the Moraxellaceae family. Other nonfermenters are discussed in Chapter 13.*

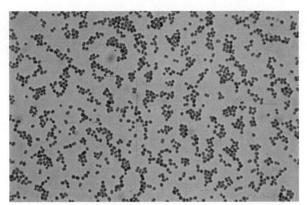

***Figure 11-16.* Gram-stained smear of *Acinetobacter baumannii* from a broth culture.** (From Winn WC Jr, et al. Koneman's Color Atlas and Textbook of Diagnostic Microbiology. 6th Ed. Philadelphia: Lippincott Williams & Wilkins, 2006.)

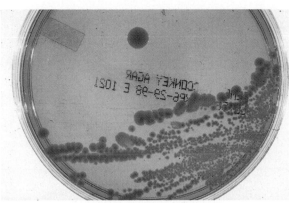

***Figure 11-17.* Colonies of *A. baumannii* on MacConkey agar.** *A. baumannii* colonies are pink to light lavender on MacConkey agar. (From Winn WC Jr, et al. Koneman's Color Atlas and Textbook of Diagnostic Microbiology. 6th Ed. Philadelphia: Lippincott Williams & Wilkins, 2006.)

colorless, slightly pink or light lavender colonies as a result of vigorous lactose oxidation (Fig. 11-17). Some strains are fastidious; they produce punctate colonies. Selective and differential media are available for isolation of *Acinetobacter* spp.

Laboratory tests. *Acinetobacter* spp. are oxidase negative, catalase positive, usually nitrate negative, and indole negative. *Acinetobacter* spp. do not ferment glucose, but some species can oxidize glucose. Those that oxidize glucose are referred to as saccharolytic species, whereas those that do not are referred to as asaccharolytic species. Most glucose-oxidizing, nonhemolytic clinical isolates are *A. baumannii*. Most nonhemolytic, glucose nonoxidizing strains are *A. lwoffii*. Most hemolytic strains are *A.*

haemolyticus. Table 11-5 summarizes various characteristics of the Gram-negative bacteria discussed in this chapter.

IDENTIFICATION OF AN UNKNOWN GRAM-NEGATIVE COCCUS, DIPLOCOCCUS, OR COCCOBACILLUS

The first step in the identification of a Gram-negative bacterium is to determine its shape, or for pleomorphic organisms, to determine its *predominant* shape. The various possibilities

TABLE 11 - 5   Characteristics of Bacteria Discussed in This Chapter

Bacteria	Oxidase	Catalase	Nitrate Reduction	Indole Production	Growth on MacConkey Agar
Neisseria spp.	+	+	+	–	–
Chromobacterium violaceum	Variable	+	+	Variable	+
Eikenella corrodens	+	– (most strains)	–	–	–
Kingella spp.	+	–	– (except for *K. denitrificans*)	–	–
Moraxella catarrhalis	+	+	Variable	–	–
Other *Moraxella* spp.	+	+	–	–	Variable
Acinetobacter spp.	–	+	–	–	+

TABLE 11 - 6	Observations and Tests of Value for Preliminary Identification of Gram-Negative Bacteria Described in This Chapter	
Cellular Morphology	**Genus/Genera**	**Observations and Test Results**
Diplococci	*Neisseria, Moraxella catarrhalis*	Oxidase positive, glucose not fermented, *Neisseria* spp. oxidize glucose but *M. catarrhalis* does not
	Acinetobacter spp.	Oxidase negative, nonmotile, glucose not fermented
Coccobacilli	*Moraxella catarrhalis*	Oxidase positive, nonmotile, glucose neither fermented nor oxidized, DNase positive
	Other *Moraxella* spp.	Oxidase positive, nonmotile, glucose neither fermented nor oxidized, DNase negative, urease negative, nitrite reduction negative
	Acinetobacter baumannii	Oxidase negative, nonmotile, glucose not fermented, glucose oxidized
	Acinetobacter lwoffii	Oxidase negative, nonmotile, glucose neither fermented nor oxidized, urease negative, nitrate reduction negative
Bacilli	*Chromobacterium violaceum*	Most strains oxidase positive, glucose fermented, purple colonies
	Acinetobacter baumannii	Oxidase negative, nonmotile, glucose not fermented, glucose oxidized
	Acinetobacter lwoffii	Oxidase negative, nonmotile, glucose neither fermented nor oxidized, urease negative, nitrate reduction negative

include cocci, diplococci, coccobacilli, and bacilli. The cellular morphology and morphologic arrangement of cells are best determined by examining a Gram-stained smear prepared from a young colony on a blood agar plate. The organism's oxidase reaction, regardless of its motility, and its ability to ferment or oxidize glucose are other important initial clues to its identity. Table 11-6 contains information about organisms discussed in this chapter. In addition to observations and tests mentioned in Table 11-6, commercial systems are available for identifying these organisms.

Chapter Review

- Most human *Neisseria* spp. are members of the indigenous flora of the upper respiratory tract and are nonpathogenic. However, *N. gonorrhoeae* and *N. meningitidis* are important pathogens that must be differentiated from other *Neisseria* spp.

- *N. gonorrhoeae* is a fastidious, oxidase-positive, Gram-negative diplococcus that requires enriched media and a 3% to 5% CO_2 atmosphere.

- *N. gonorrhoeae* is the etiologic agent of genital gonorrhea. There are many clinical manifestations of *N. gonorrhoeae* infection, including urethritis, cervicitis, proctitis, conjunctivitis, and ophthalmia neonatorum.

- β-Lactamase testing of *N. gonorrhoeae* isolates may be performed using the nitrocefin test.

- A Gram-stained smear of a urethral discharge is a highly sensitive and specific way to diagnose genital gonorrhea in symptomatic malc patients, but Gram-stained genital specimens *cannot* be used to make either a presumptive or definitive diagnosis of gonorrhea in female patients.

- The oxidation patterns of glucose, maltose, lactose, and sucrose may be used to differentiate *N. gonorrhoeae* from other *Neisseria* spp., such as *N. meningitidis* and *N. lactamica*. Of these four carbohydrates, only glucose is oxidized by *N. gonorrhoeae*.

- *N. meningitidis* is an encapsulated Gram-negative diplococcus, virtually identical in appearance to *N. gonorrhoeae*. It is the cause of meningococcal meningitis, which is often associated with crowded, stressful settings like military basic training centers and college dormitories.

- *N. meningitidis* grows well on both blood agar and chocolate agar. Unlike *N. gonorrhoeae*, it oxidizes both glucose and maltose.

- The HACEK group of organisms comprises the following fastidious Gram-negative bacilli: *Haemophilus aphrophilus/H. paraphrophilus*, *Actinobacillus actinomycetemcomitans*, *Cardiobacterium hominis*, *Eikenella corrodens*, and *Kingella* spp.

- Twitching motility is associated with *Eikenella corrodens*, *Kingella* spp., and *Acinetobacter* spp.

- *Moraxella catarrhalis* is a cause of otitis media in children.

- *Acinetobacter* spp. are aerobic, nonmotile Gram-negative coccobacilli. They are opportunistic pathogens, primarily causing infections in hospitalized, debilitated, catheterized, elderly, or immunocompromised patients.

New Terms and Abbreviations

After studying Chapter 11, you should be familiar with the following terms, which are defined within the chapter and in the Glossary at the back of the book:

Autolysis

Gonococcemia

Gonococcus (pl. gonococci)

HACEK group

Meningococcal meningitis

Meningococcemia

Meningococcus (pl. meningococci)

Nonsterile site

Ophthalmia neonatorum

Oropharyngitis

Proctitis

Sterile site

Twitching motility

References and Suggested Reading

Abbreviated Identification of Bacteria and Yeast: Approved Guideline. CLSI Document M35-A. Wayne, PA: Clinical and Laboratory Standards Institute, 2002.

Boslego JW, et al. *Neisseria meningitidis*. In: Gorbach SL, Bartlett JG, Blacklow NR, eds. Infectious Disease. 3rd Ed. Philadelphia: Lippincott Williams & Wilkins, 2004.

Evangelista AT, et al. Rapid systems and instruments for the identification of bacteria. In: Manual of Commercial Methods in Clinical Microbiology. Washington, DC: ASM Press, 2002.

Ghanem K, Zenilman JM. *Neisseria gonorrhoeae*. In: Gorbach SL, Bartlett JG, Blacklow NR, eds. Infectious Disease. 3rd Ed. Philadelphia: Lippincott Williams & Wilkins, 2004.

Ghanem KG, et al. Gonorrhea. In: Gorbach SL, Bartlett JG, Blacklow NR, eds. Infectious Disease. 3rd Ed. Philadelphia: Lippincott Williams & Wilkins, 2004.

Janda WM, Knapp JS. *Neisseria* and *Moraxella catarrhalis*. In: Murray PR, Baron EJ, Jorgensen JH, Pfaller MA, Yolken RH, eds. Manual of Clinical Microbiology. 8th Ed. Washington, DC: ASM Press, 2003.

Methods for Antimicrobial Dilution and Disk Susceptibility Testing of Infrequently Isolated or Fastidious Bacteria: Proposed Guideline. CLSI Document M45-P. Wayne, PA: Clinical and Laboratory Standards Institute, 2002.

Murphy TF. Miscellaneous Gram-negative cocci: other *Neisseria, Moraxella,* and *Kingella* Species. In: Gorbach SL, Bartlett JG, Blacklow NR, eds. Infectious Disease. 3rd Ed. Philadelphia: Lippincott Williams & Wilkins, 2004.

Nerad JL, Black S. Miscellaneous Gram-negative bacilli: *Acinetobacter, Cardiobacterium, Actinobacillus, Chromobacterium, Capnocytophaga,* and others. In: Gorbach SL, Bartlett JG, Blacklow NR, eds. Infectious Disease. 3rd Ed. Philadelphia: Lippincott Williams & Wilkins, 2004.

Protection of Laboratory Workers from Occupationally Acquired Infections: Approved Guideline. 3rd Ed. CLSI Document M29-A3. Wayne, PA: Clinical and Laboratory Standards Institute, 2005.

Schreckenberger PC, Wong JD. Algorithms for identification of aerobic Gram-negative bacteria. In: Murray PR, Baron EJ, Jorgensen JH, Pfaller MA, Yolken RH, eds. Manual of Clinical Microbiology. 8th Ed. Washington, DC: ASM Press, 2003.

Von Graevenitz A, et al. *Actinobacillus, Capnocytophaga, Eikenella, Kingella, Pasteurella,* and other fastidious or rarely encountered Gram-negative rods. In: Murray PR, Baron EJ, Jorgensen JH, Pfaller MA, Yolken RH, eds. Manual of Clinical Microbiology. 8th Ed. Washington, DC: ASM Press, 2003.

 On the CD-ROM

- Additional Self-Assessment Exercises
- Case Study
- Puzzle

Self-Assessment Exercises

Match the organism in the left column to the best description or corresponding infection in the right column.

1. _____ *N. gonorrhoeae*   A. Ophthalmia neonatorum

2. _____ *N. meningitidis*   B. Produces acid from both glucose and maltose

3. _____ *E. corrodens*   C. Causes otitis media in children

4. _____ *M. catarrhalis*   D. Member of the HACEK group

5. True or false: *N. meningitidis* will grow on blood agar.

6. True or false: Gram-stained genital specimens can be used for definitive diagnosis of gonorrhea in female patients.

7. True or false: *N. gonorrhoeae* may produce β-lactamase.

8. All *Neisseria* spp. are positive for which one of the following enzymes?

   A. Oxidase

   B. Coagulase

   C. Amylase

   D. Lipase

9. Which of the following media would not support the growth of *N. gonorrhoeae*?

   A. Chocolate agar

   B. Thayer-Martin agar

   C. Martin-Lewis agar

   D. MacConkey agar

10. While examining a Gram-stained blood specimen from a 70-year-old male patient, a clinical microbiology laboratory professional notices extracellular, kidney-shaped diplococci. The isolate grows well on blood agar and chocolate agar. The colonies on blood agar are gray to white, small, opaque, smooth, and dry looking. The technician notices that the colonies can be easily slid across the surface of the agar. What is the presumptive identification of this isolate?

    A. *N. gonorrhoeae*

    B. *N. meningitidis*

    C. *M. catarrhalis*

    D. *Acinetobacter* sp.

CHAPTER 12

Gram-Negative Bacilli: The Family Enterobacteriaceae

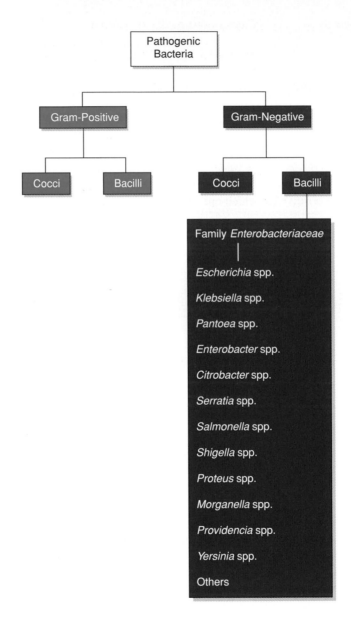

Chapter Outline

Medical Importance of the Family Enterobacteriaceae

Phenotypic Characteristics of Members of the Family Enterobacteriaceae

Laboratory Methods Used to Isolate and Identify Members of the Family Enterobacteriaceae
- Media Used to Isolate Members of the Family Enterobacteriaceae
- Identification of an Unknown Gram-Negative Bacillus

Selected Lactose-Fermenting Members of the Family Enterobacteriaceae

- *Escherichia coli*
- Enterohemorrhagic *E. coli* Serotypes
- Genus *Klebsiella*
- Genera *Pantoea* and *Enterobacter*
- Genus *Citrobacter*
- Genus *Serratia*

Selected Non-Lactose-Fermenting Members of the Family Enterobacteriaceae

- Genus *Salmonella*
- Genus *Shigella*
- Genus *Proteus*
- *Morganella morganii*
- Genus *Providencia*
- Genus *Yersinia*

LEARNING OBJECTIVES

After studying this chapter, you should be able to:

☞ Define the terms introduced in this chapter (e.g., *coliforms, deamination, decarboxylation*)

☞ Identify the clinically significant species in the family Enterobacteriaceae

☞ Relate the clinical or medical importance of the Enterobacteriaceae family

☞ Name the four genera of Enterobacteriaceae that are most often involved in infections of the gastrointestinal tract

☞ List the phenotypic characteristics of the Enterobacteriaceae (e.g., facultative anaerobe)

☞ Identify the key biochemical reactions characteristic of all Enterobacteriaceae

☞ State the selective and differential media commonly used to isolate and identify members of the family Enterobacteriaceae

☞ Outline the steps taken and observations made to identify an unknown aerobic Gram-negative bacillus

☞ Given the key biochemical reactions of an unknown member of the Enterobacteriaceae family, correctly identify the isolate

☞ Match a member of the family Enterobacteriaceae to its appropriate description or disease

☞ Given an inoculated and incubated tube of triple-sugar iron or Kligler iron agar, correctly identify and record the reactions in the tube

☞ Given an inoculated tube of triple-sugar iron agar, explain the reactions that have occurred in the tube, including which sugars have been or have not been fermented and reasons for blackening of and gas in the medium

☞ Identify positive and negative reactions for the following biochemical tests: decarboxylase, urease, indole, methyl red, Voges-Proskauer, citrate, o-nitrophenyl-β-D-galactopyranoside, and 4-methylumbelliferyl-β-D-glucuronide

☞ Explain the meaning of the term *serotypes*, and discuss the various surface antigens and the role of various serotypes in disease

☞ State the criteria specified by Clinical and Laboratory Standards Institute for the abbreviated identification of *Escherichia coli* and *Proteus* spp.

☞ Differentiate between *Salmonella* and *Shigella* spp., based on their growth on selective and differential media and their biochemical reactions

☞ Discuss the virulence factors of *E. coli, Salmonella* spp., and *Shigella* spp., including the ability to colonize, adherence factors, toxin production, and invasion of tissues of each

☞ Identify the causative organism for the following diseases: shigellosis, traveler's diarrhea, salmonellosis, typhoid fever, and plague

☞ Name the pathogen that is the most common cause of urinary tract infections

☞ Describe the clinical significance, colonial and cellular morphology, and key biochemical reactions of *Yersinia pestis*

Bubonic and pneumonic plagues. Contaminated meat recalls. Septicemia. Urinary tract infections. Traveler's diarrhea. Typhoid fever. What do these topics have in common? All are associated with some of the Gram-negative bacilli (GNB) described in this chapter.

The GNB most commonly isolated from clinical specimens are members of the family Enterobacteriaceae (often referred to here simply as the family or as Enterobacteriaceae). In distant second place are members of a group of GNB referred to as nonfermenters (see Chapter 13). Thus, if a Gram-negative bacillus is isolated from a clinical specimen, the odds are that when it is identified in the clinical microbiology laboratory, it will turn out be a member of one of these two groups. You should keep in mind, however, that not all GNB isolated from clinical specimens are members of either of these two groups (see Chapters 11 and 14).

The prefix *entero-* refers to the gastrointestinal (GI) tract. Thus, the name Enterobacteriaceae implies that members of this family are bacteria having some association with the GI tract. Some members of the family are indigenous microflora of the colon, and of these, most are opportunistic pathogens. Other members of the family (e.g., *Shigella* and *Salmonella* spp.) are not indigenous microflora; they are virtually always pathogenic when ingested. Members of the family Enterobacteriaceae are sometimes referred to as enteric bacilli, but it is important to remember that the GI tract contains many species of bacilli that are not members of the family. Although there are literally hundreds, perhaps even thousands, of species within the Enterobacteriaceae family, the following are the most clinically significant species (listed in the order in which they are discussed in this chapter):

- *Escherichia coli*
- *Klebsiella* spp.
- *Pantoea agglomerans* (previously called *Enterobacter agglomerans*)
- *Enterobacter* spp.
- *Citrobacter* spp.
- *Serratia* spp.
- *Salmonella* spp.
- *Shigella* spp.
- *Proteus* spp.
- *Morganella morganii*
- *Providencia* spp.
- *Yersinia* spp.

In this book, the discussion of Enterobacteriaceae is limited to the members of the family just listed. The names of some other members of the family can be found on the CD-ROM.

The names of Enterobacteriaceae family members are almost constantly in flux. Members are often moved from one genus to another and renamed based on the results of various molecular techniques (e.g., DNA-DNA hybridization and 16S rRNA sequencing). Names often vary from one reference book to another. Organism names found in this chapter are based on information in the eighth edition of the *Manual of Clinical Microbiology* (see "References and Suggested Reading").

MEDICAL IMPORTANCE OF THE FAMILY ENTEROBACTERIACEAE

Enterobacteriaceae are found in soil, water, and the intestinal tracts of humans and animals. They are associated with various human diseases, including abscesses, GI tract infections, meningitis, pneumonia, septicemia, urinary tract infections (UTIs), and wound infections. They are among the most common causes of **nosocomial (hospital-acquired) infections.** According to Farmer (see "References and Suggested Reading"), members of the family Enterobacteriaceae

may account for 80% of clinically significant isolates of GNB and 50% of clinically significant bacteria in clinical microbiology laboratories. They account for nearly 50% of septicemia cases, more than 70% of urinary tract infections, and a significant percentage of intestinal infections. . . . Because of the severity of these infections, prompt isolation, identification, and susceptibility testing of Enterobacteriaceae isolates are essential.

Most extraintestinal infections—infections that occur outside the GI tract—are caused by *Escherichia coli*, *Klebsiella pneumoniae*, *K. oxytoca*, *Proteus mirabilis*, *Pantoea agglomerans*, *Enterobacter aerogenes*, the *Enterobacter cloacae* complex, and *Serratia marcescens*. The most common types of extraintestinal infections caused by these organisms, in decreasing order of frequency of occurrence, are UTIs (primarily cystitis), respiratory infections, wound infections, bloodstream infections, and infections of the central nervous system. Most GI tract infections are caused by organisms in four genera—*Escherichia*, *Salmonella*, *Shigella*, and *Yersinia*—although other members of the family have also been implicated in diarrheal diseases. *Salmonella* spp., *Shigella* spp., and certain diarrheagenic (diarrhea-causing) serotypes of *E. coli* (discussed later in the chapter) are called enteric pathogens.

PHENOTYPIC CHARACTERISTICS OF MEMBERS OF THE FAMILY ENTEROBACTERIACEAE

The following phenotypic characteristics are common to all members of the family Enterobacteriaceae:

- Straight Gram-negative bacilli or coccobacilli, ranging from 0.3 to 1.0 μm wide by 0.6 to 6.0 μm long. When Gram-stained, all Enterobacteriaceae look alike (Fig. 12-1); thus, cell morphology will not be discussed for individual genera or species, except to comment on some unique feature.

- Facultative anaerobes

- Non–spore forming

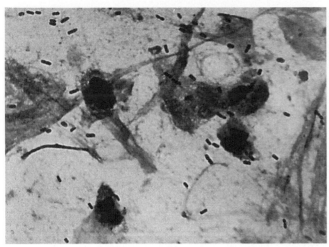

Figure 12-1. **Gram-stained bronchial brush specimen, from which *Escherichia coli* and *Klebsiella pneumoniae* were isolated.** Because these species have the same morphological appearance in a Gram-stained smear, it is impossible to distinguish between them. (From Marler LM, Siders JA, Allen SD. Direct Smear Atlas. Philadelphia: Lippincott Williams & Wilkins, 2001.)

- Biochemically active

- Capable of fermenting glucose

- Catalase positive (except *Shigella dysenteriae*)

- Oxidase negative (except *Plesiomonas shigelloides*[1])

- Capable of reducing nitrate to nitrite (nitrate reduction is discussed later in the chapter)

- Capable of growing on MacConkey agar

Essentials

Family Enterobacteriaceae

- Also known as enteric bacilli

Members of the Enterobacteriaceae family cannot be differentiated from each other by their appearance in a Gram-stained smear. They all look alike.	• Gram-negative bacilli • Glucose fermenters • Grow on MacConkey agar • Oxidase negative • Nitrate positive

Most members of the family are motile by peritrichous flagella, but some (e.g., *Klebsiella* and *Shigella* spp., and some strains of *Escherichia* and *Salmonella*) are nonmotile. All grow well on MacConkey agar (MAC), some as lactose fermenters (producing pink colonies on MAC) and some as lactose nonfermenters (producing colorless colonies on MAC; see Fig. 6-13). For some inexplicable reason, lactose nonfermenters are most often referred to as non–lactose fermenters.

CAUTION **Beware of Similar-Sounding Terms.** Organisms that ferment lactose are referred to as **lactose fermenters (LFs)** and those that do *not* ferment lactose are referred to as **non–lactose fermenters (NLFs).** Do not confuse the term *non–lactose fermenter* with the term **nonfermenter.** Whereas a non–lactose fermenter is an organism that lacks the ability to ferment lactose, a nonfermenter is an organism lacking the ability to ferment *any* sugars. As discussed in Chapter 13, organisms lacking the ability to catabolize (break down) a particular sugar by fermentative pathways (biochemical pathways that do not involve oxygen) may be able to catabolize that sugar by oxidative pathways (biochemical pathways that do involve oxygen).

LABORATORY METHODS USED TO ISOLATE AND IDENTIFY MEMBERS OF THE FAMILY ENTEROBACTERIACEAE

Media Used to Isolate Members of the Family Enterobacteriaceae

Members of the family grow well on nutrient media. Initial clues to the fermentative capabilities of an isolate are gained from its appearance on certain selective and differential plated media (Table 12-1 and Figs. 12-2 through 12-7). Additional information concerning the appearance of Enterobacteriaccae colonies on differential media can be found on the CD-ROM.

Identification of an Unknown Gram-Negative Bacillus

Initial clues in identifying an unknown Gram-negative bacillus are observations of growth or no growth of the organism on media included in the primary setup (see examples that follow). Assume that the primary setup included a blood agar plate, a chocolate agar plate, a MAC plate, and a phenylethyl alcohol agar (PEA) plate. (Recall from Chapter 8 that blood agar supports growth of most bacterial pathogens; chocolate agar supports growth of all bacteria that grow on blood agar and some fastidious organisms that do not grow on blood agar; MAC is selective for Gram-negative bacteria; and PEA is selective for Gram-positive bacteria.)

---

[1]*In this book, all members of the family Enterobacteriaceae are considered to be oxidase negative. Although* Plesiomonas shigelloides *is currently classified as an Enterobacteriaceae member, it will probably be removed from the family in the near future. See Chapter 14 for a brief discussion of* P. shigelloides, *which is only rarely isolated from clinical specimens.*

TABLE 12 - 1	Special Selective and Differential Media Used to Isolate Members of the Family Enterobacteriaceae	
Medium	**Selective**	**Differential**
Bismuth sulfite agar; has a light green color	Yes; inhibits most Gram-positive and Gram-negative bacteria; used primarily in public health laboratories to isolate *Salmonella* spp.	Yes; *Salmonella enterica* serotype Typhi colonies are black and surrounded by a black or brownish black zone; by reflected light, the zone exhibits a metallic sheen; other *Salmonella* colonies produce black or green colonies; any *Shigella* strains that grow produce brownish colonies with depressed centers
Brilliant green agar; has a brownish green color	Yes; inhibits most Gram-positive and Gram-negative bacteria; used primarily in public health laboratories to isolate *Salmonella* spp.	Yes; typical *Salmonella* colonies are slightly pink-white surrounded by a brilliant red zone; any lactose or sucrose fermenting organisms that grow produce a yellow-green colony surrounded by an intense yellow-green zone
Eosin methylene blue (EMB) agar; purple with a greenish orange cast, opalescent	Yes; inhibits most Gram-positive bacteria and Gram-negative bacteria other than enteric pathogens	Yes; strong lactose and/or sucrose fermenters, like *E. coli*, produce blue-black colonies having a greenish metallic sheen; weaker LFs (e.g., *Enterobacter, Klebsiella, Serratia*) produce pink (sometimes mucoid) colonies at 18 to 24 hours and purple colonies between 24 and 48 hours; NLFs (e.g., *Proteus, Salmonella, Shigella*) produce translucent amber-colored or colorless colonies
Hektoen enteric agar; green with a yellowish cast	Yes; inhibits Gram-positive bacteria and Gram-negative bacteria other than enteric pathogens	Yes; rapid LFs (e.g., *E. coli*) are moderately inhibited, and colonies are salmon pink to orange surrounded by a zone of bile precipitate; *Salmonella* and *Proteus* spp. produce blue-green colonies with or without black centers (as a result of H_2S production); *Shigella* colonies are greener than *Salmonella* colonies and are moist and raised
MacConkey agar (MAC) agar; has a light pink color	Yes; inhibits Gram-positive bacteria and some Gram-negative bacteria	Yes; strong LFs (e.g., *E. coli, Klebsiella, Enterobacter*) produce bright pink-to-red colonies surrounded by a pink zone of precipitated bile; slow/weak LFs (e.g., *Citrobacter, Providencia, Serratia*) produce colorless or slightly pink colonies after 24 to 48 hours; NLFs (e.g., *Proteus, Salmonella, Shigella*) produce transparent/colorless colonies
Salmonella-Shigella (S-S) agar; has an red-orange color	Yes; inhibits Gram-positive and most Gram-negative bacteria; used primarily for isolation of *Salmonella* and *Shigella* spp.	Yes; *Shigella, Salmonella,* and other NLFs produce opaque, generally smooth, translucent, or transparent colonies; any LFs that grow produce reddish, mucoid, or black-centered colonies

(continued)

TABLE 12 - 1	(Continued)	
Medium	**Selective**	**Differential**
Xylose lysine desoxycholate (XLD) agar; red color	Yes; inhibits Gram-positive bacteria and Gram-negative bacteria other than enteric pathogens	Yes; LFs produce bright yellow to yellow-red colonies; some *Proteus* spp. also produce yellow colonies, some with black centers; *Salmonella* colonies are red, most with black centers; *Shigella*, *Providencia*, and some *Proteus* spp. produce translucent/colorless or red colonies

LF, lactose fermenter; NLF, non–lactose fermenter.

Example 1

If the organism grows on chocolate agar but on none of the other plates included in the primary setup, the organism is probably fastidious (perhaps *Haemophilus influenzae*; see Chapter 14).

Example 2

If the organism grew on blood agar, chocolate agar, and MAC but not on PEA, this pattern would be consistent with a nonfastidious Gram-negative organism. The next consideration is whether its growth on MAC indicates it to be an LF or an NLF. LF colonies on MAC are pink, whereas NLF colonies on MAC are colorless. If it is an LF, the organism is most likely a member of the family Enterobacteriaceae, and the organism would be inoculated into an appropriate minisystem (see Fig. 8-20). If the organism is an NLF and its growth on blood agar appears as a thin film or waves

> Lactose fermenters produce pink colonies on MAC, whereas non–lactose fermenters produce colorless colonies on MAC.

(known as swarming), the unknown is probably a *Proteus* sp. If the organism is an NLF and no swarming is observed, the next step would be to perform an oxidase test (see Chapter 9).

Recall that all Enterobacteriaceae are oxidase negative. Thus, if the isolate is oxidase positive, it cannot be a member of the family Enterobacteriaceae. The fact that an isolate is oxidase negative, however, is insufficient proof that the isolate is a member of the Enterobacteriaceae family, because some other GNB (e.g., some nonfermenters; see Chapter 13) are also oxidase negative. At this point, the oxidase-negative isolate can be inoculated into a tube of triple-sugar iron (TSI) agar or Kligler iron agar (KIA), as described next, either prior to or simultaneously with inoculation of an appropriate minisystem. TSI and KIA tubes are primarily used as a preliminary screen for enteric pathogens like *Salmonella* and *Shigella*.

> It is important to remember that all members of the family Enterobacteriaceae are oxidase negative.

TSI tube. As the name implies, TSI agar contains three sugars: lactose (10 parts), sucrose (10 parts), and glucose (1 part). The medium also contains a pH indicator (phenol red)

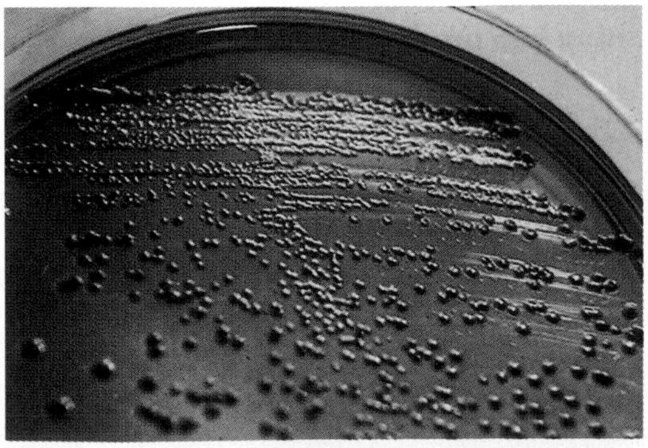

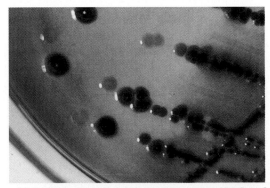

Figure 12-2. **Colonies of a lactose or sucrose fermenter on an Eosin methylene blue (EMB) plate.** Notice the characteristic metallic green sheen. (From Winn WC Jr, et al. Koneman's Color Atlas and Textbook of Diagnostic Microbiology. 6th Ed. Philadelphia: Lippincott Williams & Wilkins, 2006.)

Figure 12-3. **Colonies of a lactose fermenter (dark colonies) and a non–lactose fermenter (nonpigmented colonies) on EMB agar.** (From Winn WC Jr, et al. Koneman's Color Atlas and Textbook of Diagnostic Microbiology. 6th Ed. Philadelphia: Lippincott Williams & Wilkins, 2006.)

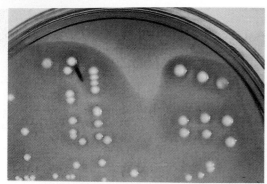

Figure 12-4. Colonies of a lactose fermenter on xylose-lysine-deoxycholate (XLD) agar. Acid production caused the color of the medium to change from pink to yellow. (From Winn WC Jr, et al. Koneman's Color Atlas and Textbook of Diagnostic Microbiology. 6th Ed. Philadelphia: Lippincott Williams & Wilkins, 2006.)

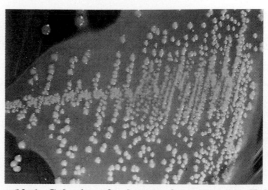

Figure 12-6. Colonies of a lactose fermenter on Hektoen enteric agar. Acid production caused the color of the medium to change from green to yellow. (From Winn WC Jr, et al. Koneman's Color Atlas and Textbook of Diagnostic Microbiology. 6th Ed. Philadelphia: Lippincott Williams & Wilkins, 2006.)

and ferrous sulfate to detect hydrogen sulfide (H_2S) production. An unknown Gram-negative bacillus is inoculated into a TSI tube to determine the following:

- Can the organism ferment glucose, and if so, can it also ferment lactose and/or sucrose?

- Is gas produced as a byproduct of fermentation?

- Does the organism produce H_2S?

A TSI tube has a slant portion and a butt (or deep) portion, and the uninoculated medium is red, meaning it is alkaline (Fig. 12-8A). The slant portion is aerobic, and the butt portion is relatively anaerobic. Inoculating bacteria into a TSI tube involves the following steps:

Step 1: Selecting a well-isolated colony of the organism to be tested and touching the top of the colony with the tip of a long, straight, sterile inoculating needle.

Step 2: Removing the cap and inoculating the butt portion of the medium by stabbing the needle through the center of the medium until it reaches the bottom of the tube.

Step 3: Withdrawing the needle from the butt portion and then, with the needle, inoculating the surface of the slant, using a zigzag motion. Recap the tube, but leave the cap loose.

Step 4: Incubating the inoculated tube at 35°C for 18 to 24 hours in a non-CO_2 incubator.

Following incubation, there are several possibilities:

Possibility 1

Both the slant and the butt are yellow (acid), with bubbles and/or cracks in the agar and/or separation of the agar from the sides and/or bottom of the tube. No blackening of the medium is apparent. *Explanation:* Yellowing of the butt indicates glucose fermentation. Yellowing of the slant indicates that the organism fermented lactose and/or sucrose, in addition to glucose. Bubbles and/or cracks in the agar or separation of the agar from

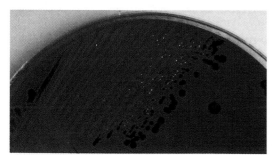

Figure 12-5. Colonies of a non–lactose fermenter on XLD agar. Black pigmentation resulted from hydrogen sulfide (H_2S) production. (From Winn WC Jr, et al. Koneman's Color Atlas and Textbook of Diagnostic Microbiology. 6th Ed. Philadelphia: Lippincott Williams & Wilkins, 2006.)

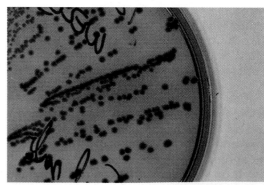

Figure 12-7. Colonies of a non–lactose fermenter on Hektoen enteric agar. (From Winn WC Jr, et al. Koneman's Color Atlas and Textbook of Diagnostic Microbiology. 6th Ed. Philadelphia: Lippincott Williams & Wilkins, 2006.)

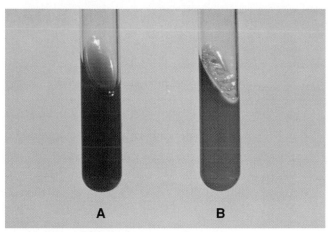

***Figure 12-8.* Tubes containing triple sugar iron (TSI) medium. A.** Uninoculated tube. **B.** Inoculated tube showing an A/A reaction. (Courtesy of the CDC.)

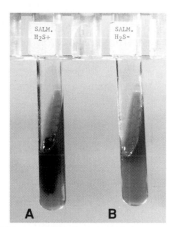

Figure 12-9. TSI reactions. **A.** K/A H_2S^+ reaction. **B.** K/A reaction. (Courtesy of M. M. Galton and the CDC.)

the sides and/or bottom of the tube indicate that gas (usually CO_2 and H_2) was formed during fermentation. Reactions are abbreviated by placing the slant reaction over the butt reaction (slant/butt). *A* means acid, *K* means alkaline, and *G* means that gas was produced during glucose fermentation.[2] Thus, the symbol for possibility 1 is A/AG. If gas had *not* been produced, the symbol would be A/A (Fig. 12-8B). The absence of blackening of the medium means that ferrous sulfide and H_2S were *not* produced. Most lactose-fermenting members of the Enterobacteriaceae family would produce either the A/A or A/AG reaction in a TSI tube.

Possibility 2

The slant is red and the butt is yellow. There is no evidence of gas formation. Some blackening of the medium appears in the butt or at the interface of the slant and the butt. *Explanation:* Yellowing of the butt indicates glucose fermentation. (Actually, the medium throughout the tube [both butt and slant] was yellow at some point during incubation of the tube. However, because the organism did not ferment either lactose or sucrose, the slant reverted back to red [alkaline] because of aerobic oxidation of the fermentation products.) Blackening of the medium indicates formation of ferrous sulfide, which is black, and H_2S, which is colorless. (Note: Sometimes blackening will occur throughout the entire butt, obscuring the yellow color. Nonetheless, the butt should be interpreted as being acid. *Question*: If the butt is black and no yellow can be seen, how do you know that the butt is acid? *Answer*: Because, except in very rare situations, production of ferrous sulfide can only occur in an acidic environment.

If the organism is oxidase negative and the butt is black, acid was most likely produced in the butt.) The symbol for possibility 2 is K/A H_2S^+ (Fig. 12-9A). Some non-lactose-fermenting members of the Enterobacteriaceae family would produce this reaction.

Possibility 3

The slant is red and the butt is yellow. No gas formation or blackening of the medium is evident. *Explanation:* Yellowing of the butt indicates glucose fermentation. (Actually, the medium throughout the tube [both butt and slant] was yellow at some point during incubation of the tube. However, because the organism did not ferment either lactose or sucrose, the slant reverted back to red [alkaline] because of aerobic oxidation of the fermentation products.) The symbol for possibility 3 is K/A (Fig. 12-9B). Some non-lactose-fermenting members of the family Enterobacteriaceae would produce this reaction.

Possibility 4

Both the slant and butt are red. There is no evidence of gas formation or blackening of the medium. *Explanation:* The organism was unable to ferment any of the three sugars; in other words, the organism is a nonfermenter. Neither gas nor H_2S were produced. The symbol for possibility 3 is K/K or K/NC, with *NC* meaning that no change occurred in the butt. Nonfermenters, such as *Pseudomonas aeruginosa* (see Chapter 13), would produce this reaction. (Note: The K/K reaction is similar in appearance to an uninoculated tube. Thus, verification that growth actually occurred in the tube is necessary before the result of K/K is reported.)

---

[2]*Sometimes a circle around the letter* A *is used to indicate that gas was produced during fermentation of glucose. However, in this book, the letter* G *indicates that gas was produced.*

Ways to Remember TSI Reactions of Enterobacteriaceae. Jarreau et al. (see "References and Suggested Reading") have suggested the following ways to remember the TSI reactions of members of the family Enterobacteriaceae:

TSI Reaction	Term to Remember (in bold)	Organisms That Produce This Reaction
A/A	**SEEK** shelter when the sun (A slant = yellow) is over the desert (A butt = yellow)	**S** for *Serratia*, **E** for *E. coli*, **E** for *Enterobacter*, **K** for *Klebsiella*
A/A H_2S^+	Wear a **CAP** to protect yourself from the H_2S geyser when the sun is over the desert	**C** for *Citrobacter*, **A** for *Arizona* (not described in this chapter), **P** for *Proteus*
K/A H_2S^+	A **CASE** of exploding firecrackers smells like H_2S when the moon (K = red) is over the desert	**C** for *Citrobacter*, **A** for *Salmonella enterica* subspecies *arizonae*, **S** for *Salmonella*, **E** for *Edwardsiella* (not described in this chapter)
K/A	**SCiPPSY** the coyote howls at the moon over the desert	**S** for *Shigella*, **Ci** for *Citrobacter*, **P** for *Providencia*, **P** for *Proteus*, **S** for *Salmonella*, **Y** for *Yersinia*

KIA tubes. The primary difference between tubes of KIA and TSI is the formulation of the media. Whereas TSI contains three sugars (glucose, lactose, and sucrose), KIA contains two sugars (1 part of glucose to 10 parts of lactose). KIA tubes are inoculated and incubated in the same manner as TSI tubes. Reactions caused by most (but not all) members of the family Enterobacteriaceae in KIA tubes are similar to the reactions produced in TSI tubes.

Possibility 1

The organism ferments both glucose and lactose. Gas may or may not be produced. The symbol for this possibility is A/A or A/AG (Fig. 12-10A, B), which is characteristic for lactose-fermenting members of the Enterobacteriaceae family (e.g., *E. coli*, *Enterobacter* spp., *Klebsiella* spp.).

Possibility 2

The organism ferments glucose but not lactose and does not produce H_2S. The symbol for this possibility is K/A (Fig. 12-10C), which is characteristic for some non-lactose-fermenting members of the family Enterobacteriaceae (e.g., *Shigella*). Because *Yersinia enterocolitica* ferments sucrose but not lactose, it will give an A/A reaction in TSI but a K/A reaction in KIA.

Possibility 3

The organism ferments glucose, but not lactose, and produces H_2S. The symbol for this possibility is K/A H_2S^+ (Fig.12-10D), which is characteristic for some non-lactose-fermenting Enterobacteriaceae (e.g., *Citrobacter*, *Proteus*, and *Salmonella* spp.).

Possibility 4

The organism ferments neither glucose nor lactose and does not produce H_2S. The symbol for this possibility is

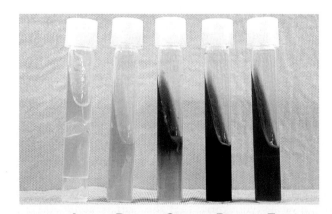

A   B   C   D   E

Figure 12-10. **Reaction patterns in Kligler iron agar tubes. A.** A/A gas. **B.** A/A. **C.** K/A. **D.** K/A H_2S^+. **E.** K/K. (From Winn WC Jr, et al. Koneman's Color Atlas and Textbook of Diagnostic Microbiology. 6th Ed. Philadelphia: Lippincott Williams & Wilkins, 2006.)

All members of the family Enterobacteriaceae produce an A/A or K/A reaction in either KIA or TSI. Any Gram-negative bacillus that produces a K/K reaction in either KIA or TSI cannot be a member of the family.

K/K (Fig. 12-10E), which is characteristic for nonfermenters like *Pseudomonas aeruginosa*. **Any Gram-negative bacillus producing the K/K reaction in either KIA or TSI cannot be a member of the family Enterobacteriaceae (recall that they all ferment glucose).** Thus, after a screening with either KIA or TSI, an isolate producing the K/K reaction would be inoculated into a minisystem designed for identification of GNB other than members of the Enterobacteriaceae family.

Most of today's clinical microbiology laboratories use some type of rapid manual or automated biochemical- or enzyme-based system to identify oxidase-negative GNB. Many of the commercially available kits incorporate tests that were, for many years, each performed separately. Examples of these tests are fermentation of various carbohydrates; tests for the presence of the enzymes, lysine, ornithine, and arginine decarboxylase; urease production; nitrate reduction; IMViC reactions; H_2S production; and the MUG test.

Decarboxylase enzymes. Lysine, ornithine, and arginine are 3 of the 20 naturally occurring amino acids found in proteins. All amino acids have the same general structure, which is illustrated in Figure 12-11. One end of the amino acid molecule is referred to as the amino end, and the other is the acid end. Organisms can use an amino acid as an energy source if they possess enzymes that break off either the amino end or the acid end of the molecule.[3] Decarboxylase enzymes cause the acid end of the molecule to break off—a process known as **decarboxylation**—yielding an alkaline amine and carbon dioxide. (Although not being discussed here, breaking off the amino end of the molecule, which requires a deaminase enzyme, is called deamination.)

For the decarboxylation test, two tubes are used, both of which contain glucose, but only one of which contains the amino acid being tested. Lysine will be used here, as an example. Following inoculation of both tubes, the broth in each tube is overlaid with mineral oil to maintain anaerobic conditions. The broth is purple or red to begin with. In the

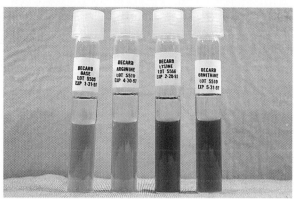

Figure 12-12. Decarboxylase test. The test organism was inoculated into four tubes of Møller decarboxylase medium. The tube on the left was a control tube, containing no amino acid. The other three tubes (from left to right) contained arginine, lysine, and ornithine. Following inoculation, mineral oil was added to the tubes, which were then incubated. This organism is arginine negative, lysine positive, and ornithine positive. (From Winn WC Jr, et al. Koneman's Color Atlas and Textbook of Diagnostic Microbiology. 6th Ed. Philadelphia: Lippincott Williams & Wilkins, 2006.)

initial phase of incubation, the media in both tubes turn yellow as a result of fermentation of glucose and subsequent production of acid. (Remember that all members of the family Enterobacteriaceae can ferment glucose.) Once the broth has become acidic, decarboxylation can take place if the organism being tested possesses the appropriate decarboxylase enzyme (lysine decarboxylase, in this example). If decarboxylation occurs, alkaline conditions result, and the medium reverts back from yellow to its original purple or red color. Thus, if the control tube is yellow and the amino acid-containing tube is purple or red, the test result is positive; the organism is lysine decarboxylase positive. If both tubes are yellow, the test result is negative; the organism is lysine decarboxylase negative. Some decarboxylase results are shown in Figure 12-12.

Urease production. Urease is an enzyme that causes the breakdown (hydrolysis) of urea into ammonia and carbon dioxide (Fig. 12-13). Ammonia, being alkaline, causes an increase in the pH of the broth. Tests designed to detect urease incorporate a pH indicator (phenol red) that changes color when alkaline conditions are produced. Thus, change in the color of the broth from the original yellow to red constitutes a

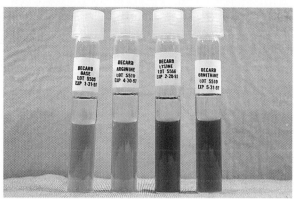

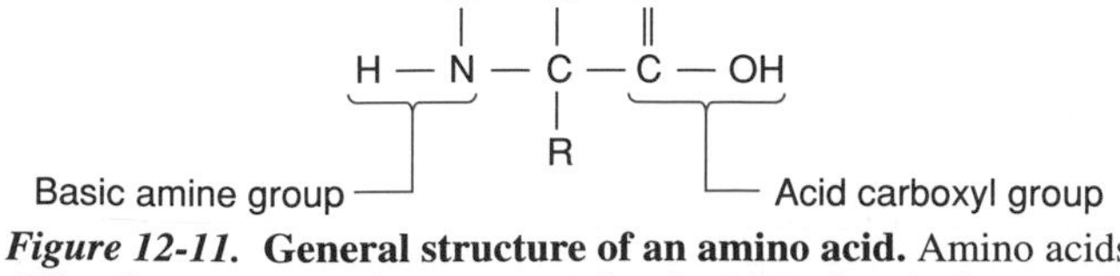

Figure 12-11. General structure of an amino acid. Amino acids differ from one another as a result of which chemical group is located at the "R" position.

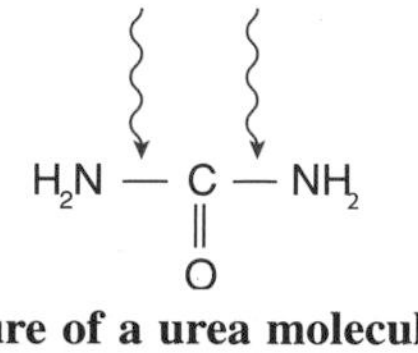

Basic amine group / Acid carboxyl group

Figure 12-13. Structure of a urea molecule, showing points of attack by urease.

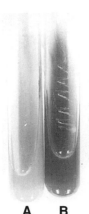

A   B

Figure 12-14. **Urease test.** Two Christensen's urea slants, illustrating a negative test result (**A**) and a positive test result (**B**). (From Winn WC Jr, et al. Koneman's Color Atlas and Textbook of Diagnostic Microbiology. 6th Ed. Philadelphia: Lippincott Williams & Wilkins, 2006.)

positive test result. (In some versions of the urease test, a bright pink color is produced; Fig. 12-14.)

Nitrate reduction. Some bacteria possess enzymes that enable them to reduce nitrate. Reduction of nitrate involves the addition of electrons and hydrogen ions, and the release of energy. The first step in the reduction of nitrate leads to the production of nitrite, but reduction of nitrate can yield many end products, depending on how many electrons are ultimately added. The end product varies from one bacterial species to another. The nitrate reduction test, details of which can be found in Appendix A, is actually a two-step procedure, as illustrated in Figure 12-15.

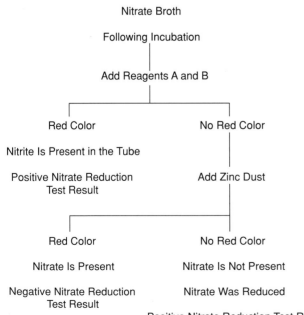

Nitrate Broth

Following Incubation

Add Reagents A and B

Red Color   No Red Color

Nitrite Is Present in the Tube

Positive Nitrate Reduction   Add Zinc Dust
Test Result

Red Color   No Red Color

Nitrate Is Present   Nitrate Is Not Present

Negative Nitrate Reduction   Nitrate Was Reduced
Test Result

Positive Nitrate Reduction Test Result

Figure 12-15. **Nitrate reduction test.**

Following inoculation and incubation of the nitrate medium, the first step is to add two different reagents (known as reagents A and B) to the tube to determine if nitrate was reduced to nitrite. Formation of a red color indicates that nitrite is present in the tube; thus, the organism is nitrate reduction positive, and testing is over (Fig. 12-16). However, if the test result is negative (no red color and thus no nitrite present in the tube), the second step is to add zinc dust to the tube to determine if nitrate is still present. The presence of nitrate (formation of a red color, following the addition of zinc dust) confirms a negative nitrate reduction result. However, the absence of a red color at this point indicates that nitrate was reduced *beyond* nitrite, sometimes as far as nitrogen gas; this constitutes a positive nitrate reduction result.

IMViC reactions. In the acronym IMViC, the *I* is for indole, *M* is for methyl red, *V* is for Voges-Proskauer, and *C* is for citrate. The lowercase *i* has no significance. IMViC reactions were originally used in water testing[4] to differentiate *E. coli* from other lactose-fermenting Enterobacteriaceae family members (e.g., *Enterobacter*

> IMViC reactions can be used to differentiate *Enterobacter aerogenes, E. cloacae,* and *Klebsiella pneumoniae* from *E. coli.*

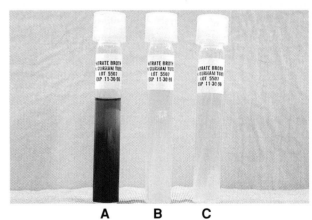

A   B   C

Figure 12-16. **Nitrate reduction test, prior to the addition of zinc dust. A.** A positive nitrate reduction test result (red color) following the addition of reagents A and B. **B.** This medium did not turn red, but the smaller inverted tube within the medium (known as a Durham tube) contains a gas bubble. The presence of the gas bubble constitutes a positive nitrate reduction test result; nitrate was reduced all the way to nitrogen gas. When zinc dust is added to this tube, the medium will not turn red. **C.** This tube did not turn red, and the Durham tube does not contain gas. When zinc dust is added to this tube, the medium will turn red, indicating that nitrate is still present in the medium. This constitutes a negative nitrate reduction test result. (From Winn WC Jr, et al. Koneman's Color Atlas and Textbook of Diagnostic Microbiology. 6th Ed. Philadelphia: Lippincott Williams & Wilkins, 2006.)

---

[4]*One of the tests used to determine if water is potable (drinkable) is the coliform count. **Coliforms** are lactose-fermenting members of the family Enterobacteriaceae, including* E. coli, Enterobacter *spp., and* Klebsiella *spp.*

TABLE 12 - 2	IMViC Test Results for *Escherichia coli, Enterobacter aerogenes, Enterobacter cloacae*, and *Klebsiella pneumoniae*			
Organism	Indole Production	Methyl Red Test	Voges-Proskauer Test	Citrate Utilization
E. coli	+	+	−	−
E. aerogenes	−	−	+	+
E. cloacae	−	−	+	+
K. pneumoniae	−	−	+	+

aerogenes, E. cloacae, and *Klebsiella pneumoniae*), which look alike on primary culture media. The presence of *E. coli* in the water would indicate fecal contamination, whereas the presence of *Enterobacter* and *Klebsiella* probably would not, since they are widespread in soil and vegetation. Three or four tubes can be used for IMViC testing: one tube of tryptophan broth for the indole test, one or two tubes of MRVP broth for the methyl red and Voges-Proskauer tests, and one Simmons citrate agar slant for the citrate utilization test.

The **indole test** is actually a test to determine if the organism possesses several enzymes collectively referred to as tryptophanase. In the presence of tryptophanase, tryptophan is broken down (deaminated) into indole, pyruvic acid, ammonia, and energy. Thus, following incubation of the organism with tryptophan, the presence of indole in the tube is evidence that the organism possesses tryptophanase. The immediate development of a red color following the addition of yellow Kovac reagent indicates the presence of indole (a positive test result). No red color indicates the absence of indole (a negative test result).

To perform both the methyl red and Voges-Proskauer tests, a tube of MRVP broth is inoculated with one drop of a 24-hour brain heart infusion broth culture of the organism to be tested. Incubation at 35°C to 37°C lasts for at least 48 hours. The broth is split into two aliquots (portions): a 5-mL aliquot for the methyl red test, and a 1-mL aliquot for the Voges-Proskauer test. (Alternatively, two tubes of MRVP broth can be inoculated.)

Methyl red test. Five or 6 drops of methyl red reagent are added to the 5-mL aliquot. The immediate formation of a bright red color in the broth indicates a pH of 4.4 or lower, demonstrating mixed acid fermentation; this is a positive test result. A red-orange color indicates a weakly positive test result, and a yellow color represents a negative test result.

Voges-Proskauer test. To the 1-mL aliquot are added 2 drops of potassium hydroxide (KOH) solution and then 6 drops of α-naphthol solution. After a thorough shaking, the mixture is observed for 5 to 10 minutes and repeatedly shaken (oxygen speeds the reaction). A red color indicates

that acetoin was formed; this is a positive test result. A yellow color indicates a negative test result.

The **citrate utilization test** determines the ability of an organism to use sodium citrate as its sole carbon source and inorganic ammonium salts as its only nitrogen source. The slant portion of a Simmons citrate agar tube is inoculated with the organism to be tested. Incubation at 35°C to 37°C lasts up to 7 days. Growth on the medium and a change in the color of the medium from green to blue is a positive test result. Absence of growth is a negative test result.

Table 12-2 shows the IMViC test results for *E. coli, Enterobacter aerogenes, E. cloacae*, and *Klebsiella pneumoniae*. Figure 12-17 shows the IMViC results for *E. coli* and *Enterobacter/Klebsiella*.

MUG test. The MUG test is a fluorogenic assay to detect the presence of the enzyme β-glucuronidase. A disk containing 4-methylumbelliferyl-β-D-glucuronide (MUG) is dampened with water, the organism to be tested applied, and the disk incubated at 35°C for up to 2 hours. Then a long-wave ultraviolet light is shined on the disk. Blue fluorescence indicates that the substrate was hydrolyzed to 4-methylumbelliferyl; this constitutes a positive test result. No fluorescence is a negative test result. *E. coli* is MUG positive.

SELECTED LACTOSE-FERMENTING MEMBERS OF THE FAMILY ENTEROBACTERIACEAE

Escherichia coli

Clinical significance. Although there are at least five species of *Escherichia, E. coli* is the species most often isolated from human clinical specimens. *E. coli* is commonly found in the indigenous GI flora of humans and animals. The *E. coli*

> *Escherichia coli* is very commonly isolated from clinical specimens. It is the most commonly isolated member of the Enterobacteriaceae family.

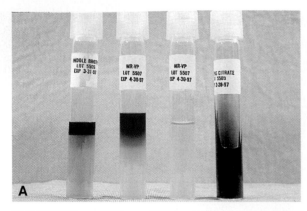

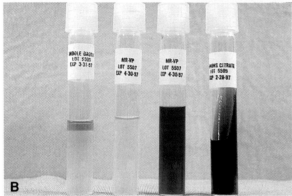

Figure 12-17. **IMViC test results. A.** IMViC test results for *E. coli*: indole +, methyl red +, Voges-Proskauer −, citrate −. **B.** IMViC test results for *Enterobacter/Klebsiella*: indole −, methyl red −, Voges-Proskauer +, citrate +. (From Winn WC Jr, et al. Koneman's Color Atlas and Textbook of Diagnostic Microbiology. 6th Ed. Philadelphia: Lippincott Williams & Wilkins, 2006.)

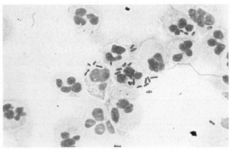

Figure 12-18. ***Escherichia coli* in a Gram-stained urine sediment; from a patient with cystitis.** In addition to the Gram-negative bacilli, notice the numerous polymorphonuclear leukocytes (PMNs). (From Winn WC Jr, et al. Koneman's Color Atlas and Textbook of Diagnostic Microbiology. 6th Ed. Philadelphia: Lippincott Williams & Wilkins, 2006.)

strains and serotypes[5] found in the human GI tract are opportunistic pathogens, usually causing problems only when they gain access to a site other than the GI tract (e.g., urinary bladder, bloodstream, wound). These *E. coli* serotypes are the most common cause of UTIs (Fig. 12-18) and are very common causes of septicemia and nosocomial infections.

> *E. coli* is the most common cause of UTIs and a very common cause of nosocomial infections and septicemia.

Other serotypes of *E. coli*, referred to as enterovirulent *E. coli* serotypes or diarrheagenic (diarrhea-causing) *E. coli* serotypes, cause GI disease when they are ingested by humans (these serotypes are discussed later in the chapter).

Virulence factors. Like all Gram-negative bacteria (except *Mycoplasma* spp.[6]), *E. coli* produces endotoxin. Other virulence factors include pili, a cytotoxin, and enterotoxins.

Drug resistance. Resistance to antimicrobial agents varies from strain to strain. **When considered to be clinically significant, isolates of all members of the family Enterobac-** teriaceae should routinely undergo antimicrobial susceptibility testing.

Clues to *E. coli* Identification

Cellular morphology. Recall that all members of the family Enterobacteriaceae look alike in Gram-stained preparations (see Fig. 12-1). *E. coli* is generally nonencapsulated, but some strains produce capsules or extracellular slime. *E. coli* strains are usually motile by peritrichous flagella.

Colonial morphology. On blood agar, *E. coli* colonies are smooth, dull gray, and 2 to 3 mm in diameter. (Note: Most members of the family Enterobacteriaceae have this appearance on blood agar; exceptions being encapsulated *Klebsiella* and *Enterobacter* spp.,

> Encapsulated strains of *Klebsiella* and *Enterobacter* spp. produce mucoid colonies.

which produce mucoid colonies.) On MAC, lactose-positive *E. coli* colonies are pink to red, flat, dry, and 2 to 3 mm in diameter; they are usually surrounded by a darker pink area of precipitated bile salts. Lactose-negative strains of *E. coli* produce colorless colonies on MAC that are 2 to 3 mm in diameter. Colonies on Hektoen enteric agar and xylose-lysine-deoxycholate (XLD) agar are yellow.

Laboratory tests. *E. coli* produces an A/AG reaction on TSI and KIA. Clinical and Laboratory Standards Institute (CLSI) Document M35-A (see "References and Suggested Reading") states that an isolate can be identified as *E. coli* (with more than 95% likelihood) if it meets the following criteria:

- GNB
- Hemolytic, nonswarming colonies
- Spot indole positive
- Oxidase negative

---

[5] *Recall from Chapter 2 that **strains** of a given species differ from each other because of differences in phenotypic characteristics, such as the enzymes that they produce. **Serotypes** of a given species differ from each other because of differences in their surface molecules (surface antigens). Sometimes, as is true for* E. coli, *different serotypes of a given species cause different diseases.*

[6] *Recall that endotoxin (also known as lipid A) is the lipid portion of lipopolysaccharide, a component of the cell walls of Gram-negative bacteria.*

TABLE 12 - 3	Categories of Enterovirulent *E. coli* Serotypes
Category	**Comments**
Shiga toxin–producing *E. coli* (STEC); also called enterohemorrhagic *E. coli* (EHEC)	These *E. coli* serotypes cause hemorrhagic colitis and hemolytic-uremic syndrome; there are dozens of different STEC serotypes, including serotypes O157:H7 and O157:nonmotile, which are the most frequently identified diarrheagenic *E. coli* serotypes in North America
Enterotoxigenic *E. coli* (ETEC)	These *E. coli* serotypes are a major cause of childhood diarrhea in developing countries; a very common, if not the most common, cause of traveler's diarrhea
Enteropathogenic *E. coli* (EPEC)	These *E. coli* serotypes causes severe, prolonged, and nonbloody diarrhea, vomiting, and fever in infants and young children; has caused outbreaks in day care centers and nurseries
Enteroinvasive *E. coli* (EIEC)	These *E. coli* serotypes cause watery, occasionally bloody diarrhea; quite rare in the United States
Enteroaggregative *E. coli* (EaggEC)	These *E. coli* serotypes have caused diarrhea in children in Chile, Mexico, Kenya, India, and Japan

If the isolate meets these criteria except that it is non-hemolytic on blood agar, it can be identified as *E. coli* if it is (1) a lactose fermenter on MAC or Eosin methylene blue (EMB), and (2) pyrrolidonyl arylamidase (PYR) negative. If the isolate meets the CLSI criteria except that it is non-hemolytic on blood agar and a non–lactose fermenter on MAC or EMB, it can be identified as *E. coli* if it is MUG positive. (Note: *E. coli* O157:H7, described next, is MUG negative.)

Essentials

Escherichia coli

- Motile Gram-negative bacillus

- Lactose-fermenting member of the Enterobacteriaceae family; pink colonies on MAC

- Many serotypes are opportunistic pathogens; enterovirulent serotypes are always pathogens

- The most common cause of urinary tract infections and very common causes of septicemia and nosocomial infections

- A/A reaction on TSI and KIA, with or without gas

- IMViC results: indole positive, MR positive, Voges-Proskauer negative, citrate negative

- Oxidase negative, nitrate positive

- PYR negative, MUG positive

Enterohemorrhagic *E. coli* Serotypes

As mentioned earlier, certain serotypes of *E. coli*, referred to as enterovirulent or diarrheagenic *E. coli* serotypes, cause GI disease when they are ingested by humans. The five categories of enterovirulent or diarrheagenic *E. coli* serotypes are listed in Table 12-3.

 STUDY AID

What's in a Name? Antigens located on an organism's capsule are called K antigens; those located on an organism's cell wall are called O or somatic antigens; and those located on an organism's flagella are called H antigens. Thus, **O157:H7** is an alphanumeric designation for a particular serotype of *E. coli*; it possesses an antigen designated 157 on its cell wall, and an antigen designated 7 on its flagella (Fig. 12-19).

> Serotypes O157:H7 and O157:nonmotile are the most frequently identified diarrheagenic *E. coli* serotypes in North America. Their presence in meat is a primary cause of the meat recalls that make the news.

Sorbitol-containing MAC (SMAC) plates can be used for isolation of O157 Shiga toxin–producing *E. coli* (STEC) strains. Unlike most other *E. coli* strains, O157 STEC strains

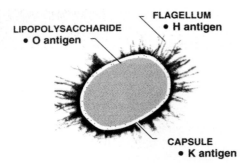

Figure 12-19. **Location of O, H, and K antigens on an *E. coli* cell.** (From Strohl WA, Rouse H, Fisher, BD. Lippincott's Illustrated Reviews: Microbiology. Philadelphia: Lippincott Williams & Wilkins, 2001.)

do not ferment D-sorbitol overnight. Thus, any D-sorbitol nonfermenting (colorless colonies) *E. coli* strains growing on SMAC are suspect. A variety of commercial immunoassays are available for detecting the presence of STEC strains in stool specimens, enrichment broths of stool specimens, and colonies. O157 and non-O157 STEC antisera and latex reagents are available.

> *E. coli* O157:H7 is the primary enterohemorrhagic *E. coli* serotype in the U.S.

Genus *Klebsiella*

Clinical significance. *Klebsiella* spp. colonize the human nasopharynx and GI tract. All species but especially *K. pneumoniae* cause nosocomial infections, including urinary tract, bloodstream, lower respiratory tract, cardiovascular, wound, ear, nose, and throat infections (Fig. 12-20). *K. oxytoca* can be isolated from blood, urine, respiratory tract specimens, and stool. *K. rhinoscleromatis* and *K. ozaenae* cause chronic granulomatous diseases of the upper respiratory tract, occurring most often in tropical areas. *K. rhinoscleromatis* causes rhinoscleroma (affecting the nose, trachea, and larynx), and *K. ozaenae* causes atrophic rhinitis (affecting the nose).

Drug resistance. Extended-spectrum β-lactamases (effective against extended-spectrum β-lactam agents) are produced by strains of most clinically significant Enterobacteriaceae, but they are most prevalent in strains of *K. pneumoniae*. *K. pneumoniae* strains also produce restricted-spectrum β-lactamases (effective against aminopenicillins and carboxypenicillins) and cephalosporinase.

Clues to *Klebsiella* spp. Identification

Cellular morphology. *Klebsiella* cells are encapsulated, whereas most other members of the family are nonencapsulated. Some *Klebsiella* strains are nonencapsulated.

Colonial morphology. On blood agar, *K. pneumoniae* colonies are mucoid and 3 to 4 mm in diameter (Fig. 12-21). On MAC, *K. pneumoniae* colonies are pink (LF), mucoid (usually), and 3 to 4 mm in diameter. Colonies on Hektoen enteric agar and XLD are yellow.

> *Klebsiella* cells are encapsulated, resulting in very mucoid colonies.

Laboratory tests. Many commercial minisystems are available for identifying *Klebsiella* spp. and other members of the family Enterobacteriaceae. *K. pneumoniae* IMViC reactions are shown in Table 12-2. Some tests of value in differentiating *Klebsiella* spp. from each other are shown in Table 12-4.

ONPG test. The compound o-nitrophenyl-β-D-galactopyranoside (ONPG) is structurally similar to lactose. The ONPG test is used to determine the ability of an organism to

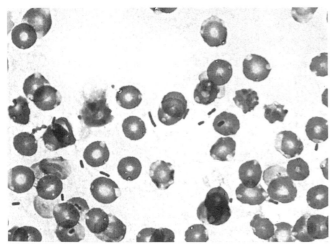

Figure 12-20. ***Klebsiella pneumoniae* in a Gram-stained blood specimen.** (From Marler LM, Siders JA, Allen SD. Direct Smear Atlas. Philadelphia: Lippincott Williams & Wilkins, 2001.)

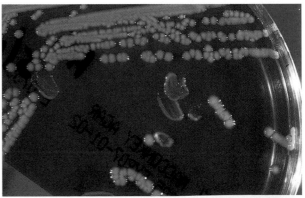

Figure 12-21. **Large, mucoid, glistening pink colonies on a MacConkey agar plate, typical of the colonies produced by many *Klebsiella* and *Enterobacter* spp.** (From Winn WC Jr, et al. Koneman's Color Atlas and Textbook of Diagnostic Microbiology. 6th Ed. Philadelphia: Lippincott Williams & Wilkins, 2006.)

TABLE 12 - 4 Tests of Value in Differentiating *Klebsiella* spp.

Klebsiella spp.	Indole	Ornithine decarboxylase	Voges-Proskauer	ONPG
K. pneumoniae	–	–	+	+
K. oxytoca	+	–	+	+
K. ozaenae	–	–	–	Variable
K. rhinoscleromatis	–	–	–	–

ONPG, *o*-nitrophenyl-β-*D*-galactopyranoside.

ferment lactose by detecting the enzyme β-galactosidase. In the presence of β-galactosidase, ONPG (which is colorless) is hydrolyzed into galactose and o-nitrophenol (which is yellow). Development of a yellow color is interpreted as a positive test result (Fig. 12-22). Tablets impregnated with ONPG are available commercially. The ONPG test is used primarily for members of the family Enterobacteriaceae and is especially useful for detecting late lactose fermenters (bacteria that ferment lactose more slowly than organisms such as *E. coli*; usually requiring more than 24 hours of incubation to be lactose positive).

Essentials

Klebsiella spp.

- Nonmotile Gram-negative bacilli
- Opportunistic pathogens that live in the intestinal tract
- Lactose-fermenting members of the Enterobacteriaceae family; pink colonies on MAC
- Encapsulated strains produce mucoid colonies

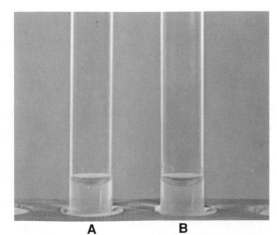

***Figure 12-22.* ONPG test. A.** Positive test result. **B.** Negative test result. (MacFaddin JF. Biochemical Tests for Identification of Medical Bacteria. Baltimore: Williams and Wilkins, 1976.)

- A/AG reaction on TSI and KIA; usually abundant gas
- IMViC results: indole negative, methyl red negative, Voges-Proskauer positive, citrate positive
- Oxidase negative, nitrate positive

Genera *Pantoea* and *Enterobacter*

Clinical significance. *Pantoea* and *Enterobacter* spp. are widely distributed in nature, being found in human and animal feces, soil, sewage, dairy products, meat, fish, and vegetation. They cause nosocomial infections, including urinary tract, bloodstream, lower respiratory tract, cardiovascular, central nervous system, wound, ear, nose, and throat infections. Some of the more clinically significant species include *Pantoea agglomerans, Enterobacter aerogenes, E. cloacae, E. gergoviae, E. sakazakii, E. taylorae,* and *E. asburiae.*

Drug resistance. Inducible β-lactamase resistance is a problem with *Enterobacter* spp. Some second- and third-generation cephalosporins and broad-spectrum penicillins are powerful β-lactamase inducers.

Clues to *Pantoea* and *Enterobacter* spp. Identification

Colonial morphology. On blood agar, *Enterobacter* colonies are smooth and 3 to 4 mm in diameter. Colonies on MAC are pink (LF) and 2 to 4 mm in diameter; colonies may be mucoid, but not as mucoid as *Klebsiella* colonies. Colonies on Hektoen enteric agar and XLD are yellow. *E. sakazakii* and some strains of *P. agglomerans* produce bright-to-pale yellow-pigmented colonies. Yellow pigmentation may be enhanced by incubation at 25°C.

Laboratory tests. *Enterobacter aerogenes* and *E. cloacae* IMViC reactions are shown in Table 12-2. Decarboxylase and carbohydrate fermentation reactions are of value in differentiating *Enterobacter* spp. *P. agglomerans* is referred to as being triple-decarboxylase negative, referring to the fact that it is lysine-, arginine-, and ornithine decarboxylase negative. Many commercial minisystems are available for identifying *P. agglomerans* and *Enterobacter* spp.

Essentials

Pantoea and *Enterobacter* spp.

- Gram-negative bacilli, usually motile
- Opportunistic pathogens that live in the intestinal tract
- Lactose-fermenting members of the family Enterobacteriaceae; pink colonies on MAC
- Encapsulated strains produce mucoid colonies
- A/A reaction on TSI and KIA, with or without gas (usually abundant gas)
- IMViC results: indole negative, methyl red negative, Voges-Proskauer positive, citrate positive
- Oxidase negative, nitrate positive

Genus *Citrobacter*

Clinical significance. There are about a dozen *Citrobacter* spp. They are part of the intestinal microflora of humans and animals and are found in soil, water, sewage, and food. They cause disease primarily in debilitated hospital patients. *Citrobacter freundii* is the most commonly isolated and most antibiotic-resistant species. It is a cause of nosocomial urinary tract and wound infections, pneumonia, septicemia, and meningitis. Other species include *C. amalonaticus* (UTIs and septicemia) and *C. koseri* (UTIs, wound infections, pneumonia, septicemia; meningitis in infants).

Clues to *Citrobacter* spp. Identification

Colonial morphology. *Citrobacter* spp. are late lactose fermenters (requiring more than 24 hours of incubation to be lactose positive). However, colonies of *Citrobacter freundii* on MAC are pink at 18 to 24 hours, resembling *E. coli*. Colonies of other *Citrobacter* spp. on MAC are usually colorless after 24 hours of incubation but are light pink after 48 hours. Colonies are colorless on Hektoen enteric agar and red, yellow, or colorless on XLD, with or without black centers.

Laboratory tests. *Citrobacter* spp. can be differentiated from *E. coli* and some other members of the family Enterobacteriaceae by their ability to use citrate as their sole carbon source (hence the name *Citro*bacter). (Note: Certain *Enterobacter*, *Klebsiella*, *Providencia*, *Salmonella*, and *Serratia* spp. are also citrate positive.) Other features of value for identification of *Citrobacter* spp. are (1) they are lysine decarboxylase negative, and (2) they do not produce acetylmethylcarbinol. *C. freundii* produces an A/AG H$_2$S$^+$ reaction in KIA. Many commercial minisystems are available for identifying *Citrobacter* spp.

Essentials

Citrobacter spp.

- Motile Gram-negative bacilli
- Opportunistic pathogens that live in the intestinal tract
- Late lactose-fermenting members of the Enterobacteriaceae family; pink colonies on MAC at 48 hours
- Can use citrate as their sole carbon source (citrate positive)
- A/AG reaction on TSI and KIA; H$_2$S positive
- IMViC results: indole variable, methyl red positive, Voges-Proskauer negative, citrate positive
- Oxidase negative, nitrate positive

Genus *Serratia*

Clinical significance. *Serratia* spp. are widely distributed in nature, primarily in soil and water. Most infections caused by *Serratia* spp. are nosocomial infections. The most commonly isolated species is *S. marcescens*. Although most strains of *S. marcescens* are nonpigmented, some produce a red pigment. *S. marcescens* causes a wide variety of infections, including UTIs; respiratory tract, eye, and postoperative wound infections; otitis externa; septicemia; endocarditis; arthritis; osteomyelitis; and meningitis. Less commonly isolated species of *Serratia* are *S. odoriferae*, *S. plymuthica*, and *S. rubidaea*.

Clues to *Serratia* spp. Identification

Colonial morphology. *Serratia* spp. are late lactose fermenters. On MAC, colonies of *Serratia* spp. are colorless after 24 hours of incubation; colonies of most strains are still colorless at 48 hours. Some strains of *S. marcescens* produce a red pigment, as do most strains of *S. rubidaea* and *S. plymuthica*; colonies may be entirely red or may have only a red center. The red pigment is called prodigiosin. On MAC, the red pigmentation can be mistaken for lactose fermentation. Colonies are colorless on Hektoen enteric agar and yellow or colorless on XLD.

> Some *Serratia* strains produce red-pigmented colonies.

Laboratory tests. Many commercial minisystems are available for identifying *Serratia* spp.

Essentials

Serratia spp.

- Motile Gram-negative bacilli
- Late lactose-fermenting members of the family Enterobacteriaceae; may or may not produce pink colonies on MAC at 48 hours

- Can use citrate as their sole carbon source (citrate positive)

- A/A reaction on TSI and KIA, with or without gas

- IMViC results: indole negative, methyl red variable, Voges-Proskauer variable (*S. marcescens* is Voges-Proskauer positive), citrate positive

- Oxidase negative, nitrate positive

SELECTED NON-LACTOSE-FERMENTING MEMBERS OF THE FAMILY ENTEROBACTERIACEAE

Genus *Salmonella*

The taxonomy of *Salmonella* spp. changes frequently. Currently, two species are recognized: *S. enterica* and *S. bongori*. What can be confusing is that *S. enterica* has six subspecies and more than 2,500 serotypes. One serotype—*S. enterica* serotype Typhi (formerly *S. typhi* and usually indicated as simply *Salmonella* serotype Typhi)—is the cause of typhoid fever. The two most common serotypes isolated in the United States are *S. enterica* serotypes Typhimurium and Enteritidis.

> *Salmonella* serotype Typhi causes typhoid fever.

Salmonella spp. have the following characteristics:

- Aerobic or facultatively anaerobic

- Usually motile

- Non–spore forming

- Urease negative (helps to distinguish *Salmonella* from *Proteus* spp.)

- Most species produce abundant H_2S (*Salmonella* serotype Typhi produces little or none)

- Most species produce gas in glucose-containing media (*Salmonella* serotype Typhi does not)

- Most species produce lysine and ornithine decarboxylase (*Salmonella* serotype Typhi does not produce ornithine decarboxylase)

- Most species do not ferment sucrose

Clinical significance. Most of the *Salmonella* serotypes cause salmonellosis—an intestinal infection accompanied by diarrhea, fever, and abdominal cramps. The symptoms may last a week or longer. Less common manifestations, especially in immunocompromised patients, are osteomyelitis, UTI, and septicemia. Transmission occurs by ingestion of foods of animal origin (e.g., eggs, unpasteurized milk, poultry) or nonanimal origin, by ingestion of contaminated water, by direct contact with animals (especially reptiles), and occasionally by human contact. Typhoid fever is a serious, sometimes fatal bloodstream infection accompanied by high fever and headache. Death is usually the result of septic shock. Transmission of typhoid fever is from person to person or by ingestion of fecally contaminated food and water. Diseases similar to typhoid fever are caused by *Salmonella* serotypes Paratyphi A, B, and C.

> Many serotypes of *S. enterica* are the cause of a diarrheal disease known as salmonellosis.

Virulence factors. *Salmonella* spp. possess pili, which enable the bacteria to adhere to intestinal epithelial cells. Secreted proteins promote phagocytosis of the bacterial cells by the epithelial cells. *Salmonella* cells can survive within phagocytes by mechanisms not completely understood. The endotoxin produced by *Salmonella* spp. is the cause of death in patients with systemic infection. *Salmonella* serotype Typhi produces virulence (Vi) antigen, which apparently protects the organism from the actions of complement.

Drug resistance. Antimicrobial therapy is not recommended for treatment of *Salmonella* gastroenteritis (salmonellosis). However, treatment with the appropriate antimicrobial agent can be crucial for patients with invasive *Salmonella* infections. Drug resistance in *Salmonella* isolates has been steadily increasing. Some isolates are multidrug resistant.

Clues to *Salmonella* spp. Identification

Colonial morphology. Enrichment broths (e.g., tetrathionate broth, tetrathionate broth with brilliant green, Selenite broth, Gram-negative broth) are used for maximal recovery of *Salmonella* from fecal specimens. Selective and differential media of value in isolating *Salmonella* include MAC, EMB, XLD, *Salmonella-Shigella* agar, and Hektoen enteric agar. Colonies on blood agar are smooth and 2 to 3 mm in diameter; they may have a greenish color resulting from H_2S production. Colonies on MAC are colorless (NLF), flat, and 2 to 3 mm diameter. Colonies on Hektoen enteric agar are green to black and colonies on XLD are red with black centers.

Laboratory tests. Most *Salmonella* isolates produce a K/AG H_2S^+ reaction on TSI and KIA. *Salmonella* serotype Typhi usually produces a K/A reaction, with only a small amount of blackening (H_2S production) at the site of the stab and within the stab line. Lysine iron agar is a useful screening medium, because most *Salmonella* isolates are lysine decarboxylase positive and produce H_2S. Various commercial systems are available for identification of *Salmonella* isolates. Serotyping of *Salmonella* isolates for epidemiologic purposes is usually performed in reference laboratories, using group- and type-specific antisera. *Salmonella* spp. are serotyped based on their O (somatic) antigens, Vi antigen (a capsular antigen), and H (flagellar) antigens.

Essentials

Salmonella spp.

- Gram-negative bacilli, usually motile

- Cause a diarrheal disease known as salmonellosis; *Salmonella* serotype Typhi causes typhoid fever

- Non-lactose-fermenting members of the Enterobacteriaceae family; colorless colonies on MAC

- K/A reaction on TSI and KIA, with or without gas; most species H_2S positive

- IMViC results: indole negative, methyl red positive, Voges-Proskauer negative, citrate variable

- Oxidase negative, nitrate positive, urease negative

Genus *Shigella*

Clinical significance. Genetically, *Shigella* spp. are virtually identical to *E. coli*. The four subgroups or serogroups (often referred to as species) of *Shigella* are

- *Shigella dysenteriae* (subgroup/serogroup A),

- *Shigella flexneri* (subgroup/serogroup B),

- *Shigella boydii* (subgroup/serogroup C), and

- *Shigella sonnei* (subgroup/serogroup D).

Shigella spp. cause a diarrheal disease known as shigellosis or bacillary dysentery. The diarrhea may be bloody or nonbloody. Humans and other large primates are the only natural reservoirs of *Shigella* spp. Transmission is from person to person or by ingestion of fecally contaminated food or water. Shigellosis is common in developing countries, where it can occur in epidemic proportions. *Shigella* spp. are common causes of traveler's diarrhea. Most cases of shigellosis in developing countries are caused by *S. dysenteriae* and *flexneri* (in that order). Most shigellosis in the United States and other developed countries is caused by *S. sonnei* and *S. flexneri* (in that order). Shigellosis is usually a self-limited disease; thus, antibiotics are unnecessary for uncomplicated cases.

> *Shigella* spp. cause a diarrheal disease known as shigellosis.

Virulence factors. Surface proteins called invasion plasmid antigens promote adherence to and phagocytosis by epithelial cells of the intestinal mucosa. Other proteins enable ingested *Shigella* to move from one host cell to another. Within the host cells, *Shigella* are protected from phagocytes and other host defense mechanisms. Infected host cells die. *S. dysenteriae* produces several toxins, including Shiga toxin (a cytotoxin) and enterotoxins. Shiga toxin may be the cause of the hemolytic-uremic syndrome sometimes associated with *S. dysenteriae* infection.

Clues to *Shigella* spp. Identification

Cellular morphology. *Shigella* cells are nonmotile, whereas most other members of the family (except *Klebsiella* spp. and some strains of *Escherichia* and *Salmonella*) are motile.

Colonial morphology. Gram-negative broth or selenite broth is often used as an enrichment medium to isolate *Shigella* (and *Salmonella*) spp. When *Shigella* is suspected, stool specimens are inoculated onto MAC and XLD or Hektoen enteric agar. On all these media, *S. dysenteriae* colonies will be smaller than colonies of other *Shigella* spp. *Salmonella-Shigella* agar inhibits some strains of *Shigella*. On blood agar, *Shigella* colonies are smooth and 2 to 3 mm in diameter. Colonies on MAC are colorless (NLF), flat, and 2 to 3 mm diameter. Colonies are green on Hektoen enteric agar and colorless on XLD.

Laboratory tests. A K/A reaction is seen on TSI and KIA, with no gas or H_2S production. Motility, urease, and lysine decarboxylase tests are negative. Several commercial systems are available for identification of *Shigella* spp. Table 12-5 lists some of the ways in which *Shigella* spp. can be differentiated from *E. coli*.

Biochemical test results of value in distinguishing among *Shigella* spp. are (1) the inability of *S. dysenteriae* to ferment mannitol, (2) production of ornithine decarboxylase by *S. sonnei*, (3) that *S. sonnei* are ONPG positive, and (4) the ability of most *S. sonnei* strains to ferment lactose after several days of incubation. Differentiation among *Shigella* species is usually accomplished by immunological methods, using group- and type-specific antisera.

Essentials

Shigella spp.

- Nonmotile Gram-negative bacilli

- Cause a diarrheal disease known as shigellosis

- Non-lactose-fermenting members of the family Enterobacteriaceae; colorless colonies on MAC

- K/A reaction on TSI and KIA, with or without gas (usually without)

- IMViC results: indole variable, methyl red positive, Voges-Proskauer negative, citrate negative

- Oxidase negative, nitrate positive

Genus *Proteus*

Clinical significance. *Proteus* spp. are found in the human GI tract, soil, water, and sewage. They are associated with UTIs, pneumonia, wound infections, septicemia, and meningitis. *P. mirabilis* is the most commonly isolated species.

TABLE 12 - 5	Tests Used to Differentiate *Shigella* spp. from *E. coli*	
Test	E. coli	Shigella spp.
Motility	+	−
Glucose fermentation within 24 hours	+	−
Gas from glucose fermentation	+	− (with rare exceptions)
Lactose fermentation within 24 hours	+ (most strains)	−
Lysine decarboxylase	+	−

Drug resistance. *P. mirabilis* is susceptible to a wider variety of agents than is *P. vulgaris* (Table 12-6), underscoring the need to differentiate between these two species.

Clues to *Proteus* spp. Identification

Colonial morphology. *P. mirabilis* and *P. vulgaris* (sometimes) swarm in waves on blood agar and chocolate agar, covering the entire surface of the plate (Fig.12-23). They produce colorless (NLF), flat, 2- to-3-mm-diameter colonies on MAC; sometimes slightly swarming; having a foul smell. Colonies on Hektoen enteric agar are colorless. Colonies on XLD are yellow or colorless, with or without black centers.

> *Proteus* spp. produce swarming growth on blood agar plates.

Laboratory tests. CLSI Document M35-A states that an isolate can be identified as a *Proteus* sp. (with more than 95% likelihood) if it meets the following criteria:

- Gram-negative bacillus
- Swarming growth
- Indole positive = *Proteus vulgaris*

- Indole negative = *Proteus mirabilis* if ampicillin sensitive (ampicillin-resistant isolates can be reported as indole-negative *Proteus*, or isolates can be further tested; *P. mirabilis* is indole negative, maltose negative, and ornithine positive; *P. penneri* is indole negative, maltose positive, and ornithine negative)

Proteus, *Morganella*, and *Providencia* spp. are the only members of the Enterobacteriaceae family that produce phenylalanine deaminase. Many commercial minisystems are available for identifying *Proteus* spp.

Phenylalanine deaminase (PAD) test. Phenylalanine is an amino acid. The enzyme phenylalanine deaminase causes the deamination of phenylalanine to phenylpyruvic acid. The PAD test detects the formation of phenylpyruvic acid. After the organism is grown on a phenylalanine agar slant, 4 or 5 drops of ferric chloride reagent are added to the agar slant, with rotation of the tube to dislodge the surface colonies. The immediate appearance of an intense green color indicates the presence of phenylpyruvic acid, which is interpreted as a positive test result (Fig. 12-24).

TABLE 12 - 6	Differences in Susceptibility Patterns Between *Proteus* spp.	
Proteus spp.	Usually Susceptible To	Usually Resistant To
P. mirabilis	Aminoglycosides, amoxicillin, ampicillin, cephalosporins, imipenem, piperacillin, trimethoprim-sulfamethoxazole	Nitrofurantoin, tetracycline
P. vulgaris	Aminoglycosides, aztreonam, broad-spectrum cephalosporins, cefepime, cefoxitin, imipenem	Amoxicillin, ampicillin, cefazolin, cefoperazone, cefuroxime, piperacillin

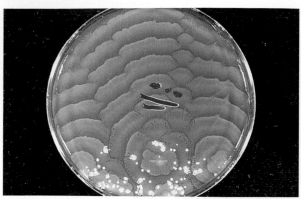

***Figure 12-23.* Waves of a swarming *Proteus* species on the surface of a chocolate agar plate.** Some of the growth has been scraped off near the center of the plate. (From Winn WC Jr, et al. Koneman's Color Atlas and Textbook of Diagnostic Microbiology. 6th Ed. Philadelphia: Lippincott Williams & Wilkins, 2006.)

Essentials

Proteus spp.

- Motile Gram-negative bacilli, sometimes highly motile

- Opportunistic pathogens that live in the intestinal tract

- Often produces swarming growth on blood agar

- Non-lactose-fermenting members of the Enterobacteriaceae family; colorless colonies on MAC

- K/A reaction on TSI and KIA, with or without gas (usually with); H_2S positive

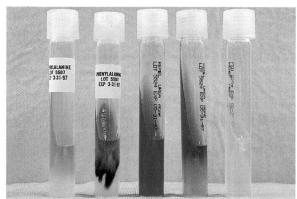

***Figure 12-24.* Phenylalanine deaminase (PAD) and urease test results.** The two tubes to the left show negative (light yellow) and positive (dark green) PAD test results. The three tubes to the right are Christensen's urea agar slants, which, from left to right, show a strong positive result (pink throughout the medium), a weak positive result (a pink slant), and an uninoculated control (yellow throughout the medium). Strong positive urease results are produced by *Proteus*, *Morganella*, and *Providencia* spp., whereas weak positive urease results are produced by *Klebsiella* spp. and some *Enterobacter* spp. (From Winn WC Jr, et al. Koneman's Color Atlas and Textbook of Diagnostic Microbiology. 6th Ed. Philadelphia: Lippincott Williams & Wilkins, 2006.)

- *Proteus vulgaris* is indole positive; *Proteus mirabilis* is indole negative

- Oxidase negative, nitrate positive

- PAD positive

Morganella morganii

Clinical significance. *M. morganii* is closely related to *Proteus* spp. and was once classified as *Proteus morganii*. It may be associated with nosocomial UTIs; respiratory tract, genitourinary, and wound infections; septicemia; diarrhea; and meningitis. Drug-resistant strains are common.

Clues to *M. morganii* Identification

Colonial morphology. On blood agar, *M. morganii* colonies are flat and 2 to 3 mm in diameter, with no swarming. Colonies on MAC are colorless (NLF), flat, and 2 to 3 mm diameter, with no swarming. Colonies are colorless on Hektoen enteric agar and red or colorless on XLD.

Laboratory tests. *M. morganii* is PAD positive. Many commercial minisystems are available for identifying *M. morganii*.

> Neither *Morganella morganii* nor *Providencia* spp. produce swarming growth.

Essentials

Morganella morganii

- Motile Gram-negative bacillus

- Non-lactose-fermenting member of the family Enterobacteriaceae; colorless colonies on MAC

- K/AG reaction on TSI and KIA; H_2S negative

- IMViC results: indole positive, methyl red positive, Voges-Proskauer negative, citrate negative

- Oxidase negative, nitrate positive

- PAD positive

Genus *Providencia*

Clinical significance. *Providencia* spp. include *P. alcalifaciens*, *P. hembachae*, *P. rettgeri*, *P. rustigiani*, and *P. stuartii*. They primarily cause infections in debilitated hosts. Infections include UTIs, pneumonia, postoperative and burn-wound infections, septicemia, and meningitis.

Clues to *Providencia* spp. Identification

Colonial morphology. On blood agar, *Providencia* colonies are flat and 2 to 3 mm in diameter, with no swarming.

Colonies on MAC are colorless (NLF), flat, and 2 to 3 mm in diameter, with no swarming. Colonies are colorless on Hektoen enteric agar and yellow or colorless on XLD.

Laboratory tests. *Providencia* spp. are PAD positive. Many commercial minisystems are available for identifying *Providencia* spp.

Essentials

Providencia spp.

- Motile Gram-negative bacilli

- Non-lactose-fermenting members of the family Enterobacteriaceae; colorless colonies on MAC

- K/A reaction on TSI and KIA, with or without gas (usually without); H$_2$S negative

- IMViC results: indole positive, methyl red positive, Voges-Proskauer negative, citrate positive

- Oxidase negative, nitrate positive

- PAD positive

Genus *Yersinia*

Clinical significance. *Yersinia* spp. and the diseases that they cause are shown in Table 12-7. Because *Y. pestis* is considered a potential bioterrorism agent, it is also discussed in Chapter 26.

Yersinia pestis, the cause of plague, is a potential bioterrorism and biological warfare agent.

Virulence factors. *Yersinia* spp. possess adhesins (which promote attachment), antiphagocytic proteins, and proteins that mediate phagocytosis of the bacteria by host cells. *Y. pestis* also produces an antiphagocytic capsule, coagulase, and fibrinolysin and can bind or store hemin. *Y. enterocolitica* produces an enterotoxin.

Clues to *Yersinia* spp. Identification

Cellular morphology. *Yersinia* spp. are GNB or coccobacilli. Cells are plump and 0.5 to 0.8 μm wide by 1.0 to 3.0 μm long. *Y. pestis* has a characteristic bipolar ("safety pin") appearance in clinical material when stained with Giemsa, Wright, Wright-Giemsa, Wayson, or methylene blue stains (see Fig. 18-6); it usually does not have this appearance when Gram stained (Fig. 12-25). (Note: Bipolar staining is not limited to *Y. pestis*; other *Yersinia* spp., *Pasteurella* spp., and other GNB can exhibit this staining characteristic.) Gram-stained broth cultures reveal single cells, pairs, and short chains. *Y. pestis* is nonmotile. Other *Yersinia* spp. are motile (peritrichous) at 22°C to 30°C but nonmotile at 37°C. The optimal growth temperature of *Yersinia* spp. is 25°C to 28°C.

Colonial morphology. *Y. pestis* is slow growing. On primary plates, *Y. pestis* may be masked by more rapidly growing organisms. On solid media, *Y. pestis* produces pinpoint, gray-white, translucent colonies at 24 hours, often too small to be seen with the naked eye. At 48 hours, colonies are 1 to 2 mm in diameter, gray-white to slightly yellow, and opaque. After 48 hours, *Y. pestis* colonies are nonhemolytic on blood agar (Fig. 12-26), smooth or mucoid on brain heart infusion agar, and colorless on MAC. When examined using an ×4 objective, colonies have a raised, irregular, "fried egg" appearance that

TABLE 12 - 7 *Yersinia* spp. and the Diseases They Cause

Yersinia spp.	Diseases
Yersinia enterocolitica	Prefers cool temperatures. Usually acquired by ingestion of contaminated food or water, but some infections have resulted from contaminated blood and blood products. Has caused ileocecal inflammation (diarrhea, fever, abdominal pain; can be mistaken for appendicitis), mesenteric lymphadenitis, polyarthritis, septicemia, wound infections, and meningitis.
Yersinia pestis	The etiologic agent of plague (once referred to as the "black death"); a zoonosis transmitted by rat fleas. There are three types of plague: (1) pneumonic plague, which is highly infectious and transmitted from person to person; (2) bubonic plague, in which buboes (swollen lymph nodes) are produced; and (3) septicemic plague, which can lead to septic shock and death.
Yersinia pseudotuberculosis	Primarily an animal pathogen; rarely infects humans. Usually acquired by ingestion of contaminated food or water. Causes localized GI infection and a scarlet fever–like disease, with high fever, arthritis, and rash. Endotoxemia may occur.

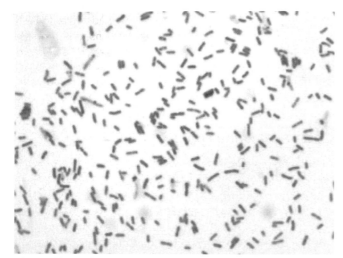

Figure 12-25. **Gram-stained *Yersinia pestis*.** (Courtesy of Larry Stauffer, Oregon State Public Health Laboratory, and the CDC.)

becomes more prominent with age. Older colonies have been described as having a shiny "hammered copper" surface.

In undisturbed broth cultures, *Y. pestis* grows in clumps that are described as flocculent or stalactite in appearance. (The term *stalactite* refers to icicle-like calcium carbonate deposits that hang down from the roofs of caves.) At 24 hours, the clumps hang along the side of the tube. After 24 hours, the growth settles to the bottom of the tube (described as "cotton fluff"). (Note: Clumped growth in unshaken or unmixed broth cultures in not unique to *Y. pestis*; some strains of *Y. pseudotuberculosis* and *Streptococcus pneumoniae* can exhibit this growth characteristic.)

On blood agar, *Y. enterocolitica* colonies are smooth and less than 1 mm in diameter. *Y. enterocolitica* produces colorless (NLF), pinpoint or flat colonies on MAC that are

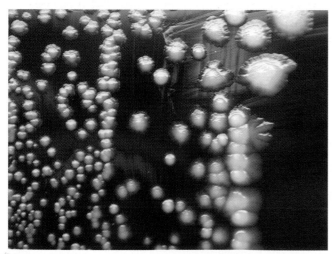

Figure 12-26. **Y. pestis colonies on sheep blood agar, after 72 hours of incubation.** Notice the "fried egg" morphology of the colonies, which is especially evident on the right side of this photograph. (Courtesy of Larry Stauffer, the Oregon State Public Health Laboratory, and the CDC.)

less than 1 mm in diameter (colonies may be colorless to peach); salmon color colonies on Hektoen enteric agar; and yellow or colorless colonies on XLD. Cefsulodin-Irgasan-novobiocin (CIN) medium is a selective and differential medium for the isolation and differentiation of *Yersinia* spp. from clinical specimens and foods.

CIN agar. CIN medium inhibits most bacteria, but a concentration of 4 µg of cefsulodin will permit growth of *Y. enterocolitica*, *Y. pseudotuberculosis*, and *Y. pestis*. After 48 hours at 25°C to 30°C, *Y. enterocolitica* colonies are 2 mm in diameter and have a bulls-eye appearance (a red center surrounded by a transparent zone). *Y. pseudotuberculosis* does not produce bulls-eye colonies. *Aeromonas* spp. (see Chapter 14) also grow on CIN agar, producing colonies with a pink center and an uneven clear apron.

Laboratory tests. *Yersinia* spp. are more metabolically active at 25°C to 30°C than at 35°C. After 2 to 5 days of incubation at 25°C to 30°C, *Y. pestis* is nonmotile, esculin positive, ornithine decarboxylase negative, oxidase negative, catalase positive, urease negative, and indole negative. *Y. pestis* ferments glucose without producing gas. In TSI, it yields a K/A reaction. *Y. enterocolitica* and *Y. pseudotuberculosis* are motile if incubated below 30°C, nonmotile at 35°C, and urease positive. See Table 12-8 for a summary of biochemical test reactions.

According to the American Society for Microbiology (http://www.asm.org/), any isolate from the respiratory tract, blood, or lymph nodes that has the following characteristics should be suspected of being *Y. pestis*:

- Bipolar-staining bacillus (using Wright-Giemsa stain) on direct smear

- Pinpoint colony at 24 hours on sheep blood agar

- NLF, but may not be visible on MAC or EMB at 24 hours

- Oxidase negative

- Urease negative

- Catalase positive

- Growth often better at 28°C

SAFETY TIP

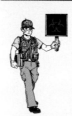

CLSI-Recommended Safety Precautions. *CLSI Document M29-A3 (see "References and Suggested Reading") recommends biosafety level 2 (BSL-2) practices, containment equipment, and facilities for handling potentially infectious clinical material, and BSL-3 practices and facilities for manipulations with a high potential for aerosol or droplet formation. Vaccination is available and recommended for anyone working with* Y. pestis*–infected rodents and other highly infectious material.*

TABLE 12 - 8 Biochemical Characteristics of *Yersinia* spp.[a]

Test	Y. pestis	Y. enterocolitica	Y. pseudotuberculosis
Indole	−	Variable (50% of strains +)	−
Urease	−	Variable (most strains +)	+
Ornithine decarboxylase	−	+	−
Esculin hydrolysis	Variable (50% of strains are +)	Variable (most strains −)	+

[a] After 2 days of incubation at 35°C.

Essentials

Yersinia pestis

- Nonmotile Gram-negative bacillus

- The causative agent of plague

- A potential bioterrorism agent

- Has a characteristic bipolar (safety pin) appearance in clinical material, when stained with Giemsa, Wright, Wright-Giemsa, Wayson, or methylene blue stains

- Slow growing; pinpoint, gray-white, translucent colonies at 24 hours; at 48 hours, colonies are 1 to 2 mm in diameter, gray-white to slightly yellow, and opaque; growth is often better at 28°C

- Colonies have a raised, irregular, fried-egg appearance that becomes more prominent with age

- Non-lactose-fermenting member of the family Enterobacteriaceae; colorless colonies on MAC

- K/AG reaction on TSI and KIA

- IMViC results: indole negative, methyl red positive, Voges-Proskauer negative, citrate negative

- Oxidase negative, nitrate positive, urease negative, catalase positive

Table 12-9 summarizes key characteristics of members of the family Enterobacteriaceae.

TABLE 12 - 9 Summary of Key Characteristics of Members of the Family Enterobacteriaceae

Genus or Species	Key Characteristics
Escherichia coli	LF, KIA = A/AG, IMViC = +/+/−/−
Klebsiella pneumoniae	LF, KIA = A/AG, nonmotile, urease +, IMViC = −/−/+/+
Enterobacter spp.	LF, KIA = A/AG, IMViC = −/−/+/+
Citrobacter freundii	LF, KIA = A/AG H_2S +, PYR +
Serratia marcescens	LF, KIA = K/AG, red pigmented colonies
Salmonella spp.	NLF, KIA = K/AG H_2S +, PYR negative
Shigella spp.	NLF, KIA = K/A, nonmotile, catalase −
Proteus spp.	NLF, KIA = K/AG H_2S +, swarming on blood agar, strongly urease +, PAD +
Morganella morganii	NLF, KIA = K/AG, strongly urease +, PAD +
Providencia spp.	NLF, KIA = K/A or K/AG, strongly urease +, PAD +
Yersinia spp.	NLF, KIA = K/K, motile at 22°C, nonmotile at 35°C

KIA, Kligler iron agar; IMViC, indole, methyl red, Voges-Proskauer, citrate; LF, lactose fermenter; NLF, non–lactose fermenter.

Chapter Review

- Members of the family Enterobacteriaceae include the following genera: *Escherichia, Klebsiella, Enterobacter, Citrobacter, Serratia, Salmonella, Shigella, Proteus, Morganella, Providencia,* and *Yersinia.*

- Members of the family Enterobacteriaceae are Gram-negative bacilli associated with the GI tract. Many members are indigenous microflora of the colon and are opportunistic pathogens. Others, like *Salmonella* and *Shigella* spp., are virtually always pathogenic when ingested.

- All members of the Enterobacteriaceae family ferment glucose, are oxidase negative, and reduce nitrate.

- Members of the Enterobacteriaceae family may possess three categories of antigenic determinants that can be used for serologic identification: O or somatic antigens, K or capsular antigens, and H or flagellar antigens.

- Identification of a Gram-negative bacillus begins with observations of growth or no growth on selective or differential media included in the primary setup.

- *E. coli* is the species of *Escherichia* most often isolated from human clinical specimens.

- Like all bacteria possessing the Gram-negative cell wall structure, members of the family Enterobacteriaceae produce endotoxin. Other virulence factors associated with the family include pili, cytotoxins, and enterotoxins.

- Lactose-fermenting members of the Enterobacteriaceae family produce pink colonies on MacConkey agar, whereas non-lactose-fermenting members produce colorless colonies.

- *Klebsiella* spp., particularly *K. pneumoniae*, are common causes of nosocomial infections.

- *Citrobacter* spp. differ from *E. coli* in that they can use citrate as their sole carbon source.

- Most *Salmonella* serotypes cause salmonellosis, an intestinal infection causing diarrhea, fever, and abdominal cramps. *Salmonella* serotype Typhi is the cause of typhoid fever.

- The four serogroups or species of *Shigella* are *S. dysenteriae, S. flexneri, S. boydii,* and *S. sonnei.*

- *Shigella* spp. cause a diarrheal disease known as shigellosis or bacillary dysentery. They are a common cause of traveler's diarrhea.

- *Proteus mirabilis* and *P. vulgaris* (sometimes) are swarmers, in that they spread in wavelike fashion over the entire surface of an agar plate.

- Many commercial biochemical tests are available for identifying members of the family Enterobacteriaceae.

- *Yersinia pestis* is a slow growing Gram-negative bacillus or coccobacillus. It has a characteristic bipolar or safety pin appearance in clinical material when stained with Giemsa, Wright, Wright-Giemsa, Wayson, or methylene blue stains. *Y. pestis* is a potential bioterrorist agent and is the cause of plague.

Winn et al. (see "References and Suggested Reading") suggest that students remember the following key facts regarding members of the family Enterobacteriaceae:

- Hydrogen sulfide–positive members of the family include *Citrobacter freundii, Edwardsiella tarda* (not discussed in this chapter), *Proteus mirabilis, Proteus vulgaris,* and *Salmonella* spp.

- Voges-Proskauer-positive members of the family include *Enterobacter* spp., *Hafnia* spp. (not discussed in this chapter), *Klebsiella* spp., *Pantoea* spp., and *Serratia* spp.

- PAD-positive members of the family include *Morganella* spp., *Proteus* spp., and *Providencia* spp.

- Members of the family that are nonmotile at 35°C to 37°C include *Klebsiella* spp., *Shigella* spp., and *Yersinia* spp. (motile at 22°C).

New Terms and Abbreviations

After studying Chapter 12, you should be familiar with the following terms, which are defined within the chapter and in the Glossary at the back of the book:

Coliforms

Deamination

Decarboxylation

Enterovirulent E. coli

IMViC reactions

Lactose fermenter (LF)

Nonfermenter

Non–lactose fermenter (NLF; also referred to as a lactose nonfermenter)

Nosocomial infections

References and Suggested Reading

Abbreviated Identification of Bacteria and Yeast: Approved Guideline. CLSI Document M35-A. Wayne, PA: Clinical and Laboratory Standards Institute, 2002.

Bopp CA, et al. *Escherichia, Shigella,* and *Salmonella*. In: Murray PR, Baron EJ, Jorgensen JH, Pfaller MA, Yolken RH, eds. Manual of Clinical Microbiology. 8th Ed. Washington, DC: ASM Press, 2003.

Farmer JJ III. Enterobacteriaceae: introduction and identification. In: Murray PR, Baron EJ, Jorgensen JH, Pfaller MA, Yolken RH, eds. Manual of Clinical Microbiology. 8th Ed. Washington, DC: ASM Press, 2003.

Isenberg HD, D'Amato RF. Enterobacteriaceae. In: Gorbach SL, Bartlett JG, Blacklow NR, eds. Infectious Disease. 3rd Ed. Philadelphia. Lippincott Williams & Wilkins, 2004.

Jarreau P, et al. Clinical Laboratory Science Review: A Bottom Line Approach. 3rd Ed. New Orleans: Louisiana State University Health Science Center Foundation, 2005.

Keusch GT. *Shigella*. In: Gorbach SL, Bartlett JG, Blacklow NR, eds. Infectious Disease. 3rd Ed. Philadelphia: Lippincott Williams & Wilkins, 2004.

Kim AY, et al. *Salmonella*: pathogenesis and vaccines. In: Gorbach SL, Bartlett JG, Blacklow NR, eds. Infectious Disease. 3rd Ed. Philadelphia: Lippincott Williams & Wilkins, 2004.

Murray PR, Baron EJ, Jorgensen JH, Pfaller MA, Yolken RH, eds. Manual of Clinical Microbiology. 8th Ed. Washington, DC: ASM Press, 2003.

Protection of Laboratory Workers from Occupationally Acquired Infections: Approved Guideline-Third Edition. CLSI Document M29-A3. Wayne, PA: Clinical and Laboratory Standards Institute, 2005.

Winn WC Jr, et al. Koneman's Color Atlas and Textbook of Diagnostic Microbiology. 6th Ed. Philadelphia: Lippincott Williams & Wilkins, 2006.

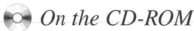 ## On the CD-ROM

- *E. coli* O157:H7 Outbreaks
- Enterobacteriaceae in Depth
- Appearance of Enterobacteriaceae Colonies on Differential Media
- Additional Self-Assessment Exercises
- Case Study
- Puzzle

Self-Assessment Exercises

Match the organism in the left column with its corresponding description or disease in the right column.

1. _____ *E. coli*   A. Cause of typhoid fever

2. _____ *Salmonella typhi*   B. Serotype O157:H7

3. _____ *Yersinia pestis*   C. Encapsulated; produces mucoid colonies

4. _____ *Klebsiella* spp.   D. Cause of plague

5. _____ *Citrobacter* spp.   E. K/A H$_2$S +

6. True or false: *Klebsiella pneumoniae* has a characteristic bipolar or safety pin appearance when Gram stained.

7. The prefix *entero-* refers to the

   A. gastrointestinal system.

   B. respiratory system.

   C. urogenital system.

   D. circulatory system.

8. All members of the Enterobacteriaceae family have the following characteristics *except*

   A. capable of fermenting glucose.

   B. capable of fermenting lactose.

   C. capable of reducing nitrate.

   D. oxidase negative.

9. An unknown organism grew on blood agar, chocolate agar, and MAC, but not on PEA. It produced pink colonies on MAC. What information can be reported at this point, based on these observations?

   A. The organism is a Gram-positive lactose fermenter.

   B. The organism is a Gram-negative, fastidious, non–lactose fermenter.

   C. The organism is a Gram-negative lactose fermenter.

   D. The organism is a Gram-positive non–lactose fermenter.

10. What three reactions can be determined by observing the butt portion of a TSI tube?

    A. _____

    B. _____

    C. _____

CHAPTER 13

Gram-Negative Bacilli: Nonfermenters

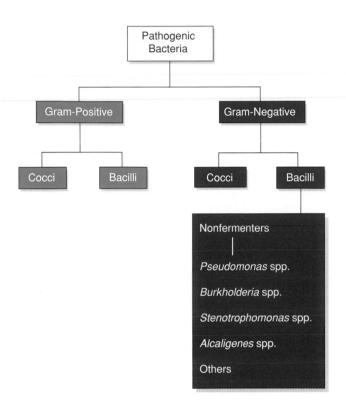

Chapter Outline

Medical Importance of Nonfermenters

Phenotypic Characteristics of Nonfermenters

Identification of an Unknown Gram-Negative Bacillus

Laboratory Methods Used to Identify Nonfermenters

Selected Nonfermenters
- Genus *Pseudomonas*
- Genus *Burkholderia*
- Genus *Stenotrophomonas*
- Genus *Alcaligenes*
- Miscellaneous Nonfermenters

LEARNING OBJECTIVES

After studying this chapter, you should be able to:

☛ Define the terms introduced in this chapter (e.g., *fermentative pathway, fermenter, nonfermenter*)

☛ Describe the general characteristics of the nonfermentative Gram-negative bacilli

☛ Explain the major difference between the metabolic pathways used by fermentative organisms and those used by nonfermentative organisms

☛ Given a description of an unknown nonfermenter, identify it by its biochemical reactions and morphological characteristics

- State the clinical significance of the following nonfermenters: *Alcaligenes* spp., *Stenotrophomonas* spp., and *Burkholderia* spp.

- Compare and contrast the phenotypic characteristics of the nonfermenters and members of the family Enterobacteriaceae

- List the initial clues that indicate a Gram-negative bacillus is a nonfermenter, rather than a member of the Enterobacteriaceae family

- State the purpose of oxidation-fermentation (O-F) tests

- Given the results of an O-F test, state whether the organism tested is an oxidizer, a fermenter, or a nonoxidizer of a particular carbohydrate

- State the characteristics common to all *Pseudomonas* spp.

- Describe the clinical significance of *Pseudomonas aeruginosa*, including its distribution in nature, role in nosocomial infections, sources of infection, and virulence factors

- Discuss the laboratory identification of *P. aeruginosa*, including its cellular and colonial morphology, reaction in triple-sugar iron (TSI) agar, odor, key biochemical reactions, and any pigments produced

- Discuss the important characteristics for laboratory identification of nonfermentative Gram-negative bacilli other than *P. aeruginosa*, including cellular and colonial morphology, TSI reaction, odor, and key biochemical reactions

- Given cellular and colonial morphology and biochemical test results, differentiate *P. aeruginosa* from other Gram-negative bacilli

Hospital-acquired infections. Pneumonia. Burn wound and urinary tract infections. Swimmer's ear. These diseases are associated with some of the Gram-negative bacilli (GNB) described in this chapter.

A nonfermenter is an organism that lacks the ability to catabolize (break down) carbohydrates by fermentative pathways. If a nonfermenter is able to catabolize a specific carbohydrate, it does so by a metabolic pathway other than fermentation. This chapter describes GNB that are nonfermenters. Their inability to ferment glucose is the primary way by which nonfermenters differ from members of the

> A nonfermenter is an organism that lacks the ability to catabolize (break down) carbohydrates by fermentative pathways.

family Enterobacteriaceae. Recall that *all* members of that bacterial family are able to ferment glucose.

CAUTION

Beware of Similar Sounding Terms. Do not confuse the term *nonfermenter* with *non–lactose fermenter*. As discussed in Chapter 12, the term *non–lactose fermenter* is used to describe an organism that cannot ferment *lactose*. A nonfermenter, on the other hand, is an organism that cannot ferment *any* carbohydrates.

Some authorities define a nonfermenter as a Gram-negative bacillus that grows on the slant portion of Kligler iron agar (KIA) or triple-sugar iron (TSI) agar but neither grows nor produces acid in the butt portion of these media (Fig. 13-1). KIA and TSI media are discussed in Chapter 12. As stated by Winn et al. (see "References and Suggested Reading"), "The dividing line between what is a 'nonfermenter' and what may otherwise be designated a 'fastidious,' 'unusual,' or 'miscellaneous' non-glucose-fermenting GNB is based more on convention than on well-defined genetic or phenotypic characteristics."

Recall from Chapter 12 that the GNB most commonly isolated from clinical specimens are members of the family Enterobacteriaceae and nonfermenters. Thus, whenever a Gram-negative bacillus is isolated, it will most likely turn out to be a member of one or the other of those groups. Keep in mind, however, that GNB that are *not* members of these two categories can also be isolated

> The two major groups of GNB isolated from clinical specimens are members of the family Enterobacteriaceae and nonfermenters.

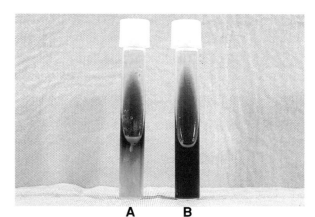

A   **B**

Figure 13-1. **Kligler iron agar (KIA) results. A.** Tube showing K/A reaction (alkaline slant, acid butt) was inoculated with a lactose-negative member of the family Enterobacteriaceae. **B.** The tube showing K/K reaction (alkaline slant, alkaline butt) was inoculated with a nonfermenter. (From Winn WC Jr, et al. Koneman's Color Atlas and Textbook of Diagnostic Microbiology. 6th Ed. Philadelphia: Lippincott Williams & Wilkins, 2006.)

from clinical specimens. These other GNB are discussed in Chapters 14 through 17.

MEDICAL IMPORTANCE OF NONFERMENTERS

Collectively, nonfermenters represent an extremely important group of pathogens. They cause a wide variety of significant, sometimes fatal infections, including pneumonia, septicemia, and urinary tract and burn wound infections. Additional information about these diseases is contained in subsequent sections of this chapter that focus on individual species.

PHENOTYPIC CHARACTERISTICS OF NONFERMENTERS

Table 13-1 lists some of the most important characteristics of nonfermenters and compares them with characteristics of members of the family Enterobacteriaceae. It is important to keep these differences in mind. Additional characteristics of nonfermenters will be discussed in sections of this chapter that describe specific organisms.

Essentials

Nonfermenters

- Gram-negative bacilli
- Do not ferment glucose
- Variable growth on MacConkey agar
- Oxidase variable
- Nitrate variable

IDENTIFICATION OF AN UNKNOWN GRAM-NEGATIVE BACILLUS

Recall from Chapter 12 that the initial clues to the identification (speciation) of any bacterium include that organism's pattern of growth on the primary setup—the various media into and onto which the clinical specimen was inoculated. *Pattern of growth* refers to the media on which the organism grew and the media on which the organism did not grow. Several examples are presented here:

Example 1

If the organism grew on phenylethyl alcohol (PEA) agar but not on MacConkey agar (MAC), you would know that the organism is Gram positive. This can be confirmed by Gram staining a portion of one of the colonies.

Example 2

If the organism grew on MAC but not on PEA, you would know that the organism is Gram negative. This can be confirmed by Gram staining a portion of one of the colonies.

Consider an organism that grew on MAC but not PEA, and a Gram stain revealed that the organism is a Gram-negative bacillus. GNB are identified (speciated) by learning about their phenotypic characteristics, especially clues to the enzymes that they possess. One of the first tests to be performed on a Gram-negative bacillus that has been isolated from a clinical specimen is the oxidase test (see Chapter 11).

TABLE 13 - 1	Phenotypic Differences Between Nonfermenters and Members of the Family Enterobacteriaceae	
Characteristic	**Nonfermenters**	**Members of the Family Enterobacteriaceae**
Fermentation of glucose	−	+
Nitrate reduction	Variable[a]	+
Oxidase production	Variable	−
Growth on MacConkey agar	Variable	+

[a] *Variable* means that some nonfermenters are positive for this characteristic and others are negative.

Example 1

If the organism is **oxidase negative,** it *may* be a member of the family Enterobacteriaceae. (As shown in Table 13-1, *all* members of the family Enterobacteriaceae are oxidase negative.) Various types of miniaturized biochemical test systems (minisystems) are available to identify members of this family (see Chapter 12). However, the organism may *not* be a member of the Enterobacteriaceae family. It is possible that it is an oxidase-negative nonfermenter. (Table 13-1 shows that some nonfermenters are oxidase positive and some are oxidase negative.)

Example 2

If the Gram-negative bacillus is **oxidase positive,** it *cannot* be a member of the family Enterobacteriaceae. It *may* be a nonfermenter. Methods used to identify nonfermenters are discussed in the next section.

LABORATORY METHODS USED TO IDENTIFY NONFERMENTERS

Listed here are some of the initial clues that an unknown Gram-negative bacillus is a nonfermenter:

- It does *not* ferment glucose.

- It is oxidase positive.

- It is nitrate reduction negative.

- It does *not* grow on MAC.

Recall from information contained in Chapter 12 that a Gram-negative bacillus having *any* of these characteristics *cannot* be a member of the family Enterobacteriaceae.

Although nonfermenters are unable to ferment glucose, they may or may not be able to oxidize glucose. Oxidation-fermentation (O-F) tests, described in the next section, are frequently used to determine which carbohydrates an unknown Gram-negative bacillus is able to catabolize, and by what type(s) of pathway(s) it is able to do so. The O-F test pattern of an isolate provides important clues to its identity.

> If an organism is able to catabolize a particular substrate, it may do so by a fermentative pathway, an oxidative pathway, or both.

O-F test. An organism may or may not be able to catabolize (break down) a specific carbohydrate, depending on the enzymes that the organism possesses. If an organism is capable of catabolizing a particular carbohydrate, it may be able to do so by oxidative or fermentative biochemical pathways, or both. (Oxygen participates in oxidative pathways but not in fermentative pathways.) With respect to a particular carbohydrate, there are three possibilities:

Possibility 1

The organism possesses the enzymes necessary to catabolize the carbohydrate by fermentative pathways (fermentatively). In the O-F test, such an organism is said to be a fermenter of that particular carbohydrate.

Possibility 2

The organism possesses the enzymes necessary to catabolize the carbohydrate by oxidative pathways (oxidatively), but lacks the enzymes necessary to catabolize the carbohydrate fermentatively. In the O-F test, such an organism is said to be an oxidizer of that particular carbohydrate.

Possibility 3

The organism cannot catabolize the carbohydrate at all, because it lacks the necessary enzymes. In the O-F test, such an organism is said to be a nonoxidizer (or nonutilizer) of that particular carbohydrate.

> With respect to a particular substrate, an organism may be a fermenter, an oxidizer, or a nonoxidizer (nonutilizer) of that substrate.

The O-F test is designed to determine whether an organism is an oxidizer, a fermenter, or a nonoxidizer of particular carbohydrates. The test requires the use of two tubes of semisolid agar for each carbohydrate being tested. Each tube contains the carbohydrate being tested. Commonly tested carbohydrates are glucose, maltose, lactose, and mannitol. Glucose is usually tested first, and if the organism is an oxidizer of glucose, then the other sugars are tested. In the following discussion, glucose is used as an example.

Using an inoculating needle, each tube is inoculated with the test organism by stabbing the medium several times, halfway to the bottom of the tube. After inoculation, the medium in one tube is overlaid (covered) with sterile mineral oil or melted paraffin (Fig. 13-2). This prevents air from coming in contact with the medium. Any chemical reactions that occur in this tube occur anaerobically (in the absence of oxygen). This tube is known as the closed tube or covered tube.

The medium in the other tube is not overlaid and thus remains exposed to air. This tube is known as the open tube. Both tubes are incubated at 35°C and examined daily for several days. Catabolic reactions occurring in either tube result in the production of acid, which lowers the pH of the

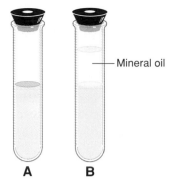

Figure 13-2. **Inoculated oxidation-fermentation (O-F) tubes prior to incubation. A.** Open tube. **B.** Closed tube.

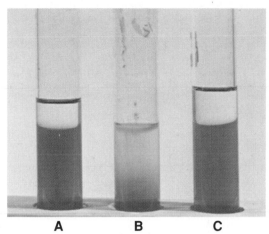

Figure 13-3. **O-F results produced by an oxidizer. A.** Uninoculated closed tube. **B.** Inoculated open tube (the yellow color indicates that acid was produced). **C.** Inoculated closed tube (no acid has been produced). (From MacFaddin JF. Biochemical Tests for Identification of Medical Bacteria. Baltimore: Williams and Wilkins, 1976.)

medium and causes the pH indicator to shift color. Possible O-F glucose reactions are shown in Table 13-2. The O-F results of an oxidizer are shown in Figure 13-3, and the O-F results of a fermenter are shown in Figure 13-4. Table 13-3 contains carbohydrate oxidation results for the nonfermenters described in this chapter.

CAUTION

Beware of Similar-Sounding Terms. Do not confuse the terms *oxidase*, *oxidation*, *oxidative pathway*, and *oxidizer*. *Oxidase* is an abbreviated name for cytochrome oxidase, an enzyme that participates in the electron transport chain. *Oxidation* is the loss of an electron, as opposed to reduction, which is the gain of an electron. An *oxidative pathway* is a biochemical pathway in which oxygen participates. An *oxidizer* is an organism that can break down a substrate oxidatively (via an oxidative pathway) but not fermentatively (via a fermentative pathway).

Other tests and observations of value in the identification of nonfermenters are the motility test, flagella stain (to determine the number and position of flagella), pigment production, oxidase, urease, indole production, growth at 4°C, growth at 42°C, citrate, acetamide, gelatin, esculin hydrolysis, and susceptibility to penicillin, vancomycin, and colistin.

SELECTED NONFERMENTERS

Genus *Pseudomonas*

Pseudomonas spp. (pseudomonads) are straight or slightly curved GNB. They range from 0.5 to 1.0 μm in width by 1.5 to 5 μm in length. The following characteristics are common to all *Pseudomonas* spp.:

- Aerobic (although some strains can grow under anaerobic conditions)

- Non–spore forming

- Motile by one or more polar flagella

TABLE 13 - 2	Possible Oxidation-Fermentation Glucose Test Reactions	
Color of the Medium in the Open Tube	**Color of the Medium in the Closed Tube**	**Interpretation**
Yellow	Green	The organism is an oxidizer of glucose; it can catabolize glucose oxidatively, but not fermentatively
Yellow	Yellow	The organism is a fermenter of glucose; it can catabolize glucose in both the presence and absence of oxygen
Green	Green	The organism is a nonoxidizer (or nonutilizer) of glucose; it cannot catabolize glucose

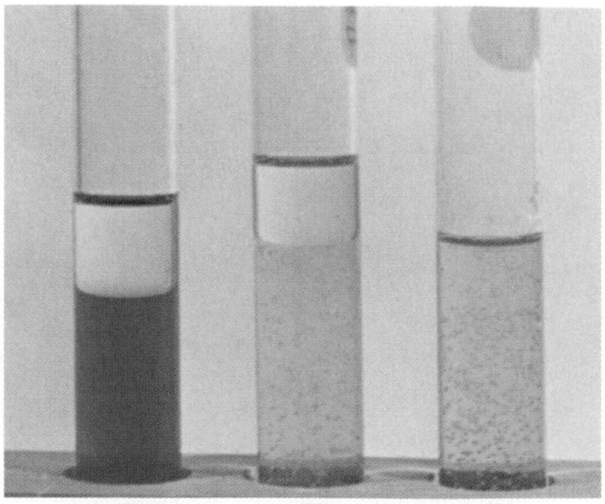

Figure 13-4. **O-F results produced by a fermenter. A.** Uninoculated closed tube. **B.** Inoculated closed tube (acid has been produced). **C.** Inoculated open tube (acid has been produced). (From MacFaddin JF. Biochemical Tests for Identification of Medical Bacteria. Baltimore: Williams and Wilkins, 1976.)

- Catalase positive

- Oxidase positive (exceptions are *P. luteola* and *P. oryzihabitans*)

- Non–lactose fermenters on MAC

- Most species can degrade glucose oxidatively (recall that they are nonfermenters and thus cannot degrade glucose fermentatively)

- Most species are nitrate positive

Pseudomonas spp. can be divided into two groups, based on production or nonproduction of a fluorescent yellow-green or yellow-brown pigment called pyoverdin. Pyoverdin fluoresces under short-wave ultraviolet light. *Pseudomonas* spp. that produce pyoverdin are referred to as the fluorescent group, which includes *P. aeruginosa*, *P. fluorescens*, *P. putida*, *P. veronii*, and *P. monteilii*. *Pseudomonas* spp. that do not produce pyoverdin are referred to as the nonfluorescent group,

TABLE 13 - 3   Carbohydrate Oxidation Results for Nonfermenters Described in This Chapter

Organism (Number of Strains Tested)	Percentage of Strains That Oxidize the Substrate							
	Glu	Fru	Xyl	Lac	Suc	Mal	Man	Arab
Pseudomonas aeruginosa (201)	97		90	0	0	0	70	
P. fluorescens (155)	100		100	24	48	2	53	
P. putida (16)	100		100	25	0	31	25	
P. veronii (8)	100	100	100		100		100	
P. monteilii (10)	100	100	0	0	0	0	0	
P. stutzeri (28)	96		93	0	0	100	89	
P. mendocina (4)	100		75	0	0	0	0	
P. pseudoalcaligenes (34)	9	79	18	0	0	0	0	
P. alcaligenes (26)	0	0	0	0	0	0	0	
P. luteola (34)	100		100	3	12	100	76	
P. oryzihabitans (36)	100		100	14	25	97	100	
Burkholderia pseudomallei (unknown)	>90		>90	>90	V	>90	>90	<10
Stenotrophomonas maltophilia (228)	85		35	60	63	100	0	

Arab, arabinose; Fru, fructose; Glu, glucose; Lac, lactose; Mal, maltose; Man, mannitol; Suc, sucrose; V, variable (some strains are oxidizers; some are not); Xyl, xylose.

Source: Kiska DL, Gilligan PH. *Pseudomonas.* In: Murray PR, Baron EJ, Jorgensen JH, Pfaller MA, Yolken RH, eds. Manual of Clinical Microbiology. 8th Ed. Washington, DC: ASM Press, 2003.

TABLE 13 - 4	Clinical Significance of *Pseudomonas* spp. Other Than *P. aeruginosa*
Pseudomonas spp.	**Clinical Significance**
P. fluorescens	Occasional cause of transfusion-related and catheter-related septicemia
P. putida	Occasional cause of transfusion-related and catheter-related septicemia
P. veronii	Very rare cause of infection
P. monteilii	Very rare cause of infection
P. stutzeri	Rare cause of infection in immunosuppressed and hospitalized patients; has caused septicemia, meningitis, pneumonia, osteomyelitis, and endophthalmitis
P. mendocina	Very rare cause of infection
P. alcaligenes	Very rare cause of infection
P. pseudoalcaligenes	Very rare cause of infection
P. luteola	Rare cause of infections, including septicemia, cellulitis, osteomyelitis, peritonitis, endocarditis, and meningitis
P. oryzihabitans	Has caused septicemia, peritonitis, cellulitis, abscesses, wound infections, and meningitis

which includes *P. stutzeri*, *P. mendocina*, *P. alcaligenes*, *P. pseudoalcaligenes*, *P. luteola*, and *P. oryzihabitans*.

Pseudomonads are widely distributed in nature; they are found in soil, water, plants, and various moist settings in hospitals. *Pseudomonas* spp., especially *P. aeruginosa*, are frequent causes of nosocomial infections, especially in debilitated and immunosuppressed patients. Table 13-4 contains information about the clinical significance of *Pseudomonas* spp. other than *P. aeruginosa*. The clinical significance of *P. aeruginosa* is described in the next section.

Pseudomonas aeruginosa

Clinical significance. According to Ohl and Pollack (see "References and Suggested Reading"), "Approximately 15% of all Gram-negative clinical isolates are non-glucose-fermenting Gram-negative rods; of these, more than two thirds are *Pseudomonas aeruginosa*." These authors also state that "*P. aeruginosa* is isolated from clinical sources more often than all other *Pseudomonas* species combined and is more often associated with clinical disease."

P. aeruginosa colonizes moist places within hospitals, such as sinks, water faucets, whirlpool baths, and inhalation equipment. It can even survive in soap and weak disinfectant solutions. Although *P. aeruginosa* is not considered a member of the human indigenous microflora, it often colonizes hospitalized patients. It is a frequent cause of nosocomial infections, such as pneumonia, urinary tract infections,

septicemia, and burn wound infections. Respiratory infections caused by *P. aeruginosa* are common in cystic fibrosis patients and are the primary cause of death among these patients. *P. aeruginosa* also causes community-acquired infections, such as folliculitis, otitis externa and otitis media, eye infections, and traumatic wound infections.

Virulence factors. Pili enable attachment of the bacterial cells to epithelial cells. The mucoid exopolysaccharide (slime) produced by mucoid strains of *P. aeruginosa* also enables it to attach to host cells and may prevent phagocytosis. Various exotoxins and exoenzymes (including hemolysins) cause destruction of host tissue and inhibit phagocyte activity. Proteases not only cause tissue destruction but also destroy antibodies and complement.

Drug resistance. *P. aeruginosa* is resistant to many antimicrobial agents, especially those used to treat infections caused by members of the family Enterobacteriaceae.

Clues to *P. aeruginosa* Identification

Cellular morphology. On Gram-stained smears, *P. aeruginosa* cannot be distinguished from other nonfermenters or members of the Enterobacteriaceae family (Fig. 13-5). Microcolonies of mucoid strains of *P. aeruginosa* can be observed in the sputum of cystic fibrosis patients. Microcolonies appear as clusters of thin GNB surrounded by more darkly staining Gram-negative, amorphous material.

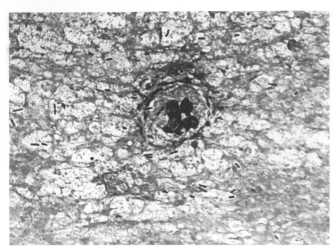

Figure 13-5. **Gram-stained sputum specimen containing** *Pseudomonas aeruginosa* **cells.** *P. aeruginosa* cannot be differentiated from any other nonfermenters or members of the family Enterobacteriaceae by its Gram-stained appearance. (From Marler LM, Siders JA, Allen SD. Direct Smear Atlas. Philadelphia: Lippincott Williams & Wilkins, 2001.)

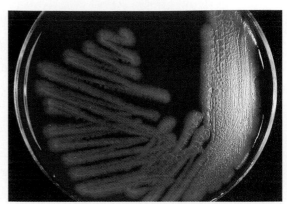

Figure 13-7. ***P. aeruginosa*** **colonies on blood agar after 24 hours of incubation at 35°C.** *P. aeruginosa* colonies have a spreading periphery, are frequently β-hemolytic, and have a fruity odor. A metallic sheen can be seen in areas of heaviest growth, as well as a scaly appearance, which has been described as an "alligator skin" morphology. (From Winn WC Jr, et al. Koneman's Color Atlas and Textbook of Diagnostic Microbiology. 6th Ed. Philadelphia: Lippincott Williams & Wilkins, 2006.)

Colonial morphology. Recall that *P. aeruginosa* is a member of the fluorescent group of pseudomonads and as such produces pyoverdin. It also produces other water-soluble, diffusible pigments, including a blue pigment called pyocyanin. When pyocyanin combines with pyoverdin, the characteristic greenish or blue-green color of *P. aeruginosa* is produced. Other pigments produced by some *P. aeruginosa* strains are pyorubin (red) and pyomelanin (brown). Note that all the pigment names contain *pyo-*, referring to pus. The color of the pus that is associated with a *P. aeruginosa* infection is determined by the pigment(s) being produced by that particular strain. These diffusible pigments are especially noticeable on lightly colored media such as

Mueller-Hinton agar (Fig. 13-6). Some strains are non-pigmented. *P. aeruginosa* colonies are usually spreading and flat, with serrated edges and a metallic sheen (Fig. 13-7). Some strains produce other colony types, including smooth, gelatinous, dwarf, and mucoid colonies. Strains producing mucoid colonies are frequently isolated from sputum specimens of cystic fibrosis patients (Fig. 13-8).

> Most *P. aeruginosa* strains produce colonies having a characteristic blue-green color.

Laboratory tests. *P. aeruginosa* produces a K/NC reaction (alkaline slant/no change in butt) on TSI agar. Growth at

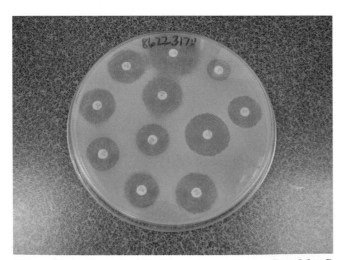

Figure 13-6. **Characteristic blue-green color produced by** ***P. aeruginosa*** **on Mueller-Hinton agar.** (Courtesy of Dr. Robert Fader.)

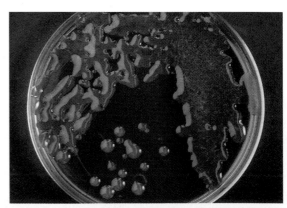

Figure 13-8. **An extremely mucoid and runny strain of** ***P. aeruginosa*** **growing on MacConkey agar.** This appearance is typical of *P. aeruginosa* strains isolated from sputum specimens of cystic fibrosis patients. (From Winn WC Jr, et al. Koneman's Color Atlas and Textbook of Diagnostic Microbiology. 6th Ed. Philadelphia: Lippincott Williams & Wilkins, 2006.)

42°C and hydrolysis of acetamide are characteristics of value in distinguishing *P. aeruginosa* (growth at 42°C positive, acetamide positive) from other *Pseudomonas* spp. (growth at 42°C negative [most strains], acetamide negative).

Acetamide utilization. This test determines the ability of an organism to use acetamide as its sole source of carbon. The slant portion of an acetamide agar tube is inoculated with the test organism. Deamination of acetamide causes the release of ammonia (alkaline), which causes the medium to change color (from pale yellow-orange to bright pink) caused by an increase in pH.

Clinical and Laboratory Standards Institute (CLSI) Document M35-A (see "References and Suggested Reading") states that an isolate can be identified as *P. aeruginosa* (with a >95% likelihood) if it meets the following criteria:

- Gram-negative bacillus

- Oxidase positive

- Typical odor (described as being fruity, similar to Concord grapes, or like a wine cellar or corn tortillas)

- Typical colonial morphology (metallic or pearlescent, rough, green pigmented, or extremely mucoid)

> *Pseudomonas aeruginosa* has a characteristic odor, often described as being fruity or like corn tortillas.

Except for the typical smell of *P. aeruginosa*, rare *Aeromonas* isolates may resemble *P. aeruginosa*. The spot indole test can be used to differentiate *P. aeruginosa* (indole negative) from *Aeromonas* (indole positive).

Various commercial systems are available to identify *P. aeruginosa* and other *Pseudomonas* spp. (Table 13-5 and Fig. 13-9), although some systems do not perform well with species other than *P. aeruginosa* and. *P. stutzeri*.

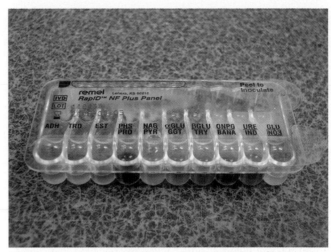

Figure 13-9. **Commercial system for identifying *Pseudomonas* spp. and other oxidase-positive GNB.** This system—the RapID NF Plus Panel—is sold by Remel. (Courtesy of Dr. Robert Fader.)

Pseudomonas aeruginosa is the nonfermenter most commonly isolated from clinical specimens. *Acinetobacter* spp. are the second most commonly isolated nonfermenters. *Acinetobacter* spp. are described in Chapter 11.

> *P. aeruginosa* and *Acinetobacter baumannii* are the two most commonly isolated nonfermenters.

Essentials

Pseudomonas aeruginosa

- Motile, Gram-negative bacillus having the same morphology as other nonfermenters and members of the family Enterobacteriaceae

TABLE 13 - 5	Commercial Systems Used to Identify *Pseudomonas* spp.
System	**Manufacturer**
API 20NE	bioMérieux Inc. (http://www.biomerieux.com/)
Crystal E/NF	BD Biosciences (http://www.bdbiosciences.com/)
MicroScan W/A Neg Combo panels	Dade Behring (http://www.dadebehring.com/)
N/F and RapID NF Plus	Remel (http://www.remelinc.com/)
Vitek GNI+ and Vitek 2 GN	bioMérieux Inc.

Source: Kiska DL, Gilligan PH. *Pseudomonas.* In: Murray PR, Baron EJ, Jorgensen JH, Pfaller MA, Yolken RH, eds. Manual of Clinical Microbiology. 8th Ed. Washington, DC: ASM Press, 2003.

- Resistant to many antimicrobial agents

- Can survive in soap and weak disinfectant solutions

- Nonfermenter (does not ferment glucose)

- Produces characteristic pigments (pyoverdin and pyocyanin)

- Has a characteristic fruity odor

- Catalase, oxidase, and nitrate positive

- Non–lactose fermenter on MAC

Other *Pseudomonas* spp.

Important characteristics of *Pseudomonas* spp. other than *P. aeruginosa* are shown in Table 13-6.

Genus *Burkholderia*

The genus *Burkholderia* consists of more than 20 species, but only two—*B. cepacia* and *B. pseudomallei*—are commonly associated with human infections. In the past, both of these species were classified in the genus *Pseudomonas*. *Burkholderia* spp. are found in water, soil, and vegetation. Infection usually results from inhalation of the organism or contact of contaminated soil or water with cut or abraded skin.

    Burkholderia spp. share the following characteristics:

- Gram-negative bacilli

- Non–spore forming

- Motile (except for *B. mallei*)

- Catalase positive

- Growth on MAC

TABLE 13 - 6	Important Characteristics of *Pseudomonas* spp. Other Than *P. aeruginosa*[a]
Pseudomonas spp.	**Important Characteristics**
P. fluorescens	Oxidase positive, no distinctive morphology or odor, most strains nitrate negative, nitrate positive strains do not reduce nitrate to nitrogen gas, gelatinase positive, growth at 4°C, no growth at 42°C
P. putida	Oxidase positive, no distinctive morphology or odor, nitrate negative, gelatinase negative, no growth at 4°C, no growth at 42°C
P. veronii	Oxidase positive, nitrate positive (reduces nitrate to nitrogen gas), no growth at 42°C
P. monteilii	Oxidase positive, nitrate negative, no growth at 42°C
P. stutzeri	Distinctive dry, buff-to-brown-colored, wrinkled colonies that can pit or adhere to the agar surface; oxidase positive; nitrate positive (reduces nitrate to nitrogen gas); growth at 42°C (most strains)
P. mendocina	Smooth, unwrinkled, flat, brownish yellow colonies; oxidase positive; nitrate positive (reduces nitrate to nitrogen gas); growth at 42°C
P. alcaligenes	No distinctive colonial morphology, does not produce pigments, oxidase positive, about 50% of strains nitrate positive, nitrate positive strains do not reduce nitrate to nitrogen gas, no growth at 42°C
P. pseudoalcaligenes	No distinctive colonial morphology, does not produce pigments, oxidase positive, nitrate positive (but does not reduce nitrate to nitrogen gas), growth at 42°C
P. luteola	Rough, wrinkled, adherent colonies; rarely, smooth colonies; nondiffusible yellow pigment; oxidase negative; most strains nitrate positive; nitrate positive strains do not reduce nitrate to nitrogen gas; growth at 42°C
P. oryzihabitans	Rough, wrinkled, adherent colonies; rarely, smooth colonies; nondiffusible yellow pigment; oxidase negative; nitrate negative; no growth at 42°C (most strains)

[a]See Table 13-3 for carbohydrate oxidation results.

Burkholderia cepacia

Clinical significance. *Burkholderia cepacia* (also referred to as *B. cepacia* complex) causes several nosocomial infections, including septicemia (particularly in patients with indwelling catheters), surgical and burn wound infections, septic arthritis, pneumonia, meningitis, peritonitis, and urinary tract infections. *B. cepacia* is a common cause of lower respiratory tract infections in cystic fibrosis patients; such infections are often fatal. In patients with chronic granulomatous disease, *B. cepacia* is a very common cause of septicemia and pneumonia and is the second leading cause of death.

Drug resistance. *B. cepacia* is one of the most drug-resistant organisms encountered in the clinical microbiology laboratory (CML). It is intrinsically resistant to most β-lactam agents and aminoglycosides. Antimicrobial susceptibility testing should include trimethoprim-sulfamethoxazole, ceftazidime, chloramphenicol, levofloxacin, meropenem, minocycline, and ticarcillin-clavulanic acid.

> *Burkholderia cepacia* is one of the most drug-resistant organisms encountered in the CML.

Clues to *B. cepacia* Identification

Cellular morphology. *B. cepacia* resembles *Pseudomonas* spp. in Gram-stained smears.

Colonial morphology. *B. cepacia* grows well on most media, including MAC, although it may take 3 days before colonies are seen on selective media. *B. cepacia* selective agar (BCSA) is the medium of choice for recovery of *B. cepacia* from respiratory tract specimens from cystic fibrosis patients. BCSA contains antimicrobial agents that inhibit growth of most strains of *P. aeruginosa*. On blood agar and BCSA, *B. cepacia* colonies are smooth and slightly raised; occasional strains are mucoid. On MAC, *B. cepacia* colonies are punctate and tenacious; they become dark pink to red after 4 to 7 days of incubation as a result of lactose oxidation. Many strains of *B. cepacia* produce a bright yellow pigment when grown on iron-containing media (such as TSI agar). *B. cepacia* has a characteristic earthy or dirtlike odor.

Laboratory tests. Several commercial minisystems are available for identification of *B. cepacia*. Cellular fatty acid analysis and molecular diagnostic procedures are also available.

Essentials

Burkholderia cepacia

- Motile, Gram-negative bacillus having the same morphology as other nonfermenters and members of the family Enterobacteriaceae

- One of the most drug-resistant organisms encountered in the CML

- Nonfermenter (does not ferment glucose)

- Weakly oxidase positive

- Produces punctate, tenacious colonies on MAC, which become dark pink to red after 4 to 7 days of incubation as a result of lactose oxidation

- Has a characteristic earthy or dirtlike odor

Burkholderia pseudomallei

Clinical significance. *B. pseudomallei* causes melioidosis, which may be asymptomatic or may cause acute, subacute, or chronic illness, leading to death in some cases. Pneumonia is the most common presentation, but *B. pseudomallei* may also cause septicemia and infections of the genitourinary tract and central nervous system. Chronic respiratory tract infections can resemble tuberculosis. The organism may lie dormant for many years and then become reactivated. Melioidosis occurs in tropical and subtropical areas worldwide but is most prevalent in Southeast Asia and northern Australia.

 CAUTION

Beware of Similar-Sounding Terms. Do not confuse ***Burkholderia pseudomallei*** with ***Burkholderia mallei***. *B. pseudomallei* causes melioidosis in humans, whereas *B. mallei* causes glanders in horses, mules, donkeys, and occasionally goats, sheep, dogs, and cats. Glanders involves increased nasal mucous secretion, lung and nasal lesions, and enlargement of the glands of the lower jaw. Although animal-to-human transmission of glanders is possible, glanders is a rare disease in humans. Both *B. mallei* and *B. pseudomallei* are potential bioterrorism agents and, as such, are discussed in Chapter 26.

> *Burkholderia mallei* and *B. pseudomallei* are potential bioterrorism and biological warfare agents.

Drug resistance. *B. pseudomallei* is susceptible to many antimicrobial agents in vitro, but, as with many nonfermenters, in vitro results are not always consistent with in vivo outcomes. Trimethoprim-sulfamethoxazole and the fluoroquinolones are the most commonly prescribed agents.

Clues to *B. pseudomallei* Identification

Cellular morphology. In direct Gram-stained smears of clinical specimens, *B. pseudomallei* often appears as a short Gram-negative bacillus with bipolar ("safety pin") staining.

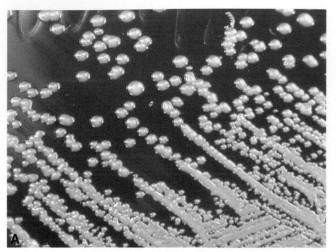
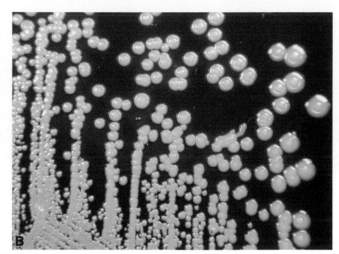

Figure 13-10. **Burkholderia pseudomallei colonies on sheep blood agar. A.** At 48 hours of incubation. **B.** At 72 hours of incubation. (Courtesy of Larry Stauffer, Oregon State Public Health Laboratory, and the Centers for Disease Control and Prevention.)

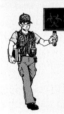

SAFETY TIP

"No Sniff" Tip. To avoid infection, do not sniff plates or broth cultures suspected of containing B. pseudomallei, *and perform all work in a biosafety cabinet.*

Colonial morphology. Like *B. cepacia*, *B. pseudomallei* grows well on most media, including MAC. It produces small, smooth colonies in the first 1 or 2 days, which change in appearance with extended incubation (Fig. 13-10), ultimately becoming dry, wrinkled colonies which are similar in appearance to *Pseudomonas stutzeri* (Fig. 13-11). A selective medium called Ashdown medium is preferred over MAC for isolation of *B. pseudomallei*. On Ashdown medium, *B. pseudomallei* colonies become deep pink as a result of absorption of neutral red dye from the medium. Clinical specimens can be inoculated into an enrichment medium containing Ashdown agar and colistin. *B. pseudomallei* produces a pronounced earthy odor, which is quite evident when the incubator door is opened.

Laboratory tests. Key identifying features for *B. pseudomallei* are oxidase positive, produces gas from nitrate, possesses two or more polar flagella, and arginine dihydrolase positive. Commercial minisystems, immunodiagnostic procedures, and molecular diagnostic procedures are available for identification of *B. pseudomallei*.

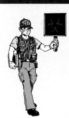

SAFETY TIP

CLSI-Recommended Safety Precautions. CLSI Document M29-A3 (see "References and Suggested Reading") recommends biosafety level 2 (BSL-2) practices, containment equipment, and facilities for all activities using known or potentially infectious body fluids, tissues, and cultures. Gloves should be worn when handling infected animals, during their necropsy, and when there is the likelihood of direct skin contact with infectious materials. Additional primary containment and personnel precautions, such as those described for BSL-3, may be indicated for activities with a high potential for aerosol or droplet production, and for activities involving production quantities or concentrations of infectious materials.

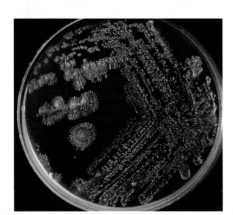

Figure 13-11. **Characteristic dry, wrinkled colonies of *Pseudomonas stutzeri* on blood agar.** CML professionals should suspect *P. stutzeri* whenever they encounter an oxidase-positive, nonfermenting, Gram-negative bacillus that produces this type of colony on blood agar. (From Winn WC Jr, et al. Koneman's Color Atlas and Textbook of Diagnostic Microbiology. 6th Ed. Philadelphia: Lippincott Williams & Wilkins, 2006.)

Essentials

Burkholderia pseudomallei

- Motile, short, Gram-negative bacillus, often having a bipolar, or safety pin, appearance on staining

- Cause of melioidosis

- Potential bioterrorism agent

- Nonfermenter (does not ferment glucose)

- Oxidase and nitrate positive

- Non–lactose fermenter on MAC

- Produces a pronounced earthy odor

Genus *Stenotrophomonas*

Of the two species in the genus *Stenotrophomonas*—*S. maltophilia* and *S. Africana*—only *S. maltophilia* is described here. Previous names for *S. maltophilia*, seen in older microbiology books, are *Pseudomonas maltophilia* and *Xanthomonas maltophilia*.

Clinical significance. *S. maltophilia* is a commonly encountered opportunistic pathogen. It causes nosocomial infections such as septicemia, pneumonia, endocarditis, urinary tract infections, meningitis, wound infections, conjunctivitis, keratitis, and peritonitis.

Drug resistance. *S. maltophilia* is resistant to several antimicrobial agents, including β-lactam agents, aminoglycosides, quinolones, and carbapenems. It is usually susceptible to trimethoprim-sulfamethoxazole, used alone or in combination with minocycline or ticarcillin-clavulanic acid. Antimicrobial susceptibility testing should be performed using microbroth dilution, agar dilution, or Etest methods. Interpretation inconsistencies have been reported when *S. maltophilia* is tested using the disk diffusion method. If plates are incubated at 35°C, trimethoprim-sulfamethoxazole results should be read at 24 hours and all other drugs read at 48 hours. Alternatively, plates can be incubated at room temperature for 48 hours before results are read.

Clues to *S. maltophilia* Identification

Cellular morphology. On Gram staining, *S. maltophilia* cannot be differentiated from other nonfermenters.

Colonial morphology. On blood agar, *S. maltophilia* colonies are rough, dull yellow, dark tan, or lavender-green and have an ammonia odor (Fig. 13-12). *S. maltophilia* is DNase positive, which is a key feature for identification of this organism. A clear zone around colonies on DNase medium is indicative of DNase activity. Clearing of the medium may take up to 72 hours. When toluidine blue DNase agar is used, a positive result is a pink zone around colonies on a blue medium.

Laboratory tests. Other key identifying features include oxidase negative, negative or late oxidation of glucose, very intense oxidation of maltose (hence, the specific epithet *maltophilia*), lysine decarboxylase positive, and a tuft of polar flagella. *S. maltophilia* has a characteristic cellular fatty acid profile.

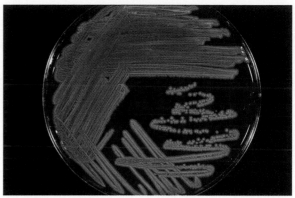

***Figure 13-12. Stenotrophomonas maltophilia* colonies on blood agar.** *S. maltophilia* colonies may be dull yellow (as shown here), dark tan, or lavender-green, depending on the age of the colonies and incubation conditions. (From Winn WC Jr, et al. Koneman's Color Atlas and Textbook of Diagnostic Microbiology. 6th Ed. Philadelphia. Lippincott Williams & Wilkins, 2006.)

Genus *Alcaligenes*

Clinical significance. Clinically significant *Alcaligenes* species include *A. faecalis* and CDC *Alcaligenes*–like group 1. Of the two species, *A. faecalis* is isolated more frequently from clinical specimens. Both species can be found in water, soil, and moist areas within the hospital environment. *A. faecalis* is an occasional cause of nosocomial infections, such as urinary tract infections, pneumonia, and septicemia. CDC *Alcaligenes*–like group 1 has been isolated from various specimens, including blood, urine, knee joint, brain abscess, and bronchial washings.

Drug resistance. *A. faecalis* has been reported to be resistant to ampicillin, aztreonam, and gentamicin, with variable susceptibility to other antimicrobial agents.

Clues to *Alcaligenes* spp. Identification

Cellular morphology. On Gram staining, *A. faecalis* and CDC *Alcaligenes*–like group 1 cannot be differentiated from other nonfermenters. They are motile by peritrichous flagella.

Colonial morphology. *A. faecalis* produces white colonies having a thin, spreading, irregular edge (Fig. 13-13). Strains of *A. faecalis* that were previously called *A. odorans* produce a characteristic green-apple odor and cause a greenish discoloration of blood agar.

> Associate a green-apple odor with *Alcaligenes faecalis*.

Laboratory tests. *A. faecalis* and CDC *Alcaligenes*–like group 1 are classified as oxidase positive, indole negative, asaccharolytic nonfermenters. *A. faecalis* can reduce nitrite but not nitrate. CDC *Alcaligenes*–like group 1 can reduce both nitrate and nitrite.

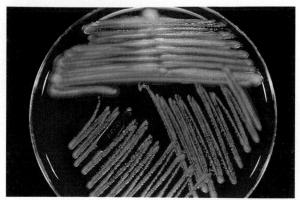

Figure 13-13. White, glistening colonies of *Alcaligenes faecalis* on blood agar after 48 hours of incubation at 35°C. Older colonies tend to spread at the periphery and turn the agar a green-apple color. (From Winn WC Jr, et al. Koneman's Color Atlas and Textbook of Diagnostic Microbiology. 6th Ed. Philadelphia: Lippincott Williams & Wilkins, 2006.)

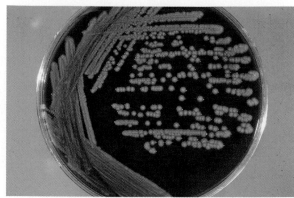

Figure 13-14. *Chryseobacterium indologenes* colonies on blood agar. *C. indologenes* colonies are deep yellow to orange after 48 hours of incubation, particularly when incubated at 30°C. (From Winn WC Jr, et al. Koneman's Color Atlas and Textbook of Diagnostic Microbiology. 6th Ed. Philadelphia: Lippincott Williams & Wilkins, 2006.)

Miscellaneous Nonfermenters

Genus *Chryseobacterium*

Clinical significance. *Chryseobacterium* spp. are found in soil, vegetation, and water (including tap water). *C. indologenes* is isolated more frequently than other *Chryseobacterium* spp. but only rarely has clinical significance. It has caused septicemia in hospitalized patients with indwelling medical devices. *C. meningosepticum* is more important clinically; it has caused septicemia and meningitis in neonates (hence, the specific epithet *meningosepticum*) and occasionally, pneumonia and septicemia in adults. Other *Chryseobacterium* spp. are thought to have no clinical significance.

Drug resistance. *Chryseobacterium* spp. are inherently resistant to some drugs used to treat Gram-negative infections (e.g., aminoglycosides, β-lactam antibiotics, tetracyclines, and chloramphenicol) but are often susceptible to drugs used to treat Gram-positive infections (e.g., rifampin, clindamycin, erythromycin, sparfloxacin, trimethoprim-sulfamethoxazole, vancomycin).

Clues to *Chryseobacterium* spp. Identification

Cellular morphology. Cells of *C. meningosepticum* and *C. indologenes* are thinner in their central regions than at their ends. Filamentous forms are sometimes observed. *C. meningosepticum* is nonmotile, but *C. indologenes* is motile.

Colonial morphology. At 24 hours of incubation, *C. meningosepticum* colonies are smooth and fairly large (1 to 2 mm in diameter), with a faint yellow color (may not be evident at 24 hours). Colonies of *C. indologenes* are deep yellow as a result of production of a yellow pigment called flexirubin (Fig. 13-14). *Cryseo-* is from the Greek word *chrysos*, meaning "gold." *Chryseobacterium* spp. grow poorly, if at all, on MAC.

> Associate *Chryseobacterium indologenes* with yellow colonies.

Laboratory tests. Unlike most nonfermenters, *Chryseobacterium* spp. are indole positive, but because the indole reaction is weak, the more sensitive Ehrlich method is recommended. *Chryseobacterium* spp. are catalase positive, oxidase positive, esculin positive, gelatinase positive, and hydrogen sulfide (H_2S) positive by the lead acetate paper method. They have characteristic cellular fatty acid patterns.

Other genera of nonfermenters include *Achromobacter*, *Acidovorax*, *Brevundimonas*, *Comamonas*, *Ochrobactrum*, *Oligella*, and *Ralstonia*. Information about these genera can be found on the CD-ROM.

Chapter Review

- Nonfermenters are organisms that lack the ability to catabolize (break down) sugars by fermentative pathways. The inability to ferment glucose is the primary way in which nonfermenters differ from members of the family Enterobacteriaceae. Recall that all members of that family ferment glucose.

- The most commonly isolated nonfermenters include the genera *Pseudomonas*, *Acinetobacter* (described in Chapter 11), *Burkholderia*, *Stenotrophomonas*, and *Alcaligenes*.

- Key clues that an isolate is a nonfermenter rather than a member of the family Enterobacteriaceae are (1) it does not ferment glucose, (2) it is oxidase positive, (3) it is nitrate reduction negative, and (4) it does not grow on MAC. Any one of these would serve as a clue that the organism is not a member of the Enterobacteriaceae family.

- O-F tests are used to determine which carbohydrates an unknown Gram-negative bacillus is able to catabolize and by what pathway(s): oxidative, fermentative, or both.

- Oxygen participates in oxidative pathways but does not participate in fermentative pathways.

- *Pseudomonas* spp. are important nonfermentative GNB that are aerobic, non–spore forming, catalase positive, oxidase positive, and non–lactose fermenters on MAC. *Pseudomonas* spp. are widely distributed in nature and frequently cause nosocomial infections in debilitated and immunosuppressed patients.

- *Pseudomonas aeruginosa* is a frequent cause of nosocomial and community-acquired infections. It possesses several virulence factors, including pili and exotoxins, and produces a blue pigment called pyocyanin. Its odor is fruity or like corn tortillas, and it produces an K/NC reaction on TSI.

- Strains of *Alcaligenes faecalis* that were previously called *A. odorans* produce a characteristic green-apple odor and cause a greenish discoloration of blood agar.

- *Chryseobacterium indologenes* has bright yellow colonies.

New Terms and Abbreviations

After studying Chapter 13, you should be familiar with the following terms, which are defined within the chapter and in the Glossary at the back of the book:

Fermentative pathway

Fermenter

Nonfermenter

Nonoxidizer

Oxidative pathway

Oxidizer

Pyocyanin

Pyoverdin

References and Suggested Reading

Abbreviated Identification of Bacteria and Yeast: Approved Guideline. CLSI Document M35-A. Wayne, PA: Clinical and Laboratory Standards Institute, 2002.

Gilligan PH, et al. *Burkholderia*, *Stenotrophomonas*, *Ralstonia*, *Brevundimonas*, *Comamonas*, *Delftia*, *Pandoraea*, and *Acidovorax*. In: Murray PR, Baron EJ, Jorgensen JH, Pfaller MA, Yolken RH, eds. Manual of Clinical Microbiology. 8th Ed. Washington, DC: ASM Press, 2003.

Kiska DL, Gilligan PH. *Pseudomonas*. In: Murray PR, Baron EJ, Jorgensen JH, Pfaller MA, Yolken RH, eds. Manual of Clinical Microbiology. 8th Ed. Washington, DC: ASM Press, 2003.

Ohl CA, Pollack M. *Pseudomonas aeruginosa* and related bacteria. In: Gorbach SL, Bartlett JG, Blacklow NR, eds. Infectious Disease. 3rd Ed. Philadelphia: Lippincott Williams & Wilkins, 2004.

Protection of Laboratory Workers from Occupationally Acquired Infections: Approved Guideline. 3rd Ed. CLSI Document M29-A3. Wayne, PA: Clinical and Laboratory Standards Institute, 2005.

Winn WC Jr, et al. Koneman's Color Atlas and Textbook of Diagnostic Microbiology. 6th Ed. Philadelphia: Lippincott Williams & Wilkins, 2006.

On the CD-ROM

- A Closer Look at Nonfermenters

- Additional Self-Assessment Exercises

- Case Study

- Puzzle

Self-Assessment Exercises

Match the description or characteristic in the left column with the appropriate organism in right column.

1. _____ Odor like grapes or corn tortillas   A. *S. maltophilia*

2. _____ Cause of glanders   B. *P. aeruginosa*

3. _____ Cause of melioidosis   C. *B. pseudomallei*

4. _____ DNase positive   D. *B. mallei*

5. Which of the following is *not* a characteristic of *all Pseudomonas* spp.?

   A. Nonmotile

   B. Non–spore forming

   C. Catalase positive

   D. Non–lactose fermenter on MAC

6. True or false: Nonfermenters are unable to ferment glucose.

7. True or false: Respiratory infections with *P. aeruginosa* are common in cystic fibrosis patients.

8. True or false: When performing an O-F test, if an organism possesses the enzymes necessary to catabolize a carbohydrate oxidatively but lacks the enzymes required to catabolize the carbohydrate fermentatively, it is said to be an oxidizer of that carbohydrate.

9. Which of the following organisms is an aerobic, opportunistic, Gram-negative pathogen that produces rough, lavender-green colonies on blood agar and has an ammonia-like odor?

   A. *B. mallei*

   B. *B. pseudomallei*

   C. *P. aeruginosa*

   D. *S. maltophilia*

10. A CML professional isolated an aerobic Gram-negative bacillus from the sputum of a cystic fibrosis patient. The colonies were small and mucoid looking. The isolate was found to be catalase positive, oxidase positive, non–lactose fermenting, and produced a blue-green pigment on Mueller-Hinton agar. What is the most likely identification of this organism?

   A. *S. maltophilia*

   B. *P. aeruginosa*

   C. *B. mallei*

   D. *E. coli*

CHAPTER 14

Fastidious and Miscellaneous Gram-Negative Bacilli

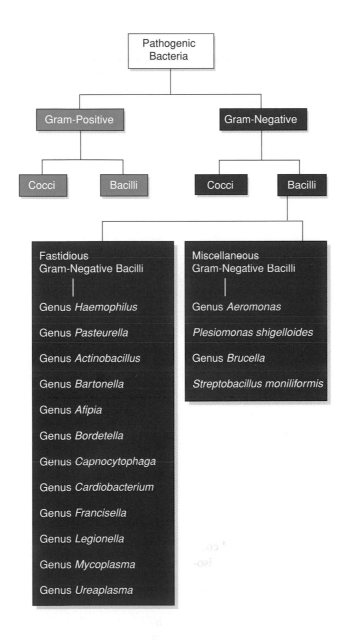

- Genus *Francisella*
- Genus *Legionella*
- Bacteria That Lack Cell Walls

Miscellaneous Gram-Negative Bacilli
- Genus *Aeromonas*
- *Plesiomonas shigelloides*
- Genus *Brucella*
- *Streptobacillus moniliformis*

chapter, including the presence or absence of a cell wall, cellular morphology, Gram reaction, growth (media) requirements, genome characteristics, virulence factors, drug resistance, and colonial morphology

☛ Name two bacteria frequently found together in the same infection

☛ Given a patient's signs and symptoms and clinical microbiology results, select the fastidious Gram-negative bacillus most likely to be involved

LEARNING OBJECTIVES

After studying this chapter, you should be able to:

☛ Define the terms introduced in this chapter (e.g., *biofilm, V factor, X factor*)

☛ When provided with key observations and test results, identify the fastidious Gram-negative bacilli discussed in the chapter

☛ Given a disease caused by a fastidious Gram-negative bacillus (e.g., whooping cough), identify the causative organism

☛ Describe the HACEK group of organisms in terms of the genera included, where they are found in the body as indigenous microflora, and involvement in endocarditis

☛ List the major phenotypic characteristics of the following genera: *Haemophilus, Pasteurella, Actinobacillus, Bartonella, Afipia, Bordetella, Capnocytophaga, Cardiobacterium, Francisella, Legionella, Aeromonas, Brucella, Streptobacillus, Mycoplasma,* and *Ureaplasma*

☛ State the X- and V-factor requirements for the major species of *Haemophilus* and specify the chemical natures of the X and V factors

☛ Outline the specimen requirements, cellular and colonial morphology, growth requirements, media for isolation, specific laboratory tests, and related diseases for the following organisms: *Haemophilus influenzae, H. aegyptius, H. ducreyi, Pasteurella multocida, Actinobacillus actinomycetemcomitans, Bartonella bacilliformis, B. pertussis, Cardiobacterium hominis, Francisella tularensis, Legionella pneumophila, Aeromonas veronii, A. hydrophila, Brucella abortus, B. melitensis, B. suis, B. canis,* and *Streptobacillus moniliformis*

☛ Differentiate *Mycoplasma* and *Ureaplasma* spp. from the other Gram-negative bacilli discussed in the

Meningitis. Ear and sinus infections. Whooping cough. Endocarditis. Tularemia. Legionnaires disease. Trench fever. These are some of the diseases that are caused by the Gram-negative bacilli described in this chapter.

Recall from Chapter 3 that fastidious ("fussy") bacteria are difficult (in some cases, impossible) to grow in the laboratory because of their demanding nutritional requirements and/or other characteristics. Fastidious bacteria described in this chapter include *Haemophilus, Pasteurella,* and *Actinobacillus* spp., all of which are in the family Pasteurellaceae. Other fastidious bacteria described in this chapter (in alphabetical order) are members of the genera *Afipia, Bartonella, Bordetella, Capnocytophaga, Cardiobacterium, Francisella,* and *Legionella*.

The term **HACEK,** introduced in Chapter 11, stands for *Haemophilus, Actinobacillus, Cardiobacterium, Eikenella,* and *Kingella*. These genera are grouped together because they are found as indigenous microflora of the oral cavity and can cause a certain type of endocarditis. Endocarditis caused by HACEK bacteria is characterized by (1) symptoms that last 2 weeks to 6 months before a diagnosis is made, (2) large, friable (easily crumbled) vegetative growths on native (natural) or prosthetic (artificial) heart valves, and (3) a tendency to form clots. These organisms typically show slow growth (up to 6 days) in blood cultures. According to Nerad and Black (see "References and Suggested Reading"), "Patients with prosthetic valve endocarditis caused by . . . members of the HACEK group . . . generally have a more favorable outcome than patients with a non-HACEK Gram-negative bacilli infection. . . . Specifically, they have less mortality and do not require valve replacement as often." *Eikenella* and *Kingella* were described in Chapter 11. The other HACEK organisms (*Haemophilus, Actinobacillus,* and *Cardiobacterium*) are described in this chapter. Additionally, several nonfastidious Gram-negative bacilli that have not been previously discussed are described at the end of this chapter.

> It is important to remember what the acronym HACEK stands for and that organisms in the HACEK group cause a similar type of endocarditis.

FASTIDIOUS GRAM-NEGATIVE BACILLI

Genus *Haemophilus*

Haemophilus spp. share the following characteristics:

- Gram-negative bacilli (ranging from coccobacilli to filamentous rods)

- Nonmotile

- Non–spore forming

- Facultative anaerobes

- Fastidious; they require one or both of the accessory growth factors, called X factor and V factor, for in vitro growth (these factors are described later in the chapter)

- Nitrate reduction positive

- Most are members of the indigenous microflora of the oral cavity and/or upper respiratory tract (an exception is *Haemophilus ducreyi*)

The *Haemophilus* spp. associated with humans include *H. influenzae, H. parainfluenzae, H. aegyptius, H. haemolyticus, H. parahaemolyticus, H. segnis, H. aphrophilus, H. paraphrophilus,* and *H. ducreyi.*

Haemophilus influenzae

Clinical significance. Historically, *H. influenzae* has been one of the three major causes of bacterial meningitis (do you recall the other two?).[1] However, in the United States, the incidence of *H. influenzae*–caused meningitis has been reduced dramatically since Hib vaccine became available. *Hib* stands for *H. influenzae* capsular type b, which was the serotype that caused most cases of bacterial meningitis in children. Worldwide, *H. influenzae* remains a major cause of meningitis. *H. influenzae* is the most common cause of purulent bacterial conjunctivitis (pink eye), the second most common cause of otitis media (*Streptococcus pneumoniae* is the most frequent cause), and a common cause of sinusitis and lower respiratory tract infections. Addi-

> *Haemophilus influenzae* is an important human pathogen. It causes a wide variety of invasive diseases, including meningitis, septicemia, epiglottitis, and pneumonia. It does not cause influenza.

tionally, *H. influenzae* can cause acute epiglottitis (obstructive laryngitis), septicemia, septic arthritis, osteomyelitis, cellulitis, and pericarditis. Figure 14-1 summarizes the diseases caused by *H. influenzae.* **It is important to note that**

H. influenzae does not cause influenza. *H. influenzae* colonizes the nasopharynx of some healthy individuals (referred to as *H. influenzae* carriers).

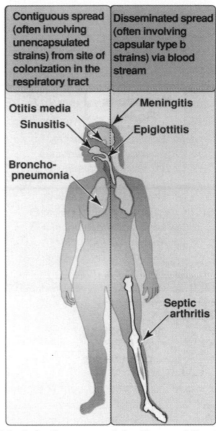

Figure 14-1. **Infections caused by *Haemophilus influenzae.*** (From Strohl WA, et al. Lippincott's Illustrated Reviews: Microbiology. Philadelphia: Lippincott Williams & Wilkins, 2001.)

 CAUTION

Beware of Misnomers. Although *Haemophilus influenzae* is a common cause of respiratory infections and *H. parainfluenzae* may occasionally be associated with respiratory infections, *neither species* causes influenza. These bacteria were named before it was discovered that influenza is actually caused by viruses.

Virulence factors. *H. influenzae* possesses a polysaccharide capsule that serves an antiphagocytic function. There are six *H. influenzae* serotypes (a through f), categorized based on the antigenic composition of the capsule. Some strains, referred to as nontypeable strains, are nonencapsulated.

Drug resistance. Many *H. influenzae* strains are resistant to ampicillin, some other β-lactam antibiotics, chloramphenicol, and tetracyclines.

Clues to *H. influenzae* Identification

Cellular morphology. *H. influenzae* cells are small bacilli that can be variable in shape. In Gram-stained cerebrospinal fluid (CSF) sediments, for example, *H. influenzae* cells are relatively

---

[1]*The three major causes of bacterial meningitis are* Haemophilus influenzae, Streptococcus pneumoniae, *and* Neisseria meningitidis *(see Chapter 11).*

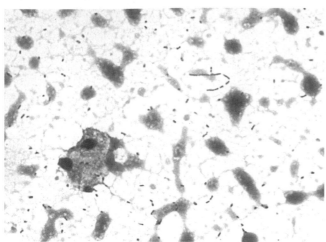

Figure 14-2. **Pleomorphic *H. influenzae* cells in a Gram-stained CSF specimen.** The cells vary from single coccobacilli to pairs of coccobacilli to short bacilli to chains of bacilli. (From Marler LM, Siders JA, Allen SD. Direct Smear Atlas. Philadelphia: Lippincott Williams & Wilkins, 2001.)

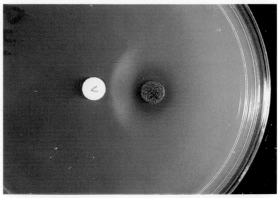

Figure 14-4. **Growth factor disk test for identification of *H. influenzae.*** The organism that was inoculated onto this plate (*H. influenzae*) is only growing in the area *between* the "V" and "X" disks, indicating that it requires both V and X factors for growth. (From Winn WC Jr, et al. Koneman's Color Atlas and Textbook of Diagnostic Microbiology. 6th Ed. Philadelphia: Lippincott Williams & Wilkins, 2006.)

pleomorphic; coccoid, coccobacillary, short rods, long rods, and filamentous forms may be observed (Fig. 14-2). Small, pleomorphic Gram-negative bacilli in Gram-stained respiratory tract specimens, in the presence of polymorphonuclear white blood cells (PMNs), are suggestive of *Haemophilus* spp. (Fig. 14-3). In Gram-stained CSF and sputum specimens, they stain very lightly with safranin and can be easily overlooked. Cells of *Haemophilus* spp. isolates are often pleomorphic in Gram-stained smears; long filamentous forms may be observed.

Colonial morphology. In vitro growth of *H. influenzae* requires the presence of both hemin—referred to as

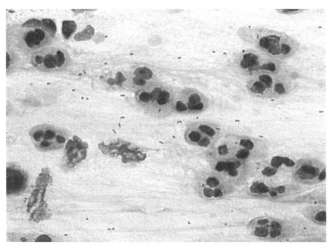

Figure 14-3. ***H. influenzae* cells in a Gram-stained sputum specimen, which also contains larger white blood cells.** The *H. influenzae* cells vary in shape from single coccobacilli to pairs of coccobacilli to short bacilli. Although some of the cells resemble *Neisseria* spp. (diplococci), recall that the adjacent sides of a *Neisseria* diplococcus are flattened. (From Marler LM, Siders JA, Allen SD. Direct Smear Atlas. Philadelphia: Lippincott Williams & Wilkins, 2001.)

X factor—and nicotinamide adenine dinucleotide or NAD—referred to as **V factor**—in the culture medium.[2] Although both X and V factors are present in sheep red blood cells, *H. influenzae* will not grow on sheep blood agar because the V factor is destroyed by enzymes in sheep blood. (Note: Depending on the age and method of preparation of the sheep blood agar, a small amount of V factor may be present.) It is important to note that *H. influenzae* will grow on horse and rabbit blood agar and on chocolate agar because X and V factors are both present in those media. Figure 14-4 illustrates the disk test that is used to demonstrate a requirement for both X and V factors. Table 14-1 shows the X-factor and V-factor requirements of *Haemophilus* spp.

> *Haemophilus influenzae* requires both X and V factors for in vitro growth. Although *H. influenzae* will not grow on sheep blood agar, it will grow on horse and rabbit blood agar and on chocolate agar.

Sheep blood agar can be used to grow *H. influenzae* if one of the following methods is used:

- A filter paper disk or strip containing V factor can be applied to the surface of the inoculated sheep blood agar plate. *H. influenzae* will grow in the immediate vicinity of the disk or strip—a phenomenon called satelliting.

- The inoculated sheep blood agar plate can be cross-streaked with a *Staphylococcus* or *Enterococcus* strain. These organisms produce V factor, which is released into the

> *H. influenzae* will not grow on sheep blood agar unless a source of V factor is provided.

---

[2] *The name X factor was probably used before the identity of this factor (heme) was known. The letter X is commonly used in algebra to represent an unknown. The V in V factor is thought to stand for vitamin. Nicotinamide is part of the structure of nicotinic acid, which is part of the vitamin B complex.*

TABLE 14 - 1	*Haemophilus* spp. Requirements for X and V Factors		
Haemophilus spp.		Requires X Factor (Hemin)	Requires V Factor (NAD)
H. influenzae		Yes	Yes
H. parainfluenzae		No	Yes
H. aegyptius (*H. influenzae* biogroup *aegyptius*)		Yes	Yes
H. haemolyticus		Yes	Yes
H. parahaemolyticus		No	Yes
H. ducreyi		Yes	No
H. segnis		No	Yes
H. aphrophilus		Yes	No
H. paraphrophilus		No	Yes

surrounding medium. *H. influenzae* will satellite in the immediate vicinity of the *Staphylococcus* or *Enterococcus* streak (Fig. 14-5).

On chocolate agar, *H. influenzae* colonies are grayish, semiopaque, smooth, and flat (Fig. 14-6). After 24 hours of incubation at 35°C to 37°C, colonies are 1 to 2 mm in diameter. Encapsulated strains of *H. influenzae* tend to grow confluently in areas of dense growth, whereas nonencapsulated strains produce nonconfluent, separate colonies. Strains isolated from patients with meningitis or epiglottitis have a pungent aroma (similar to that of *Escherichia coli*) caused by the release of indole. Non-indole-producing strains have a "mouse nest" odor.

After 24 hours of incubation, *H. parainfluenzae* colonies are flat, grayish, semiopaque, either smooth or rough and wrinkled, and up to 2 mm in diameter. Colonies of *H. aphrophilus* and *H. paraphrophilus* are rough, raised, and usually less than 1 mm in diameter. Colonies of *H. aegyptius* and *H. segnis* are smooth and less than 1 mm in diameter. After 3 days of incubation, *H. ducreyi* colonies are smooth, semitranslucent, grayish, and 0.1 to 0.5 mm in diameter. *H. ducreyi* colonies are cohesive and can be pushed intact across the agar surface.

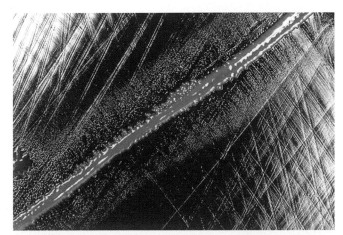

Figure 14-5. **Tiny *H. influenzae* colonies satelliting a *Staphylococcus aureus* streak on a blood agar plate.** *H. influenzae* is obtaining X factor from the red blood cells in the blood agar and V factor from the *S. aureus*. (Courtesy of Dr. Mike Miller and the Centers for Disease Control and Prevention [CDC].)

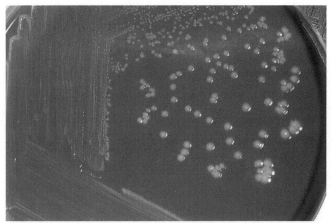

Figure 14-6. **Moist, smooth, gray *H. influenzae* colonies on chocolate agar after 24 hours of incubation at 35°C to 37°C in 5% to 7% CO_2.** (From McClatchy KD, ed. Clinical Laboratory Medicine. 2nd Ed. Philadelphia: Lippincott Williams & Wilkins, 2002.)

Laboratory tests. Presumptive identification of *H. influenzae* can be made by demonstrating a requirement for both X and V factors. However, *H. aegyptius* and *H. haemolyticus* also require both factors. *H. influenzae* and *H. aegyptius* are nonhemolytic, whereas *H. haemolyticum* is hemolytic (as the name implies). Several commercial kits are available for identifying *Haemophilus* spp. Commercial capsular antisera are available. Identification and serotyping can be accomplished using slide agglutination procedures, immunofluorescent techniques, molecular procedures, or the quellung test. (Recall from Chapter 9 that the quellung test causes the capsule to appear swollen and more readily visible.)

Clinical and Laboratory Standards Institute (CLSI) Document M35-A (see "References and Suggested Reading") states that an isolate can be identified as *H. influenzae* (with more than 95% likelihood) if it meets the following criteria:

- Isolate is from a respiratory or CSF specimen

- Small Gram-negative bacilli or coccobacilli

- Colonies are >1 mm in diameter on chocolate agar in 5% CO_2 in 24 hours, but not on sheep blood agar; or satelliting growth is evident around other colonies on sheep blood agar and a negative rapid test for porphyrin synthesis (δ-aminolevulinic acid test). (*H. haemolyticus* will produce the same results as *H. influenzae*, but it will produce β-hemolysis on rabbit or horse blood agar.)

The δ-aminolevulinic acid porphyrin test. Organisms (such as *H. influenzae*) that require hemin (X factor) for growth *lack* the enzymes necessary to synthesize porphyrins from aminolevulinic acid (ALA). To perform the ALA test, some growth is transferred from a culture plate to a piece of filter paper. ALA reagent is added to the organism on the filter paper. After 2 hours of incubation at 35°C, a long-wave ultraviolet light source is held over the spot. If porphyrins were produced from the ALA substrate, the spot will fluoresce orange-red under ultraviolet light; this is interpreted as a positive ALA test result. Lack of fluorescence is a negative test result. *H. parainfluenzae* is ALA positive, whereas *H. influenzae* is ALA negative. Commercial ALA disks are also available. Alternatively, the isolate can be grown on agar medium containing ALA. Following incubation, the growth is observed under ultraviolet light, using a Wood's lamp. Brick-red fluorescence indicates a positive test result (Fig. 14-7).

Essentials

Haemophilus influenzae

- Small Gram-negative bacilli or coccobacilli

- One of the leading causes of meningitis, ear infections, and sinus infections

- Requires both X and V factors

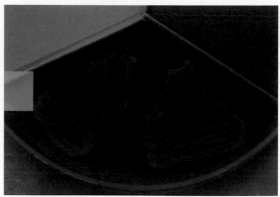

Figure 14-7. **Negative (to the left) and positive (to the right) ALA test results, using agar medium containing ALA.** The organism with the negative test result is *H. influenzae*; the organism with the positive test result is *H. parainfluenzae*. (From Winn WC Jr, et al. Koneman's Color Atlas and Textbook of Diagnostic Microbiology. 6th Ed. Philadelphia: Lippincott Williams & Wilkins, 2006.)

- Grows well on chocolate agar in 5% CO_2 in 24 hours, but not on sheep blood agar

- Will satellite around *Staphylococcus aureus* and some other colonies on sheep blood agar

- Porphyrin synthesis (δ-aminolevulinic acid test) negative

Other *Haemophilus* spp.

Key information about *Haemophilus* spp. other than *H. influenzae* can be found in Table 14-2.

Haemophilus ducreyi cells commonly appear in parallel rows of small bacilli in chains, resembling a school of fish or a railroad track (see Fig. 18-21).

Many clinical microbiology laboratories use a commercially available petri dish divided into four sections, referred to as a quad plate, to identify *Haemophilus* spp. All four sections of the quad plate available from Remel (http://www.remelinc.com/) contain beef heart infusion agar supplemented with various growth factors. The contents of the four quadrants are as follows:

> *Haemophilus aegyptius* (*H. influenzae* biogroup *aegyptius*) is the most common cause of pink eye.

> *Haemophilus ducreyi* causes a type of sexually transmitted disease known as chancroid.

> *H. ducreyi* cells are aligned in parallel chains, resembling a school of fish or a railroad track.

- Quadrant I is supplemented with hemin (X factor)

- Quadrant II is supplemented with NAD (V factor)

TABLE 14 - 2   Key Information About *Haemophilus* spp. Other Than *H. influenzae*

Haemophilus spp.	Key Information
H. parainfluenzae	The most common *Haemophilus* spp. in the indigenous microflora of the upper respiratory tract; part of the indigenous microflora of the oral cavity; colonies up to 2 mm in diameter are flat, grayish, semiopaque, and either smooth or rough and wrinkled after 24 hours of incubation
H. aegyptius (H. influenzae biogroup aegyptius)	Part of the indigenous microflora of the upper respiratory tract; associated with an acute purulent and contagious form of conjunctivitis (pink eye); especially fastidious; small (<1 mm diameter), smooth colonies
H. haemolyticus	Part of the indigenous microflora of the upper respiratory tract; hemolytic
H. parahaemolyticus	Part of the indigenous microflora of the upper respiratory tract; possibly associated with pharyngitis, lower respiratory tract infections, and oral abscesses; an occasional cause of subacute endocarditis, brain abscesses, sinusitis, arthritis, osteomyelitis, and wound and postoperative infections; strongly hemolytic (large zones of hemolysis)
H. segnis	Part of the indigenous microflora of the oral cavity; found in dental plaque; an occasional cause of subacute endocarditis, brain abscesses, sinusitis, arthritis, osteomyelitis, and wound and postoperative infections; small (<1 mm diameter), smooth colonies
H. aphrophilus	Long, slender Gram-negative bacillus; part of the indigenous microflora of the oral cavity; found in dental plaque; an occasional cause of subacute endocarditis, brain abscesses, sinusitis, arthritis, osteomyelitis, and wound and postoperative infections; rough, raised colonies, rarely exceeding 1 mm in diameter
H. paraphrophilus	Part of the indigenous microflora of the oral cavity; found in dental plaque; an occasional cause of subacute endocarditis, brain abscesses, sinusitis, arthritis, osteomyclitis, and wound and postoperative infections; rough, raised colonies, rarely exceeding 1 mm in diameter
H. ducreyi	Causes a sexually transmitted disease called chancroid, which occurs most frequently in Asia, Africa, and Latin America; especially fastidious; grows best at 33°C; in culture, produces long parallel rows of small bacilli in chains (often compared to a school of fish, railroad tracks, or a fingerprint); smooth, semitranslucent, gray, 0.1 to 0.5 mm diameter colonies on enriched chocolate agar after 3 days of incubation; cohesive colonies that can be pushed across the agar

- Quadrant III is supplemented with both hemin and NAD

- Quadrant IV is supplemented with NAD and horse blood (the horse blood provides hemin and is used to determine if the organism is hemolytic)

After inoculation of all four quadrants with a suspected *Haemophilus* sp. and incubation of the plate for 18 to 24 hours in a CO_2 incubator at 35°C to 37°C, the plate is examined for growth and hemolysis. Results are interpreted as shown in Table 14-3.

Genus *Pasteurella*

Clinical significance. *Pasteurella* spp. (pasteurellae) are widespread in the gingiva and nasopharynx of healthy and diseased animals. *P. multocida* is the species most commonly isolated from humans. Other species include *P. canis*, *P. stomatis*, and *P. dagmatis*. All four species are associated with dogs and/or cats, and human infections with these organisms usually follow dog or cat bites or scratches or the licking of skin lesions by dogs and/or cats. Diseases associated with *Pasteurella* spp. include wound infections,

TABLE 14 - 3   Interpretation of *Haemophilus* Quad Plate Results

Quadrant I	Quadrant II	Quadrant III	Quadrant IV	Interpretation
Growth	Growth	Growth	Growth, no hemolysis	*H. aphrophilus*
No growth	No growth	Growth	Growth, no hemolysis	*H. influenzae*
No growth	Growth	Growth	Growth, β-hemolysis	*H. parahaemolyticus*
No growth	Growth	Growth	Growth, no hemolysis	*H. parainfluenzae*

> Infected dog or cat bite wound or scratch? Consider *Pasteurella multocida*, although other organisms may be involved.

abscesses, septicemia, meningitis, endocarditis, arthritis, pneumonia, osteomyelitis, and peritonitis. Peritonitis in home care dialysis patients has been caused by cat bites or scratches to the dialysis tubing.

Drug resistance. Although a few β-lactamase-producing strains of *P. multocida* have been isolated, penicillin remains the drug of choice for treating *Pasteurella* infections. Pasteurellae are generally susceptible to many antimicrobial agents, but are resistant to clindamycin and amikacin.

Clues to *Pasteurella* spp. Identification

Cellular morphology. *Pasteurella* spp. (pasteurellae) are coccoid-to-small, nonmotile Gram-negative bacilli that occur singly, in pairs, or in short chains. Pleomorphism may be observed. Bipolar staining may occur, especially when Wright, Giemsa, or Wayson stain is used. *P. multocida* is encapsulated (the capsule serves an antiphagocytic function).

Colonial morphology. After 24 hours of incubation at 37°C, pasteurellae colonies on blood agar are 1 to 2 mm in diameter, convex and glistening; most species are nonhemolytic (Fig. 14-8). *P. multocida* colonies have a musty odor and, when isolated from respiratory secretions, may be mucoid and watery. Selective media containing vancomycin, clindamycin, and/or amikacin have been used to isolate pasteurellae from clinical specimens. *P. multocida* does not grow on MacConkey agar (MAC).

Laboratory tests. Pasteurellae are oxidase, catalase, indole, and nitrate positive. The oxidase reaction can be slow and weak and is more likely to be positive when the tetramethyl reagent is used (as opposed to the dimethyl reagent). Tests of value for differentiating among species are ornithine decarboxylase and carbohydrate fermentations.

Genus *Actinobacillus*

Clinical significance. There are many *Actinobacillus* spp., some of which are animal pathogens. The species associated with humans are *A. ureae*, *A. hominis*, and *A. actinomycetemcomitans*. *A. ureae* has been isolated from blood, CSF, peritoneal dialysate fluid, and respiratory tract specimens. *A. hominis* has been isolated from respiratory tract specimens and blood (rarely). *A. actinomycetemcomitans* is a part of the indigenous microflora of the oral cavity. Diseases associated with *A. actinomycetemcomitans* include HACEK-type endocarditis, soft tissue infections, periodontal disease, and peritonitis. *A. actinomycetemcomitans* may be found with *Actinomyces* spp. (see Chapter 17), particularly in soft tissue infections (see "Study Aid: What's in a Name?").

STUDY AID   What's in a Name? Who in their right mind would name an organism *Actinobacillus actinomycetemcomitans*? Excellent question! The culprit is not known, but the origin of the specific epithet, *actinomycetemcomitans*, is. It is based on this organism's being frequently isolated from

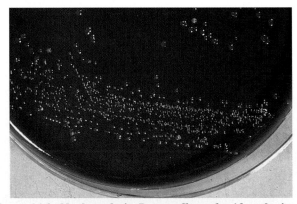

Figure 14-8. **Nonhemolytic *Pasteurella multocida* colonies on blood agar after 48 hours of incubation at 35°C to 37°C in 5% to 7% CO_2.** (From Winn WC Jr, et al. Koneman's Color Atlas and Textbook of Diagnostic Microbiology. 6th Ed. Philadelphia: Lippincott Williams & Wilkins, 2006.)

actinomycotic abscesses concomitantly (together) with members of the genus *Actinomyces*.

Virulence factors. *A. actinomycetemcomitans* produces a leukotoxin, collagenase, a β-lactamase, and endotoxin.

Drug resistance. Although some resistance to penicillin, amikacin, and macrolides has been reported, *A. actinomycetemcomitans* is susceptible to many antimicrobial agents. *A. ureae* and *A. hominis* are susceptible to most antimicrobial agents, including penicillin.

Clues to *Actinobacillus* spp. Identification

Cellular morphology. Although considered to be Gram-negative bacilli, *Actinobacillus* spp. cells may be coccoid, short (0.3 to 0.5 μm wide by 0.6 to 1.4 μm long) or longer bacilli arranged singly, in pairs, or in short chains. They are nonmotile.

Colonial morphology. *Actinobacillus* spp. are facultatively anaerobic and fastidious. Growth in the laboratory requires enriched media and is improved by incubation in a CO_2 incubator. *A. actinomycetemcomitans* colonies initially contain a central opaque dot that, on continued incubation (3 to 5 days), develops a configuration similar to a 4-to-6-point star, often likened to crossed cigars. After 24 hours of incubation at 37°C, colonies of other *Actinobacillus* spp. are 2 mm in diameter, either smooth and dome shaped or rough; they adhere to the agar surface (referred to as being sticky). Smooth colonies have a bluish hue when viewed by transmitted light. *A. actinomycetemcomitans* does not grow on

MAC. Growth of *A. actinomycetemcomitans* in blood culture media may not be evident until 3 to 6 days of incubation; extended incubation is necessary if nonautomated blood culture systems are used. In liquid media, growth occurs as discrete floccules or granules that adhere to the side and bottom of the tube. *A. actinomycetemcomitans* and *Actinomyces* spp. may both be isolated from sulfur granules.

Laboratory tests. *A. actinomycetemcomitans* is oxidase variable; catalase positive; and urease, indole, and nitrate negative. *A. actinomycetemcomitans* can easily be confused with *Pasteurella*, *Haemophilus*, and *Yersinia* spp., but none of those species produce sticky colonies.

Genus *Bartonella*

Clinical significance. The diseases caused by *Bartonella* spp. are shown in Table 14-4.

> *Bartonella* spp. are the causes of trench fever and cat scratch disease.

An estimated 25,000 cases of cat scratch disease occur annually in the United States. In typical or classical cat scratch disease, a cutaneous papule or pustule develops at the site of inoculation of the pathogen (usually the site of a cat scratch or bite). This is followed by regional lymphadenopathy and fever. Atypical cat scratch disease may involve conjunctivitis, retinitis, lymphadenitis, hepatitis, splenitis, and encephalitis.

Drug resistance. Antibiotics have been effective for treating liver and spleen infections caused by *Bartonella* spp., but not for most cases of cat scratch disease.

TABLE 14 - 4 Diseases Caused by *Bartonella* spp.

Bartonella spp.	Disease(s)
B. bacilliformis	Oroya fever (acute stage of Carrion disease; fever, bacteremia, extravascular hemolysis) and verruga peruana (the later stage of Carrion disease; nodular skin lesions); diseases of South America; transmitted by the bite of a sandfly
B. quintana	Trench fever (also known by quite a few other names); bacillary angiomatosis (involves neovascular proliferation); possibly peliosis hepatitis (involving the liver); endocarditis[a]; some HIV-associated CNS and ocular diseases; transmitted by the bite of the body louse
B. henselae	The primary cause of cat scratch disease (transmitted between cats by the cat flea); endocarditis[a]; bacillary peliosis (involving the liver and spleen); some HIV-associated CNS diseases
B. clarridgeiae	Occasional cases of cat scratch disease; possibly transmitted by ticks
B. elizabethae	Endocarditis[a]
B. vinsonii	A possible cause of endocarditis[a]

[a] The endocarditis caused by *Bartonella* spp. is similar to that caused by members of the HACEK group.
CNS, central nervous system.

Clues to *Bartonella* spp. Identification

Cellular morphology. *Bartonella* spp. are thin, short (0.6 to 1.0 μm), faintly staining Gram-negative bacilli that are often slightly curved, thus resembling *Campylobacter* or *Helicobacter* cells (see Chapter 15). *B. bacilliformis* is an intraerythrocytic pathogen. Although the extent of bacteremia is low, blood smears can on occasion be used for direct detection of *B. bacilliformis*.

Colonial morphology. *Bartonella* spp. are aerobic and highly fastidious. They grow on blood agar and chocolate agar if incubated in a CO_2 incubator, but colonies usually cannot be detected in less than 7 to 10 days. Plates should be sealed with some type of cling wrap to prevent the medium from drying out. Heart infusion agar plates containing 5% to 7% rabbit blood have been used successfully to culture *Bartonella* spp., as have blood culture bottles, biphasic culture systems, and cell cultures. (A biphasic culture system employs both liquid- and solid-culture media.) The optimal growth temperature of *B. bacilliformis* is 25°C, whereas the other species grow best at 32°C to 37°C. *B. bacilliformis* and *B. clarridgeiae* are motile by polar flagella. In a wet mount, *B. henselae* and *B. quintana* display twitching motility due to the presence of pili.

Bartonella spp. produce two distinctively different types of colonies, both of which are often present in the same culture. One type of colony is irregular, raised, whitish, rough (described as a cauliflower, molar tooth, or verrucous colony), and dry. The other colony type is smaller, circular, tan, and moist, and may pit and adhere to the agar. *B. henselae* colonies are especially adherent and have a caramel-like odor.

Laboratory tests. Immunodiagnostic and histological procedures are available for the diagnosis of some *Bartonella* infections. *Bartonella* spp. are oxidase negative (weakly positive if the Kovacs modification of the oxidase test is used), catalase negative, urease negative, and indole negative. Definitive identification can be accomplished by cellular fatty acid analysis or molecular diagnostic procedures.

Genus *Afipia*

Clinical significance. Although *Afipia* and *Bartonella* spp. share certain phenotypic characteristics, they are classified in different families. Of several known species of *Afipia*, *A. felis* is the most clinically significant. It is a facultative intracellular pathogen and an occasional cause of cat scratch disease. Recall that facultative intracellular pathogens are able to live both intracellularly and extracellularly.

STUDY AID

What's in a Name? The genus name *Afipia* is derived from AFIP, which is the acronym for the Armed Forces Institute of Pathology, where *A. felis* was first cultured. The specific epithet *felis* is based on the organism's association with cats.

Drug resistance. In vitro drug susceptibility to imipenem, aminoglycosides, and rifampin, and resistance to penicillins, cephalosporins, and quinolones have been demonstrated for *A. felis*. However, there have been too few cases of *A. felis* infection to draw conclusions about in vivo correlations.

Clues to *Afipia* spp. Identification

Cellular morphology. *Afipia* spp. are pleomorphic, weakly staining Gram-negative bacilli.

Colonial morphology. Although they are fastidious, *Afipia* spp. are less fastidious than *Bartonella* spp. Their optimal growth temperature is 30°C. *A. felis* will grow on or in solid media, blood culture bottles, biphasic culture systems, and cell cultures. At 72 hours of incubation, colonies on blood agar are grayish white, glistening, convex, and opaque. *Afipia* spp. do not grow on MAC.

Laboratory tests. *Afipia* spp. can be identified using conventional biochemical tests. They are urease and oxidase positive, unlike most *Bartonella* spp., which are urease and oxidase negative. Observations and tests of value in differentiating *Afipia felis* from *Bartonella* spp. are summarized in Table 14-5.

Genus *Bordetella*

Clinical significance. The most important disease caused by *Bordetella* spp. is pertussis (whooping cough), which is caused by *B. pertussis*. Pertussis can be a very serious disease, with violent coughing, vomiting, choking, the "whooping" sound produced as patients gasp for air, apnea (absence of breathing), anoxia (absence of oxygen from inspired gases, blood, and tissues), cyanosis (purplish discoloration of skin and mucous membranes), subconjunctival hemorrhage, umbilical and inguinal hernias, and death. Other complications of pertussis include otitis media, pneumonia (caused by secondary infection), and CNS dysfunction (rare). Acellular vaccines are available. The diseases caused by *Bordetella* spp. are summarized in Table 14-6.

> *Bordetella pertussis* causes pertussis (whooping cough), which can be a very serious, sometimes fatal disease.

Virulence factors. *B. pertussis* produces various adhesins, which enable the organism to bind to host cells. These adhesins include filamentous hemagglutinin, pertussis toxin, pertactin (a surface protein), and pili. *B. pertussis* produces endotoxin and several exotoxins, including a cytotoxin. There is evidence that *B. pertussis* can survive within macrophages.

Drug resistance. Erythromycin, azithromycin, and clarithromycin are the drugs of choice for treatment of pertussis. Trimethoprim-sulfamethoxazole and fluoroquinolones are also effective. Drug resistance does not appear to be a problem with *B. pertussis*.

TABLE 14 - 5	Observations and Tests of Value in Differentiating *Afipia felis* from *Bartonella* spp.	
Observation or Test	***Bartonella* spp.**	***A. felis***
Optimal growth temperature	35°C to 37°C, except *B. bacilliformis* (25°C to 30°C)	25°C to 30°C
Growth in nutrient broth	−	+
Flagella	− (except *B. bacilliformis* and *B. clarridgeiae*)	+
Twitching motility	− (except *B. quintana* and *B. henselae*)	−
Oxidase	− (except some strains of *B. quintana* and *B. vinsonii*)	+
Catalase	− (except *B. bacilliformis* and some strains of *B. henselae* and *B. vinsonii*)	−
Nitrate reduction	−	+
Urease	−	+

Clues to *Bordetella* spp. Identification

Cellular morphology. *Bordetella* spp. are small (0.2- to 1.0-μm) Gram-negative coccobacilli.

Colonial morphology. Properly collected nasopharyngeal aspirates (preferably) and posterior nasopharyngeal swabs are the appropriate specimens for diagnosis of pertussis. Dacron or calcium alginate swabs should be used, not cotton swabs; cotton contains substances that will inhibit growth of *B. pertussis*. Specimens should be plated immediately or placed into a suitable transport medium (e.g., Regan-Lowe transport medium, casamino acids medium, Jones-Kendrick charcoal medium, or Amies medium with charcoal).

Bordetella spp. are strictly aerobic. Their optimum growth temperature is 35°C to 37°C. With its complex nutritional requirements, *B. pertussis* is the most fastidious *Bordetella* species. Growth of *B. pertussis* is inhibited by various constituents found in routine culture media. Isolation of *B. pertussis* requires media that contain protective substances such as charcoal, blood, or starch. Preferred media

> Cotton swabs should not be used to collect nasopharyngeal specimens when whooping cough is suspected. Cotton contains substances that inhibit growth of *B. pertussis*.

TABLE 14 - 6	Diseases Caused by *Bordetella* spp.
***Bordetella* spp.**	**Disease(s)**
B. pertussis	Pertussis (whooping cough) in humans; highly contagious; vaccine available; no animal reservoir
B. parapertussis	Respiratory disease in humans similar to, but less severe than, pertussis; cough; bronchitis; can cause systemic disease in immunosuppressed patients; no animal reservoir
B. bronchiseptica	Respiratory tract pathogen of animals; rare cause of human respiratory infection
B. hinzii	Part of the respiratory tract microflora of poultry; rare cause of septicemia and respiratory infection in humans
B. holmesii	Infrequent cause of respiratory and nonrespiratory infections in humans
B. trematum	Infrequent cause of respiratory and nonrespiratory (wound, ear) infections in humans
B. avium	Causes coryza (rhinitis) in turkeys; has caused chronic otitis in humans

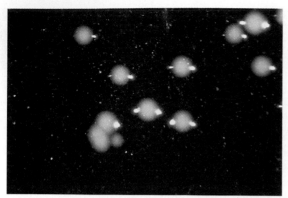

***Figure 14-9. Bordetella pertussis* colonies on charcoal horse blood medium, also known as Regan-Lowe medium.** The colonies resemble mercury droplets or pearls pushed halfway into the agar. (From Winn WC Jr, et al. Koneman's Color Atlas and Textbook of Diagnostic Microbiology. 6th Ed. Philadelphia: Lippincott Williams & Wilkins, 2006.)

for isolation of *B. pertussis* are Bordet-Gengou potato infusion medium and charcoal horse blood (CHB) medium (also known as Regan-Lowe medium). Colonies of *B. pertussis* on Bordet-Gengou medium are tiny, glistening, and translucent, surrounded by a hazy zone of hemolysis. On CHB medium, *B. pertussis* colonies are small, round, domed,

> *B. pertussis* colonies look like mercury droplets or partially imbedded pearls on CHB medium.

shiny, and silver—like mercury droplets or pearls pushed halfway into the agar (Fig. 14-9). *B. pertussis* colonies generally take at least 3 days to appear; plates should be held 7 days or longer. Other *Bordetella* spp. are less fastidious and grow on routine agars, including blood agar and MAC.

Laboratory tests. Immunofluorescent and molecular diagnostic procedures are available. *Bordetella* spp. do not ferment carbohydrates. Observations and tests of value for differentiating among *Bordetella* spp. are shown in Table 14-7.

Essentials

Bordetella pertussis

- Small (0.2- to 1.0-μm) Gram-negative coccobacilli

- Etiologic agent of whooping cough (pertussis)

- Preferred media for isolation are Bordet-Gengou potato infusion medium and CHB medium (also known as Regan-Lowe medium)

- On Bordet-Gengou medium, colonies are tiny, glistening, and translucent, surrounded by a hazy zone of hemolysis

- On CHB medium, colonies are small, round, domed, shiny, and silver—like mercury droplets or pearls pushed halfway into the agar

Genus *Capnocytophaga*

Clinical significance. The seven *Capnocytophaga* spp. are part of the indigenous microflora of humans, dogs, and cats. Diseases associated with *Capnocytophaga* spp. include dog and cat bite wound infections, periodontitis, septicemia, endocarditis, endometritis, osteomyelitis, abscesses, peritonitis, keratitis, meningitis, and arthritis. Most human infections are caused by *C. ochracea, C. sputigena,* and *C. gingivalis*. Like *A. actinomycetemcomitans, Capnocytophaga* spp. have been isolated together with *Actinomyces israelii*.

TABLE 14 - 7	**Observations and Tests of Value for Differentiating Among *Bordetella* spp.**						
***Bordetella* spp.**	**Catalase**	**Oxidase**	**Nitrate**	**Urease**	**Motility**	**Growth on Blood Agar**	**Growth on MAC**
B. pertussis	+	+	−	−	−	−	−
B. parapertussis	+	−	−	+ (24 hours)	−	+	Variable (delayed)
B. bronchiseptica	+	+	+	+ (4 hours)	+	+	+
B. hinzii	+	+	−	Variable	+	+	+
B. holmesii	+	−	−	−	−	+	+ (delayed)
B. trematum	+	−	Variable	−	+	+	+
B. avium	+	+	−	−	+	+	+

MAC, MacConkey agar.

Drug resistance. *Capnocytophaga* spp. are generally susceptible to many antimicrobial agents but resistant to aztreonam, aminoglycosides, vancomycin, trimethoprim, and polymyxin B. Some β-lactamase strains have been isolated.

Clues to *Capnocytophaga* spp. Identification

Cellular morphology. *Capnocytophaga* cells are primarily fusiform shaped (long and thin with pointed ends) and 0.4 to 0.6 μm wide by 2.5 to 7.5 μm long, but they are pleomorphic. Coccoid or spindle forms and curved filaments may also be observed (Fig. 14-10).

Colonial morphology. *Capnocytophaga* spp. are fastidious, slow growing, and facultatively anaerobic. In vitro growth requires rich media and 5% to 10% CO_2. (*Capno-* refers to CO_2. Do you remember what a capnophile is?) *Capnocytophaga* spp. grow on blood agar and chocolate agar but not on MAC. Colonies become visible after about 48 hours of incubation at 37°C. After incubating 2 to 4 days, colonies are 2 to 3 mm in diameter, convex or flat, and slightly yellow. When removed from the agar surface, a yellow pigment can be seen on the agar surface. Colonies have irregular edges and fingerlike projections (gliding or sliding motility) that appear as a thin film surrounding the central part of the colony (Fig. 14-11). The central part of the colony may have a moist, mottled, or "sweaty" appearance. Colonies adhere to the agar surface. Most species are nonhemolytic.

Laboratory tests. Most *Capnocytophaga* spp. (including *C. ochracea*, *C. sputigena*, and *C. gingivalis*) are catalase, oxidase, indole, and urease negative, and they produce negative decarboxylase tests. The *Capnocytophaga* spp. associated with infected dog and cat bite wounds (namely, *C. canimorsus* and *C. cynodegmi*) are oxidase and catalase positive.

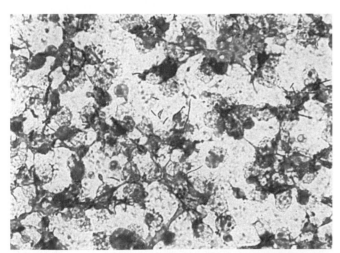

Figure 14-10. **Gram-stained blood specimen containing delicate, poorly stained Gram-negative bacilli with tapered ends.** These bacilli were later identified as *Capnocytophaga* sp., but certain *Fusobacterium* spp. also have this morphology. (From Marler LM, Siders JA, Allen SD. Direct Smear Atlas. Philadelphia: Lippincott Williams & Wilkins, 2001.)

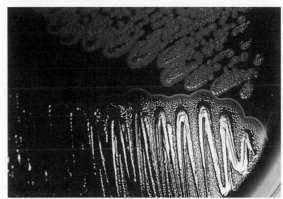

Figure 14-11. ***Capnocytophaga* colonies on blood agar after 48 hours of incubation at 35°C to 37°C in 5% to 7% CO_2.** Notice the fringes of the colonies, which illustrate the characteristic gliding motility of *Capnocytophaga* spp. (From Winn WC Jr, et al. Koneman's Color Atlas and Textbook of Diagnostic Microbiology. 6th Ed. Philadelphia: Lippincott Williams & Wilkins, 2006.)

Individual *Capnocytophaga* spp. can be differentiated by their carbohydrate fermentation and nitrate reduction test results.

Genus *Cardiobacterium*

Clinical significance. *C. hominis* is the only species in the genus *Cardiobacterium*. It is part of the indigenous microflora of the upper respiratory tract; possibly also the genitourinary and gastrointestinal tracts. *C. hominis* causes the type of endocarditis that is typical of the HACEK organisms (discussed in the opening of this chapter) but is not a common cause of endocarditis. (It is not surprising that an organism with *cardio* in its name would cause some type of heart disease.)

Drug resistance. *C. hominis* is susceptible to most antimicrobial agents but resistant to clindamycin. β-Lactamase-producing strains have been reported.

Clues to *C. hominis* Identification

Cellular morphology. *C. hominis* is a pleomorphic Gram-negative bacillus that may occur singly or in pairs, short chains, or rosette clusters (Fig. 14-12). Cells are not pleomorphic when *C. hominis* is cultured on a medium containing yeast extract. Cells are 0.75 μm wide by 1.0 to 3.0 μm long and may have a bulbous enlargement at one or both ends. Retention of crystal violet may cause irregular staining, with some cells appearing Gram positive. *C. hominis* is nonmotile.

Colonial morphology. *C. hominis* is a facultative anaerobe but does not grow well aerobically unless the air is humidified. It requires 5% to 10% CO_2 for growth. After 48 hours of incubation at 37°C, colonies on blood agar are 1 to 2 mm in diameter, circular, convex, smooth, moist, opaque, and nonhemolytic; they often pit the agar like *Eikenella corrodens* (see Chapter 11). *C. hominis* grows slowly in blood cultures. All nonautomated blood cultures should be held 2 to 3 weeks.

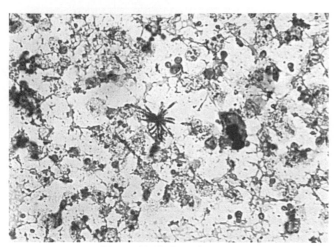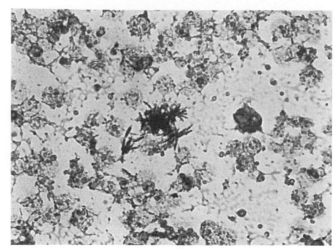

Figure 14-12. **Two Gram-stained blood specimens containing rosette clusters of *Cardiobacterium hominis* cells.** The cells are medium to long and pleomorphic, with either pointed or rounded ends. (From Marler LM, Siders JA, Allen SD. Direct Smear Atlas. Philadelphia: Lippincott Williams & Wilkins, 2001.)

Laboratory tests. *C. hominis* is oxidase positive, catalase negative, and nitrate positive. It is weakly indole positive (usually after 24 to 48 hours and extraction with xylene). *C. hominis* ferments glucose to lactic acid.

Genus *Francisella*

Clinical significance. There are two recognized species of *Francisella*: *F. tularensis* and *F. philomiragia*. *F. tularensis* is the cause of tularemia, a severe and sometimes fatal disease in humans. *F. philomiragia* is a very rare cause of human infection (primarily pneumonia). Both species are associated with the outdoor environment, small mammals, and arthropods. The most common ways in which humans become infected with *F. tularensis* are (1) contact with contaminated air, water, soil, or vegetation; (2) by handling ill or dead infected animals; and (3) from the bites of infected insects. Tularemia has been found in more than 100 species of wild animals and in at least nine species of domestic animals (including dogs and cats). Biting flies, ticks, and mosquitoes serve either as mechanical or biological vectors.[3] Infection may also occur via ingestion of contaminated water, eating contaminated food, or aerosolization.

There are four subspecies (or biovars) of *F. tularensis*, of which *F. tularensis* subsp. *tularensis* is the most virulent. It is this subspecies that is most closely associated with tularemia in North America. In the United States, most patients acquire tularemia via tick or deerfly bites or by contact with infected animals (particularly rabbits). Tick fever, deerfly fever, and rabbit fever are three of the many common names for tularemia.

F. tularensis is a facultative intracellular pathogen capable of living and multiplying within macrophages. The symptoms of tularemia depend primarily on the manner in which the patient became infected. Initial symptoms include chills, fever, headache, cough, myalgia (muscular pain), and generalized malaise. Without diagnosis and treatment, the patient may experience sweating, chills, progressive weakness, and weight loss. There are six classical forms of tularemia:

- Ulceroglandular (an ulcer develops at the site that *F. tularensis* was inoculated into the skin; lymph nodes become enlarged and painful; Fig. 14-13)

- Glandular (lymph node involvement without an ulcerative lesion)

- Oculoglandular (as a result of *F. tularensis* entering the eye)

- Oropharyngeal (pharyngitis, tonsillitis, and cervical lymphadenopathy following ingestion of *F. tularensis*)

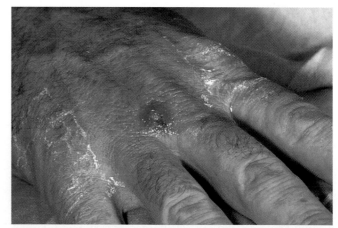

Figure 14-13. **Lesion of tularemia caused by *Francisella tularensis*.** (Courtesy of Dr. Brachman and the CDC.)

---

[3]*Arthropods may serve as either mechanical vectors or biological vectors. Mechanical vectors merely pick up the parasite at point A and drop it off at point B (like an overnight delivery service). A biological vector, on the other hand, is an arthropod in whose body the pathogen multiplies or matures (or both). Arthropod vectors are discussed more fully in Chapter 21.*

- Pneumonic (as a result of direct inhalation or secondary to hematogenous or lymphatic spread of *F. tularensis*)

- Typhoidal (septicemia; no apparent primary site of infection)

Although they are not closely related, for the following reasons the genera *Francisella* and *Brucella* (discussed later in this chapter) are often linked:

> *F. tularensis* is a potential bioterrorism and biological warfare agent and is dangerous to work with in the laboratory.

- They are similar in appearance (small Gram-negative coccobacilli).

- They produce diseases having similar symptoms.

- They produce disease in animals and humans; the human diseases they cause are zoonotic.

- Cross-reactivity occurs between antibodies produced against these two pathogens.

- Extreme care must be taken when working with these organisms in the laboratory; *F. tularensis* and *Brucella* spp. are two of the most common causes of laboratory-acquired infections.

- *Francisella* and *Brucella* spp. are potential bioterrorism agents.

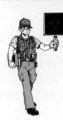

SAFETY TIP

Notification of Suspected Tularemia. Whenever a clinician suspects a case of tularemia, he or she must notify the laboratory so that (1) appropriate media can be inoculated and (2) appropriate safety measures will be taken. **F. tularensis** *is highly infectious. Clinical microbiology laboratory personnel must perform procedures, such as centrifugation and open-plate examination and manipulation of cultures, within a biosafety cabinet.*

Virulence factors. Although encapsulated, *F. tularensis* cells are phagocytized by neutrophils. However, they are able to live within the phagocytes.

Drug resistance. *F. tularensis* is resistant to natural penicillins and first-generation cephalosporins but is highly susceptible to a wide range of antimicrobial agents. Streptomycin (or gentamicin, if streptomycin is unavailable) is the drug of choice.

Clues to *F. tularensis* Identification

Cellular morphology. *F. tularensis* is a tiny (0.2 μm wide by 0.2 to 0.7 μm long), nonmotile, faintly staining Gram-negative coccobacillus (Fig. 14-14).

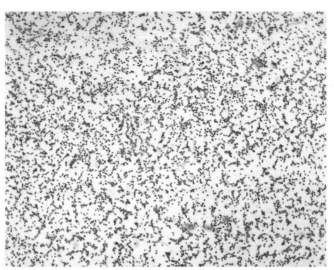

Figure 14-14. **Gram-stained** *F. tularensis* **cells.** This tiny Gram-negative coccobacillus is seen primarily as single cells. (Courtesy of Larry Stauffer, Oregon State Public Health Laboratory, and the CDC.)

Colonial morphology. *F. tularensis* is a strict aerobe that grows poorly, if at all, on most ordinary media. Optimal growth is obtained on media supplemented with sulfhydral compounds (cysteine, cystine, thiosulfate, IsoVitalex). Incorporation of antimicrobial agents (penicillin, polymyxin B sulfate, cycloheximide) in the medium suppresses growth of indigenous microflora contaminants. Optimum growth temperature is 35°C to 37°C. *F. tularensis* has a 60-minute generation time. Cultures should be observed daily for 10 to 14 days.

On chocolate agar, *F. tularensis* colonies are gray, smooth, raised, moist, and butyrous, with an entire edge. On cysteine heart blood agar supplemented with chocolatized sheep blood, growth of *F. tularensis* exhibits a prominent opalescent sheen as a result of production of hydrogen sulfide (H_2S; Fig. 14-15).

Laboratory tests. Immunological and molecular diagnostic procedures are available for diagnosing tularemia. *F. tularensis* is weakly catalase positive, is oxidase negative, and uses only a few sugars (glucose, maltose, sucrose, and glycerol) without producing gas.

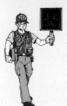

SAFETY TIP

CLSI-Recommended Safety Precautions. CLSI Document M29-A3 (see "References and Suggested Reading") recommends biosafety level 2 (BSL-2) practices, containment equipment, and facilities for activities with clinical materials of human or animal origin containing or potentially containing F. tularensis. *BSL-3 and Animal BSL-3 practices, containment equipment, and facilities are recommended for all manipulations of cultures and for experimental animal studies.*

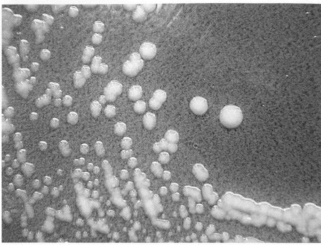

***Figure 14-15.* Colonies of *F. tularensis* on cysteine heart blood agar.** After 48 to 72 hours of incubation, colonies are 2 to 4 mm in diameter, smooth, entire, greenish white, and butyrous, with an opalescent sheen. (Courtesy of Larry Stauffer, Oregon State Public Health Laboratory, and the CDC.)

Essentials

Francisella tularensis

- Tiny (0.2 μm wide by 0.2 to 0.7 μm long), nonmotile, faintly staining Gram-negative coccobacilli

- Etiologic agent of tularemia (also known as tick fever, deerfly fever, and rabbit fever)

- Potential bioterrorism and biological warfare agent; very dangerous to work with in the laboratory

- Grows poorly, if at all, on most ordinary media; optimal growth is obtained on media supplemented with sulfhydral compounds, such as cysteine, cystine, thiosulfate, and IsoVitalex

Genus *Legionella*

Although organisms in the genus *Legionella* were unknown before 1976, there are now more than 40 named species of *Legionella*, approximately half of which can cause human disease. The first species described was *L. pneumophila*, which remains the species most commonly associated with disease in humans. The other most clinically significant *Legionella* spp. are *L. bozemanii*, *L. dumoffii*, *L. longbeachae*, and *L. micdadei*. These *Legionella* spp. cause disease ranging from a mild, self-limited, flulike illness (called Pontiac fever) to a severe type of pneumonia, to an often fatal disseminated disease. *Legionella*-associated disease (legionellosis) can either be community acquired (usually) or hospital acquired.

> *Legionella pneumophila* is the primary cause of legionellosis, a potentially serious respiratory disease.

STUDY AID **What's in a Name?** In the name *Legionella pneumophila*, the word *Legion* refers to a 1976 epidemic caused by this organism. The epidemic affected more than 200 people attending an American Legion convention in Philadelphia. The organism was present in the water that circulated through one hotel's air-conditioning system. Those who became infected had inhaled aerosols of the organism. In the specific epithet *pneumophila*, *pneumo-* refers to the lungs, and the suffix *-phil* (or *-phile*) means "to love." Thus, *Legionella pneumophila* is an organism that loves lungs. It causes a respiratory infection, which was once known as Legionnaires disease, but is now called legionellosis.

Legionella spp. are common in soil and water, including chlorinated water. They can survive over wide-ranging temperatures (0°C to 63°C), pH levels (5.0 to 8.5), and dissolved oxygen concentrations (0.2 to 15 parts per million). They colonize hot water tanks, especially when the water temperature is 40°C to 50°C. In the environment, *Legionella* spp. are commonly found in association with other microorganisms, forming what are known as **biofilms** (see the CD-ROM for a discussion of biofilms). *L. pneumophila* can infect and multiply within several species of aquatic and soil-dwelling amebas, which may serve as reservoirs.

Virulence factors. *L. pneumophila* virulence factors include endotoxin, flagella, pili, and a cytotoxin. *Legionella* spp. are facultative intracellular pathogens. *L. pneumophila* can stimulate phagocytosis, and can replicate within alveolar macrophages and probably within alveolar epithelial cells.

Drug resistance. Once the organisms are inside host cells, antimicrobial agents that cannot penetrate host cell membranes (e.g., penicillins and cephalosporins) are ineffective. Agents considered to be effective for treatment of legionellosis include erythromycin, rifampin, tetracycline, fluoroquinolones, and newer macrolide-azalides.

Clues to *Legionella* spp. Identification

Cellular morphology. *Legionella* spp. are motile, faintly staining Gram-negative bacilli, ranging in appearance from small coccobacilli to filaments up to 20 μm in length (Fig. 14-16). *Legionella* are difficult to see in Gram-stained respiratory specimens. Preferred stains are carbol fuchsin, crystal violet (with or without Lugol iodine), and silver stains (for paraffin-fixed tissues; Fig. 14-17). *L. micdadei* is weakly acid fast in tissues stained by the Kinyoun method but is not acid fast in culture. Immunofluorescent microscopy can be used to visualize *Legionella* cells in respiratory specimens.

Colonial morphology. *Legionella* spp. are fastidious, slow-growing, obligate aerobes. They do not grow well on standard culture media but will grow on chocolate agar. The primary

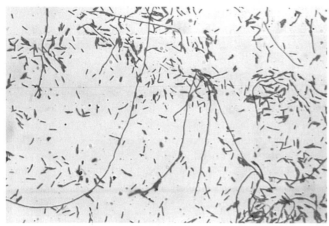

Figure 14-16. **Gram-stained *Legionella pneumophila* cells, including long chains of cells.** (Courtesy of the CDC.)

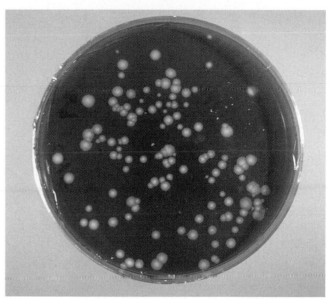

Figure 14-18. **Six-day-old *L. pneumophila* colonies on buffered charcoal yeast extract agar.** (Courtesy of Dr. Jim Feeley and the CDC.)

Legionella isolation medium is buffered charcoal yeast extract (BCYE) agar, supplemented with α-ketoglutarate, L-cysteine, and ferric pyrophosphate (Figs. 14-18 and 14-19). BCYE containing polymyxin-anisomycin-vancomycin (PAV) and inhibitory dyes should be used for contaminated specimens. Culture plates should be incubated in humidified air at 35°C to 37°C; CO_2 is not necessary. A dissecting microscope can be used to observe young colonies. On BCYE agar with PAV, *L. pneumophila* colonies will be whitish green, *L. micdadei* colonies will be blue, and contaminants (e.g., *Candida*, *E. coli*, *Staphylococcus aureus*) will be partially to completely inhibited. When examined under long-wavelength ultraviolet light, some *Legionella* colonies (excluding *L. pneumophila*) fluoresce blue-white, red, or yellow-green, depending on the species. *Legionella* spp. will not grow in conventional or automated blood culture systems.

Laboratory tests. Urinary antigen detection tests are available to detect *L. pneumophila* antigens in the urine of patients with pulmonary legionellosis. Molecular diagnostic procedures and other immunodiagnostic procedures are also available. The usual basis for identification of *Legionella* spp. includes (1) their cellular morphology (thin, weakly staining Gram-negative bacilli or filaments), (2) their requirement for cysteine, (3) their nonfermentative metabolism, and (4) serotyping by slide agglutination or direct fluorescent antibody stain. Their requirement for cysteine can be demonstrated either by inoculating BCYE agar and 5% sheep blood agar in parallel, or by inoculating BCYE agar and BCYE agar without cysteine in parallel.

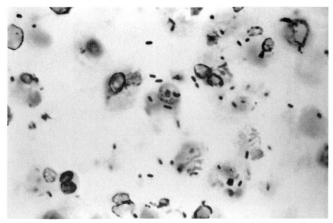

Figure 14-17. **L. pneumophila cells in a biopsied lung tissue specimen stained using a modified Dieterle silver impregnation procedure.** The bacteria stain brown to black using this staining procedure. (Courtesy of the CDC.)

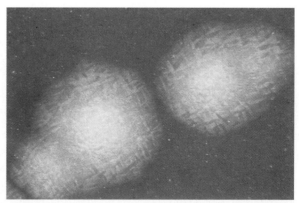

Figure 14-19. **Colonies of *L. pneumophila* on buffered charcoal yeast extract agar, as seen using a dissecting microscope.** Notice the crystalline-like interior of the colonies. (From Winn WC Jr, et al. Koneman's Color Atlas and Textbook of Diagnostic Microbiology. 6th Ed. Philadelphia: Lippincott Williams & Wilkins, 2006.)

Essentials

Legionella pneumophila

- Motile, faintly staining Gram-negative bacilli, ranging in appearance from small coccobacilli to filaments up to 20 μm in length

- One of the etiologic agents of legionellosis (Legionnaires disease)

- Requires cysteine for in vitro growth

- Does not grow well on standard culture media but will grow on chocolate agar; the primary *Legionella* isolation medium is BCYE agar, supplemented with α-ketoglutarate, L-cysteine, and ferric pyrophosphate

- Colonies on BCYE agar with PAV are whitish green

Bacteria That Lack Cell Walls

Recall from Chapter 1 that the bacterial cell wall is a rigid structure that surrounds the cell membrane and provides the cell with rigidity, shape, and protection. Virtually all bacteria possess cell walls. Notable exceptions are the bacteria described in this section—namely, *Mycoplasma* and *Ureaplasma* spp. As bacteria without cell walls, these organisms constitute a unique category within the Domain *Bacteria*.

> Reminder: Do not confuse *Mycoplasma* spp. with *Mycobacterium* spp.

> The cells of *Mycoplasma* and *Ureaplasma* spp. are pleomorphic because they do not possess cell walls.

Because they have no cell walls to define their shape, bacteria in these genera are pleomorphic (existing in various shapes).

Also, because they have no cell walls, they have no peptidoglycan to retain the crystal violet–iodine complexes that are formed during the Gram staining procedure; thus, when they stain at all, *Mycoplasma* and *Ureaplasma* spp. are Gram negative.

Mycoplasmas and ureaplasmas are tiny and have a genome that is only about one-fifth to one-half the size of most bacterial genomes. They are the simplest and smallest free-living, self-replicating procaryotes. They are pleomorphic, ranging from coccoid cells (0.2 to 0.3 μm in diameter) to tapered rods (0.1 to 0.2 μm wide by 1.0 to 2.0 μm long). Like chlamydiae, rickettsias, and viruses, mycoplasmas and ureaplasmas can pass through filters having a pore size through which most bacteria cannot pass. For this reason, they were once referred to as filterable agents. However, unlike chlamydiae, rickettsias, and viruses, mycoplasmas and ureaplasmas *can* be grown on artificial culture media. Because they have limited biosynthetic abilities, mycoplasmas and ureaplasmas require complex enriched culture media for growth. Media must contain a peptone, a sterol (such as cholesterol), preformed nucleic acid precursors (supplied by yeast extract), and a metabolite (e.g., glucose, arginine, urea). Their optimal growth temperature is 37°C.

> *Mycoplasma* and *Ureaplasma* spp. grow on especially enriched artificial media, but the colonies they produce are very small and are composed of tiny cells.

Genus Mycoplasma

Clinical significance. *Mycoplasma* spp. can be isolated from mucous membranes of the genital and upper respiratory tracts. Although there are many *Mycoplasma* spp., only three species cause human disease: *M. pneumoniae*, *M. hominis*, and *M. genitalium* (Table 14-8).

TABLE 14 - 8	Diseases Caused by *Mycoplasma* and *Ureaplasma* spp.		
Species	**Usual Habitat**	**Disease(s)**	
M. pneumoniae	Respiratory tract	Upper and lower respiratory tract infections, including pneumonia	
M. hominis	Genital tract	BV, PID, postpartum fever	
M. genitalium	Genital tract	NGU[a]; possibly PID	
Ureaplasma urealyticum	Genital tract	NGU; possibly BV and PID	

[a] Refer to "Study Aid: Nongonococcal Urethritis."

BV, bacterial vaginosis; NGU, nongonococcal urethritis; PID, pelvic inflammatory disease.

STUDY AID **Nongonococcal Urethritis.** Once upon a time, *Neisseria gonorrhoeae* was the major cause of urethritis. Cases of urethritis that were not caused by *N. gonorrhoeae* were referred to as nongonococcal urethritis (NGU). Today the major cause of NGU is *Chlamydia trachomatis*, but other organisms (e.g., *Mycoplasma genitalium* and *Ureaplasma urealyticum*) also cause NGU.

Virulence factors. *Mycoplasma* spp. are capable of adhering to and colonizing mucous membranes. Cell damage, including red blood cell damage, by *M. pneumoniae* may be caused by the H_2O_2 that it releases.

Drug resistance. Because they lack cell walls, mycoplasmas are unaffected by β-lactam antibiotics. (Recall the mechanism by which β-lactams kill bacteria: inhibition of cell wall synthesis.) Mycoplasmas are also unaffected by sulfonamides and trimethoprim because they do not synthesize folic acid. In general, mycoplasmas are susceptible to tetracyclines, aminoglycosides, and macrolides. *M. pneumoniae* is susceptible to newer fluoroquinolones, tetracyclines, and macrolides. *M. hominis* is resistant to erythromycin, rifampin, and azithromycin; some tetracycline-resistant strains have been reported. Tetracycline and doxycycline are effective against *M. genitalium*.

Clues to *Mycoplasma* spp. Identification

Colonial morphology. *Mycoplasma* spp. are facultative anaerobes. Growth of some species is enhanced by 5% to 10% CO_2. As previously mentioned, in vitro growth of mycoplasmas requires specially supplemented culture media. For example, sterols are supplied by adding serum to the media. Growth in vitro is relatively slow. *M. pneumoniae* and *M. genitalium* have generation times of 6 hours and 16 hours, respectively. On solid culture media, mycoplasmas form colonies that are often so small (15 to 600 μm in diameter) that they can only be seen by using a hand lens or low-power microscopic magnification. *M. hominis* is the only pathogenic human species that will grow on blood agar and chocolate agar, but the pinpoint translucent colonies are difficult to see. To alleviate doubt as to whether mycoplasmal colonies are present, methylene blue can be added to the agar surface. Mycoplasmal colonies will stain blue.

The colonies of some species of *Mycoplasma* (e.g., *M. hominis*) are referred to as **"fried egg" colonies,** because

> Associate fried-egg colonies with *Mycoplasma* spp.

they resemble sunny-side-up fried eggs. The colonies have an opaque granular center, which is surrounded by a flat translucent zone (Fig. 14-20). *M. pneumoniae* colonies are spherical and usually do not have the appearance of fried eggs.

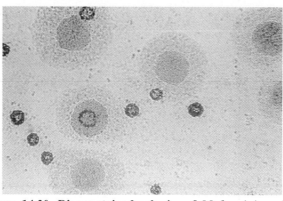

***Figure 14-20.* Dienes-stained colonies of *M. hominis* and *U. urealyticum* on Shepard's A7B differential agar.** The *M. hominis* colonies are larger, lighter in color, and have a fried egg morphology. The *U. urealyticum* colonies are smaller, darker, and more dense. (From Winn WC Jr, et al. Koneman's Color Atlas and Textbook of Diagnostic Microbiology. 6th Ed. Philadelphia: Lippincott Williams & Wilkins, 2006.)

Because of their small size, mycoplasmas usually do not produce turbidity in liquid media. A pH indicator (e.g., phenol red) is added to liquid media to detect growth (by acid production).

Laboratory tests. Immunological and molecular diagnostic procedures are available to diagnose mycoplasmal infections. Identification of mycoplasmas to species is usually accomplished in reference laboratories. Table 14-9 illustrates differences in metabolic patterns of the major *Mycoplasma* spp. and *Ureaplasma urealyticum*.

Essentials

Mycoplasma spp.

- Do not possess cell walls, causing them to be pleomorphic; they range from tiny coccoid cells (0.2 to 0.3 μm in diameter) to tapered rods (0.1 to 0.2 μm wide by 1.0 to 2.0 μm long)

- If they stain at all, they are Gram negative with the Gram staining technique

- They can be grown on artificial culture media, but they require complex enriched culture media

- On solid culture media, they form colonies that are often so small (15 to 600 μm in diameter) that they can only be seen by using a hand lens or low-power microscopic magnification

- Colonies of some species of *Mycoplasma* (e.g., *M. hominis*) are referred to as fried-egg colonies, because they resemble sunny-side-up fried eggs

Genus *Ureaplasma*

Clinical significance. *Ureaplasma urealyticum* is a common inhabitant of genitourinary mucous membranes. It can cause

TABLE 14 - 9	Metabolic Patterns of *Mycoplasma* spp. and *Ureaplasma urealyticum*		
Species	**Glucose**	**Arginine**	**Urea**
Mycoplasma pneumoniae	+	−	−
M. hominis	−	+	−
M. genitalium	+	−	−
Ureaplasma urealyticum	−	−	+

NGU, infertility, and reproductive failure, and is associated with bacterial vaginosis and pelvic inflammatory disease.

Drug resistance. *U. urealyticum* is unaffected by β-lactam antibiotics. Strains of *U. urealyticum* are usually susceptible to tetracycline and doxycycline, although some tetracycline-resistant strains have been reported.

Clues to *Ureaplasma* spp. Identification

Colonial morphology. *U. urealyticum* has a generation time of approximately 1 hour. Like *M. hominis*, it is more easily and rapidly isolated from clinical specimens than slower-growing mycoplasmas, such as *M. pneumoniae* and *M. genitalium*. Colonies are typically 15 to 60 μm in diameter, requiring magnification to be seen (see Figure 14-20).

Laboratory tests. Immunological and molecular diagnostic procedures are available to diagnose mycoplasmal infections. These are usually performed in reference laboratories. The primary characteristic that differentiates *Ureaplasma* spp. from *Mycoplasma* is its ability to hydrolyze urea, causing the release of ammonia (thus the genus name *Ureaplasma*).

MISCELLANEOUS GRAM-NEGATIVE BACILLI

The organisms described in this section do not fit neatly into any of the previously discussed categories of pathogenic Gram-negative bacilli. *Aeromonas* and *Plesiomonas* spp. are sometimes included in discussions of *Vibrio* spp. (see Chapter 15) because all are oxidase-positive fermenters and share other phenotypic similarities. However, *Vibrio* spp. are curved, whereas *Aeromonas* and *Plesiomonas* are not.

Genus *Aeromonas*

Clinical significance. *Aeromonas* spp. are found in a wide variety of freshwater ecosystems worldwide. The species associated with human infection are found in many foods, including produce, meat, and dairy products. Infection usually results from ingestion of contaminated food or water. *Aeromonas* gastroenteritis, most often caused by *A. caviae*, may be associated with diarrhea or dysentery, abdominal pain, fever, vomiting, and nausea. *A. veronii* biovar *sobria* may cause cholera-like disease, with abdominal pain, fever, and nausea. Severe infections, caused primarily by *A. hydrophila* or *A. veronii* biovar *sobria*, may include hemolytic uremic syndrome and other types of kidney disease. Wound infections, primarily caused by *A. hydrophila*, usually follow some type of traumatic injury that occurs in contact with water.

Virulence factors. *Aeromonas* spp. produce several virulence factors, including enterotoxins, hemolysins, proteases, peptidases, chondroitinase, and DNase.

Drug resistance. *Aeromonas* spp. generally are resistant to ampicillin but susceptible to ciprofloxacin, gentamicin, amikacin, tobramycin, imipenem, and trimethoprim-sulfamethoxazole.

Clues to *Aeromonas* spp. Identification

Cellular morphology. *Aeromonas* spp. are motile Gram-negative bacilli or coccobacilli, ranging from 0.3 to 1.0 μm wide and from 1.0 to 3.5 μm long (Fig. 14-21).

Colonial morphology. *Aeromonas* spp. are facultative anaerobes that grow well on culture media, including enteric media. Most clinically relevant species are hemolytic on blood agar. On modified cefsulodin-Irgasan-novobiocin (CIN) medium, *Aeromonas* colonies have a pink center and an uneven, clear apron (indistinguishable from *Yersinia enterocolitica* colonies). *Aeromonas* colonies are green on xylose-galactosidase medium. Other selective and differential media are also available for isolation of *Aeromonas* spp.

Laboratory tests. *Aeromonas* spp. are oxidase, catalase, nitrate, and indole positive. They ferment various sugars, either with or without gas production. Tests of value in differentiating *Aeromonas* species from each other are Voges-Proskauer, lysine and ornithine decarboxylase, arginine

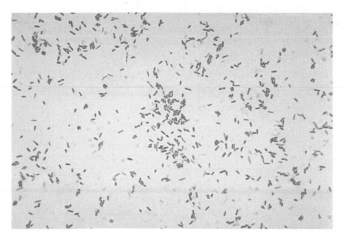

Figure 14-21. **Gram-stained *Aeromonas hydrophila* cells.** (Courtesy of W. A. Clark and the CDC.)

dihydrolase, carbohydrate fermentations and gas production, esculin hydrolysis, and cephalothin susceptibility.

Plesiomonas shigelloides

Plesiomonas shigelloides is presently classified in the Enterobacteriaceae family, but unlike other members of that family, it is oxidase positive. Thus, it seems likely that *P. shigelloides* will someday be removed from the family.

Clinical significance. *P. shigelloides* is associated with diarrheal disease and is only rarely isolated from clinical specimens. Symptoms may include diarrhea (which may either be watery or bloody), abdominal pain, dehydration, fever, and rarely, septicemia.

Virulence factors. *P. shigelloides* produces an enterotoxin, and evidence suggests that it is also able to invade and multiply within human gastrointestinal cells.

Clues to *P. shigelloides* Identification

Cellular morphology. Morphologically, *P. shigelloides* cannot be differentiated from other Gram-negative bacilli.

Colonial morphology. On blood agar, *P. shigelloides* colonies are opaque, convex, and 2 to 3 mm in diameter. On enteric plating media, colonies are typical for non–lactose and non–sucrose fermenters. On CIN medium, *P. shigelloides* colonies are opaque, and lack a pink center. (CIN, sometimes referred to as *Yersinia* selective agar, is discussed in Chapter 12. On CIN, *Y. enterocolitica* and *Aeromonas* colonies have a pink center and an opaque apron.)

Laboratory tests. Commercial biochemical systems are available for identification of *P. shigelloides* . Key test results include positive lysine, arginine, and ornithine reactions.

Genus *Brucella*

Clinical significance. *Brucella* spp. cause disease (brucellosis) in humans and a wide variety of animals. Four species

cause human brucellosis: *B. abortus*, *B. melitensis*, *B. suis*, and *B. canis*. Brucellosis is considered a zoonosis. Transmission to humans occurs via direct contact through abraded skin or mucous membranes, consumption of contaminated food products, or inhalation. Brucellosis is a worldwide health problem. Although it was once a common disease in the United States, only 120 new U.S. cases were reported to the Centers for Disease Control and Prevention in 2005. *Brucella* spp. are potential bioterrorism and biological warfare agents.

> *Brucella* spp. are potential bioterrorism and biological warfare agents and are dangerous to work with in the laboratory.

Brucellosis is associated with granulomas or abscesses in the bone marrow, liver, spleen, lymph nodes, and lungs. Other possible sites of infection include subcutaneous tissue, testes, ovary, gallbladder, kidneys, and brain. Meningitis and endocarditis may also occur.

Brucellosis is a common laboratory-acquired infection. Great care must be taken when working with *Brucella* spp. in the laboratory. All work must be performed within a biosafety cabinet. Avoid producing aerosols, and never sniff the plates.

Virulence factors. *Brucella* spp. are facultative intracellular pathogens. Although they are phagocytized by neutrophils, they resist destruction within the phagocytes.

Clues to *Brucella* spp. Identification

Cellular morphology. *Brucella* spp. are very small, nonmotile Gram-negative coccobacilli, 0.5 to 0.7 μm wide and 0.6 to 1.5 μm long (Fig. 14-22). They may be seen singly (predominantly), or in pairs, short chains, or small clusters.

Colonial morphology. *Brucella* spp. are aerobic and nonhemolytic. CO_2 incubation is required for *in vitro* growth of some strains. Their optimal growth temperature is 37°C.

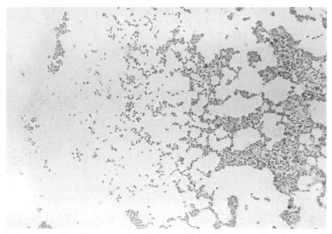

Figure 14-22. **Gram-stained *Brucella melitensis* cells.** (Courtesy of the CDC.)

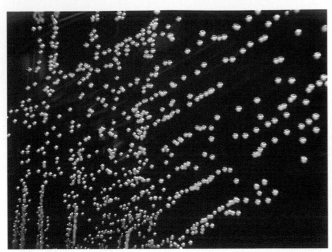

Figure 14-23. **Pinpoint, smooth, entire, translucent, non-hemolytic colonies of *Brucella melitensis* at 48 hours of incubation.** (Courtesy of Larry Stauffer, Oregon State Public Health Laboratory, and the CDC.)

Brucella spp. have a slower growth rate than most bacteria. Although most strains require complex growth media and growth is improved by the presence of serum or blood in the media, *Brucella* spp. are not considered to be nutritionally fastidious. They will grow on or in a wide range of media, including trypticase soy agar (with or without 5% sheep blood) and chocolate agar as well as brucella blood, brain heart infusion, and heart infusion agars; aerobic blood culture bottles; and biphasic bottles. Biphasic bottles, also known as Castenada bottles, contain both liquid and solid media. When growth occurs, colonies on blood agar are 0.5 to 1.0 mm in diameter, nonhemolytic, raised, and convex, with an entire edge and a smooth (usually) shiny surface (Fig. 14-23). *B. canis* does not produce smooth colonies. *Brucella* colonies rarely exceed 1 mm in diameter. Growth on MAC is variable.

Laboratory tests. Immunodiagnostic procedures are available. *Brucella* spp. are nitrate, oxidase, urease, and catalase positive. They are indole negative. Demonstration of CO_2 requirement and H_2S production are of some value in species identification. Cellular fatty acid and molecular *Brucella* identification procedures are available for use in reference laboratories.

SAFETY TIP

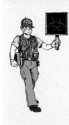

CLSI-Recommended Safety Precautions. CLSI Document M29-A3 recommends BSL-2 practices for activities with clinical specimens of human or animal origin containing or potentially containing pathogenic Brucella *spp. BSL-3 and Animal BSL-3 practices, containment equipment, and facilities are recommended for all manipulations of cultures of pathogenic* Brucella *spp.*

Essentials

Brucella spp.

- Very small, nonmotile Gram-negative coccobacilli, 0.5 to 0.7 μm wide and 0.6 to 1.5 μm long; may be seen singly (predominantly), or in pairs, short chains, or small clusters

- Cause brucellosis in humans and animals

- Potential bioterrorism and biological warfare agents; very dangerous to work with in the laboratory

- Nitrate, oxidase, urease, and catalase-positive; indole-negative

Streptobacillus moniliformis

Clinical significance. There is only one species in the genus *Streptobacillus*: *S. moniliformis*. It is found in the nasopharynx of rodents and some other animals. Most human infections result from rodent bites or the bites of animals (e.g., cats) that prey on rodents. Laboratory workers who handle rats and mice are at risk of infection. When acquired by bite, the infection is called rat bite fever. (Rat bite fever may also be caused by *Spirillum minus*, which is described in Chapter 15.) Infection may also result from ingestion of contaminated food or water. When acquired by food or water consumption, the disease is called Haverhill fever. In addition to fever, symptoms include headache, chills, myalgias, and arthralgias (joint pain), followed by development of a rash. Complications include endocarditis, myocarditis, pericarditis, meningitis, and pneumonia. *S. moniliformis* is susceptible to many antimicrobial agents. Penicillin and doxycycline are the drugs of choice.

> *Streptobacillus moniliformis is one of the causes of rat bite fever.*

 CAUTION

Do Not Confuse Rat Bite Fever with Cat Scratch Disease. Both *Streptobacillus moniliformis* and *Spirillum minus* cause infections called rat bite fever, which, as the name implies, are associated with rodent bites. The primary cause of cat scratch disease is *Bartonella henselae*, but *Bartonella clarridgeiae* and *Afipia felis* are occasional causes of this disease. All these organisms are described in this chapter, except *S. minus*, which is described in Chapter 15.

Clues to *S. moniliformis* Identification

Cellular morphology. *S. moniliformis* is a nonmotile, pleomorphic Gram-negative bacillus, usually 0.3 to 0.5 μm wide by 1.0 to 5.0 μm long. In older cultures, Gram-variable filaments as long as 100 to 150 μm may be observed, which contain granules, bulbs (central round enlargements; often in series, resembling a string of beads), and bands. Sometimes, chains and/or coccal forms can be seen. (The term *streptobacillus* means a chain of bacilli.)

Colonial morphology. *S. moniliformis* is a somewhat fastidious facultative anaerobe, preferring media containing blood or serum. Two types of colonies, referred to as eubacterial and L-phase colonies, may be observed in one culture. Eubacterial colonies (meaning "true" bacterial colonies) on blood agar are 1 to 3 mm in diameter, grayish, round, glistening, and smooth after 48 to 72 hours, when incubated in 5% to 10% CO_2 at 35°C to 37°C. L-phase colonies pit the agar and have a fried-egg appearance, with irregular outlines and coarse granular lipid globules.

(L-phase colonies are produced by cells, known as L-phase variants, with defective cell walls.) *S. moniliformis* grows well in blood cultures but is killed by a constituent of some blood culture systems, called sodium polyanetholesulfonate (SPS; Liquoid). Growth in liquid media occurs primarily as "puff balls" at the bottom of the tube. *S. moniliformis* does not grow on enteric media (selective and differential media used to isolate members of the family Enterobacteriaceae).

Laboratory tests. Biochemically, *S. moniliformis* is relatively inert. Sugar reactions are weak and delayed, without gas production. *S. moniliformis* is catalase, oxidase, indole, and nitrate negative. It can be identified using the API-ZYM system (bio-Méreiux Inc., http://www.biomereiux.com/) or by cellular fatty acid analysis.

Chapter Review

- HACEK stands for *Haemophilus*, *Actinobacillus*, *Cardiobacterium*, *Eikenella*, and *Kingella*. These organisms are grouped because they are fastidious indigenous microflora of the oral cavity that may cause a similar type of endocarditis.

- *Haemophilus* spp. are facultative anaerobes that are Gram negative, nonmotile, non–spore forming, and fastidious. They require one or both of the accessory growth factors called X factor (hemin) and V factor (nicotinamide adenine dinucleotide).

- Worldwide, *Haemophilus influenzae* is a major cause of bacterial meningitis. It is also a common cause of purulent bacterial conjunctivitis, otitis media, sinusitis, and lower respiratory tract infections. Although *H. influenzae* can cause respiratory disease, it does not cause influenza (flu), which is caused by viruses.

- *Pasteurella* spp. are widespread in the gingiva and nasopharynx of healthy and diseased animals. Most human infections are associated with dog and/or cat bites or scratches. *P. multocida* is the species most commonly isolated from human infections.

- Important *Actinobacillus* spp. associated with humans include *A. ureae*, *A. hominis*, and *A. actinomycetem-comitans*. Although considered Gram-negative bacilli, *Actinobacillus* spp. cells are short bacilli or coccoid and are arranged singly, in pairs, or in short chains.

- *Bartonella* spp. are the cause of trench fever, cat scratch disease, and other infectious diseases. They produce two types of colonies in culture.

- *Afipia* spp. are phenotypically similar to *Bartonella* spp. but are classified in a different family. *A. felis* is the most clinically significant species.

- The most important disease caused by *Bordetella* spp. is pertussis, or whooping cough, caused by *B. pertussis*. The organism produces various adhesins, which enable it to bind to host cells. Isolation of *B. pertussis* requires media (such as Bordet-Gengou or CHB) containing protective substances. On CHB, *B. pertussis* colonies may look like mercury droplets.

- *Capnocytophaga* spp. are indigenous microflora of humans, dogs, and cats. They are responsible for several diseases, most notably infections from dog and cat bite wounds.

- *Cardiobacterium hominis* is the only species in the genus *Cardiobacterium*. It causes the type of endocarditis typical of HACEK organisms.

- *Francisella tularensis* is the cause of tularemia, a severe and sometimes fatal disease. *Francisella* spp.

are associated with the outdoors, small mammals, and arthropods. In the United States, most patients acquire tularemia via tick or deerfly bites or contact with infected animals. Tularemia is also known as tick fever, deerfly fever, or rabbit fever. *F. tularensis* is highly infectious.

- Although not closely related, for several reasons, *Francisella* spp. and *Brucella* spp. are often linked together. On cysteine heart blood agar supplemented with chocolatized sheep blood, *F. tularensis* exhibits a prominent opalescent sheen resulting from H_2S production.

- *Legionella pneumophila* is the causative agent of Legionnaires disease (now called legionellosis). The organism causes respiratory infections. *Legionella* spp. are common in soil and water and can survive over a wide range of temperature. In the environment, *Legionella* spp. are commonly found in association with other microorganisms, forming biofilms.

- *Legionella* spp. are very small, motile, faintly staining Gram-negative bacilli. They are difficult to see in Gram-stained respiratory specimens. They are fastidious, slow-growing, obligate aerobes that do not grow on standard culture media. The primary isolation medium for *Legionella* spp. is BCYE agar. On that medium, *L. pneumophila* colonies are whitish green.

- *Mycoplasma* and *Ureaplasma* spp. do not possess cell walls. They are considered Gram negative. Mycoplasmas and ureaplasmas have a genome that is about one-fifth to one-half the genome size of most bacteria. They are the simplest and smallest free living, self-replicating procaryotes. They were once known as filterable agents. They require enriched culture media.

- Three species of *Mycoplasma* may cause human disease: *M. pneumoniae*, *M. hominis*, and *M. genitalium*.

- Some species of *Mycoplasma* (e.g., *M. hominis*) have colonies that look like sunny-side-up fried eggs.

- *Ureaplasma urealyticum* is a common inhabitant of the genitourinary mucous membranes, is a cause of infertility, and is associated with bacterial vaginosis and pelvic inflammatory disease.

- *Ureaplasma* spp. may be differentiated from *Mycoplasma* spp. by their ability to hydrolyze urea, with the subsequent release of ammonia.

- *Aeromonas* spp. associated with human infection are found in many foods, such as produce, meat, and dairy products. Infection usually results from ingestion of contaminated food or water. Selective and differential media are available for isolation of *Aeromonas* spp.

- Tests used to differentiate *Aeromonas* spp. from one another include Voges-Proskauer, lysine, ornithine decarboxylase, arginine dihydrolase, carbohydrate fermentations and gas production, esculin hydrolysis, and cephalothin susceptibility.

- *Brucella* spp. cause disease in humans and animals. Four species cause human brucellosis: *B. abortus, B. melitensis, B. suis,* and *B. canis. Brucella* spp. are facultative intracellular pathogens that are highly infectious.

- *Brucella* spp. are small, nonmotile, aerobic Gram-negative coccobacilli. They are slow growers, nonhemolytic, and require complex growth media. Growth is improved by the presence of serum or blood in the media.

- *Streptobacillus moniliformis* is found in the nasopharynx of rodents and other animals. Human infections result from the bites of rodents or animals that prey on rodents. It is a fastidious facultative anaerobe that grows best on media containing blood or serum. *S. moniliformis* produces two types of colonies known as eubacteria and L-phase colonies.

New Terms and Abbreviations

After studying Chapter 14, you should be familiar with the following terms, which are defined within the chapter and in the Glossary at the back of the book:

Biofilm

"Fried egg" colonies

V factor

X factor

References and Suggested Reading

Abbreviated Identification of Bacteria and Yeast: Approved Guideline. CLSI Document M35-A. Wayne, PA: Clinical and Laboratory Standards Institute, 2002.

Abbott SL. *Aeromonas*. In: Murray PR, Baron EJ, Jorgensen JH, Pfaller MA, Yolken RH, eds. Manual of Clinical Microbiology. 8th Ed. Washington, DC: ASM Press, 2003.

Chu MC, Weyant RS. *Francisella* and *Brucella*. In: Murray PR, Baron EJ, Jorgensen JH, Pfaller MA, Yolken RH, eds. Manual of Clinical Microbiology. 8th Ed. Washington, DC: ASM Press, 2003.

Dennis DT. Tularemia. In: Gorbach SL, Bartlett JG, Blacklow NR, eds. Infectious Disease. 3rd Ed. Philadelphia: Lippincott Williams & Wilkins, 2004.

Doern G. *Streptobacillus moniliformis*. In: Gorbach SL, Bartlett JG, Blacklow NR, eds. Infectious Disease. 3rd Ed. Philadelphia: Lippincott Williams & Wilkins, 2004.

Durbin WJ. *Bordetella*. In: Gorbach SL, Bartlett JG, Blacklow NR, eds. Infectious Disease. 3rd Ed. Philadelphia: Lippincott Williams & Wilkins, 2004.

Gotuzzo E, Carrillo C. *Brucella*. In: Gorbach SL, Bartlett JG, Blacklow NR, eds. Infectious Disease. 3rd Ed. Philadelphia: Lippincott Williams & Wilkins, 2004.

Huprikar SS, Bottone EJ. *Francisella tularensis*, *Pasteurella*, and *Yersinia pestis*. In: Gorbach SL, Bartlett JG, Blacklow NR, eds. Infectious Disease. 3rd Ed. Philadelphia: Lippincott Williams & Wilkins, 2004.

Kilian M. *Haemophilus*. In: Murray PR, Baron EJ, Jorgensen JH, Pfaller MA, Yolken RH, eds. Manual of Clinical Microbiology. 8th Ed. Washington, DC: ASM Press, 2003.

Loeffelholz MJ. *Bordetella*. In: Murray PR, Baron EJ, Jorgensen JH, Pfaller MA, Yolken RH, eds. Manual of Clinical Microbiology. 8th Ed. Washington, DC: ASM Press, 2003.

McCormack WM. Mycoplasmas and Ureaplasmas. In: Gorbach SL, Bartlett JG, Blacklow NR, eds. Infectious Disease. 3rd Ed. Philadelphia: Lippincott Williams & Wilkins, 2004.

Mietzner SM, Stout JE. *Legionella*. In: Gorbach SL, Bartlett JG, Blacklow NR, eds. Infectious Disease. 3rd Ed. Philadelphia: Lippincott Williams & Wilkins, 2004.

Murphy TF. *Haemophilus*. In: Gorbach SL, Bartlett JG, Blacklow NR, eds. Infectious Disease. 3rd Ed. Philadelphia: Lippincott Williams & Wilkins, 2004.

Nerad JL, Black S. Miscellaneous Gram-negative bacilli: *Acinetobacter, Cardiobacterium, Actinobacillus, Chromobacterium, Capnocytophaga*, and others. In: Gorbach SL, Bartlett JG, Blacklow NR, eds. Infectious Disease. 3rd Ed. Philadelphia: Lippincott Williams & Wilkins, 2004.

Protection of Laboratory Workers from Occupationally Acquired Infections: Approved Guideline. 3rd Ed. CLSI Document M29-A3. Wayne, PA: Clinical and Laboratory Standards Institute, 2005.

Salyers AA, Whitt DD. Bacterial Pathogenesis: A Molecular Approach. Washington, DC: ASM Press, 1994.

Stout JE, et al. *Legionella*. In: Murray PR, Baron EJ, Jorgensen JH, Pfaller MA, Yolken RH, eds. Manual of Clinical Microbiology. 8th Ed. Washington, DC: ASM Press, 2003.

Von Graevenitz A, et al. *Actinobacillus, Capnocytophaga, Eikenella, Kingella, Pasteurella*, and other fastidious or rarely encountered Gram-negative rods. In: Murray PR, Baron EJ, Jorgensen JH, Pfaller MA, Yolken RH, eds. Manual of Clinical Microbiology. 8th Ed. Washington, DC: ASM Press, 2003.

Waites KB, et al. Mycoplasma and Ureaplasma. In: Murray PR, Baron EJ, Jorgensen JH, Pfaller MA, Yolken RH, eds. Manual of Clinical Microbiology. 8th Ed. Washington, DC: ASM Press, 2003.

Welch DF, Slater LN. *Bartonella* and *Afipia*. In: Murray PR, Baron EJ, Jorgensen JH, Pfaller MA, Yolken RH, eds. Manual of Clinical Microbiology. 8th Ed. Washington, DC: ASM Press, 2003.

 On the CD-ROM

- Whooping Cough Update
- Biofilms
- Additional Self-Assessment Exercises
- Case Study
- Puzzle

Self-Assessment Exercises

1. Which of the following tests or characteristics would differentiate *Ureaplasma* spp. from *Mycoplasma* spp.?

   A. Indole

   B. Hydrolysis of ALA porphyrin

   C. Hydrolysis of urea

   D. None of the above

2. A clinical microbiology laboratory professional has isolated a small Gram-negative coccobacillus from a respiratory specimen. It is β-hemolytic on horse blood agar, nonmotile, and non–spore forming. Further testing indicates it requires both X and V factors. The most likely presumptive identification of this organism is

   A. *Haemophilus influenzae.*

   B. *H. aegyptius.*

   C. *H. haemolyticus.*

   D. *H. ducreyi.*

3. The medium most frequently used to isolate *Haemophilus* spp. is

   A. buffered charcoal yeast extract agar.

   B. Bordet-Gengou.

   C. chocolate agar.

   D. sheep blood agar.

Match the items in the column on the left with the correct description or disease in the column on the right.

4. _____ *Haemophilus ducreyi*   A. A major cause of bacterial meningitis in children

5. _____ X factor   B. Associated with dog or cat bites/scratches

6. _____ *H. influenzae* type b   C. Infectious agent of chancroid

7. _____ *Pasteurella multocida*   D. Hemin

8. _____ *Bordetella pertussis*   E. Causes whooping cough

9. On charcoal horse blood medium (also known as Regan-Lowe medium), *B. pertussis* colonies appear

A. like molar teeth.

B. like crossed cigars or a four-to-six-point star.

C. buttery.

D. like mercury droplets or small pearls imbedded in the agar.

10. Briefly explain the phenomenon of satelliting. Include a description of the phenomenon and the organisms involved.

_____

_____

_____

_____

CHAPTER 15

Curved and Spiral-Shaped Bacilli

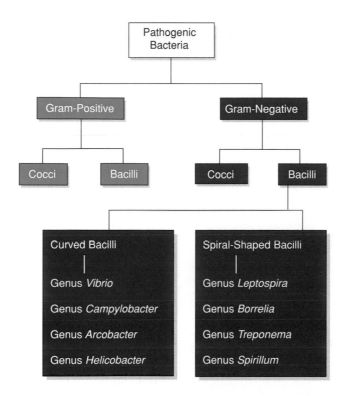

Chapter Outline

Curved Gram-Negative Bacilli
- Genus *Vibrio*
- Genus *Campylobacter*
- Genus *Arcobacter*
- Genus *Helicobacter*

Spirochetes
- Genus *Leptospira*
- Genus *Borrelia*
- Genus *Treponema*
- *Spirillum minus*

LEARNING OBJECTIVES

After studying this chapter, you should be able to:

☛ Define the terms introduced in this chapter (e.g., *chancre, endoflagella, erythema migrans*)

☛ Given a specific disease caused by a curved or spiral-shaped bacillus (e.g., leptospirosis, Lyme disease, relapsing fever), state the etiologic agent of that disease

☛ Outline the cellular morphology, colonial morphology, virulence factors, clinical significance, and laboratory tests used to identify each organism discussed in this chapter

☛ Name any selective or differential media used to isolate specific organisms discussed in the chapter

☛ Identify the organisms presented in this chapter that are associated with foodborne bacterial illnesses

☛ List the criteria for the presumptive identification of *Campylobacter* spp.

☛ Name the most appropriate specimen for the identification of each of the following: *Treponema pallidum* subsp. *pallidum, Borrelia burgdorferi, Vibrio cholerae, Campylobacter jejuni*

Cholera. Bacterial diarrhea. Septicemia. Ulcers. Leptospirosis. Lyme disease. Relapsing fever. Syphilis. Rat bite fever. These are some of the diseases caused by the curved and spiral-shaped bacilli described in this chapter.

Recall from Chapter 8 that bacteria are categorized into three general groups based on the shapes of their cells: (1) round or spherical bacteria, known as cocci; (2) rectangular or rod-shaped bacteria, known as bacilli; and (3) curved and spiral-shaped bacilli (sometimes referred to as spirilla). The third category, comprising the curved and spiral-shaped bacilli, is discussed in this chapter.

STUDY AID **Curved and Spiral-Shaped Bacilli.** Initially, the description "curved and spiral-shaped bacilli" is confusing to some people, because they associate the word "bacilli" with rod- or rectangular-shaped bacteria. However, bacilli can be straight, curved, or spiral-shaped. Organisms with straight rod-shaped cells are placed in the morphological category called bacilli. Organisms with cells that are always curved or spiral-shaped are placed in the morphological category known as the curved and spiral-shaped bacilli.

CURVED GRAM-NEGATIVE BACILLI

Genus *Vibrio*

Clinical significance. *Vibrio* spp. (vibrios) are common in saltwater environments, on and in marine animals, on plankton, and in seafood (shellfish, crabs, shrimp, and prawns). About a dozen vibrios are pathogenic for humans (Table 15-1).

The most significant of vibrio diseases, cholera, is usually acquired by drinking water contaminated with human feces or by eating food washed in contaminated water. Cholera is an acute diarrheal disease that can lead to massive fluid loss, dehydration, shock, and death. Patients produce watery stools containing whitish flecks, referred to as rice water stools. Cholera is considered one of the "great epidemic diseases." Cholera epidemics are frequently associated with natural disasters, such as hurricanes, tsunamis, and earthquakes.

> *Vibrio cholerae* is the cause of cholera, an important epidemic diarrheal disease.

Virulence factors. The primary virulence factors of *V. cholerae* are flagella, pili, and cholera toxin (an enterotoxin). *V. cholerae* also produces other adhesins and toxins. *V. parahaemolyticus* produces two types of hemolysins.

Drug resistance. Antibiotic resistance is relatively rare in vibrios compared with members of the family Enterobacteriaceae. Some strains are resistant to tetracycline (the drug of choice for treatment of cholera), ampicillin, chloramphenicol, trimethoprim, and other antimicrobial agents. Resistance patterns are useful in differentiating otherwise phenotypically similar *Vibrio* spp.

Clues to *Vibrio* spp. Identification

Cellular morphology. In general, vibrios are small (0.5 to 0.8 μm wide by 1.4 to 2.6 μm long), motile, straight, slightly curved, curved, or comma-shaped Gram-negative bacilli (Figs. 15-1 and 15-2). Some strains of *V. cholerae* O139 and *V. cholerae* non-O1, non-O139 produce a capsule, as do some strains of *V. vulnificus*.

> *V. cholerae* is a short, motile, oxidase-positive, comma-shaped Gram-negative bacillus.

Colonial morphology. Fecal specimens should be placed in Cary-Blair transport medium if a delay of more than a few

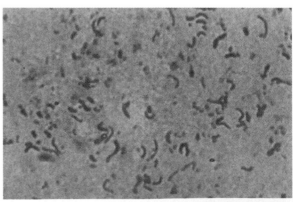

***Figure 15-1.* Gram stained appearance of *Vibrio vulnificus*.** (From Winn WC Jr, et al. Koneman's Color Atlas and Textbook of Diagnostic Microbiology. 6th Ed. Philadelphia: Lippincott Williams & Wilkins, 2006.)

TABLE 15 - 1   Human Diseases Caused by *Vibrio* spp.

Vibrio spp.	Disease(s)	Comments
V. cholerae O1; classified into 2 serotypes (Ogawa and Inaba) and 2 biotypes (classical and *eltor*)	Epidemic and pandemic cholera (mild-to-severe watery diarrhea, severe dehydration, electrolyte imbalance, nausea, vomiting, painful muscle cramps, shock, death)	The cause of many epidemics and millions of deaths; patients produce large volumes of "rice water stools" (nonbloody, clear fluid containing flecks of mucus)
V. cholerae O139	Epidemic and pandemic cholera	
V. cholerae non-O1, non-O139	Can cause sporadic, severe, watery diarrhea, but usually causes mild diarrhea, rare extraintestinal infections (septicemia, meningitis, wound infections)	
V. mimicus	Disease spectrum similar to *V. cholerae* non-O1, non-O139	Usually associated with consumption of contaminated seafood, particularly raw oysters
V. parahaemolyticus	Watery (sometimes bloody) diarrhea, nausea, vomiting, abdominal cramps, low-grade fever, chills; rarely fatal; may also cause septicemia and wound infections	Usually associated with consumption of contaminated fish or shellfish; a major cause of foodborne diarrheal illness in Japan; patients may produce either rice water stools or watery, blood-containing watery stools that are referred to as "washed meat" stools
V. fluvialis, V. furnissii, V. hollisae	Diarrhea	
V. vulnificus	Septicemia and wound infection; sometimes life threatening (*V. vulnificus* is the most common *Vibrio* sp. causing serious morbidity and mortality in the United States); rarely causes diarrhea	Septicemia usually follows consumption of contaminated raw oysters; wound infections are associated with trauma involving marine animals (e.g., cleaning fish, shelling crabs) or environments
V. damsela	Rare cause of wound infections and septicemia	
V. alginolyticus	Rare cause of wound and ear infections and septicemia	
V. metschnikovii, V. cincinnatiensis	Very rare causes of extraintestinal infections	
V. harveyi	Rare cause of wound infections	

hours between collection and processing is anticipated. The low nutrient content of Cary-Blair transport medium enhances the survival of enteric bacterial pathogens but prevents their replication. Cary-Blair medium contains sodium thioglycolate to maintain a low redox potential. Its high pH neutralizes acids produced during metabolism.

Vibrio spp. are facultative anaerobes. Most pathogenic vibrios grow well on routine culture media, such as blood agar and MacConkey agar (non–lactose fermenters), incubated at 37°C. Some strains (e.g., *V. cholerae* O1 and *V. cholerae* non-O1, non-O139) are β-hemolytic; some strains (e.g., *V. vulnificus* and others) are α-hemolytic; and some strains are non-hemolytic. In general, *Vibrio* spp. are halophilic (salt loving). The growth of most species (except *V. mimicus*) is stimulated by sodium ions (Na$^+$), with some species requiring sodium concentrations above the physiological level (0.85%). The

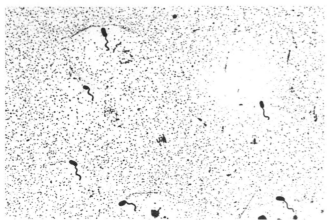

Figure 15-2. **Digitally colorized photomicrograph of** *Vibrio cholerae*, **stained with the Leifson flagella stain.** (Courtesy of Dr. William A. Clark and the Centers for Disease Control and Prevention [CDC].)

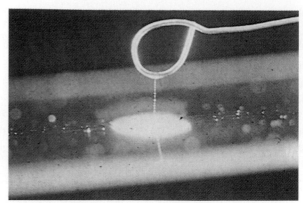

Figure 15-3. **Positive string test, which can be used to differentiate between** *V. cholerae* **(string test positive) and other** *Vibrio* **spp. (string test negative).** (From Winn WC Jr, et al. Koneman's Color Atlas and Textbook of Diagnostic Microbiology. 6th Ed. Philadelphia: Lippincott Williams & Wilkins, 2006.)

clinical microbiology laboratory should be alerted to the fact that the clinician suspects a *Vibrio* infection. Farmer et al. (see "References and Suggested Reading") have suggested comments similar to the following be added to the laboratory request slip: "*Vibrio* species suspected." "Patient ate raw oysters in New Orleans." "Patient cut foot while wading in brackish water."

Thiosulfate-citrate-bile salts-sucrose (TCBS) agar, which inhibits growth of most indigenous microflora, is a useful medium for isolation of *V. cholerae* and *V. parahaemolyticus* from stool specimens. Some *Vibrio* spp. produce smooth green colonies on TCBS agar, while others produce smooth yellow colonies (Table 15-2). Fecal specimens should also be inoculated into alkaline peptone water, which enriches growth of vibrios.

Laboratory tests. Most *Vibrio* spp. are oxidase and nitrate positive (*V. metschnikovii* is oxidase and nitrate negative). Immunodiagnostic and molecular diagnostic procedures are available for diagnosis of cholera. Commercial products are available for detection of cholera toxin. Once isolated, *Vibrio* spp. are identified using commercial identification systems. Antisera are available for identification of *V. cholerae* O1 and O139.

The string test can be used to differentiate between *Vibrio cholerae* (string test positive) and other *Vibrio* spp. (string test negative). To perform the string test, colonies from an 18- to 24-hour culture of the isolate are mixed into a drop of 0.5% sodium deoxycholate on a glass microscope slide. In a positive test, the bacterial cells are lysed by the sodium deoxycholate, and DNA is released from the cells, causing the mixture to become viscous. The tip of a wire inoculating loop is immersed into the mixture and slowly drawn away. In a positive test, a long, mucoid string will cling to the wire loop, as shown in Figure 15-3.

Essentials

Vibrio spp.

- Curved, motile, halophilic Gram-negative bacilli

- *Vibrio cholerae* causes cholera

- *Vibrio parahaemolyticus* causes diarrhea, septicemia, and wound infections

- *Vibrio vulnificus* causes septicemia and wound infections

TABLE 15 - 2	**Color of *Vibrio* Colonies on Thiosulfate-Citrate-Bile Salts-Sucrose (TCBS) Agar**
Species That Produce Green Colonies (Sucrose Negative)	**Species That Produce Yellow Colonies (Sucrose Positive)**
Vibrio mimicus, V. parahaemolyticus, V. hollisae, V. damsela, most strains of *V. vulnificus*	*Vibrio cholerae, V. alginolyticus, V. fluvialis, V. furnissii, V. harveyi, V. metschnikovii, V. cincinnatiensis,* some strains of *V. vulnificus*

- TCBS agar is useful for isolation of *Vibrio* spp.

- Oxidase positive

Genus *Campylobacter*

Clinical significance. Reservoirs of *Campylobacter* spp. (campylobacters) include cattle, sheep, pigs, poultry, and domestic pets. Human diseases caused by campylobacters are considered zoonoses (Table 15-3). Most diseases are associated with ingestion of contaminated food (primarily chickens and unpasteurized milk) or water. Allos (see "References and Suggested Reading") has stated that "*C. jejuni* and *C. coli* are the most common causes of foodborne bacterial illness in the United States and other industrialized nations."

> *Campylobacter* spp. cause most foodborne bacterial illnesses in the United States. Special precautions should be taken when preparing and eating chickens.

C. jejuni is the most common cause of sporadic bacterial enteritis in the United States, with some estimates as high as 2.5 million cases per year. (*Salmonella* and *Shigella* spp. combined account for fewer than 100,000 U.S. enteritis cases per year.) According to Nachamkin (see "References and Suggested Reading"), "*Campylobacter* species, including the common **thermophilic** (literally, "heat-loving") species *C. jejuni* and *C. coli*, should be sought in all diarrheic stools submitted to the laboratory for routine culture."

> *Campylobacter jejuni* is the most common cause of bacterial enteritis in the United States.

Virulence factors. Research studies have shown that enteric campylobacters first colonize the intestinal mucosa and then pass through the epithelial surface to underlying tissue. The pathogenic mechanisms by which this occurs are not yet understood, although motility and adherence are likely to be important virulence factors. Enterotoxins are not thought to play a role.

TABLE 15 - 3   Human Diseases Caused by *Campylobacter* spp.

Campylobacter spp.	Human Disease(s)
C. jejuni and *C. coli*	Both cause diarrheal illnesses that are clinically indistinguishable. (Many laboratories do not routinely distinguish these species.) Spectrum of illness ranging from asymptomatic to severely ill; may include fever and abdominal cramping; may mimic appendicitis. Extraintestinal infections include septicemia, hepatitis, pancreatitis, abortion and neonatal sepsis, hemolytic uremic syndrome, nephritis, prostatitis, urinary tract infection, peritonitis, myocarditis, meningitis, septic arthritis, and abscesses. Deaths caused by *C. jejuni* are rare but have been reported.
C. fetus subsp. *fetus*	Human infections are quite rare. Primarily causes extraintestinal infections, such as septicemia, septic abortion, neonatal infections, septic arthritis, abscesses, meningitis, cellulitis, urinary tract infections, endocarditis, septic thrombophlebitis, peritonitis, and salpingitis. Can also cause gastroenteritis. Causes abortion in cattle and sheep.
C. concisus	Periodontal infections, septicemia, foot ulcer, perhaps gastrointestinal infections.
C. curvus	May cause periodontal infections.
C. gracilis	Appendicitis, periodontitis, soft tissue abscesses, pulmonary infections.
C. hyointestinalis	Can cause diarrhea in humans. Causes enteritis in pigs.
C. lari	A rare cause of gastroenteritis, septicemia, and urinary tract infections.
C. mucosalis	Very rarely isolated from human specimens. Causes enteritis in lambs and pigs.
C. rectus	Periodontal infections.
C. sputorum	Abscesses.
C. upsaliensis	Human infections include gastroenteritis (watery diarrhea, abdominal cramps, low-grade fever) and septicemia. Causes acute diarrhea in dogs and cats.

Drug resistance. Erythromycin, azithromycin, and clarithromycin are the drugs of choice for treating gastrointestinal infections caused by *C. jejuni*, although ciprofloxacin or norfloxacin can be used for isolates susceptible to these drugs. Most isolates are resistant to cephalosporins and penicillins, and some strains are resistant to tetracycline, erythromycin, ciprofloxacin, and fluoroquinolones.

Clues to *Campylobacter* spp. Identification

Cellular morphology. Campylobacters are motile, curved, S-shaped, or spiral bacilli that are 0.2 to 0.9 μm wide by 0.5 to 5.0 μm long (Fig. 15-4). Following binary fission, but prior to separation from each other, a pair of curved *Campylobacter* cell rods resembles a bird in flight and is described as a "gull wing" morphology. Spherical organisms may be seen in old cultures or cultures that have been exposed to air for extended periods. Campylobacters stain weakly with safranin. Improved staining can be obtained when either carbol fuchsin or basic fuchsin is used as a counterstain. Stool specimens may or may not be bloody and fecal leukocytes may or may not be present.

> *Campylobacter* spp. are oxidase-positive, motile, slender, curved, S-shaped, or spiral bacilli. Remember the association between campylobacters and a gull wing morphology.

STUDY AID

The Significance of Fecal Leukocytes. Stained or unstained diarrheal specimens are often examined microscopically for the presence of fecal leukocytes. The presence of leukocytes in diarrheal specimens indicates an inflammatory type of diarrhea caused by invasive bacteria (e.g., enteroinvasive *Escherichia coli*, *Salmonella enteritidis*, *Shigella* spp.) or *Entamoeba histolytica* (a protozoan). Fecal leukocytes are often destroyed because of delays in transport and/or processing of the specimens. The presence of lactoferrin in diarrheal specimens is also indicative of an inflammatory type of diarrhea. The absence of leukocytes in diarrheal specimens indicates a secretory type of diarrhea, which may be caused by toxin-producing bacteria (e.g., *Bacillus cereus*, *Clostridium difficile*, enterotoxigenic *E. coli*, *V. cholerae*), viruses (e.g., Norwalk agent, rotavirus), or protozoa (e.g., *Giardia lamblia*).

Colonial morphology. Several types of enrichment broths are available to improve recovery of campylobacters from stool specimens. Campylobacters are generally microaerophilic (requiring 3% to 5% oxygen for growth), but some strains grow aerobically or anaerobically. The usual atmosphere used

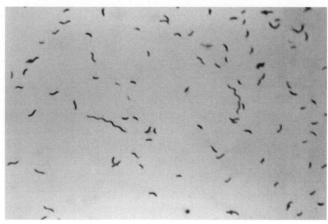

Figure 15-4. **Gram-stained *Campylobacter fetus* subsp. *fetus*, illustrating the appearance of *Campylobacter* cells.** (Courtesy of the CDC.)

to isolate campylobacters (referred to as Campy gas) contains 5% O_2, 10% CO_2, and 85% N_2. Campy gas generator packs are commercially available. Candle extinction jars (see Chapter 11) do not produce an appropriate atmosphere (too much oxygen) and should not be used for *Campylobacter* isolation. Some *Campylobacter* spp. (*C. concisus*, *C. curvus*, *C. mucosalis*, *C. rectus*, *C. sputorum*, and some strains of *C. hyointestinalis*) require hydrogen for growth. Various selective media containing antimicrobial agents (referred to as Campy media) are available for isolation of *C. jejuni* and *C. coli*. Some of these media contain blood, whereas others contain charcoal. The antimicrobial agents in these media inhibit some *Campylobacter* spp. (e.g., *C. fetus*, *C. upsaliensis*). Some campylobacters are thermophilic (preferring 42°C), some are thermotolerant (surviving at 42°C but preferring 37°C), and some are not thermotolerant (unable to survive at 42°C).

Colonial morphology of campylobacters varies depending on the type of medium being used. In general, colonies are gray, flat, irregular, and spreading (especially along the streak line) on freshly prepared media. On media having a lower moisture content, colonies are round, convex, and glistening, with little spreading. Campylobacters are nonhemolytic. Most species will not grow on MacConkey agar.

Laboratory tests. All *Campylobacter* spp. are oxidase positive, most species are nitrate positive, and most species are urease negative.

An organism can be presumptively identified as a *Campylobacter* sp. if it fulfills the following criteria:

- Growth on Campy medium, incubated at 42°C under microaerophilic conditions

- Characteristic colonial morphology (gray, mucoid, or wet colonies on Campy medium)

- Characteristic cellular morphology (curved to S-shaped Gram-negative bacilli, often having a gull wing morphology)

TABLE 15 - 4	Observations and Test Results of Value in Identifying Some *Campylobacter* spp.
***Campylobacter* spp.**	**Observations and Test Results**
C. jejuni	Growth on Campy media at 42°C but not at 25°C; oxidase, catalase, and nitrate positive; urease negative; most strains hippurate hydrolysis positive; cephalothin resistant; nalidixic acid variable
C. coli	Growth on Campy media at 42°C but not at 25°C; oxidase, catalase, and nitrate positive, urease negative; hippurate hydrolysis negative; cephalothin resistant; nalidixic acid variable
C. lari	Growth on Campy media at 42°C but not at 25°C; oxidase, catalase, and nitrate positive; urease variable; hippurate hydrolysis negative; cephalothin resistant; nalidixic acid resistant
C. upsaliensis	Growth on Campy media variable at 42°C; no growth at 25°C; oxidase and nitrate positive; catalase and urease negative; hippurate hydrolysis negative; cephalothin variable; nalidixic acid susceptible
C. fetus subsp. *fetus*	Growth on Campy media at 25°C; growth variable at 42°C; oxidase, catalase, and nitrate positive; urease negative; hippurate hydrolysis negative; cephalothin susceptible; nalidixic acid variable

- Motile

- Oxidase and catalase positive

According to Nachamkin (see "References and Suggested Reading"), "Oxidase-positive, curved Gram-negative rods that are hippurate hydrolysis positive should be reported as *C. jejuni* without further workup." Observations and test results of value in identifying some *Campylobacter* spp. are shown in Table 15-4.

Essentials

Campylobacter spp.

- Curved, motile, Gram-negative bacilli

- Gull wing morphology is often observed

- Diseases caused by *Campylobacter* spp. are considered zoonoses

- *Campylobacter* spp. are common causes of foodborne illnesses

- *C. jejuni* is the most common cause of bacterial diarrhea in the United States

- Microaerophilic and capnophilic

- Isolate using Campy agar and Campy gas at 42°C

- Oxidase positive

Genus *Arcobacter*

Clinical significance. Two *Arcobacter* spp., *A. cryaerophilus* and *A. butzleri*, may cause human disease. They were formerly classified as *Campylobacter* spp. *A. cryaerophilus* has been isolated from cattle, pigs, and sewage. Although rarely, the bacterium also has been isolated from human blood and fecal specimens. *A. butzleri* has been isolated from nonhuman primates and from fecal specimens of children with diarrhea. Some of the children also had abdominal pain, nausea, fever, chills, vomiting, and malaise. It is not known how these organisms are transmitted to humans.

Clues to *Arcobacter* spp. Identification

Cellular morphology. *Arcobacter* spp. are motile Gram-negative bacilli that may be slightly curved (*A. butzleri*), curved, S-shaped, or helical (*A. cryaerophilus*). They range in size from 0.2 to 0.9 μm wide and 1.0 to 3.0 μm long.

Colonial morphology. The ideal culture methods for *Arcobacter* spp. have yet to be determined. They have been isolated on semisolid media used to isolate *Leptospira* spp. and on Campy-CVA. They may grow aerobically at 30°C and anaerobically at 35° to 37°C. Whereas 42°C is the primary incubation temperature for recovering most campylobacters, *Arcobacter* spp. are not thermophilic and, thus, cannot be recovered at 42°C. They do not require increased hydrogen for growth, and most strains are nonhemolytic. Their colonial morphology resembles that of campylobacters. Their growth on MacConkey agar is variable.

TABLE 15 - 5 Human Infections Caused by *Helicobacter* spp.

Helicobacter spp.	Disease(s)
H. pylori	Acute gastritis (abdominal pain, nausea, vomiting), peptic and duodenal ulcers, gastric malignancy
H. heilmannii	Acute and chronic gastritis, perhaps gastric malignancy
H. fennelliae	Diarrhea, fever, bacteremia in immunosuppressed patients
H. cinaedi	Diarrhea, fever, bacteremia in immunosuppressed patients

Laboratory tests. *Arcobacter* spp. are phenotypically similar to, and difficult to differentiate from, campylobacters. (Note: Infections caused by the remaining bacteria in this chapter are usually diagnosed by nonculture methods, even though culture of most of them is possible.)

Genus *Helicobacter*

Clinical significance. More than 20 species of *Helicobacter* are found in the gastrointestinal and hepatobiliary tracts of mammals (including humans) and birds. Some of the human infections caused by *Helicobacter* spp. are shown in Table 15-5. With the exception of *H. pylori* infections, other *Helicobacter* infections are relatively uncommon. *H. pylori* is a common cause of gastritis, peptic ulcers, and gastric malignancy. Transmission of *Helicobacter* spp. is thought to occur via the fecal-oral (e.g., fecal contamination of drinking water) and oral-oral routes (e.g., kissing). Zoonotic transmission from cats and dogs to humans may also occur.

> Remember the association between *Helicobacter pylori* and ulcers.

Virulence factors. *H. pylori* produces urease, which converts urea to ammonia (alkaline) and CO_2. The ammonia neutralizes gastric acids in the immediate vicinity of the bacteria, serving to protect them long enough to invade the mucous lining of the stomach. Flagella and adhesins enable the bacteria to gain access to and bind to mucosal cells. *H. pylori* resides within mucinous crypts.

Drug resistance. *Helicobacter* infection is usually treated using a combination of clarithromycin and either amoxicillin or metronidazole, and either a proton pump inhibitor or a ranitidine-bismuth combination (the latter drugs reduce acid production in the stomach). Resistance to clarithromycin and metronidazole has been reported.

Clues to *Helicobacter* spp. Identification

Cellular morphology. *Helicobacter* spp. are motile, curved or spiral-shaped, weakly staining Gram-negative bacilli, ranging from 0.3 to 1.0 μm wide by 1.5 to 10.0 μm long.

They are easier to see when carbol fuchsin, rather than safranin, is used as the counterstain. *H. pylori* is a curved or straight bacillus in smears prepared from colonies, but appears helical or more curved in stained tissue biopsy specimens (Fig. 15-5). In biopsy specimens, *H. heilmannii* is larger and more helical than *H. pylori*.

Colonial morphology. *Helicobacter* spp. are microaerophilic. Stomach biopsy specimens should be transported to the clinical microbiology laboratory in transport media (e.g., brucella broth with 20% glycerol) and then plated immediately onto solid agar containing blood or serum. Blood-supplemented brain heart infusion, brucella, Columbia, and Skirrow's agar have been used successfully to grow *H. pylori*. Inoculated plates should be incubated at 37°C in a humid, microaerophilic

> *H. pylori* is microaerophilic, capnophilic, and oxidase, catalase, and urease positive.

(2% to 7% O_2), 5% to 10% CO_2 atmosphere. Hydrogen concentrations of 5% to 8% improve recovery. Plates may require 5 to 7 days of incubation before colonies are apparent.

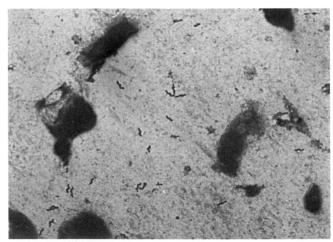

Figure 15-5. Gram-stained stomach biopsy. The Gram-negative, curved-to-spiral-shaped bacilli are suggestive of *Helicobacter pylori*. (From Marler LM, Siders JA, Allen SD. Direct Smear Atlas. Philadelphia: Lippincott Williams & Wilkins, 2001.)

Selective enriched media are available for isolation of the enterohepatic helicobacters (*H. cinaedi, H. fennelliae*). On solid culture media, *H. pylori* produces discrete, gray, translucent colonies, whereas the enterohepatic helicobacters tend to swarm, producing a thin film (*H. cinaedi, H. fennelliae*) or a thick, mucoid film. *H. pylori is* rarely isolated from blood and fecal specimens, but enterohepatic helicobacters can be isolated from such specimens.

Laboratory tests. The presence of *Helicobacter* in stomach biopsy specimens can be determined using a rapid urease test or by histological examination. The rapid urease test is performed by placing the biopsy specimen in an agar gel or onto a paper strip containing urea and a pH indicator. Production of ammonia raises the pH and causes a color change. Urea breath testing can also be performed, using ^{13}C or ^{14}C radioisotopes. The patient swallows a solution containing isotopically labeled urea. Isotopically labeled CO_2 in the patient's breath is then measured, using mass spectrometry, infrared spectroscopy, or scintillation particle-counting instruments. Immunodiagnostic procedures are available for detection of *H. pylori* antigen in fecal specimens and anti–*H. pylori* antibodies in serum. Helicobacters are oxidase positive. Most species (including *H. pylori*) are catalase positive. Gastric helicobacters are urease positive, whereas enterohepatic helicobacters are urease negative. Thus, *H. pylori* is oxidase, catalase, and urease positive.

Essentials

Helicobacter spp.

- Curved, motile Gram-negative bacilli

- *H. pylori* is a common cause of gastritis, peptic ulcers, and gastric malignancy

- Microaerophilic and capnophilic

- Oxidase positive

- *H. pylori* is urease positive

SPIROCHETES

Spirochetes are spiral-shaped bacteria. They may either be loosely coiled, such as *Borrelia* spp., or tightly coiled, such as *Leptospira*, *Treponema*, and *Spirillum* spp.

Genus *Leptospira*

Clinical significance. There are at least 12 species of *Leptospira*, with *L. interrogans* being the primary cause of leptospirosis (a zoonosis) in humans. *L. interrogans* has more than 200 serotypes (called serovars). Leptospiras cause renal infection in many types of animals (e.g., rodents, dogs, domestic farm animals). Humans usually become infected by direct or indirect contact with urine from an infected animal. Waterborne transmission has been reported (i.e., contact with water that has been contaminated with animal urine). Leptospirosis is an occupational hazard for people who have direct contact with animals (e.g., livestock farmers, veterinarians, slaughterhouse workers) or contact with the urine of an infected animal (e.g., sewer workers, septic tank cleaners, people working in rice or sugarcane fields). The usual portal of entry is through an abrasion or cut in the skin or via the conjunctiva.

Most cases of leptospirosis are subclinical or very mild, but patients may develop chills; fever; headache; myalgias; back, joint, and abdominal pain; watery eyes; stiff neck; and aseptic meningitis. The icteric or bile-related form of the disease, known as Weil disease, is associated with jaundice (yellow pigmenting of the skin and eyes), acute renal failure, pulmonary hemorrhage, and cardiac arrhythmias. Weil disease has a 5% to 15% mortality rate. A 1999 World Health Organization report indicated that leptospirosis is presumed to be the most widespread zoonosis in the world.

> Associate Weil disease with *Leptospira interrogans*.

Drug resistance. Penicillin and doxycycline are the drugs of choice to treat leptospirosis. Resistance to vancomycin and some aminoglycosides has been reported.

Clues to *Leptospira* spp. Identification

Cellular morphology. *Leptospira* spp. are flexible, tightly coiled spirochetes, approximately 0.1 μm wide (very thin) by 6 to 20 μm long, with pointed ends (Figs. 15-6 and 15-7). *Leptospira* cells possess a distinct hook at one or both ends, often making them look like a shepherd's crook (Fig. 15-8). Cells are motile as a result of two axial filaments (endoflagella, described later in the chapter); the cells may move rapidly back and forth or may spin rapidly around their long

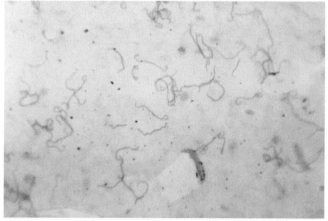

Figure 15-6. **Leptospirosis.** Liver smear stained by a silver staining technique, from a patient with a fatal case of leptospirosis. (Courtesy of Dr. Martin Hicklin and the CDC.)

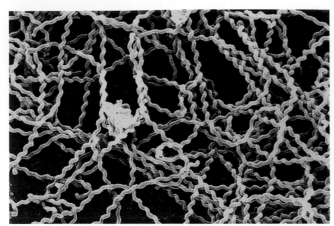

Figure 15-7. Scanning electron micrograph of a *Leptospira* sp. from culture. (Courtesy of Rob Weyant, Janice Carr, and the CDC.)

axis. *Leptospira* cells may be observed in clinical materials (e.g., blood, urine, cerebrospinal fluid, peritoneal dialysate fluid) by darkfield microscopy. Unless coated with tissue stains, the cells are too thin to be seen using a brightfield microscope.

In vitro growth. *L. interrogans* is an obligate aerobe, with an optimum growth temperature of 28°C to 30°C. It may be isolated from blood, cerebrospinal fluid, urine, or peritoneal dialysate fluids, which can be inoculated directly into a tube of semisolid agar media or a blood culture bottle at the

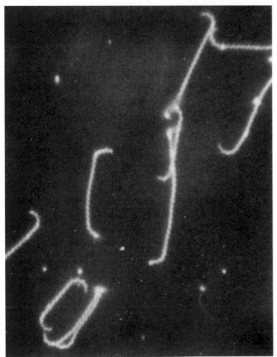

Figure 15-8. Darkfield photomicrograph of *Leptosira interrogans*. The cells possess a distinct hook at one or both ends, often making them look like a shepherd's crook. (From Volk WA, et al. Essentials of Medical Microbiology. 5th Ed. Philadelphia: Lippincott-Raven, 1996.)

patient's bedside. The preferred medium is Ellinghausen-McCullough-Johnson-Harris medium or PLM-5 medium, both of which contain 0.1% agar, oleic acid, albumin, and 5-fluorouracil. The inoculated medium should be kept sealed in the dark and incubated at 28°C to 30°C. Growth often appears as a discrete band, known as a Dinger's ring, several millimeters below the surface of the medium. Cultures are incubated for up to 13 weeks before being discarded and are examined at least weekly by darkfield microscopy.

Laboratory tests. *L. interrogans* may be identified by immunological or molecular diagnostic procedures performed in regional or national reference labs. In the microagglutination test, anti–*L. interrogans* antibodies are detected by reacting the patient's serum with a suspension of live or killed *L. interrogans*. Following incubation, the serum-antigen mixture is examined microscopically for agglutination. The microagglutination test is complicated, time consuming, and hazardous when live organisms are used.

Genus *Borrelia*

Borrelia spp. (borreliae) are highly motile spirochetes. Their flagella (referred to as endoflagella) lie between the cell membrane and an outer membrane of the cell, unlike the flagella of other motile bacteria (referred to as exoflagella), which protrude from the surface of the cell. The endoflagella connect to both ends of the cell, resulting in both corkscrew and oscillating movements of the cell. In the laboratory, borreliae grow only under microaerophilic or anaerobic conditions. There are many *Borrelia* spp., occurring in arthropods, rodents, cattle, horses, sheep, deer, fowl, and humans.

> The hard ticks (genus *Ixodes*) that transmit Lyme disease also transmit human granulocytic ehrlichiosis (see Chapter 16) and babesiosis (see Chapter 22).

Clinical significance. Human diseases caused by *Borrelia* spp. are shown in Table 15-6.

STUDY AID **Etiologic Agent Versus Vector.** If 100 randomly selected people were asked the question, "What is the cause of Lyme disease?" most would probably answer "Ticks." Not so fast! Although ticks are the arthropod vectors that transmit the bacterium that causes Lyme disease, it is the bacterium (*Borrelia burgdorferi*) that actually causes the disease. Thus, the answer to the question is *Borrelia burgdorferi*.

Lyme disease (Lyme borreliosis), caused by *Borrelia burgdorferi*, is similar to syphilis in that there are three stages of disease: (1) an early localized stage, (2) an early disseminated stage, and (3) late-stage manifestations. In stage 1, most patients develop a characteristic rash known as

TABLE 15 - 6   Human Diseases Caused by *Borrelia* spp.

Borrelia spp.	Disease	Arthropod Vector	Animal Reservoir(s)
B. burgdorferi, B. garinii, B. afzelii, and other species	Lyme disease (Lyme borreliosis)	Hard ticks	Rodents
B. recurrentis	Louseborne relapsing fever	Human body lice	Humans
B. duttonii	Tickborne relapsing fever	Soft ticks	Humans
B. hermsii, B. turicatae, B. parkeri, B. mazzottii, B. venezuelensis	American tickborne relapsing fever	Soft ticks	Rodents
Other *Borrelia* species	Tickborne relapsing fever in countries other than North and South America	Soft ticks	Rodents

erythema migrans (or erythema chronicum migrans). The center of the expanding lesion often fades to produce a bull's eye appearance (Fig. 15-9). Patients may experience low-grade fever, malaise, myalgia, stiff neck, and headache. Stage 2 follows hematogenous (via the bloodstream) dissemination of the spirochetes to various organs and tissues. Patients may feel quite ill and may experience fatigue, headache, fever, malaise, arthralgia, myalgia, and multiple secondary areas of erythema. Neurologic and cardiac involvement may also occur. The most common manifestations of stage 3 are arthritis, skin discolorations, and central nervous symptoms.

> Lyme disease is the most common vectorborne infectious disease in North America.

STUDY AID **What's in a Name?** Lyme disease or Lyme borreliosis was named for Old Lyme, Connecticut, where a small group of *Borrelia*-infected arthritis patients (12 children) were living. Although the disease was originally called Lyme arthritis, the name was changed when it was learned that organs such as the heart and nervous system could also be involved.

Relapsing fever, caused by other *Borrelia* spp., is another arthropod-borne zoonosis. It may be transmitted either by body lice (louse-borne relapsing fever, also known as epidemic relapsing fever) or ticks (tickborne relapsing fever, also known as endemic or sporadic relapsing fever). Relapsing fever is characterized by a rapid onset of symptoms, which include high fever, shaking chills, severe headache, nausea, myalgias, and severe malaise. Relapses

are common (hence the name relapsing fever), and untreated cases may be fatal.

Drug resistance. Antimicrobial therapy for Lyme disease depends on the stage of disease. Stage 1 disease is usually treated with doxycycline, amoxicillin, or cefuroxime. Disseminated infections require intravenous injections of ceftriaxone, cefotaxime, or high-dose penicillin G. Lyme arthritis is usually treated with doxycycline, intravenous cephalosporins, or penicillin G. *B. burgdorferi* is resistant to trimethoprim, sulfamethoxazole, rifampin, aminoglycosides, and quinolones. Tetracycline and erythromycin are used to treat relapsing fever.

Clues to *Borrelia* spp. Identification

Cellular morphology. *Borrelia burgdorferi* is a loosely coiled spirochete, ranging from 0.18 to 0.25 μm wide and

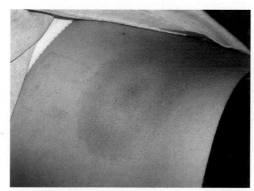

Figure 15-9. **Expanding bull's eye lesion of Lyme disease, technically known as erythema migrans.** (From Goodheart HP. Goodheart's Photoguide of Common Skin Disorders, 2nd Ed. Philadelphia: Lippincott Williams & Wilkins, 2003.)

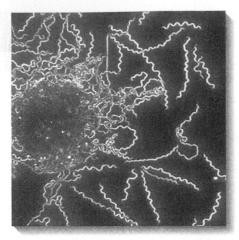

Figure 15-10. **Darkfield photomicrograph of *Borrelia burgdorferi*, from culture.** (From Strohl WA, et al. Lippincott's Illustrated Reviews: Microbiology. Philadelphia: Lippincott Williams & Wilkins, 2001.)

10 to 30 μm long (Figs. 15-10 and 15-11; see also Figs. 18-2 and 18-3). Although *B. burgdorferi* cells do stain a pale pink with the Gram stain, the cells are difficult to see using brightfield microscopy. However, the cells are easily seen using phase contrast or darkfield microscopy.

In vitro growth. The borreliae that cause relapsing fever and Lyme disease can be cultured in artificial media, but culturing is slow, time consuming, and usually performed only in reference and research laboratories. Modified Kelly medium is used, and inoculated tubes are incubated in the dark at 30°C to 33°C. *B. burgdorferi* has a generation time of 7 to 20 hours.

Laboratory tests. During febrile attacks in relapsing fever, many borreliae can be seen in a wet mount blood sample examined by darkfield or phase contrast microscopy, or a Wright- or Giemsa-stained blood smear examined by brightfield microscopy. In wet mounts, the spirochetes have a

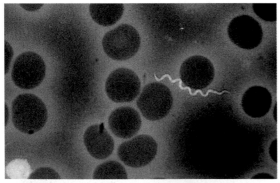

*Figure 15-11. **Borrelia* sp. in an acridine-orange–stained peripheral blood smear.** (From Winn WC Jr, et al. Koneman's Color Atlas and Textbook of Diagnostic Microbiology. 6th Ed. Philadelphia: Lippincott Williams & Wilkins, 2006.)

characteristic rotational motility. The thin and faintly stained spirochetes are difficult to see in stained blood smears. Spirochetes are rarely observed in the blood of Lyme disease patients. Immunodiagnostic procedures for detection of anti-*Borrelia* antibodies in blood are the primary ways in which Lyme disease is diagnosed. Molecular diagnostic and animal (rat, mouse, hamster) inoculation procedures (performed in reference laboratories) are also available for diagnosis of Lyme disease.

Essentials

Borrelia spp.

- Loosely coiled motile spirochetes
- *B. burgdorferi* causes Lyme disease, a tickborne zoonosis
- Lyme disease is the most common vectorborne infectious disease in North America
- Lyme disease is diagnosed using immunodiagnostic procedures
- *B. recurrentis* causes louseborne relapsing fever
- Relapsing fever is diagnosed by observation of the spirochetes in peripheral blood

Genus *Treponema*

Clinical significance. The genus *Treponema* comprises four invasive human species (Table 15-7), including *T. pallidum* subsp. *pallidum*, the cause of syphilis (Table 15-8). In addition, oral treponemes (probably nonpathologic) are found in gingival crevices, some nonpathogenic species live on skin, and other species (perhaps pathogenic) can be found in the gastrointestinal tract.

> Syphilis is caused by a spirochete named *Treponema pallidum* subsp. *pallidum*.

Virulence factors. *T. pallidum* is able to coat itself with host proteins, which may protect it from host immune responses in early stages of infection. *T. pallidum* is capable of attaching to endothelial cells (which line blood vessels) and passing through blood vessels. It can also pass through the placenta, resulting in congenital syphilis.

Drug resistance. Although penicillin has been used to treat syphilis since the introduction of the antibiotic in the 1940s, *T. pallidum* remains universally susceptible to penicillin and other β-lactam drugs.

Clues to *Treponema* spp. Identification

Cellular morphology. The pathogenic treponemes are extremely thin (about 0.18 μm), tightly coiled spirochetes

TABLE 15 - 7 Diseases Caused by *Treponema* spp.

Treponema spp.	Disease	Geographic Location
T. pallidum subsp. *pallidum*	Venereal syphilis (usually referred to simply as syphilis; see Table 15-8 for additional information)	Worldwide
T. pallidum subsp. *pertenue*	Yaws (cutaneous lesions, malaise, fever, lymphadenopathy, bone and joint lesions)	Tropical regions, Africa, South America, Caribbean, Indonesia
T. pallidum subsp. *endemicum*	Endemic syphilis (also known as bejel); oropharyngeal and cutaneous lesions, lymphadenopathy; skin, bone, and cartilage lesions	Arid regions, Africa, Middle East
T. carateum	Pinta (skin lesions, lymphadenopathy)	Semiarid warm regions, Central America, South America

that range in length from 6 to 20 μm (Fig. 15-12). They can be seen using darkfield and phase contrast microscopes (Fig. 15-13) but are too thin to be seen using brightfield microscopes. They possess endoflagella. When observed in fresh preparations, these spirochetes have a characteristic corkscrew motility (rapid rotation around the long axis), which has been described as "spinning their wheels but not going anywhere." They also flex in the center of the cell, resembling a swimmer doing the sidestroke. The pathogenic treponemes cannot be differentiated from one another by their microscopic appearance, including their electron microscopic appearance.

In vitro growth. The pathogenic treponemes are extremely fastidious and will not grow on artificial culture media. For research purposes and as a source of antigens for immunodiagnostic procedures, *T. pallidum* subsp. *pallidum* can be propagated in the testicles of live rabbits (Fig. 15-14).

> *Treponema* spp. will not grow on artificial culture media.

TABLE 15 - 8 Stages of Untreated Syphilis

Stage	When It Occurs	Manifestations
Primary syphilis	14 to 21 days following inoculation of *T. pallidum* subsp. *pallidum* into a dermal or mucous membrane site	Red painless papule that progresses into a painless ulcerated area called a chancre; most commonly found in genital, perineal, anal, or oral areas
Secondary syphilis (disseminated syphilis)	Follows hematogenous dissemination of treponemes from chancre, 4 to 10 weeks after the onset of primary syphilis	Red or reddish brown papules on the trunk and extremities, including the palms of the hands and soles of the feet; other symptoms may include lymphadenitis, malaise, sore throat, headache, weight loss, low-grade fever, muscle aches
Latent syphilis	3 to 12 weeks after the onset of secondary syphilis	Disappearance of lesions and other symptoms
Tertiary syphilis	2 to 20 years after the onset of latent syphilis	Painful granulomas (called gummata) in skin, soft tissue, bones, cartilage, liver, and testes; cardiovascular and central nervous system abnormalities

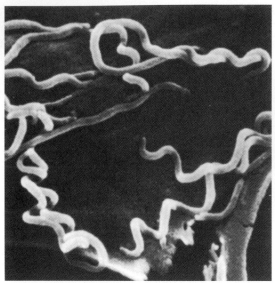

Figure 15-12. **Scanning electron micrograph of *Treponema pallidum*, from cell culture.** (From Volk WA, et al. Essentials of Medical Microbiology. 5th Ed. Philadelphia: Lippincott-Raven, 1996.)

Laboratory tests. Diagnosis of primary syphilis is accomplished by darkfield microscopic examination of freshly acquired material (containing live spirochetes) obtained from a chancre. Morphologically, *T. pallidum* subsp. *pallidum* cannot be distinguished from other human tre-

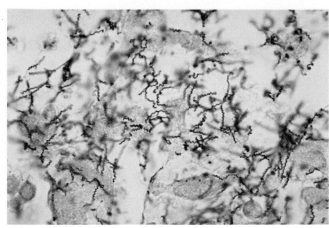

Figure 15-14. T. pallidum **in experimentally infected rabbit tissue, stained using modified Steiner silver stain.** (Courtesy of Dr. Edwin P. Ewing Jr. and the CDC.)

ponemes, but it can be recognized by its characteristic motility (described earlier). Direct fluorescent antibody tests can be used to detect *T. pallidum* in tissues and material obtained from primary or secondary lesions. Molecular diagnostic procedures are being developed. Various serologic tests are available to diagnose syphilis (see Chapter 18).

Essentials

Treponema spp.

- Tightly coiled, motile, extremely thin spirochetes
- *Treponema* spp. cause syphilis, yaws, and pinta
- *T. pallidum* subsp. *pallidum* causes syphilis
- *T. pallidum* does not grow on artificial media
- Primary syphilis is characterized by painless chancres at the sites of entry of the pathogen
- Primary syphilis is diagnosed by observation of the spirochetes using darkfield microscopy
- Immunodiagnostic procedures are used to diagnose secondary and tertiary syphilis

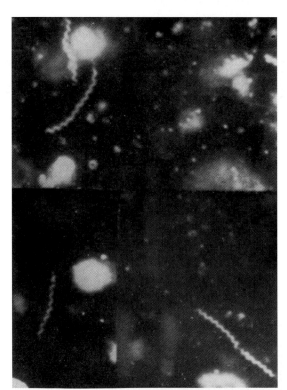

Figure 15-13. **Darkfield photomicrographs of *T. pallidum.*** (From Volk WA, et al. Essentials of Medical Microbiology. 5th Ed. Philadelphia: Lippincott-Raven, 1996.)

Spirillum minus

Clinical significance. Rat bite fever, most often caused by *Streptobacillus moniliformis* (see Chapter 14), is also caused by *Spirillum minus*, primarily in Asia. Infection is characterized by fever, chills, headache,

> **Rat bite fever may be caused by *Streptobacillus moniliformis* or *Spirillum minus*.**

lymphadenitis, and a blotchy rash. Endocarditis is a possible complication. *S. minus* infections are treatable with intramuscular injections of procaine penicillin G.

Clues to *S. minus* Identification

Cellular morphology. *S. minus* is a short, thick, tightly coiled spirochete with external flagella. Cells are 0.2 to 0.5 μm wide by 3 to 5 μm long and possess two to six spirals.

In vitro growth. *S. minus* cannot be cultured in or on artificial media.

Laboratory tests. *S. minus* may be observed by darkfield microscopy of exudates from skin lesions, lymph node aspirates, or less often, of blood. They may also be observed in Wright- or Giemsa-stained blood specimens. Immunodiagnostic and molecular diagnostic procedures are not available. However, antibodies produced against *S. minus* can cause false-positive results in immunodiagnostic tests for syphilis.

Chapter Review

- *Vibrio* spp. are common in saltwater environments, on and in marine animals, and in seafood. The most significant vibrio-related disease is cholera, which is usually acquired by ingesting contaminated drinking water or food. *V. cholerae* is a short, motile, oxidase-positive, comma-shaped Gram-negative bacillus.

- Human diseases caused by *Campylobacter* spp. are considered zoonoses. Reservoirs of *Campylobacter* spp. include cattle, sheep, pigs, poultry, and domestic pets. *Campylobacter* spp. are the most common causes of foodborne bacterial illness in the United States. *C. jejuni* is the most common cause of bacterial enteritis in the United States.

- Campylobacters are curved, S-shaped, or spiral bacilli that are motile. Isolation of campylobacters from fecal specimens requires a special medium (Campy medium), a special 2 to 7% O_2 atmosphere (Campy gas), and incubation at 42°C.

- *Helicobacter* spp. are found in the gastrointestinal and hepatobiliary tracts of mammals (including humans) and birds. *H. pylori* is a common cause of gastritis, peptic ulcers, and gastric malignancy.

- *H. pylori* is a straight bacillus in smears prepared from colonies, but is helical or curved in stained tissue specimens.

- Spirochetes are spiral-shaped bacteria and include *Borrelia*, *Leptospira*, *Treponema*, and *Spirillum* spp.

- *Leptospira interrogans* causes the zoonosis leptospirosis in humans. The icteric or bile-related form of leptospirosis is known as Weil's disease.

- Leptospiras are tightly coiled spirochetes with a hook at one or both ends. Like *Treponema* spp., they are too thin to be seen with a brightfield microscope. They can be seen using a darkfield microscope.

- *Borrelia burgdorferi* is the etiologic agent of Lyme disease, a zoonosis. It is transmitted by hard ticks (genus *Ixodes*). Lyme disease patients generally exhibit characteristic bull's eye or target lesions.

- *B. burgdorferi* is a loosely coiled spirochete that can easily be seen using phase contrast or darkfield microscopy. In Gram-stained smears, *B. burgdorferi* cells appear as very thin, faint pink, loosely coiled spirochetes.

- *Borrelia recurrentis* is an etiologic agent of relapsing fever.

- Syphilis is caused by the spirochete *Treponema pallidum* subsp. *pallidum*.

- Untreated syphilis goes through three stages—primary, secondary, and tertiary—with a latent stage occurring between stages 2 and 3.

- Treponemes are tightly coiled spirochetes that can be observed using darkfield and phase contrast microscopy. They possess endoflagella.

- Syphilis may be diagnosed by darkfield microscopic examination of fresh material from a chancre.

New Terms and Abbreviations

After studying Chapter 15, you should be familiar with the following terms, which are defined within the chapter and in the Glossary at the back of the book:

Chancre

Endoflagella

Erythema migrans

Jaundice

Thermophilic

References and Suggested Reading

Allos BM. *Campylobacter* infections. In: Gorbach SL, Bartlett JG, Blacklow NR, eds. Infectious Disease. 3rd Ed. Philadelphia: Lippincott Williams & Wilkins, 2004.

Allos BM. Campylobacters. In: Gorbach SL, Bartlett JG, Blacklow NR, eds. Infectious Disease. 3rd Ed. Philadelphia: Lippincott Williams & Wilkins, 2004.

Butler T. *Borrelia* species and *Spirillum minus*. In: Gorbach SL, Bartlett JG, Blacklow NR, eds. Infectious Disease. 3rd Ed. Philadelphia: Lippincott Williams & Wilkins, 2004.

Butler T. Relapsing fever. In: Gorbach SL, Bartlett JG, Blacklow NR, eds. Infectious Disease. 3rd Ed. Philadelphia: Lippincott Williams & Wilkins, 2004.

Dattwyler RJ, Wormser GP. Lyme disease. In: Gorbach SL, Bartlett JG, Blacklow NR, eds. Infectious Disease. 3rd Ed. Philadelphia: Lippincott Williams & Wilkins, 2004.

Farmer JJ III, et al. *Vibrio*. In: Murray PR, Baron EJ, Jorgensen JH, Pfaller MA, Yolken RH, eds. Manual of Clinical Microbiology. 8th Ed. Washington, DC: ASM Press, 2003.

Kelly PW. *Leptospira*. In: Gorbach SL, Bartlett JG, Blacklow NR, eds. Infectious Disease. 3rd Ed. Philadelphia: Lippincott Williams & Wilkins, 2004.

Kelly PW. Leptospirosis. In: Gorbach SL, Bartlett JG, Blacklow NR, eds. Infectious Disease. 3rd Ed. Philadelphia: Lippincott Williams & Wilkins, 2004.

Levett PN. *Leptospira* and *Leptonema*. In: Murray PR, Baron EJ, Jorgensen JH, Pfaller MA, Yolken RH, eds. Manual of Clinical Microbiology. 8th Ed. Washington, DC: ASM Press, 2003.

Musher DM, Baughn RE. Syphilis. In: Gorbach SL, Bartlett JG, Blacklow NR, eds. Infectious Disease. 3rd Ed. Philadelphia: Lippincott Williams & Wilkins, 2004.

Nachamkin I. *Campylobacter* and *Arcobacter*. In: Murray PR, Baron EJ, Jorgensen JH, Pfaller MA, Yolken RH, eds. Manual of Clinical Microbiology. 8th Ed. Washington, DC: ASM Press, 2003.

Nair GB, Sack DA. Vibrios. In: Gorbach SL, Bartlett JG, Blacklow NR, eds. Infectious Disease. 3rd Ed. Philadelphia: Lippincott Williams & Wilkins, 2004.

Norris SJ, et al. *Treponema* and other human host-associated spirochetes. In: Murray PR, Baron EJ, Jorgensen JH, Pfaller MA, Yolken RH, eds. Manual of Clinical Microbiology. 8th Ed. Washington, DC: ASM Press, 2003.

Parsonnet J. *Helicobacter*. In: Gorbach SL, Bartlett JG, Blacklow NR, eds. Infectious Disease. 3rd Ed. Philadelphia: Lippincott Williams & Wilkins, 2004.

Salyers AA, Whitt DD. Bacterial Pathogenesis: A Molecular Approach. Washington, DC, ASM Press, 1994.

Versalovic J, Fox JG. *Helicobacter*. In: Murray PR, Baron EJ, Jorgensen JH, Pfaller MA, Yolken RH, eds. Manual of Clinical Microbiology. 8th Ed. Washington, DC: ASM Press, 2003.

Wilske B, Schriefer ME. *Borrelia*. In: Murray PR, Baron EJ, Jorgensen JH, Pfaller MA, Yolken RH, eds. Manual of Clinical Microbiology. 8th Ed. Washington, DC: ASM Press, 2003.

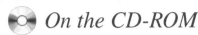 *On the CD-ROM*

- Additional Self-Assessment Exercises
- Case Study
- Puzzle

Self-Assessment Exercises

Match the items in the column on the left with the correct description or disease in the column on the right.

1. _____ reaginic antibodies

   A. Nontreponemal assay

2. _____ *Spirillum minus*

   B. The most common causes of foodborne bacterial illness in the United States

3. _____ *Vibrio parahaemolyticus*

   C. Associated with peptic ulcers

4. _____ *Campylobacter* spp.

   D. The major cause of foodborne diarrheal illness in Japan

5. _____ *Helicobacter pylori*

   E. Rat bite fever

6. True or false: "Rice water stools" are associated with *Vibrio cholerae* O1

7. True or false: Treponemes can be visualized using brightfield microscopy.

8. TCBS agar is useful for cultivating which of the following organisms?

   A. *Campylobacter* spp.

   B. *Helicobacter* spp.

   C. *Treponema* spp.

   D. *Vibrio* spp.

9. Which of the following tests could be used to differentiate between *H. pylori* and *C. jejuni*?

   A. Oxidase test

   B. Catalase test

   C. Urease test

   D. Nitrate test

10. List 4 criteria that may be used to presumptively identify an isolate as a *Campylobacter*. Include growth requirements, colonial morphology, cellular morphology, and select test results.

    A. _____

    B. _____

    C. _____

    D. _____

CHAPTER 16

Obligate Intracellular Bacteria

Chapter Outline

Genera *Chlamydia* and *Chlamydophila*

Genera *Rickettsia* and *Orientia*

Genera *Ehrlichia* and *Anaplasma*

Coxiella burnetii

☛ Name three arthropod vectors responsible for transmitting rickettsias

☛ Relate the following for *Coxiella burnetii:* cellular morphology, isolation requirements, mode of transmission to humans, biohazard risk, disease or diseases caused by the organism, and laboratory tests

LEARNING OBJECTIVES

After studying this chapter, you should be able to:

☛ Define the terms introduced in this chapter (e.g., *elementary body, intraerythrocytic pathogen, intraleukocytic pathogen*)

☛ Given a specific infectious disease, state the obligate intracellular pathogen that causes the disease

☛ Outline the cellular morphology, in vitro growth, virulence factors, clinical significance, and laboratory tests used to identify each organism described in this chapter

☛ Name any selective or differential media used to isolate specific organisms discussed in this chapter

☛ Differentiate *facultative* intracellular pathogens from *obligate* intracellular pathogens

☛ Given information about cellular morphology and laboratory test results, identify the organisms discussed in this chapter

☛ Describe the biphasic growth cycle of *Chlamydia* spp.

☛ List the human diseases caused by *Chlamydia* and *Chlamydophila* spp., *Rickettsia* spp., *Ehrlichia* spp., and *Coxiella burnetii*

☛ State how rickettsias are different from other bacteria in terms of cellular morphology, growth requirements, and laboratory tests

The terms *facultative* and *obligate intracellular pathogens* were introduced in Chapter 2. Recall that facultative intracellular pathogens are capable of both an intracellular and extracellular existence. Many facultative intracellular pathogens, but not all, can be grown in the clinical microbiology laboratory (CML) on artificial culture media. Facultative intracellular pathogens discussed in earlier chapters include *Mycobacterium tuberculosis*, *M. leprae*, *Listeria monocytogenes*, *Afipia felis*, *Francisella tularensis*, *Legionella* spp., and *Brucella* spp.

Obligate intracellular pathogens *must* live within host cells to survive and multiply. In the CML, they can be propagated in embryonated chicken eggs, laboratory animals, or cell cultures, depending on the particular pathogen. They *cannot* be grown on artificial media. Obligate intracellular bacterial pathogens discussed in this chapter include *Chlamydia*, *Chlamydophila*, *Rickettsia*, *Orientia*, *Ehrlichia*, *Anaplasma*, and *Coxiella* spp., all of which are considered to be Gram-negative bacteria.

GENERA *CHLAMYDIA* AND *CHLAMYDOPHILA*

Chlamydia and *Chlamydophila* spp., collectively referred to as chlamydiae in this chapter, have a unique developmental cycle that includes **elementary bodies (EBs)** and **reticulate bodies (RBs)** (Fig. 16-1). EBs are metabolically inactive and infectious, whereas RBs are metabolically active and noninfectious. EBs can survive in extracellular environments, whereas RBs cannot. The developmental

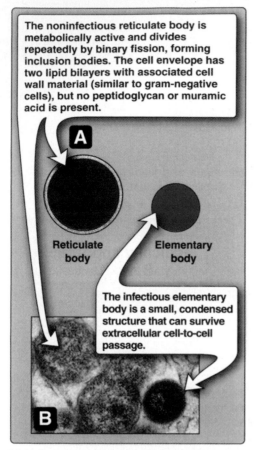

> The noninfectious reticulate body is metabolically active and divides repeatedly by binary fission, forming inclusion bodies. The cell envelope has two lipid bilayers with associated cell wall material (similar to gram-negative cells), but no peptidoglycan or muramic acid is present.

A

Reticulate body

Elementary body

> The infectious elementary body is a small, condensed structure that can survive extracellular cell-to-cell passage.

B

Figure 16-1. **Structural features of chlamydiae. A.** Schematic drawing. **B.** Transmission electron micrograph. (From Strohl WA et al. Lippincott's Illustrated Review: Microbiology. Philadelphia: Lippincott Williams & Wilkins, 2001.)

cycle of chlamydiae consists of five steps (illustrated in Fig. 16-2):

Step 1: An EB attaches to and is phagocytized by a host cell (both phagocytic and nonphagocytic cells can serve as host cells); different species and serotypes of chlamydiae invade different types of cells, such as conjunctival epithelial cells or cells of the respiratory or genital tract.

Step 2: Within a cytoplasmic vacuole, referred to as a phagosome or endosome, the EB reorganizes into an RB. This occurs 6 to 8 hours following phagocytosis of the EB.

Step 3: The RB initiates nucleic acid synthesis and divides repeatedly by binary fission. This occurs about 18 to 24 hours after phagocytosis of the EB.

Step 4: RBs then reorganize into EBs. The RB- or EB-filled vacuole is referred to as an intracytoplasmic inclusion or intracytoplasmic inclusion body (Fig. 16-3).

Step 5: At some time between 48 and 72 hours after phagocytosis of the original EB, the host cell ruptures, releasing the infectious EBs. The EBs can then infect neighboring cells.

Although they produce adenosine triphosphate (ATP) molecules, *Chlamydia* and *Chlamydophila* spp. preferentially use ATP molecules produced by host cells. This has earned them the title of "energy parasites."

> Serotypes of a given species differ from each other because of differences in their surface molecules (surface antigens). Sometimes, as is true for *Chlamydia trachomatis*, different serotypes of a given species cause different diseases.

Clinical significance. Human chlamydial diseases are shown in Table 16-1.

> Genital infection caused by *Chlamydia trachomatis* is the most common nationally notifiable infectious disease in the United States.

STUDY AID — **The Specific Epithet** *pneumoniae.* *Chlamydophila pneumoniae* is the fourth organism discussed in this book having the specific epithet *pneumoniae*. (The other three are *Streptococcus pneumoniae, Klebsiella pneumoniae,* and *Mycoplasma pneumoniae*.) It should come as no surprise that all organisms having the specific epithet *pneumoniae* cause pneumonia, although these organisms cause other diseases as well.

Drug resistance. Chlamydiae are susceptible to azithromycin, tetracyclines, macrolides, and fluoroquinolones. Aminoglycosides and cephalosporins are not effective.

Clues to *Chlamydia* and *Chlamydophila* spp. Identification

In vitro growth. Special antibiotic-containing chlamydial transport medium is available for transport of clinical specimens, which should be kept cold and transported rapidly. Frozen specimens are acceptable. Specimens should be processed immediately in the CML. Chlamydiae, especially *C. psittaci*, have been frequent causes of laboratory-acquired infections; appropriate safety precautions must be exercised when handling specimens and cultures. Although embryonated chicken eggs once were the primary method of propagating chlamydiae, cell cultures are now the primary method in CMLs. Different cell lines are used for different

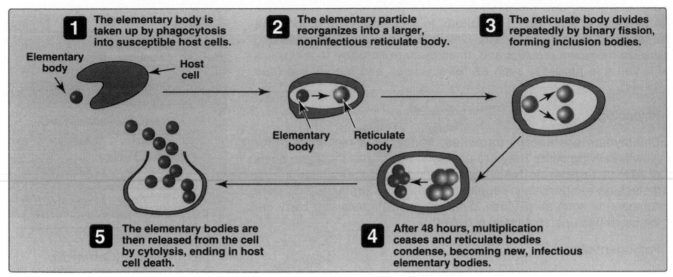

Figure 16-2. **Developmental cycle of chlamydiae.** (From Strohl WA et al. Lippincott's Illustrated Review: Microbiology. Philadelphia: Lippincott Williams & Wilkins, 2001.)

species. (Additional information about cell lines can be found on the CD-ROM.) Various stains (e.g., immunofluorescence, iodine, Giemsa stain) are available for demonstrating intracytoplasmic inclusion bodies in the inoculated cell cultures (Fig. 16-4).

Laboratory tests. In addition to culture techniques, cytological, serological, and immunodiagnostic and molecular diagnostic procedures are available for diagnosis of chlamydial infections, primarily *C. trachomatis* infections. Cytological examination reveals intracytoplasmic inclusions in clinical specimens obtained from patients with conjunctival, urethral, and cervical infections (see Fig. 16-3). Molecular diagnostic procedures include both nucleic acid hybridization and nucleic acid amplification methods.

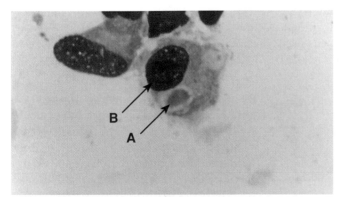

Figure 16-3. **Giemsa-stained chlamydial inclusion in cell scraping from a case of neonatal conjunctivitis. A.** Intracytoplasmic inclusion. **B.** Cell nucleus. (From McClatchy KD, ed. Clinical Laboratory Medicine. 2nd Ed. Philadelphia: Lippincott Williams & Wilkins, 2002.)

Essentials

Chlamydia and *Chlamydophila* spp.

- Obligate intracellular pathogens that produce intracytoplasmic inclusion bodies

- Biphasic developmental cycle that includes elementary bodies and reticulate bodies

- Elementary bodies are metabolically inactive and infectious

- Reticulate bodies are metabolically active and noninfectious

- Chlamydiae are considered energy parasites

- Different serotypes of *Chlamydia trachomatis* cause different diseases, including trachoma, inclusion conjunctivitis, nongonococcal urethritis, and lymphogranuloma venereum

- *Chlamydophila pneumoniae* causes respiratory diseases, including pneumonia

- *Chlamydophila psittaci* causes psittacosis, a respiratory disease

GENERA *RICKETTSIA* AND *ORIENTIA*

The genus *Rickettsia* was named for Howard T. Ricketts, a U.S. pathologist who discovered the etiologic agent and mode of transmission of "spotted fever." *Rickettsia* spp. have no connection to the disease called rickets, which is the result of a vitamin D deficiency.

TABLE 16 - 1 Human Chlamydial Diseases

Species	Disease	Comments
Chlamydia trachomatis (different serotypes [also referred to as serovars or biovars] of *C. trachomatis* cause different diseases)	Trachoma (an eye disease)	Trachoma is the most common preventable cause of blindness in the world; usually spread from child to child; flies can serve as mechanical vectors
	Nongonococcal urethritis in men and women; epididymitis in men; cervicitis, endometritis, and salpingitis in women; pneumonia in neonates	*C. trachomatis* is the most common sexually transmitted bacterial pathogen
	Inclusion conjunctivitis	
	Lymphogranuloma venereum	A sexually transmitted disease
Chlamydophila pneumoniae	Mild (often asymptomatic) pneumonia, pharyngitis, bronchitis; possible role in atherosclerosis (coronary artery disease) and stroke	
Chlamydophila psittaci	Psittacosis (a respiratory disease); also known as ornithosis	A zoonotic disease; contracted from exposure to infected avian species (e.g., psittacine birds [parrots, parakeets], turkeys); in 2005, only 16 new U.S. cases reported to the CDC

Rickettsias invade endothelial cells and vascular smooth muscle cells. They live within the cytoplasm of host cells. Rickettsias are capable of synthesizing proteins, nucleic acids, and ATP but are thought to require an intracellular environment because they possess an unusual membrane transport system. They are said to have "leaky" membranes.

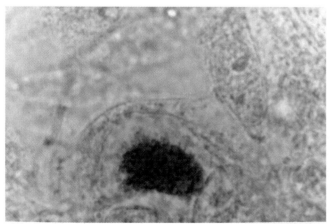

Figure 16-4. **Large, brown, iodine-stained *Chlamydia trachomatis* inclusion in McCoy cell culture.** (From McClatchy KD, ed. Clinical Laboratory Medicine. 2nd Ed. Philadelphia: Lippincott Williams & Wilkins, 2002.)

Clinical significance. Diseases caused by *Rickettsia* spp. (Table 16-2) include typhus and typhuslike diseases. All these diseases involve production of a rash. All diseases caused by *Rickettsia* species are arthropod-borne, meaning they are transmitted by arthropod vectors (carriers). Arthropods such as lice, fleas, ticks, and mites transmit the rickettsias from one host to another by their bites or waste products.

> *Rickettsia prowazekii*, the cause of Brill-Zinsser disease, epidemic typhus, and louseborne typhus, is a potential bioterrorism and biological warfare agent.

CAUTION **Beware of Similar-Sounding Terms.** Do not confuse the diseases typhus and typhoid fever. Both are systemic infections. Typical symptoms of **typhus** include severe headache, shivering and chills, high fever, malaise, and a rash. There are many forms of typhus, transmitted by a variety of arthropods (ticks, lice, fleas, larval mites). Most forms of typhus are caused by *Rickettsia* spp., but scrub typhus is caused by *Orientia tsutsugamushi*. **Typhoid fever** is

TABLE 16 - 2   Human Diseases Caused by *Rickettsia* spp.

Rickettsia spp.	Disease (Symptoms)	Geographic Region (Arthropod Vector)
R. rickettsii	Rocky Mountain spotted fever (fever, severe headache, malaise, myalgia, rash; sometimes nausea, vomiting, abdominal pain; coma; seizures; pulmonary edema; in severe cases, death)	Western Hemisphere (tick)
R. typhi	Murine typhus, endemic typhus, fleaborne typhus (cough, chest infiltrates; sometimes rash; seizures; coma; in severe cases, renal and respiratory failure)	Worldwide (flea; usually, rat flea)
R. prowazekii	Brill-Zinsser disease, epidemic typhus, louseborne typhus	Worldwide (human body louse)
R. akari	Rickettsial pox, disseminated rash, eschar at location of rickettsial inoculation	United States, eastern Europe, Korea (mite)
R. felis	Cat flea typhus	North and South America, Europe (cat flea)
R. conorii	Boutonneuse fever	Southern Europe, Africa, Middle East (tick)
Orientia tsutsugamushi (formerly *R. tsutsugamushi*)	Scrub typhus, miteborne typhus	Japan, eastern Asia, northern Australia, western and southwestern Pacific (larval mite, "chigger")

caused by *Salmonella typhi*. Symptoms of typhoid fever include continuously rising fever, septicemia, severe physical and mental depression, rose-colored spots on the chest and abdomen, abdominal swelling, and constipation. Transmission of typhoid fever is from person to person or by ingestion of fecally contaminated food or water.

Drug resistance. Doxycycline and other tetracyclines are the drugs of choice to treat infections caused by *Rickettsia* spp. and *Orientia tsutsugamushi*. Development of drug resistance in these organisms has not been a problem. Antimicrobial susceptibility testing of these organisms is not routinely performed.

> *Rickettsia rickettsii* is the cause of Rocky Mountain spotted fever (RMSF).

Clues to *Rickettsia* spp. Identification

Cellular morphology. *Rickettsia* spp. are small (0.3 to 0.5 μm wide by 1.0 to 2.0 μm long), rod-shaped or coccobacillary, weakly staining Gram-negative bacilli, with cell walls that contain lipopolysaccharide (LPS) and peptidoglycan. The cells are surrounded by a polysaccharide slime layer. *Orientia tsutsugamushi* cells have similar dimensions, but their cells walls lack LPS and peptidoglycan, they are not surrounded by a slime layer, and they do not possess flagella or pili.

In vitro growth. Because they are obligate intracellular pathogens, *Rickettsia* and *Orientia* spp. will not grow on artificial media. *Rickettsia* spp. grow well in cell cultures and embryonated chicken eggs. Cell cultures are primarily used in reference and research laboratories. *O. tsutsugamushi* is isolated by inoculating mice intraperitoneally. *Rickettsia* and *Orientia* spp. are highly infectious and all work must be performed in class II biosafety cabinets. Because of the dangers, culture techniques are performed in reference and research laboratories but not in hospital laboratories.

Laboratory tests. Several immunodiagnostic procedures are available for detecting *Rickettsia* spp. in clinical specimens, and molecular diagnostic procedures are being developed. Once isolated in cell cultures, *Rickettsia* spp. are identified primarily using immunological methods, although some reference laboratories are using molecular methods.

An older technique, known as the Weil-Felix test, used three strains of *Proteus vulgaris* bacteria as antigens to detect antirickettsial antibodies in serum. The test was based on cross-reactions between antirickettsial antibodies and *Proteus* antigens. Because the Weil-Felix test lacks sensitivity and specificity, it has been replaced in most CMLs by newer methods (e.g., an indirect immunofluorescence assay). Additional information about the Weil-Felix test is on the CD-ROM.

Essentials

Rickettsia/Orientia spp.

- Obligate intracellular Gram-negative bacilli, with leaky membranes

- Diseases caused by *Rickettsia* spp. are arthropod-borne

- *Rickettsia* spp. cause typhus and similar diseases, all of which produce a rash

- *R. rickettsii* is the cause of Rocky Mountain spotted fever

- *Orientia tsutsugamushi* is the cause of scrub typhus

GENERA *EHRLICHIA* AND *ANAPLASMA*

Clinical significance. *Ehrlichia* spp. and *Anaplasma phagocytophilum* are obligate intracellular Gram-negative bacteria. They invade various bone marrow–derived cells.[1] *Ehrlichia* spp. predominantly infect leukocytes of humans and other mammals; they are **intraleukocytic pathogens.**[2] *Ehrlichia chaffeensis* lives within human monocytes, and causes human monocytotrophic ehrlichiosis (HME), a tick-borne disease.

Anaplasma spp. infect various bone marrow–derived cells in humans, horses, cattle, sheep, goats, and dogs. *Anaplasma phagocytophilum* lives within human granulocytes, causing the tickborne disease human anaplasmosis (previously known as human granulocytic ehrlichiosis or HGE, and still often referred to as such). Details of HME and human anaplasmosis can be found on the CD-ROM.

> *Ehrlichia* and *Anaplasma* spp. are intraleukocytic pathogens.

Drug resistance. Tetracyclines, especially doxycycline, are the drugs of choice for treating HME, human anaplasmosis, and fevers of unknown origin that follow tick bites.

Clues to *Ehrlichia* and *Anaplasma* spp. Identification

Cellular morphology. *Ehrlichia* and *Anaplasma* spp. live within cytoplasmic, membrane-bound vacuoles. Both small, dense forms and larger forms are observed within the vacuole. The dense forms are 0.2 to 0.4 μm in diameter and resemble chlamydial elementary bodies. The larger forms are 0.8 to 1.5 μm in diameter and resemble chlamydial reticulate bodies. (Chlamydial elementary and reticulate bodies were described earlier in this chapter.) Elementary bodies form a pleomorphic inclusion that matures into a compact cluster of cells (a microscopic colony) called a **morula (pl. morulae)** (Fig. 16-5). The name *morula* is derived from the mulberry-like appearance of these aggregates of *Ehrlichia* cells (*morula* comes from the Latin word *morus*, meaning "mulberry"). A morula contains anywhere from a few to more than 40 *Ehrlichia* cells and ranges in size from 1 to 6 μm. Infected cells usually contain one or two morulae, but as many as 15 have been seen. *Ehrlichia* morulae stain pale blue to dark violet with various Romanowsky stains.[3]

In vitro growth. Both *Ehrlichia* and *Anaplasma* spp. can be isolated from blood specimens using leukocyte cell cultures. Inoculated cells are examined every 2 to 3 days for the

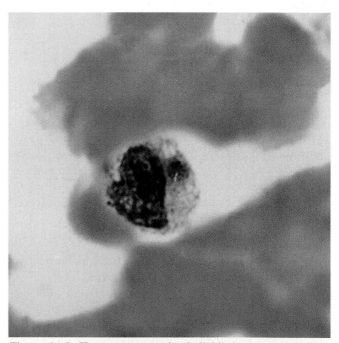

Figure 16-5. **Human monocytic ehrlichiosis.** Intracytoplasmic inclusion (morula) of *Ehrlichia chaffeensis* in a peripheral blood monocyte. The morula lies to the right of the cell nucleus. (From McClatchy KD, ed. Clinical Laboratory Medicine. 2nd Ed. Philadelphia: Lippincott Williams & Wilkins, 2002.)

---

[1]*Bone marrow–derived cells include granulocytes, monocytes, erythrocytes, and platelets.*

[2]*Ehrlichia* spp. and Anaplasma phagocytophilum *are intraleukocytic pathogens, meaning that they infect leukocytes. Some sporozoan protozoa, such as the* Plasmodium spp. *that cause human malaria and the* Babesia spp. *that cause human babesiosis, are* **intraerythrocytic pathogens,** *meaning that they live within red blood cells (erythrocytes).* Plasmodium *and* Babesia spp. *are described in Chapter 22.*

[3]*Romanowsky stains are stains that contain methylene blue and eosin. They are used to stain blood smears. Giemsa stain and Wright stain are examples of Romanowsky stains.*

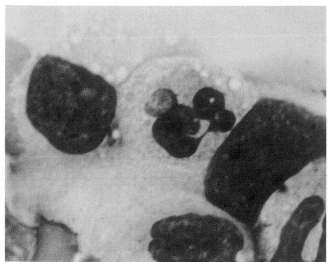

***Figure 16-6.* Human anaplasmosis (formerly called human granulocytic ehrlichiosis).** Intracytoplasmic inclusion (morula) in a Wright-stained peripheral neutrophil. The morula lies to the left of the segmented cell nucleus. (From McClatchy KD, ed. Clinical Laboratory Medicine. 2nd Ed. Philadelphia: Lippincott Williams & Wilkins, 2002.)

presence of cytoplasmic *Ehrlichia* morulae. Culturing is usually performed in reference laboratories.

Laboratory tests. Immunodiagnostic procedures and molecular diagnostic procedures are available for diagnosis of both HME and human anaplasmosis. The most widely used immunodiagnostic test for HME is an indirect fluorescent antibody (IFA) procedure, which uses *Ehrlichia*-infected cells attached to glass slides. This test is usually performed in reference laboratories.

Peripheral blood or buffy coat[4] smears from patients suspected of having HME or human anaplasmosis can be stained with Giemsa or Wright stain. Stained smears are examined microscopically for the presence of leukocytes containing cytoplasmic *Ehrlichia* morulae. The morulae are small (1 to 3 μm in diameter), round-to-oval clusters of blue or both red and blue bacteria; morulae have a stippled (dotted) appearance (Fig. 16-6). This method lacks sensitivity, however, especially for diagnosing HME.

Essentials

Ehrlichia and *Anaplasma* spp.

- Obligate intraleukocytic pathogens
- *Ehrlichia chaffeensis* lives within human monocytes and is the cause of HME
- HME is a tickborne disease

- *Anaplasma phagocytophilum* lives within human granulocytes and is the cause of human anaplasmosis
- Human anaplasmosis was previously called human granulocytic ehrlichiosis
- HME and human anaplasmosis are diagnosed by observing intracytoplasmic inclusion bodies, referred to as morulae (sing. *morula*)

COXIELLA BURNETII

Clinical significance. *Coxiella burnetii* is the only species in the genus *Coxiella*. It has been found in many animals. Transmission to humans is usually by aerosol following the birth of an infected animal (e.g., cattle, sheep, goats) but has also occurred via ingestion of contaminated milk and milk products. Tickborne transmission occurs among animals but is thought not to occur in humans. *C. burnetii* is the cause of Q fever,[5] which has both acute and chronic forms and may range from an asymptomatic infection to a severe, fatal disease. Acute Q fever can manifest itself as fever, pneumonia, hepatitis, skin eruptions, encephalitis, meningitis, myocarditis, or pericarditis. Patients often present with fever, chills, headache, myalgias, arthralgias, and cough. Unlike rickettsial diseases, Q fever does not usually present with a rash. The most common form of chronic Q fever is endocarditis; other manifestations include osteomyelitis, chronic hepatitis, and pseudotumors of the spleen and lung.

> *Coxiella burnetii* is the cause of Q fever.

Drug resistance. Tetracyclines are the drugs of choice for preventing and treating chronic Q fever. The combination of rifampin and doxycycline or rifampin and sulfamethoxazole-trimethoprim are recommended for treatment of Q fever endocarditis. Fluoroquinolones are active in vitro against *C. burnetii*, but resistant strains have been reported.

Clues to *C. burnetii* Identification

Cellular morphology. *C. burnetii* is a pleomorphic coccobacillus. Although it has a Gram-negative-type cell wall, it does not stain with the Gram staining procedure. Its developmental life cycle includes large- and small-cell variants, ranging in size from 0.2 to 0.7 μm. The small-cell variant attaches to and is ingested by a host cell (usually a macrophage). Maturation to the large cell variant occurs within a phagolysosome. (Recall that rickettsias live in the cytoplasm of infected cells.) Then sporulation begins. *C. burnetii* endospores are very resistant and can survive for long periods in the environment. In nature and in laboratory animals, *C. burnetii* exists in what is referred to as the phase I state. After numerous passages in cell culture or embryonated

[4]The term buffy coat *refers to the whitish layer of leukocytes seen above sedimented erythrocytes in a tube of centrifuged, whole, noncoagulated peripheral blood.*

[5]The disease Q fever *was given its name before the cause of the disease was known. The Q stands for "query."*

chicken eggs, it converts to the phase II state. Phase variation apparently has to do with changes in the structure of the organism's lipopolysaccharide.

In vitro growth. *C. burnetii* is an extremely infectious organism that requires great care during handling. According to Holtom and Leedom (see "References and Suggested Reading"), "a single inhaled organism is sufficient to initiate infection." *C. burnetii* can be isolated using cell cultures, the yolk sacs of embryonated chicken eggs, and laboratory animals (usually mice or guinea pigs), but because of the high risk of infection, only biosafety level 3 containment facilities should attempt its isolation.

> *Coxiella burnetii* is a potential bioterrorism and biological warfare agent; it is dangerous to work with in the laboratory.

Laboratory tests. Immunodiagnostic procedures that detect anti–*C. burnetii* antibodies in serum are the usual means of diagnosis of Q fever. The indirect fluorescent antibody test is the test of choice for diagnosis of both acute and chronic Q fever. Purified phase I and phase II *C. burnetii* cells are used as antigens. Antibodies are usually detectable 2 to 4 weeks following the onset of the disease. Molecular procedures are being developed.

Essentials

Coxiella burnetii

- Pleomorphic coccobacillus
- Obligate intracellular pathogen
- Produces endospores that are very resistant
- Transmission occurs primarily via aerosol and ingestion
- Causes Q fever
- Extremely infectious and dangerous to work with
- A potential bioterrorism and biological warfare agent
- Immunodiagnostic procedures are used to diagnose Q fever

Chapter Review

- Obligate intracellular bacterial pathogens such as *Chlamydia, Chlamydophila, Rickettsia, Orientia, Ehrlichia, Anaplasma,* and *Coxiella* spp. must live within host cells to survive and reproduce.

- *Chlamydia* and *Chlamydophila* spp., collectively referred to in this chapter as the chlamydiae, have a two-phase (biphasic) growth cycle consisting of EBs and RBs.

- Chlamydiae are called energy parasites because they preferentially use ATP molecules produced by their host cells.

- Rickettsias live within the cytoplasm of host cells. They require an intracellular environment because they possess an unusual membrane transport system—they have leaky membranes.

- All diseases caused by *Rickettsia* spp. are arthropod–borne, meaning that they are transmitted by arthropod vectors (e.g., ticks, fleas, lice).

- Diseases caused by rickettsias include typhus and typhuslike diseases, all of which are associated with a rash.

- *Rickettsia* and *Orientia* spp. do not grow on artificial media, but do grow in cell cultures and embryonated chicken eggs.

- Immunodiagnostic or molecular diagnostic techniques are available for detecting *Chlamydia, Rickettsia, Ehrlichia,* and *Anaplasma* spp.

- *Ehrlichia* spp and *Anaplasma phagocytophilum* are obligately intracellular, Gram-negative bacteria.

- *Ehrlichia* spp. predominantly infect leukocytes (white blood cells) of humans and other mammals; they are intraleukocytic pathogens. *Anaplasma phagocytophilum* infects various bone marrow–derived cells in humans, horses, cattle, sheep, goats, and dogs.

- *Coxiella burnetii* is a pleomorphic coccobacillus that does not stain with Gram staining procedures. Transmission to humans is usually by aerosol but can occur via ingestion. It is an extremely infectious agent and the cause of Q fever. Unlike rickettsial diseases, Q fever does not usually present with a rash.

New Terms and Abbreviations

After studying Chapter 16, you should be familiar with the following terms, which are defined within the chapter and in the Glossary at the back of the book:

Elementary body (EB)

Intraerythrocytic pathogen

Intraleukocytic pathogen

Morula (pl. morulae)

Reticulate body (RB)

References and Suggested Reading

Aguero-Rosenfeld ME, Dumler JS. *Ehrlichia, Anaplasma, Neorickettsia,* and *Aegyptianella.* In: Murray PR, Baron EJ, Jorgensen JH, Pfaller MA, Yolken RH, eds. Manual of Clinical Microbiology. 8th Ed. Washington, DC: ASM Press, 2003.

Brouqui P, et al. *Coxiella.* In: Murray PR, Baron EJ, Jorgensen JH, Pfaller MA, Yolken RH, eds. Manual of Clinical Microbiology. 8th Ed. Washington, DC: ASM Press, 2003.

Dumler JS. *Rickettsia rickettsii* (Rocky Mountain spotted fever). In: Gorbach SL, Bartlett JG, Blacklow NR, eds. Infectious Disease. 3rd Ed. Philadelphia: Lippincott Williams & Wilkins, 2004.

Holtom PD, Leedom JM. *Coxiella burnetii* (Q fever). In: Gorbach SL, Bartlett JG, Blacklow NR, eds. Infectious Disease. 3rd Ed. Philadelphia: Lippincott Williams & Wilkins, 2004.

Mahony JB, et al. *Chlamydia* and *Chlamydophila.* In: Murray PR, Baron EJ, Jorgensen JH, Pfaller MA, Yolken RH, eds. Manual of Clinical Microbiology. 8th Ed. Washington, DC: ASM Press, 2003.

McDade JE, Olson JG. *Rickettsia typhi* and *Rickettsia prowazekii.* In: Gorbach SL, Bartlett JG, Blacklow NR, eds. Infectious Disease. 3rd Ed. Philadelphia: Lippincott Williams & Wilkins, 2004.

Olson JG, McDade JE. *Rickettsia tsutsugamushi* and *Rickettsia akari.* In: Gorbach SL, Bartlett JG, Blacklow NR, eds. Infectious Disease. 3rd Ed. Philadelphia: Lippincott Williams & Wilkins, 2004.

Schachter J. *Chlamydia.* In: Gorbach SL, Bartlett JG, Blacklow NR, eds. Infectious Disease. 3rd Ed. Philadelphia: Lippincott Williams & Wilkins, 2004.

Sumner JW, Paddock CD. Agents of Human Ehrlichiosis. In: Gorbach SL, Bartlett JG, Blacklow NR, eds. Infectious Disease. 3rd Ed. Philadelphia: Lippincott Williams & Wilkins, 2004.

Waites KB, et al. *Mycoplasma* and *Ureaplasma*. In: Murray PR, Baron EJ, Jorgensen JH, Pfaller MA, Yolken RH, eds. Manual of Clinical Microbiology. 8th Ed. Washington, DC: ASM Press, 2003.

Walker DH, Bouyer DH. *Rickettsia*. In: Murray PR, Baron EJ, Jorgensen JH, Pfaller MA, Yolken RH, eds. Manual of Clinical Microbiology. 8th Ed. Washington, DC: ASM Press, 2003.

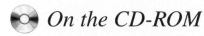

On the CD-ROM

- A Closer Look at Cell Lines
- A Closer Look at the Weil-Felix Test
- A Closer Look at HME and Human Anaplasmosis
- Additional Self-Assessment Exercises
- Case Study
- Puzzle

Self-Assessment Exercises

Match the items in the column on the left with the correct description or disease in the column on the right.

1. _____ *Ehrlichia chaffeensis*

2. _____ *Chlamydia trachomatis*

3. _____ *Coxiella burnetii*

4. _____ *Rickettsia typhi*

5. _____ *Chlamydophila psittaci*

A. Endemic typhus

B. Psittacosis or ornithosis

C. Human monocytic ehrlichiosis

D. Trachoma

E. Q fever

6. Which of the following is *not* an obligate intracellular pathogen?

A. *Rickettsia* spp.

B. *Orientia* spp.

C. *Proteus* spp.

D. *Chlamydia* spp.

7. Briefly describe the biphasic developmental cycle of *Chlamydia* spp., starting with entry of the organism into a host cell.

_____

_____

_____

8. True or false: *Ehrlichia* spp. are considered energy parasites.

9. True or false: All *Rickettsia* spp. cause diseases that usually involve a rash.

10. True or false: *Rickettsia* spp. may be isolated on routine artificial media.

CHAPTER 17

Anaerobic Bacteria

Chapter Outline

LEARNING OBJECTIVES

After studying this chapter, you should be able to:

- Define the terms introduced in this chapter (e.g., Actinomyces-*like, botulinal toxin, diphtheroid-like*)

- Describe the relationship that obligate and aerotolerant anaerobes have with oxygen and how that relationship differs from other categories of bacteria (e.g., aerobes, microaerophiles, facultative anaerobes) encountered in the clinical microbiology laboratory

- Briefly describe the two-phase theory of oxygen toxicity to anaerobes

- Explain the importance of high-quality clinical specimens for the anaerobic bacteriology laboratory, and describe appropriate specimens, collection techniques, and manner of transport

- List six acceptable and six unacceptable clinical specimens for anaerobic bacteriology

- Name three important considerations in the transport of clinical specimens for anaerobic bacteriology

- State the difference between exogenous and endogenous anaerobes, and categorize each of the following anaerobes as being either exogenous or endogenous: *Clostridium botulinum, Clostridium tetani, Bacteroides fragilis,* and *Fusobacterium nucleatum*

- List five anatomical locations of the healthy human body that would be expected to harbor anaerobic bacteria as part of the indigenous microflora at those sites

- Distinguish between the following clostridial diseases, with respect to the manner in which they are acquired: foodborne botulism, infant botulism, and wound botulism

- Identify the etiologic agents and the manner in which the following diseases are acquired: tetanus, gas gangrene, and pseudomembranous colitis

☞ Name five infectious processes or diseases that virtually always involve anaerobes of endogenous origin

☞ Outline the steps in macroscopic and microscopic examination of specimens submitted to the clinical microbiology laboratory for isolation of anaerobes

☞ Describe the type of "holding system" that could be used to prevent undue exposure of anaerobes (particularly obligate and aerotolerant anaerobes) to oxygen during the examination of clinical materials or cultures

☞ State the purpose of each of the four types of plated media routinely used in the primary setup for anaerobic bacteriology

☞ Compare and contrast the three most commonly used methods for anaerobic incubation of inoculated plates, including the advantages and disadvantages of each

☞ List the types of organisms that would be expected to grow on or in each of the media used in the primary isolation setup for anaerobic bacteriology

☞ Describe the appearance of lecithinase and lipase reactions on egg yolk agar

☞ Explain how an aerotolerance test is performed in the bacteriology laboratory, describing the media to use, the incubation environments, and how results are interpreted

☞ Differentiate between the terms *presumptive identification* and *definitive identification*

☞ Describe the features or characteristics of primary plates that would permit presumptive identification of *Clostridium perfringens, Clostridium difficile*, members of the *Bacteroides fragilis* group, and pigmented species of *Porphyromonas* and *Prevotella*

☞ State the minimal observations and/or test results required to identify the following anaerobes: a member of the *Bacteroides fragilis* group, pigmented species of *Porphyromonas* or *Prevotella, Clostridium difficile, C. perfringens, Fusobacterium mortiferum, F. necrophorum, F. nucleatum, Peptostreptococcus anaerobius, Peptoniphilus asaccharolyticus, Propionibacterium acnes*, and *Veillonella* spp.

☞ State the Gram reaction and cellular morphology of the following anaerobes: *Bacteroides* spp., *Porphyromonas* spp., *Prevotella* spp., *Clostridium perfringens, Clostridium ramosum, Fusobacterium nucleatum, Peptostreptococcus anaerobius, Veillonella* spp., *Actinomyces* spp., *Mobiluncus* spp. *Propionibacterium acnes*, and *Bifidobacterium* spp.

☞ Name two distinguishing characteristics of the genus *Clostridium*

☞ Identify four of the genera of anaerobic Gram-negative bacilli most commonly isolated from clinical specimens

☞ Name the anaerobe most commonly involved in soft tissue infectious processes and bacteremia

☞ Select the only species in the genus *Fusobacterium*, with cells that *routinely* appear fusiform in shape

☞ Identify the genus of anaerobic Gram-positive cocci and the genus of anaerobic Gram-negative cocci most frequently isolated from clinical specimens

☞ Compare and contrast biochemical-based and enzyme-based minisystems to "conventional" systems for the identification of anaerobes, including speed of identification, cost, and practicality for routine use

☞ Name two types of gas-liquid chromatography used to identify anaerobes

☞ Cite three clinical situations in which antimicrobial susceptibility testing of anaerobic isolates *should* be performed

☞ List three species of anaerobes for which susceptibility testing *should* routinely be performed whenever the isolates are deemed clinically significant

☞ Define *β-lactamases* and name several anaerobes that produce these enzymes

Many types of microorganisms are capable of surviving in anaerobic environments (i.e., environments devoid of molecular oxygen), including some species of bacteria, fungi, and protozoa. Throughout this chapter, the term *anaerobes* is used in reference to **anaerobic bacteria**—bacteria that do not require oxygen for life and reproduction. Although some species of anaerobes die when exposed to oxygen, others do not (see "Why Anaerobes Die in the Presence of Oxygen" on the CD-ROM).

Recall from Chapter 8 the various categories of anaerobes. **Obligate anaerobes** can survive only in an anaerobic environment. **Aerotolerant anaerobes** are capable of multiplication in atmospheres containing some molecular oxygen but grow best in an anaerobic environment. The concentration of oxygen that can be tolerated by aerotolerant anaerobes varies from one species to another. **Facultative anaerobes** can survive in either the presence or absence of oxygen—anywhere from 0% to 20% or 21% oxygen. Most bacteria routinely isolated from clinical specimens are facultative anaerobes, including members of the Enterobacteriaceae family, most streptococci, and most staphylococci.

. This chapter describes the role of anaerobes in disease; proper techniques for selection, collection, transport, and processing of clinical specimens for anaerobic bacteriology; and procedures for identification and antimicrobial susceptibility testing of anaerobic isolates. Although other functions and applications of anaerobes, such as agricultural and industrial applications, are important, a discussion of these aspects of anaerobic bacteriology is beyond the scope of this book.

TAXONOMIC CLASSIFICATION OF COMMONLY ENCOUNTERED, CLINICALLY SIGNIFICANT ANAEROBES

Anaerobes isolated from clinical specimens, either as true pathogens or indigenous microflora contaminants, can first be divided into those that are Gram positive and those that are Gram negative. Within each of those categories are cocci and bacilli. The Gram-positive bacilli can be divided into those capable of forming spores, called spore formers, and those that are not, called non–spore formers. This taxonomic arrangement is shown diagrammatically in Figure 17-1, along

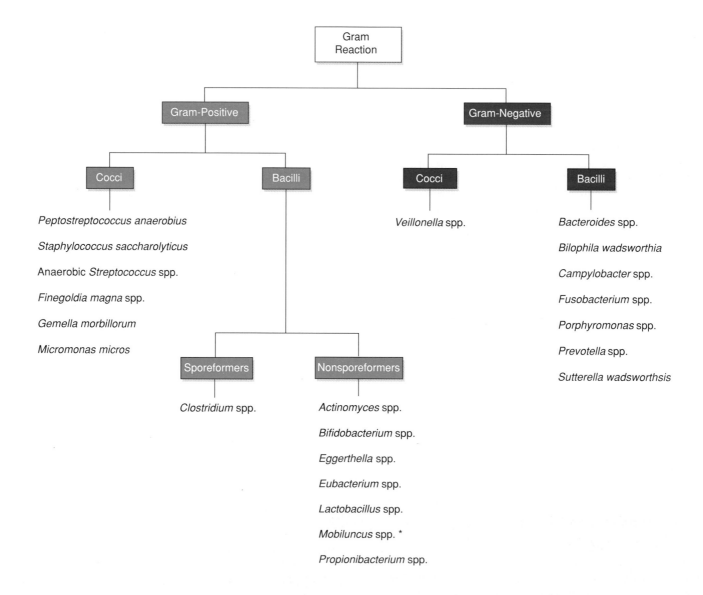

* Technically Gram-positive, but they stain Gram-negative or Gram-variable

Note: Many additional anaerobes can be isolated from clinical specimens

Figure 17-1. **Classification of commonly encountered anaerobes.**

with the names of the anaerobes most commonly encountered in clinical specimens. Some anaerobic spirochetes (*Treponema* and *Brachyspira* spp.) can be found in the indigenous microflora of the oral cavity, skin, and gastrointestinal tract. These organisms are generally considered nonpathogenic commensals and are not discussed further in this chapter.

MEDICAL IMPORTANCE OF ANAEROBES

Anaerobes are involved in many human diseases, playing an important, often major role in infectious processes of the respiratory, gastrointestinal, and female genital tracts. Anaerobes are key pathogens in brain abscesses, oral and dental diseases, actinomycosis, aspiration pneumonia, lung abscesses, chronic osteomyelitis, tetanus, botulism, gas gangrene, and numerous other infectious processes of soft tissue. In fact, certain infectious processes and diseases are so likely to involve anaerobes that, until proved otherwise, their presence should always be assumed. Examples of such infectious processes and diseases are brain abscess, oral and dental infectious processes, aspiration pneumonia, lung abscess, peritonitis, intra-abdominal abscess, infectious processes and diseases that follow bowel surgery or trauma to the bowel, endometritis, tubo-ovarian abscess, perirectal abscess, gas-forming and necrotizing infectious processes of soft tissue or muscle, and infectious processes of the lower extremities in diabetics.

Many areas of the human body are colonized with anaerobes, including the skin, upper respiratory tract, oral cavity, colon, distal urethra, and vagina. Anaerobes that are members of the body's indigenous microflora are referred to as **endogenous anaerobes,** whereas those that live in the external environment are **exogenous anaerobes.** Anaerobes in both categories are capable of causing human disease.

Generally, infectious diseases involving anaerobic bacteria follow some type of trauma to protective barriers such as the skin and mucous membranes, thus allowing endogenous anaerobes, or soil anaerobes in some cases, to gain access to deeper tissues. A clinician would usually assume that an infectious process that arises following oral, gastrointestinal, or genitourinary surgery involves anaerobes and, pending microbiology laboratory results, would probably treat the patient based on that assumption.

Diseases Caused by Anaerobes of Exogenous Origin

In the early days of clinical anaerobic bacteriology, before various technological advances, the only anaerobes recognized as human pathogens were *Clostridium* spp. that originated outside the body, usually from soil. These were the clostridia that cause diseases such as tetanus, gas gangrene,

botulism, and *Clostridium perfringens* food poisoning (all described later in the chapter). Exogenous anaerobes or their spores usually enter the body through the mouth or an open wound.

Some *Clostridium* spp. also inhabit certain body sites (e.g., the colon and vagina) as part of the indigenous microflora; thus, the origin of clostridial disease is not always outside the body. Clostridia are not the most frequently isolated anaerobes in today's clinical microbiology laboratory (CML), but they are still very important and may represent a serious medical condition when isolated.

Diseases Caused by Anaerobes of Endogenous Origin

In recent years, the anaerobes most frequently isolated from infectious processes in humans are those of endogenous origin. In other words, they are members of the patient's own indigenous microflora that somehow gained entrance to an area of the body not usually inhabited by these organisms. Table 17-1 contains information about the anaerobes that compose part of the indigenous microflora of the human body.

> The indigenous microflora of the human body includes many anaerobes.

Knowledge of the composition of the indigenous microflora at specific anatomical sites is useful for predicting the particular organisms most apt to be involved in infectious processes that arise at or adjacent to those sites. Such knowledge may also be of value to clinicians who are considering empiric antimicrobial therapy. Empiric therapy is therapy that is initiated before receipt of information from the CML.

Also, the finding of site-specific organisms at a distant and/or unusual site can serve as a clue to the underlying origin of an infectious process. For example, the isolation of oral anaerobes (e.g., *Porphyromonas* spp.) from a brain abscess may suggest communication between an oral lesion and the bloodstream.

Anaerobes of endogenous origin can contribute to an infectious disease in virtually any tissue, anatomical region, or organ of the body, provided that suitable conditions exist for colonization and penetration of the bacteria. For example, *Actinomyces* species, as well as related endogenous anaerobic bacteria (e.g., bifidobacteria, eubacteria, propionibacteria), can cause a disease called actinomycosis in the brain, orofacial region, pleuropulmonary region, or genital organs. Bacterial vaginosis is another example. That disease is thought by some investigators to involve endogenous anaerobes of the vagina—namely, curved, motile Gram-positive bacteria[1] of the genus *Mobiluncus*, especially *M. curtisii* subsp. *curtisii*.

Many of the infectious processes involving anaerobes are polymicrobial, meaning that multiple organisms are

---

[1]*Although* Mobiluncus *spp. have a Gram-positive type of cell wall, they stain pink or Gram variable with the Gram staining technique.*

TABLE 17 - 1   Anaerobes of the Indigenous Microflora

Anatomical Site	Anaerobes Found at Site
Oral cavity and upper respiratory tract	Anaerobes occurring in the highest numbers in the oral cavity are Gram-positive bacilli (*Actinomyces* and *Eubacterium* spp.), Gram-positive cocci, and Gram-negative bacilli (*Campylobacter*, *Fusobacterium*, and *Prevotella* spp.). Other anaerobes found there are *Bifidobacterium* spp. (Gram-positive bacilli), *Capnocytophaga* and *Porphyromonas* spp. (Gram-negative bacilli), and *Veillonella* spp. (Gram-negative cocci). Anaerobic spirochetes in the genus *Treponema* also inhabit the oral cavity. The predominant anaerobes inhabiting upper respiratory tract sites other than the mouth are Gram-positive cocci, Gram-positive bacilli (*Actinomyces* and *Propionibacterium* spp.), Gram-negative bacilli (*Campylobacter*, *Capnocytophaga*, *Fusobacterium*, and *Prevotella* spp.), and Gram-negative cocci (*Veillonella* spp.).
Skin	The anaerobes present in highest numbers are Gram-positive bacilli in the genus *Propionibacterium* (especially *P. acnes*). Gram-positive cocci and Gram-positive bacilli in the genus *Eubacterium* are sometimes present.
Urethra	The anaerobes present in the greatest numbers are Gram-negative bacilli (*Bacteroides*, *Prevotella*, and *Fusobacterium* spp.). Other anaerobes (e.g., Gram-positive cocci, lactobacilli, eubacteria, and clostridia) can be found in fewer numbers.
Vagina	The most common anaerobes in the cervical and vaginal secretions of healthy persons are lactobacilli (not all of which are anaerobes) and Gram-positive cocci. *Prevotella bivia* and *P. disiens* as well as curved, motile anaerobic Gram-positive bacilli in the genus *Mobiluncus* are also common members of the vaginal flora. *Clostridium* spp. from the colon can also be found in the vaginal flora because of the proximity of the vagina to the anus.
Colon	Anaerobes occurring in the highest numbers in intestinal flora are *Bacteroides*, *Bifidobacterium*, *Clostridium*, *Eubacterium*, *Lactobacillus*, and Gram-positive cocci. The most common *Bacteroides* spp. are *B. vulgatus* and *B. thetaiotaomicron*, although *B. distasonis*, *B. fragilis*, and *B. ovatus* are also quite common. The most common species of *Clostridium* are *C. ramosum* and *C. perfringens*.

> Infections involving anaerobes are frequently polymicrobial, with mixtures of bacteria acting synergistically to cause the infection.

involved in the process—generally, mixtures of obligate, aerotolerant, and facultative anaerobes. These mixtures of bacteria can act synergistically in the production of disease.

Infectious processes involving anaerobes are usually purulent—that is, they contain pus. Recall that pus contains numerous live and dead leukocytes. The absence of leukocytes at the site of an infectious process does not, however, rule out the possibility that anaerobes are contributing to the process. Some of the more serious infectious processes in humans are caused by anaerobes that produce cytotoxins and other histotoxic virulence factors that contribute to the

necrotizing process by destroying neutrophils, macrophages, and other body cells.

Factors that commonly predispose a patient to infection with endogenous and exogenous anaerobes include trauma of mucous membranes or skin, blockage of blood flow (vascular stasis), tissue necrosis, and a decrease in the oxidation-reduction (redox) potential of tissue.[2] Vascular stasis prevents oxygen from entering the site and is therefore conducive to multiplication of any anaerobes possibly present at that site. Conditions that predispose patients to anaerobic infections include human or animal bite wounds, aspiration of oral contents into the lungs, tooth extraction, oral surgery or traumatic puncture of the oral cavity, gastrointestinal tract surgery or traumatic puncture of the bowel, genital tract surgery or traumatic puncture of the genital tract, and introduction of soil into a wound.

---

[2] *The oxidation-reduction (redox) potential, expressed as E_h, of an environment is a measure of the environment's degree of oxidation or reduction. Oxidized environments have a high E_h, whereas reduced environments have a low E_h. In nature, the upper limit of E_h is about +820 millivolts (mV), whereas the lower limit is about −420 mV. Anaerobic environments, such as abscesses and necrotic tissues, could have an E_h as low as −420 mV. Well-oxygenated tissues have an E_h of about +150 mV.*

A typical scenario for an anaerobe-associated infectious process might be as follows:

1. Some condition predisposes a patient to infection, such as an automobile accident; a tooth extraction; a ruptured appendix; or oral, gynecologic, or abdominal surgery. The event causes the initial tissue damage.

2. A primary infection develops, not necessarily involving obligate or aerotolerant anaerobes. Facultative anaerobes contribute to a decrease in the redox potential at the site and to the production of anaerobic conditions. Obligate and aerotolerant anaerobes then flourish at the site.

3. Bacteria gain access to the bloodstream, where they are disseminated hematogenously (i.e., by way of the bloodstream) throughout the body.

4. At locations possibly quite distant from the original infection site, small clots develop in tiny capillaries, stopping the flow of blood and creating anaerobic conditions at those sites.

5. A septic thrombus (clot) develops at one or more of these sites.

6. An abscess forms, and organisms are disseminated hematogenously to additional sites.

7. Further complications develop, such as intravascular hemolysis, tissue necrosis, toxemia, shock, intravascular coagulation, vascular collapse, or death.

Table 17-2 contains the names of endogenous anaerobes commonly involved in human infectious diseases.

SPECIAL CONSIDERATIONS IN CLINICAL ANAEROBIC BACTERIOLOGY

Specimen Selection, Collection, and Transport

Anatomical sites that are inhabited by indigenous microflora are referred to as **nonsterile sites,** and specimens collected from such sites are called **nonsterile specimens.** A member of the indigenous microflora recovered from an inappropriate or improperly collected specimen from a nonsterile site could represent either (1) a pathogen contributing to the infectious process or (2) an indigenous microflora contaminant introduced during collection of the specimen. Neither the CML professional nor the clinician would know whether anaerobes isolated from these specimens represent contaminants or organisms actually involved in the infectious process (i.e., true pathogens).

When suspecting an infection involving anaerobes, the clinician must properly select and collect a clinical specimen and arrange for its proper and rapid transport to the CML. These steps are extremely important in the successful outcome of an anaerobic culture. The CML must disseminate written guidelines for the proper selection, collection, and transport of specimens for anaerobic bacteriology. (See Chapter 5 for a discussion of the laboratory policies and procedures manual.)

Specimens considered **unacceptable** for anaerobic culture include throat swabs and other upper respiratory tract swabs; sputum; gingival and other oral swabs; feces and rectal swabs (except for the culture of *Clostridium difficile* or *C. botulinum*); voided or catheterized urine; vaginal and cervical swabs; vaginal discharge material; and swabs of decubitus ulcers, perirectal abscesses, foot ulcers, exposed wounds, and sinus tracts. In general, any specimens collected by swabbing mucosal surfaces or skin are unacceptable for anaerobic bacteriology because they are contaminated with indigenous microflora, including endogenous anaerobes. Likewise, expectorated sputum, feces, and voided urine would all be expected to contain endogenous anaerobes.

A laboratory workup of an inappropriate specimen is a waste of time, effort, and money. Culture results must be clinically relevant; that is, they must reveal something about the patient's infection, *not* information about his or her mucosal or skin flora. CML professionals are responsible for educating persons responsible for selecting, collecting, and transporting specimens for anaerobic bacteriology. This process of education includes explaining the consequences of working up improper specimens and specimens that have been incorrectly collected or transported.

The CML must develop criteria for rejection of inappropriate specimens. These criteria, which are in the best interest of the patients, must always be developed with the knowledge, cooperation, and consent of hospital clinicians. Whenever a specimen is rejected, the CML director must explain to the requesting clinician the reasons for rejection and the consequences of working up an improper specimen. A CML professional must never discard a specimen without first talking with the clinician. Some specimens, especially those taken during surgical procedures, are impossible to replace.

Specimens that are **acceptable** for anaerobic culture are listed in Table 17-3. The best specimens for anaerobic bacteriology are aspirates collected by needle and syringe, which minimize contamination of the specimen with endogenous anaerobes.

> The best specimens for anaerobic bacteriology are aspirates collected by needle and syringe. In general, specimens collected by swabbing mucosal surfaces or skin are unacceptable because they are contaminated with indigenous microflora, including endogenous anaerobes.

TABLE 17 - 2	Endogenous Anaerobes Commonly Involved in Human Infectious Diseases
Infectious Process(es)	**Endogenous Anaerobe(s)**
Actinomycosis	*Actinomyces israelii*, other *Actinomyces* spp., *Propionibacterium propionicus*
Antibiotic-associated diarrhea and pseudomembranous colitis	*Clostridium difficile*
Bacteremia	*Propionibacterium* spp. most often represent contamination of the blood culture bottle by normal skin flora; 65–75% of clinically significant anaerobic bacteremias involve *Bacteroides* and *Fusobacterium* species; 80–90% of these are caused by the *B. fragilis* group; Gram-positive cocci are also frequently isolated
Brain abscess	Often polymicrobial; anaerobes such as *Bacteroides* spp., *Fusobacterium* spp., and Gram-positive cocci are frequently involved; clostridia, less often
Complications of Vincent angina (necrotizing ulcerative gingivitis trench mouth)	*Fusobacterium necrophorum* and anaerobic spirochetes
Endocarditis	Anaerobes are an uncommon cause; *Bacteroides* (especially *B. fragilis* group), Gram-positive cocci, and some non-spore-forming Gram-positive bacilli (*Propionibacterium acnes, Actinomyces,* and related bacteria)
Infectious processes of the eye	Gram-positive cocci, clostridia, *Bacteroides* spp., *Actinomyces* spp.
Infectious processes of the female genital tract	Anaerobes may cause disease in virtually every type of gynecologic or obstetric infectious process; Gram-positive cocci, *Bacteroides* spp., clostridia, and many other anaerobes
Intra-abdominal infectious processes	Anaerobes are frequently encountered; infections are usually polymicrobic; *Bacteroides fragilis* group, other *Bacteroides* spp., *Fusobacterium* spp., *Clostridium perfringens*, other clostridia, Gram-positive cocci
Liver abscess	Gram-positive cocci, *Bacteroides fragilis* group, other *Bacteroides, Fusobacterium necrophorum*, other fusobacteria, clostridia, *Actinomyces* spp.
Myonecrosis (gas gangrene)	*C. perfringens* (80–95% of cases), *C. novyi, C. septicum*
Oral and dental infectious processes (e.g., periodontitis)	Oral anaerobes are almost always involved; Gram-positive cocci, *Porphyromonas* spp., *Wolinella* spp., *Fusobacterium* spp.
Perineal and perirectal infectious processes	Anaerobes are commonly involved; *B. fragilis* group, other *Bacteroides* spp., *Fusobacterium* spp., clostridia, Gram-positive cocci, *Eubacterium* spp., *Actinomyces* spp.
Peritonitis	*Bacteroides* spp., Gram-positive cocci, *Fusobacterium necrophorum, Clostridium* spp.
Pleuropulmonary infectious processes	90% of cases involve anaerobes; *Porphyromonas* spp., *Fusobacterium nucleatum*, Gram-positive cocci, *Bacteroides fragilis* group, *Actinomyces* spp., *Eubacterium* spp.
Sinusitis	Anaerobes are commonly involved in chronic sinusitis; infections are often polymicrobial; *Bacteroides* spp., Gram-positive cocci, *Fusobacterium* spp.

Source: Finegold SM, George WL, Mulligon ME. Anaerobic Infections. Chicago: Year Book Medical, 1986. Table used with permission of the Colorado Association for Continuing Medical Laboratory Education, Denver, CO.

TABLE 17 - 3   Specimens Acceptable for Anaerobic Bacteriology

Site/Type of Specimen	Recommended Specimens and Methods of Collection
Abscesses	Aspirate abscess fluid via needle and syringe through disinfected, uninvolved, intact tissue
Sinus tracts or deep, draining wounds	Curettings obtained after the sinus tract and surrounding skin surface have been disinfected first with 70% alcohol and then with an iodine preparation; aspiration of pus from within the tract via a flexible plastic catheter and syringe
Oral or gingival abscesses	Aspirates or drainage collected via the external skin surface (extraoral route) are preferable; alternatively, abscess contents collected within the oral cavity via needle, following disinfection of the site
Paranasal sinus secretions	Aspirates collected by needle and syringe following disinfection of the site
Superficial ulcers (e.g., decubitus ulcers, foot ulcers in diabetics)	Curettings collected following cleaning/debridement; alternatively, aspiration of purulent material through disinfected, uninvolved skin
Respiratory tract secretions	Lung tissue, percutaneous lung or transtracheal aspirates, bronchial brushings collected via a double-lumen protected catheter, "protected" bronchoalveolar lavage, thoracentesis fluid
Female genital tract specimens	Culdocentesis, a protected sampling device, aspirates collected via needle following disinfection of the site
Specimens collected at the time of surgery	Tissue specimens placed immediately into an anaerobic transport device
Urinary tract	Urine collected by suprapubic bladder aspiration

Source: Jousimies-Somer HR, Summanen P, Baron EJ, Citron DM, Wexler HM, Finegold SM. Wadsworth-KTL Anaerobic Bacteriology Manual. 6th Ed. Belmont, CA: Star, 2002. Consult this reference for detailed instructions concerning proper disinfection and specimen collection techniques; table used with the permission of the Colorado Association for Continuing Medical Laboratory Education, Denver, CO.

Regardless of the type of specimen being submitted for anaerobic bacteriology, the specimen must be transported as rapidly as possible and with minimal exposure to oxygen. Specimens are usually collected from a warm, moist environment low in oxygen. Thus, it is important to avoid "shocking" the anaerobes by exposing them to oxygen or permitting them to dry out. In addition, the amount of time they remain at room temperature should be minimized.

Ideally, small volumes of aspirates will be injected into an oxygen-free transport tube or vial, preferably one containing prereduced, anaerobically sterilized (PRAS) transport medium. Oxygen-free transport containers are manufactured by several companies (e.g., Anaerobe Systems and BD Biosciences). Whenever such a transport system is used, care must be taken not to tip the container while the cap is removed. Because the oxygen-free gas mixture within the container is heavier than room air, it would spill from the tipped container and be displaced by room air. This would, of course, defeat the primary purpose of using such a transport system.

In the rare instances when swabs are deemed necessary, commercially available, oxygen-free swabs should be used. To prevent drying of the material during transit to the laboratory, the swab must be placed into a tube containing PRAS medium and an oxygen-free environment.

Specimen Processing

Among the various methods available for processing a specimen for anaerobic bacteriology, the emphasis is always on **speed**. It is important to remember that any anaerobes present within the specimen have been at room temperature during transit to the laboratory and may have been exposed to oxygen during specimen collection. The hope is that they have not been exposed to additional oxygen during transport and the specimen has not dried out.

Ideally, once a specimen arrives in the laboratory, it can be immediately passed into an anaerobic chamber to prevent further exposure of clinical materials to oxygen. An anaerobic chamber allows *all* steps in the processing of a specimen to be performed in an oxygen-free environment. Anaerobic chambers are described in detail in a subsequent section.

Laboratories not equipped with anaerobic chambers may use nitrogen gas holding systems (Fig. 17-2). A holding system, which may employ a jar, box, or other small chamber, allows uninoculated plates to be held under anaerobic conditions until needed and allows inoculated plates to be held under near anaerobic conditions until placed into an anaerobic chamber, jar, or bag. Care should be taken to ensure that inoculated plates do not remain in the holding jar at room temperature for extended periods. Also, because the holding jar should remain as anaerobic as possible, it is important to minimize convection currents whenever freshly inoculated plates are added to the jar.

To comply with mandatory infectious disease safety policies, appropriate safety precautions must be followed. As discussed in Chapter 4, disposable latex gloves should always be worn when handling clinical specimens containing potentially infectious agents, and use of a biosafety cabinet during processing of clinical samples is mandatory.

Processing of a clinical specimen for anaerobic bacteriology involves the steps listed in Table 17-4. The *Wadsworth-KTL Anaerobic Bacteriology Manual*, by Jousimies-Somer et al. (see "References and Suggested Reading") should be

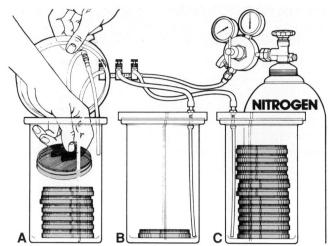

Figure 17-2. **The type of anaerobic holding jar system that could be used at the specimen-processing station in a CML not equipped with an anaerobic chamber.** The three jars contain an anaerobic atmosphere. **A and B.** Jars containing uninoculated plates. **C.** Jar containing inoculated plates being held until sufficient plates have accumulated to set up and incubate an anaerobic jar or bag. A similar holding jar system should *always* be located at the anaerobe workstation so that culture and subculture plates may be held under anaerobic conditions while they are not physically being worked on. (From Winn WC Jr, et al. Koneman's Color Atlas and Textbook of Diagnostic Microbiology. 6th Ed. Philadelphia: Lippincott Williams & Wilkins, 2006.)

TABLE 17 - 4 · Steps in the Processing of an Anaerobic Bacteriology Specimen

Step	Questions to Ask and Comments
Macroscopic examination of the specimen	Is it an appropriate specimen? Was it submitted in an appropriate container? How old is the specimen? Are the date and time of collection recorded on the accompanying request slip? Is there evidence that the specimen has dried out during transit? Does the specimen have a foul odor? Does the specimen fluoresce brick red when exposed to a Wood's lamp? (A Wood's lamp emits long-wave [366-nm] ultraviolet light.) Is the necrotic tissue or exudate black? Does the specimen contain sulfur granules? Is the specimen bloody or purulent?
Microscopic examination of the specimen, to include examination of a methanol-fixed, Gram-stained smear	This reveals the various morphological types of microorganisms present, as well as their relative numbers. Infectious processes involving anaerobes are frequently polymicrobic and complex in composition. Are leukocytes present? It is sometimes possible to make a presumptive identification of organisms based on their appearance in Gram-stained smears. The presence of certain morphotypes can serve as a guide to media selection.
Inoculation of appropriate plated and tubed media, including media specifically designed for culturing anaerobes	Discussed in the section titled "Culture Media."
Anaerobic incubation of inoculated media	Discussed in the section titled "Anaerobic Incubation."

consulted for the exact method for processing a specific type of clinical specimen.

Because Gram-negative anaerobes frequently stain a very pale pink when safranin is used as the counterstain in the Gram staining procedure, they are easily overlooked in Gram-stained smears of clinical specimens and blood cultures. To enhance the red color of Gram-negative anaerobes, a modified Gram staining procedure with 0.1% basic fuchsin as the counterstain can be used, or counterstaining with safranin can be increased to 3 to 5 minutes to make results consistent with the basic fuchsin technique.

In addition to Gram staining, some laboratories routinely examine wet mounts of clinical materials using regular transmitted light, phase contrast microscopy, or darkfield illumination. These procedures aid in detection of motile organisms and refractile spores. Acridine-orange staining and direct gas-liquid chromatography (GLC) analysis of clinical specimens are additional techniques used by some laboratories; however, these methods are not discussed here because their value is questionable.

Culture Media

The choice of media for use in the anaerobic bacteriology laboratory is an extremely important aspect of successful anaerobic bacteriology. Media that have been exposed to air for extended periods may contain toxic substances—like hydroxyl radicals, hydrogen peroxide, or superoxide anions—produced as a result of the reduction of molecular oxygen. Such media may also have redox potentials above that required for anaerobes to initiate growth.

Ideally, the medium used to culture an anaerobe has *never* been exposed to oxygen or has been exposed for only a brief time. The best medium is one that has been freshly prepared and then immediately stored under anaerobic conditions. It is, of course, not practical to prepare a fresh medium each time there is a need for it. However, a freshly prepared medium can be stored within an anaerobic chamber or anaerobic holding system until used or too dry to use.

An alternative to fresh media is the use of commercial media that have been prepared, packaged, shipped, and stored under anaerobic conditions—media not exposed to oxygen until they are inoculated, or not exposed at all when plates are inoculated within an anaerobic chamber. Such media, available from Anaerobe Systems, are prereduced and anaerobically sterilized; in other words, they are **PRAS media** (Fig. 17-3). Growth is initiated quickly on PRAS media, and many anaerobes produce sufficient growth to work with after only 24 hours of incubation.

> The ideal culture media for anaerobic bacteriology are freshly prepared media or PRAS media that have been prepared, packaged, shipped, and stored under anaerobic conditions.

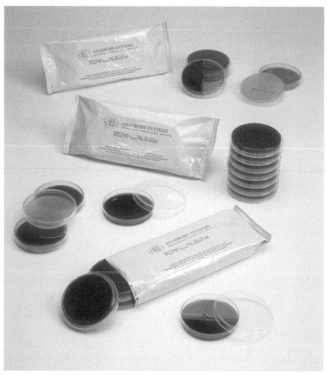

Figure 17-3. **Commercially available PRAS media for anaerobic bacteriology.** These media are prepared, packaged, shipped, and stored under anaerobic conditions. (Courtesy of Anaerobe Systems, Morgan Hill, CA.)

Another alternative is to use Oxyrase products, available from Oxyrase Inc., which can be used without an anaerobic chamber. According to the manufacturer of these products, "Oxyrase is an enzyme system that naturally, selectively, and efficiently removes oxygen from its environment."

Some CML professionals mistakenly believe that their media are performing well because they are routinely isolating *Bacteroides fragilis* and *Clostridium perfringens* from clinical specimens, and/or because their quality control strains of these particular anaerobes are growing well. However, these anaerobes are aerotolerant and will grow on media that *cannot* support the growth of strict obligate anaerobes. Routine recovery of anaerobic Gram-positive cocci, fusobacteria, and *Porphyromonas* spp. is a far better test of the suitability of media than recovery of the more aerotolerant *B. fragilis* and *C. perfringens*.

Recommendations of different authorities in the area of anaerobic bacteriology vary slightly with regard to specific media to be included in the primary setup of anaerobe cultures. The media shown in Table 17-5 are recommended in the Jousimies-Somer et al. manual (see "References and Suggested Reading").

In addition to the media listed in Table 17-5, an **egg yolk agar (EYA) plate** should be inoculated whenever clostridia are suspected, either clinically or as a result of Gram stain observations (i.e., the presence of large Gram-positive

TABLE 17 - 5	Culture Media for Anaerobic Bacteriology
Culture Medium	**Comments**
Brucella blood agar (BRU) plate	An enriched medium that, when incubated anaerobically, allows the growth of both obligate and facultative anaerobes. Contains 5% (v/v) sheep blood for enrichment and detection of hemolysis, vitamin K_1 (required by some of the pigmented *Porphyromonas* and *Prevotella* spp.), and hemin (which enhances growth of certain *Bacteroides* species, including members of the *B. fragilis* group). BRU contains no inhibitory substances. Similar excellent media (e.g., CDC anaerobe blood agar, enriched brain heart infusion blood agar, Schaedler blood agar, and FAA blood agar) are also available for recovering anaerobes from clinical specimens. The abbreviation **BRU/BA** is to be used throughout the chapter in reference to any of these acceptable anaerobic blood agars.
Bacteroides bile esculin agar (BBE) plate	Included in the primary setup mainly for the rapid isolation and presumptive identification of members of the *B. fragilis* group. Frequently, such a presumptive identification can be made after only 24 hours of incubation. BBE contains gentamicin, which inhibits most aerobic organisms, and 20% bile, which inhibits most other anaerobes. This medium supports the growth of bile-resistant *Bacteroides* species but not bile-sensitive species. Some strains of *Fusobacterium mortiferum*, *F. varium*, gentamicin-resistant members of the family Enterobacteriaceae, enterococci, pseudomonads, staphylococci, and yeast may grow to a limited extent on this medium, producing colonies much smaller than those of *Bacteroides*. Members of the *B. fragilis* group will turn the light yellow medium to brown as a result of esculin hydrolysis. BBE agar is also useful for isolation of *Bilophila wadsworthia*, which usually produces black-centered colonies on the medium because of H_2S production.
Laked blood-kanamycin-vancomycin (LKV) agar plate	Highly selective for obligately anaerobic and aerotolerant, Gram-negative bacilli, especially *Bacteroides* and *Prevotella* species. The presence of laked blood allows earlier detection of pigmented colonies of *Prevotella* spp. than does BRU/BA. Kanamycin inhibits most other Gram-negative bacilli, but yeasts and kanamycin-resistant organisms will grow on LKV. Vancomycin inhibits most Gram-positive organisms and *Porphyromonas* spp. A similar medium that substitutes paromomycin for kanamycin inhibits any kanamycin-resistant, facultatively anaerobic Gram-negative bacilli that might be present in the specimen.
Phenylethyl alcohol (PEA) agar (also called phenylethanol agar or phenethylalcohol agar) plate	The primary purpose of this medium is to inhibit facultative Gram-negative bacilli (e.g., the Enterobacteriaceae). Thus, a swarming *Proteus* species that would swarm over the surface of the BRU/BA plate would be inhibited on this medium. Most obligate anaerobes (both Gram positive and Gram negative) will grow on PEA, as will Gram-positive facultative anaerobes. PEA prevents *Clostridium septicum* from swarming.
Thioglycollate broth (THIO)	Thioglycollate broth supports the growth of most anaerobes. Anaerobes present in the broth can, however, be overgrown by more rapidly growing facultative organisms that thrive in THIO. Further, the anaerobes could be killed by toxic metabolic byproducts produced by the facultative organisms. Thus, broth cultures should *never* be relied on exclusively for the isolation of anaerobes from clinical specimens. The sole purpose of inoculating a broth medium is to provide a *backup* source of culture material. In the event of an anaerobic jar failure, for example, the broth culture could serve as a backup. Or, in the event of inhibition of growth on plated media because of antimicrobial agents present in the specimen, the broth culture could serve as a backup; the antimicrobial agents would be diluted in the broth to the point that they are no longer effective. To improve recovery of anaerobes, some manufacturers produce THIO containing supplements such as vitamin K_1 and hemin. On the day of use, THIO tubes should be placed in a boiling water bath to drive off oxygen and then cooled to 25°C to 35°C before inoculation. Chopped meat carbohydrate broth can be used in place of thioglycollate broth.

bacilli, with or without spores). EYA is useful for detecting enzymes produced by some clostridia—namely, lecithinase, lipase, and proteolytic enzymes (discussed in more detail later in the chapter).

In most CMLs, *Clostridium difficile*–associated diseases, such as antibiotic-associated diarrhea (AAD) and pseudomembranous colitis (PMC), are diagnosed by toxin assay (described later in the chapter). However, in CMLs that do not perform toxin assays, fecal specimens from patients suspected of having AAD and/or PMC can be inoculated to either a **cycloserine-cefoxitin-fructose agar (CCFA) plate** or a **cefoxitin-cycloserine-egg yolk (CCEY) agar plate.** CCFA is a selective and differential medium for recovery and presumptive identification of *C. difficile*. On CCFA, *C. difficile* produces large, yellow, ground-glass colonies, and the originally pink-colored agar turns yellow in the vicinity of the colonies. *C. difficile* colonies on CCEY agar are irregular and grayish. After some time, the colonies have white centers and fluoresce bright chartreuse under long-wave ultraviolet light. *C. difficile* colonies produce a characteristic "horse stable" odor. In addition to the thioglycollate broth and plated media to be incubated anaerobically, various plated media are inoculated and incubated in a CO_2 incubator for recovery of any aerobic organisms that might be present in the specimen.

Anaerobic Incubation

After specimens are rapidly processed and inoculated onto and into appropriate media, the inoculated plates must be incubated anaerobically at 35°C to 37°C. The three most common and most practical choices of anaerobic incubation systems for CMLs are

> Anaerobic incubation can be achieved using anaerobic jars, anaerobic bags or pouches, or anaerobic chambers.

- anaerobic chambers,

- anaerobic jars, and

- anaerobic bags or pouches.

The choice of system is influenced by several factors, including financial considerations, the number of anaerobic cultures performed, and space limitations.

Anaerobic chambers. The ideal anaerobic incubation system is an anaerobic chamber, which provides an environment free of oxygen that can be used for storing media, inoculating media, incubating cultures, and Gram staining of smears. Identification and susceptibility test systems can also be inoculated and incubated within the chamber, if necessary. Various anaerobic chambers are available commercially. Some models, called glove boxes, are fitted with airtight rubber gloves. Manufacturers of glove boxes include Coy Laboratory Products Inc. and Forma Scientific Inc. The

microbiologist inserts his or her arms into the gloves and manipulates specimens, plates, and tubes inside the chamber while wearing the gloves. Some users find the gloves bulky and difficult to work in. The gloves are often too large for their hands, manual dexterity is diminished, and the gloves frequently cause the user's hands to perspire. Some, but not all, of these problems can be overcome with experience. Traditionally, glove boxes have been constructed of flexible vinyl.

Gloveless anaerobic chambers are also available commercially (Sheldon Manufacturing Inc.). Airtight rubber sleeves that fit snugly against the user's bare forearms are used in place of gloves. This enables the microbiologist to work within an anaerobic environment with his or her bare hands. However, to comply with mandatory infectious disease safety precautions, it is recommended that thin, disposable, latex gloves be worn while clinical specimens are being processed within gloveless chambers. Subsequent manipulations may be performed without gloves.

Some gloveless models have a dissecting microscope mounted on the front of the rigid Plexiglass chamber (Fig. 17-4). This enables the user to observe colony morphology within the chamber, eliminating the need to remove plates from the chamber and eliminating exposure of the colonies to oxygen.

Anaerobic jars. For small laboratories, where the low volume of anaerobic cultures may not justify the purchase of

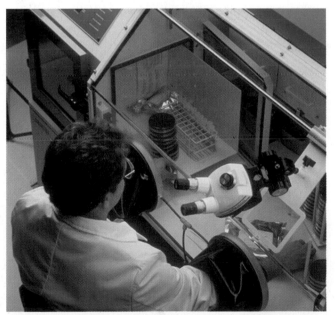

Figure 17-4. **Gloveless anaerobic chamber, manufactured by Sheldon Manufacturing Inc.** In place of rubber gloves are rubber sleeves, the ends of which fit snugly around the user's bare forearms. After the sleeves are flushed with an oxygen-free gas mixture (using foot pedals), the round port-hole-type entry doors are removed and placed inside the chamber. Instruments constantly monitor and adjust temperature and anaerobic conditions within the chamber. A high level of relative humidity is constantly maintained within the chamber. (Courtesy of Anaerobe Systems, Morgan Hill, CA.)

anaerobic chambers, alternative systems are available. These systems do not provide all the features or advantages of anaerobic chambers and, depending on the number of anaerobic cultures performed, cost analyses may reveal that, over time, a chamber is actually more cost-effective.

One such alternative is the anaerobic jar (Fig. 17-5). These jars have been used in clinical laboratories for many years, enabling even small laboratories to perform satisfactory anaerobic bacteriology. Some anaerobic jars accommodate a large number of plates as well as microtiter antimicrobial susceptibility trays and anaerobe identification strips and trays. Anaerobic jars are available from BD Biosciences, Almar, BBL, EM Science, Key Scientific, Mitsubishi, Oxoid, and other companies.

The major disadvantage of any anaerobic jar system is that the plates have to be removed from the jar for them to be examined. This, of course, exposes the colonies to oxygen, which is especially hazardous to the anaerobes during the first 48 hours of growth. A suitable anaerobic holding system should always be used in conjunction with anaerobic jars. Plates can be removed from the anaerobic jar, placed in an oxygen-free holding jar, removed one by one for rapid microscopic examination of colonies, Gram staining, and so forth, and then quickly placed into another holding jar. Plates should *never* remain in room air on the open bench.

When water is added to the GasPak envelope (BD Biosciences), two gases are generated: carbon dioxide and hydrogen. The carbon dioxide is important because some anaerobes require an increased concentration of CO_2 for growth (i.e., they are capnophiles). In the presence of a catalyst, the hydrogen generated combines with the oxygen in the jar to form water vapor.

A methylene blue indicator strip is always added to the jar to verify that an anaerobic atmosphere was truly achieved. If the catalyst performed correctly, water vapor will be present on the inside of the jar when the jar is removed from the incubator, and the indicator strip will be colorless. Some gas-generating packets contain a built-in indicator.

When using an anaerobic chamber or jar containing a reusable palladium catalyst, it is important to remember that, with time, the catalyst becomes inactivated by water and hydrogen sulfide. Thus, the catalyst must be periodically tested, cleaned, and reactivated. Reactivation is accomplished by heating the catalyst at 160°C for 2 hours. The catalyst can

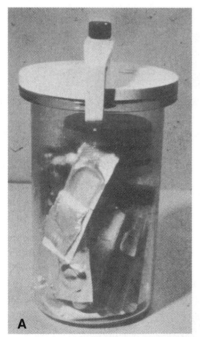
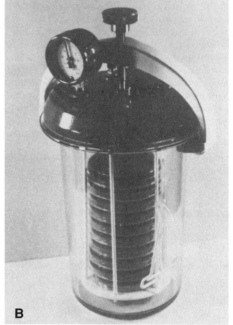

Figure 17-5. **Anaerobic jars. A.** The GasPak system (BD Biosciences). **B.** The Oxoid anaerobic jar (Oxoid USA). Inoculated plates, gas-generating envelopes, and an indicator strip are placed within the jar. Anaerobic jars contain fresh or rejuvenated catalyst pellets. Many of the commercially available gas-generating packets contain a built-in catalyst and/or indicator. Water is added to the packet, the jar is sealed, and carbon dioxide and hydrogen gases are released from the packet. If the catalyst is performing properly, the hydrogen combines with the oxygen in the jar to form water vapor. The indicator strip lets the user know that anaerobic conditions were achieved. Failure to achieve anaerobic conditions could be the result of "poisoned" catalyst or a crack in the jar, lid, or O-ring. It is important to remember that the gas-generating packets generate hydrogen gas, which is explosive. Should the catalyst not function properly, there will be hydrogen gas in the jar. Thus, the jar should never be opened in the vicinity of a Bunsen burner flame. (From Winn WC Jr, et al. Koneman's Color Atlas and Textbook of Diagnostic Microbiology. 6th Ed. Philadelphia: Lippincott Williams & Wilkins, 2006.)

be tested by flowing the anaerobic gas mixture (containing 5% hydrogen) over the catalyst in room air. If the catalyst produces heat, then it is active. If, however, no heat is produced, the catalyst should be cleaned. Cleaning is accomplished by first heating the catalyst to 200°C and then flowing the anaerobic gas mixture over the catalyst in room air while the catalyst is hot. The palladium catalyst should be reactivated after each use.

Anaerobic bags or pouches. Other alternatives to an anaerobic chamber are anaerobic bags or pouches, such as those produced by BBL, Mitsubishi, Oxoid, Hardy Diagnostics, Merck, and other companies (Fig. 17-6). These

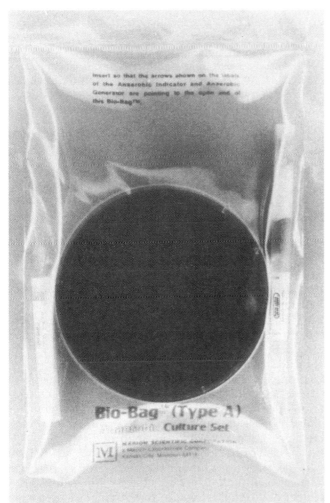

Figure 17-6. **Anaerobic bag (Bio-Bag, BD Biosciences).** After inoculated plates are added to the bag, an oxygen removal system is initiated. The bag is then tightly sealed and placed into a nonanaerobic incubator. Some bags permit observation of growth directly through the plastic, thus eliminating the need to remove plates from the bags to make such observations. Identification and susceptibility systems requiring anaerobic incubation can also be incubated within some bags. Bags can be used to transport specimens anaerobically to the laboratory. (From Winn WC Jr, et al. Koneman's Color Atlas and Textbook of Diagnostic Microbiology. 6th Ed. Philadelphia: Lippincott Williams & Wilkins, 2006.)

products are, in this chapter, collectively referred to as bags. One or two inoculated plates are placed into a bag, an oxygen removal system is activated, and the bag is sealed and incubated. Theoretically, the plates can be examined for growth without removing the plates from the bags, thereby preventing exposure of the colonies to oxygen. However, with some of the products, a water vapor film on the inner surface of the bag or the lid of the plate can sometimes obscure vision. In such cases the plates must be removed from the bag for observation of growth, and a new bag and oxygen removal system must be used whenever additional incubation is required. As with the anaerobic jar, plates must be removed from the bags before work with the colonies can proceed at the bench. Thus, an anaerobic holding jar system should always be used in conjunction with any anaerobic bag.

Bags are useful as transport devices. For example, a biopsy specimen could first be placed in a sterile Petri dish containing sterile saline. The petri dish could then be placed into one of these bags, the oxygen removal system activated, and the specimen carefully transported to the laboratory within the bag. Obviously, the petri dish should be held horizontally enroute to the laboratory to avoid spilling the contents.

Evacuation-replacement system. An alternative to an anaerobic chamber, jar, or bag is the use of an evacuation-replacement system. In such a system, air is removed from a sealed jar and replaced with an oxygen-free gas (usually N_2). The oxygen-free gas is replaced several times before finally being replaced with a gas mixture containing 80% to 90% N_2, 5% to 10% H_2, and 5% to 10% CO_2. An evacuation-replacement system produces anaerobic conditions more quickly than does an anaerobic jar or bag. One commercial evacuation-replacement system available is the Anoxomat, from Mart Microbiology BV.

WORKUP OF ANAEROBIC ISOLATES

When Should the Primary Plates Be Examined?

The first major decision in the examination of primary plates is *when* to examine them. Although plates being incubated in an anaerobic chamber can be safely examined at any time, opening an anaerobic jar or bag exposes colonies to the potentially damaging effects of oxygen.

The question is, Should jars or bags be opened after 24 or after 48 hours of incubation? Some of the slower-growing anaerobes will be too small to work with at 24 hours. However, many of the more rapidly growing pathogenic anaerobes, such as some *Clostridium* and *Bacteroides* spp., could be worked up at 24 hours, especially when appropriate PRAS media are used for the primary setup. Thus, waiting

TABLE 17 - 6 Indications of the Presence of Anaerobes

Indication	Comments
A foul odor when the anaerobic jar or bag is opened	Some anaerobes, especially *Clostridium difficile*, fusobacteria, and *Porphyromonas* spp., produce foul-smelling metabolic end products that are readily apparent when the jars or bags are opened.
Colony morphotypes that are present on the anaerobically incubated blood agar plates, but not on the CO_2-incubated blood or chocolate agar plates	These are probably anaerobes.
Good growth (gray colonies >1 mm in diameter) on the BBE plate	Indicative of members of the *Bacteroides fragilis* group.
Colonies on either the LKV or BRU/BA agar plate that fluoresce brick red under ultraviolet light or are brown to black in ordinary light	Indicative of pigmented species of *Porphyromonas* and *Prevotella*.

until 48 hours to open jars or bags could delay the identification of clinically important anaerobes by a day.

If an anaerobic holding system (described earlier) is available at the anaerobe workstation and is used in conjunction with jars or bags, exposure to oxygen will be minimized and plates can be examined as early as 24 hours. Each plate is removed from the jar or bag, *rapidly* examined for growth, and placed *immediately* into an oxygen-free holding system. Plates are then removed one-by-one from the holding system, colonies are examined quickly using a dissecting microscope, Gram-stained, and so forth, and plates are *promptly* returned to the holding system following examination. As soon as all plates are examined, those requiring additional incubation are returned to an anaerobic system and incubated for an appropriate time before reexamination of the plates.

Indications of the Presence of Anaerobes on Primary Plates

Table 17-6 contains some of the findings or observations that should alert CML professionals that anaerobes may be present on the primary plates.

Examination of Plates Included in the Primary Setup

Table 17-7 provides information concerning the examination of plates that were included in the primary setup.

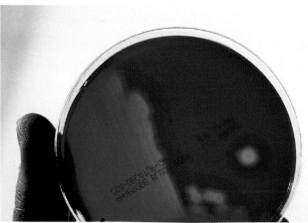

Figure 17-8. **The double zone of hemolysis produced by** *Clostridium perfringens*: **a narrow inner zone of complete hemolysis surrounded by a wider outer zone of partial hemolysis.** (From Winn WC Jr, et al. Koneman's Color Atlas and Textbook of Diagnostic Microbiology. 6th Ed. Philadelphia: Lippincott Williams & Wilkins, 2006.)

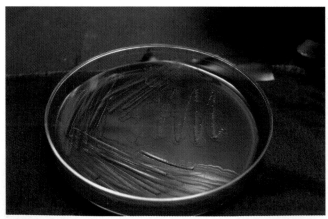

Figure 17-7. **Pitting colonies of** *Bacteroides ureolyticus*. (Courtesy of Anaerobe Systems, Morgan Hill, CA.)

TABLE 17 - 7	Examination of Plates Included in the Primary Setup

Plate	Comments
BRU/BA plate	Anaerobically incubated BRU/BA plates support the growth of facultative anaerobes, as well as anaerobes. Thus, not all colonies appearing on the plate are anaerobes. Aerotolerance testing (described later in the chapter) must be performed on each colony type to determine if it is truly an anaerobe. Table 17-8 describes procedures to be performed on each colony morphotype present on the BRU/BA agar plate. The BRU/BA agar plate should be examined for evidence of pitting, swarming, hemolysis, and discoloration of the medium (greening, browning, etc.). Pitting anaerobic Gram-negative bacilli include *Bacteroides ureolyticus*, *B. gracilis*, *Campylobacter curvus*, and *C. rectus*; pitting is depicted in Figure 17-7. Swarming anaerobic Gram-positive bacilli include *Clostridium septicum* and *C. tetani*. A double zone of hemolysis (an inner zone of complete β-hemolysis and an outer zone of partial hemolysis) is characteristic of *C. perfringens*; this double zone of hemolysis is shown in Figure 17-8. Characteristic colonies and morphologic features in Gram-stained preparations of selected anaerobes are described in Table 17-8. A BRU/BA subculture plate is inoculated for the aerotolerance test, and appropriate disks (described in a later section) are added to this subculture plate.
BBE plate	The primary purpose for including the BBE plate in the primary setup is the rapid (often 24-hour) presumptive identification of the *B. fragilis* group. If members of this group are present, the gray colonies are a minimum of 1 mm in diameter, and the originally light yellow medium is usually brown in the area around the colonies. A presumptive identification of *B. fragilis* group can be made at this point. Good growth is the result of bile resistance, and browning of the medium is caused by esculin hydrolysis. The appearance of *B. fragilis* group organisms on BBE is depicted in Figure 17-9. Although *B. vulgatus* is a member of the *B. fragilis* group, it does not hydrolyze esculin and thus does not produce a brown discoloration of the medium. Although *B. splanchnicus* is not a member of the *B. fragilis* group, it is bile resistant and esculin hydrolysis positive; thus, colonies of *B. splanchnicus* have the same appearance on BBE as members of the *B. fragilis* group. Depending on the commercial source, age, and storage conditions of the medium, other organisms (e.g., *Fusobacterium mortiferum*, *F. varium*, *Klebsiella pneumoniae*, enterococci, pseudomonads, staphylococci, yeast) may also grow on BBE. The colony size of these other organisms is less than 1 mm in diameter, and Gram staining and aerotolerance testing aid in their recognition. *Bilophila wadsworthia* produces colonies with black centers on BBE as a result of H_2S production.
LKV plate	Although most *Bacteroides* and *Prevotella* spp. grow on LKV, this medium is included in the primary isolation setup to accelerate the production of pigment by certain species of *Prevotella*. The appearance of such organisms on LKV or BRU/BA is shown in Figure 17-10. Darkening of the colonies may not always occur by 48 hours, and some strains may require up to three weeks or more before pigmentation is observed. For this reason, nonpigmented colonies on LKV or BRU/BA should always be subjected to long-wave ultraviolet light (such as a Wood's lamp). Although some pigmented species of *Porphyromonas* and *Prevotella* fluoresce colors other than brick red (e.g., brilliant red, yellow, orange, and pink-orange) and some do not fluoresce at all (e.g., *Porphyromonas gingivalis*), a brick-red (red-brown to red-orange) fluorescence allows presumptive identification of members of this group. The brick-red fluorescence of members of this group under ultraviolet light is shown in Figure 17-11. Organisms other than *Bacteroides* and *Prevotella* sometimes grow on LKV (including some yeasts); therefore, Gram staining and aerotolerance testing of colonies are absolutely necessary. Most *Porphyromonas* strains are inhibited by the vancomycin in LKV agar.
PEA plate	Essentially all anaerobes (Gram positive as well as Gram negative) grow on anaerobically incubated PEA, and in most cases, their colony appearance is identical to that on BRU/BA plates. Gram-positive facultative anaerobes also grow on PEA. The sole reason for including a PEA plate in the primary setup is to inhibit growth of Enterobacteriaceae, especially species of swarming *Proteus*. When *Proteus* is present in the specimen, it often swarms over the entire surface of the BRU/BA plate, thus making it impossible to work with other colonies. PEA inhibits the growth of *Proteus* species, permitting the CML professional to work on other colony morphotypes that are present.

(continued)

TABLE 17 - 7	Examination of Plates Included in the Primary Setup (Continued)
Plate	**Comments**
Egg yolk agar (EYA) plate	The EYA plate should be examined for lecithinase, lipase, and proteolytic reactions. Certain clostridia produce enzymes that cause these reactions, but so do a few organisms other than *Clostridium* spp. **Lecithinase reaction.** A colony of a lecithinase-positive organism is surrounded by a wide zone of opacity. This opacity is actually in the medium and is not a surface phenomenon. The appearance of the lecithinase reaction is shown in Figure 17-12. Examples of lecithinase-positive clostridia are *C. bifermentans*, *C. sordellii*, *C. perfringens*, *C. novyi* type A, and *C. baratii*. **Lipase reaction.** A colony of a lipase-positive organism is covered with an iridescent, multicolored sheen, sometimes described as resembling the appearance of oil on water or mother-of-pearl. This multicolored sheen may also appear on the surface of the agar in a narrow zone around the colony. The lipase reaction occurs only at the agar surface, unlike the lecithinase reaction, which occurs within the medium. The appearance of the lipase reaction is shown in Figure 17-13. Examples of lipase-positive clostridia are *C. botulinum*, *C. novyi* type A, and *C. sporogenes*. Other anaerobes that are lipase positive include *Fusobacterium necrophorum*, *Prevotella intermedia*, and some isolates of *P. loescheii*. **Proteolysis.** Organisms that produce proteolytic enzymes have a completely clear zone (often quite narrow) around colonies. This is best observed by holding the plate up to a strong light source and is reminiscent of the complete clearing produced by β-hemolytic organisms on BRU/BA plates.
Cycloserine-cefoxitin-fructose (CCFA) plate	If the patient is suspected of having antibiotic-associated diarrhea (AAD) or pseudomembranous colitis (PMC), a CCFA plate might have been inoculated with a fecal specimen from that patient. CCFA is a selective and differential medium for recovery and presumptive identification of *Clostridium difficile*. *C. difficile* colonies on CCFA are yellow with a ground-glass appearance, and the originally pink-colored agar is yellow in the vicinity of the colonies. The appearance of *C. difficile* on CCFA is shown in Figure 17-14. Although other organisms may grow on CCFA, their colonies are smaller than and do not resemble the characteristic colonies of *C. difficile*. Also, *C. difficile* has a characteristic horse stable–like odor, and colonies on BRU/BA fluoresce chartreuse under ultraviolet light. It is important to note that isolation of this organism from fecal specimens is not always indicative of AAD or PMC, because *C. difficile* can be part of a patient's normal gastrointestinal flora. There are more accurate ways to diagnose AAD or PMC caused by *C. difficile*, including cytotoxin assays, enzyme immunoassays, and latex agglutination procedures. It is also important to realize that *C. difficile* is not the only cause of AAD and PMC.

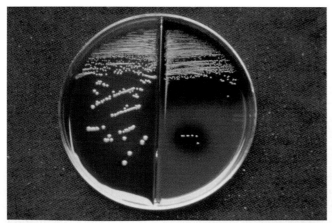

Figure 17-9. Bacteroides fragilis **growing on an LKV/BBE biplate.** Browning of the BBE agar in the vicinity of the colonies is the result of esculin hydrolysis. (Courtesy of Anaerobe Systems, Morgan Hill, CA.)

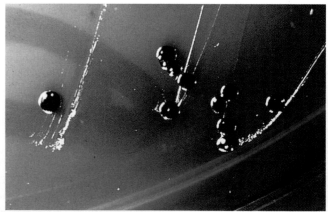

Figure 17-10. **Darkly pigmented colonies of *Prevotella melaninogenica* on blood agar after 5 days of incubation.** (From Winn WC Jr, et al. Koneman's Color Atlas and Textbook of Diagnostic Microbiology. 6th Ed. Philadelphia: Lippincott Williams & Wilkins, 2006.)

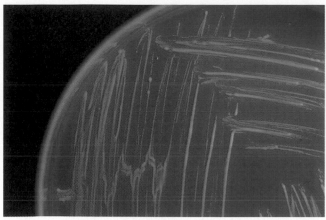

Figure 17-11. **Brick-red fluorescence of *Porphyromonas* colonies under long-wave ultraviolet light.** (Courtesy of Anaerobe Systems, Morgan Hill, CA.)

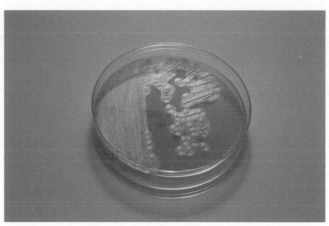

Figure 17-13. Fusobacterium necrophorum **colonies on egg yolk agar, illustrating a positive lipase reaction.** (Courtesy of Anaerobe Systems, Morgan Hill, CA.)

Processing Suspected Anaerobes

As previously mentioned, colonies growing on anaerobically incubated primary plates are only *suspected* of being anaerobes. They could be facultative anaerobes. They may, in fact, be the *same* organisms that are growing on the plates that were incubated in the CO_2 incubator. Thus, it is necessary to perform an **aerotolerance test** to confirm that they are anaerobes. In addition to aerotolerance testing, each colony morphotype[3] must be Gram stained and inoculated to a BRU/BA subculture plate. Table 17-8 summarizes the workup of each colony morphotype observed on the primary BRU/BA plate.

Aerotolerance Testing

The BRU/BA subculture plate serves as one of the plates used in the aerotolerance test. One or two additional plates are also needed. A chocolate agar plate will be incubated in a

CO_2 incubator. By marking the chocolate agar plate into sections, one plate can be used to test several different isolates. Some authorities recommend that a blood agar plate also be inoculated for incubation in a non-CO_2 incubator. This plate will enable differentiation between aerobic and capnophilic organisms. By marking the blood agar plate into sections, one plate can be used to test several different isolates.

All the aerotolerance test plates are then incubated appropriately for 24 to 48 hours. Following incubation, the aerotolerance test is interpreted in the following manner:

- Theoretically, an **anaerobe** should grow only on the anaerobically incubated BRU/BA plate. Remember, though, that some aerotolerant anaerobes, like certain *Clostridium, Actinomyces, Propionibacterium, Bifidobacterium,* and *Lactobacillus* species, are capable of growing on the CO_2-incubated chocolate agar plate. Anaerobes usually grow *better*, however, on the anaerobically incubated plate. The catalase test is useful for distinguishing

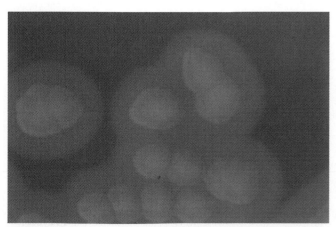

Figure 17-12. Clostridium bifermentans **on egg yolk agar, illustrating a positive lecithinase reaction.** (Courtesy of Anaerobe Systems, Morgan Hill, CA.)

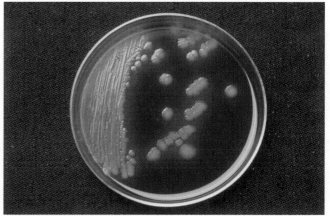

Figure 17-14. Clostridium difficile **colonies on CCFA agar.** (Courtesy of Anaerobe Systems, Morgan Hill, CA.)

---

[3]*The term* colony morphotype *refers to a colony having a particular appearance. In general, different bacterial species produce different colony morphotypes.*

TABLE 17 - 8	Procedures to Be Performed on Each Colony Morphotype Observed on the Primary BRU/BA Plate
Procedure	**Comments**
Describe colony morphology	Colonies should be examined using either a dissecting microscope or a magnifying glass. Each colony morphotype should be enumerated, described, and Gram stained, and all observations should be recorded on some type of worksheet. Growth of a particular morphotype can be semiquantitated using the terms *light*, *moderate*, or *heavy* or by using some type of coding system (e.g., 1+, 2+, 3+, 4+). Descriptions of each colony morphotype should include features such as **color or pigment** (e.g., pigmented species of *Porphyromonas* and *Prevotella* produce brown-black colonies; *Actinomyces* colonies may be red, pink, tan, yellow); **surface** (e.g., glistening, dull); **density** (e.g., opaque, translucent, transparent; members of the *B. ureolyticus* group typically have translucent to transparent colonies); **consistency** (e.g., butyrous [buttery], viscous, membranous, brittle); **form, elevation, margin** (see Chapter 8); **fluorescence** under ultraviolet light (e.g., pigmented species of *Porphyromonas* and *Prevotella* often fluoresce brick red; *F. nucleatum* and *C. difficile* fluoresce chartreuse; some species of *Veillonella* fluoresce red); **pitting of the agar** (e.g., caused by *B. ureolyticus* and *B. gracilis*); **double zone of hemolysis** (most strains of *C. perfringens* produce a narrow inner zone of complete β-hemolysis and a wider outer zone of incomplete hemolysis); **swarming** (e.g., *C. tetani* and *C. septicum* frequently swarm over the entire surface of the plate); some anaerobes have a characteristic **odor** (e.g., *C. difficile* has a horse stable odor; *P. anaerobius* has a sweet, unpleasant odor); young *Actinomyces israelii* and *Propionibacterium propionicus* colonies often appear as thin masses of wooly filaments originating at a single point (referred to as **spider colonies**); older colonies often resemble a molar tooth in appearance (**molar tooth colonies**; Fig. 17-15); some strains of *F. nucleatum* produce white **bread crumb–like colonies**; other strains produce colonies having a **ground-glass appearance** (referred to by some authors as speckled opalescence or internal flecking) when viewed under a dissecting microscope; colonies of *F. mortiferum* and *F. varium* typically have a **fried-egg appearance** (this characteristic is not specific for these organisms, however).
Prepare a Gram-stained smear of a portion of the colony; describe Gram reaction and cellular morphology	Is the organism Gram positive, Gram negative, or Gram variable? Some Gram-positive organisms (e.g., *Clostridium ramosum* and *C. clostridiiforme*) routinely stain Gram negative. Is the organism a coccus? Are the cocci arranged singly, in pairs (diplococci), in tetrads, in clusters, or in chains? Are they especially large (like *Finegoldia magna*)? Are they especially small (like *Micromonas micros* and *Veillonella* spp.)? Is the organism a bacillus? If Gram positive, are the cells branched (*Actinomyces*-like)? Are they diphtheroid in appearance (like *Propionibacterium* spp.)? Are they large (*Clostridium*-like)? Remember that not all clostridia are large. Are the ends of the cells bifurcated, or forked (like some *Actinomyces* and *Bifidobacterium* spp.)? Are the cells beaded? Is there evidence of spores? If Gram negative, are they coccobacilli? Are they curved? Are they pleomorphic? Are there bizarre forms (swellings and balloon forms)? Are they filamentous? Are they safety pin–like (bipolar staining)? Are they long and thin and tapered at the ends, or fusiform (like *Fusobacterium nucleatum*)?
Inoculate pure culture or subculture plate	A portion of the colony is inoculated to a BRU/BA subculture plate to obtain well-isolated colonies. Following anaerobic incubation, this plate serves as a pure culture of the organism.
Add appropriate disks to the pure culture or subculture plate	Based on the Gram reaction and cellular morphology of the organism, certain disks are added to the BRU/BA subculture plate prior to anaerobic incubation. The disks are placed on the heavily inoculated area of the plate—usually, the first quarter or first third of the plate, depending on the particular manner of streaking (see Fig. 17-16). The specific disks to be added are shown in Table 17-9. In many cases, disk results will enable presumptive identification of the organisms.
Set up an aerotolerance test	Described in the section titled "Aerotolerance Testing."

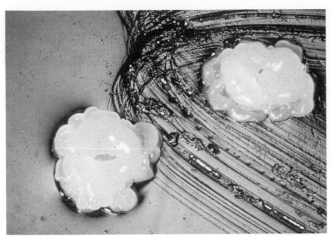

Figure 17-15. **Characteristic "molar tooth" colonies of *Actinomyces israelii*.** (From Winn WC Jr, et al. Koneman's Color Atlas and Textbook of Diagnostic Microbiology. 6th Ed. Philadelphia: Lippincott Williams & Wilkins, 2006.)

between *Bacillus* spp. (aerobic, spore-forming Gram-positive bacilli) and aerotolerant species of *Clostridium*. Most *Bacillus* spp. are catalase positive, whereas most *Clostridium* spp. are catalase negative. In addition, *Bacillus* species sporulate aerobically, whereas *Clostridium* species form spores only under anaerobic conditions.

- A **noncapnophilic, facultative organism** will grow on all three plates.

- A **capnophilic organism (capnophile)** will grow on the CO_2-incubated chocolate agar plate but not on the aerobically incubated blood agar plate. It may or may not grow on the anaerobically incubated BRU/BA plate. *Haemophilus influenzae*, for example, will grow on the BRU/BA and CO_2-incubated chocolate agar plates but not on the aerobically incubated blood agar plate.

Review of Anaerobe Processing Procedures

Whenever a colony is suspected of being an anaerobe, the colony morphology should first be described on a worksheet. A portion of the colony should then be Gram stained, and observations should be recorded. A portion of the

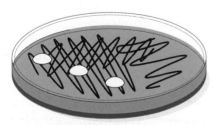

Figure 17-16. **Placement of special-potency antimicrobial disks on the BRU/BA subculture plate.**

colony must be streaked for isolation on a BRU/BA subculture plate; and based on the Gram reaction and morphology of the organism, appropriate disks are added to the BRU/BA subculture plate. Additional plates are inoculated as part of the aerotolerance test, and these are incubated appropriately. Finally, if clostridia are suspected (based on Gram stain appearance), an EYA plate should be inoculated. Remember that some aerotolerant anaerobes are capable of growing on the CO_2-incubated chocolate agar plate, and these can be confusing. However, these organisms grow better anaerobically than they do in the CO_2 atmosphere.

METHODS FOR IDENTIFICATION OF ANAEROBIC ISOLATES

Presumptive Identifications

Presumptive identifications (presumptive IDs) of microorganisms have become more popular in recent years, primarily because of increased emphasis on speed and cost reduction. Some presumptive ID methods for aerobic bacteria have already been discussed—for example, *Streptococcus pyogenes* (see Chapter 9), *Escherichia coli* and swarming species of *Proteus* (see Chapter 12), and *Pseudomonas aeruginosa* (see Chapter 13). Although many laboratories base their identifications of these organisms on presumptive ID criteria, others perform the additional procedures necessary for definitive identification (definitive ID).

Presumptive IDs of many anaerobes are also possible. As with the previously mentioned examples from the aerobic bacteriology laboratory, the decision whether presumptive IDs will suffice or definitive IDs are necessary is the responsibility of the individual laboratory. By combining readily observable colony and Gram stain features with results of simple test procedures, even small CMLs are capable of making presumptive IDs of many commonly isolated and clinically important anaerobes. It is important to remember, however, that many anaerobes *cannot* be identified using presumptive ID criteria. Definitive ID procedures are described in a subsequent section.

Because of the excellent tools available, even small CMLs can isolate anaerobes from clinical specimens, use special media, perform Gram staining, inoculate BRU/BA subculture plates, use the previously mentioned disks, and perform simple tests such as catalase, spot indole, and others described later in the chapter. As discussed in an upcoming section, it is even possible for small CMLs to perform susceptibility testing of important anaerobic isolates.

Listed here are simple observations and inexpensive tests that can be used to presumptively identify many of the anaerobes most commonly encountered in clinical specimens. Rather than using overnight tests that merely provide presumptive IDs, CML professionals might prefer to use one of the commercial identification systems that provide

same-day definitive IDs. Here the requirement for speed must be weighed against cost. The decision to use the more expensive commercial identification systems is one that must be made independently by each laboratory.

Simple Observations

- **Growth/no growth on selective media** (e.g., BBE, LKV, CCFA) and non-selective media (e.g., BRU/BA)
- **Colony morphology,** including color or pigment, surface, density, consistency, form, elevation, margin, pitting, hemolysis, swarming, and odor
- **Gram reaction and cell morphology**

Inexpensive Tests

- **Results of aerotolerance testing**
- **Fluorescence under long-wave (366-nm) ultraviolet light**
- **Special-potency antimicrobial disk results.** It is critical to use disks of the prescribed potency: a 5-μg vancomycin disk, a 10-μg colistin disk, and a 1-mg (1,000-μg)

kanamycin disk. Disks must be pressed firmly to the surface of the BRU/BA subculture plate to ensure uniform diffusion of the agent into the medium. Disk results are analyzed as shown in Table 17-10. It is important to understand that these disks give no information about antimicrobial agents that might be used for therapy.

- **Sodium polyanethol sulfonate (SPS) disk result.** As shown in Table 17-9, an SPS disk is added to the BRU/BA subculture plate whenever the Gram stain reveals the isolate to be a Gram-positive coccus. The SPS disk is especially valuable for presumptive identification of *Peptostreptococcus anaerobius*, which is susceptible to SPS.
- **Nitrate disk.** The nitrate disk is used to determine an organism's ability to reduce nitrate to nitrite. The test is a "miniaturized" version of the conventional nitrate reduction test used in the aerobic bacteriology laboratory.
- **Bile disk.** A bile disk can be used to determine an organism's ability to grow in the presence of relatively high (20%) concentrations of bile. As shown in Table 17-9, a bile disk can be added to the BRU/BA subculture plate whenever the Gram stain reveals the isolate to be a Gram-negative bacillus. Other indicators of bile resistance

TABLE 17 - 9   Disks to Add to the BRU/BA Subculture Plate

Gram Reaction and Morphology	Disk(s) to Add	Comments
Gram-positive coccus	SPS disk, nitrate disk	*SPS* is the acronym for sodium polyanethol sulfonate. This disk is useful in the presumptive identification of *Peptostreptococcus anaerobius*, which is susceptible to this substance.
Clostridium-like Gram-positive bacillus	No disks	The term *Clostridium-like* refers to large, unbranched, Gram-positive bacilli, with or without spores. (It is important to note, however, that not all clostridia are large, and not all clostridia stain Gram positive.)
Branching or diphtheroidal Gram-positive bacillus	Nitrate disk	The term *diphtheroidal* refers to organisms that morphologically resemble *Corynebacterium diphtheriae* (see Chapter 10).
Gram-negative coccus	Nitrate disk	
Gram-negative bacillus	5-μg vancomycin disk, 1-mg kanamycin disk, 10-μg colistin disk, nitrate disk, bile disk	The vancomycin, kanamycin, and colistin disks are referred to as special-potency antimicrobial disks. These disks aid in determining the *true* Gram reaction of a pink-staining bacillus. Although they are technically considered Gram-positive organisms, some clostridia routinely stain pink. If the organism is truly Gram negative, the special-potency antimicrobial disks also aid in differentiating the genus *Fusobacterium* from other genera of anaerobic Gram-negative bacilli.

	Interpretation of Special-Potency Antimicrobial Disk Results		
TABLE 17 - 10			
Vancomycin Result	**Kanamycin Result**	**Colistin Result**	**Interpretation**
Susceptible	Variable	Resistant	Probably a pink-staining Gram-positive bacillus; however, if the organism is resistant to kanamycin, it could be a *Porphyromonas* species
Susceptible	Resistant	Resistant	*Porphyromonas* species
Resistant	Resistant	Resistant	Probably a member of the *Bacteroides fragilis* group, but could be a *Prevotella* species
Resistant	Resistant	Variable	*Prevotella* species
Resistant	Resistant	Susceptible	Probably a *Prevotella* species
Resistant	Susceptible	Susceptible	Could be *Bacteroides ureolyticus*, *Bilophila wadsworthia*, or a *Fusobacterium* spp.; *Veillonella* spp. (Gram-negative cocci) will also produce these results

Table used with permission of the Colorado Association for Continuing Medical Laboratory Education, Denver, CO.

include good growth on the BBE plate and growth in 20% bile broth.

- **Catalase test.** Using a plastic, disposable inoculating loop or a wooden applicator stick, some of the growth is removed from the BRU/BA subculture plate and rubbed onto a small area of a glass microscope slide. Care must be taken not to transfer any of the agar, because sheep red blood cells contain catalase that might cause a false-positive test result. A drop of 15% aqueous hydrogen peroxide (equal parts of 30% hydrogen peroxide and type I reagent grade water) is added. The presence of gas bubbles (oxygen) indicates a positive test, whereas the absence of gas bubbles constitutes a negative test. Along with other uses, the catalase test is of value in differentiating aerotolerant strains of *Clostridium* spp. (catalase negative) from *Bacillus* spp. (catalase positive).

- **Spot indole test.** A small piece of filter paper is saturated with the spot indole reagent (1% p-dimethylaminocinnamaldehyde in 10% [v/v] concentrated HCl; DMACA). (Note: This is the only type of indole reagent to be used when testing anaerobes; this is *not* Kovac reagent.) Using an inoculating loop, some of the growth is removed from the BRU/BA subculture plate and rubbed onto the saturated area. (The growth medium must contain an adequate amount of tryptophan.) Rapid development of a blue-to-green color within 20 seconds indicates a positive test (i.e., production of indole from the amino acid tryptophan), whereas a pink-to-orange color indicates a negative test. (Note: Colonies located

less than 5 mm from different colony morphotypes should not be selected for testing. Indole can diffuse to adjacent colonies that are within 5 mm of a 2- to 3-mm-diameter colony, giving false-positive results.) Do not use growth from a plate containing a nitrate disk, as it may cause a false-negative indole result.

- **Motility test.** Motility may be determined using either very young (4 to 6 hours old) broth cultures or 24-to-48-hour-old colonies on BRU/BA. Motile Gram-negative anaerobes include *Mobiluncus* species, *Campylobacter concisus*, *C. curvus*, and *C. rectus*, among many others. Remember that *Mobiluncus* spp. are actually Gram-positive organisms, even though they stain pink with Gram staining.

- **Lecithinase and lipase reactions.** An egg yolk agar plate is used to determine the activities of these enzymes. Lecithinase and lipase reactions are of value in the identification of many species of *Clostridium*, as well as lipase-positive strains of *Prevotella intermedia*, *P. loescheii*, and *Fusobacterium necrophorum*. The opaque lecithinase reaction occurs within the medium in a relatively wide zone around colonies, whereas the lipase reaction occurs on the surfaces of colonies and on the agar surface in a relatively narrow zone around the colonies.

- **Urease test.** The ability of anaerobes to hydrolyze urea can be determined in various ways, including rapid tube, disk, and spot tests. Perhaps the easiest way to test for urease is by using Urea Differentiation Disks (Difco Laboratories). A loopful of organisms from the BRU/BA subculture plate is first suspended in a small volume of sterile water. Following addition of the urea disk, the tube is incubated for up to 4 hours. A color change from pale yellow to dark pink represents a positive test. The disk method is accurate and does not require preparation of reagents. Urease production can also be detected by anaerobic incubation of urea agar slants.

- **Oxidase test.** Kovac oxidase reagent (tetramethyl-p-phenylenediamine dihydrochloride [1% w/v]) in sterile distilled water can be used to detect the enzyme cytochrome oxidase, which is produced by a small number of anaerobes. A piece of filter paper is moistened with the reagent. With a bacteriological loop, a portion of a nonpigmented colony is rubbed onto the moistened filter paper. Development of a dark blue to purple color within 10 seconds indicates the presence of cytochrome oxidase. Formation of a white-yellow color or absence of color indicates a negative test result.

CML professionals should keep in mind that presumptive IDs are *not* definitive IDs. Because they are often based solely on morphologic characteristics and relatively few test results, presumptive IDs may be incorrect. Nevertheless, identifications based on presumptive ID criteria are rapid, relatively inexpensive, and generally correct.

> Presumptive identification of anaerobes is based on cellular and colonial morphologic characteristics and relatively few test results.

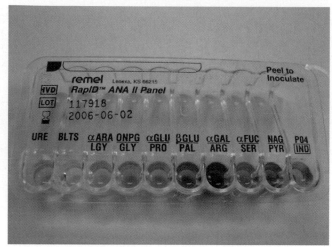

Figure 17-17. The RapID ANA II panel, manufactured by Remel, is one of the miniature anaerobe identification systems based on the presence of preexisting enzymes (i.e., enzymes already present within the organisms). Following preparation of a heavy suspension (equal to a #3 McFarland Standard) of the organism (in pure culture), the suspension is added to the wells of the panel. Inoculation can safely be performed at the bench, because further growth of organisms is not necessary. The panel is then incubated aerobically for 4 to 6 hours at 35°C to 37°C in a non-CO$_2$ incubator. Following incubation, test results are read and recorded on the manufacturer-furnished report form, after which reagents are added to appropriate wells and additional test results are read and recorded. A six-digit code number is generated, which gives the identification of the organism when the number is found in the appropriate section of the RapID ANA II Code Compendium. (Courtesy of Dr. Robert C. Fader.)

Definitive Identifications

The previous section described presumptive IDs of some of the anaerobic bacteria most commonly encountered in clinical specimens. It is important to remember that it will *not* always be possible to identify an anaerobic isolate using presumptive ID techniques. When definitive IDs of anaerobic isolates are required, CML professionals will find a wide variety of techniques available for their use (Table 17-11). Examples include PRAS and non-PRAS tubed biochemical test media, biochemical-based minisystems, preexisting enzyme-based minisystems (Fig. 17-17), GLC analysis of metabolic end products, and cellular fatty acid analysis by GLC.

It is important to remember that *none* of the commercially available biochemical-based or enzyme-based minisystems will identify *all* of the anaerobes that can potentially be isolated from clinical specimens. Many of the rapid minisystems are designed to identify the anaerobes most frequently encountered in clinical specimens and those most apt to be contributing to the infectious process. Before adopting any of these minisystems, potential users should review published evaluations, many of which are

referenced by Allen et al. (2002; see "References and Suggested Reading").

Regardless of the rapid minisystem used, it is likely that anaerobes will be encountered that can only be identified using highly sophisticated techniques employing many tubes of PRAS or non-PRAS media and/or GLC. The decision to employ time-consuming, labor-intensive procedures for identification of anaerobes of questionable clinical significance is one that must be weighed very carefully. In view of the current emphasis on cost containment in clinical laboratories, presumptive identifications might suffice, especially when susceptibility test results are also furnished. Rarely isolated organisms that are difficult and/or time consuming to identify might best be sent to reference laboratories.

The use of tubed biochemical systems and GLC procedures is often necessary at the reference laboratory level, because these laboratories frequently receive isolates that are deemed clinically significant but cannot be identified at the hospital level. Veterinary microbiology laboratories may also require tubed media and GLC to identify unique veterinary isolates not contained in the databases of the rapid minisystems.

TABLE 17 - 11 Methods for Definitive Identification of Anaerobes

Method	Comments[a]
Conventional or traditional tubed biochemical identification systems	These time-consuming and labor-intensive systems employ several to many large test tubes containing PRAS or non-PRAS biochemical test media (available from Anaerobe Systems, Randolph Biomedical, Remel, and Smith River Biologicals). Tests include, but are not limited to, various carbohydrate fermentations (e.g., arabinose, glucose, lactose, maltose, mannitol, rhamnose, salicin, sucrose, trehalose, xylose), 20% bile, catalase, esculin hydrolysis, gas production, gelatin hydrolysis, H_2S production, indole production, iron milk (proteolysis), motility, nitrate reduction, and urease. Detailed information concerning the use of these systems can be found in manuals available from the Centers for Disease Control and Prevention and the Virginia Polytechnic Institute, or the manual by Jousimies-Somer et al. (2002; see "References and Suggested Reading"). These manuals contain numerous charts used in conjunction with the PRAS and non-PRAS tubed biochemical identification systems. It is *extremely important* to remember that such charts should be relied on *only* when the test media being used have been prepared in exactly the same manner as the media used to obtain the data for the charts. For example, because of possible differences in formulations of test media, use of these charts in conjunction with some of the newer, rapid minisystems could lead to misidentifications.
Biochemical-based minisystems	Biochemical-based identification systems provide many of the same tests as the conventional systems but in the form of a small plastic strip or tray (hence, the term *minisystem*). Examples include the API 20A (bioMérieux Inc.) and Minitek Anaerobe II (BD Biosciences) systems. Biochemical-based minisystems are easier and faster to inoculate than a conventional system. Although they can be inoculated aerobically (at the bench), they require **anaerobic** incubation. The larger-model anaerobic jars and some of the commercially available bags can be used to incubate biochemical-based minisystem trays and strips if an anaerobic chamber is not available. After 24 to 48 hours of incubation, test results are read, a code number is generated for each isolate, and the numbers are looked up in a manufacturer-supplied codebook. Supplemental tests are often required, decreasing the usefulness of these systems and increasing the time for identifications by another day or two. It is also important to remember that the databases from which the codebooks were developed do not contain *all* the anaerobes that can potentially be isolated from clinical specimens and, in some cases, have not kept up with changes in organism nomenclature. Because these systems must be incubated **anaerobically**, and **require 24 to 48 hours**, many previous users have switched to the newer preexisting enzyme–based systems (described next).
Preexisting enzyme–based minisystems	These identification systems are based upon the presence of preexisting enzymes (i.e., enzymes already present in the bacterial cells). Because these minisystems do not depend on enzyme induction, there is virtually no lag time and results are available within 4 hours. The small plastic panels or cards are easy to inoculate, can be inoculated at the bench, and do not require anaerobic incubation. Most of the systems generate code numbers listed in a manufacturer-supplied codebook. As with the biochemical-based minisystems, it is important to remember that the preexisting enzyme–based systems are primarily of value for commonly isolated anaerobes. The databases from which the codebooks are developed do not contain all the anaerobes that can potentially be isolated from clinical specimens. Examples of preexisting enzyme–based minisystems include API ZYM (bioMérieux Inc.), BBL Crystal Anaerobe Identification System (Becton Dickinson Microbiology Systems), MicroScan Rapid Anaerobe Identification Panel (MicroScan Division, Baxter Healthcare Corp.), Rapid ID 32A (bioMérieux Inc.), RapID-ANA II (Remel), and the Vitek ANI Card (bioMérieux Inc.). The RapID-ANA II is shown in Figure 17-17. All these minisystems, except for the API ZYM system, provide identification tables or a database. In general, these minisystems all use the same or similar substrates. There are a number of nitrophenyl and naphthylamide compounds, which are colorless substances that produce yellow or red products, respectively, in the presence of appropriate enzymes.

TABLE 17 - 11	Methods for Definitive Identification of Anaerobes (Continued)
Method	**Comments[a]**
Tablets	Various tablets (e.g., Wee-Tabs and Add-a-Test Tablets, available from Key Scientific Co.) can be used to detect certain bacterial enzymes. These tablets have proven useful in identifying some anaerobes. According to Allen et al. (2002; see "References and Suggested Reading"), the tablets are more cost-effective than the prepackaged commercial kits when only a small battery of enzyme tests is required for identification of the organism. For detailed information concerning the use of specific tablets to identify particular anaerobes, refer to the manual by Jousimies-Somer et al. (2002; see "References and Suggested Reading").
Analysis of metabolic end products by GLC (see Fig. 8-21)	The use of GLC techniques for analysis of metabolic end products (short-chain volatile and nonvolatile fatty acids) and identification of anaerobes was pioneered by microbiologists at the Virginia Polytechnic Institute (VPI) in Blacksburg, VA. The VPI guidelines for GLC were used for many years at the Centers for Disease Control and Prevention (CDC) but with time were modified by CDC microbiologists. In today's CMLs, GLC is performed in accordance with the guidelines in the manual by Jousimies-Somer et al. and manufacturers' instructions.
Analysis of cellular fatty acids using the MIDI Sherlock System	The MIDI Sherlock Microbial Identification System, or MIDI, is a fully automated gas chromatographic system, available from MIDI Inc. It can be used to identify bacteria (including anaerobes) and certain yeasts by analysis of cellular fatty acids contained in cell membranes. Cellular fatty acids contain from 9 to 20 carbon atoms, in contrast to the short-chain volatile and nonvolatile fatty acids, which contain from 1 to 8 carbon atoms. Additional information about the MIDI system can be found in the manufacturer's literature and in Allen et al. (2002; see "References and Suggested Reading"). A number of published evaluations of the MIDI system for identification of anaerobes are referenced by Allen et al.

[a] Contact information for all companies mentioned in this chapter can be found on the CD-ROM.

CLINICAL SIGNIFICANCE AND IDENTIFICATION OF SELECTED COMMONLY ENCOUNTERED ANAEROBES

Anaerobes Isolated Most Frequently from Clinical Specimens

Although many species of anaerobes can potentially be isolated from human clinical specimens, the number of species *routinely* isolated is relatively small. Winn et al. (see "References and Suggested Reading") have reported the following organisms as the most frequently isolated and/or clinically important anaerobes encountered in properly selected and collected clinical specimens:

Gram-Negative Bacilli

Members of the Bacteroides fragilis group

Other Bacteroides spp.

Porphyromonas *and* Prevotella *spp.*

Fusobacterium *spp.*

Bilophila wadsworthia

Gram-Negative Cocci

Veillonella *spp.*

Gram-Positive Cocci

Especially Peptostreptococcus anaerobius, Finegoldia magna, Micromonas micros, Petoniphilus asaccharolyticus, *and* Anaerococcus prevotii

Non-Spore-Forming Gram-Positive Bacilli

Actinomyces *spp.*

Propionibacterium *spp.*

Bifidobacterium dentium

Eubacterium *spp.*

Spore-Forming Gram-Positive Bacilli

Certain Clostridium *species (e.g.,* C. perfringens, C. clostridioforme *group,* C. innocuum, C. ramosum, C. difficile, C. bifermentans, C. sporogenes, C. septicum, *and* C. sordellii)

Because these are the anaerobes most frequently isolated from clinical specimens, it seems logical to conclude that they are the anaerobes that CML professionals should be able to isolate and identify.

Anaerobic Gram-Positive Cocci

The human indigenous microflora contains many species of anaerobic Gram-positive cocci (GPC). Anaerobic GPC are found on skin and mucocutaneous surfaces, and in the oral cavity, upper respiratory tract, genital tract, and gastrointestinal tract. Many anaerobic GPC are isolated from clinical specimens, sometimes as contaminants and sometimes as pathogens. The anaerobic GPC that cause human infections are considered to be of endogenous origin. Numerous changes have recently occurred in the taxonomy of anaerobic GPC (consult the CD-ROM for a complete listing). For example, *Peptococcus niger* is presently the only species in the genus *Peptococcus*, and *Peptostreptococcus anaerobius* is the only species in the genus *Peptostreptococcus*. Most of the other anaerobic GPC that at one time were classified in these genera are now in the genera *Anaerococcus*, *Finegoldia*, *Micromonas*, and *Peptoniphilus*. Until these new genera are better recognized, it is acceptable to report isolates simply as anaerobic Gram-positive cocci.

Clinical significance. The most frequently isolated anaerobic GPC are *Peptostreptococcus anaerobius*, *Finegoldia magna* (formerly *Peptostreptococcus magnus*), *Peptoniphilus assacharolyticus* (formerly *Peptostreptococcus asaccharolyticus*), and *Micromonas micros* (formerly *Peptostreptococcus micros*). Anaerobic GPC are found in various clinical specimens, usually as components of mixed infections. Often, their pathogenic role is difficult to determine. Anaerobic GPC have been most commonly associated with soft tissue infections below the waist, appendicitis, and peritonitis. Decisions regarding antimicrobial therapy are often based on other organisms that are participating in the infectious process.

Clues to Anaerobic GPC Identification

Cellular and colonial morphology. Anaerobic GPC do not always appear as Gram-positive cocci in Gram-stained smears.

Some are elongated, resembling Gram-positive coccobacilli. With age, some anaerobic GPC may lose their Gram positivity. To compound matters, anaerobic Gram-negative cocci sometimes stain Gram positive. Performing the Gram stain procedure under anaerobic conditions (i.e., by performing all steps of the procedure within an anaerobic chamber) improves the results. Vancomycin susceptibility is a useful method of determining whether an anaerobic GPC is Gram positive (vancomycin susceptible) or Gram negative (vancomycin resistant). Also, anaerobic GPC are susceptible to metronidazole, whereas microaerophilic, Gram-positive cocci are not. A 5-μg metronidazole disk is used to determine metronidazole susceptibility. After 48 hours, anaerobic GPC have zones of inhibition of 15 mm or more whereas microaerophilic strains have no zones. Although metronidazole-resistant strains of anaerobic GPC have been reported, they appear to be rare.

Enriched blood agar should be used for culturing anaerobic GPC. Media preparation, age, and storage conditions are critical for the isolation of clinically significant anaerobic GPC. The size and arrangement (e.g., pairs, tetrads, chains, clusters) of the anaerobic GPC vary with growth conditions and are, therefore, not reliable criteria for identification. Gas-liquid chromatography and biochemical tests are required for definitive identification of most anaerobic GPC.

Peptostreptococcus anaerobius. P. anaerobius has a characteristic cell morphology, colony morphology, and odor. *P. anaerobius* cells are usually coccobacillary, with a diameter of 0.5 to 0.7 μm. They are often highly pleomorphic, and their cells are arranged in pairs and chains. Most strains of *P. anaerobius* form distinctive colonies that are gray with slightly raised off-white centers, opaque, and 0.5 to 2 mm in diameter after 24 hours; they usually give off a distinctive sickly sweet odor resulting from production of isocaproic acid. In addition, *P. anaerobius* is susceptible to SPS. Many authorities will identify an isolate as *P. anaerobius* if it is susceptible to SPS (zone size, 12 mm) and has the appropriate cellular and colonial morphology.

Peptoniphilus asaccharolyticus. P. asaccharolyticus has a characteristic cell morphology, colony morphology, and odor. Cell size is more uniform (0.5 to 0.9 μm in diameter) than is observed with most species of anaerobic GPC, and cells occur in clumps. When Gram stained, *P. asaccharolyticus* cells retain the crystal violet poorly and often resembling neisseriae. (Recall that a 5 μg vancomycin disk can be used to check the Gram reaction.) After 5 days of incubation, colonies are 2 to 3 mm in diameter, glistening, low convex, and usually whitish to lemon-yellow, and often have a characteristic musty odor. Most strains are indole positive, but indole-negative strains exist. The latter are difficult to identify. *Anaerococcus hydrogenalis* is also indole positive but, unlike *P. asaccharolyticus*, is alkaline phosphatase positive.

Micromonas micros. M. micros cells are usually arranged in pairs and chains but can occur in clumps when they have been cultured on solid media. *M. micros* grows very slowly on enriched blood agar to form highly characteristic colonies, having diameters of 1 mm after incubation for 5 days. Colonies are typically white (but sometimes gray), glistening, and domed and are often surrounded by a distinctive yellow-brown halo of discolored agar up to 2 mm wide. An anaerobic GPC with a milky halo around its white colonies on blood agar and very small cells (<0.6 μm in diameter) can be presumptively identified as *M. micros*. Some strains of *M. micros* are susceptible to SPS, but they generally produce smaller zones of inhibition (<12 mm).

Finegoldia magna. *F. magna* cells are larger than those of most anaerobic Gram-positive cocci, but identification of *F. magna* based on cell size alone is unreliable. It is more likely to be resistant to clindamycin than other anaerobic Gram-positive cocci.

Spore-Forming Anaerobic Gram-Positive Bacilli

Virtually all spore-forming anaerobic bacilli are classified in the genus *Clostridium*, often referred to as clostridia. As mentioned in Chapter 1, the spores produced by bacteria are technically known as **endospores**. They are thick-walled bodies formed within the bacterial cells, one endospore per cell. As is true for other bacterial endospores, clostridial spores are capable of withstanding prolonged periods of adverse environmental conditions. When conditions once again become favorable, the spores germinate, and a vegetative bacterium (i.e., one capable of growing and multiplying) emerges. Thus, endospores represent a survival mechanism.

Of the approximately 80 described *Clostridium* spp., about 30 are involved in human infections. *Clostridium* spp. cause tetanus, botulism, gas gangrene (myonecrosis), septicemia, soft tissue infections above and below the waist, appendicitis, peritonitis, pseudomembranous colitis, food poisoning, and other abdominal infections.

Clostridium spp. are defined as spore-forming anaerobic Gram-positive bacilli. However, as explained later, it seems that some *Clostridium* species "never read the book":

- Some *Clostridium* spp. are aerotolerant, with some, such as *C. carnis*, *C. histolyticum*, *C. perfringens*, *C. septicum*, and *C. tertium*, being *very* aerotolerant. The catalase test, using 15% H_2O_2, can be used to differentiate between aerotolerant species of *Clostridium*, which are catalase negative or in some cases weakly catalase positive, and *Bacillus* spp., which are spore-forming *aerobic* Gram-positive bacilli that are usually strongly catalase positive. On the other hand, some *Clostridium* spp. (e.g., *C. haemolyticum*, *C. novyi*) are among the strictest obligate anaerobes.

- Although they have a cell wall structure like other Gram-positive bacteria, some *Clostridium* spp. are difficult to stain, some appear Gram variable, and some routinely stain Gram negative. Thus, species such as *C. clostridioforme*, *C. ramosum*, and *C. innocuum* typically appear as pink-stained bacilli in Gram staining preparations. Performing the Gram staining procedure anaerobically will improve the results. Also, a 5-μg vancomycin disk can be used to differentiate Gram-positive (vancomycin-sensitive) from Gram-negative (vancomycin-resistant) bacteria. A zone of inhibition ≥10 mm around the disk is considered sensitive. However, it should be noted that some anaerobic *Gram-negative* bacilli, such as *Porphyromonas* spp. and some strains of *Prevotella melaninogenica*, are vancomycin sensitive (but they are not spore formers).

- Although all clostridia are spore formers, some species readily sporulate and others sporulate only under extremely harsh conditions. Therefore, Gram-stained smears of clinical specimens containing clostridia may or may not contain spores. Even in the absence of spores, however, Gram-positive bacilli observed on Gram-stained smears of clinical specimens should be suspected of being clostridia. With some *Clostridium* spp, such as *C. perfringens*, *C. ramosum*, *C. clostridioforme*, spores may not even be seen in Gram-stained smears of colonies from an agar plate. Ethanol or heat treatment can be used to detect sporulation, although even with these techniques, spore formation may sometimes be difficult to detect. Ethanol or heat treatment kills vegetative cells; thus, only bacteria capable of producing spores can survive such treatment. Vacuoles are sometimes mistaken for spores. A spore stain will help to differentiate them. Additionally, a particular *Clostridium* isolate will produce only one spore per cell, and the spore will be in the same location (either terminal or subterminal) in every cell. A bacterial cell may contain more than one vacuole, and vacuole locations will vary from cell to cell.

There are many ways to subdivide the clostridia. In some taxonomic schemes, they are grouped according to the location of the endospore formed within the cell. Spores are described as being either **terminal** (at the end of the cell; Fig. 17-18) or **subterminal** (at a location other than the end of the cell; Fig. 17-19). Sometimes clostridia are grouped according to various biochemical reactions, such as their ability to catabolize (break down) sugars and proteins. Species capable of catabolizing sugars are said to be saccharolytic, whereas those unable to catabolize sugars are said to be asaccharolytic. Species capable of catabolizing proteins are described as being proteolytic. Another method of categorizing clostridia involves their ability to produce the enzymes, lecithinase and lipase, as detected by using an egg yolk agar plate.

Certain clostridia have characteristics that are very useful in identification. For example, colonies of *C. difficile* have a distinctive odor reminiscent of a horse stable or barnyard.

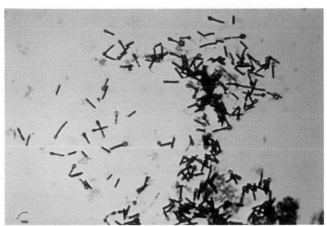

Figure 17-18. **Gram-stained *Clostridium tetani* cells.** The round, terminal spores give the cells a drumstick, lollipop, or tennis racket appearance. (From Winn WC Jr, et al. Koneman's Color Atlas and Textbook of Diagnostic Microbiology. 6th Ed. Philadelphia. Lippincott Williams & Wilkins, 2006.)

C. perfringens produces a double zone of hemolysis on blood agar, which is described in the next section.

Clostridium perfringens

Clinical significance. *Clostridium perfringens* is a common inhabitant of the colon and is the *Clostridium* sp. most frequently isolated from clinical specimens. It is the most common cause of gas gangrene, although other clostridia can also cause this disease (especially *C. novyi*, *C. septicum*, *C. histolyticum*, *C. bifermentans*, and *C. sordellii*).[4] Gas gangrene causes rapid local destruction of muscle and soft tissues, with systemic signs of toxemia and hypotension. It is

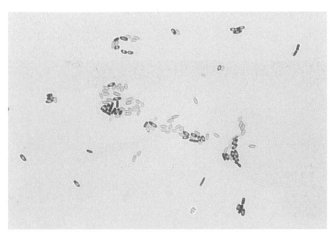

Figure 17-19. **Gram-stained *Clostridium sordellii*, illustrating ovoid subterminal spores.** (From Winn WC Jr, et al. Koneman's Color Atlas and Textbook of Diagnostic Microbiology. 6th Ed. Philadelphia: Lippincott Williams & Wilkins, 2006.)

extremely important to make the diagnosis as early as possible to stop the progression of the disease, often by amputation, and prevent further infection that might require even more extensive surgery. Finding *C. perfringens* in clinical specimens constitutes a true medical emergency, and the clinician must be notified immediately. (For an example of the Gram-stained appearance of *Clostridium* spp. in an inflammatory exudate, see Fig. 18-10.)

In addition to its role in gas gangrene, *C. perfringens* is one of the most frequent causes of food poisoning in the United States. *C. perfringens* food poisoning is caused by enterotoxin-producing strains of *C. perfringens*. The most common symptoms of *C. perfringens* food poisoning are diarrhea and moderate to severe abdominal pain, which last less than 24 hours. For food poisoning to occur, it is thought that vegetative organisms must be ingested, as opposed to spores or preformed toxin.

> *Clostridium perfringens* is the most common cause of gas gangrene and a very common cause of a relatively mild type of food poisoning.

 CAUTION

Do Not Confuse *Clostridium perfringens* Food Poisoning with Botulism. Both of these diseases are caused by *Clostridium* species. *C. perfringens* food poisoning (caused by enterotoxin-producing strains of *C. perfringens*) is a relatively mild type of food poisoning, with gastrointestinal symptoms usually lasting for only a day. Botulism, caused by neurotoxin-producing strains of *C. botulinum*, affects the central nervous system and causes a flaccid paralysis. It is the most deadly type of food poisoning.

Virulence factors. *C. perfringens* produces 12 toxins, including hemolysins, enterotoxins, and necrotizing toxins.

Clues to *Clostridium perfringens* Identification

Cellular morphology. *C. perfringens* cells are large, box-car-shaped, blunt-ended Gram-positive or Gram-variable bacilli that occur singly or in pairs (Fig. 17-20). Spores are usually not seen either in vivo or in vitro, but when present, they are large, oval, and subterminal and cause swelling of the cells.

Colonial morphology. On BRU/BA, *C. perfringens* produces large (>2 mm in diameter), gray to yellowish gray, circular, dome-shaped, glossy, translucent, spreading colonies that are usually surrounded by a **double zone of**

---

[4]*The word* gas *in* gas gangrene *refers to the pockets of gas (primarily hydrogen and nitrogen) formed in necrotic tissue, which may be detected by palpation or radiograph. It should be noted that gas production is not unique to clostridial infections. It can also be associated with infections caused by other gas-producing bacteria, such as members of the Enterobacteriaceae family, streptococci, staphylococci, and Bacteroides spp.*

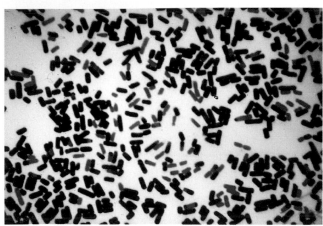

***Figure 17-20.* Gram-stained *Clostridium perfringens* cells from a 24-hour-old colony on blood agar.** Notice the lack of spores and the presence of decolorized (pink) cells. (From Winn WC Jr, et al. Koneman's Color Atlas and Textbook of Diagnostic Microbiology. 6th Ed. Philadelphia: Lippincott Williams & Wilkins, 2006.)

hemolysis. The double zone of hemolysis is an inner zone of complete hemolysis and an outer zone of partial hemolysis (see Fig. 17-8). Refrigeration of the subculture plate for 1 to 2 hours will enhance the hemolysis. *C. perfringens* is the fastest-growing clostridial species, with a generation time of less than 8 minutes under ideal conditions.

Laboratory tests. Clinical and Laboratory Standards Institute (CLSI) Document M35-A (see "References and Suggested Reading") states that an isolate can be identified as *C. perfringens* (with more than 95% likelihood) if it meets the following criteria:

• Large, boxcar-shaped, blunt-ended, anaerobic Gram-positive or Gram-variable bacilli (*C. perfringens* produces subterminal spores, but they are rarely observed and therefore need not be present to make the identification)

• Large (>2 mm diameter), irregular colonies on blood agar, surrounded by a double zone of hemolysis

• No growth on BBE

• Catalase negative

    C. perfringens is also lecithinase positive and lipase negative. *C. perfringens* food poisoning is usually diagnosed at reference laboratories or public health laboratories in any of the following three ways:

• Isolating >10^5 *C. perfringens* organisms per gram of incriminated food

• Median spore count of >10^6 *C. perfringens* organisms per gram of stool from ill people

• Isolation of the same serotype of *C. perfringens* from stools and suspected food

Essentials

Clostridium perfringens

• Large, boxcar-shaped, blunt-ended, anaerobic Gram-positive or Gram-variable bacillus; produces subterminal spores, which are rarely seen

• *Clostridium* sp. most commonly isolated from clinical specimens

• Most common cause of gas gangrene and a very common cause of a relatively mild type of food poisoning

• Produces large (>2-mm-diameter), irregular colonies on blood agar, which are surrounded by a double zone of hemolysis

• Catalase negative

• Lecithinase positive, lipase negative

Clostridium tetani

Clinical significance. *Clostridium tetani* produces a neurotoxin called **tetanospasmin,** which is the cause of the disease tetanus (sometimes referred to as lockjaw). **Tetanus is associated with a rigid, spastic type of paralysis, whereas botulism is associated with a flaccid paralysis** (Fig. 17-21). Tetanus is usually the result of *C. tetani* spores entering some type of puncture wound. Vaccines are available to prevent tetanus in animals and humans; thus, tetanus is primarily a disease of nonimmunized animals and humans. Sadly, it is estimated that the worldwide annual mortality caused by tetanus exceeds 1 million people.

> *Clostridium tetani* produces a neurotoxin called tetanospasmin, which causes the disease known as tetanus.

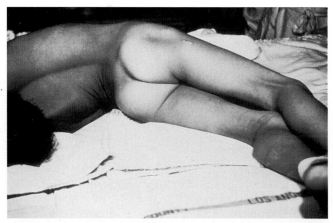

***Figure 17-21.* A patient with tetanus, displaying a body posture known as opisthotonos, caused by the neurotoxin tetanospasmin.** (Courtesy of the Centers for Disease Control and Prevention [CDC].)

Clues to *C. tetani* Identification

Cellular morphology. *C. tetani* is a slender Gram-positive bacillus that occurs singly or in pairs. Terminal spore formation results in a swelling at the tip of the bacillus, causing the organism to resemble a tennis racket, lollipop, or drumstick (see Fig. 17-18). After 24 hours of incubation or when sporulation has occurred, the cells often stain Gram negative. *C. tetani* is motile.

> The terminal spore produced by *C. tetani* causes a swelling at the tip of the cell, giving *C. tetani* cells a tennis racket, lollipop, or drumstick appearance.

Colonial morphology. *C. tetani* is rarely isolated in the CML. Diagnosis is usually established via clinical observation. When cultured, *C. tetani* colonies on BRU/BA are 4 to 6 mm in diameter, flat, irregular and rhizoid, gray, matte, translucent, and usually with a narrow zone of β-hemolysis. Often, a *C. tetani* colony swarms over the surface of a moist agar plate. Because of this swarming growth, *C. tetani* is sometimes referred to as "the *Proteus* of the anaerobe world." The swarming is quite thin and often difficult to see. (Note: When the presence of swarming growth is in doubt, scraping the agar surface with an inoculating loop will cause the growth, if present, to accumulate on the loop.)

Laboratory tests. CLSI Document M35-A (see "References and Suggested Reading") states that an isolate can be identified as *C. tetani* (with more than 95% likelihood) if it meets the following criteria:

- Anaerobic Gram-positive bacillus with a swollen terminal spore that causes the cell to resemble a tennis racquet, drumstick, or lollipop

- Slow, smoothly swarming growth on BA

- Spot indole positive, catalase negative

Essentials

Clostridium tetani

- Anaerobic Gram-positive bacillus with a swollen terminal spore, giving the cell the appearance of a tennis racquet, drumstick, or lollipop

- Produces a neurotoxin called tetanospasmin, which causes tetanus

- Rarely isolated in the CML

- Slow growth on blood agar that is smoothly swarming, quite thin, and often difficult to see; as a result of the swarming growth, *C. tetani* is sometimes referred to as "the *Proteus* of the anaerobe world"

- Spot indole positive, catalase negative

- Lecithinase variable, lipase negative or weakly positive

Clostridium botulinum

Clinical significance. *Clostridium botulinum* is the primary cause of botulism, a potentially deadly disease. It might be of interest to learn that the word *botulism* and the specific epithet *botulinum* come from *botulus*, the Latin word meaning "sausage." For centuries, botulism was associated with the consumption of sausages and other preserved meat products in Europe. Botulism is characterized by a descending flaccid paralysis and the four *D*s: **d**iplopia (double vision), **d**ysarthria (speech disturbance), **d**ysphonia (altered voice), and **d**ysphagia (difficulty swallowing). Botulism is caused by neurotoxin-producing strains of *C. botulinum*. Whereas tetanus is associated with a spastic, rigid paralysis, botulism is associated with a descending flaccid paralysis.

> Botulism is caused by neurotoxin-producing strains of *Clostridium botulinum*. Whereas tetanus is associated with a spastic, rigid paralysis, botulism is associated with a descending flaccid paralysis.

STUDY AID **Food Poisoning Caused by *Clostridium* spp.** The neurotoxin that causes botulism, called botulinal toxin, is produced in vitro by *Clostridium botulinum*. Botulism is a microbial intoxication. Other neurotoxigenic *Clostridium* spp. (*C. baratii* and *C. butyricum*) are also capable of causing botulism. The enterotoxin that causes *Clostridium perfringens* food poisoning is produced in vivo, following ingestion of *C. perfringens*–contaminated food. Although *C. perfringens* food poisoning is generally a relatively mild and self-limited gastrointestinal illness, botulism is a very serious disease that can result in a flaccid or limp type of paralysis and death.

> Botulism is a much more serious disease than *Clostridium perfringens* food poisoning.

There are three types of botulism, based on the manner in which the disease is acquired:

- **Classical foodborne botulism** results from ingestion of food containing the neurotoxin called **botulinal toxin,** produced by *C. botulinum*.

- **Wound botulism** is the result of contamination of wounds with spores of *C. botulinum*, with subsequent germination, multiplication, and production of botulinal toxin in vivo.

- **Infant botulism,** also known as intestinal botulism, follows ingestion of *C. botulinum* spores, germination, colonization of the colon, and in vivo production of botulinal toxin. Intestinal botulism is not necessarily confined to

> The three types of botulism differ in the manner in which each is acquired: classical foodborne botulism, wound botulism, and infant botulism.

infants. Both wound botulism and infant botulism differ from classical foodborne botulism in that botulinal toxin is produced and released in vivo, rather than in vitro.

Virulence factors. Almost all cases of botulism are caused by neurotoxin-producing strains of *C. botulinum*. The toxin, called botulinal toxin, has seven types, designated A, B, C, D, E, F, and G. Most cases of human botulism are caused by toxin types A, B, E, and F (the latter is the least common). The role of type G in human botulism is unclear. Types C and D cause botulism in birds and mammals other than humans.

Clues to *C. botulinum* Identification

Cellular morphology. *C. botulinum* is a Gram-variable bacillus. Cells in young cultures usually stain Gram positive, but cells in cultures older than 18 hours usually stain Gram negative. *C. botulinum* produces subterminal spores.

Colonial morphology. The colonial morphology of *C. botulinum* varies, depending on toxin type. Colonies may be raised or flat, and smooth or rough. They will show some spreading and will have an irregular edge. On EYA, they usually exhibit a pearly surface iridescence as a result of lipase positivity (Fig. 17-22). Although the toxin types that cause botulism in humans are lecithinase negative, some strains produce a yellow precipitate in EYA, with toxin type E exhibiting a wider zone of precipitation than types A and B.

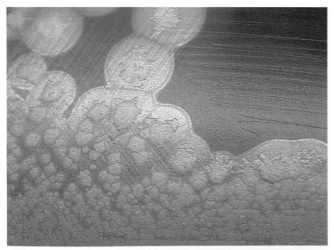

Figure 17-22. Clostridium botulinum on egg yolk agar after 72 hours of incubation. Notice the positive lipase reaction. (Courtesy of Larry Stauffer, the Oregon State Public Health Laboratory, and the CDC.)

Laboratory tests. Diagnosis of botulism is initially based on the patient's signs and symptoms, often corroborated by the patient's food history and epidemiological evidence. Laboratory confirmation of botulism, usually performed at reference and public health laboratories, involves discovering botulinal toxin in serum, feces, gastric contents, vomitus, or the implicated food; demonstrating toxicity to mice; or isolating *C. botulinum* from fecal specimens. In wound botulism, *C. botulinum* may be isolated from a wound specimen. *C. botulinum* isolates are identified by biochemical and toxin neutralization test results.

Essentials

Clostridium botulinum

- Anaerobic Gram-variable bacillus that produces a subterminal spore

- Produces a neurotoxin called botulinal toxin, which causes botulism

- The three types of botulism, classified by the manner in which the disease is acquired, are classical foodborne botulism, wound botulism, and infant botulism

- Laboratory confirmation of botulism, usually performed at reference and public health laboratories, involves discovering botulinal toxin in specimens or by isolating *C. botulinum* from fecal specimens

- Spot indole negative, catalase negative

- Lecithinase negative, lipase positive

Clostridium difficile

Clinical significance. *Clostridium difficile* is the most common, but not the sole, cause of antibiotic-associated diarrhea and pseudomembranous colitis. *C. difficile* is found as part of the normal gastrointestinal flora of many persons. Following extensive antimicrobial therapy, many organisms of the normal gastrointestinal flora other than *C. difficile* are killed, thus providing conditions (e.g., decreased competition for nutrients) that allow *C. difficile* to multiply. (Recall the discussion of superinfections in Chapter 7.)

> *Clostridium difficile* is the most common cause of antibiotic-associated diarrhea and pseudomembranous colitis, which are common infections in hospitalized patients.

Virulence factors. *C. difficile* produces two types of toxins: an enterotoxin, designated toxin A, and a cytotoxin, designated toxin B. As the population of *C. difficile* increases, the toxins reach concentrations high enough to cause disease. The enterotoxin is the primary cause of antibiotic-associated diarrhea,

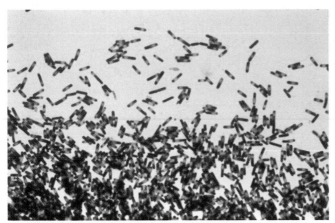

Figure 17-23. **Gram-stained** *Clostridium difficile,* **from a 72-hour old colony on blood agar.** The pink areas within cells are subterminal spores. (Courtesy of Dr. Gilda Jones and the CDC.)

whereas the cytotoxin is the primary cause of pseudomembranous colitis. *C. difficile* is a frequent cause of nosocomial (hospital-acquired) infections. Spores of *C. difficile* are frequently transmitted among hospitalized patients and are often present on the hands of hospital personnel caring for patients.

Clues to *C. difficile* Identification

Cellular morphology. *C. difficile* cells are large, straight bacilli that may produce chains (two to six cells aligned end to end; Fig. 17-23). The oval, subterminal (rarely terminal) spores cause a swelling of the cells. *C. difficile* is motile.

Colonial morphology. On BRU/BA, *C. difficile* colonies are 2 to 5 mm in diameter, circular or occasionally rhizoid, flat to low convex, grayish or whitish, matte to glossy, opaque, and nonhemolytic. On CCFA, *C. difficile* produces large, yellow, flattened, groundglass colonies, with yellowing of the usually pinkish medium around the colonies (see Fig. 17-14). *C. difficile* colonies produce a characteristic odor, described variously as smelling like cow manure, a barnyard, or a horse stable.

> *C. difficile* colonies have a distinctive odor reminiscent of a horse stable.

Laboratory tests. CLSI Document M35-A (see "References and Suggested Reading") states that an isolate can be identified as *C. difficile* (with more than 95% likelihood) if it meets the following criteria:

- Thin, anaerobic Gram-positive bacillus with rarely visible subterminal spores

- Colonies on CCFA are large, yellow, and flattened

- Colonies on blood agar fluoresce chartreuse under ultraviolet light and have a strong cow manure, barnyard-like, or horse stable odor

- Spot indole negative, catalase negative

C. difficile can be isolated from fecal specimens of healthy patients and patients with diarrheal disease caused by a pathogen other than *C. difficile*. Diagnosis of *C. difficile*–associated diseases is most often accomplished using some type of commercial enzyme immunoassay or cytotoxin tissue culture assay.

Essentials

Clostridium difficile

- Large, straight, thin, anaerobic Gram-positive bacilli that may produce chains (two to six cells aligned end to end); rarely seen oval subterminal spores cause swelling of the cells

- Produces two types of toxins: an enterotoxin, designated toxin A, and a cytotoxin, designated toxin B

- The enterotoxin is the primary cause of antibiotic-associated diarrhea, whereas the cytotoxin is the primary cause of pseudomembranous colitis

- On CCFA, *C. difficile* produces large, yellow, flattened, ground-glass colonies, with yellowing of the usually pinkish medium around the colonies

- Colonies have a characteristic odor, which has been described as similar to cow manure, a barnyard, or a horse stable

- Diagnosis of *C. difficile*–associated diseases is most often accomplished using some type of commercial enzyme immunoassay or cytotoxin tissue culture assay

- Spot indole negative, catalase negative

- Lecithinase negative, lipase negative

Other *Clostridium* spp.

Table 17-12 summarizes information of value for identification of *Clostridium* spp. *C. septicum* is isolated from serious, often fatal infections. *C. septicum* bacteremia is often associated with some type of underlying malignancy, especially colon or breast cancer, leukemia, or lymphoma. CLSI Document M35-A (see "References and Suggested Reading") states that an isolate can be identified as *C. septicum* (with more than 95% likelihood) if it meets the following criteria:

- Thin anaerobic Gram-positive bacilli with swollen, subterminal spores

- Smoothly swarming growth over the surface of a blood agar plate

- Spot indole negative, catalase negative

TABLE 17 - 12 Information of Value for Identification of *Clostridium* spp.

Category	Species	Additional Information
Lecithinase-positive, lipase-positive species	*Clostridium novyi* A	Proteolytic[a]
Lecithinase-positive, lipase-negative species	*C. baratii*	Nonproteolytic
	C. bifermentans	Chalk-white colonies with an irregular, scalloped edge; many free spores, often chaining; proteolytic; urease negative; indole positive
	C. limosum	Proteolytic
	C. perfringens	Double zone of hemolysis; boxcar-shaped bacilli; spores rarely seen; nonmotile; proteolytic
	C. sordellii	Proteolytic, indole positive, usually urease positive
Lecithinase-negative, lipase-positive species	*C. botulinum*	Proteolytic
	C. sporogenes	Medusa-head colonies; may swarm; subterminal and many free spores; proteolytic
Lecithinase-negative, lipase-negative, proteolytic species	*C. cadaveris*	White-gray, raised to slightly convex colonies, with an edge that is entire to slightly irregular; oval terminal spores; spot indole positive; DNase positive
	C. difficile	Creamy yellow to gray-white colonies, with an irregular coarse mottled to mosaic internal structure; colonies have a matte or dull surface; colonies fluoresce chartreuse; characteristic yellow, ground-glass colony on CCFA; characteristic horse stable odor; oval, subterminal spores; free spores may be observed; gelatin hydrolysis is slow in about half of the strains; mannitol positive
	C. hastiforme	Subterminal spores; some strains nitrate positive; does not ferment glucose
	C. histolyticum	Quite aerotolerant; oval, subterminal spores which are only produced anaerobically
	C. putrificum	Oval, terminal spores; ferments glucose
	C. septicum	Medusa-head colony, followed by heavy swarming over the surface of the agar; oval, subterminal spores; DNase positive; sucrose negative
	C. subterminale	Oval, subterminal spores; does not ferment glucose
	C. tetani	Round, terminal spores; tennis racket appearance; cells often stain Gram negative when sporulation; often swarms over the surface of the agar

TABLE 17 - 12   (Continued)

Category	Species	Additional Information
Lecithinase-negative, lipase-negative, nonproteolytic species	C. butyricum	Very large, irregular colonies, with a mottled to mosaic internal structure; oval, subterminal spores; ferments many carbohydrates, including glucose
	C. clostridioforme	Colonies resemble those of *Bacteroides fragilis* but usually have a slightly irregular edge; short, football-shaped cells that often stain Gram negative; oval, subterminal spores that distend the cells, but spores are rarely observed
	C. glycolicum	Convex, gray-white colonies with an entire to scalloped edge; subterminal and free spores; DNase positive
	C. innocuum	Gray-white to brilliant greenish colonies with a coarsely mottled to mosaic internal structure; colonies fluoresce chartreuse; nonmotile; rare, oval, terminal spores that distend the cells; cells often stain Gram negative; mannitol positive; lactose negative; maltose negative
	C. ramosum	Colonies resemble those of *Bacteroides fragilis* but usually have a slight irregular edge; colonies may fluoresce red; long, thin, palisading bacilli that often stain Gram negative; tiny, oval, terminal spores, but spores are rarely observed; nonmotile; mannitol positive
	C. tertium	Quite aerotolerant; oval, terminal spores produced only anaerobically

[a]Proteolytic species are gelatin hydrolysis positive; nonproteolytic species are gelatin hydrolysis negative.

CLSI Document M35-A also states that an isolate can be identified as *C. sordellii* (with more than 95% likelihood) if it meets the following criteria:

- Thin anaerobic Gram-positive bacilli with subterminal spores

- Large, lobate, irregular, slowly swarming, flat colonies with serpentine edges

- Spot indole positive, rapid urease positive, catalase negative

Non-Spore-Forming Anaerobic Gram-Positive Bacilli

The non-spore-forming anaerobic Gram-positive bacilli (hereafter referred to as NSF anaerobic GPB) is a heterogenous group. They have varying morphologies, ranging from short rods to long, branching filaments. Although many species of NSF anaerobic GPB can be isolated from clinical specimens, the most common are *Actinomyces*, *Bifidobacterium*, *Eggerthella*, *Eubacterium*, *Lactobacillus*, *Mobiluncus*, *Propionibacterium*, and *Pseudoramibacter* spp.

Clinical significance. In general, NSF anaerobic GPB and coccobacilli have been most commonly associated with head and neck infections, respiratory infections, soft tissue infections above and below the waist, appendicitis, peritonitis, and other abdominal infections.

The disease actinomycosis is most often caused by *Actinomyces israelii* and *Propionibacterium propionicum*, although it can be caused by similar NSF anaerobic GPB. When these members of the indigenous oral flora gain entrance to tissue, they can cause chronic destructive abscesses or granulomas that may eventually discharge a viscous pus. The pus often contains minute yellowish granules called sulfur granules (see Fig. 20-16). Actinomycosis commonly affects the cervicofacial area, abdomen, and thorax.

Clues to the Identification of Non-Spore-Forming Anaerobic Gram-Positive Bacilli

In most cases, it is not possible to presumptively identify NSF anaerobic GPB and coccobacilli. Biochemical tests, enzyme tests, and/or gas-liquid chromatography are required to identify virtually all NSF anaerobic GPB.

Exceptions are *Propionibacterium acnes* and *Eggerthella lenta* (formerly *Eubacterium lentum*; discussed later).

***Actinomyces* spp.** *Actinomyces* spp. are primarily involved in infections of the head and neck, miscellaneous skin soft tissue and bone infections both above and below the waist, and appendicitis. *Actinomyces* spp. are straight to slightly curved rods, ranging in size from short rods to long filaments. The shorter rods may have clubbed ends and may be seen in diphtheroid arrangements, short chains, or small clusters. (The term *diphtheroid* refers to an organism that morphologically resembles *Corynebacterium diphtheriae*.) Longer rods and straight or wavy filaments may be branched. Although *Actinomyces* spp. are Gram positive, irregular staining may cause a beaded or banded appearance. The typical beaded, branching, filamentous Gram-stained appearance of an *Actinomyces* species is depicted in Figure 17-24; this is the appearance that is often referred to as ***Actinomyces*-like.** Members of the genus *Actinomyces* are seldom obligate anaerobes. Some are quite fastidious, requiring special vitamins like vitamin K_1, certain amino acids, and hemin for adequate growth.

***Propionibacterium* spp.** *Propionibacterium* spp. are pleomorphic rods that may be coccoid, diphtheroidal (resembling *Corynebacterium diphtheriae*), or club shaped. The rods may be bifurcated (forked) or branched.

Propionibacterium acnes is the most common anaerobe in the indigenous microflora of the skin and is thus a common contaminant of blood cultures (much like *Staphylococcus epidermidis*). However, like *S. epidermidis*, *P. acnes* can also cause subacute bacterial endocarditis and bacteremia, although less often than *S. epidermidis*, and is thus not always a contaminant. As its name implies, *P. acnes* plays a role in the development of acne.

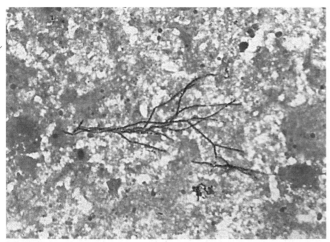

Figure 17-24. **Grain-stained facial drainage specimen, illustrating the beaded, branched, filamentous morphology referred to as *Actinomyces*-like.** (From Marler LM, Siders JA, Allen SD. Direct Smear Atlas. Philadelphia: Lippincott Williams & Wilkins, 2001.)

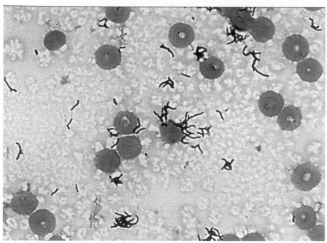

Figure 17-25. **Gram-stained blood specimen containing *Propionibacterium acnes*, illustrating diphtheroid-like morphology.** (From Marler LM, Siders JA, Allen SD. Direct Smear Atlas. Philadelphia: Lippincott Williams & Wilkins, 2001.)

The Gram-stained appearance of *P. acnes* is shown in Figure 17-25; this is the morphology that is often referred to as **diphtheroid-like,** diphtheroidal, or a diphtheroid appearance. On blood agar, *P. acnes* colonies are punctiform to 0.5 mm in diameter, circular, and glistening, with an entire to pulvinate margin. Although the colonies are initially white to gray, they become yellowish tan with age. In peptone-yeast-glucose (PYG) broth, cells are 0.3 to 1.3 μm wide by 1.0 to 10 μm long, club shaped, with or without metachromatic granules, and possibly arranged in "Chinese letter" configurations. Most strains of *P. acnes* are indole positive, catalase positive, and nitrate positive. Indole-negative and catalase-negative strains of *P. acnes* exist, and some strains can grow in 5% to 10% CO_2.

CLSI Document M35-A (see "References and Suggested Reading") states that an isolate can be identified as *P. acnes* (with more than 95% likelihood) if it meets the following criteria:

- Pleomorphic, coryneform anaerobic Gram-positive bacilli

- Small (1 to 2 mm in diameter), opaque, enamel-white, circular colonies on blood agar

- No growth on BBE

- Spot indole positive, catalase positive (with 15% H_2O_2)

***Eubacterium* and *Eggerthia* spp.** Eubacteria are common members of the indigenous microflora of the colon. *Eubacterium* and *Eggerthia* spp. may be observed as either uniform or pleomorphic Gram-positive rods. They may be coccoid, diphtheroidal, or filamentous and may range in width from thin to plump.

On blood agar, *Eggerthia lenta* (formerly *Eubacterium lentum*) colonies are 0.5 to 2.0 mm in diameter, circular, raised to low convex, smooth, dull to shiny, with an entire to erose edge. Some strains fluoresce red under long-wave ultraviolet light (Woods lamp). To observe the fluorescence, it may be necessary to (1) hold the plate very close to the Woods lamp, (2) tilt the plate at various angles to find the optimal angle, and (3) reincubate the plate for one or more days. In PYG broth, cells are 0.2 to 0.4 μm wide by 0.2 to 2.0 μm long, occurring singly or in pairs and short chains. Pleomorphic, coryneform NSF anaerobic GPB that are indole negative and nitrate positive can be identified as *E. lenta*. Most strains are catalase negative.

***Bifidobacterium* spp.** *Bifidobacterium* spp. are named for their bifurcated (forked) appearance, but they are highly variable in their appearance and, thus, are not always bifurcated.

Anaerobic Gram-Negative Cocci

Clinical significance. Although other anaerobic Gram-negative cocci (anaerobic GNC), such as *Acidaminococcus* and *Megasphaera* spp., can be isolated from clinical specimens, only *Veillonella* spp. are considered to be clinically significant. *Veillonella* spp. are common inhabitants of the mouth, gastrointestinal tract, and vagina, and when isolated, most often represent contaminants. They are most commonly associated with head and neck infections, and soft tissue infections above and below the waist.

Clues to *Veillonella* spp. Identification

Cellular morphology. *Veillonella* spp. are small (<0.5 μm in diameter) anaerobic GNC, usually arranged in clusters or diplococci. Recall that some anaerobic GPC, such as *Peptoniphilus asaccharolyticus* and *P. indolicus*, are easily decolorized and may appear to be Gram negative. A 5-μg vancomycin disk can be used to confirm that anaerobic GNC are truly Gram negative. Anaerobic GNC are resistant to vancomycin, whereas anaerobic GPC are susceptible.

Colonial morphology. Colonies of *Veillonella* spp. on blood agar are small, convex, grayish white, and translucent to transparent, with entire edges. They often fluoresce red under long-wave ultraviolet light.

Laboratory tests. CLSI Document M35-A (see "References and Suggested Reading") states that an isolate can be identified as a *Veillonella* sp. (with more than 95% likelihood) if it meets the following criteria:

- Tiny anaerobic GNC or diplococci

- Small (0.5 to 1.0 mm diameter), transparent-to-opaque colonies on BRU/BA that fluoresce brick-red under ultraviolet light

- No growth on BBE agar

- Indole negative and nitrate positive (nitrate-negative strains do exist)

Anaerobic Gram-Negative Bacilli

Many species of anaerobic Gram-negative bacilli (anaerobic GNB) inhabit the body. They are part of the indigenous microflora of the mouth as well as the upper respiratory, gastrointestinal, and geritourinary tracts. Anaerobic GNB are the anaerobes most commonly encountered in clinical infections. They are isolated from more than 50% of all specimens from which anaerobes are isolated. The anaerobic GNB most commonly isolated from clinical specimens include *Bacteroides*, *Porphyromonas*, *Prevotella*, *Fusobacterium*, *Campylobacter*, *Sutterella*, and *Bilophila* spp., all of which are discussed in this section.

Bacteroides fragilis Group

One of the most important genera of anaerobic Gram-negative bacilli is the genus *Bacteroides*. *Bacteroides* spp. have received a great deal of publicity over the years because of their frequent involvement in infectious processes and their resistance to antimicrobial agents. Taxonomically, the genus *Bacteroides* can be divided into species that are bile resistant and those that are bile sensitive (Table 17-13). Many anaerobes that were previously classified as bile-sensitive *Bacteroides* spp. have been reclassified into the genera *Porphyromonas* and *Prevotella*, which are discussed later.

Clinical significance. Members of the *Bacteroides fragilis* group are the most frequently encountered anaerobes in clinical specimens. They are most commonly associated with septicemia, soft tissue infections below the waist, appendicitis, peritonitis, and other abdominal infections. Members of the *B. fragilis* group tend to be more virulent and drug resistant than most other anaerobes. The two most important members of the group are *B. fragilis* and *B. thetaiotaomicron* because of their frequent occurrence in clinical infection and their resistance to antimicrobial agents.

> Members of the *Bacteroides fragilis* group are the most frequently encountered anaerobes in clinical specimens. They tend to be more virulent and drug resistant than most other anaerobes.

Drug resistance. Penicillin-resistant strains of *B. fragilis* and other members of the *B. fragilis* group have been encountered for many years, but there have also been reports of resistance to numerous other antimicrobial agents among isolates of this group. Members of the *B. fragilis* group were the first anaerobes reported to produce β-lactamases—enzymes capable of inactivating penicillins and cephalosporins.

Clues to *B. fragilis* Group Identification

Cellular morphology. Members of the *B. fragilis* group are anaerobic Gram-negative coccobacilli or straight bacilli of variable length, sometimes forming filaments.

TABLE 17 - 13   *Bacteroides* spp.

Bile-Resistant Species	Bile-Sensitive Species
***Bacteroides fragilis* group**	*B. capillosus* (some strains are bile resistant)
B. caccae	*B. forsythus* (recently reclassified as *Tannerella forsythensis*)
B. distasonis[a]	*B. ureolyticus*
B. eggerthii	
B. fragilis	
B. merdae[a]	
B. ovatus	
B. stercoris	
B. thetaiotaomicron	
B. uniformis	
B. vulgatus	
Other *Bacteroides* species	
B. coagulans	
B. putredinis (some strains are bile-sensitive)	
B. pyogenes	
B. splanchnicus	
B. tectus	

Source: Jousimies-Somer HR, Summanen P, Baron EJ, Citron DM, Wexler HM, Finegold SM. Wadsworth-KTL Anaerobic Bacteriology Manual. 6th Ed. Belmont, CA: Star, 2002.
[a] Will probably be removed from the *B. fragilis* group.

Colonial morphology. Members of the *B. fragilis* group produce colonies >1 mm in diameter on BBE agar and cause browning of the medium as a result of esculin hydrolysis. Table 17-14 describes the appearance of various *B. fragilis* group members on BRU/BA.

Laboratory tests. An anaerobic GNB or coccobacillus that is resistant to all three special-potency antimicrobials (vancomycin, kanamycin, and colistin) is most likely a member of the *B. fragilis* group, but it might be a *Prevotella* sp. (discussed later in the chapter). However, if the isolate is also growing on the BBE plate, indicating that it is bile resistant, it can be presumptively identified as a member of the *B. fragilis* group. (*Prevotella* spp. are bile

> Members of the *B. fragilis* group are resistant to all three of the special-potency antimicrobials: vancomycin, kanamycin, and colistin.

sensitive.) It is important to identify members of the *B. fragilis* group to the species level because of species-to-species variability in both virulence and drug resistance. Table 17-14 contains additional information about members of the *B. fragilis* group. The Gram-stained appearance of typical members of the *Bacteroides fragilis* group are shown in Figure 17-26.

CLSI Document M35-A (see "References and Suggested Reading") states that an isolate can be identified as a member of the *B. fragilis* group (with more than 95% likelihood) if it meets the following criteria:

- Anaerobic GNB
- Large (>1 mm diameter), convex colonies on blood agar and LKV agar

> Members of the *B. fragilis* group are bile resistant and esculin hydrolysis positive.

- Large, convex, dark (gray or black) colonies on BBE agar

TABLE 17 - 14	Presumptive Identification of Members of the *Bacteroides fragilis* Group

Species	Colonial Morphology on BRU/BA	Spot Indole	Catalase	Comments
B. fragilis	1 to 3 mm in diameter, circular, low convex, entire edge, translucent to semiopaque, concentric rings when viewed by obliquely transmitted light; some strains hemolytic	−	+	
B. vulgatus	1 to 2 mm in diameter, circular, convex, entire edge, grayish, semiopaque, nonhemolytic	−	+ (most strains)	Can be presumptively identified as *B. vulgatus* if indole negative, catalase positive, and esculin negative (no browning of the BBE medium); some strains of *B. vulgatus* are esculin positive
B. distasonis	Pinpoint to 0.5 mm in diameter, circular, convex, entire, gray-white, smooth, translucent to opaque, some strains α-hemolytic	−	+ (most strains)	
B. merdae (rarely isolated)	0.5 to 1.0 mm in diameter, circular to slightly irregular, convex, entire edge, white, shiny and smooth, rabbit blood is slightly hemolyzed	−	− (most strains)	α-Fucosidase negative
B. caccae		−	−	α-Fucosidase positive
B. theta-iotaomicron	Punctiform, circular, convex, entire edge, whitish, shiny, semiopaque, soft, nonhemolytic	+	+	Can be presumptively identified as *B. thetaiotaomicron* if indole positive and catalase positive
B. uniformis	0.5 to 2.0 mm diameter, circular, low convex, entire, gray to white, translucent to slightly opaque, usually nonhemolytic but some strains produce a slight greening of the agar	+	− (most strains)	
B. ovatus	0.5 to 1.0 mm in diameter, circular, convex, entire edge, pale buff, semiopaque, may have a mottled appearance, nonhemolytic	+	− (most strains)	
B. stercoris (rarely isolated)	0.5 to 1.0 mm in diameter, circular, convex, entire edge, shiny, smooth, transparent to translucent, β-hemolytic	+	−	

Source: Mangels JI. Anaerobic bacteriology. In: Essential Procedures for Clinical Microbiology. Washington, DC: ASM Press, 1998. Engelkirk PG, et al. Principles and Practice of Anaerobic Bacteriology. Belmont, CA: Star, 1992.

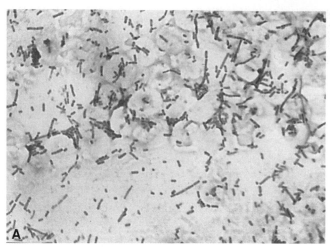
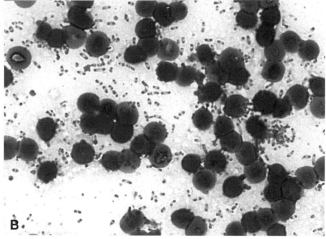

Figure 17-26. **Appearance of typical members of the** *Bacteroides fragilis* **group in Gram-stained blood specimens.** Vacuoles, irregular staining, and "safety pin" forms are common. **A.** *Bacteroides fragilis.* **B.** *Bacteroides vulgatus.* (From Marler LM, Siders JA, Allen SD. Direct Smear Atlas. Philadelphia: Lippincott Williams & Wilkins, 2001.)

Essentials

Bacteroides fragilis Group

- Anaerobic Gram-negative coccobacilli or straight bacilli of variable length, sometimes forming filaments; often vacuolated and bipolar staining

- The most frequently encountered anaerobes in clinical specimens; *B. fragilis* is the most common species of anaerobic bacteria isolated from soft tissue infectious processes and bacteremia

- More virulent and drug resistant than most other anaerobes

- Produce large (>1-mm-diameter) convex colonies on blood agar and LKV agar

- Bile resistant, esculin hydrolysis positive

- Produce large, convex, dark (gray or black) colonies on BBE agar

Bilophila wadsworthia and the *Bacteroides ureolyticus* Group

Clinical significance. *Bilophila wadsworthia* is most commonly associated with appendicitis and peritonitis. Members of the *B. ureolyticus* group are less commonly associated with soft tissue infections below the waist.

Clues to *Bilophila wadsworthia* and the *Bacteroides ureolyticus* Group Identification

Laboratory tests. An anaerobic GNB or coccobacillus that is vancomycin resistant, kanamycin-sensitive, and colistin-sensitive, could be a member of the *Bacteroides ureolyticus*

group (nitrate positive), *Bilophila wadsworthia* (nitrate positive), or a *Fusobacterium* sp. (nitrate negative). The *B. ureolyticus* group comprises *B. ureolyticus*, *B. gracilis*, *Campylobacter curvus*, *C. rectus*, and *C. consisus*. The key feature of members of this group is that they produce pitting colonies (see Fig. 17-7). However, not all strains of *Campylobacter* spp. will pit agar, and even pitting strains will produce a variety of colony types on a given plate. Table 17-15 contains information about the *B. ureolyticus* group and *B. wadsworthia*. *Fusobacterium* spp. are discussed in a later section.

> The key feature of the *Bacteroides ureolyticus* group is that they produce pitting colonies.

CLSI Document M35-A (see "References and Suggested Reading") states that an isolate can be identified as *Bilophila wadsworthia* (with more than 95% likelihood) if it meets the following criteria:

- Anaerobic, Gram-negative bacillus (regular rods to filaments)

- Tiny (<1.0-mm-diameter) translucent colonies on BA

> On BBE agar, *Bilophila wadsworthia* colonies have a black center as a result of H₂S production.

- Translucent colonies with black centers (caused by hydrogen sulfide [H_2S] production) on BBE agar at 72 hours

- Strongly catalase positive (with 15% H_2O_2), spot indole negative

CLSI Document M35-A states that an isolate can be identified as *Bacteroides ureolyticus* (with more than 95% likelihood) if it meets the following criteria:

TABLE 17 - 15	Presumptive Identification of *Bilophila wadsworthia* and the *Bacteroides ureolyticus* Group				
Species	**Agar Pitting**	**Motility**	**Urease**	**Strong Oxidase**	**Comments**
Bilophila wadsworthia	–	–	+ (most strains)	–	Bile resistant; produces fish eye colonies (clear colonies with black centers) on BBE; catalase positive
B. ureolyticus	+ (most strains)	–	+	Variable	Agar pitting, urease positive, isolates can be presumptively identified as *B. ureolyticus*
B. gracilis	+ (most strains)	–	–	–	
C. curvus and *C. rectus*	– (most strains)	+	–	–	
C. concisus	– (most strains)	+	–	+	

- Tiny anaerobic Gram-negative bacilli or coccobacilli

- Flat, translucent, pitting colonies on blood agar

- No growth on BBE agar

- Catalase negative (with 15% H_2O_2), urease positive, indole negative

Porphyromonas and *Prevotella* spp.

Clinical significance. *Porphyromonas* and *Prevotella* spp. can be divided into those that produce pigmented colonies and those that do not (Table 17-16). Pigmented colonies may be buff, tan, brown, or black. *Porphyromonas* spp. of animal origin are included as they may be isolated from animal bite infections. *Porphyromonas* spp. are most commonly associated with soft tissue infections below the waist, appendicitis, and peritonitis. *Prevotella* spp. are most commonly associated with head and neck infections, soft tissue infections above and below the waist, and appendicitis.

Clues to *Porphyromonas* and *Prevotella* spp. Identification

Pigmented species of *Porphyromonas* and *Prevotella* produce colonies ranging in color from buff to tan to brown to black (see Fig. 17-10). Pigment production usually occurs within 3 to 14 days but may take as long as 21 days. Plated media containing laked blood are frequently used in an attempt to enhance pigmentation. Brick-red fluorescence of colonies under long-wave ultraviolet light can also be used

to presumptively identify these species (see Fig. 17-11), but the fluorescence usually disappears as pigment develops.

> *Porphyromonas* spp. and many *Prevotella* spp. produce brown-black pigmented colonies, which fluoresce a brick-red color before becoming darkly pigmented.

Table 17-17 contains information regarding presumptive identification of the three most commonly isolated *Porphyromonas* spp. If the isolate is an anaerobic GNB or coccobacillus that is vancomycin susceptible, kanamycin resistant, and colistin resistant, the organism could be a pink-staining Gram-positive bacillus or a *Porphyromonas* sp. The CML professional would try performing the Gram stain under anaerobic conditions. If the organism is still Gram negative, the CML professional would assume the isolate to be a *Porphyromonas* sp. and attempt to identify it using information found in Table 17-17.

Laboratory tests. CLSI Document M35-A (see "References and Suggested Reading") states that an isolate can be identified as a *Porphyromonas* sp. (with more than 95% likelihood) if it meets the following criteria:

- Tiny anaerobic Gram-negative coccobacilli

- Black-pigmented colonies on BRU/BA or small translucent or opaque colonies that fluoresce brick red under long-wave ultraviolet light

- No growth on LKV agar or BBE agar

- Spot indole positive

TABLE 17 - 16 *Porphyromonas* and *Prevotella* spp.

Pigmented Species	Nonpigmented Species
Porphyromonas spp.	**Porphyromonas spp.**
P. asaccharolytica	P. catoniae
P. canoris (animal origin)	**Prevotella spp.**
P. cangingivalis (animal origin)	P. bivia
P. cansulci (animal origin)	P. buccae
P. circumdentaria (animal origin)	P. buccalis
P. crevioricanis (animal origin)	P. dentalis
P. endodontalis	P. disiens
P. gingivalis (some strains of animal origin)	P. enoeca
P. gingivicanis (animal origin)	P. heparinolytica
P. levii (animal origin)	P. oralis
P. macacae (animal origin)	P. oris
Prevotella spp.	P. oulorum
P. corporis	P. veroralis
P. denticola	P. zoogleoformans
P. intermedia	
P. loescheii	
P. melaningogenica	
P. nigrescens	
P. pallens	
P. tannerae	

Source: Jousimies-Somer HR, Summanen P, Baron EJ, Citron DM, Wexler HM, Finegold SM. Wadsworth-KTL Anaerobic Bacteriology Manual. 6th Ed. Belmont, CA: Star, 2002.

TABLE 17 - 17 Presumptive Identification of *Porphyromonas* spp.

Porphyromonas species	Arginine	α-Fucosidase	Trypsin	N-Acetyl-β-Glucosamidase	Fluorescence Under Ultraviolet Light
P. asaccharolytica	+ (most strains)	+	−	−	+
P. endodontalis	− (most strains)	−	−	−	+
P. gingivalis	+	−	+	+	−

Source: Mangels JI. Anaerobic bacteriology. In: Essential Procedures for Clinical Microbiology. Washington, DC: ASM Press, 1998.

CLSI Document M35-A states that an isolate can be identified as a *Prevotella* sp. (with more than 95% likelihood) if it meets the following criteria:

- Tiny anaerobic Gram-negative coccobacilli

- Black-pigmented colonies on BRU/BA and LKV agar or small translucent or opaque colonies that fluoresce brick red under long-wave ultraviolet light

- No growth on BBE agar

- Report *Prevotella* sp. if spot indole negative; report *Prevotella intermedia* if spot indole positive

An anaerobic GNB or coccobacillus that is vancomycin resistant, kanamycin resistant, and colistin sensitive or resistant is most likely a *Prevotella* sp. As previously mentioned, not all *Prevotella* spp. produce pigmented colonies. If the isolate *is* producing pigmented colonies, the information in Table 17-18 can be used to presumptively identify it.

Essentials

Pigmented *Porphyromonas* and *Prevotella* spp.

- Tiny anaerobic Gram-negative bacilli or coccobacilli

- Both will grow on BRU/BA, but *Porphyromonas* spp. do not grow on LKV because of vancomycin sensitivity; neither grows on BBE

- Produce pigmented colonies that range in color from buff to tan to brown to black; pigment production usually occurs within 3 to 14 days but may take as long as 21 days; plated media containing laked blood are frequently used in an attempt to enhance pigmentation

- Brick-red fluorescence of colonies under long-wave ultraviolet light can also be used to presumptively identify these species, but the fluorescence usually disappears as pigment develops

- *Porphyromonas* spp. are indole positive; most *Prevotella* spp. are indole negative

Fusobacterium spp.

Clinical significance. *Fusobacterium* spp. are most commonly associated with head and neck infections, respiratory infections, soft tissue infections above and below the waist, appendicitis, and peritonitis.

Clues to *Fusobacterium* spp. Identification

Cellular morphology. The term **fusiform,** which means long, thin, and tapered at the ends, is frequently associated with the genus *Fusobacterium*. These cells are sometimes described as being spindle shaped. It is

> Not all *Fusobacterium* spp. are fusiform in shape. Some species are quite pleomorphic.

Species	Color of Pigmented Colonies	Indole	Lipase	Esculin	Comments
P. melaninogenica	Tan to buff	−	−	− (most strains)	
P. denticola	Tan to buff	−	−	+	Can be presumptively identified as *P. denticola*
P. loescheii	Tan to buff	−	− (most strains); some strains weakly +	−	Can be presumptively identified as *P. loescheii* if indole negative and lipase positive
P. corporis	Black	−	−	−	
P. intermedia	Black	+	+ (most strains)	−	Can be presumptively identified as *P. intermedia* if indole positive and lipase positive
P. bivia	Variable	−	−	−	

TABLE 17 - 18 Presumptive Identification of Pigmented *Prevotella* spp.

Source: Mangels JI. Anaerobic bacteriology. In: Essential Procedures for Clinical Microbiology. Washington, DC: ASM Press, 1998.

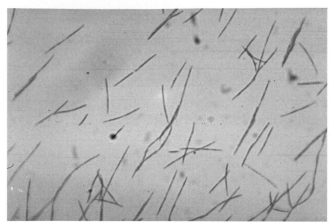

Figure 17-27. **Gram-stained appearance of *Fusobacterium nucleatum* subsp. *fusiforme*.** Notice the fusiform, spindle shape of the cells. (Courtesy of Dr. V. R. Dowell Jr. and the CDC.)

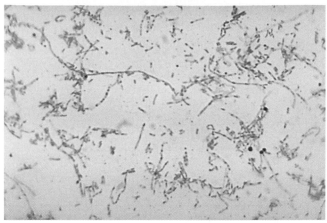

Figure 17-29. **Gram-stained appearance of *Fusobacterium necrophorum*.** (Courtesy of Dr. V. R. Dowell Jr. and the CDC.)

important to note, however, that (1) only one subspecies of *F. nucleatum* has cells that are consistently fusiform in shape, and (2) bacteria that are fusiform in shape are not necessarily fusobacteria (e.g., *Bacteroides gracilis, B. forsythus,* and microaerophilic *Capnocytophaga* species).

Fusobacterium nucleatum subspecies *fusiforme* is the only *Fusobacterium* that *routinely* exists as long, thin Gram-negative rods that are tapered (pointed) at the ends. The Gram-stained appearance of *F. nucleatum* subsp. *fusiforme* is depicted in Figure 17-27.

Although some cells of certain other fusobacteria (e.g., *F. gonidiaformans, F. naviforme, F. necrophorum) may* be fusiform shaped, these species and most other *Fusobacterium* spp. are pleomorphic. In fact, certain species, such as *F. mortiferum,* can be extremely pleomorphic, exhibiting globular forms, swellings, and other bizarre shapes. The Gram-stained appearances of *F. mortiferum* and *F. necrophorum* are illustrated in Figures 17-28 and 17-29, respectively.

Laboratory tests. An anaerobic GNB or coccobacillus that is vancomycin resistant, kanamycin sensitive, and col-

istin sensitive could be a member of the *Bacteroides ureolyticus* group (nitrate positive), *Bilophila wadsworthia* (nitrate positive), or a *Fusobacterium* sp. (nitrate negative). (*B. wadsworthia* and the *B. ureolyticus* group were discussed earlier in the chapter.) *Fusobacterium* spp. can be presumptively identified using the criteria in Table 17-19.

> *Fusobacterium* spp. are resistant to vancomycin but susceptible to the other two special-potency antimicrobials: kanamycin and colistin.

CLSI Document M35-A (see "References and Suggested Reading") states that an isolate can be identified as *F. nucleatum* (with more than 95% likelihood) if it meets the following criteria:

- Thin, pointed, fusiform anaerobic Gram-negative bacilli
- Opalescent or bread crumb–like colonies on BA
- No growth on BBE agar
- Spot indole positive

ANTIMICROBIAL SUSCEPTIBILITY TESTING OF ANAEROBES

Traditionally, the isolation, identification, and susceptibility testing of obligate anaerobes have been quite slow compared with those of the other groups of bacteria. As a result, antimicrobial therapy of anaerobe-associated infectious processes was frequently initiated on an **empiric basis**—that is, when clinicians suspected the presence of anaerobes, they selected an antimicrobial agent they *thought* would be effective. Although not a very scientific approach, empiric therapy undoubtedly saved many lives.

Anaerobe susceptibility patterns were once thought to be quite predictable, but the results of numerous studies have provided evidence refuting that predictability. Resistance has

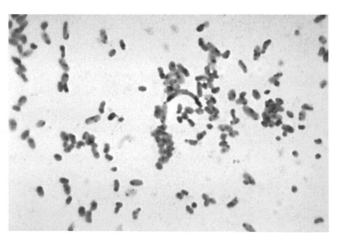

Figure 17-28. **Gram-stained appearance of *Fusobacterium mortiferum*.** (Courtesy of Dr. V. R. Dowell Jr. and the CDC.)

TABLE 17 - 19	Presumptive Identification of Clinically Significant *Fusobacterium* spp.				
Species	**Cellular Morphology**	**Colonial Morphology**	**Indole**	**Bile Resistant**	**Comments**
F. nucleatum	Slender, tapered cells	Bread crumb–like, speckled	+	No	Can be presumptively identified as *F. nucleatum* if indole positive and cells are fusiform
F. gonidiaformans		Smooth	+	No	
F. necrophorum	Large bacilli, rounded ends, bizarre shapes	Umbonate with greening of the blood agar	+	No (most strains)	Can be presumptively identified as *F. necrophorum* if lipase positive
F. naviforme	Boat shaped	Mottled	+	No	
F. varium	Large bacilli, rounded ends	Smooth, fried egg colonies	most strains +	Yes	Can be presumptively identified as *F. varium* if indole negative, bile resistant, and esculin negative
F. mortiferum	Bizarre shapes, including round bodies	Fried-egg colonies	–	Yes	Can be presumptively identified as *F. mortiferum* if esculin positive
F. russi	Large, rounded ends	Smooth	–	No	Can be presumptively identified as *F. russi* if indole negative and bile-sensitive

Source: Mangels JI. Anaerobic bacteriology. In: Essential Procedures for Clinical Microbiology. Washington, DC: ASM Press, 1998.

been detected to virtually all the drugs traditionally considered to have excellent activity against anaerobes. Thus, clinicians can no longer assume susceptibility of anaerobes to these agents.

Significant antimicrobial resistance has been demonstrated in members of the *B. fragilis* group, other *Bacteroides* spp., *Bilophila wadsworthia*, *Sutterella wadsworthensis*, and *Porphyromonas*, *Prevotella*, *Fusobacterium*, *Clostridium*, *Propionibacterium* spp., and anaerobic Gram-positive cocci. Resistance patterns among these anaerobes often vary greatly from one hospital to another and from one geographical area to another. Thus, clinicians at one institution cannot rely on resistance data generated at another institution.

As stated in CLSI Document M11-A7 (see "References and Suggested Reading"), "The recent and varied trends in antibiotic resistance, the spread of resistance genes, and the potential for poor clinical outcomes when using an ineffective antibiotic argue strongly for more susceptibility testing

of anaerobic organisms." Antimicrobial susceptibility testing of anaerobes must be performed in accordance with CLSI guidelines.

When Should Susceptibility Testing of Anaerobes Be Performed?

In CLSI Document M11-A7, the CLSI Working Group on Susceptibility Testing of Anaerobic Bacteria (hereafter referred to as the CLSI Working Group) reports three major reasons for susceptibility testing of anaerobic isolates:

1. "To assist in the management of infection in individual patients with serious or life-threatening infections"

2. "To periodically monitor local and regional resistance patterns so that such information is available as a guide for empiric antimicrobial choice"

3. "To determine patterns of susceptibility of anaerobes to new antimicrobial agents as they are approved for treatment of infections involving anaerobes"

The CLSI Working Group further states that "the major indications for testing clinical isolates are situations in which decisions about the selection of agents are critical because of the:

- known resistance of a particular organism or species

- persistence of the infection despite adequate treatment with an appropriate therapeutic regimen

- difficulty in making empiric decisions based on precedent

- confirmation of appropriate therapy for severe infections or for those that may require long-term therapy"

Antimicrobial susceptibility testing should be limited to isolates considered clinically significant. The CLSI Working Group cites "examples of specific infections from which isolates should be tested: brain abscess, endocarditis, osteomyelitis, joint infection, infection of prosthetic devices or vascular grafts, and bacteremia." In addition, "isolates from normally sterile body fluids should be tested unless they are believed to be contaminants."

Because many anaerobe-associated infectious processes are polymicrobial, it is frequently difficult to decide *which* anaerobic isolates to perform susceptibility testing on. The CLSI Working Group suggests that anaerobes recognized as highly virulent and/or for which susceptibility to the antimicrobial agent(s) commonly used for treatment cannot be predicted should be considered for testing. These include *Bilophila wadsworthia*, *Sutterella wadsworthensis*, and some species of *Bacteroides*, *Prevotella*, *Fusobacterium*, and *Clostridium.*

Specific Antimicrobial Agents to Be Tested

As stated by the CLSI Working Group, "Selection of the most appropriate antimicrobial agents to test and report routinely is a decision made best by each clinical microbiology laboratory in consultation with the infectious disease practitioners and the hospital pharmacy." CLSI Document M11-A7 suggests groupings of antimicrobial agents that can be considered when testing specific anaerobes.

Susceptibility Testing Options

CLSI Document M11-A7 describes two methods for antimicrobial susceptibility testing of anaerobes, and anyone performing susceptibility testing of anaerobes should strictly adhere to the protocols described in that publication.

Reference agar dilution procedure (Wadsworth method). This method requires a large number of agar plates, one plate for each test concentration of each antimicrobial agent to be tested. Standardized suspensions of organisms to be tested are inoculated onto the surface of each plate. A large number of isolates can be inoculated simultaneously, using some type of replicating device (such as the Steer's replicator; see Fig. 7-3). The plates are incubated anaerobically at 35°C to 37°C for 42 to 48 hours. The lowest concentration of each antimicrobial agent that inhibits growth of an organism is reported as the minimal inhibitory concentration (MIC) of that agent. The agar dilution method is usually reserved for institutions testing large numbers of isolates simultaneously and is not a very practical technique for use in smaller CMLs. Nonetheless, the agar dilution method is considered the "gold standard"; therefore, the results achieved with any other method must compare favorably with those achieved using the agar dilution method.

The broth microdilution procedure. CLSI Document M11-A7 suggests that this method be used only for testing members of the *B. fragilis* group. The broth microdilution procedure uses plastic microtiter trays or plates. Each well contains a particular concentration of an antimicrobial agent. One isolate is tested per tray. Inoculated trays are incubated anaerobically at 35°C to 37°C for 46 to 48 hours. The MIC endpoint is the concentration where no growth, or the most significant reduction of growth, is observed.

Although other susceptibility testing procedures are commercially available, they are neither described in Document M11-A7 nor endorsed by the CLSI. It is the responsibility of the U.S. Food and Drug Administration, not the CLSI, to approve or clear commercial devices for use in the United States. Examples of commercially available products include the concentration gradient diffusion system (the Etest) and broth microdilution systems. Before using any of these systems, CML professionals must confirm that results achieved with the system are comparable to those achieved using one of the CLSI reference methods.

β-LACTAMASE TESTING

As discussed in Chapter 7, β-lactamases are enzymes that destroy the β-lactam ring of penicillins (penicillinases) and cephalosporins (cephalosporinases), thus rendering these antibiotics ineffective. The first anaerobes shown to produce β-lactamases were members of the *Bacteroides fragilis* group, but it is now known that many different anaerobes produce these enzymes.

According to Jousimies-Somer et al. (2002; see "References and Suggested Reading"), the following anaerobes have been reported to produce β-lactamases:

- Members of the *Bacteroides fragilis* group

- *Prevotella* spp.

- *Bilophila wadsworthia*

- *Fusobacterium* spp.

- *Clostridium* spp.

The ability of an anaerobe to produce β-lactamase can be determined using simple commercially available methods, such as the nitrocefin disk assay (Cefinase, BD Bioscience) and the S1 chromogenic cephalosporin disk (International BioClinical Inc.). The absence of β-lactamase does not necessarily mean that an organism is susceptible to β-lactam antibiotics. Anaerobes can be resistant to such agents by mechanisms other than β-lactamases. For example, penicillin resistance can occur as a result of alteration of the number or type of penicillin-binding proteins. Alternatively, resistance can occur as a result of blocked penetration of the drug into the active site via alteration of the bacterial outer-membrane pores, or porins. Anaerobes known to be resistant to β-lactam drugs by mechanisms other than production of β-lactamases include *Bacteroides gracilis*, *Bilophila wadsworthia,* and some strains of *Bacteroides distasonis* and *B. fragilis*. **Thus, β-lactamase testing may be used as an adjunct to susceptibility testing but never as a replacement for such testing.**

Chapter Review

- Anaerobes do not require molecular oxygen for life and reproduction, but species vary in their ability to withstand oxygen and its toxic reduction products.

- Anaerobes are found in specific environmental niches: soil, freshwater and saltwater mud, and many anatomical sites in the bodies of animals and humans.

- Although anaerobes exist as part of the indigenous microflora of animals, they can also be involved in serious diseases of humans and animals.

- Knowledge of the composition of the indigenous microflora at specific anatomical sites is useful for predicting the particular organisms most apt to be involved in infectious processes that arise at or adjacent to those sites, as well as the antimicrobial agents most likely to be of value in empiric antimicrobial therapy. The finding of site-specific organisms at a distant and/or unusual site can serve as a clue to the underlying origin of an infectious process.

- Anaerobes occurring in the highest numbers in the microflora of the oral cavity are Gram-positive bacilli (*Actinomyces* and *Eubacterium* spp.), Gram-positive cocci, and Gram-negative bacilli (*Campylobacter*, *Fusobacterium*, *Porphyromonas*, and *Prevotella* spp.). An oral origin should be suspected when oral anaerobes such as *Fusobacterium nucleatum* or pigmented species of *Porphyromonas* are recovered from the bloodstream or from abscesses far distant from the oral cavity.

- The predominant anaerobes inhabiting various sites in the upper respiratory tract other than the mouth are Gram-positive cocci, Gram-positive bacilli (*Actinomyces* and *Propionibacterium* spp.), Gram-negative bacilli (*Campylobacter*, *Capnocytophaga*, *Fusobacterium*, and *Prevotella* spp.), and Gram-negative cocci (*Veillonella* spp.).

- The anaerobes present in highest numbers as indigenous skin flora are *Propionibacterium* spp. (especially *P. acnes*) and, less often, Gram-positive cocci.

- The anaerobes colonizing the distal urethra in the greatest numbers are Gram-negative bacilli: *Bacteroides*, *Fusobacterium*, and *Prevotella* species.

- About 50% of the bacteria in cervical and vaginal secretions are anaerobes, the most common being lactobacilli (not all of which are anaerobes) and Gram-positive cocci. *Prevotella bivia, P. disiens,* and *Mobiluncus* spp. are common anaerobic members of the vaginal flora.

- The anaerobes that are present in the highest numbers in the intestinal flora are species of *Bacteroides,* *Bifidobacterium, Clostridium, Eubacterium, Lactobacillus,* and Gram-positive cocci. *Bacteroides* species are the most common anaerobes in the colon, outnumbering *Escherichia coli* by about 1,000 to 1. In the colon, the most common *Bacteroides* species are *B. vulgatus* and *B. thetaiotaomicron.*

- Anaerobes that are involved in human diseases may originate either *outside* the body (exogenous origin) or *within* the body (endogenous origin). Those of exogenous origin are usually members of the genus *Clostridium,* many species of which are found in soil. Anaerobes of endogenous origin, on the other hand, are members of the indigenous microflora—organisms living on or in the human body.

- Anaerobes of endogenous origin can contribute to infectious processes and diseases in virtually any tissue or any organ of the body. These processes are usually polymicrobial and purulent. However, some necrotic processes involve histotoxic anaerobes that produce cytotoxins capable of causing necrosis of neutrophils, macrophages, and cells of various tissues.

- Certain infectious processes and diseases virtually always involve anaerobes. These include brain and lung abscesses, oral and dental infectious processes, bacterial aspiration pneumonia, peritonitis, intra-abdominal abscess, infectious processes that follow bowel surgery or trauma to the bowel, endometritis, tubo-ovarian abscess, perirectal abscess, gas-forming or necrotizing infectious processes of soft tissue or muscle, and infectious processes of the lower extremities of diabetics.

- Proper selection, collection, and transport of specimens are essential for good anaerobic bacteriology. The quality of anaerobic bacteriology performed in any laboratory can be only as good as the quality of specimens received.

- Processing of a specimen for anaerobic bacteriology includes a macroscopic examination of the specimen, a microscopic examination of the specimen, inoculation of appropriate plated and tubed media, and anaerobic incubation of inoculated media. Each step is critical to the successful recovery of clinically relevant anaerobes from specimens.

- Important characteristics to note during the macroscopic examination of a specimen include its odor, color, turbidity, and fluorescence, in addition to the presence of blood, leukocytes, or sulfur granules.

- Recommended modifications to the conventional Gram staining procedure include methanol fixation in place of heat fixation, counterstaining with safranin for 3 to 5 minutes rather than one minute, or substitution of basic fuchsin for safranin as the counterstain.

These modifications improve the morphology of organisms and host cells present in the specimen and cause Gram-negative bacteria to stain more darkly.

- The ideal media for use in the anaerobic bacteriology laboratory are (1) freshly prepared media; (2) media that have been stored under anaerobic conditions since their preparation; and (3) media that have been manufactured, packaged, shipped and stored under anaerobic conditions (known as PRAS media).

- Recommended plated media for use in the primary setup of specimens for anaerobic bacteriology are BRU, PEA, BBE, and LKV agar, or acceptable alternatives. In addition, specimens should be inoculated to additional media that will be incubated in a CO_2 incubator or in air.

- Anaerobic incubation of inoculated plates can be accomplished using an anaerobic chamber or anaerobic jars or bags. Although anaerobic chambers are recommended for use in laboratories doing a high volume of anaerobic bacteriology, jars and bags have proven to be acceptable alternatives for smaller laboratories.

- Processing a colony suspected to be an anaerobe includes (1) describing the colony, (2) preparing and examining a Gram stain from it, (3) inoculating a pure culture or subculture plate, and (4) performing an aerotolerance test.

- In the aerotolerance test, obligate anaerobes will grow on the anaerobically incubated BRU/BA plate, but not on the CO_2 incubated chocolate agar plate or the aerobically incubated blood agar plate. Although some aerotolerant anaerobes can grow on a CO_2 incubated chocolate agar plate, they will grow better on an anaerobically incubated BRU/BA plate.

- Among the simple observations and inexpensive tests used to presumptively identify anaerobic isolates are growth or no growth on selective media, colony morphology, Gram reaction and cell morphology, aerotolerance testing, fluorescence, special-potency antimicrobial disk, SPS disk, nitrate disk, bile disk, spot indole test, catalase test, urease test, motility test, and oxidase test.

- Many techniques are available for definitively identifying anaerobic isolates. Examples include PRAS and non-PRAS tubed biochemical test media, biochemical-based minisystems, preexisting enzyme-based minisystems, gas-liquid chromatographic analysis of metabolic end-products, and cellular fatty acid analysis by GLC.

- Anaerobes are taxonomically divided into those that produce endospores and those that do not. All spore-forming anaerobic bacilli are members of the genus *Clostridium*. Although all clostridia form spores, spores are not always seen in clinical specimens containing clostridia or pure cultures of the organisms.

- The most frequently isolated and or clinically important anaerobes encountered in properly selected and collected clinical specimens are members of the *Bacteroides fragilis* group, *Porphyromonas* and *Prevotella* spp., *Fusobacterium nucleatum* and *Fusobacterium necrophorum*, anaerobic cocci (e.g., *Peptostreptococcus anaerobius* and *Finegoldia magna*), *Actinomyces israelii*, and certain *Clostridium* species (e.g., *C. perfringens*, *C. ramosum*, *C. clostridioforme*, *C. septicum*, and *C. difficile*).

- The most frequently isolated anaerobic GPC are *Peptostreptococcus anaerobius*, *Finegoldia magna* (formerly *Peptostreptococcus magnus*), *Peptoniphilus assacharolyticus* (formerly *Peptostreptococcus asaccharolyticus*), and *Micromonas micros* (formerly *Peptostreptococcus micros*). Most anaerobic Gram-negative cocci encountered in clinical specimens are *Veillonella* spp.

- *Clostridium perfringens* causes a relatively mild type of food poisoning but is also the most common cause of gas gangrene.

- *Clostridium tetani* causes tetanus, *Clostridium botulinum* causes botulism, and *Clostridium difficile* is the most common cause of antibiotic-associated diarrhea and pseudomembranous colitis.

- *Bacteroides* and *Fusobacterium* species are the most commonly encountered anaerobic Gram-negative bacilli.

- Members of the *B. fragilis* group include *B. caccae*, *B. distasonis*, *B. eggerthii*, *B. fragilis*, *B. merdae*, *B. ovatus*, *B. stercoris*, *B. thetaiotaomicron*, *B. uniformis*, and *B. vulgatus*. *B. fragilis* is the most common species of anaerobic bacteria isolated from soft tissue infectious processes and bacteremia.

- *Porphyromonas* species are asaccharolytic, bile-sensitive Gram-negative bacilli, most of which produce brown-black pigmented colonies. Species of *Porphyromonas* include *P. asaccharolytica, P. endodontalis,* and *P. gingivalis.* Some *Prevotella* spp. also produce brown-black–pigmented colonies.

- *F. nucleatum* subsp. *fusiforme* is the only *Fusobacterium* that routinely exists as long, thin Gram-negative bacilli with tapered ends. Although some cells of certain other fusobacteria (e.g., *F. gonidiaformans, F. naviforme, F. necrophorum*) may be fusiform shaped, these species and most other *Fusobacterium* species are pleomorphic.

- Antimicrobial resistance occurs among many different anaerobes and involves many different antimicrobial agents. Especially resistant anaerobes include members of the *Bacteroides fragilis* group, *B. gracilis*, *Clostridium ramosum*, and *Fusobacterium varium*.

- The major indications for performing susceptibility testing of anaerobes are (1) to determine patterns of susceptibility of anaerobes to *new* antimicrobial agents, (2) to monitor susceptibility patterns periodically in medical centers, (3) to monitor susceptibility patterns periodically in local communities and hospitals, and (4) to assist in the management of infectious processes in patients when appropriate.

- Many different anaerobes produce β-lactamases, including the *Bacteroides fragilis* group, *Clostridium* spp., *Fusobacterium* spp., and *Prevotella* spp. Some anaerobes (e.g., *Bacteroides gracilis*, *Bilophila wadsworthia*, and some *B. distasonis* and some *B. fragilis* strains) are resistant to β-lactam drugs by mechanisms other than production of β-lactamases.

New Terms and Abbreviations

After studying Chapter 17, you should be familiar with the following terms, which are defined within the chapter and in the Glossary at the back of the book:

Actinomyces-like

Botulinal toxin

Diphtheroid-like

Endogenous anaerobe

Exogenous anaerobe

Fusiform

Nonsterile sites

Nonsterile specimens

PRAS media

Tetanospasmin

References and Suggested Reading

Abbreviated Identification of Bacteria and Yeast: Approved Guideline. CLSI Document M35-A. Wayne, PA: Clinical and Laboratory Standards Institute, 2002.

Allen SD, et al. Anaerobic bacteriology. In: Truant AL, ed. Manual of Commercial Methods in Clinical Microbiology. Washington, DC: ASM Press, 2002.

Allen SD, et al. *Clostridium*. In: Murray PR, Baron EJ, Jorgensen JH, Pfaller MA, Yolken RH, eds. Manual of Clinical Microbiology. 8th Ed. Washington, DC: ASM Press, 2003.

Allen SD, et al. Current issues and problems in dealing with anaerobes in the clinical laboratory. Contemp Issues Clin Microbiol 1995;15:333–364.

Bartlett JG. Anaerobic bacteria. In: Gorbach SL, Bartlett JG, Blacklow NR, eds. Infectious Disease. 3rd Ed. Philadelphia: Lippincott Williams & Wilkins, 2004.

Bartlett JG. Anaerobic cocci. In: Gorbach SL, Bartlett JG, Blacklow NR, eds. Infectious Disease. 3rd Ed. Philadelphia: Lippincott Williams & Wilkins, 2004.

Bartlett JG. *Clostridium difficile*–associated diarrhea and colitis. In: Gorbach SL, Bartlett JG, Blacklow NR, eds. Infectious Disease. 3rd Ed. Philadelphia: Lippincott Williams & Wilkins, 2004.

Bartlett JG. *Clostridium tetani*. In: Gorbach SL, Bartlett JG, Blacklow NR, eds. Infectious Disease. 3rd Ed. Philadelphia: Lippincott Williams & Wilkins, 2004.

Citron DM, Hecht DW. Susceptibility test methods: anaerobic bacteria. In: Murray PR, Baron EJ, Jorgensen JH, Pfaller MA, Yolken RH, eds. Manual of Clinical Microbiology. 8th Ed. Washington, DC: ASM Press, 2003.

Engelkirk PG, et al. Principles and Practice of Anaerobic Bacteriology. Belmont, CA: Star, 1992.

Finegold SM. Anaerobic Gram-negative rods: *Bacteroides, Prevotella, Porphyromonas, Fusobacterium, Bilophila, Sutterella, Tannerella*. In: Gorbach SL, Bartlett JG, Blacklow NR, eds. Infectious Disease. 3rd Ed. Philadelphia: Lippincott Williams & Wilkins, 2004.

Finegold SM, George WL, Mulligon ME. Anaerobic Infections. Chicago: Year Book Medical, 1986.

Gorbach SL. *Clostridium perfringens* and other clostridia. In: Gorbach SL, Bartlett JG, Blacklow NR, eds. Infectious Disease. 3rd Ed. Philadelphia: Lippincott Williams & Wilkins, 2004.

Hatheway CL, Bartlett JG. *Clostridium botulinum*. In: Gorbach SL, Bartlett JG, Blacklow NR, eds. Infectious Disease. 3rd Ed. Philadelphia: Lippincott Williams & Wilkins, 2004.

Holdeman LV, et al. VPI Anaerobe Laboratory Manual. 4th Ed. Blacksburg, VA: Virginia Polytechnic Institute and State University, 1977 (updated 1987).

Jousimies-Somer HR, et al. *Bacteroides, Porphyromonas, Prevotella, Fusobacterium*, and other anaerobic Gram-negative bacteria. In: Murray PR, Baron EJ, Jorgensen JH, Pfaller MA, Yolken RH, eds. Manual of Clinical Microbiology. 8th Ed. Washington, DC: ASM Press, 2003.

Jousimies-Somer HR, Summanen P, Baron EJ, Citron DM, Wexler HM, Finegold SM. Wadsworth-KTL Anaerobic Bacteriology Manual. 6th Ed. Belmont, CA: Star, 2002.

Koneman EW, et al. Color Atlas and Textbook of Diagnostic Microbiology. 5th Ed. Philadelphia: Lippincott-Raven Publishers, 1997.

Lombard GL, Dowell VR Jr. Gas Liquid Chromatography and Analysis of the Acid Products of Bacteria. Atlanta: Centers for Disease Control, 1982.

Mangels JI. Anaerobic bacteriology. In: Essential Procedures for Clinical Microbiology. Washington, DC: ASM Press, 1998.

Methods for Antimicrobial Susceptibility Testing of Anaerobic Bacteria: Approved Standard. 6th Ed. CLSI Document M11-A7. Wayne, PA: Clinical and Laboratory Standards Institute, 2007.

Moncla BJ, Hillier SL. *Peptostreptococcus*, *Propionibacterium*, *Lactobacillus*, *Actinomyces*, and other non-spore-forming anaerobic Gram-positive bacteria. In: Murray PR, Baron EJ, Jorgensen JH, Pfaller MA, Yolken RH, eds. Manual of Clinical Microbiology. 8th Ed. Washington, DC: ASM Press, 2003.

Winn WC Jr, et al. Koneman's Color Atlas and Textbook of Diagnostic Microbiology. 6th Ed. Philadelphia: Lippincott Williams & Wilkins, 2006.

 ## *On the CD-ROM*

- Why Anaerobes Die in the Presence of Oxygen

- Indications of Anaerobe Involvement in Human Diseases

- Recap of Bacteria Discussed in Chapters 9 Through 17

- Additional Self-Assessment Exercises

- Case Study

- Puzzle

Self-Assessment Exercises

1. Define the following terms:

    A. Aerotolerant anaerobe: _____

    B. Facultative anaerobe: _____

    C. Obligate anaerobe: _____

2. The toxicity of oxygen to anaerobes is thought to occur in a two-stage process: a bacteriostatic phase (first phase) and a bactericidal phase (second phase). Briefly describe what happens in each phase. (Note: The answer to this question can be found on the CD-ROM.)

    A. First phase: _____

    B. Second phase: _____

3. Give the Gram reaction (Gram positive or Gram negative) and morphologic appearance of each of the following anaerobes (e.g., *Propionibacterium acnes* is a Gram-positive diphtheroid).

	Gram Reaction	Morphology
A. *Bacteroides fragilis*	_____	_____
B. *Clostridium perfringens*	_____	_____
C. *Fusobacterium nucleatum*	_____	_____
C. *Peptostreptococcus anaerobius*	_____	_____
E. *Veillonella* spp.	_____	_____
F. *Bacteroides ureolyticus*	_____	_____
G. *Actinomyces* spp.	_____	_____
H. *Mobiluncus* spp.	_____	_____
I. *Bifidobacterium* spp.	_____	_____

4. True or false: All spore-forming anaerobic bacilli are classified as *Clostridium* species.

5. True or false: It is easy to recognize *Clostridium* species in Gram-stained smears of clinical specimens because they always stain blue and always contain spores.

6. Name five species in the *Bacteroides fragilis* group.

    A. _____

    B. _____

    C. _____

    D. _____

    E. _____

D. _____

E. _____

7. True or false: The anaerobes most often involved in infectious diseases are from endogenous sources.

8. The following specimens have been received in the laboratory for anaerobic culture. Indicate which of these specimens are acceptable (**A**), and which are unacceptable (**U**) for routine anaerobic bacteriology.

_____ A. Voided urine

_____ B. Blood

_____ C. Cerebrospinal fluid

_____ D. Feces

_____ E. Catheterized urine

_____ F. Synovial fluid

_____ G. Swab containing material from oral abscess

_____ H. Swab containing pus from skin lesions

_____ I. Bone marrow

_____ J. Tissue biopsy specimen

9. List four types of solid culture media recommended for primary isolation of anaerobes from clinical specimens.

A. _____

B. _____

C. _____

D. _____

10. List five simple test results or reactions that are of value in making presumptive identifications of anaerobes.

A. _____

B. _____

C. _____

D. _____

E. _____

CHAPTER 18

Laboratory Diagnosis of Selected Bacterial Infections

Chapter Outline

LEARNING OBJECTIVES

After studying this chapter, you should be able to:

☞ Define the terms introduced in this chapter (e.g., *fasciae, fasciitis, gangrene*)

☞ Name at least one infectious disease and associated bacterial pathogen for each body site discussed in this chapter (e.g., cardiovascular system, eyes, ears)

☞ Discuss the criteria for blood cultures to include number of specimens to collect, amount of blood, and time intervals

☞ Given a particular type of clinical specimen (e.g., skin) identify potential pathogens, and indigenous microflora and/or contaminants, as appropriate

- Relate the importance of the Gram stain in the identification of bacterial infections and disease processes, and discuss the significance of polymorphonuclear leukocytes, "clue" cells, and other types of cells

- Differentiate between gangrene and gas gangrene

- For each body site discussed, describe the following aspects of diagnosing bacterial infections: clinical specimen required, any specimen preservation and transport requirements, Gram-stain observations, any screening tests, media necessary for isolation of the pathogen, incubation requirements, and general laboratory diagnostic procedures

- Given a particular pathogen (e.g., *Neisseria gonorrhoeae*), identify the most appropriate media for isolation and identification of that pathogen

- Describe the special procedures used to decontaminate and digest sputum for *Mycobacterium tuberculosis* workup, including the purpose of each procedure and the reagents used

- Identify the most common bacterial causes of cystitis and pyelonephritis

- Given sufficient information, calculate the number of colony-forming units per mL of urine

- Given a patient's urine colony count results, correctly state whether a urinary tract infection is likely or unlikely

- Relate the special collection, transport, and media requirements for clinical specimens suspected of containing *Neisseria gonorrhoeae*

- State how gonorrhea is diagnosed in men and in women

- Relate the procedures for the immunodiagnosis of syphilis, and describe the type of specimen, category of the procedure (i.e., treponemal and nontreponemal), and basic principle (e.g., fluorescent antibody)

- Compare and contrast the treponemal and nontreponemal tests for syphilis, and discuss reaginic antibodies

- List the three main etiologic agents of vaginitis

- Given laboratory data from a patient suspected of having bacterial vaginosis, calculate the likelihood of the disease using the Nugent criteria

- Given an actual saline wet mount or micrograph of vaginal fluid, identify the presence of any clue cells

- Name three of the most common bacterial causes of diarrheal diseases

It would be impossible in a book of this size to describe *all* the infectious diseases caused by bacteria. Thus, only selected bacterial diseases are discussed in this chapter. Readers should keep in mind that although diseases are described in one particular section of the chapter (e.g., under cardiovascular infections or lower respiratory tract infections), often a bacterial disease has more than one clinical manifestation affecting more than one anatomical site. Gonorrhea is a good example. Though described in the section on sexually transmitted diseases of the genital tract, gonorrhea can affect many areas of the body, such as eyes, joints, muscles, skin, and throat, in addition to the genital tract.

The order in which bacterial diseases are presented in this chapter closely follows the order of clinical specimens discussed in Chapter 5. Recall that the names of many infectious diseases are defined in that earlier chapter, which also discusses the various types of clinical specimens necessary for diagnosis of those diseases, the importance of high-quality specimens, and the criteria for rejecting inappropriate or otherwise unacceptable specimens. Rather than repeat information already presented, this chapter often refers to earlier chapters for specific information concerning the manner in which bacterial pathogens are identified or speciated.

BACTERIAL INFECTIONS OF THE CARDIOVASCULAR SYSTEM

Diseases and most likely pathogens. Blood is normally sterile. The presence of bacteria in the bloodstream may represent (1) a transient bacteremia; (2) bacteremia secondary to infection at a primary site, such as the lungs; or (3) an infection of the bloodstream, known as septicemia or sepsis. Thus, many types of bacteria may be isolated from blood specimens. The most common causes of septicemia are Enterobacteriaceae, streptococci, enterococci, and staphylococci. Depending on the clinical situation, bacteremia may be continuous or intermittent.

STUDY AID   **Bacteremia Versus Septicemia.** Recall that **bacteremia** means the presence of bacteria in the bloodstream, which may or may not be caused by an infectious disease. **Septicemia,** on the other hand, is a serious disease characterized by chills, fever, prostration, and the presence of bacteria and/or their toxins in the bloodstream.

Bacteremia is usually continuous in patients with endocarditis. The most common bacterial causes of native valve endocarditis are α-hemolytic streptococci, enterococci (especially *Enterococcus faecalis*), and staphylococci (primarily

Staphylococcus aureus). Other causes are the HACEK group of aerobic Gram-negative bacilli (see Chapters 11 and 14). The most common bacterial causes of prosthetic valve endocarditis are *Staphylococcus epidermidis* and *S. aureus*. Any of these bacteria, as well as many others, can be isolated from the bloodstream. Endocarditis is discussed in greater detail later in the chapter.

Clinical specimens. Great care must be taken when collecting blood for culture. The phlebotomy or venipuncture site must be properly disinfected prior to needle insertion, using one of several available antiseptics (e.g., iodophors, tincture of iodine, chlorhexidine). The tops of blood culture bottles must be disinfected with 70% isopropyl alcohol or a phenolic before introducing the specimen. Multiple blood specimens should be drawn to detect intermittent bacteremia or to confirm or rule out contaminated cultures. Guidelines regarding collection of blood culture specimens vary from institution to institution and are based on the age of the patient, the suspected infectious disease, and the type of blood culture system used. Some proposed guidelines are presented in Table 18-1, but not all authorities are in agreement with these guidelines. Some authorities believe that the volume of blood drawn (at least 20 mL for adults) is far more critical than the timing of blood collection.

The general rule is to collect two or three blood specimens, each inoculated with at least 10 to 20 mL of blood, per 24-hour period. Specimens should be collected at intervals no closer than 3 hours, to demonstrate that the bacteremia is continuous. Specimen collection should be done before initiation of antimicrobial therapy. If antimicrobial therapy is to be initiated immediately, two specimens should be collected from different sites. Blood collected through peripheral or indwelling central venous catheters is often contaminated with members of the indigenous microflora of the skin. Additional guidelines regarding blood culture specimens are provided by Miller and by Thomson and Miller (see "References and Suggested Reading").

> The number of blood culture specimens to collect depends on the age of the patient, the suspected infectious disease, and the type of blood culture system being used.

TABLE 18 - 1 Guidelines for Collecting Blood Culture Specimens

Age Group	Suspected Clinical Condition	Specimens to Collect	Comments
Adults and adolescents	Severe septicemia, meningitis, osteomyelitis, arthritis, pneumonia	Collect 2 cultures: one 10- to 20-mL sample from each arm	Collect specimens before initiation of therapy
	Subacute bacterial endocarditis	Collect 3 cultures spaced over a 24-hour period	Collect 2 specimens at the first sign of febrile episodes; collect 3 more specimens if the first 3 are negative
	Acute bacterial endocarditis	Collect 3 cultures	Collect before initiation of therapy
	Low-grade intravascular infection	Collect 3 cultures, spaced over a 24-hour period	Space collections at least 1 hour apart; collect 2 specimens at the first sign of febrile episodes
	Bacteremia of unknown origin (when the patient is receiving therapy)	Collect 4 to 6 cultures over a 48-hour period	Collect specimens just before administration of antibiotic
	Febrile episodes	Collect no more than 3 cultures	Bear in mind that bacteremia may precede fever by 1 hour
Children		1- to 2-mL samples	2 cultures are usually adequate to diagnose bacteremia in neonates

Source: Miller JM. A Guide to Specimen Management in Clinical Microbiology. 2nd Ed. Washington, DC: ASM Press, 1999.

Specimen preservation. Transport time at room temperature should be less than 2 hours.

Contaminants. During collection, blood specimens frequently become contaminated with members of the indigenous microflora of the skin. Coagulase-negative staphylococci, especially *S. epidermidis*, are especially common contaminants.

Gram stain information. Gram staining of blood specimens at the time of collection is rarely of value. However, it can be helpful when bacteria are observed in hematology smears, as in cases of meningococcemia, *Streptococcus pneumoniae* infection, or other infections in which the concentration of bacteria in the bloodstream is very high (10^4 bacteria/mL or higher).

Screening tests. In traditional blood culture systems, bottles were examined by clinical microbiology laboratory (CML) professionals at regular intervals—at least once daily—for evidence of bacterial growth, such as hemolysis, bubbles, or turbidity. The newer systems detect gas production or other metabolic activities of any microorganisms present. Detection techniques include infrared spectroscopy, color change in an indicator, and pressure measurement.

Culture media. Modern blood culture systems, which most often are two-bottle systems, support the growth of most aerobes or anaerobes that could be present in the blood.

Laboratory diagnosis. The contents of positive blood cultures are Gram stained. If bacteria are observed, a preliminary report (often telephonic) should be sent to the clinician stating the cellular morphology, cellular arrangement, and Gram reaction of the organism(s) observed. For example, a clinician receiving a report stating "Gram-positive cocci in clusters" could assume that the organism is a *Staphylococcus* species and might initiate appropriate therapy based on that assumption (Fig. 18-1).

The contents of the positive blood culture are inoculated onto appropriate media. The types of media inoculated are most often based on the Gram stain observations. Anaerobic media should be inoculated if the cellular morphology is suggestive of a particular species of anaerobe, or when only the anaerobic bottle is positive. When no organisms are observed on Gram stain, a routine battery of media is inoculated, such as blood agar, chocolate agar, MacConkey agar (MAC), and colistin-nalidixic acid agar (CNA). Some CMLs routinely inoculate media to be incubated anaerobically. Further workup depends on the type(s) of organisms that grow on these media. For example, if a Gram-positive coccus was isolated, it would be identified using the criteria described in Chapter 9. If a lactose-fermenting Gram-negative bacillus was isolated, it would be identified using the criteria described in Chapter 12. **It is important to keep in mind that more than one pathogen may be present.**

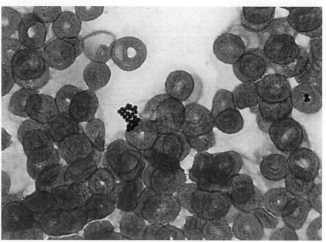

Figure 18-1. **A *Staphylococcus*-like cluster of Gram-positive cocci in a Gram-stained blood culture.** (From Marler LM, Siders JA, Allen SD. Direct Smear Atlas. Philadelphia: Lippincott Williams & Wilkins, 2001.)

Infective Endocarditis

Disease. Infective (or infectious) endocarditis is usually caused by a bacterium or a fungus. It is characterized by the presence of vegetations (bacteria and blood clots) on or within the endocardium, most commonly involving a heart valve. Abnormal or damaged valves are most susceptible to infection, although valves can become contaminated during open heart surgery. The vegetations can break loose and be transported to vital organs, where they can block arterial blood flow. Obviously, such obstructions are very serious, possibly leading to strokes, heart attacks, or death.

Pathogens. The two most common types of infective endocarditis are acute bacterial endocarditis and subacute bacterial endocarditis. Acute bacterial endocarditis is usually caused by colonization of heart valves by virulent bacteria such as *S. aureus* (the most common cause), *Streptococcus pneumoniae*, *Neisseria gonorrhoeae*, *Streptococcus pyogenes*, or *E. faecalis*. In subacute bacterial endocarditis, heart valves are infected by less virulent organisms, such as α-hemolytic streptococci of oral origin (viridans group streptococci), *S. epidermidis*, *Enterococcus* spp., or *Haemophilus* spp. Fungal endocarditis is rare, but cases of *Candida* and *Aspergillus* endocarditis do occur.

Oral streptococci can enter the bloodstream following minor or major dental procedures, oral surgery, or aggressive toothbrushing. Phlebotomy procedures and insertion of intravenous lines sometimes force organisms from the skin into the bloodstream. Intravenous drug users are at high risk of developing infective endocarditis as a result of contaminated needles, syringes, and drug solutions.

Laboratory diagnosis. Blood cultures are required for diagnosis of infective endocarditis.

Lyme Disease

Disease. Lyme disease or Lyme borreliosis is a tickborne disease characterized by three stages: (1) an early, distinctive, targetlike, red skin lesion, usually at the site of the tick bite, expanding to a diameter of 15 cm, often with a central clearing; (2) early systemic manifestations that may include fatigue, chills, fever, headache, stiff neck, muscle pain, and joint aches, with or without lymphadenopathy; and (3) neurologic abnormalities (e.g., aseptic meningitis, facial paralysis, myelitis, encephalitis) and cardiac abnormalities (e.g., arrhythmias, pericarditis) several weeks or months after the initial symptoms appear. The first U.S. cases occurred in 1975 in Lyme, Connecticut. Since then, Lyme disease has been reported in 45 states (mainly in the Mid-Atlantic, Northeast, and North Central regions), and it occurs in many other areas of the world. **Lyme disease is the most common arthropod-borne disease in the United States.**

Pathogen. The etiologic agent of Lyme disease is *Borrelia burgdorferi*, a loosely coiled Gram-negative spirochete. Ticks, rodents (especially deer mice), and mammals (especially deer) serve as reservoirs. Transmission occurs via tick bite.

Laboratory diagnosis. Lyme disease is usually diagnosed by observation of the characteristic targetlike skin lesion (see Fig. 15-9) plus immunodiagnostic procedures and polymerase chain reaction. *B. burgdorferi* can be observed in Gram-stained blood specimens and can be grown in the laboratory on a special medium—Barbour-Stoenner-Kelley medium—at 33°C (Fig. 18-2). See Chapter 15 for additional information regarding identification of *Borrelia* spp.

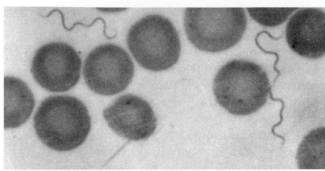

Figure 18-3. Borrelia recurrentis **in a Giemsa-stained blood specimen.** (From Binford CH, Connor DH. Pathology of Tropical and Extraordinary Diseases, vol 1. Washington, DC: Armed Forces Institute of Pathology, 1976.)

Relapsing Fever

Disease. As the name implies, relapsing fever is characterized by periods of fever that alternate with afebrile periods. The periods of fever last from 2 to 9 days, and afebrile periods last from 2 to 4 days. The number of relapses varies from 1 to 10. Relapsing fever may be transmitted either by lice or ticks. Louseborne relapsing fever usually lasts from 13 to 16 days. Tickborne relapsing fever usually lasts longer. Patients may develop a transitory petechial rash and gastrointestinal, respiratory, and/or meningeal symptoms. Relapsing fever occurs in most areas of the world. Tickborne relapsing fever occurs in the United States, whereas louseborne relapsing fever does not.

Pathogen. Louseborne relapsing fever is caused by *Borrelia recurrentis*, a Gram-negative spirochete. It is usually acquired by crushing an infected louse and subsequent entry

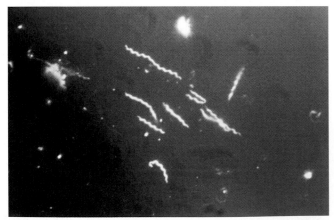

Figure 18-2. Borrelia burgdorferi, **as seen by darkfield microscopy.** (Specimen source unknown; perhaps culture.) Although they are quite thin, *Borrelia* spp. can also be seen in Gram-stained blood smears. (Courtesy of the Centers for Disease Control and Prevention [CDC].)

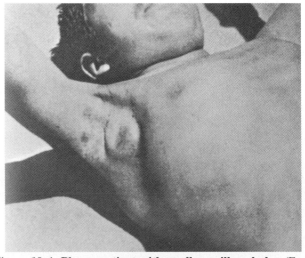

Figure 18-4. **Plague patient with swollen axillary bubo.** (From Binford CH, Connor DH. Pathology of Tropical and Extraordinary Diseases, vol 1. Washington, DC: Armed Forces Institute of Pathology, 1976.)

Historical Vignette

Plague. *During the Middle Ages, plague was referred to as the black death because of the darkened, bruised appearance of the corpses (Fig. 18-5). The blackened skin and foul smell were the result of cell necro-*

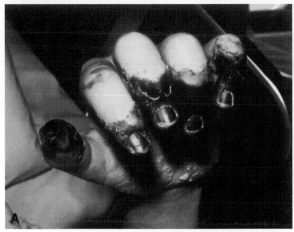
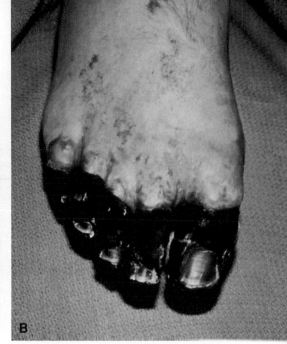

Figure 18-5. **Gangrenous hand (A) and foot (B) of patients with plague.** ([A] Courtesy of Dr. Jack Poland and the CDC. [B] Courtesy of William Archibald and the CDC.)

sis and hemorrhaging into the skin. Plague probably dates back a thousand or more years BC. In the past 2000 years, the disease has killed millions of people, perhaps hundreds of millions. Huge plague epidemics occurred in Asia and Europe, including the European plague epidemic of 1348–1350, which killed about 44% of the population (40 million of 90 million people). The last major plague epidemic in Europe occurred in 1721. Plague still occurs, but the availability of insecticides and antibiotics has greatly reduced the incidence of this dreadful disease. Human plague is very rare in the United States (only eight cases in 2005).

---

of the pathogen through the bite wound or skin abrasion. Tickborne relapsing fever is caused by other *Borrelia* spp. that usually enter the skin at the site of a tick bite.

Laboratory diagnosis. Diagnosis is usually made by observation of the pathogen in darkfield preparations of fresh blood or stained thick or thin blood films (Fig. 18-3; see Chapter 22). The organisms are usually absent from the bloodstream between relapses.

Plague

Disease. Plague is an acute, often severe zoonosis. Initial signs and symptoms may include fever, chills, malaise, myalgia, nausea, prostration, sore throat, and headache. There are three types of plague: **Bubonic plague** is named for the swollen, inflamed, and tender lymph nodes (buboes) that develop. Usually, the lymph nodes affected are those receiving drainage from the site of the bite of an infected flea (Fig. 18-4). In about 90% of cases, the inguinal (groin area) lymph nodes are involved. **Pneumonic plague,** which

is highly communicable, involves the lungs. It can result in localized outbreaks or devastating epidemics. **Septicemic plague** may cause septic shock, meningitis, or death.

Pathogen. The etiologic agent of plague is *Yersinia pestis*, a nonmotile, bipolar-staining Gram-negative coccobacillus sometimes referred to as the plague bacillus. Reservoirs include wild rodents (especially ground squirrels in the United States) and their fleas and, rarely, rabbits, wild carnivores, and domestic cats. Transmission is usually via flea bite (rodent to flea to human). Transmission may also occur as a result of handling tissues of infected rodents, rabbits, and other animals, as well as droplet transmission from person to person (in pneumonic plague).

Laboratory diagnosis. Plague is diagnosed by observation of the typical appearance of *Y. pestis* (bipolar-staining bacilli that resemble safety pins) in Gram-stained or Wright-Giemsa-stained sputum, cerebrospinal fluid, or material aspirated from a bubo (Fig. 18-6). Diagnosis can also be made by culture, biochemical tests, and immunodiagnostic

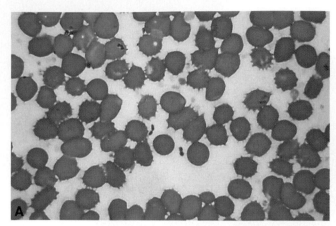
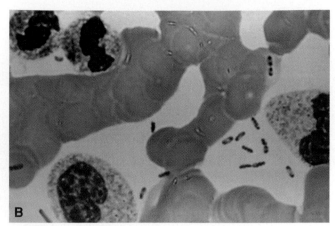

Figure 18-6. Yersinia pestis, **the etiologic agent of plague. A.** *Y. pestis* in a Gram-stained blood smear. **B.** *Y. pestis* in a Wright-stained blood smear. Notice the safety-pin appearance that results from bipolar staining. ([A] Courtesy of Dr. Jack Poland and the CDC. [B] Courtesy of the CDC.)

tests. Chapter 12 provides additional information regarding identification of *Yersinia* spp.

Tularemia

Disease. Tularemia, also known as rabbit fever, is an acute zoonosis with various clinical manifestations, depending on the portal of entry of the pathogen into the body. Tularemia most often presents as a skin ulcer (see Fig. 14-13) and regional lymphadenitis. Ingestion of the pathogen results in pharyngitis, abdominal pain, diarrhea, and vomiting. Inhalation of the pathogen results in pneumonia and septicemia, with a 30% to 60% fatality rate.

Pathogen. The etiologic agent of tularemia is *Francisella tularensis*, a small, pleomorphic Gram-negative coccobacillus. Some strains are more virulent than others. Reservoirs include wild animals (especially rabbits, muskrats, beavers), some domestic animals, and hard ticks. Transmission occurs via tick bite, ingestion of contaminated meat or drinking water, entry of organisms into a wound while skinning infected animals, inhalation of dust, or animal bites. Tularemia is not transmitted from person to person.

Laboratory diagnosis. Diagnosis is by culture, biochemical tests, and immunodiagnostic procedures. Refer to Chapter 14 for additional information regarding identification of *F. tularensis*.

Typhoid Fever

Disease. Typhoid fever, also known as enteric fever, is a systemic bacterial disease with fever, severe headache, malaise, anorexia, a rash on the trunk in about 25% of patients, nonproductive cough, and constipation. Other possible complications include bacteremia; pneumonia; gallbladder, liver, or bone infection; endocarditis; and meningitis. About 10% of untreated patients die. Worldwide an estimated 17 million cases occur annually, with approximately 600,000 deaths.

Pathogen. The etiologic agent of typhoid fever is *Salmonella enterica* subsp. *enterica* serovar Typhi (also called *Salmonella typhi* or the typhoid bacillus). *S. typhi* is a Gram-negative bacillus that releases endotoxin and produces exotoxins. A similar, but less severe, infection is caused by *Salmonella enterica* subsp. *enterica* serovar Paratyphi (also known as *Salmonella paratyphi*). Infected humans serve as reservoirs for *S. typhi* and *S. paratyphi*; rarely, domestic animals are reservoirs for *S. paratyphi*. Some people become carriers following infection, shedding the pathogens in their feces or urine (see the Chapter 2 section of the CD-ROM for the "Typhoid Mary" story.) Transmission occurs via the fecal-oral route: food or water contaminated by the feces or urine of patients or carriers, oysters harvested from fecally contaminated waters, or fecally contaminated fruits or raw vegetables. Food may become fecally contaminated via flies.

Laboratory diagnosis. Diagnosis necessitates isolation of *S. typhi* from blood, urine, feces, or bone marrow. *S. typhi* is identified by biochemical tests. Immunodiagnostic procedures are available. For additional information on identification of *Salmonella* spp., see Chapter 12.

Ehrlichiosis

Disease. Ehrlichiosis is an acute, febrile illness ranging from asymptomatic to mild to severe and life threatening. Patients usually present with acute influenza-like illness with fever, headache, and generalized malaise. Ehrlichiosis is reminiscent of Rocky Mountain spotted fever, without the rash. The estimated fatality rate is about 5%. There are two types of ehrlichiosis: human monocytotrophic ehrlichiosis (HME) and human granulocytotrophic ehrlichiosis (HGE). Cases of HME are more common than HGE cases. Most HME cases have occurred in the southeastern and mid-Atlantic states, whereas most HGE cases have occurred in states with high rates of Lyme disease (particularly, Connecticut, Minnesota, New York, and Wisconsin). In these states, the tick that transmits the HGE agent is the same tick that transmits *Borrelia burgdorferi,* the etiologic agent of Lyme disease. The two types of ehrlichiosis seem to be transmitted by different species of ticks.

Pathogens. The etiologic agents of ehrlichiosis are Gram-negative coccobacilli that are closely related to rickettsias. They are obligate intraleukocytic pathogens. *Ehrlichia chaffeensis* invades human monocytes, causing HME. *Anaplasma phagocytophilum*, which previously was an *Ehrlichia* species, invades human granulocytes, causing HGE. A canine species, *E. ewingi*, has caused a small number of human cases. Reservoirs are unknown. Transmission occurs via tick bite.

> The etiologic agents of ehrlichiosis are obligate intraleukocytic pathogens

Laboratory diagnosis. Ehrlichiosis is diagnosed using immunodiagnostic procedures and nucleic acid assays. Refer to Chapter 16 for additional information regarding identification of *Ehrlichia* and *Anaplasma* spp.

BACTERIAL INFECTIONS OF THE SKIN AND SUBCUTANEOUS TISSUES

Staphylococcal and Streptococcal Infections

Diseases and most likely pathogens. Bacterial infections of the skin include infections with multiple etiologies—such as abscesses, bite wounds, burn wounds, other types of wounds, cellulitis, decubitus ulcers, and folliculitis—and infections with specific etiologies. The latter category includes *Staphylococcus aureus* infections, such as furuncles, carbuncles, staphylococcal scalded skin syndrome, impetigo, and ecthyma,[1] and *Streptococcus pyogenes* infections, such as impetigo, ecthyma, erysipelas, and scarlet fever. It is important to understand that skin lesions and rashes can be a component of many types of infection, including gonorrhea, syphilis, meningococcemia, and rickettsial infections, which are described elsewhere in this chapter. Gas gangrene and necrotizing fasciitis are also described later in the chapter.

Clinical specimens. Whenever possible, aspirates should be submitted to the CML, rather than swabs. Swab specimens contain less material, are more apt to be contaminated with indigenous microflora of the skin, and may dry out en route to the CML. Tissue biopsy specimens are also preferable to swabs.

Specimen preservation. Aspirated material should be injected into some type of anaerobic transport vial. Tissue specimens can be transported to the CML in a sterile container or a sterile petri dish containing a sterile, moistened gauze pad. Small pieces of tissue can be moistened with a few drops of sterile, nonbacteriostatic saline to prevent the specimen from drying out. Swab specimens should be transported in an appropriate transport medium, such as Stuart or Amies.[2]

Contaminants. Specimens collected from superficial wounds, abscesses, and lesions are often contaminated with indigenous microflora of the skin. The predominant bacteria in skin microflora are coagulase-negative staphylococci (especially *S. epidermidis*), *Micrococcus* spp., diphtheroids, and *Propionibacterium* spp. (especially *P. acnes*).

Gram stain information. All wound and abscess specimens should be Gram stained. Polymorphonuclear leukocytes (PMNs) are often observed, in addition to the etiologic agent(s). Wound infections and abscesses are frequently polymicrobial infections. The presence of numerous epithelial cells, relatively few PMNs, and multiple bacterial cellular morphotypes usually indicates contamination.

Media for aerobic incubation. Impetigo, ecthyma, folliculitis, furuncles, and carbuncles are most often diagnosed clinically, and cultures are usually unnecessary. All wound and abscess specimens should be inoculated onto blood agar, chocolate agar, MAC, and CNA, at a minimum. It is very important that the CML be informed as to the type and anatomic location of a wound. Special media might be necessary to isolate the pathogen, such as a selective medium containing vancomycin, clindamycin, and/or amikacin to isolate *Pasteurella multocida* from infected dog or cat bite wounds or scratches.

> It is very important that the CML be informed of the type and anatomic location of a wound, so that appropriate media can be inoculated.

Media for anaerobic incubation. Unless no other type of specimen is possible, swab specimens are unacceptable for anaerobic bacteriology. Aspirates from wound infections and abscesses should be inoculated to a routine battery of anaerobic media, such as brucella blood agar (BRU/BA), laked blood-kanamycin-vancomycin agar (LKV), bacteroides bile esculin agar (BBE), and phenylethyl alcohol agar (PEA).

Laboratory diagnosis. Workup of isolated organisms depends on the media on which they grew, their cellular morphology, and their colonial morphology. The most commonly isolated pathogens, *S. aureus* and *S. pyogenes*, would be identified using the criteria described in Chapter 9.

---

[1] *Ecthyma is a pyogenic infection of the skin characterized by adherent crusts beneath which ulceration occurs.*

[2] *Stuart transport medium contains agar, glycerol phosphate to maintain the pH, methylene blue as a redox indicator, and sodium thioglycolate. The glycerol phosphate can be used as an energy source by some contaminants, which may then overgrow the pathogen. In Amies transport medium, a modification of Stuart medium, phosphate buffer is used in place of glycerol phosphate. Amies medium also contain salts that control the permeability of bacterial cells. Charcoal may be added to either medium to neutralize toxic metabolic products.*

Detecting Methicillin-Resistant
Staphylococcus aureus

Several methods for detection of methicillin-resistant *S. aureus* (MRSA) strains are commercially available. They include molecular diagnostic procedures, fluorescence technology, and latex agglutination. The Clinical and Laboratory Standards Institute recommends the use of a 30-mg cefoxitin disk to screen for MRSA strains (see "References and Suggested Reading").

Acne

Disease. Acne is a common condition in which pores become clogged with dried sebum, flaked skin, and bacteria, which leads to the formation of blackheads and whiteheads (collectively known as acne pimples) and inflamed, infected abscesses. Acne is most common among teenagers.

Pathogens. The etiologic agents of acne are *Propionibacterium acnes* and other *Propionibacterium* spp., all of which are anaerobic Gram-positive bacilli. Infected humans serve as reservoirs, although acne is probably not transmissible.

Laboratory diagnosis. Diagnosis is made on clinical grounds.

Anthrax

Disease. Anthrax, also known as woolsorter's disease, can affect the skin (cutaneous anthrax), lungs (inhalation or pulmonary anthrax), or gastrointestinal tract (gastrointestinal anthrax), depending on the portal of entry of the etiologic agent. In cutaneous anthrax, depressed blackened lesions called eschars form as a result of a necrotoxin (a toxin that kills cells; Fig. 18-7). Inhalation and gastrointestinal anthrax are often fatal, but cutaneous anthrax usually is not. Ordinarily, human cases in the United States are quite rare. However, 22 U.S. cases occurred in the fall of 2001 as a result of

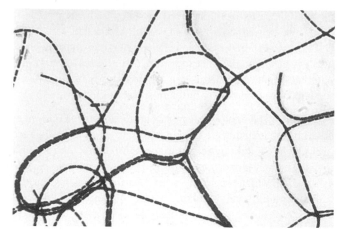

Figure 18-8. Gram-stained *Bacillus anthracis*. (Courtesy of the CDC.)

the mailing of letters that had purposely been contaminated with *B. anthracis* spores. The 22 cases included 11 cases of inhalation anthrax (5 fatal) and 11 cases of cutaneous anthrax (none fatal; see Chapter 26 for more information).

Pathogen. The etiologic agent of anthrax is *Bacillus anthracis*, an encapsulated, spore-forming, Gram-positive bacillus (Figs. 18-8 and 18-9). Reservoirs include anthrax-infected animals as well as spores that may be present in soil, animal hair, wool, animal skins and hides, and products made from them. Transmission occurs via entry of endospores through breaks in skin, inhalation of spores, or ingestion of bacteria in contaminated meat. Person-to-person transmission is very rare.

Laboratory diagnosis. Anthrax is diagnosed by isolation of *B. anthracis* from blood, lesions, or discharges and identification using biochemical- or enzyme-based tests. Immunodiagnostic procedures are available. See Chapters 10 and

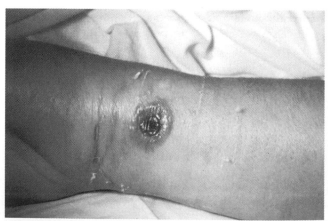

Figure 18-7. Cutaneous anthrax lesion located on the arm of a woman who worked in a wool factory. (Courtesy of Dr. Philip S. Brachman and the CDC.)

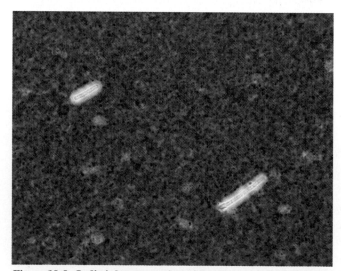

Figure 18-9. India ink preparation of *Bacillus anthracis*. Capsules can be seen as unstained "halos" around the cells. (Courtesy of Larry Stauffer, Oregon State Public Health Laboratory, and the CDC.)

26 for additional information regarding identification of *B. anthracis*.

Gas Gangrene

Disease and most likely pathogens. Gas gangrene, also known as clostridial myonecrosis, is caused by *Clostridium* spp. Although *C. perfringens* is the most common cause, other clostridia, such as *C. septicum*, *C. novyi* B, *C. histolyticum*, *C. bifermentans*, and *C. sordellii*, can also cause this condition. In gas gangrene, exotoxins, like α- and θ-toxins, and exoenzymes produced by the clostridia cause muscle and soft tissue necrosis, allowing deeper penetration by the organisms. Tissue destruction occurs rapidly, often necessitating amputation of the affected anatomic site. In its most severe forms, gas gangrene produces tissue destruction, shock, and renal failure. Chapter 17 contains additional information about gas gangrene.

> Gas gangrene is a rapidly progressing, life-threatening condition requiring immediate CML attention and prompt clinical diagnosis and treatment.

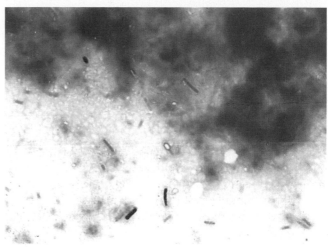

Figure 18-10. **Gram-stained smear of an aspirate from an arm wound, showing two large clostridia-like Gram-positive bacilli and numerous Gram-negative bacilli (probably decolorized clostridia).** The pink staining material in the background probably represents liquifactive necrosis caused by clostridial exotoxins and exoenzymes. (From Marler LM, Siders JA, Allen SD. Direct Smear Atlas. Philadelphia: Lippincott Williams & Wilkins, 2001.)

STUDY AID **Gangrene Versus Gas Gangrene.** The term **gangrene** refers to tissue necrosis (death) resulting from local anemia (ischemia). **Ischemia** results from an obstruction, loss, or reduction of blood supply, leading to a lack of oxygen. Gangrene may have nothing whatsoever to do with microorganisms. **Gas gangrene,** on the other hand, is *always* caused by microorganisms—specifically, *Clostridium* spp. As mentioned in Chapter 17, the clostridia produce gaseous metabolic byproducts—primarily, hydrogen and nitrogen—that accumulate in the necrotic tissues. Regardless of the cause, gangrenous tissue becomes brownish black and foul smelling.

Clinical specimens. Often the clostridia causing gas gangrene are not uniformly distributed in the affected tissues. Therefore, several tissue specimens should be collected at the site where gas gangrene is suspected. Blood cultures are positive in approximately 15% of patients with gas gangrene.

Specimen preservation. See the specimen preservation comments under the previous section titled "Staphylococcal and Streptococcal Infections."

Contaminants. Depending on the manner in which they are collected, specimens may contain indigenous skin microflora. See the contaminant comments under the previous section titled "Staphylococcal and Streptococcal Infections" for more information.

Gram stain information. Because of the rapidly progressing, life-threatening nature of gag gangrene, Gram staining

of a tissue specimen should be performed immediately on its arrival at the CML. The clinician should be notified immediately if clostridia-like Gram-positive bacilli are observed. Some of the clostridia in tissue specimens may appear as Gram-negative bacilli (Fig. 18-10). PMNs are frequently absent or low in number because of the leukocidins produced by the clostridia. Spores may or may not be observed, because sporulation by clostridia in tissue is uncommon. The presence of gas in necrotic tissue can also be caused by pathogens other than clostridia. Thus, the Gram stain may reveal pathogens such as streptococci or members of the family Enterobacteriaceae.

> Because of the serious nature of gas gangrene, the clinician should be notified immediately if clostridia-like Gram-positive bacilli are observed in Gram-stained tissue specimens.

Media for aerobic incubation. Infections that mimic gas gangrene can be caused by *S. aureus*, *S. pyogenes*, and other bacterial pathogens. Thus, the specimen should be inoculated onto blood agar, chocolate agar, MAC, and CNA plates. Inoculated plates should be incubated for 72 hours at 35°C.

Media for anaerobic incubation. In addition to a routine battery of anaerobic media (BRU/BA, LKV, BBE, PEA), an egg yolk agar (EYA) plate should be inoculated in cases of suspected gas gangrene. As discussed in Chapter 17, the EYA plate is useful for detecting proteolytic activity as well as lecithinase and lipase production. Clostridia, especially *C. perfringens*, usually produce good growth on anaerobic media after 1 to 2 days of incubation. Some CMLs also inoculate thioglycolate broth or chopped meat broth.

Laboratory diagnosis. Initial clues to the identity of *Clostridium* spp. include cellular morphology, spore shape and location, colony morphology, hemolysis pattern, and reactions on EYA. Recall from Chapter 17 that *C. perfringens* produces a double zone of hemolysis and is lecithinase-positive. *Clostridium* spp. should be identified using the criteria described in Chapter 17.

Necrotizing Fasciitis

Disease and most likely pathogens. Necrotizing fasciitis is a serious infection involving subcutaneous tissues and extensive undermining and tracking along fascial planes.[3] Most often caused by *Streptococcus pyogenes*, *Staphylococcus aureus*, or *Peptostreptococcus* spp., necrotizing fasciitis is sometimes polymicrobial. The strains of *S. pyogenes* that cause necrotizing fasciitis have been labeled "flesh-eating bacteria" by the press. These are strains that produce necrotizing enzymes that cause rapid and extensive tissue destruction. Necrotizing fasciitis is considered a medical emergency, as is gas gangrene.

> The strains of *Streptococcus pyogenes* that cause necrotizing fasciitis are often referred to as flesh-eating bacteria.

STUDY AID **Critical or Panic Values in Microbiology.** CML professionals must be aware of the observations or isolations known as "critical values" or "panic values" in clinical microbiology, and the urgent need to report these observations or isolations to the appropriate clinician. A list of critical or panic values can be found on the CD-ROM. It is important to note that positive noncontaminated blood cultures, Gram stain results suggesting gas gangrene, and detection of *Streptococcus pyogenes* in a surgical wound specimen are examples of critical or panic values that must be immediately reported to clinicians.[4]

Clinical specimens. In necrotizing fasciitis, a thin, brownish exudate usually emerges from the infected site, samples of which should be sent to the CML along with tissue samples. Blood cultures should also be sent. See the previous section titled "Bacterial Infections of the Skin and Subcutaneous Tissues" for additional information.

Specimen preservation. See the specimen preservation comments under the previous section titled "Staphylococcal and Streptococcal Infections."

Contaminants. Depending on the manner in which they are collected, specimens may contain indigenous skin microflora. See the contaminants comments under the previous section titled "Staphylococcal and Streptococcal Infections" for additional information.

Gram stain information. Gram staining of the specimen provides information about the pathogen(s) and an early clue to therapy. Observing Gram-positive cocci in chains suggests *S. pyogenes*, Gram-positive cocci in clusters suggests *S. aureus*, and mixed cellular morphotypes suggests a polymicrobial infection.

Media for aerobic incubation. See the previous section titled "Gas Gangrene."

Media for anaerobic incubation. See the previous section titled "Gas Gangrene."

Laboratory diagnosis. Workup of isolated organisms depends on the media on which they grew, their cellular morphology, and their colonial morphology. The most commonly isolated pathogens, *S. pyogenes* and *S. aureus*, can be identified using the criteria in Chapter 9.

Leprosy

Disease. Leprosy is today more commonly known as Hansen disease. There are two forms of leprosy: (1) lepromatous leprosy, characterized by numerous nodules in skin and possible involvement of the nasal mucosa and eyes (Fig. 18-11) and (2) tuberculoid leprosy, in which relatively few skin lesions occur. Peripheral nerve involvement tends to be severe, with loss of

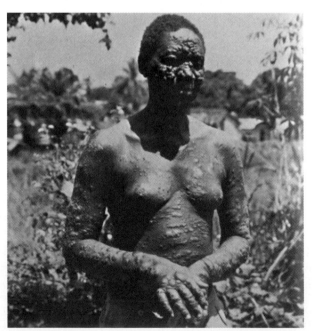

Figure 18-11. **Zairean patient with lepromatous leprosy.** (From Binford CH, Connor DH. Pathology of Tropical and Extraordinary Diseases, vol 1. Washington, DC: Armed Forces Institute of Pathology, 1976.)

---

[3] *Fasciae* (sing., *fascia*) are sheets of fibrous tissue that envelop the body beneath the skin and enclose muscles and groups of muscles. *Fasciitis* is inflammation of the fasciae.

[4] These are examples of panic values in microbiology as proposed by Isenberg (see "References and Suggested Reading"). Panic values vary somewhat from CML to CML.

sensation. Hansen disease is named for G. A. Hansen who, in 1873, discovered the bacillus that causes leprosy. Leprosy occurs primarily in warm, wet areas of the tropics and subtropics. The worldwide prevalence of leprosy was estimated to be about 1.5 million cases in 1997. Most U.S. cases involve people who emigrated from developing countries.

Pathogen. The etiologic agent of leprosy is *Mycobacterium leprae*, an acid-fast bacillus. Infected humans serve as reservoirs; *M. leprae* is present in nasal discharges and is shed from cutaneous lesions. Armadillos in Texas and Louisiana have a naturally occurring disease that is identical to experimental leprosy in those animals, suggesting that transmission from armadillos to humans is possible. The exact mode of transmission has not been clearly established. The organisms may gain entrance through the respiratory system or broken skin. Leprosy does not appear to be easily transmitted from person to person. Prolonged, close contact with an infected person seems to be necessary. The tuberculoid form of leprosy is not contagious.

Laboratory diagnosis. *M. leprae* cannot be grown on artificial culture media. It can be cultured only in laboratory animals, such as nine-banded armadillos or mouse footpads. Diagnosis is made by demonstration of acid-fast bacilli in skin smears or skin biopsy specimens. See Chapter 10 for additional information regarding identification of *M. leprae*.

> *Mycobacterium leprae* cannot be grown on artificial culture media.

Rickettsial Infections

The following rickettsial diseases are actually systemic diseases. They are being discussed here because each is associated with a skin rash.

Rocky Mountain Spotted Fever

Disease. Rocky Mountain spotted fever (RMSF) or tickborne typhus fever is a tickborne rickettsial disease characterized by sudden onset of moderate-to-high fever, extreme exhaustion (prostration), muscle pain, severe headache, chills, conjunctival infection, and maculopapular rash on extremities on about the third day, which spreads to the palms, soles, and much of the body (Fig. 18-12). In about 4 days, small purplish areas (petechiae) develop as a result of bleeding in the skin. Although uncommon, death can result. RMSF occurs in the Western Hemisphere, including all parts of the United States, especially the Atlantic seaboard.

Pathogen. The etiologic agent of RMSF is *Rickettsia rickettsii*, a Gram-negative bacterium. Like all rickettsias, *R. rickettsii* is an obligate intracellular pathogen that invades endothelial cells (cells that line blood vessels). Reservoirs include infected ticks on dogs, rodents, and other animals. Transmission occurs via the bite of an infected tick.

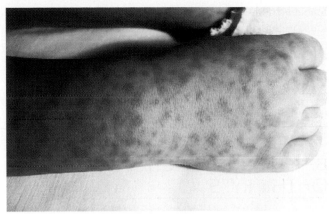

Figure 18-12. **Rocky Mountain spotted fever rash.** (Courtesy of the CDC.)

Laboratory diagnosis. Immunodiagnostic procedures are used to diagnose RMSF. Refer to Chapter 16 for additional information regarding identification of *Rickettsia* spp.

Endemic Typhus Fever

Disease. Endemic typhus fever, also known as murine typhus fever and fleaborne typhus, is an acute febrile disease that is similar to, but milder than, epidemic typhus, which is described next. Symptoms include shaking chills, headache, fever, and a faint, pink rash. Endemic typhus fever has a worldwide occurrence, but is rare in the United States.

Pathogen. The etiologic agent of endemic typhus fever is *Rickettsia typhi*, a Gram-negative bacterium. It is an obligate intracellular pathogen. Reservoirs include rats, mice, possibly other mammals, and infected rat fleas. Transmission occurs from rat to flea to human. Infected fleas defecate while feeding, and the rickettsiae in the feces are rubbed into the bite wound or other superficial abrasions.

Laboratory diagnosis. Immunodiagnostic procedures are used to diagnose endemic typhus. For additional information regarding identification of *Rickettsia* spp., see Chapter 16.

Epidemic Typhus Fever

Disease. Epidemic typhus fever or louseborne typhus is an acute rickettsial disease, often with sudden onset of headache, chills, prostration, fever, and general pains. A rash appears on the fifth or sixth day, initially on the upper trunk, followed by spread to the entire body but usually not to the face, palms, or soles. Epidemic typhus fever may be fatal if untreated. It occurs in cold climates in areas where people live under unhygienic conditions and are louse infested. In World War I, the body lice that transmitted epidemic typhus fever were referred to as "cooties" by soldiers.

Pathogen. The etiologic agent of epidemic typhus fever is *Rickettsia prowazekii*, a Gram-negative bacterium. It is an obligate intracellular pathogen. Reservoirs include infected humans and body lice. Transmission occurs from human to louse to human. Infected lice defecate while feeding and the rickettsiae in the feces are rubbed into the bite wound or other superficial abrasions.

Laboratory diagnosis. Immunodiagnostic procedures are used to diagnose epidemic typhus. Refer to Chapter 16 for additional information regarding identification of *Rickettsia* spp.

BACTERIAL INFECTIONS OF THE EYES

Diseases and most likely pathogens. The most common type of bacterial eye infection is conjunctivitis. The bacteria most often associated with conjunctivitis are *Haemophilus influenzae* (especially *H. influenzae* subsp. *aegyptius*), *Streptococcus pneumoniae, Staphylococcus aureus, Neisseria meningitidis,* and *Chlamydia trachomatis* (some serotypes of which cause inclusion conjunctivitis and others of which cause trachoma). Ophthalmia neonatorum or gonococcal conjunctivitis is caused by *Neisseria gonorrhoeae.* The most common bacterial causes of keratitis are *S. aureus, S. pneumoniae, Pseudomonas aeruginosa,* enterococci, *Streptococcus pyogenes,* Enterobacteriaceae, and *Pasteurella multocida.* The bacteria most often associated with endophthalmitis[5] are *S. aureus, P. aeruginosa, Propionibacterium acnes, Bacillus cereus, S. pneumoniae,* and *N. meningitidis.* The most common bacterial causes of periorbital cellulitis[6] are *S. aureus, S. pyogenes, S. pneumoniae, H. influenzae,* and *Clostridium* spp.

Clinical specimens. Specimens for diagnosis of bacterial eye infections include conjunctival swabs and scrapings for diagnosis of conjunctivitis, corneal scrapings for diagnosis of keratitis, vitreous fluid aspirates for diagnosis of endophthalmitis, and aspirated fluid or tissue biopsy for diagnosis of periorbital cellulitis. It is recommended that both eyes be cultured, even if only one eye appears to be infected. This can provide information regarding the presence of indigenous microflora.

Specimen preservation. Preservatives are not required. When agar plates are directly inoculated at the site of collection, inoculation should occur within 15 minutes of collection. If conjunctival swabs are properly transported to the CML, plate inoculation should occur within 2 hours of collection. Other types of eye specimens should be inoculated within 15 minutes of collection. Special media are available for transporting specimens for chlamydial culture. These specimens may be refrigerated for short delays or stored at −70°C for delays longer than 48 hours.

Contaminants. Relatively few organisms live in the area of the eye. The most common bacteria are coagulase-negative staphylococci, such as *S. epidermidis,* and diphtheroids; less commonly, saprophytic *Neisseria* spp. and viridans group

streptococci may be present. During specimen collection, care must be taken to avoid contamination of the specimen with indigenous skin microflora (see the contaminants comments in the previous section titled "Staphylococcal and Streptococcal Infections").

Gram stain information. A smear should be prepared for Gram staining. PMNs are usually present in smears obtained from conjunctivitis patients.

Media for aerobic incubation. Blood agar and chocolate agar plates should be inoculated. If ophthalmia neonatorum is suspected, an enriched or selective medium such as Thayer-Martin agar should be inoculated for isolation of *N. gonorrhoeae.* Recall that *N. gonorrhoeae* is capnophilic and borderline microaerophilic, requiring incubation in a special atmosphere (see Chapter 11).

Media for anaerobic incubation. Inoculation of anaerobic culture media is rarely necessary.

Laboratory diagnosis. Predominant colony morphotypes should be Gram stained. Further identification methods will depend on the cellular morphotype(s) observed in the Gram-stained smear. A Gram-negative diplococcus growing only on Thayer-Martin agar will most likely be identified as *N. gonorrhoeae.* Refer to Chapter 11 for additional information regarding identification of *N. gonorrhoeae.*

Diagnosis of chlamydial infections can be made by indirect fluorescent antibody staining, enzyme immunoassay, observing intracytoplasmic inclusions within epithelial cells in Giemsa-stained conjunctival smears, and cell culture (Fig. 18-13; see Figs. 16-3 and 16-4).

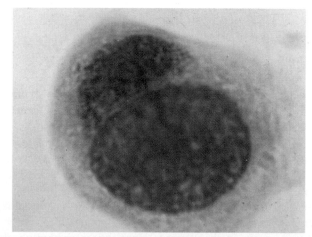

Figure 18-13. **Giemsa-stained conjunctival smear showing an epithelial cell containing an intracytoplasmic inclusion body of inclusion conjunctivitis.** The inclusion body lies above the cell nucleus. The intracytoplasmic inclusion body of inclusion conjunctivitis is morphologically indistinguishable from the inclusion body of trachoma. (From Binford CH, Connor DH. Pathology of Tropical and Extraordinary Diseases, vol 1. Washington, DC: Armed Forces Institute of Pathology, 1976.)

---

[5] *Endophthalmitis is inflammation of the tissues within the eyeball.*

[6] *Periorbital cellulitis is infection involving the superficial tissue layers anterior to the orbital septum, a fibrous membrane attached to the body cavity containing the eye and extending into the eyelids.*

Bacterial Conjunctivitis

Disease. Bacterial conjunctivitis or pink eye involves irritation and reddening of conjunctiva, edema of eyelids, mucopurulent discharge, and sensitivity to light. The disease is highly contagious.

Pathogens. The most common etiologic agents of pink eye are *Haemophilus influenzae* subsp. *aegyptius* and *Streptococcus pneumoniae*, although many other bacteria can cause pinkeye. Infected humans serve as reservoirs. Human-to-human transmission occurs via contact with eye and respiratory discharges, contaminated fingers, facial tissues, clothing, eye makeup, eye medications, ophthalmic instruments, and contact lens-wetting and lens-cleaning agents.

Laboratory diagnosis. Infections of the eye caused by bacteria (including chlamydiae) and viruses should be differentiated from allergic manifestations and irritation by microscopic examination of the exudate (oozing pus), culture of pathogens, and/or immunodiagnostic procedures. See Chapters 9 and 14 for information on identification of *S. pneumoniae* and *H. influenzae*, respectively.

Chlamydial Conjunctivitis

Disease. Chlamydial conjunctivitis is also known as inclusion conjunctivitis and paratrachoma. In neonates, acute conjunctivitis with mucopurulent discharge may result in mild scarring of conjunctivae and cornea. It may be concurrent with chlamydial nasopharyngitis or pneumonia. In adults, chlamydial conjunctivitis may be concurrent with nongonococcal urethritis.

Pathogens. The etiologic agents of chlamydial conjunctivitis are certain serotypes (serovars) of *Chlamydia trachomatis*. Infected humans serve as reservoirs. Transmission occurs via contact with genital discharges of infected people, contaminated fingers to eye, infection in newborns via infected birth canal, or nonchlorinated swimming pools (swimming pool conjunctivitis).

Laboratory diagnosis. Chlamydiae do not grow on artificial media. Diagnosis is made by cell culture and/or immunodiagnostic procedures. Refer to Chapter 16 for additional information regarding identification of *Chlamydia trachomatis*.

Trachoma

Disease. Trachoma or chlamydia keratoconjunctivitis is a highly contagious, acute or chronic conjunctival inflamma-

> **Trachoma is the leading cause of blindness in the world.**

tion of the eyes, resulting in scarring of cornea and conjunctiva, deformation of eyelids, and blindness. Trachoma is most common in poverty-stricken areas of the hot, dry Mediterranean countries and the Far East. It is the leading cause of blindness in the world. Trachoma occurs only rarely in the United States.

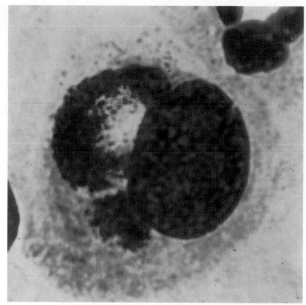

Figure 18-14. Giemsa-stained conjunctival smear showing an epithelial cell containing an intracytoplasmic inclusion body of trachoma. The inclusion body, which lies to the left of the cell nucleus, contains numerous elementary bodies of *Chlamydia trachomatis*. (From Binford CH, Connor DH. Pathology of Tropical and Extraordinary Diseases, vol 1. Washington, DC: Armed Forces Institute of Pathology, 1976.)

Pathogens. The etiologic agents of trachoma are certain serotypes (serovars) of *Chlamydia trachomatis*, a Gram-negative bacterium and obligate intracellular pathogen. Infected humans serve as reservoirs. Transmission occurs via direct contact with infectious ocular or nasal secretions or contaminated articles; the disease is also spread by flies serving as mechanical vectors (see Chapter 21).

Laboratory diagnosis. Trachoma is diagnosed by microscopic observation of intracellular chlamydial elementary bodies in epithelial cells of Giemsa-stained conjunctival scrapings or by an immunofluorescence procedure (Fig. 18-14). Alternatively, the chlamydiae can be isolated from specimens using cell culture techniques. Chapter 16 provides additional information regarding identification of *C. trachomatis*.

Gonococcal Conjunctivitis

Disease. Gonococcal conjunctivitis or gonococcal ophthalmia neonatorum is associated with an acute redness and swelling of conjunctiva and purulent discharge (Fig. 18-15). Corneal ulcers, perforation, and blindness may occur if the disease is untreated.

Pathogen. The etiologic agent of gonococcal conjunctivitis is *Neisseria gonorrhoeae*, a kidney bean-shaped Gram-negative diplococcus. *N. gonorrhoeae* is also known as gonococcus (pl. *gonococci*) or GC. Infected humans—specifically, infected maternal birth canals—serve as reservoirs.

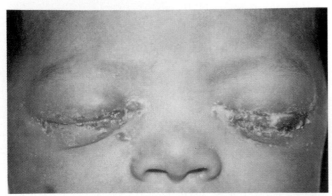

***Figure 18-15.* Gonococcal ophthalmia neonatorum.** (Courtesy of J. Pledger and the CDC.)

Transmission is via contact with the infected birth canal during delivery. Adult infection can result from finger-to-eye contact with infectious genital secretions.

Laboratory diagnosis. Gonococcal conjunctivitis is diagnosed by microscopic observation of Gram-negative diplococci in smears of purulent material and isolation of *N. gonorrhoeae* on appropriate culture media (e.g., chocolate agar or modified chocolate agar, such as Thayer-Martin agar, Martin-Lewis agar, or Transgrow). Refer to Chapter 11 for additional information regarding identification of *N. gonorrhoeae.*

BACTERIAL INFECTIONS OF THE EARS

Diseases and most likely pathogens. Recall from Chapter 5 that otitis externa is infection of the outer ear canal and otitis media is middle ear infection. The most common bacterial causes of otitis externa are *Staphylococcus aureus*, *Streptococcus pyogenes*, *Pseudomonas aeruginosa* (swimmer's ear), and *Vibrio alginolyticus*. The bacteria most often associated with otitis media are *Streptococcus pneumoniae*, *Haemophilus influenzae*, *S. pyogenes*, *Moraxella catarrhalis*, and *S. aureus*. Anaerobes are sometimes involved, especially in chronic otitis media. Most often, these are species of Gram-positive cocci, *Bacteroides*, *Porphyromonas*, *Prevotella*, and *Fusobacterium*.

Clinical specimens. Specimens collected by swab are used to diagnosis otitis externa. Middle ear fluid collected by tympanocentesis (needle puncture of the eardrum) is used for diagnosis of complicated, recurrent, or chronic persistent otitis media.

Specimen preservation. Preservatives are not required. Swab and fluid specimens should be inoculated within 2 hours of collection.

Contaminants. Swab specimens of the outer ear canal are likely to contain indigenous skin microflora (see discussion on this topic under "Bacterial Infections of the Skin and Subcutaneous Tissues"). The most common contaminants are coagulase-negative staphylococci (especially *S. epider-*

midis) and diphtheroids; *Bacillus* spp., *Micrococcus* spp., and saprophytic *Neisseria* spp. are less common. Middle ear fluid specimens are less likely to be contaminated.

Gram stain information. All ear specimens should be Gram stained.

Media for aerobic incubation. Blood agar, chocolate agar, and MAC should be inoculated for diagnosis of otitis externa. Blood agar and chocolate agar plates should be inoculated for diagnosis of otitis media. Fungi can also cause otitis externa (see Chapter 20); thus, media for fungus isolation should also be inoculated.

Media for anaerobic incubation. Because anaerobes can be involved in otitis media, routine media for anaerobic bacteriology (BRU/BA, LKV, BBE. PEA) should be inoculated with middle ear fluid.

Laboratory diagnosis. Predominant colony morphotypes should be Gram stained. Further identification methods will depend on the cellular morphotype(s) observed in the Gram-stained smear. Recall that *P. aeruginosa* possesses the distinguishing characteristics of blue-green pigment production and a fruity odor. Refer to Chapter 13 for additional information regarding identification of *P. aeruginosa.*

Additional comments. Polymerase chain reaction (PCR) assays are being developed for identification of common causes of otitis media.

BACTERIAL INFECTIONS OF THE UPPER RESPIRATORY TRACT

Group A Strep Pharyngitis

Disease and most likely pathogens. Throat swabs are usually collected to diagnose pharyngitis (sore throat) and/or tonsillitis caused by *Streptococcus pyogenes*, also known as group A strep or strep throat. Pharyngitis is commonly caused by viruses and less commonly caused by streptococci in groups B, C, and G, *Arcanobacterium haemolyticum*, *Neisseria gonorrhoeae*, and other bacteria.

Clinical specimens. Two pharyngeal swabs should be collected for diagnosis of streptococcal pharyngitis: one for culture and one for a rapid antigen detection assay, if such an assay is performed at the health care facility. If the rapid test is positive, the second swab is usually discarded, but if the rapid test is negative, an appropriate culture medium is inoculated using the second swab. If *N. gonorrhoeae* is suspected, appropriate transport devices should be inoculated (see Chapters 5 and 11).

Specimen preservation. For transport, swabs should be placed in a transport container containing Amies or modified Stuart medium. The container should be refrigerated if transport will take more than a few hours. However, do not refrigerate the specimen if *N. gonorrhoeae* is the suspected etiologic agent.

Contaminants. Throat swabs will be contaminated with indigenous nasopharyngeal microflora, which is similar to the indigenous microflora of the oral cavity. More than 300 identified species of bacteria live in the oral cavity, including viridans group streptococci and many anaerobes (e.g., spirochetes, *Actinomyces*, *Bacteroides*, *Fusobacterium*, Gram-positive cocci, *Prevotella*, *Propionibacterium*, and *Veillonella* spp.). Potential pathogens such as *Neisseria meningitidis*, *Streptococcus pneumoniae*, *H. influenzae*, and *S. aureus* may be present, but these organisms are thought not to cause pharyngitis. Some people carry small numbers of *S. pyogenes* as part of their nasopharyngeal microflora. About 25% to 30% of healthy adults harbor *S. aureus* in their anterior nares; these people are referred to as *S. aureus* carriers.

Gram stain information. Gram stains are usually not performed on routine throat swabs. For a patient with anaerobic tonsillitis (Vincent angina), a Gram stain reveals numerous fusiform Gram-negative bacilli and spirochetes. Vincent angina is discussed in greater detail later in the chapter.

Screening tests. Many rapid immunodiagnostic tests are available for diagnosis of strep throat (see Chapter 9). Test results are available within 10 to 20 minutes. A DNA probe test is also available (Gen-Probe Inc.).

Media for aerobic incubation. Routine throat swabs are usually inoculated only onto a blood agar plate. Selective media such as streptococcus selective agar are used in some CMLs. The CML must be alerted if the clinician suspects a pathogen other than *S. pyogenes* to be causing the patient's pharyngitis. For example, if the clinician suspects the cause to be *N. gonorrhoeae*, it would be necessary for the CML to inoculate a Thayer-Martin plate. If only a blood agar plate was inoculated, indigenous microflora contaminants would overgrow the fastidious *N. gonorrhoeae*. If diphtheria (discussed later in the chapter) is suspected, cysteine tellurite blood agar (or modified Tinsdale medium) and/or Loeffler serum medium should be inoculated.

> The CML must be notified if the clinician suspects a pathogen other than *Streptococcus pyogenes* to be causing the patient's pharyngitis, so that appropriate media may be inoculated.

Media for anaerobic incubation. If anaerobic tonsillitis (Vincent angina) is suspected, routine anaerobic culture media (BRU/BA, LKV, BBE, PEA) can be inoculated, although this disease is usually diagnosed by Gram stain. Vincent angina is further discussed later in the chapter.

Laboratory diagnosis. *S. pyogenes* produces characteristic colonies on blood agar: opaque, gray, pearly colonies surrounded by a zone of β-hemolysis that is relatively wide compared with the colonies (see Fig. 9-16). Positive identification of *S. pyogenes* can be accomplished using the criteria described in Chapter 9.

Additional comments. Failure to diagnose and treat group A strep can lead to serious complications, referred to as poststreptococcal sequelae. These sequelae include necrotizing fasciitis, scarlet fever, streptococcal toxic shock syndrome, rheumatic fever, and glomerulonephritis.

Epiglottitis

Disease and most likely pathogens. Epiglottitis, primarily a disease of young children, is most often caused by *H. influenzae*, and less frequently caused by *S. pneumoniae* or *S. pyogenes*. The incidence of epiglottitis caused by *H. influenzae* has decreased markedly since introduction of Hib (*H. influenzae* type b) vaccine.

Clinical specimens. Epiglottitis is a serious condition with the potential for swollen tissues to obstruct the patient's airway. **Collection of a throat swab specimen from a patient with epiglottitis is dangerous!** Touching the inflamed epiglottis with a swab could precipitate complete obstruction of the airway. When deemed necessary, collection of a throat swab should only be done by a clinician, and emergency intubation devices should be readily accessible.

Specimen preservation. The throat swab should be placed in an appropriate transport container and processed within 2 hours of collection.

Contaminants. Throat swabs will be contaminated with indigenous nasopharyngeal microflora, which could include small numbers of *H. influenzae*.

Gram stain information. Gram stains are usually not performed.

Media for aerobic incubation. Inoculate blood agar and chocolate agar plates.

Laboratory diagnosis. *H. influenzae* grows on a chocolate agar plate but not a blood agar plate (see Fig. 14-4). It is a faintly staining, somewhat pleomorphic Gram-negative coccobacillus. The isolate can be identified as *H. influenzae* using criteria discussed in Chapter 14.

Additional comments. *H. influenzae* can usually be isolated from blood cultures of patients with *H. influenzae* epiglottitis.

Diphtheria

Disease and pathogen. Diphtheria is a potentially serious upper respiratory tract disease caused by toxigenic strains of *Corynebacterium diphtheriae*. Recall from Chapter 10 that toxigenic strains produce the toxin that causes diphtheria, whereas nontoxigenic strains do not. The disease primarily involves the tonsils, pharynx, larynx, and nose, and occasionally involves other mucous membranes, skin, conjunctivae, and the vagina. The characteristic lesion is an asymmetrical adherent gray-white membrane with surrounding inflammation. Sore throat, swollen and tender cervical lymph nodes, and swelling of the neck are common. The membrane may cause airway obstruction. Diphtheria is uncommon in the United States because of the availability of an effective vaccine.

Clinical specimens. Throat and nasopharyngeal swabs (Dacron) are used to diagnose diphtheria. Both the posterior nares and posterior pharynx are swabbed.

Specimen preservation. Swabs should be processed immediately. If a delay in processing is anticipated, swabs should be sent dry in a container with desiccant, or placed in a transport tube containing Amies or Stuart medium.

Contaminants. Throat swabs will be contaminated with indigenous nasopharyngeal microflora.

Gram stain information. Gram-stained smears of specimens from patients with diphtheria should reveal Gram-positive bacilli with typical *C. diphtheriae* morphology—slightly curved, with nonparallel sides, sometimes having a club or dumbbell shape. Sometimes the cells stain unevenly. When stained with Loeffler methylene blue stain, the cells will appear as pleomorphic, beaded rods, with swollen ends, and metachromatic granules (see Fig. 10-3). Albert stain, containing toluidine blue and methyl green, will also reveal the metachromatic granules. Recall from Chapter 10 that metachromatic granules are granules within *C. diphtheriae* cells that become reddish purple when methylene blue and certain other dyes attach to them. It is important to note that other coryneform bacteria may also contain metachromatic granules.

Screening tests. Presumptive diagnosis of diphtheria is based on observation of the characteristic membrane.

Media for aerobic incubation. The CML must be alerted that diphtheria is suspected so that cysteine tellurite blood agar or modified Tinsdale medium (preferred), which are selective and differential, and/or Loeffler serum medium, which is enriched and nonselective, can be inoculated. Blood agar and chocolate agar plates should also be inoculated, because other pathogens may be causing a dual infection. All plates should be incubated for 2 days. *C. diphtheriae* grows on blood agar, and the colonies resemble γ-streptococci on day 1. However, unlike streptococci, *C. diphtheriae* colonies continue to grow and are catalase positive.

> Associate cysteine tellurite blood agar and modified Tinsdale medium with *Corynebacterium diphtheriae.*

Laboratory diagnosis. On modified Tinsdale medium, *C. diphtheriae* colonies will be dull metal gray to black as a result of telluride reduction, surrounded by a brown halo caused by cystinase activity (see Fig. 10-5). Other Gram-positive bacteria (e.g., other coryneform bacteria, staphylococci, streptococci) can also produce black colonies, but they are not surrounded by a brown halo. Loeffler serum medium enhances the production of metachromatic granules within the cells. Refer to Chapter 10 for additional information regarding identification of *C. diphtheriae.*

Sinusitis

Disease and most likely pathogens. The most common causes of sinusitis are *Haemophilus influenzae* and *Streptococcus pneumoniae.* Less frequent causes are *Streptococcus pyogenes, Moraxella catarrhalis,* and anaerobes such as *Propionibacterium acnes.* Anaerobes are especially common in cases of chronic sinusitis.

Clinical specimens. The ideal specimen for diagnosis of sinusitis is a needle aspirate collected after decontamination of the nasal cavity. Some CMLs also process secretions collected by direct sinus washes and curettage and biopsy material collected by endoscopy. Inappropriate specimens include nasal or nasopharyngeal swabs, nasopharyngeal secretions, sputum, and saliva.

Specimen preservation. Specimens should be kept moist during transport to the CML.

Contaminants. Inappropriate specimens will be contaminated with indigenous nasopharyngeal microflora.

Gram stain information. Examination of a Gram-stained smear can sometimes provide a rapid, presumptive identification of the etiologic agent(s). For example, a preponderance of Gram-positive diplococci would suggest *S. pneumoniae.* Faintly staining, somewhat pleomorphic Gram-negative coccobacilli would be suggestive of *H. influenzae.*

Media for aerobic incubation. Blood agar, chocolate agar, and MAC should be inoculated.

Media for anaerobic incubation. Anaerobic culture should be performed in cases of chronic sinusitis. A battery of routine anaerobic culture media (BRU/BA, LKV, BBE, PEA) should be inoculated.

Laboratory diagnosis. Predominant colony morphotypes should be Gram stained. Further identification methods will depend on the cellular morphotype(s) observed in the Gram-stained smear.

BACTERIAL INFECTIONS OF THE LOWER RESPIRATORY TRACT

The portion of the respiratory tract below the level of the larynx is usually protected from bacterial colonization by the actions of the epiglottis and ciliated epithelial cells. Thus, in healthy persons, the trachea, bronchi, and lungs contain only transiently inhaled microorganisms.

Lower Respiratory Tract Infections Having Multiple Etiologies

Diseases and most likely pathogens. Diseases of the lower respiratory tract and their most common bacterial etiologies are listed in Table 18-2. Note that the etiologic agents of community-acquired lower respiratory tract infections are different from those acquired in the hospital.

TABLE 18 - 2   Lower Respiratory Tract Infections

Infection	Most Common Bacterial Causes
Empyema	*Streptococcus pneumoniae*, anaerobes, viridans group streptococci, *Staphylococcus aureus*, *Streptococcus pyogenes*, Gram-negative bacilli (including Enterobacteriaceae, *Pseudomonas aeruginosa* and other nonfermenters)
Bronchitis (community acquired)	*S. pneumoniae*, *Haemophilus influenzae*, other *Haemophilus* spp., *Moraxella catarrhalis*, *S. aureus*, *Chlamydophila pneumoniae*, *Mycoplasma pneumoniae*, *Bordetella pertussis*, *S. pyogenes*
Bronchitis (hospital acquired)	Enterobacteriaceae, *S. aureus*, *P. aeruginosa* and other nonfermenters
Lung abscess	*S. aureus*, *Klebsiella pneumoniae*, *P. aeruginosa*, *S. pyogenes*, *Nocardia asteroides* complex, anaerobes (aspiration pneumonia cases)
Pneumonia (community acquired)	*S. pneumoniae*, *H. influenzae*, *M. catarrhalis*, *C. pneumoniae*, *M. pneumoniae*, *Legionella pneumophila*, *N. asteroides* complex, *Pasteurella multocida*, anaerobes (aspiration pneumonia cases); *Burkholderia cepacia* is a common respiratory pathogen in patients with cystic fibrosis
Pneumonia (hospital acquired)	Enterobacteriaceae, *S. aureus*, *P. aeruginosa* and other nonfermenters, *L. pneumophila*, anaerobes (aspiration pneumonia cases)
Tracheitis (intubated patient)	Enterobacteriaceae, *S. aureus*, *P. aeruginosa* and other nonfermenters

Source: Thomson RB, Miller JM. Specimen collection, transport, and processing: Bacteriology. In: Murray PR, Baron EJ, Jorgensen JH, Pfaller MA, Yolken RH, eds. Manual of Clinical Microbiology. 8th Ed. Washington, DC: ASM Press, 2003.

Community-acquired infections are any infections *not* acquired as a result of hospitalization.

STUDY AID **Typical Versus Atypical Pneumonia.** Patients with **typical pneumonia** experience chest pain, dyspnea (shortness of breath), fever, chills, and a productive cough (one that produces purulent sputum). Less common symptoms include anorexia, headache, nausea, diarrhea, and vomiting. Radiographic abnormalities are proportional to the physical symptoms. Common causes of typical pneumonia are *Streptococcus pneumoniae*, *Haemophilus pneumoniae*, *Staphylococcus aureus*, and viruses like influenza virus types A and B, parainfluenza viruses, and respiratory syncytial virus (RSV). Other causes are *Legionella pneumophila*, *Mycoplasma pneumoniae*, *Chlamydophila pneumoniae*, and Gram-negative bacilli. **Atypical pneumonia** has a more insidious (slower) onset than typical pneumonia. Patients present with headache, fever, cough with little sputum, and myalgia. Radiographic abnormalities are usually greater than the physical symptoms would predict. Common causes of atypical pneumonia are *M. pneumoniae*, *C. pneumoniae*, *L. pneumophila*, and viruses like influenza viruses, RSV, and adenoviruses. Other causes are *Chlamydophila psittaci*, *Pneumocystis jiroveci* (a fungus), varicella-zoster virus, and parainfluenza viruses. Note that some pathogens can produce either typical or atypical pneumonia.

Clinical specimens. Specimens acceptable for diagnosis of lower respiratory tract infections include bronchoalveolar lavage fluid, bronchial brushings, bronchial washes, alveolar lavage, endotracheal tube aspirates, transtracheal aspirates, pleural fluid, sputum, and lung biopsy specimens.

Specimen preservation. Lower respiratory tract specimens should be processed within 2 hours of collection. If there will be a delay in processing, expectorated sputum, bronchoalveolar lavage, brushings, washings, and endotracheal aspirates should be stored at 4°C and processed within 24 hours.

Contaminants. Lower respiratory tract specimens can become contaminated by oral and nasopharyngeal microflora during collection. However, the presence of these microflora in lower respiratory tract specimens does not necessarily represent contamination. Most bacterial lower respiratory tract infections follow aspiration of oropharyngeal secretions; thus, the bacteria of microflora most often are the causes of lower respiratory tract infections.

Gram stain information. All lower respiratory tract specimens should be Gram stained. Good-quality sputum specimens should contain PMNs, which should be present in greater quantities than squamous epithelial cells (refer to Chapter 5 for a discussion on this topic). Since the lower respiratory tract contains no squamous epithelial cells, their presence in sputum specimens represents contamination of the specimen with oropharyngeal secretions. Observing potential pathogens within PMNs (i.e., intracellular bacteria) is a significant finding. A preliminary report based on Gram stain observations may be of value to the clinician. For example, a Gram-stained sputum containing numerous PMNs and numerous Gram-positive diplococci is highly suggestive of pneumococcal pneumonia. Numerous PMNs and numerous Gram-positive cocci in clusters is suggestive of staphylococcal pneumonia. The presence of thin, beaded, branching Gram-positive filaments is suggestive of *Nocardia* spp.

Screening tests. To determine which sputum specimens are suitable for culture, some CMLs use the grading system developed by Bartlett (see "References and Suggested Reading"; see also Table 5.4) or one of several similar grading systems.

A coughed or induced sputum and endotracheal aspirate is likely to produce significant results if a Gram-stained smear of the specimen contains a predominant potential pathogen, abundant PMNs, and a potential pathogen within PMNs. Bronchoalveolar lavage fluid is likely to produce significant results if a predominant potential pathogen is seen in every $\times 100$ field of a Gram-stained smear of the specimen and a potential pathogen is seen within PMNs. Molecular diagnostic procedures are available for diagnosis of *M. pneumoniae* and chlamydial respiratory diseases.

Media for aerobic incubation. Lower respiratory tract specimens should be inoculated to blood agar, chocolate agar, and MAC, as a minimum. Lung biopsy specimens should also be placed in thioglycollate broth. Inoculated plates should be incubated at 35°C in a CO_2 incubator for 48 hours before being reported as negative. If legionellosis is suspected, specimens should be inoculated onto buffered charcoal yeast extract agar, with and without antimicrobial agents; inoculated plates should be incubated in humidified air at 35°C for a minimum of 5 days. Cell culture techniques are necessary for recovery of chlamydiae.

Media for anaerobic incubation. Protected bronchoscope brushings and lung tissue should be inoculated to a routine battery of anaerobic media (BRU/BA, LKV, BBE, and PEA).

Laboratory diagnosis. Cultures are likely to be significant if they yield a predominant potential pathogen. The specific steps in the workup depend on the type of potential pathogen isolated. For example, workup of a Gram-positive coccus would be as described in Chapter 9.

Tuberculosis

Diseases and most likely pathogens. Tuberculosis may be caused by any of the species in the *Mycobacterium tuberculosis* complex, but it is most often caused by *M. tuberculosis*. *M. tuberculosis* may cause primary and chronic pulmonary tuberculosis, pleuritis, lymphadenitis, tuberculosis of bones and joints, central nervous system tuberculosis, gastrointestinal tuberculosis, and pericardial tuberculosis. Widespread tuberculosis, known as miliary tuberculosis, involves many lesions throughout the body, and results from the hematogenous dissemination (via the bloodstream) of mycobacteria. Tuberculosis is one of the most important infectious diseases worldwide.

Clinical specimens. Most specimens submitted to the mycobacteriology section of the CML (commonly called the TB lab) are lower respiratory tract specimens, such as sputum, tracheal and bronchial aspirates, and bronchoalveolar lavage fluid. Other types of specimens include urine, gastric aspirates, tissues, biopsy specimens, and cerebrospinal fluid (CSF). Blood and fecal specimens from immunocompromised patients may also be received in the TB lab. Only sputum specimens, the most commonly submitted specimens for diagnosis of pulmonary tuberculosis, will be described in this section.

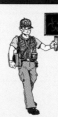

SAFETY TIP

Special Safety Precautions Required for the TB Lab. Recall from Chapter 4 that, because of the highly infectious nature of Mycobacterium tuberculosis, *staff at TB labs must follow strict safety procedures. All manipulations involving specimens and cultures, including preparation of smears, inoculation of media, opening of centrifuge cups, and sonication, must be performed in a biosafety cabinet.*

Specimen preservation. Traditionally, early morning sputum specimens are collected on 3 consecutive days. Pooled specimens—that is, a mixture of several sputum specimens collected over time—are unacceptable because of the increased likelihood of contamination. Fixatives are not required. Specimens should be refrigerated if a delay in processing of more than 1 hour is anticipated.

Contaminants. Sputum specimens are virtually always contaminated with indigenous microflora of the nasopharynx and oral cavity. For this reason, sputum specimens are treated with a decontaminant, usually 4% sodium hydroxide. Alternative reagents (e.g., Zephiran-trisodium phosphate, oxalic acid, cetylpyridinium chloride) are also available for use as decontaminants. Care must be taken, however, because harsh decontamination also kills mycobacteria. Sputum specimens can be treated with a digestion or liquefaction agent—usually, N-Acetyl-L-cysteine—to dissolve mucous, in which mycobacteria and/or contaminant bacteria might be trapped. Mycobacteria are then concentrated by centrifugation of the digestion/decontamination mixture. The sediment is used to inoculate media and for preparation of a smear for acid-fast staining.

Thus, in the TB lab, sputum specimens are digested, decontaminated, and concentrated before they are inoculated onto or into culture media. These topics are discussed in greater detail in Appendix A.

Staining information. Recall from Chapter 10 that waxes in the cell walls of mycobacteria prevent the cells from readily absorbing dyes. Gram-staining is not recommended, because mycobacteria often do not take up stain and thus appear as unstained areas or "ghosts" in Gram-stained smears. Acid-fast procedures are used to stain mycobacteria. These procedures are discussed in Chapter 10. At the conclusion of either the Kinyoun or Ziehl-Neelsen acid-fast staining procedures, mycobacteria are red and are referred to as acid-fast bacilli. Acid-fast bacilli are approximately 0.2 to 0.6 μm wide (quite slender) by 1.0 to 10 μm long and may be straight, curved, or bent. The cells may be unevenly stained, giving them a beaded appearance. Observing numerous acid-fast bacilli in acid-fast-stained sputum smears is usually sufficient for a presumptive diagnosis of tuberculosis. However, it is important to remember that cross-contamination of slides during the staining process or the presence of nontuberculous mycobacteria in the water used during the staining process may cause false-positive results. The acid-fast bacilli may be mycobacteria other than *M. tuberculosis* or bacteria other than mycobacteria (e.g., *Rhodococcus*, *Nocardia*, and *Legionella* spp.), which show various degrees of acid fastness.

Screening tests. Commercial molecular diagnostic procedures, including PCR and ribosomal RNA amplification procedures, are available for detection of *M. tuberculosis* in clinical specimens.

Media for aerobic incubation. Both selective and nonselective media are used for isolation of mycobacteria. Examples of nonselective media are Löwenstein-Jensen medium (an egg-based medium) and Middlebrook 7H11 medium (an agar-based medium). Examples of selective, antimicrobial agent-containing media are Löwenstein-Jensen-Gruft, Mycobactosel Löwenstein-Jensen, and Mitchison selective 7H11. Plates and slants should be incubated at 35°C to 37°C in an atmosphere of 5% to 10% CO_2 for 6 to 8 weeks. Recall that *M. tuberculosis* is an extremely slow-growing organism, with a generation time of approximately 20 hours. Broth media and biphasic media are also available for culturing mycobacteria, as are many automated and nonautomated commercial systems (see Chapter 10).

Laboratory diagnosis. Organisms growing on or in the media should be identified as described in Chapter 10.

Legionellosis

Disease. Legionellosis, also known as Legionnaires disease, is an acute bacterial pneumonia with anorexia, malaise, myalgia, headache, high fever, chills, and dry cough followed by a productive cough, shortness of breath, diarrhea, and pleural and abdominal pain. There is about a 40% fatality rate. Pontiac fever, an influenza-like, less severe form of legionellosis, is not associated with pneumonia or death. Legionnaires disease was first recognized as a disease following an outbreak in a Philadelphia hotel in 1976, but evidence exists that prior epidemics and deaths were caused by *Legionella* spp. Epidemics continue to occur, often associated with hotels, cruise ships, hospitals, and supermarkets. Legionellosis usually affects elderly persons; people with preexisting respiratory disease, diabetes mellitus, renal disease, or malignancy; people who are immunocompromised; or people who smoke or drink heavily.

Pathogens. The primary etiologic agent of legionellosis is *Legionella pneumophila*, a poorly staining Gram-negative bacillus. Other *Legionella* spp. and organisms within related genera can also cause the disease. As of 2003, 40 species of *Legionella* were known. Reservoirs include environmental water sources, such as ponds, lakes, and creeks; hot-water and air-conditioning systems, cooling towers, and evaporative condensers; whirlpool spas, hot tubs, shower heads, humidifiers, and tap water and water distillation systems; decorative fountains; and perhaps soil and dust. Infection occurs primarily via airborne transmission from water and possibly dust. Transmission has occurred as a result of aerosols of *Legionella* spp. that have been produced by vegetable-misting devices in supermarkets. Legionellosis is probably not transmitted from person to person.

Laboratory diagnosis. Sputum and blood specimens should be sent to the microbiology laboratory for culture and susceptibility testing. *Legionella* spp. stain poorly and require cysteine and other nutrients to grow. The recommended culture medium is buffered charcoal yeast extract agar. Immunodiagnostic procedures are available, such as antigen detection in urine. Additional information on identifying *Legionella* spp. is presented in Chapter 14.

Mycoplasmal Pneumonia

Disease. Mycoplasmal pneumonia, also known as primary atypical pneumonia, has a gradual onset with headache, malaise, dry cough, sore throat, and less often, chest discomfort. The amount of sputum the patient produces is scant at first but may increase as the disease progresses. Illness may last from a few days to a month or more. Mycoplasmal pneumonia is most common in people aged 5 to 35 years. Pneumonias produced by mycoplasmas and chlamydiae are the most common types of atypical pneumonias (i.e., pneumonias caused by organisms other than those that are the typical causes of pneumonia).

Pathogen. The etiologic agent of mycoplasmal pneumonia is *Mycoplasma pneumoniae*, a tiny Gram-negative bacterium lacking cell walls. Infected humans serve as reservoirs. Transmission occurs via droplet inhalation, usually by direct contact with an infected person or particles contaminated with nasal secretions or sputum from an ill, coughing patient.

Laboratory diagnosis. Mycoplasmal pneumonia is diagnosed by demonstration of a rise in antibody titer between acute and convalescent sera. On artificial media, *M. pneumoniae* produces tiny "fried egg" colonies, having a dense central area and a less dense periphery. Refer to Chapter 14 for additional information regarding identification of *Mycoplasma* spp.

Whooping Cough (Pertussis)

Disease and pathogen. Whooping cough (pertussis) is caused by *Bordetella pertussis*. The disease has an insidious onset, with a cough that starts as irritating and progresses to violent. Coughing spells, known as paroxysms, consist of numerous coughs without intervening inhalation, often followed by the characteristic high-pitched inspiratory whoop for which the disease is named. Paroxysms frequently end with the patient expelling clear, tenacious mucus and vomiting. Complications include pneumonia, atelectasia (loss of lung volume), seizures, encephalopathy (brain disorders), weight loss, hernias, and death. Pneumonia is the most common cause of death. *B. parapertussis* causes a respiratory disease in humans that is similar to but less severe than pertussis.

Clinical specimens. Nasopharyngeal swabs, washes, and aspirates are acceptable specimens for diagnosis of pertussis. Small-tip calcium alginate or Dacron swabs should be used because rayon or cotton may be toxic to *Bordetella* spp.

Specimen preservation. Whenever possible Regan-Lowe medium should be inoculated on site. When necessary to transport swabs, they should be transported in Amies medium with charcoal if the specimens will be processed within 24 hours. For longer delays, Regan-Lowe transport medium should be used.

Contaminants. Specimens will be contaminated with indigenous nasopharyngeal microflora.

Gram stain information. Gram staining is not usually performed.

Screening tests. Direct fluorescent antibody staining and PCR techniques are available for detecting *B. pertussis* in specimens.

Media for aerobic incubation. Inoculate specimen to Regan-Lowe charcoal agar with 10% horse blood and cephalexin. A similar medium without cephalexin should also be inoculated, because some strains of *B. pertussis* are susceptible to cephalexin. Incubate plates at 35°C in a humid atmosphere. *B. pertussis* colonies generally take at least 3 days to appear; plates should be held 7 days or longer.

Laboratory diagnosis. On Regan-Lowe medium, *B. pertussis* colonies are small, round, domed, shiny, and silver (like mercury droplets or pearls pushed halfway into the agar; see Fig. 14-9).

> Associate Regan-Lowe medium with *Bordetella pertussis*.

Refer to Chapter 14 for additional information regarding identification of *B. pertussis*.

Additional comments. Although a pertussis vaccine is available, the protection appears to decline after several years. The number of pertussis cases has been steadily rising in the United States.

BACTERIAL INFECTIONS OF THE CENTRAL NERVOUS SYSTEM

Note: Although botulism and tetanus are bacterial diseases of the central nervous system, they are not described in this chapter. Information about these diseases can be found in Chapter 17 and Appendix 1 of the CD-ROM.

Meningitis

Diseases and most likely pathogens. As explained in Chapter 5, meningitis is inflammation of the membranes that surround the brain, collectively known as the meninges. Meningitis can have many causes, including the ingestion of poisons, the ingestion or injection of drugs, a reaction to a vaccine, or it may be caused by a pathogen. If caused by a pathogen, it might be a virus, a bacterium, a fungus, or a protozoan.

The most common symptoms of meningitis are headache, fever, chills, nausea and vomiting, and photalgia (light-induced pain). Other complaints include nuchal rigidity (profound stiffness of the neck that prevents flexing of the neck), and cardiac arrhythmias. Meningitis can be either an acute or chronic disease. Acute meningitis is usually caused by bacteria. The most common causes of acute neonatal meningitis are *Streptococcus agalactiae* (group B strep), *Escherichia coli*, other members of the family Enterobacteriaceae, *Listeria monocytogenes*, and *Chryseobacterium* (*Elizabethkingia*) *meningosepticum*. The most common causes of acute meningitis in other age groups are *Neisseria meningitidis*, *Streptococcus pneumoniae*, *Haemophilus influenzae*, and *Staphylococcus aureus*. Chronic meningitis may be caused by bacteria, fungi (see Chapter 20), protozoa (see Chapter 22), helminths (see Chapter 23), or viruses (see Chapter 25). Bacterial causes of chronic meningitis include the *Nocardia asteroides* complex, *Brucella* spp., *Leptospira interrogans*, *Mycobacterium tuberculosis*, *Treponema pallidum*, and *Borrelia*

> The three most common causes of acute neonatal meningitis are *Streptococcus agalactiae* (group B strep), *Escherichia coli* and other members of the family Enterobacteriaceae, and *Listeria monocytogenes*.

> The three most common causes of meningitis in age groups other than neonates are *Neisseria meningitidis*, *Streptococcus pneumoniae*, and *Haemophilus influenzae*.

burgdorferi. Encephalitis is most often caused by viruses (see Chapter 25).

Clinical specimens. To diagnose meningitis, CSF must be obtained by lumbar puncture (spinal tap), and immediately transported to the CML.

Specimen preservation. Preservatives are not used. If the CSF specimen cannot be immediately transported to the CML, it should remain at room temperature or be placed in a 35°C incubator temporarily and processed within 2 hours of collection (preferably within 15 minutes). CSF specimens must never be refrigerated (except for viral studies; see Chapter 25).

Contaminants. The CSF of healthy persons is sterile. Care must be taken to avoid contamination of the CSF specimen with indigenous skin microflora during collection of the specimen.

Gram stain information. Because of the serious nature of meningitis, CSF specimens should be processed immediately on their receipt in the CML. CSF smears should be prepared by cytocentrifugation. Gram staining results should be reported to the clinician immediately and should include information about the types of bacteria and white blood cells observed. Observing Gram-negative diplococci would be suggestive of *N. meningitidis.* Observing Gram-positive diplococci would be suggestive of *S. pneumoniae.* Acridine-orange staining of the CSF specimen may be more sensitive than the Gram stain, but it should be followed by Gram staining to determine whether the bacterial pathogen is Gram positive or Gram negative.

> Because of the serious nature of meningitis, CSF specimens should be processed immediately on receipt at the CML.

> Results of a CSF Gram stain should be reported to the clinician immediately and should include information about the types of bacteria and white blood cells observed.

Screening tests. Antigen detection procedures are available for *S. agalactiae, S. pneumoniae, N. meningitidis, E. coli,* and *H. influenzae,* but antigen detection is much more expensive and may be less sensitive than Gram staining. Latex agglutination techniques replaced the once popular counterimmunoelectrophoresis procedures, but neither are commonly used anymore. The Limulus amoebocyte lysate assay can be used to detect endotoxin in CSF specimens, but that test also is not widely used in CMLs.

Media for aerobic incubation. Blood agar and chocolate agar should be inoculated with 0.5 mL of CSF or CSF sediment that has been resuspended in 0.5 mL of CSF following centrifugation of the specimen.

Media for anaerobic incubation. Anaerobic culture of CSF specimens is usually not routinely performed but can be done when specifically requested by the clinician. The routine battery of BRU/BA, LKV, BBE, and PEA should be used.

Laboratory diagnosis. Gram stain any organism that grows on the blood agar and chocolate agar plates. If the patient is a neonate, what appears to be a Gram-positive coccus is most likely *S. agalactiae* (see Chapter 9) or *Listeria monocytogenes* (coccobacilli; see Chapter 10). If it is a Gram-negative bacillus, it is most likely a member of the family Enterobacteriaceae (usually *E. coli*; see Chapter 12) or, much less commonly, *Chryseobacterium meningosepticum* (see Chapter 13). If the patient is a child, observing small, pleomorphic, faintly staining Gram-negative bacilli is suggestive of *H. influenzae* (see Chapter 14). In any age group, Gram-negative diplococci are suggestive of *N. meningitidis* (see Chapter 11), Gram-positive diplococci are suggestive of *S. pneumoniae* (see Chapter 9), and Gram-positive cocci in clusters are suggestive of *S. aureus* (see Chapter 9).

Additional considerations. Blood cultures should be performed on patients suspected of having meningitis. *Leptospira interrogans* can be detected in CSF during the first 10 days of acute illness by examining the sediment from centrifuged CSF by darkfield microscopy. Also, a semisolid medium such as Fletcher or Ellinghausen-McCullough-Johnson-Harris medium should be inoculated whenever leptospirosis is suspected.

BACTERIAL INFECTIONS OF THE URINARY TRACT

Diseases and most likely pathogens. In this chapter, cystitis, pyelonephritis, and ureteritis are considered urinary tract infections (UTIs). Prostatitis and urethritis are considered genital tract infections; they are discussed later in the chapter. UTIs occur more frequently in women than in men. A patient with a UTI presents with dysuria (difficulty or pain on urination), lumbar pain, fever, and chills. The latter two symptoms are more common in pyelonephritis than in cystitis.

UTIs may be acquired either within a health care setting (called nosocomial or hospital-acquired UTIs) or elsewhere (called community-acquired UTIs). UTIs are the most common type of nosocomial infection, often following urinary catheterization. Most UTIs are acquired via the ascending route, whereby the pathogen moves upward from the urethra. Far fewer UTIs occur via the descending route from the bloodstream to the kidneys. The most common causes of cystitis are Enterobacteriaceae (especially *Escherichia coli, Proteus* spp., and *Klebsiella* spp.), enterococci, *Staphylococcus saprophyticus,* and nonfermenters

> *Escherichia coli* is the most common cause of urinary tract infections—both cystitis and pyelonephritis, and both nosocomial and community-acquired UTIs.

(especially *Pseudomonas aeruginosa*). The most common causes of pyelonephritis are Enterobacteriaceae (especially *E. coli*), enterococci, and pathogens (e.g., *Staphylococcus aureus*, *Salmonella* spp.) that reach the kidneys via the bloodstream.

Clinical specimens. Clean-catch midstream urine specimens are preferred. Acceptable specimens include midstream urine, which is not clean-catch, and urine collected by suprapubic aspiration, which involves needle puncture of the urinary bladder. Urine collected via a catheter may be contaminated with indigenous urethral microflora. Urine collected via an indwelling catheter is likely to be contaminated. Urine obtained from a Foley catheter collection bag is unacceptable for culture, as are Foley catheter tips.

Specimen preservation. Unpreserved urine specimens should be processed within 2 hours of collection. If refrigerated from time of collection, specimens must be processed within 24 hours of collection. Processing of boric acid–preserved specimens should occur within 24 hours of collection.

Contaminants. The distal urethra is colonized by various bacteria, including members of the Enterobacteriaceae family (especially *E. coli*), *Lactobacillus* spp., diphtheroids, *Streptococcus* spp., *Enterococcus* spp., coagulase-negative staphylococci, *Peptostreptococcus* spp., and *Bacteroides* spp. Less common colonizers are *Mycoplasma hominis*, *Ureaplasma urealyticum*, and *Mycobacterium smegmatis*. Unless care is taken during collection, urine specimens could contain any of these organisms as contaminants.

Gram stain information. Gram staining of urine specimens can be used as a screening technique, to determine if specimens are suitable for culture. Two or more bacteria of the same morphotype per oil immersion field correlates with a colony count of 100,000 per milliliter or greater. Gram stain of urine sediment may be performed to check specimen quality. Observing three or more potential pathogens implies contamination. PMNs may be observed in urine specimens from symptomatic patients.

Screening tests. Leukocyte esterase is an enzyme produced by PMNs. A positive leukocyte esterase dipstick test on urine implies UTI. A positive nitrate dipstick test also implies infection. False-negative results are common with these dipstick tests. Several automated and semiautomated screening systems are available, including the FiltraCheck-UTI system (Meridian Diagnostics), bacterial ATP Assay (Coral Biotechnology), Bact-T-Screen (bioMérieux Inc.), Yellow IRIS system (International Remote Imaging Systems), and Cellenium System (Trek Diagnostic Systems).

Media for aerobic incubation. Inoculate blood agar and MAC plates. A **calibrated loop** is used to determine the number of **colony-forming units (CFU)** per milliliter of urine. A calibrated loop is an inoculating loop that has been manufactured to contain an exact quantity of liquid. Two types of calibrated loops are used for urine cultures: one cal-

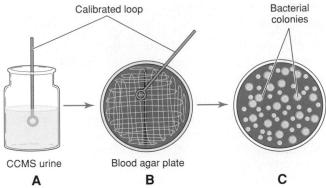

Figure 18-16. **Obtaining a urine colony count. A.** A calibrated loop is dipped into a clean-catch midstream (CCMS) urine specimen. **B.** The volume of urine contained within the calibrated loop is spread over the entire surface of a blood agar plate, which is then incubated overnight at 37°C. **C.** The colonies are counted after the plate is removed from the incubator.

ibrated to contain 0.01 mL of liquid and the other calibrated to contain 0.001 mL of liquid. It is common practice to use the 0.01-mL-calibrated loop for catheterized urine specimens and the 0.001-mL-calibrated loop for clean-catch midstream urine specimens. One calibrated loopful of urine is inoculated in such a manner as to distribute the urine (either 0.01 mL or 0.001 mL) over the entire surface of the plate. Following overnight incubation, the number of colonies on the plate are counted (Fig. 18-16).

Because each colony has theoretically been produced by a single bacterium that landed on the plate, the term *colony forming units* or *CFUs* refers to the number of live bacteria that were present in the urine at the time of plating. The number of CFUs per milliliter of urine is calculated as follows:

Colonies counted × Dilution factor = CFUs/mL

The dilution factor is 100 if the 0.01-mL loop was used and 1,000 if the 0.001-mL loop was used.

Colony count results are interpreted as shown in Table 18-3. UTIs are usually, but not always, caused by one pathogen. Thus, voided or catheterized urine cultures containing three or more colony morphotypes usually represent contamination, especially when there is no predominating organism. Various commercial agar-coated paddle systems are also available for urine culture.

Media for anaerobic incubation. Anaerobes are rare causes of UTIs. Because they are likely to be contaminated with indigenous microflora, voided or catheterized urine specimens are unacceptable for anaerobic culture. Urine specimens collected by suprapubic bladder aspiration are acceptable, but they are rarely submitted to the CML. Suprapubic bladder aspiration involves collection of urine through a needle that is inserted through the abdominal wall into the urinary bladder.

Laboratory diagnosis. If the predominant organism grew on both blood agar and MAC, it is most likely a member of the family Enterobacteriaceae because they are the most

TABLE 18 - 3 Interpretation of Urine Colony Count Results

Type of Specimen	UTI Likely	UTI Unlikely
Midstream urine from a female patient suspected of having cystitis	$>10^2$ CFU of a potential pathogen per mL; positive urine LE result	Colony count of contaminating microflora exceeds the colony count of a potential pathogen
Midstream urine from a female patient suspected of having pyelonephritis	$>10^5$ CFU of a potential pathogen per mL; positive urine LE result; Gram stain may reveal potential pathogen in PMNs and/or casts	The colony count of contaminating microflora exceeds the colony count of a potential pathogen
Midstream urine from an asymptomatic patient with bacteriuria	$>10^5$ CFU of a potential pathogen per mL; urine LE result usually negative	$<10^5$ CFU of a potential pathogen per mL; colony count of contaminating microflora exceeds the colony count of a potential pathogen
Midstream urine from a male patient suspected of having a UTI	$>10^3$ CFU of a potential pathogen per mL; positive urine LE result; Gram stain may reveal potential pathogen in PMNs and/or casts	$<10^3$ CFU of a potential pathogen per mL; colony count of contaminating microflora exceeds the colony count of a potential pathogen
Urine collected from either a female or male patient by straight catheterization	$>10^2$ CFU of a potential pathogen per mL; positive urine LE result in symptomatic patients; Gram stain may reveal potential pathogen in PMNs and/or casts	$<10^2$ CFU of a potential pathogen per mL; negative urine LE result
Urine collected from either a female or male patient by indwelling catheter	$>10^3$ CFU of a potential pathogen per mL; multiple pathogens may be present	Bacteriuria detected in asymptomatic patients; positive or negative urine LE result

Source: Thomson RB, Miller JM. Specimen collection, transport, and processing: Bacteriology. In: Murray PR, Baron EJ, Jorgensen JH, Pfaller MA, Yolken RH, eds. Manual of Clinical Microbiology. 8th Ed. Washington, DC: ASM Press, 2003.

CFU, colony-forming units; LE, leukocyte esterase test; PMN, polymorphonuclear leukocyte; UTI, urinary tract infection.

common causes of UTIs (Fig. 18-17). If the isolate ferments lactose (i.e., it produces pink colonies on MAC), it is most likely *E. coli*, the number one cause of UTIs, but it could be another lactose-fermenting member of the family (e.g., *Klebsiella* or *Enterobacter* spp.). If the isolate is a non-lactose-fermenter (i.e., it produces colorless colonies on MAC), it could be a non-lactose- or late-lactose-fermenting member of the family Enterobacteriaceae (e.g., a *Proteus, Morganella,* or *Providencia* sp.) or a nonfermenter (e.g., *Pseudomonas aeruginosa*). When an oxidase test is performed, if the organism is oxidase negative, it is most likely a member of the family Enterobacteriaceae; in that case, the criteria contained in Chapter 12 should be used to identify it. If it is oxidase-positive, identification should be attempted using the criteria in Chapter 13.

> *E. coli* is the number one cause of urinary tract infections.

If the organism grew on blood agar but not on MAC, it could either be a Gram-positive organism or a Gram-negative organism that does not grow on MAC. On Gram staining, if the isolate appears to be a Gram-positive coccus, it is most likely *Staphylococcus aureus, S. epidermidis, S. saprophyticus,* or an *Enterococcus* spp. and should be identified using criteria contained in Chapter 9. If it is a Gram-negative bacillus, identification using the criteria contained in Chapter 13 should be attempted.

Additional considerations. Because of the descending nature of the infection (i.e., blood to kidney), blood cultures should be performed for patients suspected of having pyelonephritis. Also, a stat Gram stain of the patient's urine can sometimes provide immediate preliminary identification of the pathogen. Urine from patients suspected of having leptospirosis must be inoculated into some type of special liquid medium (e.g., Fletcher medium) for culture of *Leptospira interrogans.*

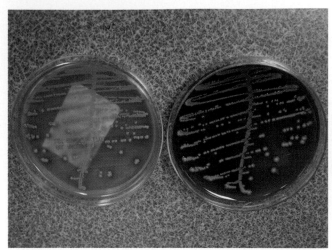

Figure 18-17. **Urine culture results. Both the MAC plate (to the left) and the blood agar plate (to the right) had been inoculated in an appropriate manner to obtain a colony count.** A bacterial pathogen, and the probable cause of the patient's urinary tract infection (UTI), is growing heavily on both plates. The colony count is >100,000 CFUs/mL. As evident from the pink colonies on the MAC plate, the isolate is a lactose fermenter and, when identified, will probably turn out to be *Escherichia coli*—the most common cause of UTIs. (Courtesy of Dr. Robert C. Fader.)

SEXUALLY TRANSMITTED BACTERIAL INFECTIONS OF THE GENITAL TRACT

Chlamydial Genital Infections

Diseases and most likely pathogens. *Chlamydia trachomatis* is considered to be the most common sexually transmitted bacterial pathogen. Different serovars[7] of *C. trachomatis* cause different diseases.

> *Chlamydia trachomatis* is considered to be the most common sexually transmitted bacterial pathogen.

Serovars D through K are the major causes of nongonococcal urethritis[8] and epididymitis in men; and cervicitis, urethritis, endometritis, and salpingitis in women. Serovars L1, L2, and L3 are associated with lymphogranuloma venereum, a sexually transmitted disease. Other serovars cause the eye diseases, trachoma and inclusion conjunctivitis.

Lymphogranuloma venereum is a relatively rare disease in the United States. The disease progresses through three stages: (1) a primary, usually painless ulcer that heals spontaneously; (2) lymphadenopathy and tenderness in regional nodes, accompanied by fever, chills, malaise, headache, and weight loss; and (3) coalescence of abscesses within lymph nodes and obstruction of lymph drainage.

Clinical specimens. *C. trachomatis* infects columnar and squamocolumnar epithelial cells. Swabs, scrapings, and small tissue samples can be used to culture chlamydiae. Because of toxicity problems, swabs with wooden shafts should not be used.

Specimen preservation. Specimens should be forwarded to the CML in special chlamydial transport media containing antimicrobial agents, and specimens must be kept cold during transport. If processing cannot be accomplished immediately, specimens should be refrigerated, or they should be frozen at −70°C if processing cannot be accomplished within 24 hours of collection. Specimens collected for immunodiagnostic or molecular diagnostic procedures should be collected, transported, and stored in accordance with manufacturers' instructions.

Contaminants. As previously mentioned, the distal urethra is colonized by various bacteria, any of which could be present in urethral swabs. Vaginal and cervical swabs will be contaminated with members of the indigenous vaginal flora, such as lactobacilli (the predominant organisms), diphtheroids, micrococci, coagulase-negative staphylococci, enterococci, streptococci, mycoplasmas, and ureaplasmas.

Screening tests. Nonculture methods of diagnosing chlamydial infections include amplified DNA probe techniques and immunoassays. PCR, transcription-mediated amplification, and strand displacement amplification can be used to detect chlamydia infection using urine specimens. For cytological examination (looking for intracytoplasmic inclusions), impression smears of tissues or scrapings are air dried, methanol fixed, and stained. Either Giemsa staining or direct fluorescent antibody staining can be used.

In vitro growth. Recall that *Chlamydia* spp. are obligate intracellular pathogens and, as such, will not grow on or in artificial culture media. Specimens are inoculated to cell cultures, usually McCoy cells.

Laboratory diagnosis. Identification of chlamydiae in cell culture involves demonstration of intracytoplasmic inclusions by immunofluorescence, iodine, or Giemsa staining procedures (see Chapter 16). An iodine-stained inclusion body is shown in Figure 16-4. Transport of specimens and culturing of *C. trachomatis* on McCoy cells is so problematic that most CMLs use nonculture methods. Refer to Chapter 16 for additional information on identifying chlamydiae.

Gonorrhea

Disease and pathogen. The etiologic agent of gonorrhea is *Neisseria gonorrhoeae*. It is important to understand that not all clinical presentations of gonorrhea involve the genital tract. Gonorrhea may present as asymptomatic mucosal infection, ophthalmia neonatorum, urethritis, proctitis, pharyngitis, epididymitis, cervicitis, Bartholin gland infection, pelvic inflammatory disease, endometritis, salpingitis, peritonitis,

---

[7] *The terms* serotypes *and* serovars *are synonymous. Serovars of a particular species differ from each other primarily as a result of differences in surface antigens. Sometimes, as in the case of* Chlamydia trachomatis *and* Escherichia coli, *different serovars of a particular species cause different diseases.*

[8] *The term* nongonococcal urethritis *refers to urethritis that is not caused by* Neisseria gonorrhoeae. *Although other organisms can cause nongonococcal urethritis,* Chlamydia trachomatis *is the major cause. Nongonococcal urethritis is more common than gonococcal urethritis.*

and disseminated gonococcal infection. Patients with disseminated gonococcal infection have myalgia (muscular pain), arthralgia (joint pain), polyarthritis (inflammation of joints), and a characteristic dermatitis—skin lesions located primarily on the extremities.

> Gonorrhea has many clinical manifestations, not just those affecting the genital tract.

Clinical specimens. Urethral discharge specimens, collected by swab, are acceptable for diagnosing gonorrheal urethritis in male patients by Gram stain and culture. Wire-shafted swabs tipped with calcium alginate or synthetic fibers should be used to collect urethral samples from asymptomatic men or male patients lacking a urethral exudate. Cotton-tipped, wooden-shafted swabs may be toxic to *N. gonorrhoeae*, especially when specimens are sent to the CML in transport medium. Swabs tipped with calcium alginate or synthetic fibers should be used to collect specimens from the uterine endocervix for diagnosis of urogenital tract gonorrhea in female patients. Specimens for molecular diagnostic procedures should be collected, transported, and stored in accordance with manufacturers' directions.

Specimen preservation. Ideally, specimens should be inoculated immediately to appropriate enriched and selective media (e.g., Thayer-Martin or Martin-Lewis medium) and incubated at 35°C in a microaerophilic and capnophilic atmosphere. If this is not possible, special transport media are available for shipment of specimens to the CML. One such transport system is the JEMBEC system with CO_2 generating tablets. JEMBEC stands for John E. Martin biological environmental chamber, named for the developer of the system.

Contaminants. As previously mentioned, the distal urethra is colonized by a variety of bacteria, any of which could be present in urethral swabs. Vaginal and cervical swabs will be contaminated with members of the indigenous vaginal flora, such as lactobacilli, diphtheroids, micrococci, coagulase-negative staphylococci, enterococci, streptococci, mycoplasmas, and ureaplasmas.

Gram stain information. Swab specimens should be rolled (not rubbed) onto glass microscope slides to preserve the integrity of any PMNs present in the specimen. For diagnosing gonorrhea in women, although Gram staining of urethral and cervical swabs is recommended, it cannot take the place of culture. In men, however, Gram staining of urethral swabs is of value for diagnosis of gonorrhea. For specimens from men, the Gram stain is considered positive *if, and only if,* intracellular Gram-negative diplococci (i.e., Gram-negative diplococci within PMNs) are observed (Fig. 18-18). Observing PMNs and only extracellular Gram-negative diplococci is considered equivocal for gonorrhea, but is often considered a significant enough finding to warrant initiation of treatment. Gram staining of swab specimens is not recommended for diagnosis of either pharyngeal gonorrhea or

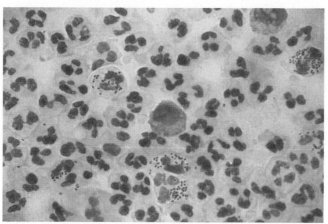

Figure 18-18. **Gram-stained urethral exudate from a male patient with gonorrhea.** Notice the numerous Gram-negative intracellular diplococci, which are sometimes referred to as GNIDs. (Courtesy of Joe Miller and the CDC.)

proctitis because of the presence of nongonococcal *Neisseria* spp. and Gram-negative diplococci and coccobacilli that resemble *Neisseria* spp. in appearance.

Screening tests. A variety of molecular diagnostic procedures are available to diagnose gonorrhea using urogenital specimens and urine. These include both nucleic acid amplification tests (e.g., polymerase chain reaction, transcription-mediated amplification, and strand displacement amplification tests) and nucleic acid hybridization tests.

Media for aerobic incubation. A highly enriched or selective medium, such as Thayer-Martin agar, must be used to isolate *N. gonorrhoeae* from nonsterile specimens. Otherwise, the fastidious gonococci will be overgrown and killed by hardier, faster-growing organisms in the specimen. Recall from Chapter 8 that Thayer-Martin agar (also Martin-Lewis agar) is a chocolate agar–based medium containing extra nutrients and several antimicrobial agents. This highly enriched medium will support the growth of even the most fastidious strains of *N. gonorrhoeae*, and the antimicrobial agents in Thayer-Martin agar inhibit growth of most indigenous microflora that are present in the clinical specimen.

The medium must be at room temperature prior to inoculation. Plates are incubated in a CO_2 incubator containing 3% to 7% CO_2 or candle extinction jar at 35°C. The incubation atmosphere should be moist. Plates should be examined at 24, 48, and 72 hours.

Laboratory diagnosis. Typical colonies of *N. gonorrhoeae* are about 0.5 mm in diameter, glistening, and raised, although various colony types, related to the extent of piliation of the bacteria, may be present on the same plate. Suspicious colonies should be Gram stained, and an oxidase test should be performed. Recall that all *Neisseria* spp. are oxidase-positive, Gram-negative diplococci. Methods for presumptive and definitive identification of *N. gonorrhoeae* are described in Chapter 11.

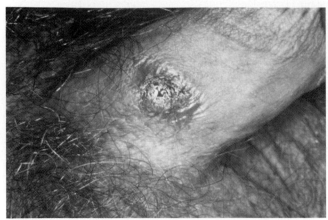

Figure 18-19. **Syphilis chancre on penile shaft.** (Courtesy of Dr. Gavin Hart, Dr. N. J. Fiumara, and the CDC.)

Syphilis

Disease and pathogen. Sexually transmitted bacterial infections involving genital ulceration include syphilis, lymphogranuloma venereum, chancroid, and granuloma inguinale. The latter two diseases are discussed later in the chapter. Syphilis is caused by a spirochete named *Treponema pallidum* subsp. *pallidum*. The various manifestations of syphilis include a painless chancre (Fig. 18-19) and inguinal lymphadenopathy in primary syphilis; rash, disseminated lymphadenopathy, fever, malaise, weight loss, and arthritis in secondary syphilis; and serious cardiovascular and neurologic problems in tertiary syphilis. Chancres develop at the site where *T. pallidum* subsp. *pallidum* entered the genital mucosa or skin through a break in the surface. They are usually firm, round, small, and painless. Chancres last 3 to 6 weeks and heal spontaneously without treatment. However, the infection may progress to the secondary stage if adequate treatment is not administered.

Clinical specimens. To diagnose primary syphilis, exudate or scrapings are obtained from the chancre. Serum is required for diagnosis of secondary and tertiary syphilis.

Specimen preservation. Material obtained from chancres for darkfield or phase contrast microscopy must be examined immediately because it is important to observe the characteristic motility of live treponemes in the specimen (Fig. 18-20). Material for the direct fluorescent antibody *T. pallidum* (DFA-TP) test can be air dried onto slides, as neither pathogen viability nor immediate examination is required. Serum specimens can be stored refrigerated for 3 to 5 days or frozen for long periods.

Contaminants. Morphologically similar, nonpathogenic spirochetes live within or near the genitalia, but their motility patterns differ from that of *T. pallidum* subsp. *pallidum*. Indigenous spirochetes can also be seen in specimens obtained from the oral cavity and lower gastrointestinal tract.

Gram stain information. *T. pallidum* subsp. *pallidum* is too thin to be seen by brightfield microscopy.

> *Treponema pallidum* is too thin to be seen in Gram-stained preparations.

Screening tests. Primary syphilis can be diagnosed using either darkfield or phase-contrast microscopy to observe treponemes in material obtained from the chancre. *T. pallidum* subsp. *pallidum* exhibits a characteristic corkscrew motility (rapid rotation about the long axis), which has been described as

> First-stage or primary syphilis can be diagnosed using either darkfield or phase contrast microscopy to observe treponemes in material obtained from chancres.

"spinning its wheels but not going anywhere." Flexing and reversal of rotation may also be observed. Treponemes can also be visualized using the DFA-TP test, which, because of the presence of indigenous spirochetes, is recommended for oral or gastrointestinal specimens. It is also sometimes possible to observe treponemes in material

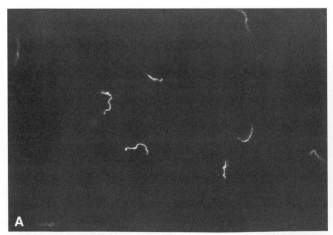

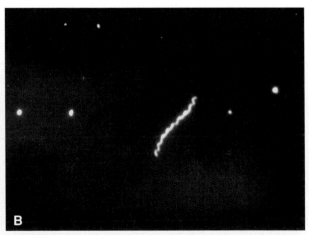

*Figure 18-20. **Treponema pallidum* as seen by darkfield microscopy. A.** ×54 magnification. **B.** ×400 magnification. (Courtesy of C. W. Hubbard and the CDC.)

TABLE 18 - 4 Serologic Procedures for the Diagnosis of Syphilis

Category	Name of Test	Discussion
Nontreponemal tests	Venereal Disease Research Laboratory (VDRL) test	Performed on serum and cerebrospinal fluid; flocculation test requiring microscopic examination
	Rapid plasma reagin (RPR) card test	Performed on serum or plasma; flocculation test; results can be read macroscopically
	Unheated serum reagin (USR) test	Performed on serum; flocculation test requiring microscopic examination
	Toluidine red unheated serum test (TRUST)	Performed on serum or plasma; flocculation test; results can be read macroscopically
Treponemal tests	Fluorescent treponemal antibody absorption (FTA-ABS) test, a fluorescence microscopy procedure	Performed on serum and CSF; an indirect fluorescent antibody technique; uses *T. pallidum* subsp. *pallidum* as antigen and fluorescein isothiocyanate–labeled antihuman immunoglobulin; spirochetes fluoresce if patient's serum or CSF contains anti-*T. pallidum* antibodies
	Fluorescent treponemal antibody-absorption double-staining (FTA-ABS DS) test; a fluorescence microscopy procedure	Performed on serum; a modified FTA-ABS test that uses two fluorescent dye–labeled reagents—an anti–human immunoglobulin and an anti–*T. pallidum* immunoglobulin
	Microhemagglutination assay for antibodies to *T. pallidum* (MHA-TP)	Performed on serum; an agglutination procedure that uses erythrocytes sensitized (coated) with *T. pallidum* subsp. *pallidum* antigens
	Treponema pallidum particle agglutination (TP-PA) test	Performed on serum; an agglutination procedure that uses gelatin particles sensitized with *T. pallidum* subsp. *pallidum* antigens

obtained from secondary syphilis skin lesions. Molecular diagnostic techniques are being developed.

Several serologic procedures are available to diagnose syphilis (Table 18-4). Serologic tests for syphilis are the only practical methods for diagnosing latent and tertiary (late) syphilis. Treponemal assays detect anti–*T. pallidum* antibodies, whereas nontreponemal assays detect what are known as reaginic antibodies. Reaginic antibodies are antibodies produced in response to lipoidal material that is released from damaged host cells and possibly also in response to lipoprotein-like material and cardiolipin released from treponemes. The reagent used in nontreponemal tests is an alcoholic solution containing cardiolipin, cho-

lesterol, and lecithin.[9] Reaginic antibodies are produced in response not only to treponemal infections but also to autoimmune diseases, pregnancy, and other conditions causing tissue damage. Thus, the presence of reaginic antibodies in a serum specimen is not specific for syphilis. Although nontreponemal assays are inexpensive and easy to perform, they lack sensitivity (in the early and late stages of syphilis) and specificity (false-positive results occur). Treponemal assays are more expensive and technically more difficult to perform. They are of greatest value in

> Several serologic procedures are available to diagnose latent and tertiary or late syphilis.

[9] Cardiolipin, cholesterol, and lecithin are lipids found in mammalian cell membranes. Antibodies to these lipids are produced as a result of cell damage and subsequent release of these lipids into the bloodstream.

distinguishing between true-positive and false-positive non-treponemal test results and for diagnosis of latent and tertiary syphilis. It is important to note that serum specimens from patients with yaws, pinta, or bejel will produce positive results when tested with serologic tests for syphilis.

> *T. pallidum* cannot be grown on or in artificial culture media.

In vitro growth. *T. pallidum* subsp. *pallidum* cannot be grown on or in artificial culture media. Rabbit inoculation is used to produce large numbers of *T. pallidum* organisms for research purposes.

Chancroid

Disease and pathogen. Chancroid is caused by *Haemophilus ducreyi*. The disease is also known as soft chancre, to distinguish it from the firm chancre of primary syphilis. The soft chancres develop at the site where *H. ducreyi* entered the genital mucosa or skin through a break in the surface. The chancres are quite painful, unlike syphilis chancres, and bleed readily. Chancroid is rare in the United States.

Clinical specimens. Swab specimens should be collected from the base of the chancre. Two swabs should be collected, one for Gram staining and the other for culture.

Specimen preservation. Ideally, swabs should be inoculated directly at the collection location or within an hour of specimen collection. Alternatively, they can be transported in a thioglycolate-hemin–based transport medium. Specimens in transport medium can be stored at 4°C.

Contaminants. Depending on the location of the chancre, specimens may be contaminated with indigenous skin, urethral, or vaginal microflora.

Gram stain information. Observing many small, pleomorphic Gram-negative bacilli and coccobacilli in chains and groupings (said to resemble schools of fish or railroad tracks) would be highly suggestive of *H. ducreyi* but are rarely seen in direct Gram-stained smears.

Media for aerobic incubation. The optimal culture media for *H. ducreyi* are those containing calf serum, charcoal, horse blood, or rabbit blood. Chocolate agar containing Iso-VitaleX (BD Biosciences) can also be used. Inoculated plates should be incubated at 33°C in an atmosphere containing 5% CO_2 and maximal humidity. If necessary, a candle extinction jar containing a moist paper towel can be used. Growth is usually apparent by 48 hours.

Laboratory diagnosis. *H. ducreyi* is a small, bipolar-staining Gram-negative bacillus or coccobacillus. The cells may be seen in parallel rows of chains, resembling a school of fish or a railroad track (Fig. 18-21). Chapter 14 contains additional information regarding identification of *H. ducreyi*.

Additional comments. Because dual infections can occur, material collected from chancres should be examined by darkfield microscopy to observe *T. pallidum*, if present.

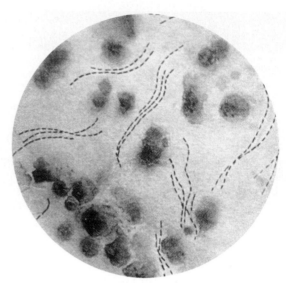

Figure 18-21. Drawing of *Haemophilus ducreyi*, illustrating the "school of fish" or "railroad track" arrangement of cells that is sometimes observed in Gram-stained preparations. (Courtesy of the CDC.)

Granuloma Inguinale

Disease and pathogen. Granuloma inguinale or ulcerative donovanosis is caused by *Calymmatobacterium granulomatis*, a pleomorphic Gram-negative bacillus having a prominent capsule. The organism has features suggestive of the family Enterobacteriaceae, especially *Klebsiella* spp., and is called *Klebsiella granulomatis* by some taxonomists. The genital lesions of granuloma inguinale appear at the site of entry of the pathogen, most often on the penis or on the labia and cervix. They are painless, beefy red, and raised. They enlarge slowly over months or even years and may reach a diameter of 5 to 20 cm. The lesions are often misdiagnosed as carcinoma. It is estimated that fewer than 100 cases occur annually in the United States.

Clinical specimens. Scrapings of the ulcerative lesion should be spread onto a glass microscope slide, air dried, methanol fixed, and stained with either Wright or Giemsa stain.

Staining information. In tissue smears, the bacteria are found in large histiocytes (fixed macrophages). Apparently, they multiply in cytoplasmic vacuoles containing hundreds of organisms liberated when the host cell ruptures. Diagnosis of granuloma inguinale is based on the observation of these bacteria-filled vacuoles, referred

> Associate Donovan bodies with *Calymmatobacterium granulomatis* and granuloma inguinale.

to as Donovan bodies, in Wright- or Giemsa-stained smears (Fig. 18-22). Host cells may contain more than one Donovan body. Donovan bodies should not be confused with the intracytoplasmic inclusions of chlamydiae, which are located in the cytoplasm of epithelial cells, or *Ehrlichia* and

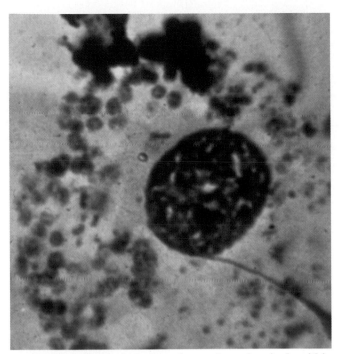

Figure 18-22. **Donovan bodies of granuloma inguinale within an infected skin cell.** Donovan bodies contain encapsulated, safety pin shaped *Calymmatobacterium granulomatis* cells. (Courtesy of Richard O. Deitrick and the CDC.)

Anaplasma, which are located in the cytoplasm of peripheral monocytes and granulocytes, respectively.

Screening tests. No immunodiagnostic or molecular diagnostic procedures are available.

In vitro growth. *C. granulomatis* does not grow on or in artificial media.

OTHER BACTERIAL INFECTIONS OF THE GENITAL TRACT

Genital tract infections and their usual bacterial etiologic agents are shown in Table 18-5. Included in the table are some of the sexually transmitted pathogens previously discussed. Female genital tract infections include bacterial vaginosis, cervicitis, endometritis, genital ulcers, ovarian abscess, salpingitis, urethritis, and vulvovaginitis. Male genital tract infections include epididymitis, genital ulcers, prostatitis, and urethritis.

Urethritis
Disease and most likely pathogens. Infections of the urethra are most often, but not always, sexually transmitted. The

TABLE 18 - 5	Bacterial Infections of the Genital Tract
Infection	**Most Likely Pathogens**
Bacterial vaginosis	Polymicrobial infection caused by a mixture of *Gardnerella*, *Mobiluncus*, *Prevotella*, *Peptostreptococcus*, and *Mycoplasma* spp.
Cervicitis	*N. gonorrhoeae*, *C. trachomatis*, perhaps *U. urealyticum*
Endometritis	Enterobacteriaceae, groups A and B streptococci, enterococci, mixed anaerobic flora
Epididymitis	*N. gonorrhoeae*, *C. trachomatis*, Enterobacteriaceae, *P. aeruginosa*, various Gram-positive cocci
Genital ulcers	*T. pallidum*, *H. ducreyi*, *C. trachomatis*
Pelvic abscess	Mixed aerobic and anaerobic flora
Prostatitis	Enterobacteriaceae, *P. aeruginosa*, enterococci
Salpingitis/oophoritis	*N. gonorrhoeae*, *C. trachomatis*, mixed anaerobic flora
Urethral syndrome	Enterobacteriaceae (especially *E. coli*), *S. saprophyticus*, *C. trachomatis*, *N. gonorrhoeae*, enterococci, nonfermenters, *Corynebacterium urealyticum*
Urethritis	*C. trachomatis*, *N. gonorrhoeae*, *U. urealyticum*
Vulvovaginitis	*N. gonorrhoeae* and *C. trachomatis* in prepubescent female patients

Source: Thomson RB, Miller JM. Specimen collection, transport, and processing: Bacteriology. In: Murray PR, Baron EJ, Jorgensen JH, Pfaller MA, Yolken RH, eds. Manual of Clinical Microbiology. 8th Ed. Washington, DC: ASM Press, 2003.

major causes of urethritis in men are *Chlamydia trachomatis*, *Neisseria gonorrhoeae*, and occasionally, *Ureaplasma urealyticum*. Urethritis not caused by *N. gonorrhoeae* is called nongonococcal urethritis, which is most commonly caused by *C. trachomatis*.

> Urethritis that is not caused by *Neisseria gonorrhoeae* is referred to as nongonococcal urethritis, the most common cause of which is *Chlamydia trachomatis*.

Urethritis caused by *C. trachomatis* is the most common form of male urethritis in the United States. Patients present with dysuria (difficulty or pain on urination) and/or a mucoid-to-watery white urethral discharge. Urethritis is the most common clinical manifestation of gonorrhea in male patients, who typically present with dysuria, frequency of urination, and a purulent yellow urethral discharge.

In female patients, urethritis most often presents as acute urethral syndrome or urethrocystitis, which affects both the urethra and the urinary bladder. The major causes are Enterobacteriaceae and *Staphylococcus saprophyticus*, and less often *C. trachomatis* and *N. gonorrhoeae*. Chlamydial genital infections and gonorrhea were discussed earlier in this chapter. Information about *S. saprophyticus*, Enterobacteriaceae, and *U. urealyticum* is presented in Chapters 9, 12, and 14, respectively.

Clinical specimens. Urethral discharge material can be collected using two swabs: one for preparation of a smear for Gram-staining and one for culture. When there is no discharge, a urethrogenital swab should be inserted about 2 cm into the urethra and left in place for a few seconds to increase absorption. If only one urethrogenital swab is collected, inoculate appropriate media first and then prepare a smear for Gram staining.

Specimen preservation. Urethral swabs should be placed into some type of swab transport system. Special transport devices are available for *N. gonorrhoeae*. The specimens should not be refrigerated. Ideally, specimens should be processed within 2 hours.

Contaminants. Recall that the distal urethra is colonized by various bacteria, any of which could be present in urethral swabs.

Gram stain information. Gonorrhea can be presumptively diagnosed in male patients when a Gram-stained smear of a urethral discharge reveals numerous PMNs and intracellular Gram-negative diplococci. A diagnosis of nongonococcal urethritis can be made when the smear reveals numerous PMNs but no Gram-negative diplococci, and *N. gonorrhoeae* is not isolated from the specimen.

Screening tests. Immunodiagnostic procedures are available for diagnosis of nongonococcal urethritis caused by *C. trachomatis*.

Media for aerobic incubation. Thayer-Martin agar should be inoculated for isolation of *N. gonorrhoeae*. Cell cultures are inoculated for isolation of *C. trachomatis* and *U. urealyticum*.

Laboratory diagnosis. Identification of *N. gonorrhoeae* and *C. trachomatis* were discussed in Chapters 11 and 16, respectively. *U. urealyticum* was discussed in Chapter 14.

Bacterial Vaginosis

Disease and most likely pathogens. The three main causes of vaginitis are the yeast *Candida albicans* (see Chapters 19 and 20), the protozoan *Trichomonas vaginalis* (see Chapter 22), and a mixture of bacteria. When caused by a mixture of bacteria, the condition is known as bacterial vaginosis. Bacterial vaginosis is a synergistic or polymicrobial infection that results when the normally predominant lactobacilli in vaginal microflora are replaced by a superinfection of high concentrations of mixtures of any or all of the following bacteria: *Gardnerella vaginalis*; anaerobes such as *Prevotella*, *Mobiluncus*, and Gram-positive cocci; and *Mycoplasma hominis*. Some women with bacterial vaginosis are asymptomatic, whereas others present with a fishy-smelling vaginal discharge. The fishy odor is caused by trimethylamine, an amine that is a metabolic product of the bacterial superinfection. Bacterial vaginosis is a risk factor for acute pelvic inflammatory disease and other upper genital tract infections. Pregnant patients with bacterial vaginosis have an increased rate of preterm low-birth-weight deliveries, amnionic fluid infections, and chorioamnionic infections.

Clinical specimens. Vaginal discharge specimens are collected by swab.

Specimen preservation. Saline wet mount examinations of freshly collected vaginal discharge specimens are usually performed in the gynecologist's office. The reason for this practice is that if the vaginal discharge is caused by infection with *T. vaginalis*, this usually highly motile protozoan dies rapidly on exposure to air and room temperature, causing it to round up and resemble a leukocyte. Saline wet mount examinations are described in Appendix A.

Contaminants. Bacterial members of the indigenous microflora of the healthy human vagina were previously discussed. Any of these organisms can be observed in Gram stains of vaginal swabs or vaginal discharge specimens.

Gram stain information. According to the criteria established by Nugent et al. (see "References and Suggested Reading"), diagnosis of bacterial vaginosis requires observation of a Gram-stained vaginal smear. Values are determined for each of the three morphotype categories, using the criteria listed at the bottom of Table 18-6, and a score is assigned for each category (listed in the last column of the table). Those scores are then totaled. Total scores of 0 to 3 are considered normal (not bacterial vaginosis). Total scores of 4 to 6 are considered intermediate (possible bacterial

TABLE 18 - 6	Nugent Criteria for Diagnosis of Bacterial Vaginosis			
Presence of *Lactobacillus* spp. Morphotypes	Presence of *Gardnerella* and *Bacteroides* spp. Morphotypes	Presence of Curved Gram-Variable Bacilli	Assigned Score
4+	0	0	0
3+	1+	1+ or 2+	1
2+	2+	3+ or 4+	2
1+	3+		3
0	4+		4

Note: Morphotype values represent the average number of bacteria having that morphotype seen per oil immersion field.

0, no bacteria of morphotype observed; 1+, <1 of morphotype present; 2+, 1 to 4 of morphotype present; 3+, 5 to 30 of this morphotype present; 4+, 30 or more of morphotype present.

vaginosis). Total scores of 7 to 10 are interpreted as bacterial vaginosis. Following are some examples:

Example 1

Each of the morphotype categories received a value of 3+. According to Table 18-6, a 3+ value for the *Lactobacillus* category yields a score of 1, 3+ value for the *Gardnerella/Bacteroides* category yields a score of 3, and a 3+ value for the curved Gram-variable bacilli category yields a score of 2. The total score is 1 plus 3 plus 2, or 6. Since a total score between 4 and 6 is considered intermediate, it is possible that this patient has bacterial vaginosis.

Example 2

The *Lactobacillus* category received a value of 4+, and each of the other categories received a value of 1+. The table shows that a 4+ value for the *Lactobacillus* category yields a score of 0, a 1+ value for the *Gardnerella/Bacteroides* category yields a score of 1, and a 1+ value for the curved Gram-variable bacilli category yields a score of 1. The total score is 0 plus 1 plus 1, or 2. A total score between 0 and 3 is considered normal, meaning that this patient does not have bacterial vaginosis.

Example 3

The *Lactobacillus* category received a value of 1+, and each of the other categories received a value of 4+.

The table shows that a 1+ value for the *Lactobacillus* category yields a score of 3, a 4+ value for the *Gardnerella/Bacteroides* category yields a score of 4, and a 4+ value for the curved Gram-variable bacilli category yields a score of 2. The total score is 3 plus 4 plus 2, or 9. A total score between 7 and 10 is considered indicative of bacterial vaginosis. Thus, according to the Nugent criteria, this patient has the disease.

Screening tests. Although examination of a Gram-stained smear of vaginal discharge material is considered the "gold standard" for diagnosis of bacterial vaginosis, the disease can also be diagnosed according to the criteria devised by Amsel et al. (see "References and Suggested Reading"). A diagnosis of bacterial vaginosis can be made if three of the following criteria are found:

- A thin, homogeneous vaginal discharge, resembling skim milk

- Vaginal pH >4.5

- A positive "whiff" test (a fishy amine odor is produced when 10% potassium hydroxide is added to a smear of a vaginal discharge specimen)

- Observance of numerous "clue" cells in a saline wet mount of the vaginal fluid; clue cells, so named because they provide a clue that the patient has bacterial vaginosis, are squamous epithelial cells coated with large numbers of bacilli and coccobacilli (Fig. 18-23); some authorities

> "Clue" cells provide a clue that the patient has bacterial vaginosis.

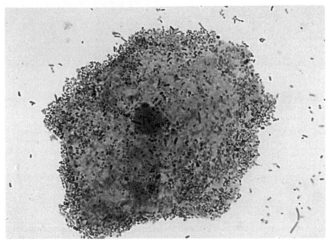

Figure 18-23. **"Clue" cell.** Finding vaginal epithelial cells coated with many Gram-positive and Gram-negative curved and straight bacilli provides a clue that the patient has bacterial vaginosis. (From Marler LM, Siders JA, Allen SD. Direct Smear Atlas. Philadelphia: Lippincott Williams & Wilkins, 2001.)

have suggested that at least 20% of the epithelial cells present should be clue cells.

It should be noted that some authorities feel that the absence of numerous bacteria of the *Lactobacillus* morphotype and the presence of an abnormally high number of bacteria having other morphotypes is more important than the presence of clue cells in the diagnosis of bacterial vaginosis.

Media for aerobic incubation. Cultures are not used to diagnose bacterial vaginosis because the bacteria causing the disease are members of the indigenous vaginal microflora.

BACTERIAL INFECTIONS OF THE ORAL CAVITY

Diseases and most likely pathogens. Periodontal diseases, gingivitis and periodontitis, are usually polymicrobial infections, with anaerobes being the primary etiologic agents. The anaerobes most often associated with periodontal diseases are black-pigmented species of *Porphyromonas* (*P. gingivalis*, *P. endodontalis*) and *Prevotella* (*P. intermedia*), *Bacteroides forsythus*, and spirochetes (*Treponema denticola*). *Actinobacillus actinomycetemcomitans*, a microaerophilic Gram-negative coccobacillus, has been associated with localized juvenile periodontitis. These are all members of normal dental plaque flora, so their isolation from oral specimens is not pathognomonic[10] for periodontal disease. When these bacteria are isolated from oral specimens, it is difficult to know whether they are involved in an infectious process or are merely contaminants.

Clinical specimens. Tissue biopsy specimens or needle aspirates are the specimens of choice. Sampling of superficial tissue surfaces should be discouraged. Additional information about specimens for diagnosis of oral infections can be found in the manual by Jousimies-Somer et al. (see "References and Suggested Reading").

Specimen preservation. Carefully collected scrapings or aspirates should be transported to the CML in some type of anaerobic transport system (see Chapter 17).

Contaminants. Virtually all oral specimens will be contaminated with indigenous oral cavity microflora. It has been estimated that the oral cavity of healthy adults is inhabited by more than 200 species of bacteria and that anaerobes outnumber aerobes by a ratio of at least 100:1. Common members of the oral cavity microflora are viridans group streptococci and anaerobes such as *Actinomyces*, *Veillonella*, *Bacteroides*, *Prevotella*, *Fusobacterium*, *Propionibacterium* spp., and anaerobic Gram-positive cocci.

Gram stain information. Gram stains are not useful.

Screening tests. The anaerobes most often associated with periodontal disease—*P. gingivalis*, *B. forsythus*, and *T. denticola*—are capable of hydrolyzing benzoyl-DL-arginine-naphthylamide (BANA). Thus, the BANA hydrolysis test can be used to diagnose an anaerobic periodontal infection. If anaerobes are shown to be present, then appropriate antimicrobial therapy (e.g., metronidazole) can be initiated. The test is of limited value, however, because these three anaerobes are also present in plaque samples from healthy persons. DNA probes and immunological assays are also available to detect the presence of these anaerobes in specimens.

Media for aerobic incubation. Inoculation of routine media for CO_2 incubation is of limited value.

Media for anaerobic incubation. Special anaerobic media (described in the manual by Jousimies-Somer et al.) should be inoculated in addition to routine anaerobic media (BRU/BA, LKV, BBE).

Laboratory diagnosis. Anaerobes isolated from oral specimens should be identified using the criteria described in Chapter 17.

Additional comments. Vincent angina is also known as Vincent disease, acute necrotizing ulcerative gingivitis, fusospirochetal disease, and trench mouth. The disease is characterized by pharyngitis, membranous exudate, foul-smelling breath, and oral ulcerations. It is a polymicrobial infection caused by *Fusobacterium necrophorum*, *Borrelia* spp., and other anaerobes. Diagnosis is usually made by examination of a Gram-stained smear. Observing PMNs, Gram-negative spirochetes, and fusiform bacilli is presumptive evidence of Vincent angina (Fig. 18-24). Routine anaerobic media (BRU/BA, LKV, BBE) should be inoculated if this condition is suspected, but culture is usually not helpful.

---

[10]*If something is pathognomic, it is indicative or characteristic of a particular disease.*

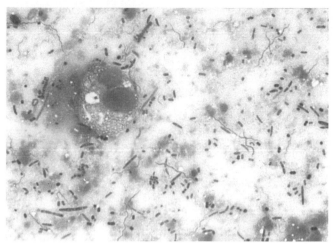

Figure 18-24. **Gram-stained material collected from an oral cavity ulcer.** The predominance of Gram-negative fusiform bacteria and spirochetes is consistent with the diagnosis of trench mouth. (From Marler LM, Siders JA, Allen SD. Direct Smear Atlas. Philadelphia: Lippincott Williams & Wilkins, 2001.)

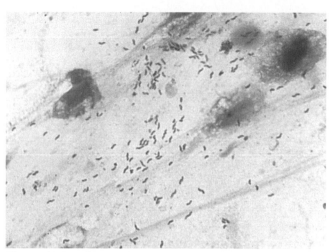

Figure 18-25. **Gram-stained stomach biopsy.** The curved-to-spiral-shaped Gram-negative bacilli suggest *Helicobacter pylori*. (From Marler LM, Siders JA, Allen SD. Direct Smear Atlas. Philadelphia: Lippincott Williams & Wilkins, 2001.)

BACTERIAL INFECTIONS OF THE GASTROINTESTINAL TRACT

Gastritis and Gastric Ulcers

Diseases and most likely pathogens. *Helicobacter pylori* has been linked to a variety of gastric and extragastric diseases. The gastric diseases include acute gastritis (inflammation of the mucosal lining of the stomach, with abdominal pain, nausea, vomiting), dyspepsia (gastric indigestion), duodenal and gastric ulcers, and gastric adenocarcinoma and lymphoma. Among the extragastric diseases are hepatic and pancreatic diseases.

Clinical specimens. Stomach biopsy specimens, collected by fiber-optic endoscopy, can be used for culture, histological examination, and performance of a rapid urease test (described later).

Specimen preservation. Stomach biopsy materials should be immediately placed into a transport medium (e.g., brucella broth with glycerol, cysteine-Albimi broth with glycerol, or Stuart medium) or sterile saline to prevent desiccation. The specimen should be transported to the CML immediately and processed within 2 hours of collection. If processing will be delayed, specimens should be refrigerated.

Contaminants. A variety of acid-tolerant bacteria may reside in the healthy stomach (e.g., *Helicobacter* spp., streptococci, staphylococci, lactobacilli, some anaerobes), but their concentrations are generally low.

Gram stain information. Biopsy specimen imprints can be stained either with a rapid Giemsa stain or Gram stain. Counterstaining with carbol fuchsin rather than safranin may make it easier to observe the bacteria. Recall that *H. pylori* are curved Gram-negative bacilli (Fig. 18-25).

Screening tests. The rapid urease test is performed by placing the stomach biopsy specimen into a tube of urea broth containing a pH indicator. Production of ammonia causes the pH indicator to turn red, confirming the presence of *H. pylori*. Agar gel–based tests and paper strip tests are also available for rapid urease testing. A noninvasive urea breath test is available, as are immunodiagnostic procedures for detection of *H. pylori* antigen.

Media for aerobic incubation. Biopsy specimens for *H. pylori* are usually productive, whereas gastric aspirates are usually nonproductive. Helicobacters grow best in freshly prepared, moist media incubated for 5 to 7 days at 37°C in an atmosphere containing 5% to 10% CO_2 and 5% to 10% O_2. Media such as brucella agar with horse blood; brain heart infusion agar with horse blood; and Skirrow agar containing horse blood, horse serum, or sheep blood have been used successfully to culture *H. pylori*. *H. pylori* will not grow on *Campylobacter* blood agar (Campy blood agar) because of the presence of antibiotics in the medium.

Laboratory diagnosis. Presumptive identification of *H. pylori* can be made if curved Gram-negative bacilli are isolated and are urease, catalase, and oxidase positive. *Helicobacter* isolates are motile; motility can be observed using phase-contrast microscopy. For more information on identification of *H. pylori*, see Chapter 15.

Diarrheal Diseases

Diseases and most likely pathogens. Diarrhea can have many causes and is a symptom in a wide variety of conditions and diseases. It can be caused by certain foods or drugs, or it may be the result of an infectious disease. If the diarrhea is the result of an infectious disease, the pathogen may be a

TABLE 18 - 7   Bacterial Causes of Diarrheal Diseases

Category	Most Common Bacterial Pathogens
Traveler's diarrhea	Enterotoxigenic, enteroaggregative, and enteroinvasive *Escherichia coli* serotypes; *Yersinia, Campylobacter, Salmonella, Shigella, Aeromonas, Plesiomonas*, and *Vibrio* spp.
Diarrhea in AIDS patients	*Salmonella, Campylobacter*, and *Shigella* spp.; *Mycobacterium avium* complex; enteroaggregative *E. coli*; *Clostridium difficile*
Food poisoning/foodborne diseases	*Staphylococcus aureus; Bacillus cereus; Clostridium perfringens; Salmonella, Shigella, Vibrio, Campylobacter*, and *Yersinia* spp.; *E. coli* O157:H7 and other Shiga toxin–producing *E. coli* serotypes; *Listeria monocytogenes*
Nosocomial diarrhea	*Clostridium difficile*

Source: Bouckenooghe AP, DuPont HL. Approach to the patient with diarrhea. In: Gorbach SL, Bartlett JG, Blacklow NR, eds. Infectious Disease. 3rd Ed. Philadelphia: Lippincott Williams & Wilkins, 2004.

virus, a bacterium, a protozoan, or a helminth. Dysentery—a severe form of diarrheal disease—may also be caused by various pathogens, including bacteria (e.g., *Shigella* spp. cause bacillary dysentery) and protozoa (e.g., amebiasis and balantidiasis; see Chapter 22). Some of the bacterial pathogens are shown in Table 18-7. Some cases of diarrhea are examples of microbial intoxications, the result of ingesting preformed toxins (such as those produced by *Staphylococcus aureus* or *Bacillus cereus*). Microbial intoxications are discussed in Appendix 1 of the CD-ROM.

Clinical specimens. To culture for bacterial pathogens, three diarrheal stool specimens should be submitted on 3 consecutive days. Generally, rectal swab specimens are recommended only for infants, but there may be other occasions (e.g., outbreaks) when rectal swabs are acceptable. Feces must be observable on rectal swabs.

Specimen preservation. If fecal specimens cannot be delivered immediately to the CML, they should be refrigerated. However, the drop in pH that occurs as fecal specimens cool inhibits growth of many *Shigella* spp. and some *Salmonella* spp. Fecal specimens should be added to Cary-Blair transport medium if a 2- to 3-hour delay is anticipated. Rectal swabs can be transported in an all-purpose transport medium such as Stuart.

Contaminants. The indigenous microflora of the healthy human colon contains more than 200 species of bacteria, most (roughly 98%) of which are anaerobes. The most common indigenous bacteria found in fecal specimens, in approximate order of frequency, are *Bacteroides, Bifidobacterium, Eubacterium*, and *Lactobacillus* spp.; members of the family Enterobacteriaceae; and *Peptostreptococcus, Streptococcus, Enterococcus*, and *Clostridium* spp.

Gram stain information. Gram stain examinations of fecal specimens are of limited value. Sometimes they can provide information on the presence or absence of fecal leukocytes and, when present, the predominance of one particular cellular morphotype.

Screening tests. A fecal leukocyte or lactoferrin test helps to differentiate inflammatory diarrhea from noninflammatory (secretory) diarrhea. To observe fecal leukocytes, a portion of a fresh fecal specimen, preferably containing mucous, is mixed with 2 drops of dilute Loeffler methylene blue on a microscope slide and examined microscopically. The presence of five or more PMNs per high-power field is indicative of mucosal inflammation. The presence of lactoferrin is a more sensitive leukocyte marker, and the test does not require a fresh specimen. Not all intestinal pathogens are invasive, however; some produce disease solely by enterotoxin production. In such cases, both fecal leukocyte and lactoferrin tests are negative. Inflammatory diarrhea is typically caused by invasive pathogens such as *Shigella, Salmonella*, enteroinvasive *Escherichia coli, Campylobacter, Yersinia enterocolitica*, and *Plesiomonas shigelloides*, or by cytotoxins produced by *Shigella, C. difficile, E. coli* O157:H7, and other Shiga toxin–producing *E. coli*.

Media for aerobic incubation. Media for isolation of routine enteric pathogens include MAC, EMB, Hektoen enteric agar, xylose-lysine-deoxycholate agar, Gram-negative and selenite F enrichment broths, SS agar (for *Shigella* and *Salmonella*), and Campy blood agar for *Campylobacter*. Refer to Chapter 12 for information regarding the appearance of enteric pathogen colonies on commonly used selective and differential media. Some CMLs also routinely inoculate blood agar and chocolate agar plates. Inoculated plates should be incubated in a non-CO_2 incubator at 35°C to 37°C for 2 days. (Incubation in a CO_2 incubator causes acidification of the medium and alters the appearance of lactose-negative organisms.) Campy blood agar plates should be incubated for 3 days at 42°C in a microaerophilic and capnophilic atmosphere containing 10% CO_2 and 5% O_2.

It is very important that the CML be notified if bacterial pathogens other than *Salmonella*, *Shigella*, or *Campylobacter* are suspected. Isolation of other pathogens (e.g., *Aeromonas*, *E. coli* O157:H7, *Vibrio*, *Yersinia*) requires special laboratory procedures. For example, cefsulodin-Irgasan-novobiocin (CIN) medium is inoculated when *Yersinia enterocolitica* is suspected; thiosulfate-citrate-bile salts-sucrose (TCBS) medium is inoculated when *Vibrio* spp. are suspected; and a sorbitol-containing medium is inoculated when *E. coli* O157:H7 is suspected.

> It is very important that the CML be notified if bacterial pathogens other than *Salmonella*, *Shigella*, or *Campylobacter* are suspected to be the cause of a patient's diarrhea, so that CML professionals can inoculate appropriate media.

> Associate CIN medium with *Yersinia enterocolitica* and TCBS medium with *Vibrio* spp.

Media for anaerobic incubation. None are required unless *Clostridium difficile* isolation is needed for epidemiologic purposes, in which case the specimen would be inoculated to CCFA and incubated anaerobically. *C. difficile* is discussed later in the chapter.

Laboratory diagnosis. The initial clues in the identification of potential pathogens are the media on which the organism grew, reactions observed on differential media, colony morphology, and, sometimes, cellular morphology (e.g., *Vibrio* and *Campylobacter* spp. are curved Gram-negative bacilli). The primary challenge to the CML professional is to decide which culture results are normal and which are abnormal. Identification criteria can be found in previous chapters (e.g., see Chapter 12 for Enterobacteriaceae and Chapter 15 for *Vibrio* and *Campylobacter* spp.). Growth on the blood agar plate can be tested for oxidase; *Aeromonas* spp. and *P. shigelloides* are both oxidase positive.

Campylobacter Enteritis

Disease. *Campylobacter* enteritis is an acute bacterial enteric disease, ranging from asymptomatic to severe, with diarrhea, nausea, vomiting, fever, malaise, and abdominal pain. The disease is usually self-limiting, lasting 2 to 5 days. Stools may contain gross or occult (hidden) blood, mucus, and white blood cells. *Campylobacter* spp. are the major cause of bacterial diarrhea in the United States.

Pathogens. The etiologic agents of *Campylobacter* enteritis are *C. jejuni* and, less commonly, *C. coli*. *Campylobacter* spp. are curved, S-shaped, or spiral-shaped Gram-negative bacilli, often having a "gull wing" morphology (a pair of curved bacilli) following cell division. They are

microaerophilic and capnophilic, and their optimal growth temperature is 42°C. Reservoirs are animals, including poultry, cattle, sheep, swine, rodents, birds, kittens, puppies, and other pets. Most raw poultry is contaminated with *C. jejuni*, thus necessitating proper methods of cleaning and disinfecting in the kitchen. Transmission occurs via ingestion of contaminated food (e.g., chicken, pork), raw milk, or water; contact with infected pets or farm animals; or contaminated cutting boards.

Laboratory diagnosis. Diagnosis depends on the recovery of *Campylobacter* spp. from stool specimens, using selective medium (Campy blood agar, which contains several antimicrobial agents to suppress growth of other bacteria), a Campy gas mixture (5% O_2, 10% CO_2, 85% N_2), and 42°C incubation. Refer to Chapter 15 for additional information regarding identification of *Campylobacter* spp.

Enterovirulent *Escherichia coli*

As previously discussed, *Escherichia coli* is a Gram-negative bacillus found in the gastrointestinal tract of all humans. The strains and serotypes of *E. coli* that are part of the indigenous microflora of the gastrointestinal tract are opportunistic pathogens. They usually cause no harm while in the gastrointestinal tract but have the potential to cause serious infections if they gain access to the bloodstream, the urinary bladder, or a wound. *E. coli* is the major cause of septicemia, urinary tract infections, and nosocomial infections.

Some strains and serotypes of *E. coli*, however, are not indigenous microflora of the human colon and always cause disease when ingested. Collectively, these strains and serotypes are referred to as enterovirulent *E. coli*. Information pertaining to two general types of enterovirulent *E. coli*—enterohemorrhagic *E. coli* and enterotoxigenic *E. coli*—is provided here.

Enterohemorrhagic E. coli Diarrhea

Disease. Enterohemorrhagic *E. coli* (EHEC) diarrhea consists of a hemorrhagic, watery diarrhea with abdominal cramping. Usually, patients have no fever or only a slight fever. About 5% of infected people (especially children younger than age 5 and the elderly) develop hemolytic-uremic syndrome, with anemia, low platelet count, and kidney failure. The first recognized outbreak of diarrhea caused by enterohemorrhagic *E. coli* (O157:H7) occurred in 1982, involving contaminated hamburger meat—hamburger meat contaminated with cattle feces. Since then several well-publicized epidemics involving the same serotype have occurred. Not all of the outbreaks involved meat; some resulted from ingestion of unpasteurized milk or apple juice, lettuce, or other raw vegetables. It has been estimated that *E. coli* O157:H7 infection accounts for as many as 73,000 cases of illness and 60 deaths in the United States each year.

Pathogens. *E. coli* O157:H7 (a serotype that possesses a cell wall antigen designated O157 and a flagellar antigen designated H7) is the most commonly involved EHEC serotype. Other EHEC serotypes include O26:H11, O111:H8, and O104:H21. These are all Gram-negative bacilli that produce potent cytotoxins called Shiga-like toxins—named for their close resemblance to Shiga toxin, produced by *Shigella dysenteriae*. Reservoirs include cattle and infected humans. Transmission occurs via the fecal-oral route: inadequately cooked, fecally contaminated beef; unpasteurized milk; person-to-person contact; or fecally contaminated water.

Laboratory diagnosis. *E. coli* O157:H7 infection should be suspected in any patient with bloody diarrhea. Stool specimens should be inoculated onto sorbitol MacConkey agar. Colorless, sorbitol-negative colonies should then be assayed for O157 antigen using commercially available antiserum. Other immunodiagnostic procedures are available.

Enterotoxigenic E. coli Diarrhea

Disease. Enterotoxigenic *E. coli* (ETEC) diarrhea, also known as traveler's diarrhea, causes a profuse, watery diarrhea with or without mucus or blood; vomiting; and abdominal cramping. Dehydration and low-grade fever may occur. Enterotoxigenic strains of *E. coli* are the most common cause of traveler's diarrhea worldwide and a common cause of diarrheal disease in children from developing countries.

Pathogens. ETEC diarrhea is caused by many different serotypes of enterotoxigenic *E. coli* that produce either a heat-labile toxin, a heat-stable toxin, or both. Infected humans serve as reservoirs. Transmission occurs via the fecal-oral route: ingestion of fecally contaminated food or water.

Laboratory diagnosis. ETEC diarrhea is diagnosed by isolation of the organism from stool specimens, followed by demonstration of enterotoxin production, DNA probe techniques, or immunodiagnostic procedures. These procedures are usually not routinely performed in CMLs.

Salmonellosis

Diseases. Salmonellosis is a gastroenteritis caused by *Salmonella* spp. and characterized by sudden onset of headache, abdominal pain, diarrhea, nausea, and sometimes vomiting. Dehydration may be severe. Salmonellosis may develop into septicemia or localized infection in any tissue of the body.

Pathogens. Gastrointestinal salmonellosis is caused by members of the family Enterobacteriaceae currently named *Salmonella enterica* (of which there are more than 2,000 serotypes or serovars). These Gram-negative bacilli invade intestinal cells, release endotoxin, and produce cytotoxins and enterotoxins. About 200 of the *S. enterica* serotypes cause gastrointestinal salmonellosis in the United States.

The most commonly reported serotypes are *S. enterica* subsp. *enterica* serovar *typhimurium* (also known as *Salmonella typhimurium*) and *S. enterica* subsp. *enterica* serovar *enteritidis* (also known as *Salmonella enteritidis*). Reservoirs include a wide range of wild and domestic animals, such as poultry, swine, cattle, rodents, reptiles (e.g., pet iguanas and turtles), pet chicks, dogs, and cats. Infected humans (e.g., patients, carriers) are also reservoirs. Transmission occurs via ingestion of contaminated food (e.g., eggs, unpasteurized milk, meat, poultry, or raw fruits or vegetables); fecal-oral transmission from person to person; food handlers; or contaminated water supplies.

Laboratory diagnosis. Stool specimens should be submitted to the microbiology laboratory for culture and susceptibility testing. *Salmonella* spp. are non–lactose fermenters and thus produce colorless colonies on MAC. Biochemical tests are used for identification, and commercially available antisera are used for serotyping. Refer to Chapter 12 for additional information regarding identification of *Salmonella* spp.

Shigellosis

Disease. Shigellosis, also known as bacillary dysentery, is an acute bacterial infection of the lining of the small and large intestine, producing diarrhea (as many as 20 bowel movements a day) with blood, mucus, and pus. Other symptoms include nausea, vomiting, cramps, and fever. Sometimes toxemia (toxins in the blood) and convulsions occur in children. Other serious complications, such as hemolytic-uremic syndrome, may occur. Worldwide shigellosis is estimated to cause approximately 600,000 deaths per year, with about two-thirds of the cases and most of the deaths occurring among children younger than 10 years of age.

Pathogens. The etiologic agents of shigellosis are *Shigella dysenteriae*, *S. flexneri*, *S. boydii*, and *S. sonnei*. They are nonmotile Gram-negative bacilli that are members of the Enterobacteriaceae family. A plasmid is associated with toxin production and virulence. Relatively few (10 to 100) organisms are required to cause disease. Infected humans serve as reservoirs. People become infected by direct or indirect fecal-oral transmission from patients or carriers; fecally contaminated hands or fingernails; or fecally contaminated food, milk, or drinking water; flies can transfer organisms from latrines to food.

Laboratory diagnosis. Leukocytes will be present in stool specimens. Fresh fecal or rectal swab specimens should be immediately inoculated into Gram-negative enrichment broth and onto a solid medium (such as MacConkey, XLD, or Hektoen enteric agar). *Shigella* spp. produce colorless colonies on MAC because they are non–lactose fermenters. They are also non–xylose fermenters. Identification includes culture and biochemical and immunodiagnostic procedures. Refer to Chapter 12 for additional information regarding the identification of *Shigella* spp.

Cholera

Disease. Cholera is an acute bacterial diarrheal disease with profuse watery stools, occasional vomiting, and rapid dehydration. If untreated, circulatory collapse, renal failure, and death may occur. More than 50% of untreated people with severe cholera die. Cholera occurs worldwide, with periodic epidemics and pandemics. A recent Western Hemisphere cholera pandemic started in Peru in 1991; by 1994, more than 950,000 cases had been reported in 21 countries in the Western Hemisphere. Most U.S. cases involve the ingestion of raw or undercooked seafood (e.g., oysters) from the coastal waters of Louisiana or Texas.

Pathogens. The etiologic agents of cholera are certain biotypes of *Vibrio cholerae* serogroup 01. These are curved (comma-shaped) Gram-negative bacilli that secrete an enterotoxin (a toxin that adversely affects cells in the intestinal tract) called choleragen. Other *Vibrio* spp. (*V. parahaemolyticus, V. vulnificus*) also cause diarrheal diseases. Vibrios are halophilic (salt loving) and thus are found in marine environments. Reservoirs include infected humans and aquatic reservoirs (copepods and other zooplankton). Transmission occurs via the fecal-oral route: contact with feces or vomitus of infected people, ingestion of fecally contaminated water or foods (especially raw or undercooked shellfish and other seafood), or mechanical transmission by flies.

Laboratory diagnosis. Rectal swabs or stool specimens should be inoculated onto TCBS agar; different *Vibrio* spp. produce different reactions on this medium. Biochemical tests are used to identify the various species. Biotyping is accomplished using commercially available antisera. Refer to Chapter 15 for additional information regarding the identification of *Vibrio* spp.

> Associate TCBS medium with *Vibrio* spp.

Clostridium difficile–Associated Diseases

Diseases and most likely pathogen. *Clostridium difficile* (often referred to simply as C. dif) is a spore-forming anaerobic Gram-positive bacillus. It is a member of the indigenous colonic microflora in about 2% to 3% of healthy, nonhospitalized adults. Hospitalized patients frequently become colonized with *C. difficile* as a result of the presence of the organism in the hospital environment. It is estimated that about 20% to 30% of hospitalized patients are colonized with *C. difficile*.

C. difficile is the major cause of conditions known as antibiotic-associated diarrhea (AAD) and pseudomembranous colitis (PMC), which frequently occur in patients following antibiotic therapy. *C. difficile* is the most common cause of hospital-acquired diarrhea and virtually always the cause of PMC. It does not seem to matter for what condition the patient was receiving antibiotics, which antibiotics the patient was receiving, the dosage, or the route of administration.

Antibiotics that have a profound effect on colonic flora, such as cephalosporins, ampicillin, amoxicillin, and clindamycin, are the drugs most frequently implicated.

The following scenario illustrates how antibiotic therapy can lead to AAD and PMC:

Step 1: Relatively small numbers of *C. difficile* are present in the indigenous microflora of a hospitalized patient's colon prior to the initiation of antibiotic therapy. *C. difficile* produces two toxins: an enterotoxin called toxin A and a cytotoxin called toxin B. Some strains produce only toxin B. When relatively few *C. difficile* cells are present in the colon, the concentration of these toxins is not high enough to cause disease.

Step 2: When the patient receives antibiotics, colonic bacteria susceptible to those antibiotics are killed. The strain of *C. difficile* colonizing the patient's colon is resistant to those antibiotics. (In other cases, *C. difficile* spores from the hospital environment enter the patient's intestinal tract when the level of antibiotic drops below an inhibitory concentration.)

Step 3: A superinfection of *C. difficile* occurs as a result of the decreased competition in the colon for space and nutrients. Recall from Chapter 7 that a superinfection is an overgrowth or population explosion of an organism that is usually present at a particular anatomical site in a much lower number.

Step 4: As a result of the superinfection of *C. difficile*, sufficient quantities of toxins A and B are present to cause disease. Toxin A is thought to be the cause of AAD and toxin B the cause of PMC.

In PMC, multiple elevated, yellowish white, 5- to 10-mm-diameter plaques develop on the mucosal lining of the colon. With time, the lesions coalesce, large sections of the mucous lining slough off, and a pseudomembrane develops. The pseudomembrane is composed of inflammatory cells and sloughed mucosal epithelial cells. Sloughing of the epithelial cells causes bleeding.

Clinical specimens. A single freshly passed diarrheal specimen is the preferred specimen for both *C. difficile* culture and toxin assay. Rectal swabs can be used for culture, but usually the amount of fecal material is not sufficient for use in toxin assays.

Specimen preservation. Specimens should be transported in tightly sealed, leakproof containers without transport medium and, ideally, should be processed within 2 hours of collection. Specimens for culture can be refrigerated for up to 2 days or frozen. Specimens for toxin assay may be refrigerated for up to 3 days or frozen at −70°C (*not* at −20°C) for longer periods.

Contaminants. The indigenous microflora of the healthy human colon contains more than 200 species of bacteria, most (approximately 98%) of which are anaerobes. This includes some *Clostridium* spp. Even *C. difficile* can be isolated from fecal specimens of healthy persons.

Screening tests. Endoscopy can help to detect anatomic changes in the colon, but the procedure is unpleasant and expensive. Fecal leukocyte and lactoferrin tests are often positive in patients with *C. difficile*–associated diseases. A tissue culture assay can be used to detect *C. difficile* cytopathic toxin B, but test results are not available for 3 or 4 days, and many CMLs do not perform the test. Several immunoassays to detect toxin A or toxins A and B, varying widely in sensitivity and specificity, are commercially available. Immunoassay results are available much sooner than with the tissue culture assay. Molecular diagnostic procedures are being developed.

Media for aerobic incubation. *C. difficile* is an anaerobe.

Media for anaerobic incubation. Culture is usually not necessary for diagnosis of *C. difficile*–associated diseases. If culture is desired, fecal or rectal swab specimens must be inoculated to a selective medium, such as CCFA, which is incubated anaerobically at 35°C to 37°C for 24 to 48 hours. The presence of *C. difficile* in fecal or rectal swab specimens does not necessarily mean that the organism is causing disease. *C. perfringens* has been reported to be a much less common cause of AAD than *C. difficile*.

Laboratory diagnosis. *C. difficile* will produce large, yellowish-to-white, circular-to-irregular, flat, ground-glass colonies on CCFA and will have a horse stable–like odor. The originally pink-colored agar turns yellow in the vicinity of the colonies. *C. difficile* colonies on CCFA may fluoresce chartreuse under ultraviolet light. Gram staining of the organisms reveals thin, even-sided Gram-positive to Gram-variable bacilli that are 0.5 μm wide by 3 to 5 μm long. Subterminal spores may be seen. See Chapter 17 for additional information regarding identification of *C. difficile*. A recap of bacterial diseases discussed in this chapter can be found on the CD-ROM.

Chapter Review

- Blood is normally sterile. The presence of bacteria in the bloodstream may represent a transient bacteremia, bacteremia secondary to infection at a primary site, or an infection of the bloodstream known as septicemia.

- Bacterial infections of the skin include those with multiple etiologies, such as wounds, abscesses, and ulcers, and those with specific etiologies, such as erysipelas.

- Bacterial infections of the subcutaneous tissues include leprosy, gas gangrene, and necrotizing fasciitis.

- The most common type of bacterial eye infection is conjunctivitis, which may be caused by *Haemophilus influenzae* subsp. *aegyptius*, *Streptococcus pneumoniae*, *Staphylococcus aureus*, *Neisseria meningitidis*, or *Chlamydia trachomatis*.

- Bacterial infections of the ear include otitis externa and otitis media.

- Bacterial infections of the upper respiratory tract include group A strep pharyngitis (strep throat), epiglottitis, diphtheria, and sinusitis.

- Lower respiratory bacterial infections include empyema, bronchitis, pneumonia, tracheitis, tuberculosis, and lung abscess.

- Bacterial meningitis is a serious infection of the central nervous system that may be acute or chronic.

- The major causes of neonatal meningitis are *Streptococcus agalactiae* (group B strep), *Escherichia coli* and other members of the family Enterobacteriaceae, and *Listeria monocytogenes*.

- The major causes of meningitis in adolescents and adults are *Neisseria meningitidis*, *Streptococcus pneumoniae*, and *Haemophilus influenzae*.

- Bacterial infections of the urinary tract include cystitis, pyelonephritis, and ureteritis. UTIs may be nosocomial or community-acquired infections.

- Sexually transmitted bacterial infections of the genital tract include chlamydial genital infections, gonorrhea, syphilis, chancroid, and granuloma inguinale.

- The three main causes of vaginal infection are the yeast *Candida albicans*, the protozoan *Trichomonas vaginalis*, and a mixture of bacteria. When the infection is caused by a mixture of bacteria, the condition is known as bacterial vaginosis.

- Bacterial infections of the oral cavity include periodontal diseases like gingivitis and periodontitis. These diseases are usually polymicrobial, with anaerobes being the primary etiologic agents.

- Gastrointestinal tract bacterial infections include gastritis and gastric ulcers, diarrheal diseases, and *Clostridium difficile*–associated diseases.

New Terms and Abbreviations

After studying Chapter 18, you should be familiar with the following terms, which are defined within the chapter and in the Glossary at the back of the book:

Fasciae (sing. fascia)

Fasciitis

Gangrene

Gas gangrene

Ischemia

Reaginic antibody

Serovars

References and Suggested Reading

Amsel R, et al. Nonspecific vaginitis. Am J Med 1983;74:14–22.

Bartlett RC. A plea for clinical relevance in microbiology. Am J Clin Pathol 1974;61:867–872.

Baum J, Barza M. Infections of the eye. In: Gorbach SL, Bartlett JG, Blacklow NR, eds. Infectious Disease. 3rd Ed. Philadelphia: Lippincott Williams & Wilkins, 2004.

Bouckenooghe AP, DuPont HL. Approach to the patient with diarrhea. In: Gorbach SL, Bartlett JG, Blacklow NR, eds. Infectious Disease. 3rd Ed. Philadelphia: Lippincott Williams & Wilkins, 2004.

Ghanem KG, et al. Gonorrhea. In: Gorbach SL, Bartlett JG, Blacklow NR, eds. Infectious Disease. 3rd Ed. Philadelphia: Lippincott Williams & Wilkins, 2004.

Gorbach SL. Gas gangrene and other clostridial skin and soft tissue infections. In: Gorbach SL, Bartlett JG, Blacklow NR, eds. Infectious Disease. 3rd Ed. Philadelphia: Lippincott Williams & Wilkins, 2004.

Granato PA. Pathogenic and indigenous microorganisms of humans. In: Murray PR, Baron EJ, Jorgensen JH, Pfaller MA, Yolken RH, eds. Manual of Clinical Microbiology. 8th Ed. Washington, DC: ASM Press, 2003.

Heymann DL, ed. Control of Communicable Diseases Manual. 18th Ed. Washington, DC: American Public Health Association, 2004.

Isenberg HD. Collection, transport, and manipulation of clinical specimens and initial laboratory concerns. In: Isenberg HD, ed. Essential Procedures for Clinical Microbiology. Washington, DC: ASM Press, 1998.

Jousimies-Somer HR, Summanen P, Baron EJ, Citron DM, Wexler HM, Finegold SM. Wadsworth-KTL Anaerobic Bacteriology Manual. 6th Ed. Belmont, CA: Star, 2002.

Loesche WJ. Dental infections. In: Gorbach SL, Bartlett JG, Blacklow NR, eds. Infectious Disease. 3rd Ed. Philadelphia: Lippincott Williams & Wilkins, 2004.

Miller JM. A Guide to Specimen Management in Clinical Microbiology. 2nd Ed. Washington, DC: ASM Press, 1999.

Musher DM, Baughn BE. Syphilis. In: Gorbach SL, Bartlett JG, Blacklow NR, eds. Infectious Disease. 3rd Ed. Philadelphia: Lippincott Williams & Wilkins, 2004.

Nugent RP, et al. Reliability of diagnosing bacterial vaginosis is improved by a standardized method of Gram stain interpretation. J Clin Microbiol 1991;29:297–301.

Performance Standards for Antimicrobial Disk Susceptibility Testing: 17th Informational Supplement. CLSI Document M100-17. Wayne, PA: Clinical and Laboratory Standards Institute, 2007.

Ronald A, Alfa MJ. Chancroid, lymphogranuloma venereum, and granuloma inguinale. In: Gorbach SL, Bartlett JG, Blacklow NR, eds. Infectious Disease. 3rd Ed. Philadelphia: Lippincott Williams & Wilkins, 2004.

Schachter J. Chlamydial infections of the genital tract. In: Gorbach SL, Bartlett JG, Blacklow NR, eds. Infectious Disease. 3rd Ed. Philadelphia: Lippincott Williams & Wilkins, 2004.

Thomson RB, Miller JM. Specimen collection, transport, and processing: Bacteriology. In: Murray PR, Baron EJ, Jorgensen JH, Pfaller MA, Yolken RH, eds. Manual of Clinical Microbiology. 8th Ed. Washington, DC: ASM Press, 2003.

 On the CD-ROM

- Critical Values/Panic Values in Clinical Microbiology
- Recap of Bacterial Diseases Discussed in Chapter 18
- Additional Self-Assessment Exercises
- Case Studies
- Puzzle

Self-Assessment Exercises

For questions 1–4, match the bacterial infection/disease in the left column with its associated body site.

1. _____ Gonorrhea   A. Gastrointestinal tract

2. _____ Gas gangrene   B. Urinary tract

3. _____ Cystitis   C. Genital tract

4. _____ Antibiotic-associated diarrhea   D. Subcutaneous tissues

5. List three common bacterial causes of septicemia:

   A. _____

   B. _____

   C. _____

6. "Clue" cells are one of the criteria used to diagnose

   A. gonorrhea.

   B. bacterial vaginosis.

   C. tuberculosis.

   D. antibiotic-associated diarrhea.

7. True or false: All clinical presentations of gonorrhea involve the genital tract.

8. To determine whether a patient has a urinary tract infection, appropriate media were inoculated using a 0.01-mL calibrated loop. After incubation, the CML professional counted 150 CFUs. What is the number of CFUs/mL?

   A. 150 CFUs/mL

   B. 1,500 CFUs/mL

   C. 15,000 CFUs/mL

   D. 150,000 CFUs/mL

9. For each of the following suspected bacterial infections, list at least one medium used to isolate the suspected pathogen.

   A. Gonorrhea   _____

   B. Tuberculosis   _____

   C. Antibiotic-associated diarrhea   _____

10. True or false: Good-quality sputum specimens should contain PMNs in greater quantities per microscopic field than squamous epithelial cells.

CHAPTER 19

Introduction to Medical Mycology

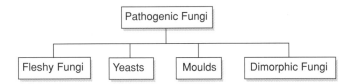

Chapter Outline

Fungal Reproduction

Classification of Fungi

General Mycology Laboratory Methods
- Specimen Processing
- Inoculation of Media

Fleshy Fungi and the Diseases They Cause

Yeasts
- Description
- Human Diseases Caused by Yeasts
- Identifying Yeasts

Moulds
- Description
- Human Diseases Caused by Moulds
- Identifying Moulds

Dimorphic Fungi
- Description
- Human Diseases Caused by Dimorphic Fungi
- Identifying Dimorphic Fungi

Immunodiagnostic Procedures

Molecular Diagnostic Procedures

Antimicrobial Susceptibility Testing of Fungi

LEARNING OBJECTIVES

After studying this chapter, you should be able to:

☞ Define the terms introduced in this chapter (e.g., *aerial hyphae, aseptate hyphae, blastoconidia*)

☞ Identify where fungi are classified in the five-kingdom and three-domain systems of classification and the term used to describe the study of fungi

☞ Name three ways fungi can reproduce

☞ Differentiate between sexual spores and asexual spores, and give examples of each

☞ Name the four categories of fungi that cause human diseases

☞ Identify three types of specimens that are processed more frequently in the mycology section of the clinical microbiology laboratory than in the bacteriology section

☞ Describe the use of each of the following in the processing of mycology specimens: KOH prep, calcofluor white, Gram stain, and India ink prep; describe the purpose and basic procedure for each

☞ Identify the types of media used in the mycology section and the requirements for incubation of fungal cultures

☞ Describe the general characteristics of yeasts to include morphology and methods of reproduction

☞ Name three yeasts of medical importance

☞ **Name five criteria by which yeasts can be identified**

☞ **Relate how yeast can be differentiated from bacteria on a Gram-stained smear**

☞ **Describe the germ tube test for the identification of yeasts; include a description of germ tubes, the purpose of the procedure, and the general procedure**

☞ **Differentiate between a yeast and a mould with regard to colonial growth and appearance**

☞ **Given a cross-section diagram of a mould colony, identify its structures**

☞ **Given a particular mould, correctly describe its texture and topography, using the terminology presented in the chapter**

☞ **Name the microscopic clues used to assist in the identification of a mould**

☞ **Name three examples of human diseases caused by dimorphic fungi**

☞ **List two other types of laboratory methodologies, besides culture, that can be used to diagnose fungal infections**

In the five-kingdom system of classification, fungi (sing. *fungus*) are in a kingdom by themselves, appropriately called the Kingdom Fungi. In the three-domain system of classification, fungi are included in the Domain *Eucarya*, along with all other eucaryotic organisms. The study of fungi is called mycology, and a person who studies fungi is called a mycologist. **Medical mycology** is the study and use of methods for the diagnosis of human fungal infections.

The overall responsibility of the mycology section of the clinical microbiology laboratory (CML) is to assist clinicians in the diagnosis of fungal infections, also known as **mycoses.** In the mycology section, various types of clinical specimens are processed, fungal pathogens are isolated, and tests are performed to identify the fungal pathogens. Although susceptibility testing of fungi is not currently performed in most CMLs, it is likely that such testing will become routine in the near future.

> Fungi are eucaryotic organisms. The study of fungi is called mycology.

> Fungal infections are called mycoses (sing. *mycosis*).

FUNGAL REPRODUCTION

Depending on the particular species, fungi can reproduce by budding, hyphal extension, or the formation of spores. Fungal spores are very resistant structures that can be carried great distances by air currents. They are resistant to heat, cold, acids, bases, and other chemicals. Many people are allergic to fungal spores. The two general categories of fungal spores are sexual spores and asexual spores.

> One way fungi reproduce is by producing spores. The two general types of spores are sexual spores and asexual spores.

Sexual spores. Sexual spores are produced as a result of the fusion of two gametes—thus, the fusion of two nuclei. Fungi are classified primarily by the types of sexual spores they produce or the types of structures on which or within which spores are produced. Examples of sexual spores are zygospores, ascospores, oospores, and basidiospores; the names are based on the manner in which the spores are produced. Zygospores are produced by the fusion of morphologically identical cells, whereas oospores are produced by the fusion of two morphologically different cells. Ascospores are produced within baglike structures called asci (sing. *ascus*), which are contained within a larger structure called a cleistothecium.

> Sexual fungal spores are produced as a result of the fusion of gametes—thus, the fusion of nuclei. Fungi are classified primarily by the types of sexual spores they produce or the types of structures on which or within which spores are produced.

Asexual spores. Asexual spores are *not* produced by the fusion of gametes. They are produced in two general ways (Fig. 19-1). If produced within a saclike structure, known as

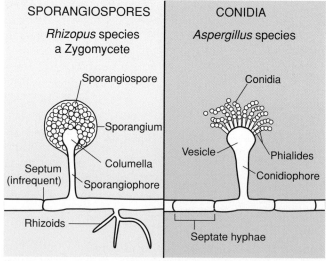

Figure 19-1. Asexual reproduction in *Rhizopus* and *Aspergillus* spp., illustrating the structures within and on which asexual spores are produced. (From Winn WC Jr, et al. Koneman's Color Atlas and Textbook of Diagnostic Microbiology. 6th Ed. Philadelphia: Lippincott Williams & Wilkins, 2006.)

a sporangium, they are called **sporangiospores.** When they are not produced within a sporangium, they are referred to as **conidia (sing.** *conidium*). Blastoconidia, chlamydoconidia, and arthroconidia

> Asexual fungal spores are known as conidia. Blastoconidia, chlamydoconidia, and arthroconidia are examples of conidia.

are examples of conidia. Blastoconidia are yeast cells, produced by budding. Chlamydoconidia, also known as chlamydospores, are thickened and enlarged conidia found within, on the side of, or at the tip of hyphae. Arthroconidia are thickened and enlarged conidia that form within hyphae and are released by the lysis of adjacent hyphal cells.

Some species of fungi produce *both* asexual and sexual spores. Fungi that have both a sexual form and an asexual form are known as **perfect fungi.** The sexual form is referred to either as the perfect state or the teleomorph. The asexual stage is known as the imperfect state or the anamorph. Frequently, the two forms have different names, which can be confusing. For example, *Ajellomyces dermatitidis* is the sexual form of *Blastomyces dermatitidis*. This particular fungus grows at 37°C as a yeast, the imperfect stage, and at 25°C as a mould, the perfect state. To further compound matters, the anamorph and teleomorph stages of perfect fungi are often taxonomically classified in different subdivisions.

CLASSIFICATION OF FUNGI

Sometimes fungi are incorrectly referred to as plants. They are *not* plants. One way in which fungi differ from plants

> One way fungi differ from plants and algae is that they are not photosynthetic. Fungi possess neither chlorophyll nor other photosynthetic pigments.

and algae is that they are not photosynthetic; fungi possess neither chlorophyll nor other photosynthetic pigments. The cell walls of algal and plant cells contain cellulose (a polysaccharide), but cellulose is not found in the cell walls of medically important

> Fungal cell walls contain chitin, a polysaccharide not found in the cell walls of any other microorganisms.

fungi. Fungal cell walls contain chitin, a polysaccharide not found in the cell walls of any other microorganisms. Chitin is also found in the exoskeletons of arthropods.

The classification of fungi changes periodically, and different taxonomists classify fungi in different ways. According to Beneke and Rogers (see "References and Suggested Reading"), medically important fungi are contained within five phyla, referred to as subdivisions by some fungal taxonomists (Table 19-1).

For discussion purposes, the fungi that cause human diseases have been divided into four categories:

1. Fleshy fungi
2. Yeasts
3. Moulds
4. Dimorphic fungi

As discussed in Chapter 20, mycoses can be categorized in accordance with the part(s) of the body afflicted. The four categories are (1) superficial mycoses, (2) cutaneous mycoses, (3) subcutaneous mycoses, and (4) systemic or generalized mycoses.

GENERAL MYCOLOGY LABORATORY METHODS

Specimen Processing

Types of specimens. The types of clinical specimens processed in the mycology section are essentially the same types processed in the bacteriology section, including blood, cerebrospinal fluid (CSF), urine, and tissue specimens. However, three types of

> Nail clippings, hair clippings, and skin scrapings are more frequently submitted to the mycology section of the CML than to the bacteriology section.

specimens are more frequently processed in the mycology section of the CML than in the bacteriology section: nail clippings, hair clippings, and skin scrapings. Additional information regarding mycology specimens is presented in Chapter 20.

Potassium hydroxide preparation (KOH prep). Specimens such as skin scrapings and nail and hair clippings are usually examined using the KOH prep. The potassium hydroxide serves as a clearing agent, dissolving keratin in the specimen, making it easier to observe any fungal elements (e.g., hyphae and yeast cells) that might be present. Hair clippings, nail clippings, and skin scrapings all contain keratin. The specimen is placed in 1 or 2 drops of

> Keratin is dissolved during the KOH prep, making it easier to observe any fungal elements that may be present in the specimen. The potassium hydroxide is considered a clearing agent.

10% KOH on a microscope slide, a coverslip is added, and the preparation is gently heated by either using a slide warmer or passing the slide several times through a Bunsen burner flame. The preparation is then examined microscopically.

Calcofluor white/KOH prep. Clinical specimens can be examined using a fluorescent brightener called calcofluor

TABLE 19 - 1   Phyla Containing Medically Important Fungi

Phylum or Subdivision	Type of Hyphae[a]	Asexual Reproduction	Sexual Reproduction	Medical Importance
Zygomycota (or Zygomycotina), comprises lower fungi: common bread moulds and other fungi that cause food spoilage	Aseptate	By means of sporangia-containing spores (sporangiospores), sporangioles, or conidia	Results in the formation of thick-walled, spherical spores (called zygospores)	Bread moulds such as *Rhizopus, Mucor,* and *Absidia* spp. can cause disease which is called zygomycosis (older terms are *mucormycosis* and *phycomycosis*)
Ascomycota (or Ascomycotina) comprises some higher fungi: most pathogenic fungi with a known perfect state, such as certain yeasts and some fungi that cause plant diseases (e.g., Dutch elm disease)	Septate	By means of budding cells, cell division, arthroconidia, chlamydoconidia, and conidiophores bearing conidia	Results in the formation of an ascus, which usually contains 8 ascospores	Cause of mycetomas
Basidiomycota (or Basidiomycotina) comprises some higher fungi, including some yeasts, some fungi that cause plant diseases, and the large fleshy fungi that live in the woods (e.g., mushrooms, toadstools, puffballs)	Septate	Unknown	Results in the formation of a club-shaped basidium, which usually bears 4 basidiospores on its surface	Some fleshy fungi (e.g., *Amanita* spp.) produce mycotoxins that, when ingested, can cause human disease
Deuteromycota (or Deuteromycotina; also known as Fungi Imperfecti) comprises some higher fungi, including fungi having no mode of sexual reproduction or whose mode of sexual reproduction is not known	Yeasts or septate hyphae, if filamentous	Conidia are produced either by budding or fragmentation of hyphae	None	Yeasts such as *Candida, Cryptococcus, Trichosporon, Malassezia*; moulds such as *Epidermophyton, Coccidioides, Sporothrix, Aspergillus, Alternaria, Penicillium*

[a]Septate hyphae contain cross walls or septa; the cytoplasm within these hyphae is partitioned into cells. Aseptate hyphae do not contain septa; the cytoplasm within these hyphae is multinucleated and is not partitioned into cells.

> Fungal elements fluoresce when examined using a calcofluor white/KOH prep.

white, mixed with KOH. The calcofluor white binds to chitin in fungal cell walls, and the KOH serves as a clearing agent, making it easier to observe any fungi that are present. A portion of the specimen is added to a drop containing both calcofluor white and 10% KOH, and then a glass coverslip is added. After 5 minutes, the preparation is examined using a fluorescent microscope equipped with the appropriate exciter and barrier filters. Fungal elements fluoresce either a blue-white or apple green, depending on the filter setup.

Unless they are overdecolorized, most fungal elements (e.g., yeast cells and hyphae) stain blue with the Gram staining procedure. The terms *Gram positive* and *Gram negative* are reserved for bacteria.

Gram stain. Specimens may also be examined microscopically following Gram staining. Unless they are overdecolorized, most fungal elements (e.g., yeast cells and hyphae) stain blue with the Gram staining procedure.

India ink prep. An India ink prep is of value in the presumptive diagnosis of cryptococcal meningitis and is usually performed on CSF specimens. However, an India ink prep is sometimes performed on sputum, blood, or urine. A drop of the specimen is placed on a microscope slide and mixed with a drop of India ink. Then a coverslip is added, and the preparation is examined microscopically. The presence of budding, encapsulated yeasts (Fig. 19-2) is interpreted as a presumptive or tentative diagnosis of cryptococcosis (cryptococcal meningitis if the specimen was CSF). Culture and identification by biochemical tests are necessary for definitive diagnosis, because other yeasts (e.g., *Rhodotorula* spp. and other *Cryptococcus* spp.) may also produce capsules.

The India ink prep is of value for a rapid, presumptive diagnosis of cryptococcosis, which is caused by the encapsulated yeast *Cryptococcus neoformans*.

Inoculation of Media

The most common type of plated medium used in the mycology section is Sabouraud dextrose agar. With its low pH

(5.6), this medium is selective for fungi. At such a low pH, bacteria likely to be found in clinical specimens do not grow but most fungi grow well. Other types of plated media used in the mycology section include brain-heart infusion agar with or without added blood and/or antibiotics, Sabhi agar with or without added antibiotics, potato dextrose and potato flakes agars with or without added antibiotics, and dermatophyte test medium, Mycosel agar, and mycobiotic agar for isolation of dermatophytes.[1]

Associate Sabouraud dextrose agar with the mycology section.

The antibacterial agents most commonly added to mycology media are chloramphenicol and gentamicin, although penicillin and streptomycin are also used. Cycloheximide, a drug that inhibits nonpathogenic fungi, is sometimes added to mycology media. Sheep blood agar plates or slants are often used for isolation of yeasts and the yeast phase of dimorphic fungi (discussed later). Primary plates for isolation of fungi are usually incubated at 25°C to 30°C (preferably at 30°C). Because fungi have longer generation times than bacteria, cultures must be kept for longer periods, generally 3 to 4 weeks, and measures must be taken to prevent cultures from drying.

It is important to remember that most fungi that cause human infections are present in the environment and thus may represent contaminants when isolated. Because of the potential for contamination of specimens or culture media with fungal spores from the environment, the ideal way to confirm a fungal infection is to observe fungal elements in the affected tissue(s).

The ideal way to confirm a fungal infection is to observe fungal elements in the affected tissue(s).

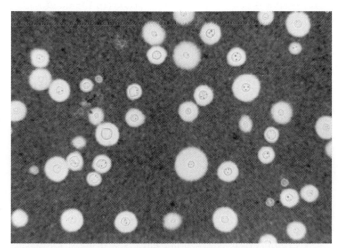

Figure 19-2. Photomicrograph of encapsulated *Cryptococcus neoformans* cells in an India ink preparation. (From Winn WC Jr, et al. Koneman's Color Atlas and Textbook of Diagnostic Microbiology. 6th Ed. Philadelphia: Lippincott Williams & Wilkins, 2006.)

FLESHY FUNGI AND THE DISEASES THEY CAUSE

The large fungi encountered in forests, such as mushrooms, toadstools, puffballs, and bracket fungi, are collectively referred to as **fleshy fungi.** Obviously, they are not microorganisms. Some are large enough to trip over. A mushroom consists of a fruiting body (the part of the organism that sticks up from the ground) and an extensive series of long, thin, intertwined, cytoplasmic filaments called **hyphae (sing. hypha).** Many mushrooms are edible, but others, including some that resemble edible fungi, are

The word *mycology* is derived from the Greek word *mykes*, meaning "mushroom." Usually, the prefix *myco-* pertains to fungi. There are exceptions, however, including mycobacteria and mycoplasmas.

---

[1] The term dermatophytes *refers to a group of moulds that cause infections of tissues containing keratin, such as skin, hair, and nails. Examples of dermatophytes include* Epidermophyton, Microsporum, *and* Trichophyton *spp.*

extremely toxic and may cause permanent liver and/or brain damage or death if ingested. The toxins that fungi produce are referred to as **mycotoxins,** and the microbial intoxications that they cause are called **mycotoxicoses (sing. *mycotoxicosis*).** Refer to the Appendix 1 section of the CD-ROM for additional information about mycotoxicoses. Because the CML does not play a role in the diagnosis of diseases caused by fleshy fungi, this group of fungi will not be discussed further in the chapter.

YEASTS

Description

Yeasts are microscopic, eucaryotic, single-celled (unicellular) organisms that lack hyphae. Individual yeast cells, sometimes referred to as **blastospores** or **blastoconidia,** can only be observed using a microscope. Most yeasts are oval or round, but some are elongate or irregular in shape. Although yeasts usually reproduce by budding (Fig. 19-3), they occasionally do so by hyphal extension or by a type of spore formation. Budding is a process whereby a yeast cell (referred to as a mother cell) pinches off a part of itself to produce what is referred to as a daughter cell.

> The primary way in which yeasts reproduce is by budding. A string of elongated, connected buds is called a pseudohypha (pl. *pseudohyphae*). A pseudohypha resembles a hypha in appearance but is *not* a hypha.

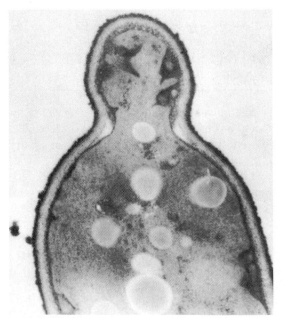

***Figure 19-3.* Longitudinal section of a budding yeast cell.** (From Lechavalier HA, Pramer D. The Microbes. Philadelphia: Lippincott, 1970.)

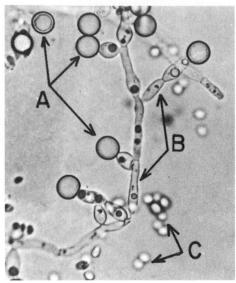

***Figure 19-4.* Culture of *Candida albicans*. A.** Chlamydospores. **B.** Pseudohyphae. **C.** Budding yeast cells or blastospores. (From Davis BD, et al. Microbiology. 4th Ed. Philadelphia: Harper & Row, 1987.)

Sometimes a string of elongated, connected buds is formed; this string of buds is called a **pseudohypha (pl. *pseudohyphae*).** A pseudohypha resembles a hypha in appearance, but it is *not* a hypha (Fig. 19-4). Some yeasts produce thick-walled, sporelike structures called chlamydospores (or chlamydoconidia).

Human Diseases Caused by Yeasts

Most pathogenic yeasts are classified as Deuteromycota, or Fungi Imperfecti. Yeasts such as *Candida albicans* and *Cryptococcus neoformans* are common human pathogens. *Candida albicans* is an opportunistic yeast that lives harmlessly on the skin and mucous membranes of the mouth, gastrointestinal tract, and genitourinary tract. However, when conditions cause a reduction in the number of indigenous bacteria at these anatomical locations, *C. albicans* flourishes, leading to yeast infections of the mouth (**thrush**), skin, and vagina (yeast vaginitis). This type of local infection may become a focal site from which the organisms invade the bloodstream to become a generalized or systemic infection in many internal areas (referred to as candidiasis). *C. albicans* is the yeast and fungus most frequently isolated from human clinical specimens. Other *Candida* spp. also cause human disease.

> *Candida albicans* is the yeast and fungus most frequently isolated from human clinical specimens.

Cryptococcus neoformans causes a disease known as cryptococcosis, which may be a respiratory infection or an infection of the central nervous system. Other *Cryptococcus* spp. are very rare causes of human disease. Some of the other yeasts of medical importance are listed in Table 19-2.

TABLE 19 - 2	Yeasts of Medical Importance
Genus	**Diseases**
Blastoschizomyces	Onychomycosis (nail infection), endocarditis
Candida	Oral and esophageal candidiasis, vaginitis, cystitis, endocarditis, meningitis, multifocal disseminated disease
Cryptococcus	Pulmonary infection, meningitis, disseminated infection involving skin, bones, and joints
Hansenula	Catheter-related infections
Malassezia	Dermatological diseases, rare systemic infections
Rhodotorula	Septicemia, meningitis, systemic infections, peritonitis, catheter-related infections
Saccharomyces	Rare cause of oral infection, vaginitis, empyema
Trichosporon	Hair infection (white piedra), skin lesions, disseminated infection

Prothecosis is a rare human infection that is caused by an alga—a *Prototheca* sp. Although not a yeast, this alga is sometimes mistaken for one. It grows on fungal media and can be identified using yeast identification methods. Additional information about *Prototheca* can be found in Chapter 20.

Identifying Yeasts

Direct examination of a specimen by KOH prep, calcofluor white, Gram stain, or India ink not only can alert CML professionals to the presence of yeast cells in the specimen but also can provide initial clues to their identity, such as these:

- Size and shape of the yeast cells
- Method of attachment of buds
- Presence of a capsule
- Thickness of the cell wall
- Presence of pseudohyphae or hyphae

Most yeasts grow well on commonly used mycological and bacteriological media, producing colonies by 24 to 72 hours. On plated media, yeasts produce colonies that look much like bacterial colonies (Fig. 19-5). In fact, it is sometimes impossible to distinguish a yeast colony from a bacterial colony merely by macroscopic observation. The quickest way to differentiate between yeast and bacterial colonies is a wet mount. A small portion of the colony is transferred to a drop of water or saline on a microscope slide, a coverslip is added, and the preparation is examined microscopically. Yeasts can be distinguished from bacteria by their size and shape. Usually oval shaped and larger than bacteria, ranging from 2 to 60 µm in diameter, yeast cells are often observed in the process of budding. Bacteria do not produce buds.

Yeast and bacterial colonies can also be differentiated by

> A wet mount can be used to distinguish between yeasts and bacteria. Yeast cells are usually oval shaped and larger than bacteria, ranging from 2 to 60 µm in diameter. Often yeast cells are observed in the process of budding; bacteria do not produce buds.

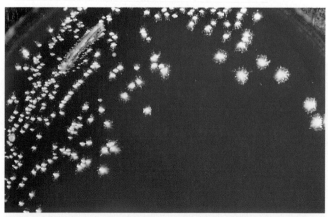

***Figure 19-5.* Colonies of the yeast *Candida albicans* on a blood agar plate.** The footlike extensions from the margins of the colonies are typical of this species. (From Winn WC Jr, et al. Koneman's Color Atlas and Textbook of Diagnostic Microbiology. 6th Ed. Philadelphia: Lippincott Williams & Wilkins, 2006.)

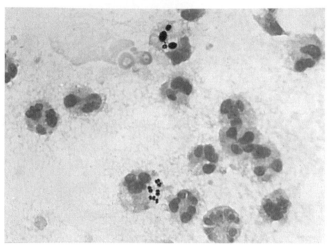

Figure 19-6. **Gram-stained wound aspirate, illustrating the size differences among yeasts, bacteria, and white blood cells.** Included in this photomicrograph are numerous white blood cells (red objects), two blue-stained budding yeast cells (top), and several Gram-positive cocci (small blue spheres at the bottom). (From Marler LM, Siders JA, Allen SD. Direct Smear Atlas. Philadelphia: Lippincott Williams & Wilkins, 2001.)

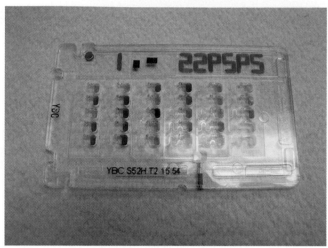

Figure 19-7. **Vitek YBC Card, a commercial system for the identification of yeasts, manufactured by bioMerieux Inc.** (Courtesy of Dr. Robert C. Fader.)

examining a Gram-stained smear of the colony, but the Gram staining procedure takes longer to perform than a wet mount. Remember that yeasts (like all fungi) stain dark blue to purple in the Gram staining procedure (Fig. 19-6).

Yeast colonies are usually moist, smooth, and creamy, but they can be glabrous, membranous, or mucoid. In terms of color, yeast colonies may be hyaline (colorless, transparent), white to cream, brightly colored, or darkly pigmented.

A wet mount of a yeast colony can provide the same information as might have been obtained in the direct examination of the specimen (previously listed). An India ink prep can be performed to determine if the yeast is encapsulated. A Gram stain of the colony can ensure that the colony is pure (i.e., not a mixture of bacteria and yeasts).

Although cellular and colonial morphology provide some clues to the identification of yeasts, they are primarily identified using a series of biochemical tests—carbohydrate assimilations and fermentations—usually, by inoculating a commercial minisystem designed for yeast identification. Various minisystems for yeast identification are commercially available (Table 19-3); one is illustrated in Figure 19-7.

> Yeasts are primarily identified using a series of biochemical tests—carbohydrate assimilations and fermentations—usually, by inoculating a commercial yeast identification minisystem.

Germ tube test. Another test of value in yeast identification is the germ tube test. Germ tubes are filamentous hyphal outgrowths from blastoconidia (Fig. 19-8). Twenty-four- to 48-hour-old colonies from Sabouraud dextrose agar or blood agar are inoculated into a test substrate such as fetal bovine serum, and the suspension is incubated at 37°C for 3 hours. The preparation is then examined microscopically for the presence of germ tubes. It is the high protein content of serum that induces germ tube formation. Clinical and Laboratory Standards Institute (CLSI) Document M35-A (see "References and Suggested Reading") states that a properly interpreted, positive germ tube test can be used to identify *C. albicans* if the germ tubes are produced within 3 hours. Germ tubes produced after 3 hours of incubation should be disregarded. It

> A properly interpreted, positive germ tube test can be used to identify *Candida albicans*, if the germ tubes are produced within 3 hours. Not all strains of *C. albicans* produce germ tubes, however.

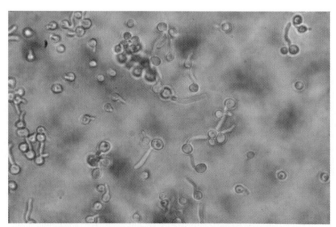

Figure 19-8. **Photomicrograph showing germ tubes of *C. albicans*.**

TABLE 19 - 3	Examples of Commercially Available Minisystems for Yeast Identification	
Method Type	**Minisystem (arranged alphabetically)**	**Manufacturer**
Nonautomated	API 20 C	bioMérieux Inc. (http://www.biomerieux.com/)
	API Candida System	bioMérieux Inc.
	API ID32C	bioMérieux Inc.
	API Yeast-Ident	bioMérieux Inc.
	Auxacolor System	Bio-Rad Laboratories (www.bio-rad.com)
	Candifast	International Microbio (www.int-microbio.com)
	Fungichrom I	International Microbio
	Fungifast Twin	International Microbio
	Identicult-Albicans	PML Microbiologicals Inc. (www.pmlmicro.com)
	Mycotube	Roche (http://www.roche.com/)
	RapID Yeast Plus/IDS YeastPlus Panel	Innovative Diagnostic Systems/Remel (http://www.remelinc.com/)
	Uni-Yeast-Tek	Remel
	YeastStar	CLARC Laboratories
Automated	MIS	Microbial ID Inc. (www.microbialid.com)
	Rapid Yeast Identification Panel	Dade Behring (http://www.dadebehring.com/)
	YBC, YST	bioMérieux Inc.
	YT Microplate	Biolog Inc. (http://www.biolog.com/)

Source: Wolk DM, Roberts GD. Commercial methods for identification and susceptibility testing of fungi. In: Manual of Commercial Methods in Clinical Microbiology. Washington, DC: ASM Press, 2002.

should be noted that not all strains of *C. albicans* produce germ tubes. It is also important to notice whether or not there is a constriction at the junction of the yeast cell and the germ tube. No constrictions are observed with *C. albicans*, but they are observed with *C. tropicalis*. It is important not to confuse germ tubes with pseudohyphae, which, as previously mentioned, are strings of elongated buds. Details of the germ tube test are contained in Appendix A.

Other tests of value in identifying yeasts are urease and rapid nitrate tests, morphology on cornmeal–Tween 80 agar, and phenol oxidase detection. A presumptive identification of *Candida* sp. can be made if blastoconidia (yeast cells) and pseudohyphae are observed in cornmeal–Tween 80 agar preparations. Additionally, *C. albicans* produces chlamydospores on cornmeal–Tween 80 agar. *Cryptococcus neo-formans* produces phenol oxidase on substrates containing caffeic acid, causing colonies on niger seed (bird-seed) agar to turn maroon red to dark brown in 2 to 5 days (Fig. 19-9).

> *Cryptococcus neoformans* produces phenol oxidase on substrates containing caffeic acid, causing colonies on niger seed (birdseed) agar to turn maroon red to dark brown in 2 to 5 days.

Some laboratories use chromogenic differential culture media (e.g., CHROMagar) to assist in the identification of yeasts, especially *C. albicans*, which produces yellow-green to blue-green colonies on CHROMagar (Fig. 19-10).

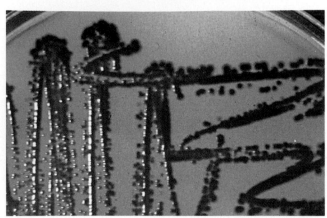

Figure 19-9. **Maroon red pigmentation of *Cryptococcus neoformans* colonies on niger seed (birdseed) agar.** (From Winn WC Jr, et al. Koneman's Color Atlas and Textbook of Diagnostic Microbiology. 6th Ed. Philadelphia: Lippincott Williams & Wilkins, 2006.)

MOULDS

Description

Moulds[2] are multicellular, eucaryotic, filamentous forms of fungi. The hyphae in a mould interweave to form a matlike colony. Almost everyone has seen mould colonies, sometimes in places where they are not wanted, like in refrigerators or growing on the surface of bread, cheese, or jam. The mildew growing in a shower is a collection of mould colonies.

The technical term for a mould colony is a **mycelium (pl. mycelia).** Some of the hyphae within the mycelium are above the surface on which the mycelium is growing. These hyphae are referred to as **aerial hyphae** or, because spores are produced on them, as **reproductive hyphae.** The longer the aerial hyphae, the fuzzier the appearance of the mycelium. The nutrient-absorbing hyphae that lie beneath the surface on which the mycelium is growing are called **vegetative hyphae.** Some moulds have **septate hyphae,** meaning that the cytoplasm is divided into cells by clearly visible cross walls (septa), whereas other moulds have **aseptate hyphae.** Although aseptate hyphae *usually* contain no septa, septa may be present in areas of damage and near reproductive structures. Observing whether a particular mould has septate or aseptate hyphae is an important clue to its identification. Figure 19-11 illustrates aerial, vegetative, septate, and aseptate hyphae.

> A mould colony (mycelium) is composed of hyphae. Some hyphae, called aerial hyphae, extend into the air, whereas others, called vegetative hyphae, lie beneath the surface of whatever the colony is growing on. Observing whether a particular mould has septate or aseptate hyphae is an important clue to its identification.

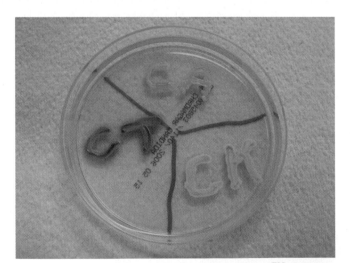

Figure 19-10. Candida **spp. on CHROMagar**™ *Candida* **medium, which is manufactured by BBL.** Yeasts were inoculated to this plate in such a way that their growth would form the abbreviations of their names. CA stands for *Candida albicans*, which produces light- to medium-green colonies on this medium. CK stands for *Candida krusei*, which produces light rose to pink colonies with a whitish border. CT stands for *Candida tropicalis*, which produces dark blue to metallic-blue colonies, with or without halos. (Courtesy of Dr. Robert C. Fader.)

Human Diseases Caused by Moulds

Fungal infections are especially common in immunosuppressed individuals. Patients most apt to develop fungal infections are those who are HIV infected, have received organ or tissue transplants, are undergoing cancer chemotherapy, or have received corticosteroids. Many of these patients are infected with fungi referred to as opportunistic fungi—fungi that usually do not cause serious infections in healthy, immunocompetent individuals. A properly functioning cellular immune system (see Chapter 3) is the key to resistance to fungal infections. Persistent fungal infections in a patient are often the result of impaired cell-mediated immunity.

The term **phaeohyphomycosis** refers to an infection caused by a fungus having dark hyphae, which result in a dark or black mycelium. Such moulds are referred to as **dematiaceous fungi.** The term **hyalohyphomycosis** refers to an infection caused by a fungus that produces colorless or transparent hyphae. Such moulds are referred to as **hyaline fungi.**

> Dematiaceous fungi are moulds having dark hyphae, resulting in a dark or black mycelium. Hyaline fungi are moulds that produce colorless or transparent hyphae.

Moulds can cause infections in many parts of the body. As previously mentioned, and described further in Chapter 20, they can cause superficial, cutaneous, subcutaneous, and systemic mycoses.

---

[2] *The term used for filamentous fungi may be spelled with or without a u. Mycologists tend to favor* mould, *because the word is derived from the Norse word* mowlde, *meaning "fuzzy." Mold, on the other hand, is derived from the French word* molde, *meaning "shape" or "form." As Dr. Fungus (http://www.doctorfungus.org/) points out, "If you make gelatin in a mold, a mould might then grow on the gelatin in your mold."*

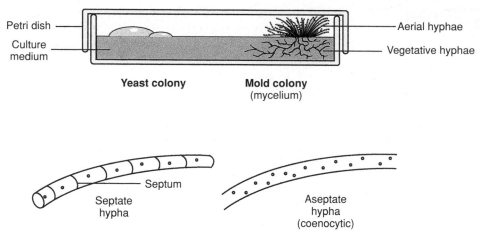

Figure 19-11. **Fungal colonies and terms relating to hyphae.**

Identifying Moulds

In the mycology section of the CML, moulds are identified primarily by a combination of growth rate and macroscopic and microscopic observations. Moulds are classified as *rapid growers* if the mycelium matures in 5 days or less; as *intermediate growers* if the mycelium matures in 6 to 10 days; and *slow growers* if it takes 11 or more days for the mycelium to mature. Some moulds and dimorphic fungi take up to 8 weeks to produce identifiable mature colonies.

> Moulds are identified or speciated primarily by growth rate and macroscopic and microscopic observations. Biochemical test results are usually *not* used to identify moulds.

Macroscopic observations useful for speciating moulds include the color of the mould colony (both front and reverse sides), its texture, and its topography. *Dematiaceous* moulds are those that produce dark (olive-green, brown, or black) colonies. Other moulds are *hyaline* (colorless) or pastel. Terms used to describe texture and topography are shown in Table 19-4. Note that biochemical test results are usually *not* used to identify moulds.

> Macroscopic observations of the color, texture, and topography of mould colonies are part of the identification process.

TABLE 19 - 4   Terms Used to Describe Mould Colonies

Terms Used to Describe Texture	Terms Used to Describe Topography
Cottony (or wooly or floccose): mycelium has long aerial hyphae	**Flat**
Velvety: mycelium has short aerial hyphae	**Rugose:** the mycelium has grooves that radiate out from the center
Granular (or powdery): mycelium resembles granulated or powdered sugar, due to heavy spore (conidia) production	**Folded:** the mycelium has random folds
Glabrous: mycelium is leathery or waxy in appearance	**Umbonate:** mycelium has a raised, buttonlike center (an "outie")
	Crateriform: mycelium has a sunken (craterlike) center (an "innie")
	Verrucose: mycelium has rough knobs (warts) on the surface
	Cerebriform: mycelium surface is irregular (brainlike) in appearance

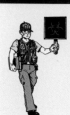
Tease mount. Microscopic observations include determining whether the hyphae are septate or aseptate and observing the types of structures within or on which spores are produced. To examine a mould microscopically, a tease mount is prepared. First, a small portion of the mycelium, containing both aerial and vegetative hyphae, is transferred to a drop of lactophenol cotton blue (LPCB) stain on a glass microscope slide. Sterile, straight teasing needles (also known as dissecting needles) are used to gently pull (tease) the piece of mycelium apart; this must be done carefully so as not to disrupt or damage the tiny structures that will be used as clues to identify the mould. LPCB stain contains lactic acid, phenol, and cotton blue. The lactic acid preserves morphology; the phenol kills the organisms, so that the preparation will not be infectious; and the cotton blue stains the mycelial structures blue. A glass coverslip is then added, and the tease mount preparation is examined under the microscope.

Alternatives to the tease mount preparation are cellulose tape preparations and slide cultures. All of these methods are described in Appendix A.

Microscopic examination can provide the following clues to a mould's identity:

- Whether the hyphae are septate or aseptate
- Type(s) of sexual and/or asexual spores (conidia) that the mould produces
- Type of structure on or within which the conidia are produced
- Whether both macroconidia (large conidia) and microconidia (small conidia) are produced

The microscopic appearance of several moulds is diagrammatically depicted in Figure 19-12.

DIMORPHIC FUNGI

Description

Some fungi, including some human pathogens, can live as either yeasts or moulds, depending on growth conditions. This phenomenon is called **dimorphism**—a term that means "two shapes"—and the organisms are referred to as **dimorphic fungi** (Fig. 19-13). When grown in vitro at body temperature (37°C), dimorphic fungi exist as unicellular yeasts and produce yeast colonies.

> When grown at 25°C, dimorphic fungi exist as moulds, but when grown at 37°C, they exist as yeasts.

Within the human body (in vivo), dimorphic fungi exist as yeasts. However, when grown in vitro at room temperature (25°C), dimorphic fungi exist as moulds, producing mould colonies (mycelia).

Human Diseases Caused by Dimorphic Fungi

Dimorphic fungi acting as etiologic agents of human disease include the following:

- *Blastomyces dermatitidis*: North American blastomycosis
- *Coccidioides immitis*: coccidioidomycosis
- *Histoplasma capsulatum*: histoplasmosis
- *Paracoccidioides brasiliensis*: paracoccidioidomycosis, or South American blastomycosis
- *Penicillium marneffei*: focal and systemic infections
- *Sporothrix schenckii*: sporotrichosis

In addition, *Candida* spp. can produce blastospores (yeast cells), pseudohyphae (strings of elongated buds), or true hyphae in vivo, but the various forms are not temperature dependent.

Identifying Dimorphic Fungi

Dimorphism can be demonstrated in the CML by converting the mould form of the fungus to the yeast form, using brain-heart infusion agar with blood (or some other type of special medium) and 37°C incubation. This procedure is useful for *B. dermatitidis*, *P. marneffei*, and *S. schenckii*, but does not work as well for *C. immitis* or *H. capsulatum*. *C. immitis* does not convert to a yeast form but will form spherules with special media or animal inoculation. *H. capsulatum* takes a long time (3 to 5 weeks) to

> In some cases, dimorphism can be demonstrated in the CML by converting the mould form of the fungus to the yeast form, using brain-heart infusion agar with blood, or some other type of special medium, and 37°C incubation.

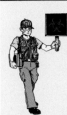

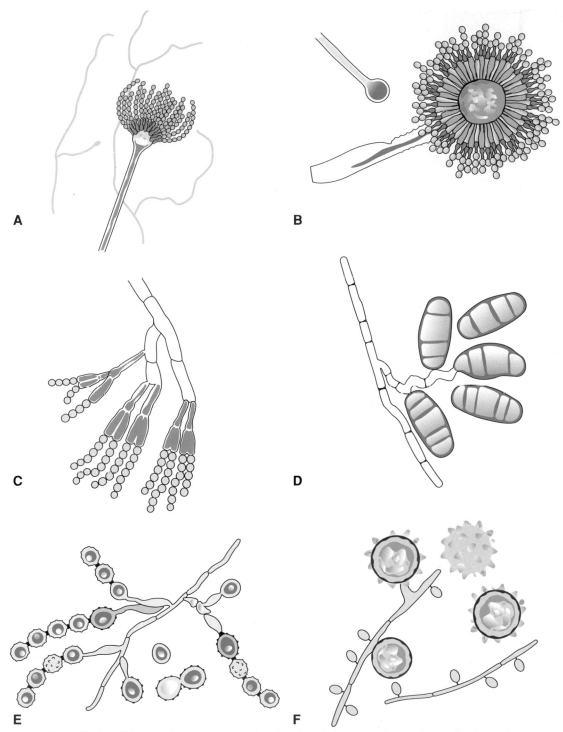

***Figure 19-12.* Microscopic appearance of various fungi. A.** *Aspergillus fumigatus.* **B.** *Aspergillus flavus.* **C.** *Penicillium* sp. **D.** *Curvularia* sp. **E.** *Scopulariopsis* sp. **F.** *Histoplasma capsulatum.* (From Winn WC Jr, et al. Koneman's Color Atlas and Textbook of Diagnostic Microbiology. 6th Ed. Philadelphia: Lippincott Williams & Wilkins, 2006.)

convert when blood agar slants are used to keep the medium moist. Once an isolate has been identified as a dimorphic fungus, it is speciated using a combination of macroscopic and microscopic observations. Some CMLs use molecular diagnostic procedures for confirmation of dimorphic fungi (as discussed later in the chapter).

IMMUNODIAGNOSTIC PROCEDURES

Recall that immunodiagnostic procedures (IDPs) are laboratory procedures used to diagnose various diseases (including

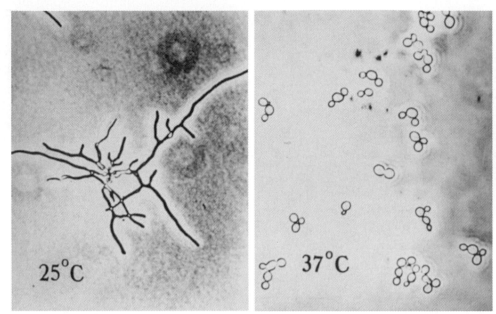

Figure 19-13. **Dimorphism.** These photomicrographs illustrate the dimorphic fungus *Histoplasma capsulatum* grown at 25°C and 37°C. (From Schaechter M, Engleberg NC, Eisenstein BI, Medoff G, eds. Mechanisms of Microbial Disease. 3rd Ed. Philadelphia: Lippincott Williams & Wilkins, 1999.)

infectious diseases), using the principles of immunology. IDPs for the diagnosis of infectious diseases detect either antigens or antibodies in clinical specimens. Several mycology IDPs are commercially available for detection of *Aspergillus, B. dermatitidis, Candida albicans, Cryptococcus neoformans, Coccidioides immitis, H. capsulatum,* and *P. brasiliensis* antigens, but they are not widely used in CMLs. When testing is performed properly, detection of cryptococcal antigen in CSF and serum is an excellent method of diagnosing cryptococcosis. Both latex agglutination tests and enzyme immunoassays are available commercially.

Immunodiagnostic procedures that detect complement-fixing antibodies are of value in the diagnosis of infections with systemic fungi. CSF yields positive results if the infection is current. The titer increases in disseminated disease and decreases with effective treatment. Latex and immunodiffusion tests are also of value in acute infections. These tests are of limited value in immunosuppressed patients, partly because of their diminished ability to produce antibodies and partly because of the rapid progression of infection in these patients.

MOLECULAR DIAGNOSTIC PROCEDURES

Relatively few molecular diagnostic procedures are commercially available for the diagnosis of fungal infec-

tions. They are primarily used in research and reference laboratories. One such system of DNA probes (Accuprobe by Gen-Probe; http://www.gen-probe.com/) can be used for culture confirmation of *H. capsulatum, B. dermatitidis, Coccidioides immitis,* and *Cryptococcus neoformans.*

ANTIMICROBIAL SUSCEPTIBILITY TESTING OF FUNGI

In most CMLs, antimicrobial susceptibility testing is currently performed on bacterial pathogens but *not* on fungal pathogens. However, with the increasing number of fungi—both yeasts and moulds—that are becoming resistant to antifungal agents, it is likely that antifungal susceptibility testing will become a routine procedure in the near future. Some of the newer antifungal agents can be used when fungi show resistance to the older agents. The CLSI has published approved standards for broth dilution susceptibility testing of yeasts and filamentous fungi, and an approved guideline for disk diffusion susceptibility testing of yeasts (see "References and Suggested Reading"). Commercial methods (e.g., colorimetric, spectrophotometric, and agar diffusion methods) that yield results comparable to the CLSI methods are also available.

Chapter Review

- Medical mycology is the study of fungi that cause human diseases.

- Depending on the particular species, fungi reproduce by budding, hyphal extension, or the formation of spores. The two general categories of spores are sexual spores and asexual spores.

- Zygospores, oospores, ascospores, and basidiospores are examples of sexual spores.

- Sporangiospores and conidia are examples of asexual spores. Blastoconidia, chlamydoconidia, and arthroconidia are examples of conidia.

- Fungi are not plants. They possess neither chlorophyll nor other photosynthetic pigments. Fungal cell walls contain a polysaccharide called chitin.

- The fungi that cause human diseases are divided into four categories: fleshy fungi, yeasts, moulds, and dimorphic fungi.

- Specimens processed in the mycology section of the CML include all the types typically handled in the bacteriology section, with the addition of hair clippings, nail clippings, and skin scrapings.

- Some of the methods used to process fungal specimens include KOH, calcofluor white, and India ink preparations.

- The types of plated media used in the mycology section, which differ from those used in the bacteriology section, include Sabouraud dextrose agar with or without antibiotics, brain-heart infusion agar with or without added blood and/or antibiotics, potato dextrose agar, and dermatophyte test medium.

- The toxins that fungi produce are referred to as mycotoxins, and the microbial intoxications that they cause are called mycotoxicoses.

- Most pathogenic yeasts are classified as Deuteromycota or Fungi Imperfecti. Yeasts such as *Candida albicans* and *Cryptococcus neoformans* are common human pathogens.

- Methods of identifying yeasts include KOH prep, calcofluor white, Gram stain, India ink, Germ tube test, and biochemical tests.

- Moulds are multicellular, eucaryotic, filamentous forms of fungi consisting of long, thin, intertwined, cytoplasmic filaments called hyphae.

- Observing whether a particular mould has septate or aseptate hyphae is an important clue to its identification. Methods used to identify moulds include growth rate and macroscopic and microscopic observations.

- Fungi that can live either as yeasts or moulds are known as dimorphic fungi.

- Examples of dimorphic fungi that cause human disease are *Blastomyces dermatitidis*, *Coccidioides immitis*, and *Histoplasma capsulatum*.

- Dimorphism can be demonstrated in the CML by converting the mould form of the fungus to the yeast form, using brain-heart infusion agar with blood, incubated at 37°C.

- Immunodiagnostic procedures that detect antibodies are of value in diagnosing infections with systemic fungi.

New Terms and Abbreviations

After studying Chapter 19, you should be familiar with the following terms, which are defined within the chapter and in the Glossary at the back of the book:

Aerial hyphae

Aseptate hyphae

Blastoconidia

Blastospores

Dematiaceous fungi

Dimorphic fungi

Dimorphism

Fleshy fungi

Hyalohyphomycosis

Hyaline fungi

Hypha (pl. hyphae)

Medical mycology

Mycelium (pl. mycelia)

Mycosis (pl. mycoses)

Mycotoxicosis (pl. mycotoxicoses)

Mycotoxin

Perfect fungi

Phaeohyphomycosis

Pseudohypha (pl. pseudohyphae)

Septate hyphae

Sporangiospores

Thrush

Vegetative hyphae

References and Suggested Reading

Beneke ES, Rogers AL. Medical Mycology and Human Mycoses. Belmont, CA: Star, 1996.

Fromtling RA, et al. Taxonomy, classification, and morphology of fungi. In: Murray PR, Baron EJ, Jorgensen JH, Pfaller MA, Yolken RH, eds. Manual of Clinical Microbiology. 8th Ed. Washington, DC: ASM Press, 2003.

LaRocco MT. Reagents, stains, and media: mycology. In: Murray PR, Baron EJ, Jorgensen JH, Pfaller MA, Yolken RH, eds. Manual of Clinical Microbiology. 8th Ed. Washington, DC: ASM Press, 2003.

Merz WG, Roberts GD. Algorithms for detection and identification of fungi. In: Murray PR, Baron EJ, Jorgensen JH, Pfaller MA, Yolken RH, eds. Manual of Clinical Microbiology. 8th Ed. Washington, DC: ASM Press, 2003.

Method for Antifungal Disk Diffusion Susceptibility Testing of Yeasts: Approved Guideline. CLSI Document M44-A. Wayne, PA: Clinical and Laboratory Standards Institute, 2004.

Protection of Laboratory Workers from Occupationally Acquired Infections; Approved Guideline. 3rd Ed. CLSI Document M29-A3. Wayne, PA: Clinical and Laboratory Standards Institute, 2005.

Reference Method for Broth Dilution Antifungal Susceptibility Testing of Filamentous Fungi: Approved Standard. CLSI Document M38-A. Wayne, PA: Clinical and Laboratory Standards Institute, 2002.

Reference Method for Broth Dilution Antifungal Susceptibility Testing of Yeasts: Approved Standard. 2nd Ed. CLSI Document M27-A2. Wayne, PA: Clinical and Laboratory Standards Institute, 2002.

Sutton DA. Specimen collection, transport, and processing: mycology. In: Murray PR, Baron EJ, Jorgensen JH, Pfaller MA, Yolken RH, eds. Manual of Clinical Microbiology. 8th Ed. Washington, DC: ASM Press, 2003.

Wolk DM, Roberts GD. Commercial methods for identification and susceptibility testing of fungi. In: Manual of Commercial Methods in Clinical Microbiology. Washington, DC: ASM Press, 2002.

 ## On the CD-ROM

- Additional Self-Assessment Exercises
- Puzzle

Self-Assessment Exercises

1. Briefly describe what is meant by a dimorphic fungus and how to determine if a fungus is dimorphic.

   _____

   _____

2. Which of the following is an example of an asexual spore?

   A. Zygospore

   B. Ascospore

   C. Blastoconidium

   D. None of the above

3. True or false: Fungi that have both a sexual and asexual form of reproduction are known as perfect fungi.

4. True or false: Fungi are included in the same kingdom as plants.

5. Which of the following procedures is used to better observe fungal structures by dissolving keratin in the specimen?

   A. KOH prep

   B. Gram stain

   C. Tease preparation

   D. India ink prep

6. Which of the following statements about fungi is *false*?

   A. Fungi are eucaryotic organisms, classified in the Domain *Fungi*.

   B. Fungi are not photosynthetic.

   C. Fungal cell walls contain chitin, a substance not found in the cell walls of any other microorganisms.

   D. Fungal elements usually stain blue with the Gram staining procedure.

7. Which of the following fungi is most frequently isolated from human clinical specimens?

   A. *Cryptococcus neoformans*

   B. *Malassezia furfur*

   C. *Trichosporon* spp.

   D. *Candida albicans*

8. Briefly describe how yeasts can be differentiated from bacteria using a Gram-stained smear.

_____

9. Mould colony hyphae that lie above the surface of whatever the colony is growing on are known as

_____.

10. Name three general criteria by which mould colonies are identified.

A. _____

B. _____

C. _____

CHAPTER 20

Laboratory Diagnosis of Selected Fungal Infections

Chapter Outline

Superficial Mycoses

Cutaneous, Hair, and Nail Mycoses

Subcutaneous Mycoses
- Mycetomas
- Chromoblastomycosis
- Sporotrichosis
- Protothecosis

Systemic Mycoses
- Fungal Infections of the Lower Respiratory Tract
- Fungal Infections of the Central Nervous System
- Fungal Infections of the Genitourinary System

LEARNING OBJECTIVES

After studying this chapter, you should be able to:

☞ Define the terms and abbreviations introduced in this chapter (e.g., *actinomycetoma, chitin, dermatophytes*)

☞ Given a description, prepared specimen, and/or color photograph of a microscopic fungal structure, identify the fungus

☞ Name the four categories of mycoses presented in this chapter and the area of the body where infection occurs

☞ Name the specimen of choice for recovery of the fungal infections discussed in this chapter

☞ List the groups of patients especially at risk of developing fungal infections

☞ Given a particular fungal infection, such as tinea versicolor or coccidioidomycosis, categorize it as to type of mycosis (e.g., cutaneous, subcutaneous)

☞ Given a description of a fungal infection, including any macroscopic and/or microscopic observations, identify the fungus involved

☞ Given a microscopic view of a fungus, identify it as being septate or aseptate and dematiaceous or nondematiaceous

☞ Describe the type of clinical specimens used to diagnose a fungal infection based on the category of mycoses (e.g., clinical specimens used to diagnose superficial mycoses include skin scrapings and hair)

☞ Identify the fungus having a morphology described as "spaghetti and meatballs"

☞ Given a photograph of a direct mount of hair, differentiate between ectothrix, endothrix, and favic fungal infections

☞ Describe the colonial and microscopic appearance of the following fungi: *Hortaea werneckii, Piedraia hortae, Trichosporon beigelii, Malassezia furfur*, and *Microsporum* spp.

☞ Describe the general laboratory workup of a potential fungal pathogen

☞ Differentiate between *Trichosporon* and *Trichophyton* species of moulds, and name the category of mycosis caused by each and specific examples of infections

☞ Name at least three dermatophytes commonly encountered in the clinical laboratory

☞ State some of the general characteristics (e.g., site infected, severity) of subcutaneous and systemic mycoses

☞ Give two or three examples of subcutaneous and systemic mycoses

☞ Describe mycetomas, or maduromycoses, including clinical presentation and possible etiologic agents

☞ Given a list of pathogenic fungi, identify those that are dimorphic

Fungal infections are known as mycoses (sing. *mycosis*). The discussion of mycoses in this chapter is divided into the following four categories:

- Superficial mycoses

- Cutaneous, hair, and nail mycoses

- Subcutaneous mycoses

- Systemic mycoses, also known as generalized or deep-seated mycoses

Sometimes a particular fungal infection may progress through several or even all of these stages. Although fungi can also cause eye and ear infections, endocarditis, and sinusitis, those types of mycoses are not discussed in this chapter.

Spores of some pathogenic fungi may be inhaled with dust from contaminated soil or dried bird or bat feces (guano), or they may enter through wounds of the hands or feet. If the spores are inhaled into the lungs, they may germinate there to cause a respiratory infection similar to tuberculosis. Examples of deep-seated pulmonary infections are blastomycosis, coccidioidomycosis, cryptococcosis, and histoplasmosis. In each case, the pathogens may invade further to cause widespread systemic infections, especially in immunosuppressed patients.

As mentioned in Chapter 19, the types of fungi that cause human mycoses are yeasts, moulds, and dimorphic fungi. With roughly more than 200 fungi acting as etiological agents of human illness, it is impossible to discuss all the disease-causing fungi in a book of this size. Therefore, this chapter focuses on a few of the most frequently encountered fungal pathogens and the diseases they cause. Some of the many additional fungi involved in opportunistic infections are mentioned on the CD-ROM.

> The types of fungi that cause infectious diseases are yeasts, moulds, and dimorphic fungi.

Many of the fungi that infect humans are referred to as opportunistic fungi. These are fungi of relatively low or limited virulence that usually cause disease only in debilitated or immunosuppressed patients. Nonetheless, infections caused by these fungi can, in some cases, be fatal. Because of the number and variety of fungal spores present in the air, it is sometimes difficult to determine if a fungal isolate is a contaminant or is actually causing disease. Following are some questions to ask when attempting to distinguish between a pathogen and a contaminant:

- Was the fungus isolated in pure culture? A pure culture indicates that the fungus is most likely a pathogen rather than a contaminant.

- How many colonies of the fungus are on the plate? Multiple colonies indicate that the fungus is most likely a pathogen rather than a contaminant.

- Is the fungus growing on the streak lines? If so, the fungus is most likely a pathogen rather than a contaminant.

- Is the fungus present in more than one culture from that patient on the same day? If so, the fungus is most likely a pathogen rather than a contaminant.

- Can the fungus be recovered from the same site in cultures taken on different days? If so, the fungus is most likely a pathogen rather than a contaminant.

Did you know that bread moulds can cause human disease, even death? Inhalation of spores of common bread moulds, like *Rhizopus* and *Mucor* spp., by an immunosuppressed patient can lead to a respiratory disease called **zygomycosis.** Older terms for this disease are mucormycosis and phycomycosis. Following infection, the mould can become disseminated throughout the patient's body and lead to death.

Winn et al. (see "References and Suggested Reading") list the following groups of patients as being especially at risk of developing fungal infections:

- Immunosuppressed and leukopenic patients

- Transplant recipients

- Patients with intravascular or prosthetic devices

- Cancer patients, especially those with leukemia and lymphoma and those receiving chemotherapy

- Patients with debilitating immunologic and metabolic disorders, such as systemic lupus erythematosus or diabetes, or alcohol or IV drug abusers

- Recipients of corticosteroids, cytotoxic agents, or prolonged antibiotic therapy

- People who have traveled to or live in regions of the world where fungal infections are endemic

- People whose activities or occupations bring them into contact with infected animals, contaminated materials, or aerosols of dust containing fungal spores

SUPERFICIAL MYCOSES

Diseases and most likely pathogens. Superficial mycoses are fungal infections of the outermost areas of the human body—the outer surface of hair shafts and the outermost, nonliving layer of the skin (the epidermis). Specific infections include otomycosis, black piedra,

> Superficial mycoses include otomycosis, black piedra, white piedra, pityriasis versicolor, and tinea nigra.

white piedra, pityriasis versicolor, and tinea nigra, each of which is briefly described here.

Otomycosis is a type of otitis externa, an infection of the outer ear canal. Many different moulds may cause otomycosis,

> Otomycosis is a fungal infection of the outer ear canal.

including *Aspergillus*, *Penicillium*, *Mucor*, and *Rhizopus* spp. Less commonly, a dermatophyte (described later in the chapter) is the cause. Bacteria such as *Micrococcus*, *Staphylococcus*, *Streptococcus*, *Proteus*, and *Pseudomonas* spp. can cause otitis externa, which can be mistaken for otomycosis.

Black piedra is a fungal infection of scalp hair and less commonly, eyebrows, eyelashes, and pubic hair. It is character-

> The mould *Piedraia hortae* is the cause of black piedra, a hair infection.

ized by discrete, hard, gritty, dark brown or black nodules of various size and shape that firmly adhere to hair shafts. The cause of black piedra is the mould *Piedraia hortae*.

White piedra is a fungal infection of mustache, beard, pubic, and axilla hair. It is characterized by soft, pigmented (white, yellowish, beige, or

> The hair infection white piedra is most frequently caused by the mould *Trichosporon beigelii*.

greenish) nodules of various sizes on hair shafts. The nodules, which may be discrete or coalescent, are more easily separated from hair shafts than are *P. hortae* nodules. White piedra is caused by *Trichosporon* spp., primarily *T. beigelii*.

Tinea versicolor or pityriasis versicolor is a ringworm infection that affects the skin of the chest or back and, less commonly,

> The primary causes of the skin infection, tinea versicolor or pityriasis versicolor, are moulds in the *Malassezia furfur* complex.

the arms, thighs, neck, and face. Tinea versicolor is characterized by irregular, pigmented (light brown, yellow brown, brown, or red) or at times unpigmented

scaly patches. A Wood's lamp, which emits ultraviolet light, can be used to locate all areas of infection, which fluoresce a pale yellow under ultraviolet light. The primary causes of tinea versicolor are moulds in the *Malassezia furfur* complex.

STUDY AID **Ringworm.** The term *ringworm* is used in reference to some of the superficial and cutaneous mycoses, which more correctly are known as tinea infections. Be aware that diseases referred to as ringworm have absolutely *nothing* to do with worms. The term most likely arose long before fungi were known to be the cause of these lesions. Some of the lesions are circular and raised,

> Ringworm infections are fungal infections that have nothing to do with worms.

prompting early speculation that a worm lay coiled beneath the skin surface.

Tinea nigra is a ringworm infection of the palm of the hands and, less commonly, the neck and feet. It is characterized by flat, sharply marginated, brown-to-black, nonscaly macular lesions. Tinea nigra is caused by the mould *Hor-taea werneckii*.

> Tinea nigra, a ringworm infection of the skin, is caused by the mould *Hortaea werneckii*.

Clinical specimens. Depending on the location of the infection, clinical specimens include skin scrapings, hair clippings, ear canal debris, and exudate, if present. Before the skin is scraped, it should be swabbed with 70% alcohol to remove any bacteria present. Cellulose (Scotch) tape can also be used to remove portions of infected epidermis. Hair samples should be collected from areas of scaling or hair loss, or areas where the hairs fluoresce under a long-wave ultraviolet light source (e.g., Wood's lamp).

Contaminants. Specimens are often contaminated with bacteria of the indigenous microflora of skin.

Screening tests. Skin scrapings and hair hafts can be examined using a 10% potassium hydroxide preparation (KOH prep) or calcofluor white staining. If fungi are present, hyphae, conidiophores and conidia, or sporangiophores and sporangiospores may be observed, depending on the species causing the infection. Ear canal debris should also be Gram stained. Cellulose tape specimens can be placed on a microscope slide, sticky side down, onto a drop of lactophenol cotton blue stain for microscopic examination.

Media to be inoculated. Sabouraud dextrose agar. It should be noted that most superficial mycoses are diagnosed clinically and by microscopic examination of specimens; they are rarely cultured.

SAFETY TIP

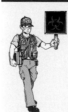

CLSI-Recommended Safety Precautions. As mentioned in Chapter 19, the Clinical and Laboratory Standards Institute (see "References and Suggested Reading") recommends that mould colonies be examined in a biosafety cabinet, not only to prevent contamination of the laboratory environment with spores but also because of the possibility that they might be colonies of systemic fungi such as Blastomyces dermatitidis, Coccidioides immitis, *or* Histoplasma capsulatum.

Laboratory diagnosis. Fungal colonies (mycelia) should be examined via a tease mount or cellulose tape mount

TABLE 20 - 1	Superficial Mycoses: Summary of Macroscopic and Microscopic Observations	
Species and Disease It Causes	**Macroscopic Observations**	**Microscopic Observations**
Piedraia hortae, black piedra	Slow grower; greenish brown to black colony; heaped in the center with a flat periphery; glabrous to cerebriform; short, dark aerial hyphae; sometimes produces a reddish brown diffusible pigment on the agar	Dark, thick-walled, septate hyphae, with numerous chlamydoconidia or enlarged irregular cells; asci and ascospores may be present but usually are not seen
Trichosporon spp., white piedra	Rapid grower; white to cream colored, slimy, soft colony that later becomes finely wrinkled, raised in the center, darker, and more firmly attached to the agar	Hyaline hyphae, arthroconidia, and blastoconidia; no asci
Malassezia furfur, tinea or pityriasis versicolor	Culture is not necessary for diagnosis; colonies are cream colored, glossy or rough, and raised, later becoming tan to brownish, dull, and dry	Colonies contain oval budding cells with a broad-based isthmus; elongate hyphae are rarely seen, although short hyphae are; sometimes has a "spaghetti and meatballs" appearance
Hortaea werneckii, tinea nigra	Slow grower; colonies have a moist, shiny olive to greenish black, yeastlike appearance; older colonies (2 weeks) are less moist and are dark green with grayish aerial hyphae	Black, yeastlike colonies contain blastoconidia or budding cells that have developed laterally from dark hyphal cells; blastoconidia may form clusters along the hyphae; short conidiophores along the sides of hyphae produce chains or clusters of 1-to-2-celled dark conidia; older hyphae may lack spores

and lactophenol cotton blue. The presence of any conidiophores, conidia, sporangiophores, sporangiospores, and septate or aseptate hyphae are noted. Species identification is based on macroscopic observations (colony features) and microscopic observations. Table 20-1 contains information useful in identifying common etiologic agents of superficial mycoses. Photographs of nodules, colonies, and hyphae can be found in the books by Beneke and Rogers and by Winn et al. (see "References and Suggested Reading").

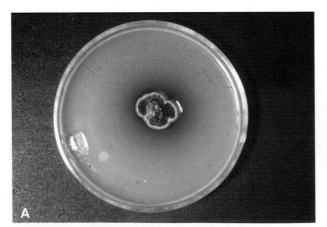
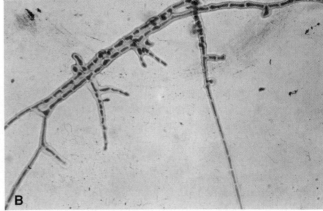

Figure 20-1. **Colony (A) and hyphae (B) of *Piedraia hortae*, the cause of black piedra.** (Courtesy of Dr. Lucille K. Georg and the Centers for Disease Control and Prevention [CDC].)

Diagnosis of otomycosis. Otomycosis is diagnosed by direct examination and culture of exudate and epithelial cells obtained from the ear canal. Direct examination of the specimen by KOH prep should reveal hyphae and may reveal conidiophores and conidia or sporangiophores and sporangiospores. Because otitis externa can be caused by bacteria, the specimen should also be Gram stained. Sabouraud agar slants or plates should be inoculated and held for 2 to 3 weeks. Fungal colonies should be examined by tease mount or cellophane tape preparation. Various observations that serve as clues to identification include septate or aseptate hyphae, conidiophores and conidia, and sporangiophores and sporangiospores.

Diagnosis of black piedra. Black piedra nodules are composed of compact masses of dark, branched, septate, thick-walled hyphae that are 4 to 8 μm in diameter. Also visible are round-to-oval asci containing aseptate ascospores that are hyaline, curved, and fusiform. Hair clippings are examined by KOH prep and inoculated to Sabouraud dextrose agar with and without cycloheximide. The mycelium of *P. hortae* is greenish brown to black, raised or flat in the center, and glabrous to cerebriform (Fig. 20-1A). The hyphae are dark and thick walled, and the septa are close together (Fig. 20-1B). Numerous chlamydoconidia, enlarged irregular cells, and possibly asci and ascospores may be observed.

Diagnosis of white piedra. Microscopic examination of squashed white piedra nodules reveals intertwined, hyaline, septate hyphae that break up into oval or rectangular arthroconidia 2 to 4 μm in diameter. Occasional blastoconidia may be seen. *T. beigelii* is sensitive to cycloheximide. Colonies of *T. beigelii* are initially cream colored, slimy, and soft, but with age the colonies become finely wrinkled, raised in the center, darker, and more firmly attached to the agar. Microscopically, hyaline hyphae, arthroconidia, and blastoconidia may be observed, but not asci.

Diagnosis of tinea versicolor. Microscopic examination of infected skin cells reveals short, septate, occasionally

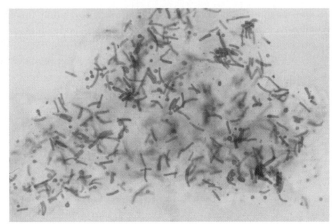

Figure 20-2. **"Spaghetti and meatball" appearance of** *Malassezia furfur* **in a skin scraping.** (Courtesy of Dr. Lucille K. Georg and the CDC).

branching, 2.5-to-4-μm-diameter hyphae and clusters of thick-walled, oval or round, unicellular, 4-to-8-μm-diameter cells, some of which may be budding.

> Associate a spaghetti-and-meatball appearance with *Malassezia furfur* and tinea versicolor.

This mix of hyphae and oval-to-round cells has been described as a "spaghetti and meatball" appearance (Fig. 20-2). Culture is usually not necessary for diagnosis. Culture media must contain lipids, usually olive oil.

Diagnosis of tinea nigra. Microscopic examination of infected cells reveals light brown to dark green, branched, septate, 1.5- to 5-μm-diameter hyphae. Swollen cells and chlamydoconidia are also present. *H. werneckii* grows slowly on Sabouraud dextrose agar (with or without cycloheximide and chloramphenicol), developing moist, shiny black, yeastlike colonies that reach a maximum size after 2 weeks. Older colonies are less moist and become dark green with grayish aerial hyphae (Fig. 20-3A). Microscopically, the

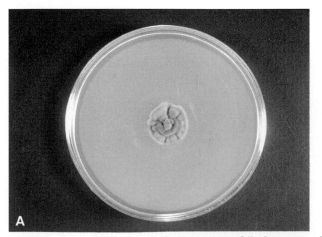

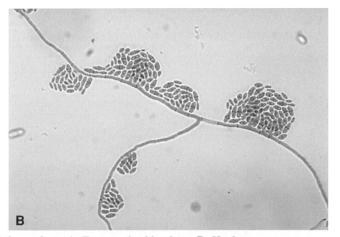

Figure 20-3. Hortaea werneckii, **the cause of tinea nigra. A.** Four-week-old colony. **B.** Hyphae and conidia. ([A] Courtesy of Dr. Lucille K. Georg and the CDC. [B] Courtesy of Dr. Libero Ajello and the CDC.)

colony contains blastoconidia or budding cells that have developed laterally from the dark hyphal cells. The blastoconidia may form clusters along the hyphae (Fig. 20-3B). Short conidiophores on the sides or tips of the hyphae produce chains or clusters of one-to-two-celled dark conidia.

CUTANEOUS, HAIR, AND NAIL MYCOSES

Diseases and most likely pathogens. Fungal infections of the living layers of skin (the dermis), hair shafts, and nails—commonly called tinea infections or ringworm infections—are caused by a group of moulds collectively referred to as dermatophytes. Dermatophytes include *Epidermophyton* spp., *Microsporum* spp., and *Trichophyton* spp. Tinea infections are named in accordance with the part of the anatomy infected (Table 20-2; Figs. 20-4 through 20-6).

CAUTION **Beware of Similar-Sounding Names.** *Trichosporon* and *Trichophyton* are two genera of moulds. *Trichosporon* spp. cause infections of the external surfaces of hair shafts known as white piedra. *Trichophyton* spp. are dermatophytes that cause various cutaneous and hair infections, referred to as tinea or ringworm infections.

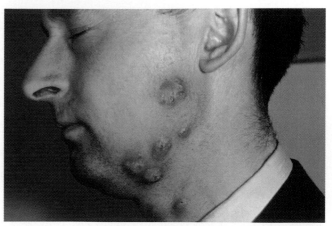

Figure 20-4. **Tinea barbae, ringworm of the bearded areas of the face and neck, also known as barber's itch.** (Courtesy of the CDC.)

Fungal infections of hair shafts are classified as ectothrix, endothrix, or favic infections (Table 20-3). A patient with tinea capitis is shown in Figure 20-5.

Clinical specimens. Skin scrapings, nail clippings, or hair clippings are used, depending on the site of infection. Hair and skin scrapings infected with some *Microsporum* spp. (see Table 20-3) fluoresce a bright yellowish green when examined using a Wood's lamp.

Contaminants. Specimens may be contaminated with members of the indigenous microflora of the skin.

TABLE 20 - 2	Tinea Infections	
Infection	**Anatomical Site(s) Affected**	**Most Common Cause (Dermatophyte)**[a]
Tinea barbae (see Fig. 20-4)	Beard and moustache	*Trichophyton verrucosum, T. mentagrophytes* complex
Tinea capitis (see Fig. 20-5)	Scalp, eyebrows, eyelashes	*T. tonsurans, Microsporum canis*
Tinea corporis	Face, trunk, and major limbs	Any dermatophyte; chronic lesions of the trunk and extremities are usually caused by *T. rubrum*
Tinea cruris	Groin, perineal and perianal areas	*T. rubrum, Epidermophyton floccosum*
Tinea favosa (also called favus)	Scalp	*T. schoenleinii*
Tinea pedis (see Fig. 20-6)	Soles and between toes	*T. mentagrophytes* complex, *T. rubrum*
Tinea manuum	Palms	*Microsporum gypseum, T. verrucosum, M. canis*
Tinea unguium (also known as onychomycosis)	Nails	*T. rubrum*

[a]Some authorities feel that the species listed have no particular predilection for a specific body site.

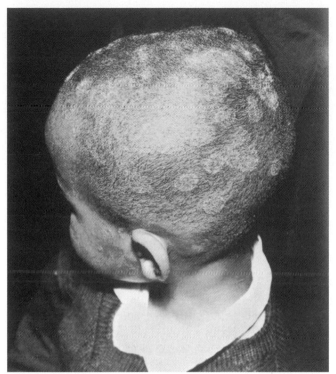

Figure 20-5. **Tinea capitis, presenting as multiple patches of alopecia (hair loss) and scaling.** (From Binford CH, Connor DH. Pathology of Tropical and Extraordinary Diseases, vol 2. Washington, DC: Armed Forces Institute of Pathology, 1976.)

Screening tests. Specimens should be examined using a KOH prep, or a KOH prep with calcofluor white staining. Calcofluor white binds to the chitin in fungal cell walls, resulting in a bright green or blue fluorescence. In Figure 20-7, a KOH prep of a skin scraping has revealed a fungal hypha. Figure 20-8 illustrates a case of endothrix infection.

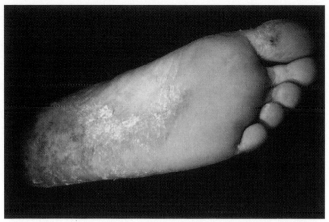

Figure 20-6. **Tinea pedis, ringworm of the foot, also known as athlete's foot.** (Courtesy of the CDC.)

Media to be inoculated. Specimens should be pressed into the surface of Sabouraud dextrose agar with chloramphenicol and cycloheximide, such as Mycosel or mycobiotic agar. Dermatophyte test medium (DTM) can also be used. Dermatophytes cause an increase in pH, which causes DTM to turn red. Plates should be held for at least 2 weeks.

Laboratory diagnosis. Moulds that are isolated are identified by a combination of macroscopic and microscopic observations. The dermatophytes most commonly encountered in CMLs in the United States are

- *Trichophyton tonsurans,*
- *Trichophyton rubrum,*
- *Trichophyton mentagrophytes,*
- *Microsporum canis,* and
- *Epidermophyton floccosum.*

TABLE 20 - 3	Categories of Hair Infections	
Category	**Description**	**Most Common Cause**
Ectothrix infections	Arthroconidia appear as a sheath around the hair shaft or as chains on the surface of the hair shaft; ectothrix infection by some dermatophytes causes the hairs to fluoresce yellowish green under an ultraviolet light source (Wood's lamp)	Dermatophytes that cause infected hairs to fluoresce: *Microsporum audouinii*, *M. canis, M. ferrugineum*. Causes of nonfluorescent ectothrix infections: *M. gypseum* complex, *M. praecox*, *Trichophyton megninii*, *T. mentagrophytes* complex, *T. verrucosum*
Endothrix infections	Chains of arthroconidia fill the insides of shortened hair stubs; no fluorescence under a Wood's lamp	*T. soudanense, T. tonsurans, T. violaceum*
Favic infections	Hyphae, air bubbles, tunnels, and fat droplets occur within hair shafts; hairs fluoresce dull green under a Wood's lamp	*T. schoenleinii*

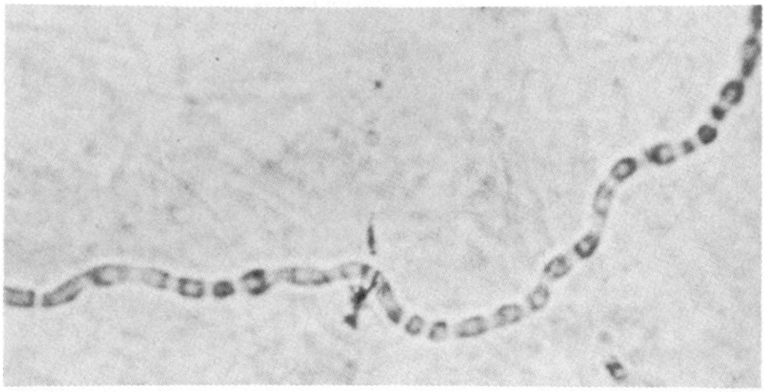

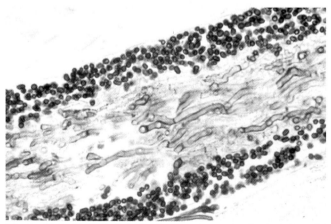

Figure 20-7. **Fungal hypha, as seen in a KOH prep of a skin scraping.** The hypha appears to be breaking up into arthroconidia. (From Winn WC Jr, et al. Koneman's Color Atlas and Textbook of Diagnostic Microbiology. 6th Ed. Philadelphia: Lippincott Williams & Wilkins, 2006.)

In general, *Trichophyton* spp. produce many microconidia but few, if any, macroconidia. When produced, the macroconidia are thin walled and smooth. Criteria of value in speciating *Trichophyton* spp. are the size and arrangement of the microconidia, production of pigment, urease activity, type of hair infection they cause (endothrix or ectothrix), and their growth patterns on *Trichophyton* differential agars (media with and without thiamine and niacin). Commonly isolated *Trichophyton* spp. are shown in Figures 20-9 through 20-11.

In general, *Microsporum* spp. produce many macroconidia but few, if any, microconidia. Macroconidia are multicelled, with a thick, spiny, or bumpy cell wall. Species identification is based primarily on differences in the morphology of the macroconidia. For example, the cross walls or septa within a macroconidium are often likened to seats in

Figure 20-8. **Endothrix infection.** In this longitudinal section of a Gomori methenamine silver–stained hair shaft, hyphae are seen in the center of the shaft and conidia at the periphery. (From Winn WC Jr, et al. Koneman's Color Atlas and Textbook of Diagnostic Microbiology. 6th Ed. Philadelphia: Lippincott Williams & Wilkins, 2006.)

a canoe. The macroconidia of different species of *Microsporum* (and other dermatophytes) contain different numbers of "seats." When present, the microconidia are small, hyaline, tear-drop or elliptical in shape, and attached to the sides of the hyphae. *Microsporum canis* and *M. gypseum* are illustrated in Figures 20-12 and 20-13.

In general, *Epidermophyton* spp. produce club-shaped, smooth-walled, 2-to-4-celled macroconidia that are formed either singly from hyphae or, more characteristically, in clusters of two or three. A key feature in the identification of *Epidermophyton* spp. is the absence of microconidia. *Epidermophyton floccosum* is illustrated in Figure 20-14.

At this point, a review of Figures 20-9 through 20-14 might be helpful. What differences appear among the objects depicted in these drawings? Noticing the differences is a significant step in understanding how microscopic observations aid in the identification of moulds. However, it is also important to keep in mind that only a few of the most commonly isolated moulds are discussed here. Many additional moulds can cause cutaneous, hair, or nail infections, and in some cases, the morphological differences among them are very subtle.

SUBCUTANEOUS MYCOSES

Subcutaneous mycoses are fungal infections of the dermis and underlying tissues. They are more severe than superficial and cutaneous mycoses. Subcutaneous mycoses are usually the result of some type of traumatic introduction of the fungal pathogen into the skin. The infection may remain localized, may slowly spread to surrounding tissue, and, in some cases, may spread via lymphatic channels or the bloodstream (rarely). Subcutaneous mycoses can be quite grotesque in appearance. Examples of subcutaneous mycoses are mycetomas, chromoblastomycosis, and sporotrichosis. Each of these categories are discussed in this section.

> Subcutaneous mycoses are fungal infections of the dermis and underlying tissues. Mycetomas, chromoblastomycosis, and sporotrichosis are examples of subcutaneous mycoses.

Mycetomas

Diseases and most likely pathogens. Mycetomas, also known as maduromycoses, are chronic granulomatous infections that involve the feet (usually), hands, or other areas of the body. Granulomatous infections, or granulomas, are nodular inflammatory lesions containing a variety of phagocytic cells. Mycetomas usually involve enlargement, deformity, sinus drainage, and bone destruction. Some mycetomas, such as Madura foot, are rather grotesque in appearance (Fig. 20-15). The terms *maduromycosis* and

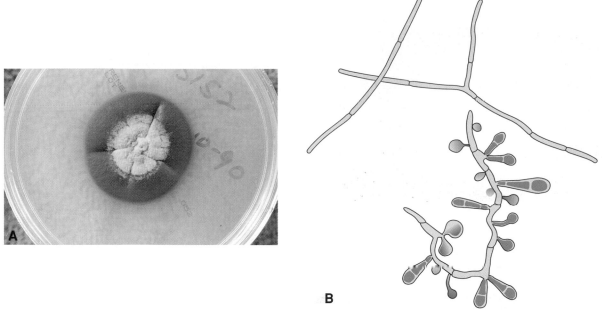

Figure 20-9. Trichophyton tonsurans. **A.** *T. tonsurans* colony after 14 days of incubation on Sabouraud dextrose agar. The surface tends to be granular with radial grooves (rugae), and most strains produce some shade of yellow-brown pigment. **B.** Drawing of the club-shaped and spherical conidia that form laterally on delicate, hyaline hyphae. (From Winn WC Jr, et al. Koneman's Color Atlas and Textbook of Diagnostic Microbiology. 6th Ed. Philadelphia: Lippincott Williams & Wilkins, 2006.)

Madura foot are derived from the name of an Indonesian island, Madura. Mycetomas most commonly occur in tropical and subtropical regions where shoes are not worn. The fungal agents enter the skin through traumatic wounds and penetrating injuries.

Pus from mycetoma lesions often contain grains or granules that vary in color. There are two general categories of mycetomas, depending on the nature of the etiologic agent: (1) **eumycotic mycetomas,** which are caused by fungi, and (2) **actinomycotic mycetomas,** which are caused

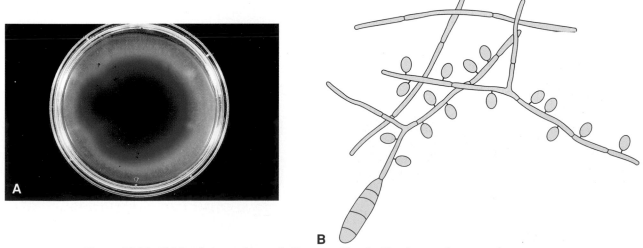

Figure 20-10. Trichophyton rubrum. **A.** Reverse side of a *T. rubrum* colony growing on potato dextrose agar. The deep wine-red pigmentation that is characteristic of this species is particularly intense when the organism is grown on potato dextrose or cornmeal agar. **B.** Drawing of the tiny "birds on a fence" conidia that form on the sides of the hyphae. (From Winn WC Jr, et al. Koneman's Color Atlas and Textbook of Diagnostic Microbiology. 6th Ed. Philadelphia: Lippincott Williams & Wilkins, 2006.)

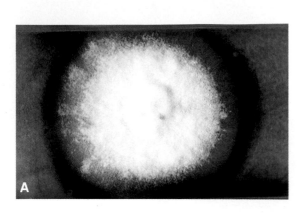

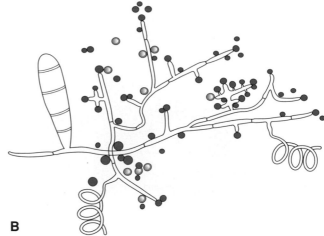

B

Figure 20-11. Trichophyton mentagrophytes. **A.** Fluffy variant of *T. mentagrophytes* growing on Sabouraud dextrose agar. Certain strains of *T. mentagrophytes* produce a reddish pigmentation (as seen here), but the color is never as intense as is seen with *T. rubrum* growing on potato dextrose or cornmeal agar. **B.** Drawing of tiny, spherical conidia arranged in loose clusters. (From Winn WC Jr, et al. Koneman's Color Atlas and Textbook of Diagnostic Microbiology. 6th Ed. Philadelphia: Lippincott Williams & Wilkins, 2006.)

by funguslike bacteria (actinomycetes). Table 20-4 contains information about the etiologic agents of mycetomas and the color of the granules they produce.

Clinical specimens. Pus, curettings, and biopsy specimens are acceptable for diagnosis of mycetomas. Curettings are scrapings that have been collected by using a sharp-edged instrument known as a curette. Pus may be obtained either from draining fistulas or by needle and syringe.[1] Specimens

should be transported to the CML in sterile shallow bottles or petri dishes.

Screening tests. Specimens should be examined for the presence of granules that typically are 0.5 to 2 mm in diameter. Granules should be crushed in a drop of 10% KOH or lactophenol cotton blue stain on a glass microscope slide and then examined microscopically. Microscopic examination reveals that the granules are composed of either colorless or

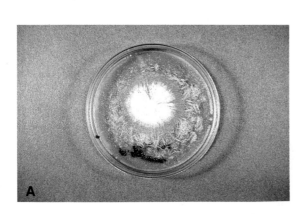

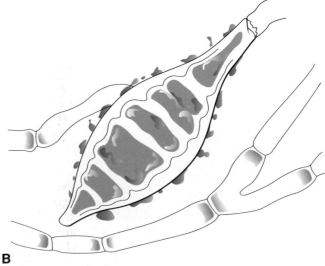

B

Figure 20-12. Microsporum canis. **A.** *M. canis* colony after 5 days of incubation. Colonies of *M. canis* may be fluffy or granular if conidia production is heavy. The lemon-yellow apron or margin surrounding the colony is typical of this species. **B.** Drawing of a multicelled macroconidium. Notice the spindle shape, thick spiny wall, cross septations, and tapered tip. (From Winn WC Jr, et al. Koneman's Color Atlas and Textbook of Diagnostic Microbiology. 6th Ed. Philadelphia: Lippincott Williams & Wilkins, 2006.)

[1]*A fistula is an abnormal passage from one epithelial surface to another.*

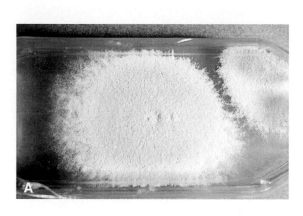
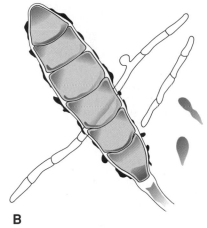

Figure 20-13. Microsporum gypseum. **A.** Powdery, off-yellow *M. gypseum* colony after 6 days of incubation. Because *M. gypseum* sporulates more heavily than *M. canis*, its colonies tend to be more granular than those of *M. canis*. **B.** Drawing of a multicelled macroconidium. Notice the thick, spiny wall, cross septations, and rounded terminal cell. (From Winn WC Jr, et al. Koneman's Color Atlas and Textbook of Diagnostic Microbiology. 6th Ed. Philadelphia: Lippincott Williams & Wilkins, 2006.)

pigmented septate hyphae (in the case of fungal agents) *or* branching bacteria (Fig. 20-16). Fungal hyphae are 2 to 5 μm in diameter, whereas the branching bacteria are only about 1 μm in diameter. The yellow or yellowish granules produced by some actinomycetes are referred to as sulfur granules.

Media to be inoculated. Aspirates may be directly inoculated onto Sabouraud dextrose agar, but granules from draining fistulas should first be washed in a sterile saline or antibiotic solution to reduce contamination. Cultures are incubated at both 30°C and 37°C. Because some of the fungal agents are slow growing, cultures should be held for 3 to 4 weeks.

Laboratory diagnosis. Fungal isolates are identified by a combination of macroscopic and microscopic observations. Because eucaryotic mycetoma may be caused either by hyaline or dematiaceous moulds, the colonies may either be light colored or dark. Recall from Chapter 19 that the term *hyalohyphomycoses* refers to fungal infections caused by hyaline fungi—fungi that produce colorless or transparent hyphae. Some of the hyaline moulds that cause eucaryotic mycetoma—*Acremonium* spp., *Aspergillus flavus*, *Fusarium* spp., and *Pseudoallescheria boydii*—are discussed in this section. In the United States, the most common cause of mycetoma is *P. boydii*. It is important to understand that the

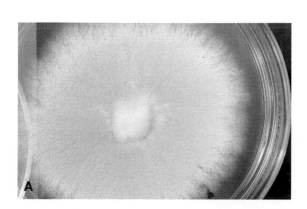
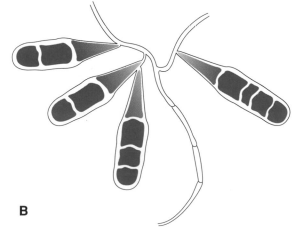

Figure 20-14. Epidermophyton floccosum. **A.** *E. floccosum* colony after 6 days of incubation. This colony is more fluffy than granular because microconidia are not produced by *Epidermophyton* spp. Although the colony shown here has an off-yellow pigmentation, classic *E. floccosum* colonies are described as khaki green. **B.** Drawing of the elongated, cylindrical-shaped macroconidia of *E. floccosum*, illustrating their smooth walls and transverse septa. (From Winn WC Jr, et al. Koneman's Color Atlas and Textbook of Diagnostic Microbiology. 6th Ed. Philadelphia: Lippincott Williams & Wilkins, 2006.)

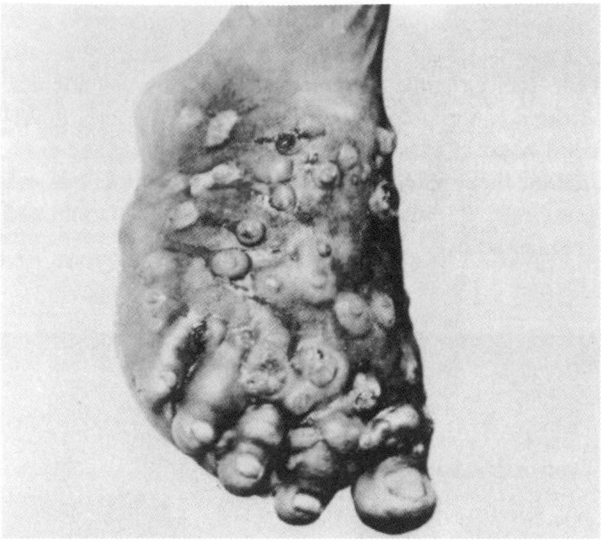

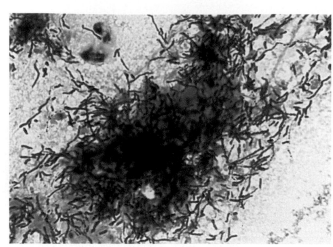

Figure 20-15. **Mycetoma of the foot (Madura foot).** (From Binford CH, Connor DH. Pathology of Tropical and Extraordinary Diseases, vol 2. Washington, DC: Armed Forces Institute of Pathology, 1976.)

Figure 20-16. **Gram-stained, crushed sulfur granule composed of branched, beaded, filamentous Gram-positive bacteria suggestive of *Actinomyces* spp.** (From Marler LM, Siders JA, Allen SD. Direct Smear Atlas. Philadelphia: Lippincott Williams & Wilkins, 2001.)

hyaline fungi mentioned here can also cause infections other than mycetoma.

The term *phaeohyphomycoses* refers to fungal infections caused by dematiaceous fungi—fungi having dark-pigmented hyphae. Dematiaceous moulds that cause mycetoma are discussed later in the section titled "Chromoblastomycosis." It is important to understand that the term *phaeohyphomycosis* is not limited to mycetoma. Dematiaceous fungi can also cause

many other types of infections, including sinusitis, keratitis, endocarditis, and pneumonia.

***Acremonium* spp.** *Acremonium* spp. tend to produce rather delicate mycelia, which appear smooth or glabrous, as opposed to the more wooly or granular mycelia of other hyaline moulds. The mycelia may be white or various shades of light pastel green and yellow (Fig. 20-17A). On microscopic

TABLE 20 - 4   Most Common Etiologic Agents of Mycetomas[a]

Category	Color of Granules in Pus	Possible Etiologic Agent
Eumycotic mycetoma	White	*Acremonium* spp., *Aspergillus nidulans, Cylindrocarpon destructans, Fusarium* spp., *Neotestudina rosatii, Polycytella hominis, Pseudoallescheria boydii, Pseudochaetosphaeronema larense*
	Black	*Corynespora cassicola, Curvularia* spp., *Exophiala jeansellmei, Leptosphaeria* spp., *Madurella* spp., *Pyrenochaeta romeroi*
Actinomycotic mycetoma	White	*Nocardia asteroides*
	White yellow	*Actinomadura madurae*
	White to yellow	*Nocardia brasiliensis*
	Yellow	*Streptomyces somaliensis*
	Garnet red	*Actinomadura pelletieri*

[a]Aerobic actinomycetes are discussed in Chapter 10, and anaerobic actinomycetes are discussed in Chapter 17.

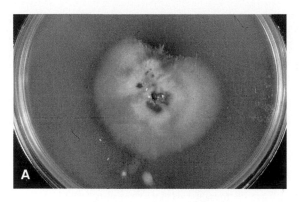

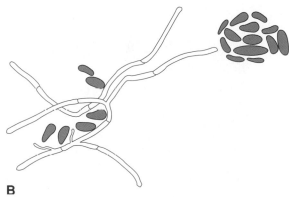

B

***Figure 20-17. Acremonium* spp. A.** *Acremonium* colony after 5 days of incubation on Sabouraud dextrose agar. *Acremonium* colonies usually have a smooth, almost yeastlike appearance because of the extremely delicate nature of the hyphae and spore-producing structures. Colonies may be light pastel yellow, light green, or peach red. **B.** Drawing of a delicate conidiophore supporting a loose cluster of elliptical conidia arranged in a diphtheroidal pattern. (From Winn WC Jr, et al. Koneman's Color Atlas and Textbook of Diagnostic Microbiology. 6th Ed. Philadelphia: Lippincott Williams & Wilkins, 2006.)

observation of slide cultures, the microconidia of *Acremonium* spp. are elongated and arranged in loose clusters, described as a crisscross formation or having a diphtheroidal appearance (Fig. 20-17B).

Aspergillus flavus. *Aspergillus flavus* colonies are granular to wooly and yellow, yellow-green, or yellow-brown (Fig. 20-18A). *Flavus* is Latin for "yellow." Microscopically, *A. flavus* resembles a dandelion that is in the process of producing seeds or a daisy head. Chains of conidia arise from either a single or double row of phialides, covering the entire surface of a central spherical vesicle (Fig. 20-18B). **Phialides** are conidia-producing cells.

> Microscopically, the fruiting bodies of *Aspergillus* spp. resemble dandelions in the process of producing seeds—the kind that children blow on to make the white seeds drift off.

***Fusarium* spp.** The mycelia of *Fusarium* spp. are generally cottony or wooly, with a distinctive lavender, rose-red, or magenta surface and reverse-side pigmentation (Fig. 20-19A). *Fusarium* spp. produce both microconidia and macroconidia. The microconidia resemble those of *Acremonium* spp. The characteristic macroconidia are the key to identification of *Fusarium* spp. They are long, sickle shaped, and multicellular, resembling green-bean pods or bananas (Fig. 20-19B). The terminal cell, called the foot cell, has a small, hairlike extension.

Pseudallescheria boydii. Colonies of *P. boydii* develop rapidly. Initially, they are cottony white with aerial hyphae, but later, as a result of conidia production, they become gray and then brown. Older colonies have a gray-to-black reverse side. A slide mount reveals moderately large, septate hyphae, with long or short conidiophores, each terminated by a single oval-to-pear-shaped pigmented conidium (Fig. 20-20). Note: Unless cleistothecia are observed, this

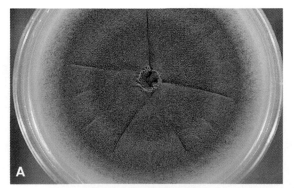

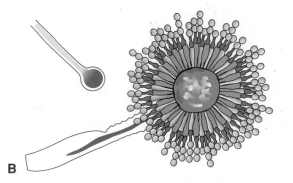

B

Figure 20-18. Aspergillus flavus. A. *A. flavus* colony on Sabouraud dextrose agar. The texture of mature *A. flavus* colonies is usually granular as a result of conidia production. Some shade of yellow is characteristic. **B.** Drawing of a central spherical vesicle, supporting a double row of phialides that arise from the entire surface of the vesicle. (From Winn WC Jr, et al. Koneman's Color Atlas and Textbook of Diagnostic Microbiology. 6th Ed. Philadelphia: Lippincott Williams & Wilkins, 2006.)

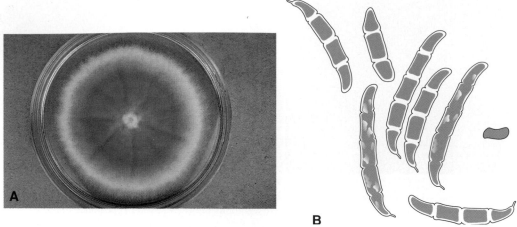

Figure 20-19. ***Fusarium*** **sp. A.** *Fusarium* sp. colony after 6 days of growth on Sabouraud dextrose agar. *Fusarium* should be suspected when a rapidly growing granular or fluffy rose-red, lavender, or purple colony is observed. **B.** Drawing of the characteristic long, multicelled, canoe- or boat-shaped macroconidia. (From Winn WC Jr, et al. Koneman's Color Atlas and Textbook of Diagnostic Microbiology. 6th Ed. Philadelphia: Lippincott Williams & Wilkins, 2006.)

fungus should be called *Scedosporium apiospermum*, rather than *P. boydii*. Cleistothecia are brown, 100 to 200 μm long, and develop around the periphery of the colony. They mature by 10 days.

Chromoblastomycosis

Disease and most likely pathogens. Chromoblastomycosis or chromomycosis is a chronic, spreading fungal infection of the skin and subcutaneous tissues, usually afflicting a lower extremity. Progression to surrounding tissues is slow, over a period of years, eventually producing large bumpy or even cauliflower-like masses and blockage of the flow of lymph. Chromoblastomycosis is primarily a disease of rural, barefooted agricultural workers in tropical regions.

Direct examination. Microscopic examination of scrapings or biopsy material reveals large, brown, thick-walled, rounded cells. Confirmation of the diagnosis is made by biopsy and attempted culture of the fungal pathogen.

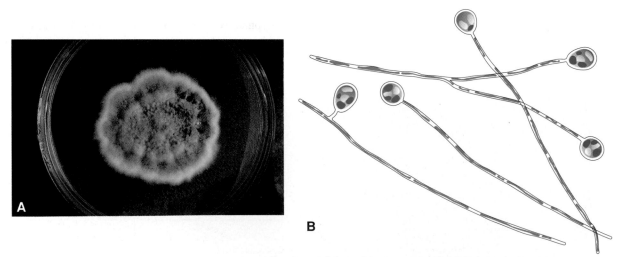

Figure 20-20. ***Scedosporium apiospermum*** **(the anamorphic form of *Pseudallescheria boydii*).** **A.** Five-day-old colony on Sabouraud dextrose agar. *S. apiospermum* colonies are a characteristic "house mouse" gray color, with a silky or fluffy surface on which tiny water droplets appear. Rapidly growing mould colonies that are mouse-gray color should be suspected of being *S. apiospermum*. **B.** Straight, narrow, lollipop-like conidiophores. (From Winn WC Jr, et al. Koneman's Color Atlas and Textbook of Diagnostic Microbiology. 6th Ed. Philadelphia: Lippincott Williams & Wilkins, 2006.)

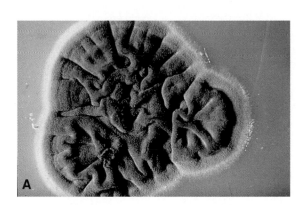

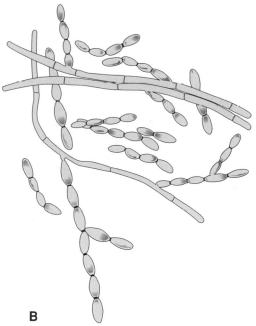

Figure 20-21. Cladosporium **spp. A.** Environmental strain of a *Cladosporium* spp., a dematiaceous mould. This particular strain produces a dark green mycelium, with a suedelike surface and numerous rugae (grooves). Environmental strains of *Cladosporium* spp. may be green, gray, gray-brown, or brown-black. **B.** Drawing of cladosporium-type sporulation. Freely branching hyphae give rise to long chains of dark-staining, elliptical conidia separated by delicate scars known as dysjunctors. (From Winn WC Jr, et al. Koneman's Color Atlas and Textbook of Diagnostic Microbiology. 6th Ed. Philadelphia: Lippincott Williams & Wilkins, 2006.)

Laboratory diagnosis. Dematiaceous fungi that cause mycetoma and chromoblastomycosis include *Cladophialophora* (*Cladosporium*), *Phialophora*, *Fonsecaea*, *Exophiala*, and *Wangiella* spp. (Figs. 20-21 through 20-23). Mycelia of dematiaceous fungi are dark, but they vary in color, and their textures may be wooly, downy or hairlike, or similar to suede or leather. Species are primarily differentiated by their mode of conidia formation, the structure of conidiophores and phialides, and the morphology and arrangement of their conidia.

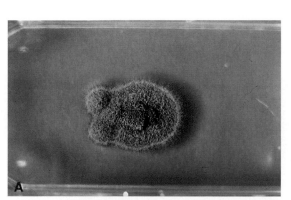

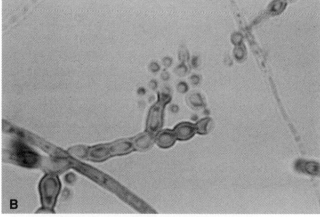

Figure 20-22. Phialophora verrucosum. **A.** *P. verrucosum* colony after 14 days of incubation. This strain has a dark gray-black hue with a hairlike texture. **B.** Phialophora-type sporulation of the type seen in *P. verrucosum.* Ball-like clusters of spherical to oval-shaped, yellow-pigmented conidia emerge from urn-shaped phialides. The elongated terminal portion of each phialide causes the structure to resemble a vase or soda bottle. Not all *Phialophora* spp. have bottlelike phialides. (From Winn WC Jr, et al. Koneman's Color Atlas and Textbook of Diagnostic Microbiology. 6th Ed. Philadelphia: Lippincott Williams & Wilkins, 2006.)

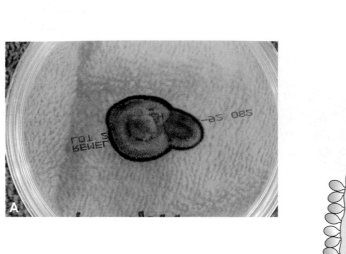

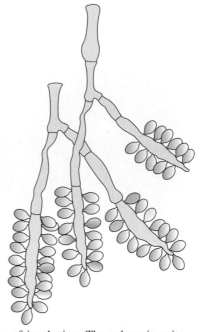

B

Figure 20-23. Fonsecaea pedrosoi. A. Colony after 16 days of incubation. The colony is quite small, with typical dark brown-black pigmentation. This strain has a flat, almost suedelike consistency. **B.** Drawing of rhinocladiella-type sporulation, as seen in some strains of *F. pedrosoi.* Elliptical conidia are produced singly, directly, and laterally in compact rows from the sides of conidiophores. (From Winn WC Jr, et al. Koneman's Color Atlas and Textbook of Diagnostic Microbiology. 6th Ed. Philadelphia: Lippincott Williams & Wilkins, 2006.)

Sporotrichosis

Disease. Sporotrichosis is a fungal disease that typically affects the skin of an extremity. The disease starts as a nodule but develops into a series of nodules that may soften and ulcerate. Systemic complications are rare.

Pathogen. Sporotrichosis is caused by a dimorphic fungus named *Sporothrix schenckii.* It is usually acquired by introduction of the organism through the skin (traumatic implantation) when the skin is pricked by thorns or barbs, by slivers of wood, or when handling sphagnum moss or hay. Sporotrichosis is an occupational disease of farmers, gardeners, and horticulturists.

> Remember that *Sporothrix schenckii* is a dimorphic fungus. It exists as a yeast within the human body (37°C) but grows as a mould at room temperature.

Clinical specimens. Diagnosis of sporotrichosis is confirmed by stain and culture of a biopsy. The pathogen is

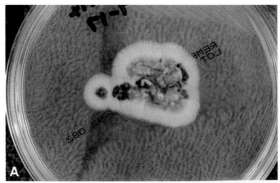

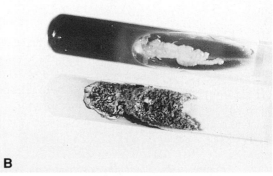

Figure 20-24. Sporothrix schenckii. A. Smooth, gray-brown yeast colony. As a result of extremely delicate sporulation, *S. schenckii* colonies appear more yeastlike than mouldlike, even when grown at 25°C to 30°C. Colonies darken with prolonged incubation, with some strains becoming almost jet-black. **B.** *S. schenckii* growing in two tubes of brain-heart infusion agar, the yeast form in the top tube and the mould form in the bottom tube. (From Winn WC Jr, et al. Koneman's Color Atlas and Textbook of Diagnostic Microbiology. 6th Ed. Philadelphia: Lippincott Williams & Wilkins, 2006.)

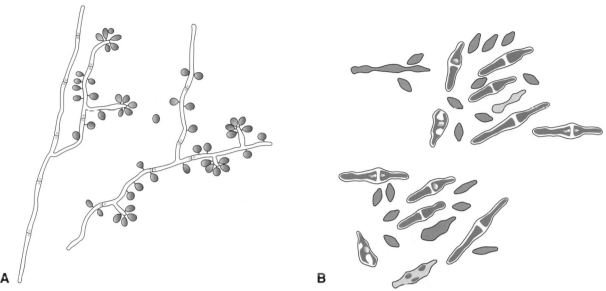

Figure 20-25. S. schenckii. A. Drawing of the microscopic appearance of the mould form of *S. schenckii*. Careful examination reveals an extremely short, thin structure by which each conidium is attached to a conidiophore. **B.** Drawing of the yeast forms of *S. schenckii*, some of which are in an elongated, two-celled stage described as a "cigar body" form. (From Winn WC Jr, et al. Koneman's Color Atlas and Textbook of Diagnostic Microbiology. 6th Ed. Philadelphia: Lippincott Williams & Wilkins, 2006.)

rarely observed on direct smears. Biopsy material should be stained with fungal stains. Pus or exudate rarely yields the pathogen.

Laboratory diagnosis. When grown at 30°C, *S. schenckii* colonies are initially smooth but may become tough and wrinkled or folded with age. When mature, dark, fuzzy, aerial hyphae develop. Colonies are initially gray-white but turn buff, brown, or brown-black with age (Fig. 20-24A). When incubated at 37°C, *S. schenckii* produces yeastlike colonies that may turn dark brown or black when mature (Fig. 20-24B).

Microscopic examination of the mould form of *S. schenckii* reveals delicate, hyaline, septate hyphae bearing small, oval, hyaline, smooth conidia. The conidia arise from delicate conidiophores located on the sides or tips of the hyphae. Sometimes the conidia are arranged in a daisylike cluster at the tip of a conidiophore (Fig. 20-25A). Fine focus should reveal an extremely thin, hairlike structure between the conidiophore and the conidium. (The genus name *Sporothrix* is based on these tiny hairlike structures: *thrix* is Greek for "hair.") The yeast forms tend to be oval or elliptical, often with a single bud (Fig. 20-25B).

Protothecosis

Disease and pathogen. Protothecosis is not a fungal disease but a rare illness caused by an alga. The disease is being discussed here because the etiologic agents of protothecosis—*Prototheca* spp.—are sometimes isolated in the mycology section of the CML and are sometimes confused with fungi. Unlike most algae, the cells of *Prototheca* spp. do not contain chloroplasts. For this reason, *Prototheca* spp. are referred to as achloric algae. They are found in soil and water.

> Protothecosis is a rare disease caused by an alga. The etiologic agents, *Prototheca* spp., can be isolated in the mycology section and can be confused with fungi.

Prototheca spp. can enter wounds, especially those located on the feet, producing a small subcutaneous lesion that can progress to a crusty, warty-looking lesion. Severe subcutaneous infections are rare, but they do occur (Fig. 20-26). If the organism enters the lymphatic system, it may cause a debilitating, sometimes fatal infection, especially in immunosuppressed patients. Fatal infections are extremely rare.

In stained tissue sections, *Prototheca* spp. appear as ovoid or spherical cells, ranging in size from 3 to 15 μm. The parent cell divides asexually by septation to form two, four, eight, or more internal spores (Fig. 20-27). The spores are discharged when the parent cell ruptures.

Laboratory diagnosis. *Prototheca* spp. can be grown in the laboratory. They produce yeastlike, white to cream-colored colonies that may be dull, moist, or mucoid in appearance. Individual cells of *Prototheca* spp. may be round, oval, or cylindrical. Unlike yeasts, they do not reproduce by budding. Some commercial miniaturized biochemical test systems (minisystems) for the identification of yeasts can be used to identify *Prototheca* spp.

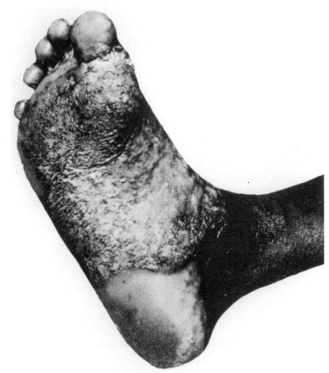

Figure 20-26. **Protothecosis, of 5 years' duration.** (From Binford CH, Connor DH. Pathology of Tropical and Extraordinary Diseases, vol 2. Washington, DC: Armed Forces Institute of Pathology, 1976.)

SYSTEMIC MYCOSES

Systemic mycoses, which are also known as generalized or deep-seated mycoses, are the most serious types of fungal infections. They are fungal infections of internal organs of the body, sometimes affecting two or more organ systems simultaneously—for example, simultaneous infection of the respiratory system and the bloodstream, or simultaneous infection of the respiratory tract and the central nervous system. The most common causes of systemic mycoses are dimorphic fungi; opportunistic moulds like *Aspergillus*, *Penicillium*, and some bread moulds; and yeasts like *Candida albicans* and *Cryptococcus neoformans*.

Fungal Infections of the Lower Respiratory Tract

Pulmonary Zygomycosis

Disease and pathogens. The term *zygomycosis* (formerly *mucormycosis* or *phycomycosis*) refers to a disease caused by one of the many fungi in the class Zygomycetes. These fungi, collectively referred to as zygomycetes, are widely distributed in soil and vegetative matter. Most commonly, humans become infected with zygomycetes by inhaling

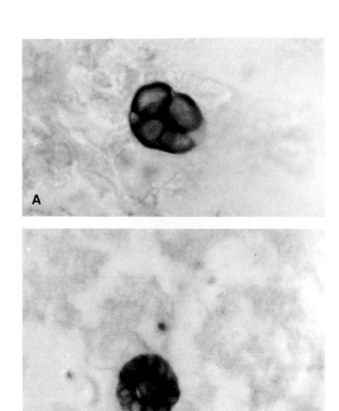

Figure 20-27. *Prototheca* **cells in stained tissue specimens.** **A.** Cell containing internal spores. **B.** Some cells develop a distinct and characteristic morular pattern.

airborne spores, although ingestion and direct inoculation through traumatic breaks in the skin and mucous membranes can also lead to infection. Although these fungi are being discussed in a section on lower respiratory diseases, it is important to keep in mind that they cause diseases with a wide range of clinical manifestations. Examples of other clinical syndromes caused by members of the Zygomycetes class include sinusitis, cerebral infection, cutaneous disease, gastrointestinal disease, and disseminated disease, which can involve virtually every organ.

The class Zygomycetes consists of two orders that contain human pathogens: Mucorales and Entomophthorales. Only members of the order Mucorales are described here. The most important members of the order Mucorales are in the genera *Mucor*, *Rhizopus*, and *Absidia*. These fungi are often referred to as bread moulds because they are responsible for the white or gray fuzzy growth seen on foods such as bread and cheese. The fuzziness is a result of aseptate aerial

> Zygomycetes have aseptate hyphae. However, in the laboratory, zygomycete hyphae can become sparsely septate in older cultures.

hyphae. (Recall from Chapter 19 that the cytoplasm of aseptate hyphae is *not* divided into individual cells by cross walls or septa.) In the laboratory, however, hyphae can become sparsely septate in older cultures. Spores called sporangiospores are produced in saclike structures called sporangia (sing. *sporangium*) at the tips of sporangiophores.

Laboratory diagnosis. Diagnosis of zygomycosis can be made by microscopic observation of distinctive ribbon-like, broad, aseptate hyphae in tissue sections and by culture of biopsy tissues. The hyphae range from 3 to 25 μm in width. Isolation alone is insufficient, because members of the Mucorales order are common contaminants. Members of the class Zygomycetes are rapid growers. They have been referred to as lid lifters because they can completely fill a petri dish with a wooly mycelium in 48 to 72 hours. Microscopic examination reveals broad, aseptate hyphae and sporangia.

> Zygomycetes are rapid growers. They have been called lid lifters because in 48 to 72 hours they can completely fill a petri dish with a wooly mycelium.

The next thing to note is whether or not the isolate is producing rhizoids—tiny rootlike structures present in some species. *Rhizopus* and *Absidia* spp. possesses rhizoids, but *Mucor* spp. do not. Rhizoids may either be nodal or internodal. Nodal rhizoids, such as those seen in *Rhizopus* spp., arise from hyphae at a point immediately adjacent to sporangiophores (Fig. 20-28). Internodal rhizoids, as seen in

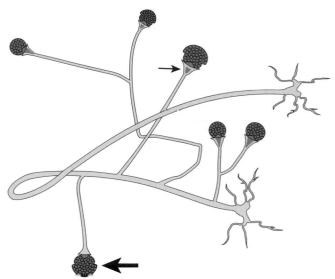

Figure 20-29. Photomicrograph of an *Absidia* sp. Notice the internodal rhizoids and the typical funnel-like expansion (*small arrow*) at the tip of each sporangiophore into a structure known as the apophysis (*large arrow*). Also notice the branching of some of the sporangiophores. (From Winn WC Jr, et al. Koneman's Color Atlas and Textbook of Diagnostic Microbiology. 6th Ed. Philadelphia: Lippincott Williams & Wilkins, 2006.)

Absidia spp., arise from points along the hyphae that are between the sporangiophores (Fig. 20-29). As previously mentioned, *Mucor* spp. do not produce rhizoids.

Bronchopulmonary Aspergillosis

Disease and pathogens. *Aspergillus* spp. are ubiquitous in nature, meaning that they are found virtually everywhere. They are present in soil, decaying vegetation, and various types of organic matter, such as piles of leaves or compost piles. Inhalation of spores can lead to sinusitis or lower respiratory infection (Fig. 20-30 and 20-31). Invasive aspergillosis can affect the eyes, heart, kidneys, skin, and other organs. Invasive infection is most commonly caused by *A. flavus*, *A. fumigatus*, *A. nidulans*, *A. niger*, and *A. terreus*.

Screening tests. Diagnosis of bronchopulmonary aspergillosis can be made by radiograph, isolation by culture, skin testing, and immunodiagnostic procedures.

Laboratory diagnosis. *Aspergillus* spp. are rapid growers, forming colonies within 3 to 5 days. Young colonies are cottony, but the colony surface becomes sugary or granular as conidia are produced. Because *Aspergillus* spores are found throughout the environment, they are commonly isolated in the laboratory as contaminants.

Aspergillus flavus. *A. flavus* has been previously described, in the section on eucaryotic mycetoma (see Fig. 20-18).

Aspergillus fumigatus. *A. fumigatus* colonies are granular to cottony and usually blue-green, green-gray, or green-brown

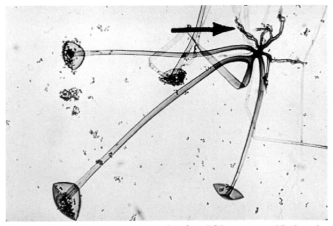

Figure 20-28. Photomicrograph of a *Rhizopus* sp. Notice the nodal rhizoids (*arrow*) and the typical collapsed umbrella shape of the sporangia following the release of sporangiospores. These sporangia are sometimes referred to as collapsed or postmature sporangia. (From Winn WC Jr, et al. Koneman's Color Atlas and Textbook of Diagnostic Microbiology. 6th Ed. Philadelphia: Lippincott Williams & Wilkins, 2006.)

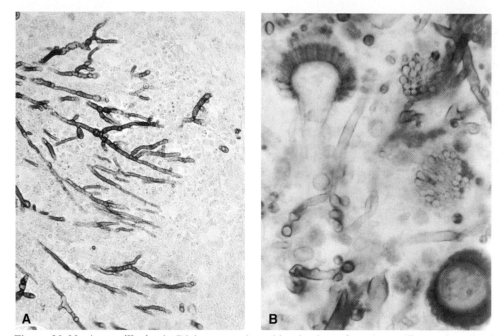

***Figure 20-30.* Aspergillosis. A.** Dichotomous branching hyphae of an *Aspergillus* sp. in stained lung tissue. **B.** *Aspergillus* hyphae and characteristic conidiophores (fruiting bodies) in stained material from a pulmonary abscess. (From Binford CH, Connor DH. Pathology of Tropical and Extraordinary Diseases, vol 2. Washington, DC: Armed Forces Institute of Pathology, 1976.)

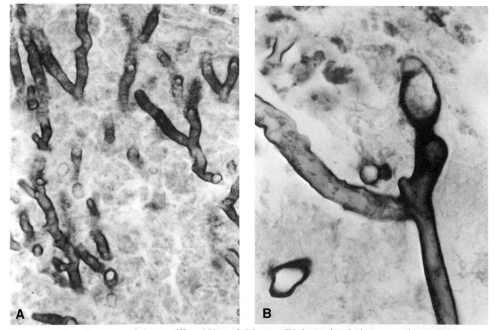

***Figure 20-31.* Hyphae of *Aspergillus* (A) and *Mucor* (B) in stained tissue sections.** These photomicrographs were taken at the same magnification. Notice the difference in the diameter of the hyphae. Hyphae of most *Aspergillus* spp. are septate and usually less than 10 μm in diameter, whereas hyphae of *Mucor* spp. and most other zygomycetes are nonseptate and greater than 10 μm in diameter. (From Binford CH, Connor DH. Pathology of Tropical and Extraordinary Diseases, vol 2. Washington, DC: Armed Forces Institute of Pathology, 1976.)

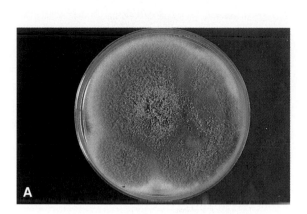

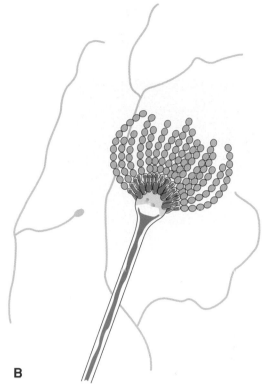

Figure 20-32. Aspergillus fumigatus. **A.** Five-day-old *A. fumigatus* colony on Sabouraud dextrose agar. The outer margin often appears as a white apron, as can be seen here. **B.** Drawing of the fruiting head of *A. fumigatus*, with long, inwardly curving chains of conidia arising from a single row of phialides located on the top half of a club-shaped vesicle. (From Winn WC Jr, et al. Koneman's Color Atlas and Textbook of Diagnostic Microbiology. 6th Ed. Philadelphia: Lippincott Williams & Wilkins, 2006.)

(Fig. 20-32A). Microscopically, the relatively long (300 to 500 μm) conidiophores arise from a segment of a septate hypha known as a foot cell. The fruiting head of *A. fumigatus* has a single row of phialides over the upper half of a club-shaped vesicle (Fig. 20-32B). Spherical, usually smooth conidia arise from the phialides in long chains that tend to curve inward.

Aspergillus niger. The surface of a mature *A. niger* colony is covered with a dense aggregate of jet-black conidia, causing a characteristic peppered effect (Fig. 20-33A). The color of *A. niger* colonies is caused by pigmented aerial hyphae, as opposed to colonies of dematiaceous fungi whose color is caused by pigmented vegetative hyphae. The reverse side of an *A. niger* colony is buff or yellow-gray, whereas the reverse side of a dematiaceous fungus colony is jet-black. Microscopically, dense sporulation is observed on *A. niger*, with conidia often covering the entire surface of the vesicle (Fig. 20-33B). Conidia arise from a double row of phialides.

Aspergillus terreus. Colonies of *A. terreus* are granular; buff, brown, or orange-brown; with radial grooves called **rugae** (Fig. 20-34A).[2] As with *A. fumigatus*, *A. terreus* sporulation occurs from the top half of a club-shaped vesicle. However,

A. terreus vesicles are smaller than those of *A. fumigatus*, a double row of phialides is present, and the phialides are much longer than those of *A. fumigatus* (Fig. 20-34B). *A. terreus* also produces tiny, smooth, spherical microconidia that are attached laterally to vegetative hyphae.

Penicilliosis

Diseases and pathogens. The only true pathogen in the genus *Penicillium* is *P. marneffei*, which is a common cause of opportunistic infections in AIDS patients in Southeast Asia. Infections are usually disseminated, involving lungs, liver, and skin. *P. marneffei* is unique among *Penicillium* spp., in that it is a dimorphic fungus. It produces yeastlike cells in tissues and rich media at 37°C.

Although several other *Penicillium* spp. have been reported as the cause of lung infection, endocarditis, fungemia, peritonitis, urinary tract infection, and disseminated infections, isolation of a *Penicillium* sp. usually represents contamination.

Laboratory diagnosis. Presumptive diagnosis of *P. marneffei* infection can be made by demonstration of yeastlike, oval, or cylindrical cells in Wright-stained smears from skin lesions or

---

[2] *The grooves that radiate outward from the center of a mould colony are called rugae (sing. ruga). A mould colony possessing rugae is described as being rugose.*

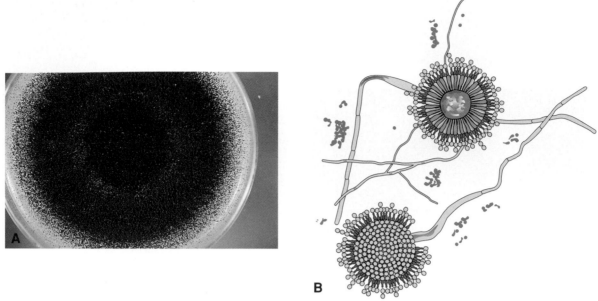

Figure 20-33. Aspergillus niger. **A.** *A. niger* colony after 4 days of incubation on Sabouraud dextrose agar. A deep brown or black, densely stippled surface is characteristic of *A. niger*, caused by pigmented aerial hyphae. The reverse side of an *A. niger* colony is light gray or buff. **B.** Drawing of the fruiting head of *A. niger*. (From Winn WC Jr, et al. Koneman's Color Atlas and Textbook of Diagnostic Microbiology. 6th Ed. Philadelphia: Lippincott Williams & Wilkins, 2006.)

biopsy specimens. The cells are 3 to 6 μm long, and may have a cross wall. *P. marneffei* colonies are granular to fluffy, depending on the degree of sporulation, and possess a distinct white apron or margin (Fig. 20-35). *P. marneffei* can be suspected if its wine-red pigment is observed diffusing into the agar. Immunodiagnostic and molecular diagnostic procedures are available to diagnose *P. marneffei* infection.

Colonies of other *Penicillium* spp. are granular and usually blue-green (Fig. 20-36A), although yellow and yellow-brown variants are sometimes seen. Microscopically, the

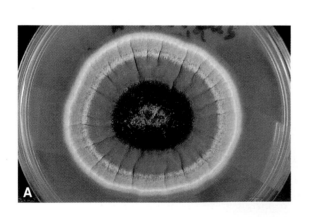

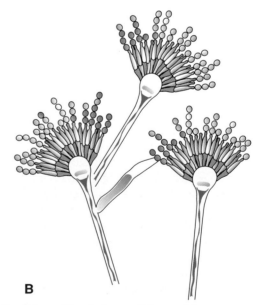

Figure 20-34. Aspergillus terreus. **A.** *A. terreus* colony after 6 days of incubation on Sabouraud dextrose agar. *A. terreus* colonies typically have a granular surface and some shade of yellow or brown pigmentation. Radiating rugae are often seen, and concentric zones of light and dark pigmentation are not unusual. **B.** Drawing of the fruiting structure of *A. terreus*. Chains of conidia arise from a double row of phialides over the upper half of a swollen vesicle. (From Winn WC Jr, et al. Koneman's Color Atlas and Textbook of Diagnostic Microbiology. 6th Ed. Philadelphia: Lippincott Williams & Wilkins, 2006.)

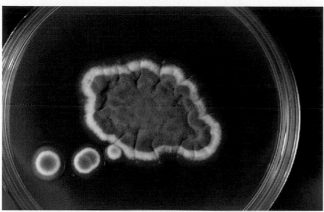

Figure 20-35. Penicillium marneffei **colony after 4 days of incubation on Sabouraud dextrose agar.** Notice the red pigmentation of a portion of the colony. Leaching of the red pigment has caused the agar to turn a light wine-red color. (From Winn WC Jr, et al. Koneman's Color Atlas and Textbook of Diagnostic Microbiology. 6th Ed. Philadelphia: Lippincott Williams & Wilkins, 2006.)

> Microscopically, the fruiting bodies of *Penicillium* spp. resemble paintbrushes.

chains of conidia emanating from the blunt tips of phialides. The conidia are spherical and regular in size, and stain evenly.

Pulmonary Cryptococcosis

Cryptococcosis is caused by the yeast *Cryptococcus neoformans*. Although cryptococcosis starts as a lung infection, it usually spreads via the bloodstream to the brain. The disease is described in a later section of this chapter titled "Cryptococcal Meningitis." Figure 20-37 depicts a *Cryptococcus* sp. in a Gram-stained bronchoalveolar lavage.

Coccidioidomycosis

Disease. Coccidioidomycosis starts as a respiratory infection, with fever, chills, cough, and rarely, pleuritic pain. The primary infection may heal completely or may progress to the disseminated form of the disease, which is often fatal. Disseminated coccidioidomycosis may include lung lesions and abscesses throughout the body, especially in subcutaneous tissues, skin, bone, and the central nervous system. Other tissues and organs, such as inguinal lymph nodes, liver, kidneys, thyroid gland, heart, pituitary gland, esophagus, and pancreas, may be involved.

typical brushlike penicillus can be observed (Fig. 20-36B). The penicillus is composed of conidiophores that branch at their ends, with

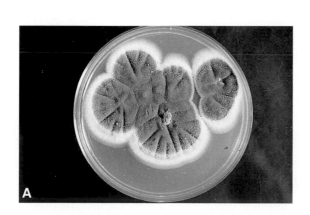

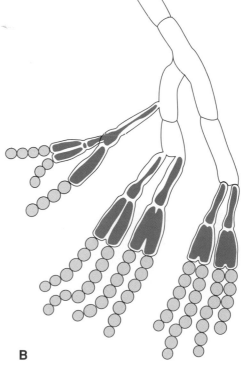

Figure 20-36. Penicillium sp. **A.** Typical blue-green color appears after 5 days of incubation on Sabouraud dextrose agar. Notice the granular surface, radial grooves (rugae), and white apron or margin. **B.** Drawing of brushlike penicillus produced by branching conidiophores and chains of spherical conidia. (From Winn WC Jr, et al. Koneman's Color Atlas and Textbook of Diagnostic Microbiology. 6th Ed. Philadelphia: Lippincott Williams & Wilkins, 2006.)

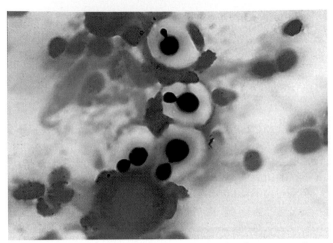

Figure 20-37. **Gram-stained bronchoalveolar lavage specimen containing four darkly stained, narrow-necked, budding yeasts, suggestive of a *Cryptococcus* sp.** The negatively stained halos surrounding the yeast cells are dense polysaccharide capsules. (From Marler LM, Siders JA, Allen SD. Direct Smear Atlas. Philadelphia: Lippincott Williams & Wilkins, 2001.)

Pathogen. Coccidioidomycosis is caused by *Coccidioides immitis*, a dimorphic fungus. It exists as a mould in soil and on culture media (25°C), where it produces arthrospores (arthroconidia; Fig. 20-38). In tissues, it appears as spherical cells called spherules that reproduce by endospore formation.

Arthrospores are present in soil in arid and semiarid areas of the Western Hemisphere: in the United States from California to southern Texas, and in Mexico, Central America, and South America. *C. immitis* is transmitted by inhalation of arthrospores, especially during wind and dust storms; it is not directly transmissible from person to person or animal to human. *C. immitis* arthrospores have potential use as a bioterrorism agent.

> *Coccidioides immitis* is a dimorphic fungus. It causes the disease coccidioidomycosis.

Clinical specimens. Specimens for the diagnosis of coccidioidomycosis include sputum, pus, urine, cerebrospinal fluid (CSF), and biopsy materials.

Screening tests. Spherules may be seen on direct examination of clinical specimens (Fig. 20-39). The spherules range from 20 to 200 μm in diameter. They contain endospores that, when mature, are 2 to 4 μm in diameter. Skin tests and immunodiagnostic procedures are also available.

Media to be inoculated. *C. immitis* can be isolated on Sabouraud dextrose agar or blood agar with or without chloramphenicol and cycloheximide. Better sporulation is achieved on modified cornmeal agar, glucose yeast extract agar, or yeast extract phosphate medium.

Laboratory diagnosis. The mycelia are gray-white and weblike or hairlike (Fig. 20-40). On sheep blood agar, the

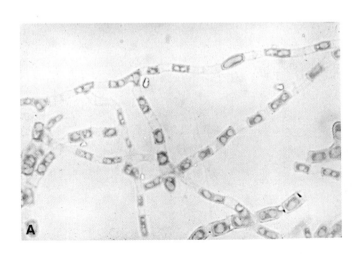

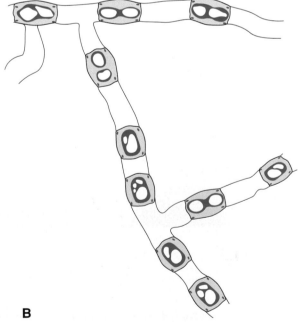

B

Figure 20-38. **Barrel-shaped arthrospores of *Coccidioides immitis*.** Photomicrograph (**A**) and drawing (**B**) show stained arthrospores separated by pale-staining empty spaces. (From Winn WC Jr, et al. Koneman's Color Atlas and Textbook of Diagnostic Microbiology. 6th Ed. Philadelphia: Lippincott Williams & Wilkins, 2006.)

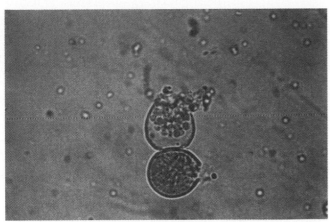

Figure 20-39. **Spherules of *C. immitis*.** The spherules contain endospores, many of which can be seen escaping from the ruptured upper spherule. (From Winn WC Jr, et al. Koneman's Color Atlas and Textbook of Diagnostic Microbiology. 6th Ed. Philadelphia: Lippincott Williams & Wilkins, 2006.)

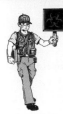

SAFETY TIP

Caution Required When Working with **Coccidioides immitis.** *The mould form of C. immitis is highly infectious. All work must be performed in a biosafety level 2 (BSL-2) or BSL-3 facility. All work involving fluffy mould colonies must be performed in a biosafety cabinet.* **Never sniff mould colonies.**

colonies may appear dark green-black as a result of absorption of hemoglobin pigments. When grown at 30°C, the hyphae are delicate and break up into barrel-shaped arthroconidia. The arthroconidia of *C. immitis* are separated by empty spaces. DNA probes are available for identification of *C. immitis*.

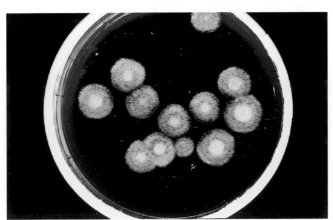

Figure 20-40. **Gray-white colonies of *C. immitis* on sheep blood agar after 7 days of incubation.** Notice the delicate, hairlike texture. (From Winn WC Jr, et al. Koneman's Color Atlas and Textbook of Diagnostic Microbiology. 6th Ed. Philadelphia: Lippincott Williams & Wilkins, 2006.)

Histoplasmosis

Disease. Histoplasmosis is a systemic mycosis of varying severity, ranging from asymptomatic to acute to chronic. The primary lesion is usually in the lungs. The acute disease involves malaise, fever, chills, headache, myalgia, chest pains, and a nonproductive cough (i.e., no sputum produced). Histoplasmosis is the most common systemic fungal infection in AIDS patients.

Pathogen. Histoplasmosis is caused by *Histoplasma capsulatum* var. *capsulatum*, a dimorphic fungus that grows as a mould in soil and as a yeast in animal and human hosts. Reservoirs include warm, moist soil containing a high organic content and bird droppings, especially chicken droppings but also bat droppings in caves and around starling, blackbird, and pigeon roosts. Transmission occurs via inhalation of conidia

> *Histoplasma capsulatum* is a dimorphic fungus. It causes the disease histoplasmosis.

(asexual spores) from soil. Bulldozing and excavation may produce aerosols of spores. Histoplasmosis is the most common systemic fungal disease in the United States, occurring primarily in the Ohio, Mississippi, and Missouri River valleys.

STUDY AID **What's in a Name?** Although the name *Histoplasma capsulatum* would lead one to think that this organism is encapsulated, it is not. In tissue sections, the *H. capsulatum* cells, often clustered within macrophages, are surrounded by a clear space, making it appear that they are encapsulated. When you think of encapsulated yeasts, think of *Cryptococcus neoformans*.

Clinical specimens. Specimens for the diagnosis of histoplasmosis include ulcer exudates, bo.ne marrow, sputum, and blood, and biopsies of ulcers, liver, lymph nodes, or lung.

Screening tests. *H. capsulatum* yeasts may be observed in Giemsa- or Wright-stained smears of ulcer exudates, bone marrow, sputum, and blood. Figure 20-41 illustrates what *H. capsulatum* looks like in a Gram-stained preparation. Special stains can be used to demonstrate the organism in biopsies of ulcers, liver, lymph nodes, or lung. Skin tests and immunodiagnostic procedures are available. Immunodiagnostic procedures can detect anti-*Histoplasma* antibodies in serum and *Histoplasma* antigens in serum and urine.

Media to be inoculated. Specimens may be inoculated onto brain-heart infusion agar with blood, yeast extract phosphate agar, of Sabouraud brain-heart-infusion agar with or without chloramphenicol or penicillin and streptomycin.

Laboratory diagnosis. *H. capsulatum* produces mould colonies when incubated at room temperature and yeast

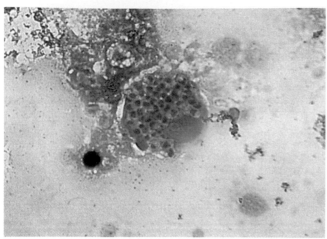

Figure 20-41. Gram-stained bronchoalveolar lavage. A macrophage contains numerous 2-to-4-μm-diameter yeast cells that are consistent in appearance with *Histoplasma capsulatum.* (From Marler LM, Siders JA, Allen SD. Direct Smear Atlas. Philadelphia: Lippincott Williams & Wilkins, 2001.)

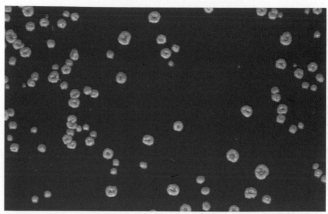

Figure 20-43. Small, yellowish yeast colonies of *H. capsulatum* on sheep blood agar incubated at 37°C. When this organism is incubated at room temperature, it produces mould colonies (see Fig. 20-42). (From Winn WC Jr, et al. Koneman's Color Atlas and Textbook of Diagnostic Microbiology. 6th Ed. Philadelphia: Lippincott Williams & Wilkins, 2006.)

colonies when incubated at body temperature. The mould form of *H. capsulatum* may take 10 to 30 days to grow on culture media, although heavy concentrations of organisms can produce mycelia as early as 5 days following inoculation. *H. capsulatum* produces a delicate weblike or hairlike mycelium that is initially white but turns gray or gray-brown with age (Fig. 20-42A). Microscopic examination of the colony reveals large, roughened or spiked macroconidia, ranging from 10 to 20 μm in diameter (Fig. 20-42B). Small, oval microconidia may be observed in young cultures; they appear in a sleevelike arrangement on the sides of delicate hyphae. DNA probes are available for identification of *H. capsulatum* mould colonies.

Conversion from the mould form to the yeast form can sometimes be accomplished in the laboratory. *H. capsulatum*

yeast colonies are typically smooth, yellow-white, and somewhat glistening and have a pasty consistency (Fig. 20-43). The individual yeast cells are 2 to 4 μm in diameter and may show a single bud connected by a delicate filament.

Blastomycosis

Disease. Blastomycosis is a granulomatous mycosis primarily affecting the lungs, skin, bone, and/or genitourinary tract. Pulmonary blastomycosis may either be acute or chronic. Extrapulmonary involvement follows the pneumonia and hematogenous dissemination of the pathogen. Cutaneous lesions begin as erythematous papules that later become verrucous, crusted, or ulcerated. Untreated disseminated or chronic pulmonary blastomycosis can lead to

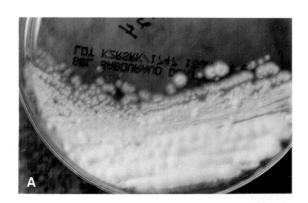

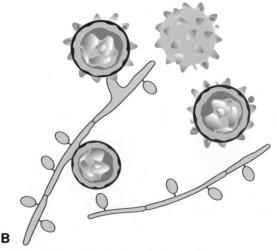

Figure 20-42. *Histoplasma capsulatum*. A. White, weblike, 25-day-old colonies of *H. capsulatum* on brain-heart infusion agar incubated at 30°C. **B.** Drawing showing both macroconidia and microconidia. (From Winn WC Jr, et al. Koneman's Color Atlas and Textbook of Diagnostic Microbiology. 6th Ed. Philadelphia: Lippincott Williams & Wilkins, 2006.)

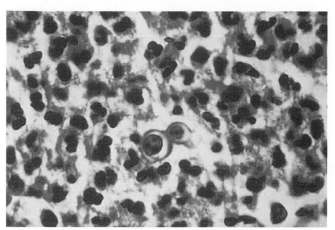

Figure 20-44. **Budding *Blastomyces dermatitidis* cell in skin tissue, surrounded by numerous neutrophils.** Notice the broad-based bud. (Courtesy of the CDC.)

death. Blastomycosis is relatively uncommon in the United States, occurring primarily in the states adjacent to the Mississippi and Ohio River valleys.

Pathogen. Blastomycosis is caused by *Blastomyces dermatitidis*, a dimorphic fungus. It grows as a yeast in tissue or enriched culture media at 37°C and as a mould at room temperature (25°C). Moist soil serves as a reservoir. Transmission occurs via inhalation of dust containing conidia.

Laboratory diagnosis. Diagnosis of blastomycosis can be made by finding characteristic *B. dermatitidis* yeast forms in smears of sputum or material obtained from lesions. The yeasts produce broad-based buds, and the parent cell with its connected bud frequently has a figure-eight or dumbbell shape (Fig. 20-44). Colonies are produced slowly (10 to 30 days) in primary culture at 30°C, except in heavy infections

when they may be produced in a week. *B. dermatitidis* mould colonies are gray-white to light buff, with delicate, silky, weblike or hairlike aerial hyphae (Fig. 20-45A). When mould colonies are examined microscopically, delicate (1- to 2-µm-diameter), hyaline, septate hyphae are seen, bearing 1- to 4-µm-diameter, lollipop-like conidia (Fig. 20-45B).

An intermediate prickly stage may be seen during the laboratory conversion of the mould stage to the yeast stage (Fig. 20-46A). The colonies then become more yeastlike. They are small, entire, slightly convex, and smooth and may by off-yellow or buff colored. Aerial spikes protruding from the surface resemble hairs standing on end. Microscopically, the yeast forms are large (10 to 15 µm in diameter) and characteristically have a single bud attached to the parent cell by a broad base (Fig. 20-46B). Immunodiagnostic tests are available. DNA probes are available for identification of *B. dermatitidis*.

Pneumocystis Pneumonia

Disease. Pneumocystis pneumonia (PCP), or interstitial plasma cell pneumonia, is an acute-to-subacute pulmonary disease found in malnourished, chronically ill children; premature infants; and immunosuppressed patients, such as those with AIDS. PCP is a common contributory cause of death in AIDS patients. *Pneumocystis* causes an asymptomatic infection in immunocompetent people (people whose immune systems are functioning properly). Immunosuppressed patients have fever, difficulty in breathing, rapid breathing, dry cough, cyanosis, and pulmonary infiltration of alveoli with frothy exudate. PCP is usually fatal in untreated patients.

Pathogen. The etiologic agent of PCP is *Pneumocystis jiroveci* (formerly *Pneumocystis carinii*). This organism has both protozoal and fungal properties. It was classified as a protozoan for many years but is currently classified as a

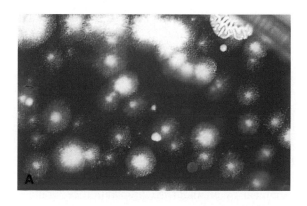

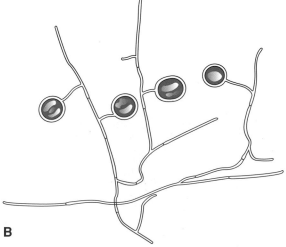

B

Figure 20-45. **B. dermatitidis. A.** Weblike colonies of *B. dermatitidis* after 5 days of incubation at room temperature on sheep blood agar. **B.** Drawing of the microscopic appearance of *B. dermatitidis*, with its lollipop-like conidia. (From Winn WC Jr, et al. Koneman's Color Atlas and Textbook of Diagnostic Microbiology. 6th Ed. Philadelphia: Lippincott Williams & Wilkins, 2006.)

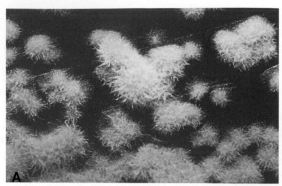
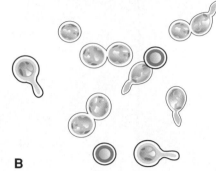

Figure 20-46. B. dermatitidis. **A.** Intermediate, prickly-stage colonies of *B. dermatitidis*, as observed during the 37°C mould-to-yeast conversion. **B.** Drawing of budding *B. dermatitidis* yeast cells. Notice the broad-based buds and dumbbell shapes. (From Winn WC Jr, et al. Koneman's Color Atlas and Textbook of Diagnostic Microbiology. 6th Ed. Philadelphia: Lippincott Williams & Wilkins, 2006.)

nonfilamentous fungus. Infected humans serve as reservoirs. The mode of transmission is unknown—perhaps direct contact, perhaps transfer of pulmonary secretions from infected to susceptible persons, perhaps airborne.

Laboratory diagnosis. Diagnosis of PCP is made by demonstration of *Pneumocystis* in material from bronchial brushings, open lung biopsy, lung aspirates, or smears of tracheobronchial mucus by various staining methods (Fig. 20-47). *P. jiroveci* cannot be cultured.

Fungal Infections of the Central Nervous System

Cryptococcal Meningitis

Disease. Cryptococcosis starts as a lung infection but spreads via the bloodstream to the brain. It usually presents as a subacute or chronic meningitis. Infection of the lungs,

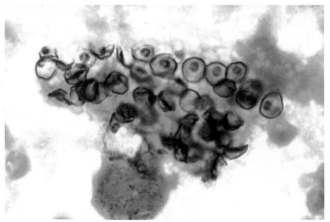

Figure 20-47. Pneumocystis **cysts in a methenamine silver-stained smear of material collected by bronchoalveolar lavage.** (Courtesy of Dr. Russell K. Byrnes and the CDC.)

kidneys, prostate, skin, and bone may also occur. Cryptococcosis is a common infection in AIDS patients.

Pathogens. Cryptococcosis can be caused by three subspecies of *Cryptococcus neoformans*, an encapsulated yeast. The capsule enables *C. neoformans* to adhere to mucosal surfaces and avoid phagocytosis by white blood cells. Reservoirs include pigeon nests; pigeon, chicken, turkey, and bat droppings; and soil contaminated with bird droppings. Growth of *C. neoformans* is stimulated by the alkaline pH and high nitrogen content of bird droppings. Transmission occurs by inhalation of yeasts, often projected into the air by sweeping or excavation. Cryptococcosis is not transmitted from person to person or animal to human.

CAUTION

Beware of Similar-Sounding Names. Do not confuse *Cryptococcus neoformans* (a yeast) with *Cryptosporidium parvum* (a protozoan). Likewise, do not confuse **cryptococcosis** (a yeast infection) with **cryptosporidiosis** (a protozoan infection). *Cryptosporidium parvum* and cryptosporidiosis are described in Chapter 22.

Clinical specimens. Specimens for isolation of *C. neoformans* include CSF, sputum, urine, and pus.

Screening tests. Cryptococcal meningitis is often diagnosed by observing encapsulated, budding yeasts in CSF specimens examined by an India ink preparation (Fig. 20-48). Details of the India ink preparation are contained in Appendix A. Yeasts may also be observed in sputum, urine, and pus examined by an India ink preparation or Gram stain (see Fig. 20-37). A sensitive cryptococcal antigen detection test is also recommended.

Media to be inoculated. Sabouraud dextrose agar or sheep blood agar may be used. Media containing cycloheximide should not be used, however, because cycloheximide

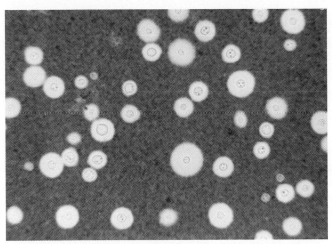

Figure 20-48. **Unstained, spherical, irregular-sized, encapsulated cells of *Cryptococcus neoformans*, as seen in an India ink preparation.** The dark background consists of India ink particles. (From Winn WC Jr, et al. Koneman's Color Atlas and Textbook of Diagnostic Microbiology. 6th Ed. Philadelphia: Lippincott Williams & Wilkins, 2006.)

inhibits growth of *C. neoformans*. Growth on sheep blood agar usually occurs within 36 to 72 hours. Encapsulated strains produce mucoid colonies (Fig. 20-49), but not all strains of *C. neoformans* are encapsulated.

Laboratory diagnosis. Nonpigmented, mucoid yeast colonies are suggestive of *C. neoformans*. The individual yeast cells are irregularly sized, ranging from 4 to 10 μm in diameter. The spherical cells are surrounded by a thick polysaccharide capsule, which may be up to 10 μm thick. Thus, if the capsule is included in the measurement, cells may be up to 20 μm in diameter. Pseudohyphae are not produced in cornmeal agar preparations. Confirmation of *C. neoformans* can be achieved using niger seed (birdseed) agar or a commercially available caffeic acid–impregnated filter paper strip. *C. neoformans* produces phenol oxidase enzyme, which results in production of melanin when the organism is grown on

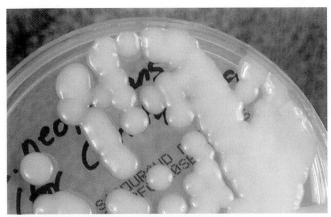

Figure 20-49. **Mucoid colonies of *C. neoformans* on Sabouraud dextrose agar after 4 days of incubation.** (From Winn WC Jr, et al. Koneman's Color Atlas and Textbook of Diagnostic Microbiology. 6th Ed. Philadelphia: Lippincott Williams & Wilkins, 2006.)

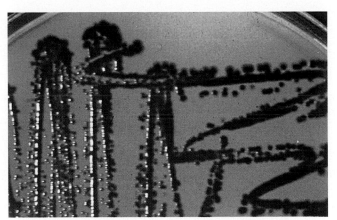

Figure 20-50. ***C. neoformans*** **producing colonies colored dark maroon red to brown on niger seed (birdseed) agar.** (From Winn WC Jr, et al. Koneman's Color Atlas and Textbook of Diagnostic Microbiology. 6th Ed. Philadelphia: Lippincott Williams & Wilkins, 2006.)

caffeic acid agar or niger seed agar. Thus, when it is grown on these media, *C. neoformans* produces colonies pigmented dark maroon red to brown (Fig. 20-50), whereas other *Cryptococcus* spp. do not. Immunodiagnostic procedures are available for detection of antigen in serum and CSF.

CLSI Document M35-A (see "References and Suggested Reading") states that a spherical, budding yeast producing nonpigmented, mucoid or nonmucoid colonies on Sabouraud agar or blood agar can be identified as *C. neoformans* if it produces a positive phenol oxidase test result using a commercial caffeic acid disk. The CLSI cautions that false-positive results can occur if the disk is overmoistened and that test results are less accurate when colonies for testing have been removed from a glucose-containing medium, such as Sabouraud dextrose agar. *C. neoformans* is also urease positive, but so too are other yeasts.

Fungal Infections of the Genitourinary System

Yeast Vaginitis

Disease and most likely pathogens. An abnormal vaginal discharge is one of the most common reasons why women visit clinicians. The discharge may be caused by vaginal infection (vaginitis) or cervical infection (cervicitis). Cervicitis is most often caused by *Neisseria gonorrhoeae* (see Chapter 11) or *Chlamydia trachomatis* (see Chapter 16). Vaginal infection is most often caused by *Candida albicans*, a yeast; *Trichomonas vaginalis*, a protozoan (see Chapter 22); or a mixture of bacteria. When caused by a mixture of bacteria, the condition is referred to as bacterial vaginosis, which is discussed in Chapter 18.

When caused by *Candida albicans* or some other *Candida* sp., the condition is referred to as yeast vaginitis or vaginal candidiasis. *C. albicans* causes about 85% to 90% of yeast vaginitis. Other *Candida* spp., such as *C. glabrata*, *C. krusei*, *C. tropicalis*, and *C. pseudotropicalis*, can also cause yeast vaginitis. Most *Candida* spp. exist in two forms: (1) blastospores (budding yeast cells), which are capable of attaching to and colonizing the surface of epithelial cells, and (2) a germinated form with hyphae, which are capable of invasion of the superficial epithelium. Typical symptoms of yeast vaginitis are vulvar pruritus (itching), a burning sensation, dysuria, and a white discharge. Vulvar erythema (redness) and rash sometimes occur.

Although *Candida* spp. are being described in this section, it is important to understand that they may be involved in various infectious processes in addition to vaginitis. These conditions include oral infection (thrush), skin rash, and disseminated *Candida* infection (disseminated candidiasis). Candidiasis of the tongue is shown in Figure 20-51.

Laboratory diagnosis. Yeast vaginitis can be diagnosed by microscopic examination of a saline wet mount of vaginal discharge material, in which yeasts and hyphae may be observed. The vaginal discharge material should also be cultured. *Candida* spp. grow well on blood agar and Sabouraud dextrose agar. CHROMagar *Candida* can also be of value in the isolation and tentative identification of *Candida* spp. (see Fig. 19-10). It is also important to keep in mind that the vaginal microflora of up to 25% of healthy women can contain *Candida* spp. Although *C. albicans* is the yeast and fungus most commonly isolated from clinical specimens, it is sometimes isolated as a pathogen and sometimes isolated as a contaminant.

> *Candida albicans* is the yeast and fungus most commonly isolated from clinical specimens—sometimes isolated as a pathogen and sometimes isolated as a contaminant.

Candida spp. can usually be identified using a commercial yeast identification minisystem. Also of value in the identification of *C. albicans* is the germ tube test (see Chapter 19). Not all strains of *C. albicans* are germ tube positive, however, and another *Candida* sp.—*C. dubliniensis*—is also germ tube positive. *C. tropicalis* can produce germ tube–like structures, but there are several ways to distinguish *C. tropicalis* from *C. albicans* in the germ tube test:

- *C. tropicalis* cells are larger than *C. albicans* cells.

- With *C. albicans*, there is no constriction at the point where the germ tube–like structure joins the blastospore,

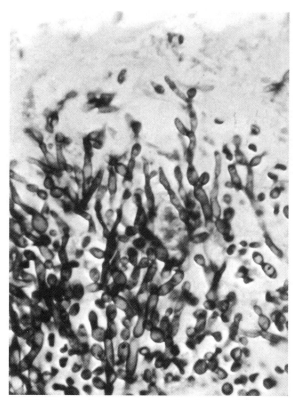

Figure 20-51. **Blastospores, pseudohyphae, and hyphae of a *Candida* sp. are present in this stained tissue specimen from a patient with candidiasis of the tongue.** (From Binford CH, Connor DH. Pathology of Tropical and Extraordinary Diseases, vol 2. Washington, DC: Armed Forces Institute of Pathology, 1976.)

unlike with *C. tropicalis*, which has a definite constriction at the juncture.

- Only about 15% of *C. tropicalis* cells produce the germ tube–like structures, whereas most *C. albicans* cells produce germ tubes.

CLSI Document M35-A (see "References and Suggested Reading") states that yeast colonies less than 48 hours old on a blood-containing medium that exhibit mycelial starlike projections (referred to as feet) can be identified as *C. albicans* (see Fig. 19-5). On rare occasions, *C. tropicalis* displays a fringed type of colony after 24 hours that may be mistaken for feet.

Chapter Review

- The four categories of mycoses described in this chapter are (1) superficial mycoses; (2) cutaneous, hair, and nail mycoses; (3) subcutaneous mycoses; and (4) systemic mycoses.

- The types of fungi that cause human mycoses are certain yeasts, moulds, and dimorphic fungi.

- Many of the fungi that infect humans are opportunistic fungi.

- Superficial mycoses are fungal infections of the outermost areas of the body, such as the epidermis and outer surfaces of hair shafts.

- Cutaneous, hair, and nail mycoses involve the dermis, internal and external portions of hair shafts, and fingernails and toenails. This group of infections is caused by moulds that are collectively referred to as dermatophytes. They include *Epidermophyton*, *Microsporum*, and *Trichophyton* spp.

- Fungal hair infections may be ectothrix, endothrix, or favic infections.

- Subcutaneous mycoses are fungal infections of the dermis and underlying tissues. They are more severe than superficial and cutaneous mycoses.

- Mycetomas, or maduromycoses, are chronic granulomatous infections that involve the feet, hands, or other areas of the body.

- Specimens from mycetoma lesions may contain granules composed of either colorless or pigmented, septate hyphae (in the case of fungal agents) *or* branching bacteria. Referred to as sulfur granules, they are yellowish particles or clumps produced by some actinomycetes.

- Systemic mycoses, also known as generalized or deep-seated mycoses, are the most serious type of fungal infections. They involve the internal tissues and organs of the body.

- The most common causes of systemic mycoses are dimorphic fungi; opportunistic moulds like Aspergillus, *Penicillium*, and bread moulds; and yeasts such as *Candida albicans* and *Cryptococcus neoformans*.

- Dimorphic fungi exist in one form in tissues and a different form when grown in vitro at room temperature. *Coccidioides immitis*, *Histoplasma capsulatum*, and *Blastomyces dermatitidis* are examples of dimorphic fungi.

- Some fungi, such as the mould form of *C. immitis*, are highly infectious. Work involving these fungi should be performed in a BSL-2 or BSL-3 facility.

New Terms and Abbreviations

After studying Chapter 20, you should be familiar with the following terms, which are defined within the chapter and in the Glossary at the back of the book:

Actinomycetoma

Chitin

Dermatophytes

Ectothrix infection

Endothrix infection

Eumycetoma

Favic infection

Macroconidium (pl. macroconidia)

Microconidium (pl. microconidia)

Mycetoma

Phialide (pl. phialides)

Ringworm

Zygomycosis

References and Suggested Reading

Abbreviated Identification of Bacteria and Yeast: Approved Guideline. CLSI Document M35-A. Wayne, PA: Clinical and Laboratory Standards Institute, 2002.

Beneke ES, Rogers AL. Medical Mycology and Human Mycoses. Belmont, CA: Star, 1996.

Heymann DL, ed. Control of Communicable Diseases Manual. 18th Ed. Washington, DC:, American Public Health Association, 2004.

Protection of Laboratory Workers from Occupationally Acquired Infections: Approved Guideline. 3rd Ed. CLSI Document M29-A3. Wayne, PA: Clinical and Laboratory Standards Institute, 2005.

Winn, WC Jr, et al. Koneman's Color Atlas and Textbook of Diagnostic Microbiology. 6th Ed. Philadelphia: Lippincott Williams & Wilkins, 2006.

Wolk DM, Roberts GD. Commercial methods for identification and susceptibility testing of fungi. In: Murray PR, Baron EJ, Jorgensen JH, Pfaller MA, Yolken RH, eds. Manual of Clinical Microbiology. 8th Ed. Washington, DC: ASM Press, 2003.

 ## On the CD-ROM

- Additional Fungi That Cause Opportunistic Infections
- Fungi in the News
- Additional Self-Assessment Exercises
- Case Studies
- Puzzle

Self-Assessment Exercises

Match the fungal infection or disease in the left column with the appropriate causative agent in the right column.

1. _____ Histoplasmosis

2. _____ Coccidioidomycosis

3. _____ Sporotrichosis

4. _____ Tinea pedis

A. *C. immitis*

B. *H. capsulatum*

C. *T. rubrum*

D. *S. schenckii*

For questions 5–10, identify both the fungal infection and the causative agent.

5. This disease is a superficial mycosis affecting hair. It is characterized by discrete, hard, gritty nodules that are dark brown to black and adhere to hair shafts. The causative agent has branched, septate, thick-walled hyphae and round-to-oval asci containing aseptate ascospores.

   Fungal infection: _____

   Causative agent: _____

6. This mycosis is a ringworm infection that primarily affects the skin of the chest or back. Microscopically, the causative agent is characterized by short, septate hyphae and clusters of thick-walled oval or round unicellular cells. It is frequently described as having a "spaghetti and meatballs" appearance.

   Fungal infection: _____

   Causative agent: _____

7. This mycosis starts as a lung infection but usually spreads via the bloodstream to the brain, where it usually presents as a subacute or chronic meningitis. Specimens typically submitted for diagnosis include CSF, sputum, urine, or pus, and the organism appears as a spherical, budding, encapsulated yeast. On Sabouraud dextrose agar, it produces nonpigmented mucoid or nonmucoid colonies.

   Fungal infection: _____

   Causative agent: _____

8. Name two genera of dematiaceous fungi that cause mycetoma and chromoblastomycosis.

   A. _____

   B. _____

9. Name two dimorphic fungi that cause human disease.

A. _____

B. _____

10. Name three dermatophytes commonly encountered in the mycology section of the CML.

A. _____

B. _____

C. _____

SECTION V

Parasitic Infections

CHAPTER 21

Introduction to Medical Parasitology

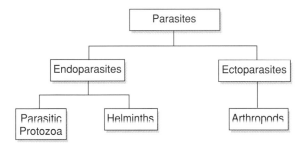

Chapter Outline
Terms and Definitions

Overview of Parasitic Protozoa

Overview of Helminths

Overview of Medically Important Arthropods

LEARNING OBJECTIVES
After studying this chapter, you should be able to:

- Define the terms introduced in this chapter (e.g., *accidental host, biological vector, blepharoplast*)

- Differentiate between the following: ectoparasites and endoparasites, definitive hosts and intermediate hosts, facultative parasites and obligate parasites, mechanical vectors and biological vectors

- State the four categories of protozoa based on differences in their modes of locomotion

- Name the two major categories of helminths

- Identify the three stages in a typical helminth life cycle

- State four ways in which arthropods may be involved in human infectious diseases

- Name the category of arthropod that transmits a specified infectious disease (e.g., mosquitoes transmit viral encephalitis)

TERMS AND DEFINITIONS

Medical parasitology is the study of parasites that cause human diseases. Although parasitology is considered a branch of microbiology, not all organisms studied in a parasitology course are microorganisms. In fact, of the three categories of organisms studied in a parasitology course (parasitic protozoa, helminths, and arthropods), only one category (parasitic protozoa) contains microorganisms. Thus, in this book, parasitic protozoa are discussed in greater detail than are helminths and arthropods.

Parasitism is a symbiotic relationship that is of benefit to one party or symbiont (the parasite) at the expense of the other party (the host).[1] Although many parasites cause disease, some do not. Even if a parasite is not causing disease, it is depriving the host of nutrients; therefore, parasitic relationships are always considered detrimental to the host. The focus of this chapter is on parasites that cause human disease.

Parasites are defined as organisms that live *on* or *in* other living organisms (hosts), at whose expense they gain some

---

[1]Symbiosis is the living together or close association of two dissimilar organisms (i.e., two species). The three major types of symbiotic relationships are commensalism, mutualism, and parasitism. A commensal relationship benefits one party (symbiont) but is of no consequence to the other (i.e., neither beneficial nor harmful). A mutual relationship is a benefit to both parties; that is, it is mutually beneficial.

advantage. In addition to parasites of humans, there are many types of plant parasites (i.e., parasites of plants) and many types of animal parasites (i.e., parasites of animals).

Parasites that live outside the host's body are referred to as **ectoparasites,** whereas those living inside the host are called **endoparasites.** Arthropods such as mites, ticks, and lice are examples of ectoparasites. Parasitic protozoa and helminths are examples of endoparasites.

> Parasites are organisms that live *on* or *in* other living organisms (hosts), at whose expense they gain some advantage. Parasites that live outside the host's body, like mites and ticks, are ectoparasites, whereas those living inside the host, like protozoa and helminths, are endoparasites.

The life cycle of a particular parasite may involve one or more hosts. If more than one host is involved, the **definitive host** is the one harboring the adult or sexual stage of the parasite or the sexual phase of the life cycle. The **intermediate host** harbors the larval or asexual stage of the parasite or the asexual phase of the life cycle. Parasite life cycles range from simple to complex. There are one-host parasites, two-host parasites, and three-host parasites. Knowing the life cycle of a parasite enables epidemiologists and other health care professionals to control the parasitic infection through intervention at some point in the life cycle. In addition, parasitic infections are most often diagnosed by observing a particular life cycle stage in a clinical specimen.

An **accidental host** is a living organism that can serve as a host in a particular parasite's life cycle but is not a *usual* host in that life cycle. Some accidental hosts are **dead-end hosts,** from which the parasite cannot continue its life cycle.

> The definitive host harbors the adult or sexual stage of the parasite or the sexual phase of the parasite's life cycle. The intermediate host harbors the larval or asexual stage of the parasite or the asexual phase of the life cycle.

A **facultative parasite** is an organism that can be parasitic but does not have to live as a parasite. It is capable of living an independent life, apart from a host. The free-living amebas that can cause keratoconjunctivitis (a severe eye infection) and primary amebic meningoencephalitis are examples of facultative parasites. An **obligate parasite,** on the other hand, has no choice; to survive, it must be a parasite. Most parasites that infect humans are obligate parasites.

> Facultative parasites are organisms that *can* be parasitic but are also capable of a free-living existence. Obligate parasites have no choice; to survive, they must be parasites.

Parasitology is the study of parasites in general, and a **parasitologist** is someone who studies parasites. As previously stated, any upper division or graduate-level parasitology course would be divided into three areas of study: the study of parasitic protozoa, the study of helminths, and the study of arthropods.

The overall responsibility of the parasitology section of the clinical microbiology laboratory (CML) is to assist clinicians in the diagnosis of parasitic diseases—primarily, parasitic infections caused by endoparasites such as parasitic protozoa (see Chapter 22) and helminths (see Chapter 23).

In general, parasitic infections are diagnosed by observing and recognizing various parasite life cycle stages in clinical specimens. Because of the extremely small size of some of these life cycle stages (e.g., amebic cysts and *Cryptosporidium* oocysts), finding them in specimens represents one of the greatest challenges faced by microbiologists.

> In general, parasitic infections are diagnosed by observing and recognizing various parasitic life cycle stages in clinical specimens.

OVERVIEW OF PARASITIC PROTOZOA

In the five-kingdom system of classification of living organisms, protozoa are in the Kingdom Protista. Some taxonomists prefer to place protozoa in a kingdom by themselves—the Kingdom Protozoa (Table 21-1). Most protozoa are unicellular, but some are multicellular (colonial) protozoa. Protozoa are classified taxonomically by their mode of locomotion. **Amebas** move by means of pseudopodia (literally, "false feet"). **Flagellates** move by means of whiplike flagella. **Ciliates** move by means of hairlike cilia. Protozoa classified as *Sporozoa* (**sporozoans**) have no pseudopodia, flagella, or cilia and therefore exhibit no motility.

> Protozoa are classified taxonomically by mode of locomotion. Some move by means of pseudopodia, others by flagella, others by cilia, and some are nonmotile.

Not all protozoa are parasitic. For example, many of the pond water protozoa (e.g., *Paramecium* and *Stentor* spp.) studied in introductory biology and microbiology courses are not parasites. Some protozoa are facultative parasites, capable of a free-living, nonparasitic existence but also able to become parasites when they accidentally gain entrance to the body. *Acanthamoeba* spp. and *Naegleria fowleri* are examples of facultative parasites. These free-living amebas normally reside in soil or water but can cause serious diseases when they gain entrance to the eyes or the nasal

TABLE 21 - 1	Taxonomy of Human Protozoal Parasites (Kingdom Protozoa)[a]		
Phylum	**Mode of Locomotion**	**Examples of Protozoa in the Phylum**	
Amoebozoa (amebas)	Pseudopodia	*Acanthamoeba, Balamuthia, Entamoeba* spp.	
Ciliophora (ciliates)	Cilia	*Balantidium coli*	
Metamonada (intestinal flagellates)	Flagella	*Giardia lamblia*	
Parabasalia (intestinal and related flagellates)	Flagella	*Dientamoeba fragilis, Trichomonas vaginalis*	
Euglenozoa (flagellates possessing kinetoplasts[b])	Flagella	*Leishmania, Trypanosoma* spp.	
Percolozoa (flagellated amebas[c])	Flagella and pseudopodia	*Naegleria fowleri*	
Sporozoa	Possess no organelles of locomotion	*Cryptosporidium, Toxoplasma, Cyclospora, Babesia, Plasmodium* spp.	

Source: Cox FEG. Taxonomy and classification of human parasites. In: Murray PR, Baron EJ, Jorgensen JH, Pfaller MA, Yolken RH, eds. Manual of Clinical Microbiology. 8th Ed. Washington, DC: ASM Press, 2003.

[a]The classification of protozoa is very controversial; for example, not all taxonomists agree that protozoa should be placed in a separate kingdom.

[b]A **kinetoplast** is the darkly staining part of a large DNA-containing mitochondrion, found in the cytoplasm of certain protozoa (e.g., *Leishmania* and *Trypanosoma* spp.). It is located adjacent to the basal body or **blepharoplast** at the base of a flagellum.

[c]Flagellated amebas are also called ameboflagellates. In its free-living state, *Naegleria fowleri* exists either as an ameba or a flagellate but is found only as an ameba in host tissues.

mucosa. From the nasal mucosa, they travel via the olfactory nerve into the brain and cause diseases affecting the central nervous system. Most protozoal parasites of humans are obligate parasites.

The various procedures used to diagnose protozoal infections are performed in the parasitology section of the CML. On occasion, laboratory personnel working in other parts of the clinical pathology division may also observe parasites. For example, personnel working in the hematology laboratory may observe malarial parasites within red blood cells while examining stained peripheral blood smears. Because protozoa are tiny, protozoal infections are most often diagnosed by microscopic examination of body fluids, tissue specimens, or feces. Peripheral blood smears are usually stained with Giemsa stain, whereas fecal specimens are stained with trichrome, iron hematoxylin, or acid-fast stains. Most protozoal infections are diagnosed by observing trophozoites, cysts, oocysts, or spores in the specimen.

The **trophozoite** is the motile, feeding, dividing stage in a protozoan's life cycle, whereas **cysts, oocysts,** and spores are dormant stages. In some ways, protozoal cysts, oocysts, and spores are similar to bacterial spores. Protozoal infections are primarily acquired by ingestion or inhalation of

cysts, oocysts, or spores. Only rarely do trophozoites serve as the infective stages. Parasitic protozoa are rarely cultured in the CML. The role of the CML in the diagnosis of selected protozoal infections is described in Chapter 22.

> The trophozoite is the motile, feeding, dividing stage in the protozoal life cycle, and the cyst, oocyst, and spore are dormant stages. Protozoal infections are most often acquired by ingestion or inhalation of dormant stages.

OVERVIEW OF HELMINTHS

The word **helminth** means parasitic worm. Although helminths are not microorganisms, the various procedures used to diagnose helminth infections are performed in the parasitology section of the CML. These procedures often involve the observation of microscopic stages—eggs and larvae—in the life cycles of these parasites. Helminths infect humans, other animals, and plants, but only helminth infections of humans are discussed here. The helminths that infect humans are always endoparasites.

TABLE 21 - 2	Taxonomy of Human Helminth Parasites (Kingdom Animalia)	
Phylum	**Class**	**Examples of Helminths in the Class**
Nemathelminthes (nematodes; roundworms)	Adenophorea	*Trichinella, Trichuris* spp.
	Secernentea	*Ancylostoma, Necator, Ascaris, Dracunculus, Brugia, Loa, Wuchereria, Onchocerca, Enterobius, Strongyloides* spp.
Platyhelminthes (flatworms)	Digenea (trematodes, flukes)	*Schistosoma, Fasciola, Fasciolopsis, Opisthorchis, Paragonimus* spp.
	Cestoidea (Cestoda, cestodes, tapeworms)	*Diphyllobothrium, Dipylidium, Hymenolepis, Hymenolepis, Taenia, Echinococcus* spp.

Source: Cox FEG. Taxonomy and classification of human parasites. In: Murray PR, Baron EJ, Jorgensen JH, Pfaller MA, Yolken RH, eds. Manual of Clinical Microbiology. 8th Ed. Washington, DC: ASM Press, 2003.

> Helminths—parasitic worms—are divided into roundworms (nematodes) and flatworms. Flatworms are further divided into tapeworms (cestodes) and flukes (trematodes).

Helminths are multicellular, eucaryotic organisms in the Kingdom Animalia. The two major divisions of helminths are roundworms (phylum Nemathelminthes or Nematoda; **nematodes**) and flatworms (phylum Platyhelminthes). The flatworms are further divided into tapeworms (class Cestoidea or Cestoda; **cestodes**) and flukes (class Digenea or Trematoda; **trematodes**). Table 21-2 contains additional information on helminth taxonomy.

The typical helminth life cycle comprises three stages: the *egg*, the *larva*, and the *adult* worm. Adults produce eggs, from which larvae emerge, and the larvae mature into adult worms. Adult nematodes are either male or female. Cestodes and many trematodes are hermaphroditic, meaning that adult worms contain both male and female reproductive organs. Thus, it only takes one worm to produce fertile eggs.

> The typical helminth life cycle comprises three stages: the *egg*, the *larva*, and the *adult* worm.

The host that harbors the larval stage is called the **intermediate host,** whereas the host that harbors the adult worm is called the **definitive host.** Sometimes helminths have more than one intermediate host or more than one definitive host. The fish tapeworm, for example, is what is known as a three-host parasite, having one definitive host (human) and two intermediate hosts (the *Cyclops* genus of freshwater crustaceans and a freshwater fish) in its life cycle (Fig. 21-1). Fleas serve as the intermediate host in the life cycle of the dog tapeworm, whereas dogs, cats, and humans serve as definitive hosts.

Helminth infections are primarily acquired by ingesting a larva-containing egg, although some larvae are injected into the body via the bite of infected insects, and others enter the body by penetrating skin. Helminth infections are usually diagnosed by observing (1) whole worms or segments of worms in clinical specimens (usually, fecal specimens) or (2) larvae or eggs of helminths in stained or unstained clinical specimens.

> Helminth infections are usually diagnosed by observing (1) whole worms or segments of worms in clinical specimens—most often, fecal specimens—or (2) larvae or eggs of helminths in stained or unstained clinical specimens.

Only rarely are helminths cultured in the CML. The role of the CML in the diagnosis of selected helminth infections is described in Chapter 23.

OVERVIEW OF MEDICALLY IMPORTANT ARTHROPODS

There are many classes of arthropods, but only three are studied in a parasitology course: *insects* (class Insecta), *arachnids* (class Arachnida), and certain *crustaceans* (class Crustacea). The insects studied include lice, fleas, flies, mosquitoes, and reduviid bugs. Arachnids include mites and ticks. Crustaceans include crabs, crayfish, and certain *Cyclops* spp. that may serve as intermediate hosts. Arthropods may be involved in human infectious diseases in any of four ways, as shown in Table 21-3.

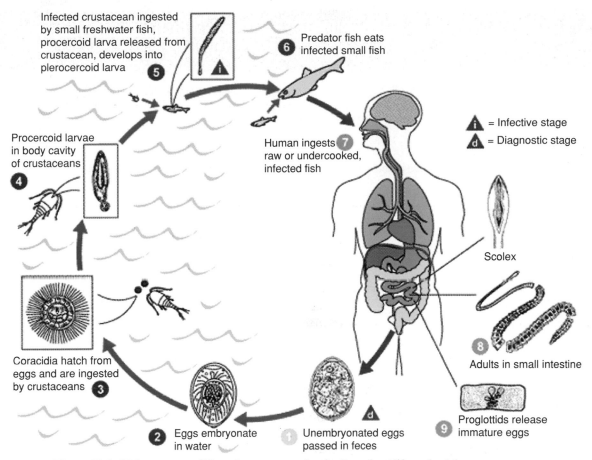

Infected crustacean ingested by small freshwater fish, procercoid larva released from crustacean, develops into plerocercoid larva **5**

6 Predator fish eats infected small fish

▲ i = Infective stage

▲ d = Diagnostic stage

Procercoid larvae in body cavity of crustaceans **4**

Human ingests **7** raw or undercooked, infected fish

Scolex

Coracidia hatch from eggs and are ingested by crustaceans **3**

8 Adults in small intestine

2 Eggs embryonate in water

1 Unembryonated eggs passed in feces

9 Proglottids release immature eggs

Figure 21-1. **Fish tapeworm life cycle—an example of a three-host life cycle.** A human serves as the definitive host, harboring the adult worm. A *Cyclops* sp. (crustacean) serves as the first intermediate host, harboring the procercoid larva. A freshwater fish serves as the second intermediate host, harboring the plerocercoid (the infective stage). (Courtesy of the Centers for Disease Control and Prevention, Division of Parasitic Diseases.)

TABLE 21 - 3	Arthropod Involvement in Human Diseases
Type of Involvement	**Example(s)**
Cause of the disease	Scabies, a disease in which microscopic mites live in subcutaneous tunnels and cause intense itching
Intermediate host in the life cycle of a parasite	Flea in the life cycle of the dog tapeworm; beetle in the life cycle of the rat tapeworm; *Cyclops* spp. in life cycle of the fish tapeworm; tsetse fly in the life cycle of African trypanosomiasis; *Simulium* blackfly in the life cycle of onchocerciasis; mosquito in the transmission of filariasis
Definitive host in the life cycle of a parasite	Female *Anopheles* mosquito in the life cycle of malarial parasites
Vector (either mechanical or biological) in the transmission of an infectious disease	Oriental rat flea in the transmission of plague; tick in the transmission of Rocky Mountain spotted fever and Lyme disease; louse in the transmission of epidemic typhus

TABLE 21 - 4	**Arthropods That Serve as Vectors of Human Infectious Diseases**

Vectors	Disease(s)
Blackflies (*Simulium* spp.)	Onchocerciasis (river blindness) (H)
Cyclops spp.	Fish tapeworm infection (H), guinea worm infection (H)
Fleas	Dog tapeworm infection (H), endemic typhus (B), murine typhus (B), plague (B)
Lice	Epidemic relapsing fever (B), epidemic typhus (B), trench fever (B)
Mites	Rickettsial pox (B), scrub typhus (B)
Mosquitoes	Dengue fever (V), filariasis (elephantiasis) (H), malaria (P), viral encephalitis (V), yellow fever (V)
Reduviid bugs	American trypanosomiasis (Chagas disease) (P)
Sandflies (*Phlebotomus* spp.)	Leishmaniasis (P)
Ticks	Babesiosis (P), Colorado tick fever (V), ehrlichiosis (B), Lyme disease (B), relapsing fever (B), Rocky Mountain spotted fever (B), tularemia (B)
Tsetse flies (*Glossina* spp.)	African trypanosomiasis (P)

B, bacterial; H, helminthic; P, protozoal; V, viral.

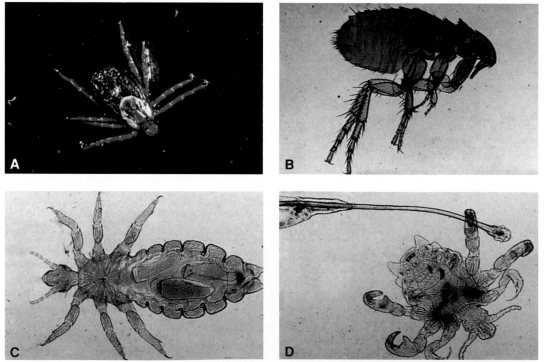

Figure 21-2. **Arthropod ectoparasites and vectors of human infectious diseases. A.** *Dermacentor andersoni,* the wood tick; one of the tick vectors of Rocky Mountain spotted fever. **B.** *Xenopsylla cheopis,* the oriental rat flea; the vector of plague and endemic typhus. **C.** *Pediculus humanus,* the human body louse; a vector of epidemic typhus. **D.** *Phthirus pubis,* the pubic louse; because of its appearance, it is also known as the crab louse. (From Winn WC Jr. et al. Koneman's Color Atlas and Textbook of Diagnostic Microbiology, 6th ed. Philadelphia: Lippincott Williams & Wilkins, 2006.)

Historical Vignette

The Mosquito, a Persistent and Deadly Foe. *"No animal on earth has touched so directly and profoundly the lives of so many human beings. For all of history, and all over the globe, she has been a nuisance, a pain, and an angel of death. The mosquito has killed great leaders, decimated armies, and decided the fate of nations. All this, and she is roughly the size and weight of a grape seed." (From the Preface to Mosquito: A Natural History of Our Most Persistent and Deadly Foe, by Andrew Spielman and Michael D'Antonio [New York: Hyperion, 2001].)*

Arthropods may serve as mechanical or biological vectors in the transmission of certain infectious diseases. **Mechanical vectors** merely pick up the parasite at point A and drop it off at point B, similar to an overnight delivery service. For example, a housefly could pick up parasite cysts on the sticky hairs of its legs while walking around on animal feces in a meadow. The fly might then come through an open kitchen window and drop off the parasite cysts while walking on a pie cooling on the counter. A **biological vector,** on the other hand, is an arthropod in whose body the pathogen multiplies or matures (or both). Many arthropod vectors of human diseases are biological vectors. A particular arthropod may serve as both a host and a biological vector. Table 21-4 lists some arthropods that serve as vectors of human infectious diseases, and several disease-causing arthropods are depicted in Figure 21-2.

CML professionals are rarely called on to identify arthropods. The various techniques and criteria used to identify arthropods are beyond the scope of this book.

Chapter Review

- Parasites are defined as organisms that live *on* or *in* other living organisms (hosts), at whose expense they gain some advantage—usually, by depriving the host of nutrients.

- Parasites that live outside the host's body are referred to as ectoparasites, whereas those living inside the host are called endoparasites.

- The definitive host harbors the adult or sexual stage of the parasite or the sexual phase of the life cycle. The intermediate host harbors the larval or asexual stage of the parasite or the asexual phase of the life cycle.

- A facultative parasite can be parasitic but does not have to live as a parasite. It is capable of living an independent life, apart from a host. An obligate parasite has no choice; to survive, it must be parasitic.

- In general, parasitic infections are diagnosed by observing and recognizing various parasitic life cycle stages in clinical specimens.

- Protozoa are classified taxonomically by their mode of locomotion. Amebas move by means of pseudopodia. Flagellates move via whiplike flagella. Ciliates move using hairlike cilia. Sporozoans are nonmotile.

- The motile, feeding, dividing stages in protozoal life cycles are called trophozoites. Cysts, oocysts, and spores are examples of dormant stages. Protozoal infections are most often acquired by ingestion or inhalation of dormant stages. Only rarely are trophozoites the infective stage.

- Helminths are parasitic worms. They are divided into roundworms (nematodes) and flatworms. Flatworms are further divided into tapeworms (cestodes) and flukes (trematodes).

- Helminth infections are usually diagnosed by observing eggs, larvae, whole worms, or segments of worms in clinical specimens.

- Mites, ticks, fleas, lice, mosquitoes, and biting flies are example of arthropods that can serve as vectors in the transmission of infectious diseases, including parasitic infections.

- A particular arthropod may be the actual cause of an infectious disease, or it may serve as an intermediate host, a definitive host, a mechanical vector, or a biological vector.

- Mechanical vectors merely pick up the parasite at one location and drop it off at another. A biological vector is an arthropod in whose body the pathogen multiplies or matures or both.

New Terms and Abbreviations

After studying Chapter 21, you should be familiar with the following terms, which are defined within the chapter and in the Glossary at the back of the book:

Accidental host

Biological vector

Blepharoplast

Cestodes

Ciliates

Cyst

Dead-end host

Definitive host

Ectoparasite

Endoparasite

Facultative parasite

Flagellates

Helminth

Host

Intermediate host

Kinetoplast

Mechanical vector

Medical parasitology

Nemathelminthes

Obligate parasite

Parasite

Parasitism

Parasitologist

Parasitology

Platyhelminthes

Sporozoans

Trematodes

Trophozoite

References and Suggested Reading

Cox FEG. Taxonomy and classification of human parasites. In: Murray PR, Baron EJ, Jorgensen JH, Pfaller MA, Yolken RH, eds. Manual of Clinical Microbiology. 8th Ed. Washington, DC: ASM Press, 2003.

 On the CD-ROM

- Tickborne Diseases in the United States
- Additional Self-Assessment Exercises
- Puzzle

Self-Assessment Exercises

1. Briefly define *parasite*. _____

2. Define *definitive host*. _____

_____

3. Define *facultative parasite*. _____

_____

4. List the three categories of motile protozoa and their mode of locomotion.

A. _____ move by _____

B. _____ move by _____

C. _____ move by _____

5. Briefly describe what a parasite cyst is.

_____

6. Name two human parasites in the category of parasites known as flagellates.

A. _____

B. _____

7. What are the three major stages in the life cycle of a helminth?

A. _____

B. _____

C. _____

8. True or false: The helminths that infect humans are always endoparasites.

9. True or false: The host that harbors the larval stage is called the definitive host.

10. Which of the following is an example of an intestinal flagellate:

A. *Entamoeba histolytica*

B. *Balantidium coli*

C. *Trypanosoma cruzi*

D. *Giardia lamblia*

CHAPTER 22

Laboratory Diagnosis of Selected Protozoal Infections

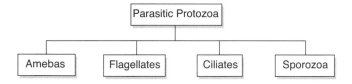

Chapter Outline

Clinical Specimens Required for the Diagnosis of Protozoal Infections

Laboratory Methods Used to Diagnose Protozoal Infections
- Processing Blood Specimens
- Processing Stool Specimens
- Processing Genitourinary Specimens
- Processing Aspirates
- Processing Cerebrospinal Fluid
- Culture Methods
- Immunodiagnostic Procedures
- Molecular Diagnostic Procedures

Selected Protozoal Infections
- Protozoal Infections of the Cardiovascular System
- Protozoal Infections of the Skin and Mucous Membranes
- Protozoal Infections of the Eyes
- Protozoal Infections of the Central Nervous System
- Protozoal Infections of the Genitourinary Tract
- Protozoal Infections of the Gastrointestinal Tract

LEARNING OBJECTIVES

After studying this chapter, you should be able to:

☛ Define the terms and abbreviations introduced in this chapter (e.g., *amastigote, ameboflagellate, ameboma*)

☛ Given a description, permanent stained smear, or color photograph of a protozoan, correctly identify the parasite

☛ Given a list of parasites, identify each as an ameba, flagellate, ciliate, or sporozoan parasite

☛ Name the specimen of choice for recovery of the parasites discussed in the chapter

☛ Given a permanent stained smear, prepared slide, or photograph, differentiate a potential pathogenic parasite from an artifact

☛ Briefly describe the life cycle of a malarial parasite, and specify the stage that is infective to humans and the stages that must be ingested during the mosquito's blood meal for the life cycle to continue

☛ Discuss the clinically significant signs and symptoms of malaria, including the type of cyclic paroxysm and characteristic life cycle stages (e.g., trophozoites, number of merozoites, ring forms, schizonts)

☛ Given a particular anatomic site, name the most probable protozoal infection and parasite that causes the infection

☛ List the advantages and disadvantages of the various stool preservatives

☛ Compare and contrast the flotation and sedimentation concentration methods for parasites

☛ Given a particular parasite, name the corresponding disease and geographic distribution

Clinical microbiology laboratory (CML) professionals assist clinicians in the diagnosis of protozoal infections. Table 22-1 provides an overview of the protozoal infections described in this chapter (no attempt has been made to

TABLE 22 - 1   Selected Protozoal Infections of Humans

Anatomical Location	Infection	Protozoan That Causes the Infection
Cardiovascular system	African trypanosomiasis (African sleeping sickness)	Subspecies of *Trypanosoma brucei* (F)
	American trypanosomiasis (Chagas disease)	*Trypanosoma cruzi* (F)
	Babesiosis	*Babesia* spp. (S)
	Malaria	*Plasmodium* spp. (S)
Skin and mucous membranes	Leishmaniasis	*Leishmania* spp. (F)
Eyes	Amebic eye infections	*Acanthamoeba* spp. (A)
	Toxoplasmosis	*Toxoplasma gondii* (S)
Central nervous system	African trypanosomiasis (African sleeping sickness)	Subspecies of *Trypanosoma brucei* (F)
	Granulomatous amebic encephalitis (GAE)	*Acanthamoeba* spp. (A)
	Primary amebic meningoencephalitis (PAM)	*Naegleria fowleri* (A)
Genitourinary system	Trichomoniasis	*Trichomonas vaginalis* (F)
Gastrointestinal tract	Amebiasis	*Entamoeba histolytica* (A)
	Balantidiasis	*Balantidium coli* (C)
	Cryptosporidiosis	*Cryptosporidium parvum* (S)
	Cyclosporiasis	*Cyclospora* spp. (S)
	Giardiasis	*Giardia lamblia* (F)

A, ameba; C, ciliate; F, flagellate; S, sporozoan.

include all protozoal infections of humans). Laboratory techniques used to diagnose protozoal infections are performed in the parasitology section of the CML.

It is very important to remember that a patient may be infected with more than one parasite, depending on where he or she has lived and/or traveled. Thus, a CML professional should continue to examine a specimen after discovering a particular parasite. Even though many of the protozoal infections described in this chapter are not endemic diseases in the United States, people emigrating from other countries or U.S. residents returning from travel to foreign countries could be infected with one or more of these parasites.

> It is very important to remember that a patient may be infected with more than one parasite, depending on where he or she has lived and/or traveled. Thus, a CML professional should continue to examine specimens after observing a particular parasite.

CLINICAL SPECIMENS REQUIRED FOR THE DIAGNOSIS OF PROTOZOAL INFECTIONS

Clinical specimens commonly used to diagnose protozoal infections are listed in Table 22-2.

LABORATORY METHODS USED TO DIAGNOSE PROTOZOAL INFECTIONS

In general, protozoal infections are diagnosed by observing and recognizing various parasite life cycle stages, such as trophozoites, cysts,

> In general, protozoal infections are diagnosed by observing and recognizing various parasite life cycle stages, such as trophozoites, cysts, oocysts, and spores.

TABLE 22 - 2	Clinical Specimens Commonly Used to Diagnose Protozoal Infections

Clinical Specimen	Infection(s)
Aspirates from cutaneous ulcers	Cutaneous leishmaniasis
Blood (plasma)	African trypanosomiasis, American trypanosomiasis
Blood (red blood cells)	Malaria, babesiosis
Blood (white blood cells; buffy coat preparations)	Toxoplasmosis, visceral leishmaniasis
Bone marrow	Visceral leishmaniasis
Brain tissue	Granulomatous amebic encephalitis (GAE), primary amebic meningoencephalitis (PAM), toxoplasmosis
Cerebrospinal fluid	African trypanosomiasis, GAE, PAM, toxoplasmosis
Duodenal contents	Giardiasis
Eye specimens (biopsy, corneal scrapings, contact lens)	Acanthamebic infection (keratitis, corneal ulceration), toxoplasmosis
Intestinal contents collected by sigmoidoscopy	Amebiasis
Liver aspirates, biopsy specimens	Amebiasis, visceral leishmaniasis
Lymph node aspirates	African trypanosomiasis, American trypanosomiasis, visceral leishmaniasis
Material obtained from mucocutaneous lesions (aspirates, biopsy specimens)	Mucocutaneous leishmaniasis
Serum (for immunodiagnostic procedures)	Amebiasis, American trypanosomiasis, leishmaniasis, toxoplasmosis
Skin specimens (scrapings, aspirates, or biopsy specimens from skin lesions)	Cutaneous leishmaniasis
Splenic aspirates, biopsy specimens	Visceral leishmaniasis
Sputum	Respiratory cryptosporidiosis (rare)
Stool	Amebiasis, balantidiasis, *Blastocystis hominis* infection, cryptosporidiosis, cyclosporiasis, *Dientamoeba fragilis* infection, giardiasis, *Isospora belli* infection, microsporidial infection
Tissue biopsy specimens (various tissues)	American trypanosomiasis, microsporidial infection, toxoplasmosis
Urogenital specimens (vaginal discharge, urethral discharge, prostatic secretion)	Trichomoniasis

oocysts, and spores. CML professionals must be able to identify protozoa by the characteristic appearance (e.g., size, shape, internal details) of stained or unstained life cycle stages.

Processing Blood Specimens

Although it is possible to observe some parasites by microscopic examination of fresh, whole blood, permanent stained blood smears—sometimes referred to as blood films—are necessary for species identification. Both thick and thin blood smears can be prepared from either whole, fresh blood or anticoagulated blood. When anticoagulated blood is used, the preferred anticoagulant is ethylenediamine tetraacetic acid. Thick smears enable examination of a greater quantity of blood than do thin smears. Used to screen for parasites, thick smears are more apt to demonstrate a low parasitemia. Thin smears are used to identify parasites based on their characteristic features—features that often become distorted in the thick smear. The Centers for Disease Control and Prevention (CDC) recommends that two sets of smears be prepared (i.e., two thick and two thin smears of each specimen). Instructions for preparing thick and thin blood smears can be found in Appendix A.

Staining the blood smears. The CDC recommends that only one set of smears be stained. The unstained duplicates are valuable should a problem occur during the staining process and/or if smears are later sent to a reference laboratory. Blood smears may be stained with Giemsa (recommended), Wright, or Wright-Giemsa stain. If Giemsa stain is used, the thin smears must first be fixed with methanol. Wright and Wright-Giemsa stains contain a fixative as well as the dyes. Schüffner dots—the prominent pink-red-stained granules seen in infected red blood cells—cannot be seen when Wright or Wright-Giemsa stain is used.

Microscopic examination of stained thick blood smears. The CDC recommends that stained thick smears be examined in the following manner:

Step 1: First screen the whole smear at a low magnification (×10 or ×20 objective lens) to detect large parasites such as microfilaria.

Step 2: Examine the smear using the ×100 oil immersion objective lens. Select an area that is well stained, free of stain precipitate, and well populated with white blood cells (10 to 20 white blood cells per field).

Step 3: If parasites are observed, make a tentative species determination on the thick blood smear, and then move to the thin smear to confirm your impression. Usually, the thin smear is the appropriate sample on which to base your species identification.

Step 4: The College of American Pathologists recommends that when malaria is suspected but no parasites are observed on the thick smear, at least 300 fields, each containing approximately 20 white blood cells, be screened before calling a thick smear negative. In this case, the laboratory report would state, "No parasites found (NPF)."

Protozoa are sought at the feathered end of the stained thin smear, where the erythrocytes are drawn out into a single layer of cells (Fig. 22-1). Screening of the slide starts with a ×100 total magnification and ends with a ×1000 total magnification.

Processing Stool Specimens

Stool specimens may be either fresh (with no added preservatives) or preserved. Live, motile trophozoites can only be

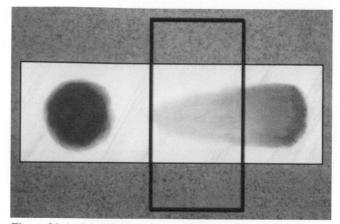

Figure 22-1. **Stained thick and thin blood smears on the same slide.** The boxed area indicates the feathered end of the stained thin smear, where the erythrocytes are drawn out into a single layer of cells and where protozoa should be sought. (Courtesy of Steven Glenn, Centers for Disease Control and Prevention [CDC], Laboratory Training and Consultation Division.)

observed in fresh specimens. Many commercial transport devices are available that contain stool preservatives. Preservatives include formalin, polyvinyl alcohol, sodium acetate-acetic acid-formalin, Schaudinn's fluid, and merthiolate (thimerosal)-iodine-formalin. Advantages and disadvantages of the various stool preservatives are summarized in Table 22-3.

Stool specimens containing barium are unacceptable because this opaque, chalky substance can obscure the presence of intestinal protozoa. Other substances and medications that interfere with the detection of intestinal protozoa include mineral oil, bismuth, antibiotics such as metronidazole and tetracyclines, antimalarial agents, and certain antidiarrheal preparations.

Stool specimens are examined both macroscopically and microscopically. During the macroscopic examination, the consistency of the stool is noted, as are the presence of blood or mucus. Terms such as *liquid, soft,* or *formed* are used to describe the consistency of the stool. Nonpreserved liquid specimens should be examined within 30 minutes of passage; semiformed, within 1 hour of passage; and formed, within 24 hours of passage. Trophozoites are most likely to be observed in liquid specimens.

For many years, examination of stool specimens for the presence of parasites has been referred to as the **O&P examination,** with *O* standing for *ova* (eggs) and *P* standing for *parasite* stages other than eggs. When written on a laboratory request slip, *O&P* means to examine the specimen for any evidence of parasite life cycle stages. In the case of protozoa, this would mean evidence of trophozoites, cysts, oocysts, or spores. (Spores are produced by microsporidia, which are discussed briefly on the CD-ROM.)

TABLE 22 - 3	Advantages and Disadvantages of Various Stool Preservatives	
Preservative	**Advantages**	**Disadvantages**
Formalin	Protozoan cysts and oocysts are preserved well; concentrated sediment can be used for most immunodiagnostic methods; does not contain mercury compounds	Trophozoites are not preserved well; not a good preservative for preparation of permanent stained smears; cannot be used for molecular diagnostic procedures and some immunoassays
Polyvinyl alcohol (PVA)	Good preservation of protozoan trophozoites and cysts; can be used for concentration techniques and preparation of permanent stained smears; suitable for molecular diagnostic procedures	*Giardia* cysts are not concentrated as well as with formalin fixatives; either trichrome or iron hematoxylin stain can be used for permanent stained slides; cannot be used for immunodiagnostic procedures; contains mercury compounds (hence disposal problems); modified PVA preservatives are available without mercury compounds
Sodium acetate-acetic acid-formalin	Can be used for concentration techniques, preparation of permanent stained smears, and most immunodiagnostic methods; does not contain mercury compounds	Poor adhesive properties; protozoal morphology in permanent stained slides is better when iron hematoxylin stain is used rather than trichrome stain
Schaudinn fluid	Excellent preservation of protozoan trophozoites and cysts	Not recommended for concentration procedures; poor adhesive qualities with liquid and mucoid specimens; either trichrome or iron hematoxylin stain can be used for permanent stained slides; contains mercury compounds
Merthiolate (thimerosal) iodine-formalin	Both fixes and stains; protozoa can be identified in wet mounts; thimerosal is a mercury compound	Not very good for preparation of permanent stained smears; polychrome IV stain should be used; morphology of organisms on permanent stained smears is generally not as good as with Schaudinn fluid or PVA

The O&P examination of stool specimens consists of three steps:

Step 1: A direct wet mount examination of the specimen. Assuming that the specimen is fresh, this would enable the observation of live, motile trophozoites. Performing a direct wet mount examination on preserved specimens is unnecessary because the preservative kills any trophozoites present. The direct wet mount is prepared by mixing about 2 mg of stool with a drop of 0.85% saline and covering the preparation with a coverslip. The preparation is then examined using the low ($\times$10) and high dry ($\times$40) objectives. Because protozoan trophozoites are very pale and transparent, low-intensity lighting should be used. Following a direct wet mount examination using saline, a drop of Lugol or D'Antoni iodine can be placed at the edge of the coverslip, or a new preparation may be prepared in iodine. It is important that a saline prep be examined first, because iodine kills any trophozoites present.

Step 2: A wet mount examination of the specimen, following some type of concentration procedure, with or without the use of iodine as a stain. As the name implies, the purpose of a concentration procedure is to concentrate any parasite life cycle stages present in the stool specimen. The two general types

> Examination of fecal specimens in the parasitology section is referred to as an O&P examination and consists of three steps: (1) a wet mount examination of the specimen, (2) a wet mount examination of the specimen following some type of concentration procedure, and (3) examination of a permanent stained smear of the specimen.

> The best morphological detail of protozoa is seen on permanently stained specimens. The trichrome staining procedure is the easiest and most reproducible of the staining procedures.

of concentration procedures are sedimentation and flotation procedures. Sedimentation procedures, such as the formalin ethyl acetate method, involve centrifugation of the specimen, after which the sediment is examined for parasite life cycle stages. With flotation procedures, such as the zinc sulfate method, parasite life cycle stages are usually found in the surface film that develops at the top of the preparation, but the sediment should also be examined. Large helminth eggs do not always float when flotation procedures are used.

Step 3: Examination of a permanent stained smear of a fresh or preserved specimen. This is the most important step in finding and identifying protozoa. The two most commonly used stains are the trichrome and iron hematoxylin stains.

A modified acid-fast staining method can be used to identify any coccidia (e.g., *Cryptosporidium parvum*, *Cyclospora cayetanensis*) that might be present in the specimen.

In addition to protozoan life cycle stages, microscopic examinations of stool specimens may reveal red blood cells, white blood cells, Charcot-Leyden crystals (elongated crystalline structures derived from eosinophils), and various objects that can be mistaken for parasite life cycle stages; the latter are referred to as artifacts (see the CD-ROM). Microscopes should be equipped with a calibrated ocular micrometer, because the size of a protozoan life cycle stage, such as a cyst or oocyst, is often an important identifying characteristic. Ocular micrometers and their calibration are discussed in Appendix A.

Processing Genitourinary Specimens

Vaginal and urethral discharge material and prostatic secretions are usually examined for the presence of *Trichomonas vaginalis* by a saline wet mount (as discussed later in the chapter). Various methods for culturing *T. vaginalis* are also available but are not commonly used in CMLs.

Processing Aspirates

Fine-needle aspirates of cysts and abscesses may be stained and examined for amebas using trichrome stain, *Toxoplasma gondii* using Giemsa stain, *Cryptosporidium parvum* and microsporidia using the modified trichrome stain, and *C. parvum* using an acid-fast staining procedure. Bone marrow aspirates can be stained with Giemsa stain and examined for *Plasmodium* spp. and amastigotes of *Trypanosoma cruzi* and *Leishmania* spp. Bronchoscopy aspirates may be examined for *T. gondii*, *C. parvum*, and microsporidia. Duodenal aspirates are examined for *Giardia lamblia*, *C. parvum*, and microsporidia.

Processing Cerebrospinal Fluid

Cerebrospinal fluid (CSF) sediment can be stained with Giemsa for trypanosomes or trypomastigotes, *T. gondii*, amebas, and microsporidia; with trichrome or calcofluor for amebas; or with acid-fast stain, calcofluor, or modified trichrome (chromotrope stain) for microsporidia. An agar/bacterial overlay method can be used to culture CSF for amebas such as *Naegleria* and *Acanthamoeba* spp., in which *Escherichia coli* is used as "food" for the amebas. However, *Balamuthia* amebas cannot be cultured in this manner.

Culture Methods

Culture of protozoa is rarely performed in CMLs. Although culture methods are available for *Entamoeba histolytica*, *Naegleria fowleri*, *Acanthamoeba* spp., *Trichomonas vaginalis*, *Toxoplasma gondii*, *Trypanosoma cruzi*, and *Leishmania* spp., these procedures are usually only performed in reference and research laboratories. When any of these protozoa are grown in vitro by themselves (i.e., no other microorganisms are present in the culture), the cultures are known as **axenic cultures.** When cultured together with another organism, the cultures are referred to as **monoxenic cultures.** When cultured with a mixture of other microorganisms, the cultures are referred to as **xenic cultures.**

Immunodiagnostic Procedures

Several immunodiagnostic procedures (IDPs) have been developed over the years for the diagnosis of parasitic infections—both protozoal and helminth infections. Antibody detection procedures have been developed for the diagnosis of African trypanosomiasis, amebiasis, babesiosis, Chagas disease, cryptosporidiosis, giardiasis, leishmaniasis, malaria, and toxoplasmosis. Antigen detection procedures have been developed for detection of *C. parvum*, *E. histolytica*, *G. lamblia*, microsporidia, and *T. vaginalis*. Relatively few of these parasitology IDPs are in routine use in CMLs, however, primarily because of problems related to sensitivity, specificity, expense, and the difficulty of interpreting results.

The most commonly used parasitology IDPs in CMLs are enzyme immunoassays for the detection of *Giardia* and

Cryptosporidium antigens in fecal specimens. The major disadvantages of most of the parasitology IDPs is that they detect only one or two parasites and fail to detect less common or exotic parasites. Because the patient may be infected with additional parasites, IDPs do not take the place of a thorough microscopic stool examination.

Molecular Diagnostic Procedures

Various molecular diagnostic procedures have been developed for the diagnosis of parasitic infections, but they are primarily used in research and reference laboratories. Molecular diagnostic procedures have been developed for African and American trypanosomiasis, amebiasis, cryptosporidiosis, giardiasis, leishmaniasis, microsporidial infections, malaria, and toxoplasmosis. Polymerase chain reaction procedures for detection of *G. lamblia*, *Cryptosporidium* sp., *Cyclospora cayetanensis*, microsporidia, and *Entamoeba histolytica* or *E. dispar* are performed in the Division of Parasitic Diseases at the CDC.

SELECTED PROTOZOAL INFECTIONS

Protozoal Infections of the Cardiovascular System

Although certain protozoal infections are diagnosed by observing protozoal life cycle stages in blood specimens, it is important to understand that these infections also involve other anatomical sites. Protozoal infections diagnosed by observing protozoal life cycle stages in blood specimens are summarized in Table 22-4.

Malaria

Disease. Malaria is a systemic sporozoan infection with malaise, fever, chills, sweating, headache, and nausea. The frequency with which the cycle of chills, fever, and sweating is repeated is referred to as periodicity, which depends on the particular species of malarial parasite causing the infection. The intermittent bouts of chills and fevers are sometimes referred to as **paroxysms.** In addition to these symptoms, falciparum malaria may be accompanied by cough, diarrhea, respiratory distress, shock, renal or liver failure, pulmonary or cerebral edema, coma, or death.

Geographic occurrence. Malaria is one of the most important infectious diseases in the world. It is a major health problem in many tropical and subtropical countries, with an estimated 300 million to 500 million cases and 1.5 million to 2.7 million deaths annually. About 90% of all malaria cases occur in Africa, where approximately 1 million children die from malaria each year. Recall from Chapter 2 that, in the United States, certain illnesses are designated as nationally notifiable infectious diseases and that newly diagnosed cases of these diseases must be reported to the CDC. Four parasitic diseases, all caused by parasitic protozoa, are reportable: malaria, giardiasis, cryptosporidiosis, and cyclosporiasis. A discussion of U.S. malaria cases is on the CD-ROM.

> Malaria is one of the most important infectious diseases in the world, causing an estimated 300 million to 500 million cases and 1.5 million to 2.7 million deaths annually.

Parasites. Malaria is caused by four species of the genus *Plasmodium*: *P. vivax*, *P. falciparum*, *P. malariae*, and *P. ovale*. These are **intraerythrocytic** sporozoan parasites, meaning that they live within erythrocytes, or red blood cells (RBCs). Worldwide *P. vivax* malaria is the most common type of malaria, *P. falciparum* malaria is the most deadly, and *P. ovale* malaria is the least common. Infection caused by *P. vivax* or *P. ovale* causes chills and fever every 48 hours and is referred to as tertian malaria. *P. malariae* infection causes chills and fever every 72 hours and is referred to as quartan malaria. *P. falciparum* periodicity varies from 36 to 48 hours. Mixed infections—that is, infections involving

TABLE 22 - 4	Examples of Protozoal Infections Diagnosed by Examining Stained Blood Smears	
Infection	**Observation Required for Diagnosis**
African trypanosomiasis	Extracellular trypomastigotes
American trypanosomiasis	Extracellular trypomastigotes
Babesiosis	Intraerythrocytic protozoa
Malaria	Intraerythrocytic protozoa

Four species of *Plasmodium* cause human malaria: *P. vivax, P. falciparum, P. malariae,* and *P. ovale.*

The *Plasmodium* life cycle is complex, involving an *Anopheles* mosquito as the definitive host and a human as the intermediate host.

The life cycle of malarial parasites is depicted in Figure 22-2

more than one *Plasmodium* spp.—occur in certain geographic areas. Drug-resistant strains of *P. falciparum* are common.

Plasmodium spp. have a complex life cycle involving a female *Anopheles* mosquito, the liver and erythrocytes of an infected human, and many life cycle stages.

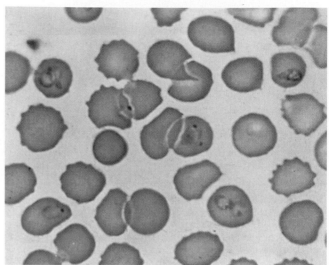

Figure 22-3. **Giemsa-stained peripheral blood smear showing** ***Plasmodium falciparum*** **trophozoites within red blood cells.** (From Binford CH, Connor DH. Pathology of Tropical and Extraordinary Diseases, vol 1. Washington, DC: Armed Forces Institute of Pathology, 1976.)

and described in detail on the CD-ROM. Most human infection occurs as a result of injection of sporozoites into the bloodstream by an infected female *Anopheles* mosquito while taking a blood meal. However, infection may also occur as a result of blood transfusion or the use of contaminated needles or syringes. Congenital transmission of malaria has also been documented.

Laboratory diagnosis. Malaria is diagnosed by observation and identification of intraerythrocytic *Plasmodium* parasites in Giemsa-stained blood smears (Fig. 22-3). The drawings in Figures 22-4 through 22-7 depict malarial parasites as seen in thin blood smears. Information regarding the appearance of malarial parasites in thick blood smears is contained on the CD-ROM. Table 22-5 lists the identifying features of the three most common causes of human malaria. Immunodiagnostic and molecular diagnostic procedures have been developed, but are not generally available in CMLs.

Malaria is diagnosed by finding and identifying intraerythrocytic *Plasmodium* parasites in stained blood smears.

For additional information on identifying *Plasmodium* spp., refer to the CD-ROM.

Essentials

Plasmodium **spp.**

• Four species cause human malaria: *P. vivax, P. falciparum, P. ovale, P. malariae*

• Intraerythrocytic sporozoan parasites

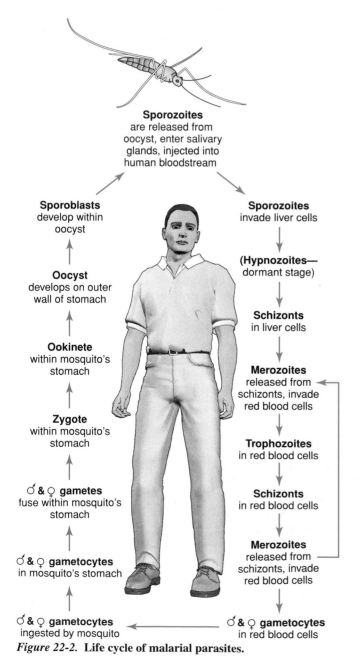

Sporozoites
are released from oocyst, enter salivary glands, injected into human bloodstream

Sporoblasts
develop within oocyst

Oocyst
develops on outer wall of stomach

Ookinete
within mosquito's stomach

Zygote
within mosquito's stomach

♂ & ♀ **gametes**
fuse within mosquito's stomach

♂ & ♀ **gametocytes**
in mosquito's stomach

♂ & ♀ **gametocytes**
ingested by mosquito

Sporozoites
invade liver cells

(Hypnozoites—
dormant stage)

Schizonts
in liver cells

Merozoites
released from schizonts, invade red blood cells

Trophozoites
in red blood cells

Schizonts
in red blood cells

Merozoites
released from schizonts, invade red blood cells

♂ & ♀ **gametocytes**
in red blood cells

Figure 22-2. **Life cycle of malarial parasites.**

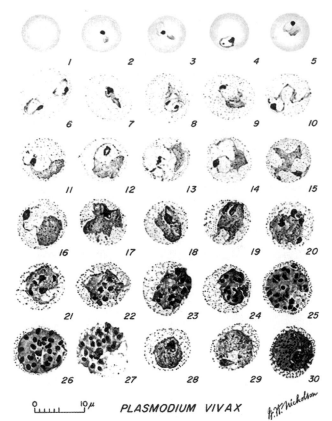

Figure 22-4. **Life cycle stages of *Plasmodium vivax* that can be observed in a thin blood smear. 1.** Normal RBC. **2–6.** Young ring-stage trophozoites. **7–18.** Mature trophozoites. **19–27.** Schizonts. **28–29.** Macrogametocytes (female gametocytes). **30.** Microgametocyte (male gametocyte). (Drawings by G. H. Nicholson. Courtesy of the CDC, Division of Parasitic Diseases.)

- Transmitted by the bite of infected *Anopheles* mosquitoes

- Mosquitoes are definitive hosts, and humans are intermediate hosts

- Malaria is diagnosed by observing trophozoites, sporozoites, or gametocytes in stained blood smears

Babesiosis

Disease. Babesiosis is a sporozoan disease that may include fever, chills, myalgia, fatigue, jaundice, and anemia. It is potentially severe and sometimes fatal, especially in splenectomized and elderly people. Patients may be simultaneously infected with *Borrelia burgdorferi*, the etiologic agent of Lyme disease (see Chapter 15), which is transmitted by the same species of ticks.

Geographic occurrence. Babesiosis is an endemic disease in many parts of the world, including Europe, Mexico, and the United States. Most U.S. cases occur in New York and New England.

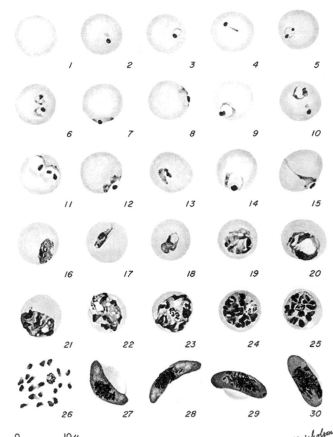

Figure 22-5. **Life cycle stages of *Plasmodium falciparum* that can be observed in a thin blood smear. 1.** Normal RBC. **2–10.** Young ring-stage trophozoites. **11–18.** Mature trophozoites. **19–26.** Schizonts. **27–28.** Mature macrogametocytes (female gametocytes). **29–30.** Mature microgametocytes (male gametocytes). (Drawings by G. H. Nicholson. Courtesy of the CDC, Division of Parasitic Diseases.)

Parasites. Babesiosis is caused by *Babesia microti* and other *Babesia* spp., including *B. divergens* in Europe. Like the malaria parasites, *Babesia* spp. are intraerythrocytic sporozoa (i.e., they live within erythrocytes, or RBCs). Reservoirs include rodents for *B. microti* and cattle for *B. divergens*. Transmission occurs by tick bite and rarely, by blood transfusion.

> Babesiosis is caused by sporozoan parasites in the genus *Babesia*. Because *Babesia* spp. are intraerythrocytic parasites, they are sometimes mistaken for malarial parasites.

Laboratory diagnosis. Babesiosis is diagnosed by observation and identification of intraerythrocytic *Babesia* parasites in Giemsa-stained blood smears (Fig. 22-8). They resemble the early trophozoite or "ring" forms of malarial parasites—particularly, *Plasmodium falciparum*—and thus must be differentiated from malarial parasites. In its early

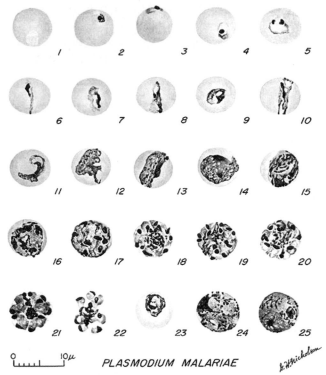

Figure 22-6. **Life cycle stages of *Plasmodium malariae* that can be observed in a thin blood smear. 1.** Normal RBC. **2–5.** Young ring-stage trophozoites. **6–13.** More mature trophozoites. **14–22.** Schizonts. **23.** Developing gametocyte. **24.** Macrogametocyte (female gametocyte). **25.** Microgametocyte (male gametocyte). (Drawings by G. H. Nicholson. Courtesy of the CDC, Division of Parasitic Diseases.)

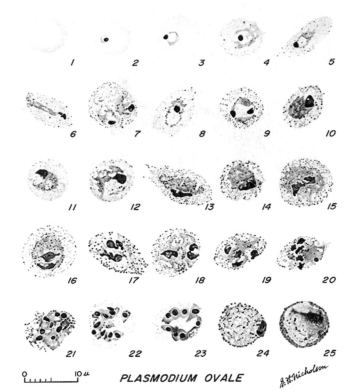

Figure 22-7. **Life cycle stages of *Plasmodium ovale* that can be observed in a thin blood smear. 1.** Normal RBC. **2–5.** Young ring-stage trophozoites. **6–15.** More mature trophozoites. **16–23.** Schizonts. **24.** Macrogametocyte (female gametocyte). **25.** Microgametocyte (male gametocyte). (Drawings by G. H. Nicholson. Courtesy of the CDC, Division of Parasitic Diseases.)

form, a *Babesia* parasite contains very little cytoplasm and a very small nucleus or chromatin dot. (**Chromatin** is the DNA-containing portion of a protozoan nucleus.) Mature forms may possess one or two chromatin dots. Unlike in malaria, *Babesia* infected RBCs are neither enlarged nor pale, they do not contain stippling, and malarial pigment is never seen. A tetrad formation, referred to as a Maltese cross, is sometimes seen (see Fig. 22-8). Immunodiagnostic and molecular diagnostic procedures have been developed but are not generally available in CMLs.

> Babesiosis is diagnosed by finding and identifying intraerythrocytic *Babesia* parasites in stained blood smears.

Essentials

Babesia spp.

- Intraerythrocytic sporozoan parasites
- Cause babesiosis
- Transmitted by the bite of infected ticks

- Babesiosis is diagnosed by observation and identification of intraerythrocytic *Babesia* parasites in stained blood smears

- Intraerythrocytic ring forms can be confused with malarial parasites

African Trypanosomiasis (African Sleeping Sickness)

Disease. African trypanosomiasis is a systemic disease caused by flagellated protozoa in the bloodstream, known as **hemoflagellates.** Early stages of the disease include a painful chancre at the site of a tsetse fly bite, fever, intense headache, insomnia, lymphadenitis, anemia, local edema, and rash. Later stages of the disease include body wasting, falling asleep, coma, and death if untreated. The later stages of the disease have given rise to the name African sleeping sickness or simply sleeping sickness.

Geographic occurrence. African trypanosomiasis is transmitted by the tsetse fly (genus *Glossina*), so the disease occurs only in tropical Africa where tsetse flies are found. It is estimated that more than 300,000 people have African trypanosomiasis and that about 66,000 people die each year from the disease.

TABLE 22 - 5	Identification Features of the Three Most Common Causes of Human Malaria		
Species	**Trophozoites**	**Schizonts**	**Gametocytes**
Plasmodium vivax (see Fig. 22-4)	Trophozoites in all stages may be observed. Young trophozoites occupy less than one-third of the diameter of the infected RBC. Older trophozoites have flowing or ameboid cytoplasm. Infected RBCs tend to be somewhat irregular in shape, enlarged and pale, with prominent pink-red-staining granules called Schüffner dots. Finely granular, brownish malarial pigment may be abundant in the infected RBCs.	Mature schizonts contain 12 to 14 or more merozoites, usually >13.	Gametocytes are large (half the diameter of the RBC or larger) and circular. Finely granular, brownish malarial pigment may be abundant in the infected RBCs.
Plasmodium falciparum (see Fig. 22-5)	Early ring forms are small, occupying more than one-third of the diameter of the RBC. Multiple ring forms may be observed within a RBC. Some ring forms may have two nuclei. Heavy infections involve >20% of the RBCs. Appliqué or accole forms may be seen, in which the ring forms are flattened out against the inner surface of the RBC's cell membrane. More developed trophozoites are usually observed only in fulminant infections. Infected RBCs are not enlarged and do not contain Schüffner dots.	Schizonts are rarely observed, except in fulminant infections.	Observation of characteristic banana-shaped or sickle-shaped gametocytes is diagnostic for *P. falciparum* malaria.
Plasmodium malariae (see Fig. 22-6)	Some developing trophozoites extend from one side of the RBC cell membrane to the other; these are referred to as "band forms." Infected RBCs are neither enlarged nor pale, and they do not contain Schüffner dots. Coarse or chunky, brownish malarial pigment may be abundant in the infected RBCs.	Mature schizonts contain 6 to 12 merozoites, arranged in a circular rosette pattern.	RBCs containing gametocytes are not enlarged.

Source: Winn WC Jr, et al. Koneman's Color Atlas and Textbook of Diagnostic Microbiology. 6th Ed. Philadelphia: Lippincott Williams & Wilkins, 2006.

RBC, red blood cell.

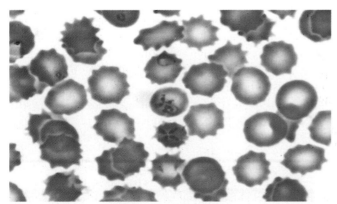

***Figure 22-8.* Intraerythrocytic *Babesia* parasites in a Wright-Giemsa-stained peripheral blood smear.** The parasites are sometimes arranged in pairs, resembling rabbit ears, or in tetrads, resembling a Maltese cross. (From Winn WC Jr, et al. Koneman's Color Atlas and Textbook of Diagnostic Microbiology. 6th Ed. Philadelphia: Lippincott Williams & Wilkins, 2006.)

Parasites. Two subspecies of *Trypanosoma brucei* cause African trypanosomiasis. *T. brucei* subsp. *gambiense*, in western and central Africa, causes most cases of sleeping sickness; the disease may last several years. *T. brucei* subsp. *rhodesiense*, in eastern Africa, causes a more rapidly fatal form of African trypanosomiasis; the disease is usually lethal within weeks or a few months without treatment. Infected humans serve as reservoirs of *T. brucei* subsp. *gambiense*, whereas wild animals and domestic cattle are the primary reservoirs of *T. brucei* subsp. *rhodesiense*. The tsetse fly becomes infected when it ingests blood that contains the trypanosomes. The parasites then multiply and mature within the infected tsetse fly. Humans

> African trypanosomiasis is caused by flagellated protozoa in the genus *Trypanosoma*, and is transmitted by a tsetse fly.

become infected when mature trypanosomes (trypomastigotes) are injected into the bloodstream as the infected tsetse fly takes a blood meal.

Laboratory diagnosis. African trypanosomiasis is diagnosed by observing and identifying trypomastigotes in blood, lymph node aspirates, or CSF. The trypomastigotes are long (30 μm or more) and slender with a long polar flagellum (Fig. 22-9). A parasite concentration technique, such as capillary tube centrifugation, is usually required to detect *T. brucei* subsp. *gambiense* but is usually not necessary to detect *T. brucei* subsp. *rhodesiense*. IDPs have been developed but are generally not available in CMLs.

> African trypanosomiasis is diagnosed by observing and identifying trypomastigotes in blood, lymph node aspirates, or CSF.

Essentials

Subspecies of *Trypanosoma brucei*

- Hemoflagellates

- Cause African trypanosomiasis

- *T. brucei* subsp. *gambiense* causes most cases of African sleeping sickness

- *T. brucei* subsp. *rhodesiense* causes a more rapidly fatal form of African trypanosomiasis

- Transmitted by the bite of infected tsetse flies (genus *Glossina*)

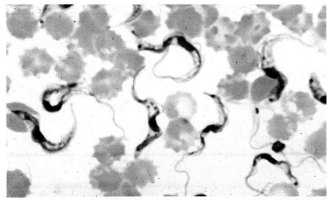

Figure 22-9. **Extracellular trypomastigotes in a Wright-stained peripheral blood smear of a patient with African trypanosomiasis.** Each trypomastigote has a centrally located nucleus and a posterior kinetoplast. A flagellum arises near the kinetoplast, extends along the outer edge of an undulating membrane, and projects as a free flagellum at the anterior end of the cell. (From Winn WC Jr, et al. Koneman's Color Atlas and Textbook of Diagnostic Microbiology. 6th Ed. Philadelphia: Lippincott Williams & Wilkins, 2006.)

> - African trypanosomiasis is diagnosed by observing and identifying trypomastigotes in blood, lymph node aspirates, or CSF

American Trypanosomiasis (Chagas Disease)

Disease. American trypanosomiasis is also known as Chagas disease, in honor of Carlos Chagas, who described the entire life cycle of *Trypanosoma cruzi* in 1909. In the acute stage of the disease, patients may present with an inflammatory response at the site of a reduviid bug bite, fever, malaise, lymphadenopathy, hepatomegaly (enlarged liver), and splenomegaly (enlarged spleen), although it may be asymptomatic. Chronic irreversible complications include heart damage, arrhythmias, enlarged esophagus (megaesophagus), and enlarged colon (megacolon). Life-threatening meningoencephalitis may occur.

Geographical occurrence. Chagas disease occurs primarily in South America, Central America, and Mexico, although a few cases have been reported in the United States (by bug bite or blood transfusion). As increasing numbers of infected people enter the country from endemic areas, concern is growing in the United States about the safety of the blood supply. Currently, U.S. donor blood is not routinely screened for the presence of *T. cruzi*. It is estimated that between 16 million and 18 million people have Chagas disease and that about 50,000 people die each year from the disease.

Parasite. The etiologic agent of American trypanosomiasis is *T. cruzi*, which occurs in two stages: a hemoflagellate, which is the trypomastigote form, and a nonmotile, intracellular parasite, which is the **amastigote** form. Reservoirs include humans and more than 150 species of domestic and wild animals, including dogs, cats, rodents, carnivores, and primates. The vectors of American trypanosomiasis are rather large insects known as bugs (see "Study Aid: Bugs"). They are known by many names, including reduviid bugs, triatome bugs, kissing bugs, assassin bugs, and cone-nosed bugs (Fig. 22-10). A bug becomes infected when it takes a blood meal from an infected animal. Then, as it takes a blood meal or feeds at the corner of a sleeping person's eye, the bug defecates. The person becomes infected by rubbing the insect feces—which contain the parasite—into the bite wound or eye. The characteristic unilateral swelling of the eyelid that occurs after *T. cruzi* is rubbed into the eye is called Romaña sign (Fig. 22-11). Transmission by blood transfusion and organ transplantation also occurs.

> Chagas disease or American trypanosomiasis is caused by the flagellated protozoan *Trypanosoma cruzi* and is transmitted by a reduviid bug.

> Associate Romaña sign with American trypanosomiasis (Chagas disease).

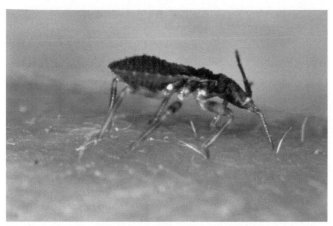

Figure 22-10. **A reduviid bug, the vector of American trypanosomiasis.** (Courtesy of the CDC and the World Health Organization.)

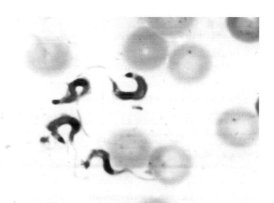

Figure 22-12. **Extracellular trypomastigotes in a Wright-stained peripheral blood smear of a patient with American trypanosomiasis.** Notice the characteristic *C* or *U* shape of the stained trypomastigotes and the large, darkly stained, dotlike kinetoplast at the posterior tip of each trypomastigote. A flagellum arises near the kinetoplast, extends along the outer edge of an undulating membrane, and projects as a free flagellum at the anterior end of the cell. (From Winn WC Jr, et al. Koneman's Color Atlas and Textbook of Diagnostic Microbiology. 6th Ed. Philadelphia: Lippincott Williams & Wilkins, 2006.)

STUDY AID

Bugs. Some people refer to all, or most, insects as bugs, but only one category of insects (class Insecta) actually contains bugs. Technically, true bugs are in the order Hemiptera. Included in this order are bed bugs, reduviid bugs, several types of water bugs, and many plant bugs.

those of *T. brucei*, the trypomastigotes of *T. cruzi* are usually *C* or *U* shaped in permanent stained smears and have a large oval kinetoplast at the posterior end. As mentioned in Chapter 21, a kinetoplast is part of a large DNA-containing mitochondrion. IDPs have been developed but are generally not available in CMLs.

> American trypanosomiasis is diagnosed by observing and identifying trypomastigotes in blood or amastigotes in blood or tissue or lymph node biopsies.

Laboratory diagnosis. American trypanosomiasis is diagnosed by observation of trypomastigotes in blood (Fig. 22-12) or amastigotes in blood or tissue (especially cardiac muscle) or lymph node biopsies (Fig. 22-13). Although they resemble

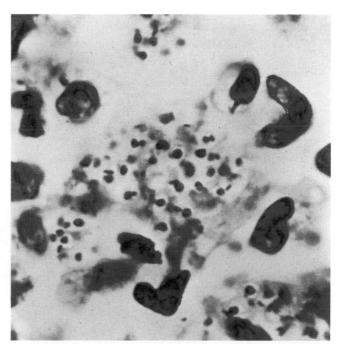

Figure 22-13. **Numerous red-stained amastigotes of *Trypanosoma cruzi*.** Each amastigote contains a large nucleus and a rod-shaped kinetoplast. The amastigote of *T. cruzi* is indistinguishable from the amastigote of *Leishmania* spp. (From Binford CH, Connor DH. Pathology of Tropical and Extraordinary Diseases, vol 1. Washington, DC: Armed Forces Institute of Pathology, 1976.)

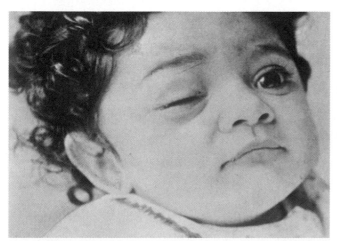

Figure 22-11. **Romaña sign.** The swelling around the right eye of this child is a characteristic sign of Chagas disease. (From Binford CH, Connor DH. Pathology of Tropical and Extraordinary Diseases, vol 1. Washington, DC: Armed Forces Institute of Pathology, 1976.)

> Xenodiagnosis is a method of diagnosing Chagas disease by allowing uninfected reduviid bugs to take blood meals from the person suspected of having the disease.

An interesting diagnostic procedure known as **xenodiagnosis** is performed in endemic countries, primarily South America. In this procedure, sterile (uninfected) laboratory-raised reduviid bugs are allowed to take blood meals from persons suspected of having Chagas disease. The bugs are then taken to a laboratory. After 30 to 60 days, feces from the bugs are periodically checked microscopically for the presence of the parasite. Finding trypomastigotes in the bug feces indicates that the bugs became infected when they ingested the person's blood and thus confirms the diagnosis of Chagas disease. Xenodiagnosis is not performed in the United States.

Essentials

Trypanosoma cruzi

- Hemoflagellate

- Causes American trypanosomiasis (also known as Chagas disease)

- Transmitted by infected reduviid bugs (the parasite is present in bug feces); can also be transmitted by blood transfusion

- Associate Romaña sign and xenodiagnosis with Chagas disease

- Chagas disease is diagnosed by observing motile trypomastigotes in blood or nonmotile amastigotes in blood or tissue (especially cardiac muscle) or lymph node biopsies

Protozoal Infections of the Skin and Mucous Membranes

Leishmaniasis

Disease. There are three forms of leishmaniasis: cutaneous, mucocutaneous (or mucosal), and visceral. The cutaneous form starts with a papule that enlarges into a craterlike ulcer (Fig. 22-14). Individual ulcers may coalesce, causing severe tissue destruction and disfigurement. Visceral leishmaniasis, also known as kala-azar, is characterized by fever, enlarged liver and spleen, lymphadenopathy, anemia, leukopenia, and progressive emaciation and weakness. Death may result in untreated cases (Fig. 22-15).

Geographic occurrence. Leishmaniasis occurs in many regions of the world, including Pakistan, India, China, the Middle East, Africa, South America, Central America, and Mexico; cases have also occurred in south central Texas. It is estimated that between 1.5 million and 2 million people have leishmaniasis and that about 57,000 people die each year from the disease.

Parasites. Leishmaniasis is caused by various species of flagellated protozoa in the genus *Leishmania*. The nonmotile, intracellular form of the parasite is called an amastigote. The motile, extracellular form of the parasite is called a promastigote. Reservoirs include infected humans, domestic

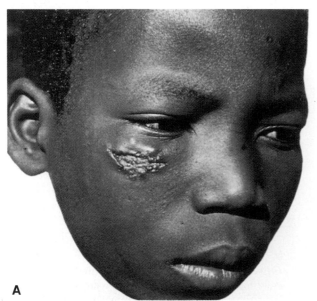

A

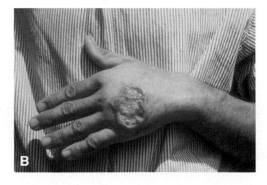

B

Figure 22-14. **Patients with cutaneous leishmaniasis.** ([A] From Binford CH, Connor DH. Pathology of Tropical and Extraordinary Diseases, vol 1. Washington, DC: Armed Forces Institute of Pathology, 1976. [B] Courtesy of Dr. D.S. Martin and the CDC.)

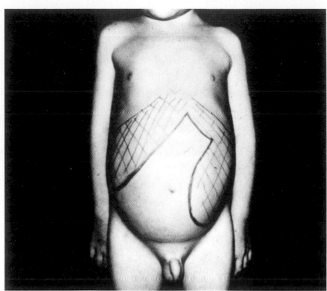

Figure 22-15. **Visceral leishmaniasis patient with hepatosplenomegaly.** Enlarged liver (outlined on the patient's right and left sides) and spleen (outlined on the patient's left side, beneath the left lobe of the liver). (From Binford CH, Connor DH. Pathology of Tropical and Extraordinary Diseases, vol 1. Washington, DC: Armed Forces Institute of Pathology, 1976.)

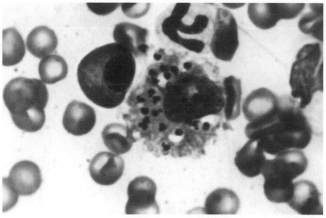

Figure 22-16. *Leishmania donovani* **amastigotes within a macrophage in a bone marrow smear from an infected dog.** (Courtesy of Dr. Francis W. Chandler and the CDC.)

possess a single anterior flagellum. An intradermal test, called the Montenegro test, and immunodiagnostic and molecular diagnostic procedures are also available. In the Montenegro test, an antigen derived from promastigotes is injected into the skin.

Diagnosis of visceral leishmaniasis is made by culture of biopsy specimens or aspirates, or by demonstration of intracellular amastigotes—called **Leishman-Donovan bodies**—in stained smears from the bone marrow, spleen, liver, lymph node, or blood. A PCR technique is available but is not generally available in CMLs.

> Visceral leishmaniasis is diagnosed by culture of biopsy specimens or aspirates or by demonstration of intracellular amastigotes—called Leishman-Donovan bodies—in stained smears from bone marrow, spleen, liver, lymph node, or blood.

Essentials

Leishmania spp.

- Tissue flagellates; many species

- Cause cutaneous, mucocutaneous (or mucosal), and visceral leishmaniasis; the latter form of the disease is also known as kala azar

- Many animal reservoirs

- Usually transmitted via the bite of an infected sandfly; rarely, by blood transfusion

- Diagnosis is usually made by microscopic identification of the nonmotile amastigote form in stained preparations from lesions; some diagnoses obtained by

> Leishmaniasis is caused by various species of flagellated protozoa in the genus *Leishmania* and is usually transmitted via the bite of an infected sandfly.

dogs, and various wild animals. Leishmaniasis is principally a zoonosis and is usually transmitted via the bite of an infected sandfly. Transmission by blood transfusion and person-to-person contact has been reported.

Laboratory diagnosis. Diagnosis of cutaneous and mucocutaneous leishmaniasis is made by microscopic identification of the amastigote form in stained preparations from lesions (Fig. 22-16) or by culture of the extracellular promastigote form on suitable media. Culture is rarely performed in CMLs. In stained preparations, amastigotes are seen within macrophages and close to disrupted cells. Amastigotes are small (3.0 to 5.0 μm in diameter), round or oval bodies containing large nuclei and small kinetoplasts. Promastigotes are long (10 to 15 μm) and slender and

> Diagnosis of cutaneous and mucocutaneous leishmaniasis is made by microscopic identification of the amastigote form in stained preparations from lesions or by culture of the extracellular promastigote form on suitable media.

> Associate the Montenegro skin test with cutaneous and mucocutaneous leishmaniasis.

cultures of the motile extracellular promastigote form, and some by IDPs

- In stained preparations, amastigotes are seen within macrophages and close to disrupted cells

- Associate the Montenegro skin test and Leishman-Donovan bodies with leishmaniasis

Protozoal Infections of the Eyes

Protozoal infections of the eyes include conjunctivitis and keratoconjunctivitis (inflammation of the cornea and conjunctiva) caused by amebas in the genus *Acanthamoeba*, and toxoplasmosis caused by the sporozoan *Toxoplasma gondii*. Although toxoplasmosis is described in this section of the chapter, there are many manifestations of toxoplasmosis in addition to ocular disease. Ocular manifestations of toxoplasmosis occur primarily in immunosuppressed patients, in whom the infection can lead to removal of the infected eyeball (enucleation). Amebic conjunctivitis and keratoconjunctivitis can also result in enucleation.

Amebic Eye Infections

Disease. Amebic conjunctivitis and keratoconjunctivitis are amebic infections causing inflammation of the conjunctiva, corneal ulcers, pus formation, and severe pain. These infections can lead to loss of vision. The disease process is more rapid if corneal abrasions are present.

Geographic occurrence. Amebic eye infections occur in many countries on all continents.

> Amebic eye infections, such as amebic conjunctivitis and keratoconjunctivitis, are caused by several species of amebas in the genus *Acanthamoeba*. These amebas are facultative parasites, capable of either a free-living or a parasitic existence.

Parasites. Amebic eye infections are caused by several species of amebas in the genus *Acanthamoeba*. Because these amebas are capable of either a free-living or a parasitic existence, they are referred to as facultative parasites. The amebas enter the eye from ameba-contaminated waters. Infections have occurred primarily in people who wear soft contact lenses and have used nonsterile, homemade cleaning or wetting solutions or have become infected in ameba-contaminated spas or hot tubs.

SAFETY TIP

Avoiding Amebic Eye Infections. To help prevent amebic eye infections, people who wear soft contact lenses should not wear their lenses while swimming or in hot tubs and should strictly follow manufacturers' instructions regarding care and cleaning of the lenses.

Laboratory diagnosis. Amebic eye infections are diagnosed by microscopic examination of scrapings, swabs, or aspirates of the eye, or by culture on media seeded with *Escherichia coli* bacteria or another member of the family Enterobacteriaceae. The bacteria on the media serve as food for the amebas.

> Amebic eye infections are diagnosed by microscopic examination of scrapings, swabs, or aspirates of the eye, or by culture on media seeded with *Escherichia coli* or related bacteria.

Toxoplasmosis

Disease. Toxoplasmosis is a systemic sporozoan infection that, in immunocompetent people, may be asymptomatic or resemble infectious mononucleosis. However, serious disease, even death, may occur in immunodeficient persons; diseases typically involve the central nervous system, eyes (chorioretinitis), lungs, muscles, or heart. Cerebral toxoplasmosis is common in AIDS patients. Infection during early pregnancy may lead to fetal infection, causing death of the fetus or serious birth defects (e.g., brain damage).

Geographic occurrence. Toxoplasmosis occurs worldwide.

Parasite. The cause of toxoplasmosis is *Toxoplasma gondii*, an intracellular sporozoan. Definitive hosts include cats and other felines that usually acquire infection by eating infected rodents or birds. Intermediate hosts include rodents, birds, sheep, goats, swine, and cattle. Humans usually become infected by eating infected raw or undercooked meat (usually pork or mutton) containing the cyst form of the parasite or by ingesting oocysts that have been shed in the feces of infected cats. Oocysts may be present in food or water contaminated by feline feces. Children may ingest oocysts from sandboxes containing cat feces. Infection can also be acquired transplacentally, by blood transfusion, or by organ transplantation.

> Toxoplasmosis is caused by *Toxoplasma gondii*, an intracellular sporozoan. Humans usually become infected by eating infected raw or undercooked meat containing the cyst form of the parasite or by ingesting oocysts that have been shed in the feces of infected cats.

SAFETY TIP

Avoiding Toxoplasmosis. Prevention of toxoplasmosis can be achieved by cooking meats thoroughly, covering sandboxes when not in use, wearing gloves when gardening or cleaning a cat's litter box, disposing of cat feces and litter

daily (before the parasite becomes infective) in the toilet or by burying deeply, and washing hands after handling cats. In addition, pregnant women should avoid litter boxes, soil contaminated with cat feces, and eating rare or raw meat.

> **Laboratory diagnosis.** Toxoplasmosis is typically diagnosed using IDPs. Other diagnostic methods include demonstration of the parasite in stained biopsy or necropsy specimens, or isolation of *T. gondii* using laboratory animals or cell culture.

Laboratory diagnosis. Toxoplasmosis is typically diagnosed using IDPs. Other diagnostic methods include demonstration of the parasite in stained body tissues or fluids obtained by biopsy or necropsy, and isolation of *T. gondii* using laboratory animals or cell culture.

Essentials

Toxoplasma gondii

- An intracellular sporozoan parasite

- Causes a systemic infection called toxoplasmosis

- Definitive hosts include cats and other felines; intermediate hosts include rodents, birds, sheep, goats, swine, and cattle

- Humans usually become infected by eating infected raw or undercooked meat that contains the cyst form of the parasite or by ingesting oocysts that have been shed in the feces of infected cats; infection can also be acquired transplacentally, by blood transfusion, or by organ transplantation

- Toxoplasmosis is usually diagnosed using IDPs

- Other diagnostic methods include demonstration of the parasite in stained body tissues or fluids obtained by biopsy or necropsy, and isolation of *T. gondii* using laboratory animals or cell culture

Protozoal Infections of the Central Nervous System

Protozoal infections of the central nervous system (CNS) include African trypanosomiasis and toxoplasmosis (both of which were discussed earlier in the chapter), primary amebic meningoencephalitis, and granulomatous amebic encephalitis.

Primary Amebic Meningoencephalitis

Disease. Primary amebic meningoencephalitis (PAM) is an amebic disease causing inflammation of the brain and meninges, sore throat, severe frontal headache, hallucinations, nausea, vomiting, high fever, and stiff neck. Death occurs within 10 days, usually on day 5 or 6.

Geographic occurrence. PAM has been reported worldwide.

Parasites. The most common cause of PAM is *Naegleria fowleri*, an **ameboflagellate.** These organisms are either amebas or free-living flagellates in water and soil but exist only as amebas within a host. Usually, they enter the nasal passages of a person diving and/or swimming in ameba-contaminated water, such as ponds, lakes, "the old swimming hole," thermal springs, hot tubs, spas, and public swimming pools. After the amebas colonize the nasal tissues, they invade the brain and meninges by traveling along the olfactory nerves.

> **SAFETY TIP**
>
> *Avoiding Primary Amebic Meningoencephalitis. To avoid PAM, people should not dive into or swim in stagnant water, especially lakes and ponds where infection is known or presumed to have been acquired. Proper chlorine levels should always be maintained in swimming pools, spas, and hot tubs.*

Laboratory diagnosis. PAM is diagnosed by microscopic examination of wet mount preparations of fresh CSF. Because they are colorless and transparent, amebas are difficult to see in wet mounts unless the microscope light is turned very low. Phase contrast microscopy is helpful. *Naegleria* trophozoites may become flagellated after a few hours in water. Smears of CSF sediment can be stained with Wright, Wright-Giemsa, Giemsa, or trichrome stain. Leukocytes and amebas are similar in appearance. Unfortunately, most cases of PAM are diagnosed after the patient's death through observation of amebas in stained sections of brain tissue.

> Amebas are difficult to see in CSF and, when seen, may be mistaken for white blood cells.

Granulomatous Amebic Encephalitis

Disease. Granulomatous amebic encephalitis (GAE) is a granulomatous disease of the brain and meninges of immunocompromised patients. The term *granulomatous* means "having the characteristics of a granuloma." A **granuloma** is a nodular inflammatory lesion, containing compactly grouped phagocytic cells, such as epithelioid cells, giant cells, and macrophages.

Geographic occurrence. This disease occurs throughout the world.

Parasite. GAE is caused by environmental amebas in the genera *Acanthamoeba* and *Balamuthia*. Usually, these amebas enter the body through a skin lesion and make their way to the CNS via the bloodstream.

Laboratory diagnosis. Diagnosis of GAE is made by microscopic examination of wet mounts or stained smears of CSF. *Acanthamoeba* spp. can be cultured on nonnutrient agar seeded with *E. coli* or another member of the family Enterobacteriaceae. The Web site of the CDC's Division of Parasitic Diseases (http://www.dpd.cdc.gov/dpdx) or a parasitology textbook should be consulted for information on methods of differentiating among species of *Naegleria*, *Acanthamoeba*, and *Balamuthia*.

Protozoal Infections of the Genitourinary Tract

Trichomoniasis

Disease. Trichomoniasis is a sexually transmitted protozoal disease affecting both males and females. The disease is usually symptomatic in women, causing vaginitis with a profuse, thin, foamy, malodorous, greenish yellow discharge. It has been estimated that trichomoniasis accounts for approximately one-third of the cases of vaginitis in the United States (another third is caused by *Candida albicans* and another third by bacteria). In women, trichomoniasis may also present as urethritis or cystitis. Although rarely symptomatic in men, trichomoniasis may lead to prostatitis, urethritis, or infection of the seminal vesicles. Persons with trichomoniasis often also have other sexually transmitted diseases, especially gonorrhea.

Geographic occurrence. Trichomoniasis occurs worldwide.

Parasite. *Trichomonas vaginalis*, a flagellate, is the cause of trichomoniasis (Fig. 22-17). Infected humans are the only reservoirs. Transmission is by direct contact with vaginal and urethral discharges of infected people during sexual intercourse (Fig. 22-18). Because this organism exists only in the fragile trophozoite stage (there is no cyst stage), it cannot survive long outside the human body.

Laboratory diagnosis. Vaginitis caused by *T. vaginalis* can be diagnosed by performing a saline wet mount examination (described in Appendix A) of freshly collected vaginal discharge material and observing the motile trophozoites (Fig. 22-19). The specimen must be fresh because the trophozoites die shortly after specimen collection, become more spherical, and then cannot be differentiated from white blood cells. Trophozoites are 5 to 15 μm wide by 7.0 to 23 μm long. They possess a pointed axostyle that protrudes from the posterior end,[1] an undulating membrane approximately half the length of the trophozoite, and four anterior flagella that are too thin to be seen with a compound light microscope. The flagella and undulating membrane cause the organism to be in constant motion. Culture procedures are also available but are rarely performed in CMLs. *T. vaginalis* trophozoites are sometimes seen in urine and Papanicolaou (Pap) smears. Diagnosis of trichomoniasis in males can be accomplished by performing a saline wet mount of urethral discharge material or prostatic secretions.

> Trichomoniasis is a sexually transmitted protozoal disease caused by *Trichomonas vaginalis*, a flagellated protozoan. Although the name of the organism suggests that trichomoniasis is a disease affecting females, it is important to remember that the disease affects both genders.

> Trichomoniasis is usually diagnosed by microscopic examination of vaginal and urethral discharge material or prostatic secretions.

Essentials

Trichomonas vaginalis

- A flagellate that has no cyst form

- Causes a sexually transmitted disease called trichomoniasis

- Trichomoniasis is usually symptomatic in females and asymptomatic in males

- Humans are the only hosts; transmission typically occurs by direct contact with vaginal and urethral discharges of infected people

- Vaginitis caused by *T. vaginalis* is usually diagnosed by performing a saline wet mount examination of freshly collected vaginal discharge material and observing motile trophozoites

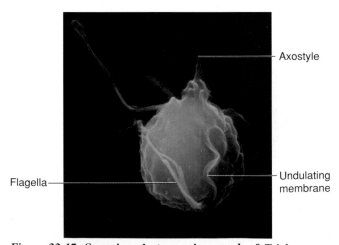

Axostyle

Flagella

Undulating membrane

Figure 22-17. **Scanning electron micrograph of *Trichomonas vaginalis*.** (Courtesy of Dr. S. Erlandsen.)

---

[1] An axostyle is an internal, elongate, supporting rod or tubule that runs the length of certain protozoa, frequently projecting from the posterior end. Examples of parasitic protozoa with axostyles are Trichomonas vaginalis and Giardia lamblia.

Trichomoniasis
(Trichomonas vaginalis)

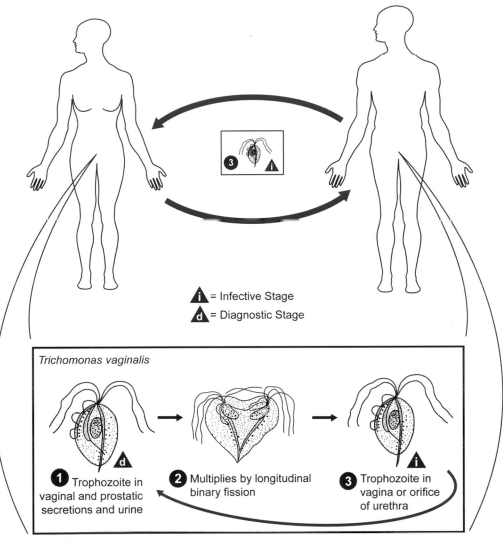

i = Infective Stage
d = Diagnostic Stage

Trichomonas vaginalis

1 Trophozoite in vaginal and prostatic secretions and urine

2 Multiplies by longitudinal binary fission

3 Trophozoite in vagina or orifice of urethra

Figure 22-18. **Trichomoniasis.** *T. vaginalis* resides in the female lower genital tract and the male urethra and prostate (**1**), where it replicates by binary fission (**2**). *T. vaginalis* is transmitted among humans, its only known host, primarily by sexual intercourse. (Courtesy of the CDC, Division of Parasitic Diseases.)

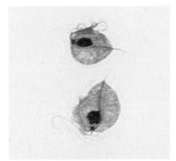

Figure 22-19. **Giemsa-stained *T. vaginalis* trophozoites from in vitro culture.** (Courtesy of the CDC, Division of Parasitic Diseases.)

- Diagnosis of trichomoniasis in males can be accomplished by performing a saline wet mount of urethral discharge material or prostatic secretions

- Culture techniques are available but are rarely used

Protozoal Infections of the Gastrointestinal Tract

Of the many protozoal infections of the gastrointestinal (GI) tract, only amebiasis, balantidiasis, cryptosporidiosis, cyclosporiasis, and giardiasis are discussed here. The latter

TABLE 22 - 6	Intestinal Protozoal Infections Diagnosed by Examining Stool Specimens
Infection	**Observation Required for Diagnosis**
Amebiasis	Trophozoites (amebas) and/or cysts
Balantidiasis	Trophozoites and/or cysts
Cryptosporidiosis	Oocysts
Cyclosporiasis	Oocysts
Giardiasis	Trophozoites and/or cysts

three diseases are nationally notifiable infectious diseases in the United States (see the Chapter 2 section of the CD-ROM for information regarding the incidence of these diseases in the United States). Table 22-6 summarizes how some important intestinal protozoal infections of humans are diagnosed.

Amebiasis, Amebic Dysentery, Amebic Abscesses, Amebomas

Disease. Amebiasis or amebic dysentery is a protozoal gastrointestinal infection that may be asymptomatic, mild, or severe and is often accompanied by dysentery, fever, chills, bloody or mucoid diarrhea or constipation, and colitis. The amebas may invade mucous membranes of the colon, forming abscesses and **amebomas,** which are granulomas sometimes mistaken for carcinoma. Amebas also may be disseminated via the bloodstream to extraintestinal sites, leading to abscesses of the liver, lung, brain, or other organs (Fig. 22-20). Depending on their location, untreated extraintestinal amebic abscesses can be fatal.

Geographic occurrence. Amebiasis occurs worldwide.

Parasite. Amebiasis is caused by *Entamoeba histolytica.* Like all amebas, *E. histolytica* has two stages: the cyst stage, which is the dormant, infective stage, and the motile, metabolically active, reproducing trophozoite stage. Reservoirs include symptomatic or asymptomatic humans and fecally contaminated food or water. Transmission occurs in one of several ways: (1) via ingestion of fecally contaminated food or water containing cysts, (2) by flies transporting cysts from feces to food, (3) via the fecally soiled hands of infected food handlers, (4) by oral-anal sexual contact, or (5) by anal intercourse involving multiple sex partners.

> Amebiasis or amebic dysentery is a protozoal gastrointestinal infection caused by the ameba *Entamoeba histolytica.*

Laboratory diagnosis. Amebic dysentery is diagnosed by microscopic observation of *E. histolytica* trophozoites and/or cysts in stained smears of fecal specimens. Amebic trophozoites and cysts are only 1 or 2 μm in diameter and thus are difficult to find in permanent stained smears of fecal material. It is also necessary for CML professionals to be able to differentiate *E. histolytica* from other pathogenic and nonpathogenic intestinal amebas, some of which are shown in Figure 22-21 and are briefly discussed on the CD-ROM.

> Amebic dysentery is diagnosed by microscopic observation of *E. histolytica* trophozoites and/or cysts in stained smears of fecal specimens.

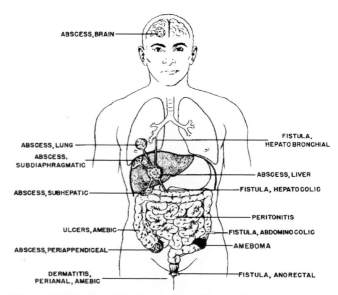

Figure 22-20. **Complications of amebiasis.** (From Binford CH, Connor DH. Pathology of Tropical and Extraordinary Diseases, vol 1. Washington, DC: Armed Forces Institute of Pathology, 1976.)

AMEBAE

	Entamoeba histolytica	Entamoeba hartmanni	Entamoeba coli	Entamoeba polecki[1]	Endolimax nana	Iodamoeba bütschlii	Dientamoeba fragilis[2]
Trophozoite							
Cyst							No cyst

[1]Rare, probably of animal origin
[2]Flagellate

Scale: | 0   5   10 μm

Adapted from Brooke and Melvin, 1964

Figure 22-21. **Drawings of amebas that can be observed in human fecal specimens.** (Courtesy of the CDC, Division of Parasitic Diseases.)

White blood cells, pollen grains, partially digested vegetative matter, and other artifacts are sometimes misidentified as ameba trophozoites and cysts (see the CD-ROM). The trophozoites and cysts of *E. histolytica* are shown in Figures 22-22 and 22-23, respectively. Nonpathogenic strains of *E. histolytica*, called *E. dispar*, are identical in appearance to the pathogenic strains, with one exception: *E. histolytica* trophozoites may contain ingested RBCs, whereas *E. dispar* trophozoites do not. The presence of RBCs within trophozoites indicates invasive amebiasis, but ingested RBCs are not always present. Immature cysts of *E. histolytica* contain one nucleus, a glycogen mass, and several darkly staining chromatoidal bars having smooth, rounded edges.

> When observed in fecal smears, trophozoites containing ingested RBCs are virtually always indicative of an invasive strain of *E. histolytica.*

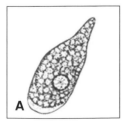 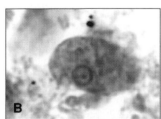 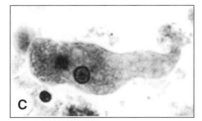 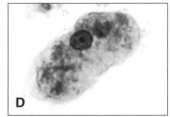

Figure 22-22. **Trophozoites of *Entamoeba histolytica* or *E. dispar*.** The trophozoites of these two species are identical in appearance. Only when ingested RBCs are observed can pathogenic *E. histolytica* be distinguished from nonpathogenic *E. dispar*. **A.** Line drawing. **B, C, and D.** Stained trophozoites, each possessing a typical-appearing single nucleus, containing a centrally located karyosome (chromatin mass) and uniformly distributed peripheral chromatin. It should be noted that the nuclei of *E. histolytica* and *E. dispar* do not always have this typical appearance. The cytoplasm has a granular or ground-glass appearance. (Courtesy of the CDC, Division of Parasitic Diseases.)

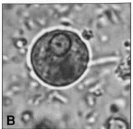
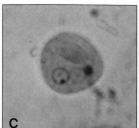
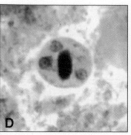
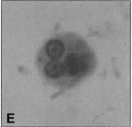

A   B   C   D   E

Figure 22-23. **Cysts of *E. histolytica* or *E. dispar*. A.** Line drawing. **B and C.** Cysts in iodine-stained wet mounts. **D and E.** Cysts in permanent stained preparations. The cysts are usually spherical and often have a halo, as seen in B and C. Mature cysts have four nuclei. The cyst in B appears uninucleate, while two to three nuclei are visible in the focal planes in C, D, and E. The nuclei have characteristically centrally located karyosomes and fine, uniformly distributed peripheral chromatin. The cysts in C, D, and E contain chromatoid bodies; the one in D is particularly visible, with typically blunted ends. *E. histolytica* cysts are usually 12 to 15 μm in diameter. (Courtesy of the CDC, Division of Parasitic Diseases.)

Cysts may contain one, two, or four nuclei. Mature cysts range from 10 to 20 μm in diameter and may or may not contain chromatoidal bars. Physical features of *E. histolytica* trophozoites and cysts enable differentiation from most other pathogenic and nonpathogenic amebas found in stool specimens.

Nonpathogenic amebas that may be observed in human fecal specimens include *Entamoeba coli*, *Entamoeba hartmanni*, *Iodamoeba bütschlii*, and *Endolimax nana*. CML professionals must be able to differentiate the trophozoites and cysts of these species from those of *E. histolytica* and *E. dispar*. Information about these nonpathogenic amebas can be found on the CD-ROM.

IDPs are available for the diagnosis of amebiasis, but these procedures are performed primarily at reference laboratories.

Essentials

Entamoeba histolytica

- An intestinal ameba

- Causes amebiasis (amebic dysentery); amebas may invade mucous membranes of the colon, forming abscesses and granulomas called amebomas; amebas may be also be disseminated via the bloodstream to extraintestinal sites, leading to abscesses of the liver, lung, brain, and other organs

- Reservoirs include symptomatic or asymptomatic humans and fecally contaminated food or water

- Transmission most often occurs by ingestion of fecally contaminated food or water containing cysts

- Amebic dysentery is diagnosed by microscopic observation of tiny *E. histolytica* trophozoites and/or cysts in stained smears of fecal specimens; *E. histolytica*

must be differentiated from other pathogenic and nonpathogenic intestinal amebas, as well as artifacts that resemble trophozoites or cysts

- When observed in fecal smears, trophozoites containing ingested RBCs are virtually always indicative of an invasive strain of *E. histolytica*

Balantidiasis

Disease. Balantidiasis is a protozoal gastrointestinal infection of the colon causing diarrhea or dysentery, colic, nausea, and vomiting.

Geographic occurrence. Although seen worldwide, balantidiasis is rare in the United States.

Parasite. Balantidiasis is caused by *Balantidium coli*, a ciliated protozoan. *B. coli* is the only ciliate that causes disease in humans. Balantidiasis occurs more commonly in pigs than in humans. Reservoirs include pigs and anything that might be contaminated with pig feces (e.g., drinking water). Transmission most often occurs via ingestion of *B. coli* cysts in fecally contaminated food or water.

> *Balantidium coli* is the only ciliated protozoan that causes human infection. Transmission most often occurs via ingestion of *B. coli* cysts in fecally contaminated food or water.

Laboratory diagnosis. Balantidiasis is diagnosed by observing and identifying *B. coli* trophozoites or cysts in fecal specimens (Figs. 22-24 and 22-25), which may also contain blood and mucus. Trophozoites are large (40 to 70 μm wide by 50 to 100 μm long), oval, and covered with

> Balantidiasis is diagnosed by observing and identifying *Balantidium coli* trophozoites or cysts in fecal specimens, which may also contain blood and mucus.

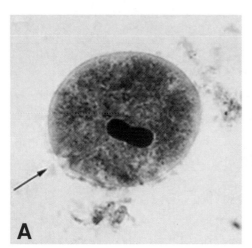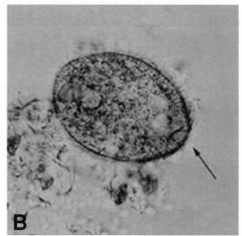

Figure 22-24. **Trophozoites of *Balantidium coli*. A.** A darkly stained macronucleus can be seen in this trophozoite. The arrow is pointing to its cytostome (primitive mouth). **B.** The macronucleus is visible in this trophozoite, as are short cilia on the trophozoite's surface. The arrow is pointing to its cytostome. (Courtesy of the CDC, Division of Parasitic Diseases.)

short cilia that are barely visible with the compound light microscope. Cysts are large (50 to 70 μm in diameter) and spherical with two nuclei—a macronucleus and a micronucleus. The micronucleus is often difficult to see, but the large, kidney-shaped macronucleus is always visible and is considered a diagnostic feature.

Essentials

Balantidium coli

- An intestinal ciliate

- The only ciliate that causes disease in humans

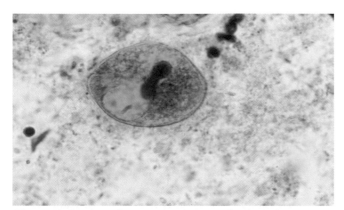

Figure 22-25. ***B. coli*** **cyst.** The darkly stained macronucleus is clearly visible. The tiny micronucleus, adjacent to and just left of the macronucleus, can barely be seen. (To compare the size of this macronucleus with that of a micronucleus, see Fig. 22-26.) (From Winn WC Jr, et al. Koneman's Color Atlas and Textbook of Diagnostic Microbiology. 6th Ed. Philadelphia: Lippincott Williams & Wilkins, 2006.)

- Causes a dysenteric disease called balantidiasis

- Reservoirs include pigs and anything that might be contaminated with pig feces (e.g., drinking water)

- Transmission usually occurs via ingestion of *B. coli* cysts in fecally contaminated food or water

- Balantidiasis is diagnosed by observing and identifying relatively large *B. coli* trophozoites or cysts in fecal specimens; the trophozoites and cysts contain two nuclei (a macronucleus and a micronucleus)

Cryptosporidiosis

Disease. Cryptosporidiosis is a gastrointestinal infection caused by a coccidial protozoan. Coccidia are classified in the phylum Sporozoa. Other coccidial parasites of humans are in the genera *Cyclospora*, *Isospora*, and *Sarcocystis* (Fig. 22-26). Cryptosporidiosis may be asymptomatic or may cause diarrhea, cramping, and abdominal pain. Less common symptoms include malaise, fever, anorexia, nausea, and vomiting. The disease may be prolonged, fulminant, and fatal in immunosuppressed patients. Children under 2 years of age, animal handlers, travelers, homosexuals, and day care center workers are particularly likely to be infected. Outbreaks in day care centers are common. Outbreaks have also been associated with drinking water, recreational use water, and drinking unpasteurized apple cider contaminated with cattle feces. The largest waterborne outbreak that has ever occurred in the United States was the 1993 cryptosporidiosis

> The largest waterborne disease outbreak that has ever occurred in the United States was cryptosporidiosis.

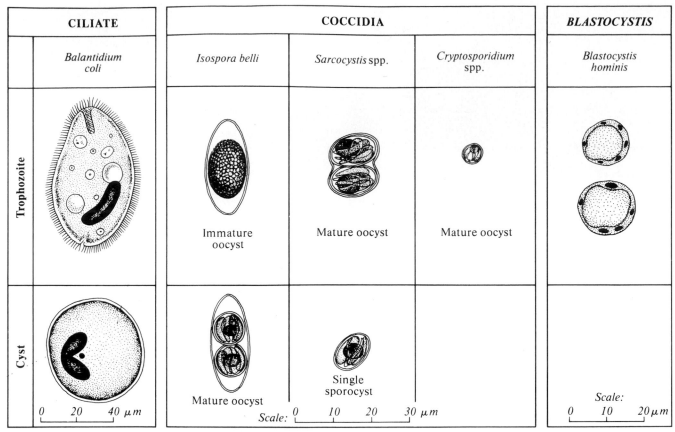

CILIATE	COCCIDIA			BLASTOCYSTIS
Balantidium coli	*Isospora belli*	*Sarcocystis* spp.	*Cryptosporidium* spp.	*Blastocystis hominis*

Figure 22-26. **Intestinal protozoa of humans other than amebas and flagellates.** See text for discussions of *Balantidium coli* and *Blastocystis hominis* and the CD-ROM for discussions of *Isospora* and *Sarcocystis* spp. (Courtesy of the CDC, Division of Parasitic Diseases.)

outbreak in Milwaukee, Wisconsin, which affected more than 400,000 people. Cryptosporidiosis can also be a respiratory disease, but only rarely.

Geographic occurrence. This disease has been reported worldwide.

Parasite. Cryptosporidiosis results from ingestion of oocysts of *Cryptosporidium parvum*, a coccidian. Reservoirs include infected humans, cattle, and other domestic animals. The parasite infects intestinal epithelial cells and produces oocysts that pass in the feces. The oocysts can survive for long periods under adverse environmental conditions and are highly resistant to the chemicals used to purify drinking water. Fecal-oral transmission may occur from person to person, from animal to person, or via ingestion of contaminated water or food.

> Cryptosporidiosis is a gastrointestinal infection caused by *Cryptosporidium parvum*, a coccidial protozoan. The disease is usually acquired by ingestion of oocysts, which are transmitted from person to person, from animal to person, or via ingestion of contaminated water or food.

Laboratory diagnosis. Cryptosporidiosis can be diagnosed by microscopic observation of small (4-to-6-μm-diameter) acid-fast oocysts in stained smears of fecal specimens (Fig. 22-27). Sporozoites may or may not be seen within the oocysts. Sensitive and specific IDPs are also widely used.

> Cryptosporidiosis can be diagnosed by microscopic observation of small (4-to-6-μm-diameter) acid-fast oocysts in stained smears of fecal specimens.

Essentials

Cryptosporidium parvum

- A coccidial protozoan, classified in the phylum Sporozoa

- Causes a diarrheal disease known as cryptosporidiosis

- Cryptosporidiosis results from ingestion of oocysts of *C. parvum*

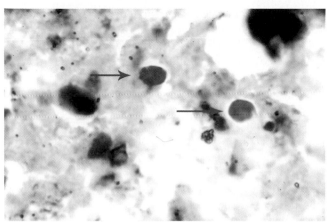

Figure 22-27. **Acid-fast stained** *Cryptosporidium* **oocysts** (***arrows***). (From Winn WC Jr, et al. Koneman's Color Atlas and Textbook of Diagnostic Microbiology. 6th Ed. Philadelphia: Lippincott Williams & Wilkins, 2006.)

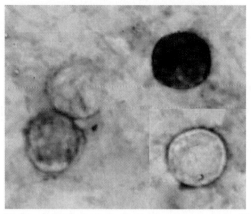

Figure 22-28. **Acid-fast stained** *Cyclospora* **oocysts.** Note that the staining is variable among the four oocysts. (Courtesy of the CDC, Division of Parasitic Diseases.)

- Reservoirs include infected humans, cattle, and other domestic animals

- Fecal-oral transmission may occur from person to person, animal to person, or via ingestion of contaminated water or food

- Cryptosporidiosis can be diagnosed by microscopic observation of small (4-to-6-μm-diameter) acid-fast oocysts in stained smears of fecal specimens; IDPs are also widely used

Cyclosporiasis

Disease. Cyclosporiasis is a coccidial gastrointestinal infection causing watery diarrhea (six or more stools per day), nausea, anorexia, abdominal cramping, fatigue, and weight loss. The diarrhea lasts between 9 and 43 days in immunocompetent patients and months in immunocompromised patients.

Geographic occurrence. Cyclosporiasis has been diagnosed in Asia, the Caribbean, Mexico, Peru, and the United States.

Parasite. Cyclosporiasis results from ingestion of oocysts of *Cyclospora cayetanensis*, a coccidian. Reservoirs include fecally contaminated water sources and produce that has been rinsed with fecally contaminated water. Transmission is primarily waterborne, but outbreaks have involved contaminated raspberries, basil, and lettuce.

> Cyclosporiasis is a coccidial gastrointestinal infection caused by ingestion of oocysts of *Cyclospora cayetanensis*. Transmission is primarily waterborne, but outbreaks have involved ingestion of contaminated raspberries, basil, and lettuce.

Laboratory diagnosis. Diagnosis of cyclosporiasis is made by microscopic observation of the 8-to-10-μm-diameter acid-fast oocysts (Fig. 22-28), which are about twice the size of *Cryptosporidium* oocysts. An ocular micrometer is quite useful here. The oocysts have a much thicker wall than *Cryptosporidium parvum* oocysts, and the contents are more granular than *C. parvum* oocysts. *Cyclospora* oocysts autofluoresce a bright green to intense blue under ultraviolet fluorescence when examined using the types of filters commonly used for calcofluor white staining.

> Diagnosis of cyclosporiasis is made by microscopic observation of the acid-fast oocysts that are 8 to 10 μm in diameter, about twice the size of *Cryptosporidium* oocysts.

Blastocystis hominis Infection

Disease. The pathogenicity of *Blastocystis hominis* remains controversial. Large numbers of *B. hominis* forms have been found in the stools of patients with diarrhea, when no other causative agent has been recovered. It may cause recurrent watery diarrhea without fever, abdominal pain, anorexia, vomiting, and weight loss, especially in immunosuppressed patients.

Geographic occurrence. Infection with *B. hominis* occurs worldwide.

Parasite. The taxonomic status of *B. hominis* remains controversial. Once thought to be a yeast, it has most recently been classified as an ameba. It extends and retracts pseudopodia, ingests bacteria, and has no cell wall.

Laboratory diagnosis. The morphology of *B. hominis* is quite variable. They are irregularly sized spherical cells ranging from <5 to 15 μm in diameter. The cells possess a homogeneous-staining central body (usually green or red

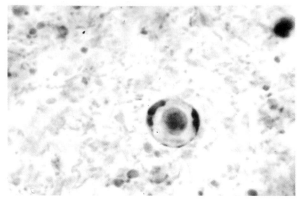

Figure 22-29. **Trichrome-stained *Blastocystis hominis*.** (From Winn WC Jr, et al. Koneman's Color Atlas and Textbook of Diagnostic Microbiology. 6th Ed. Philadelphia: Lippincott Williams & Wilkins, 2006.)

when stained with trichrome stain) that occupies 70% or more of the cell. The nuclear material may be scattered in undefined fragments between the central body and the cell membrane (Fig. 22-29; see Fig. 22-26) or may appear as one or two elongated masses arranged in a bipolar distribution. When present in a stool specimen, they should be reported as being rare, few, moderate, or many. Five or more per high-power field is considered moderate to many.

Giardiasis

Disease. Giardiasis is a protozoal infection of the duodenum (the uppermost portion of the small intestine) and may be asymptomatic, mild, or severe. Patients experience diarrhea; loose, pale, malodorous, fatty stools; abdominal cramps; bloating; abdominal gas; fatigue; and possibly weight loss.

Geographic occurrence. This disease occurs worldwide.

Parasite. Giardiasis is caused by *Giardia lamblia* (also called *Giardia intestinalis*), a flagellated protozoan. Trophozoites attach by means of a ventral sucker to the mucosal lining of the duodenum. Trophozoites and/or cysts are expelled in feces. Reservoirs include infected humans, possibly beavers and other wild and domestic animals that have consumed water containing *Giardia* cysts, and fecally contaminated drinking water and recreational water. Transmission occurs via the fecal-oral route, usually by ingestion of cysts

> Giardiasis is a diarrheal disease caused by *Giardia lamblia* (also called *Giardia intestinalis*), a flagellated protozoan. Transmission occurs via the fecal-oral route, usually by ingestion of cysts in fecally contaminated water or foods, or from person to person by soiled hands to mouth (as occurs in day care centers).

in fecally contaminated water or food, or from person to person by soiled hands to mouth (as occurs in day care centers). Large community outbreaks have resulted from consumption of treated but unfiltered water. Filtration is necessary because the concentrations of chlorine used in routine water treatment do not kill *Giardia* cysts, especially in cold water. Smaller outbreaks have involved contaminated food, person-to-person transmission in day care centers, and fecally contaminated recreational water (e.g., swimming and wading pools).

Laboratory diagnosis. Giardiasis is diagnosed by microscopic observation of trophozoites and/or cysts in stained smears of fecal specimens or duodenal aspirates. A string test is also available for collection of duodenal fluids. CML professionals must be able to differentiate *Giardia* trophozoites and cysts from those of other pathogenic and nonpathogenic flagellates that may be present in human fecal specimens (Fig. 22-30). The characteristic teardrop-shaped *Giardia* trophozoite is 5 to 15 μm wide by 10 to 20 μm long. It contains two nuclei, which give the trophozoite the appearance of a face

> Giardiasis is diagnosed by microscopic observation of trophozoites and/or cysts in stained smears of fecal specimens or duodenal aspirates. Associate the appearance of "a face looking back at you" with the trophozoites of *G. lamblia*.

(Fig. 22-31)—it appears to be looking up at the person observing it microscopically. The *Giardia* trophozoite is commonly described as resembling an owl face, a clown face, or an old man with glasses. Trophozoites contain two curved median bodies and possess eight flagella that are too thin to be seen using a compound light microscope. Cysts are round to oval, 7 to 10 μm wide by 11 to 14 μm long. They possess two or four nuclei, axostyles, and two or four median bodies (Fig. 22-32). Sensitive IDPs are also available.

Essentials

Giardia lamblia

- Also known as *Giardia intestinalis*
- Intestinal flagellate
- Causes a diarrheal disease called giardiasis
- Giardiasis is diagnosed by observing characteristic trophozoites and/or cysts in stool specimens
- Teardrop-shaped trophozoites contain two nuclei, causing the trophozoite to resemble a face
- Round-to-oval cysts contain two or four nuclei

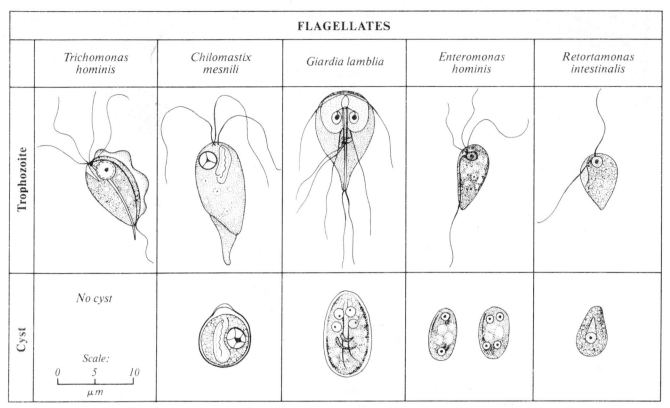

Figure 22-30. Intestinal flagellates. Of the protozoa pictured here, only *Giardia lamblia* is considered to be pathogenic. (Courtesy of the CDC, Division of Parasitic Diseases.)

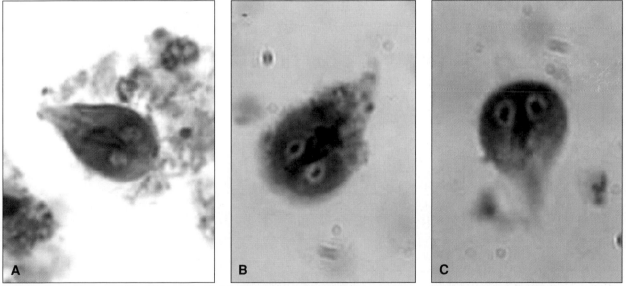

Figure 22-31. Three *Giardia lamblia* trophozoites. The two nuclei resemble eyes, thus making the trophozoite look like a face. (Courtesy of the CDC, Division of Parasitic Diseases.)

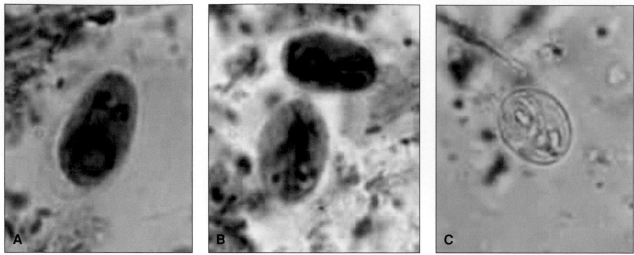

Figure 22-32. **Cysts of *G. lamblia*.** The cysts shown here contain two nuclei, but *G. lamblia* cysts may contain four nuclei. (Courtesy of the CDC, Division of Parasitic Diseases.)

Dientamoeba fragilis Infection

Disease. *Dientamoeba fragilis* causes persistent to intermittent diarrhea, abdominal pain, anorexia, fatigue, nausea, and weight loss or insufficient weight gain.

Geographic occurrence. This type of infection occurs worldwide.

Parasite. Although its name would suggest that it is an ameba, *D. fragilis* is classified as a flagellate. Flagella are not observed with the compound light microscope, however. *D. fragilis* exists only as a trophozoite and, as such, is quite fragile (hence its name). It is generally accepted that *D. fragilis* trophozoites can be transmitted from host to host within the egg of the pinworm *Enterobius vermicularis*.

Laboratory diagnosis. Because of its fragile nature, permanent stained smears of fixed stool specimens should be used to observe *D. fragilis* trophozoites. When seen in wet mounts, it possesses relatively broad-lobed, clear pseudopodia. In permanent smears, it has an ameboid appearance and ranges from 5 μm to 12 μm in diameter. Either one or two nuclei are present, usually two. The nuclear chromatin typically is fragmented into three to five granules, and there is no peripheral chromatin on the nuclear membrane. Remember that *D. fragilis* has no cyst stage.

> *Dientamoeba fragilis* is "fragile" because it has no cyst stage.

Chapter Review

- It is important to remember that patients may be infected with more than one parasite, so once a parasite is found, the CML professional should continue to look for other possible parasites.

- Parasitic protozoa include amebas, ciliates, flagellates, and sporozoan parasites.

- Specimens commonly used to diagnose protozoal infections include aspirates, blood, stool, bone marrow, tissue, CSF, biopsy specimens, duodenal contents, lesions, serum, skin scrapings, intestinal contents, and urogenital discharge material.

- In general, protozoal infections are diagnosed by observing and recognizing parasite life cycle stages by specific characteristics such as size, shape, and internal details.

- Both thick and thin blood smears should be used to identify blood parasites such as malaria. Thick and thin blood smears may be stained with Giemsa, Wright-Giemsa, or Wright stains.

- Stool may be examined by using either fresh or preserved specimens. Commercial transport containers are available that contain stool preservatives, each of which has particular advantages and disadvantages. Stool specimens are examined both macroscopically and microscopically.

- The O&P examination of a stool specimen consists of a direct wet mount, a wet mount of a concentrated specimen, and an examination of a permanent stained smear of a fresh or preserved specimen.

- Because size is an important identifying characteristic of many parasites, microscopes should be equipped with an ocular micrometer to measure the size of various life cycle stages.

- Molecular diagnostic procedures are becoming increasingly available to diagnose parasitic infections.

- American trypanosomiasis is also known as Chagas disease and is caused by a flagellate known as *Trypanosoma cruzi*.

- Some parasitic diseases, such as Chagas disease, malaria, and babesiosis, may be transmitted by blood transfusion.

- Human malaria is a systemic sporozoan infection transmitted by four species of *Plasmodium*: *P. vivax*, *P. falciparum*, *P. malariae*, and *P. ovale*. The parasite is transmitted by the bite of an infected female *Anopheles* mosquito.

- Malaria is diagnosed by observation of the intraerythrocytic *Plasmodium* parasite in stained blood smears.

- There are three forms of leishmaniasis: cutaneous, mucocutaneous, and visceral.

- Toxoplasmosis is caused by *Toxoplasma gondii*, an intracellular sporozoan.

- The cause of primary amebic meningoencephalitis (PAM) is *Naegleria fowleri*, a free-living ameboflagellate.

- Trichomoniasis is a sexually transmitted protozoal disease of men and women. It is caused by *Trichomonas vaginalis*, a flagellate.

- Intestinal protozoal infections include amebiasis, balantidiasis, cryptosporidiosis, cyclosporiasis, and giardiasis.

- Amebiasis is caused by *Entamoeba histolytica*. Transmission can occur via ingestion of fecally contaminated food or water containing cysts, by flies transporting cysts from feces to food, via fecally soiled hands of food handlers, or by any sexual contact involving risk of fecal contamination.

- *Balantidium coli* is a ciliated protozoan. It is the only ciliate that causes disease in humans.

- Coccidial parasites are in the phylum Sporozoa and include the human parasitic genera, *Cryptosporidium*, *Cyclospora*, *Isospora*, and *Sarcocystis*.

- Giardiasis is caused by *Giardia lamblia*, a flagellated protozoan that can be recognized by its characteristic cyst or trophozoite stages. The appearance of the trophozoite stage is frequently likened to a monkey's face, an owl's face, or an old man with glasses. Transmission is by the fecal-oral route.

New Terms and Abbreviations

After studying Chapter 22, you should be familiar with the following terms, which are defined within the chapter and in the Glossary at the back of the book.

Amastigote

Ameboflagellate

Ameboma

Chromatin

Chromatoidal bar

Cytostome

Gametocyte

Granuloma

Hemoflagellate

Intraerythrocytic parasite

Karyosome

Leishman-Donovan bodies

Merozoite

Oocyst

Paroxysm

Schizont

Sporozoite

Trypomastigote

Xenodiagnosis

References and Suggested Reading

Cox FEG. Taxonomy and classification of human parasites. In: Murray PR, Baron EJ, Jorgensen JH, Pfaller MA, Yolken RH, eds. Manual of Clinical Microbiology. 8th Ed. Washington, DC: ASM Press, 2003.

Garcia LS. Diagnostic medical parasitology. In: Manual of Commercial Methods in Clinical Microbiology. Washington, DC: ASM Press, 2002.

Garcia LS. Practical Guide to Diagnostic Microbiology. Washington, DC: ASM Press, 1999.

Garcia LS, et al. Algorithms for detection and identification of parasites. In: Murray PR, Baron EJ, Jorgensen JH, Pfaller MA, Yolken RH, eds. Manual of Clinical Microbiology. 8th Ed. Washington, DC: ASM Press, 2003.

Garcia LS, et al. Specimen collection, transport, and processing: parasitology. In: Murray PR, Baron EJ, Jorgensen JH, Pfaller MA, Yolken RH, eds. Manual of Clinical Microbiology. 8th Ed. Washington, DC: ASM Press, 2003.

Heymann DL, ed. Control of Communicable Diseases Manual. 18th Ed. Washington, DC: American Public Health Association, 2004 (with 2006 update).

Winn WC Jr, et al. Koneman's Color Atlas and Textbook of Diagnostic Microbiology. 6th Ed. Philadelphia: Lippincott Williams & Wilkins, 2006.

 ## On the CD-ROM

- A Closer Look at Coccidia and Microsporidia
- A Closer Look at Artifacts in Stool Specimens
- A Closer Look at the Malarial Parasite Life Cycle
- Malaria in the United States
- Appearance of Malarial Parasites in Thick Blood Smears
- Speciation of Malarial Parasites
- A Closer Look at Nonpathogenic Intestinal Amebas
- Additional Self-Assessment Exercises
- Case Studies
- Puzzle

Self-Assessment Exercises

Match the parasitic infection or disease in the left column with the appropriate parasite in the right column.

1. _____ Chagas disease

2. _____ Toxoplasmosis

3. _____ Primary amebic meningoencephalitis

4. _____ Giardiasis

5. _____ Malaria

A. *Plasmodium* spp.

B. *Trypanosoma cruzi*

C. *Giardia lamblia*

D. *Toxoplasma gondii*

E. *Naegleria fowleri*

List the most appropriate specimen to be used for diagnosis of the following parasitic infections:

6. Malaria _____

7. Amebiasis _____

8. Giardiasis _____

9. True or false: *Giardia lamblia* is a ciliated protozoan parasite.

10. True or false: Live, motile trophozoites can only be observed in fresh specimens.

CHAPTER 23

Laboratory Diagnosis of Selected Helminth Infections

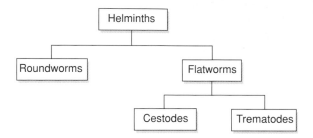

Chapter Outline

Clinical Specimens Required for the Diagnosis
of Helminth Infections

Laboratory Methods Used to Diagnose Helminth Infections
- Blood Specimens
- Stool Specimens
- Skin Snips
- Culture and Hatching Procedures
- Immunodiagnostic Procedures
- Molecular Diagnostic Procedures

Selected Helminth Infections
- Helminth Infections of the Cardiovascular System
- Helminth Infections of the Skin
- Helminth Infections of the Muscles and Subcutaneous
  Tissues
- Helminth Infections of the Eyes
- Helminth Infections of the Respiratory System
- Helminth Infections of the Central Nervous System
- Helminth Infections of the Gastrointestinal Tract,
  Including the Liver

LEARNING OBJECTIVES

After studying this chapter, you should be able to:

- Define the terms introduced in this chapter (e.g.,
  ascites, autoinfection, Calabar swellings)

- Given a description, prepared specimen, and/or color
  photograph of a helminth, correctly identify the parasite

- Given a list of helminths, identify each of them as a
  nematode, trematode, or cestode

- Describe how humans acquire a particular helminth

- Name the specimen of choice for diagnosing diseases
  caused by helminths discussed in the chapter

- Given a prepared slide or photograph, differentiate a
  potentially pathogenic parasite from an artifact

- Discuss the clinically significant signs and symptoms
  of the helminth infections discussed in this chapter

- Given a particular anatomic site, name the most
  probable helminth infections and parasites

- Given a particular parasitic infection, name the
  corresponding disease and geographic distribution

- Given a patient's laboratory results, signs, and
  symptoms, identify the most likely parasite

- Given a type of specimen (e.g., blood), list the
  methods available to diagnose a helminth infection

- Given a helminth infection, identify the appropriate
  vector, if any

Helminths—parasitic worms—are multicellular animals.
Although some stages in their life cycles are microscopic,
helminths are *not* microorganisms. Nonetheless, helminths
are studied in a parasitology course, and parasitology is

considered a subdiscipline of microbiology. Clinical microbiology laboratory (CML) professionals are expected to assist clinicians in the diagnosis of helminth infections. Table 23-1 provides an overview of the helminth infections described in this chapter. No attempt has been made to include all helminth diseases of humans. Laboratory techniques used to diagnose helminth infections are performed in the parasitology section of the CML.

It is important to keep in mind that patients may be infected with more than one species of helminth, depending on where they have lived and/or traveled. Even though many of the helminth infections described in this chapter are not endemic diseases in the United States, people emigrating from other countries or U.S. residents returning from travel to endemic countries could be infected.

> Depending on where they have lived and/or traveled, patients may be infected with more than one species of helminth.

CLINICAL SPECIMENS REQUIRED FOR THE DIAGNOSIS OF HELMINTH INFECTIONS

Clinical specimens commonly used to diagnose helminth infections are listed in Table 23-2.

LABORATORY METHODS USED TO DIAGNOSE HELMINTH INFECTIONS

Helminth infections are usually diagnosed by observing and recognizing the various life cycle stages—eggs, microfilariae, larvae, adult worms—in clinical specimens. Helminths are identified by the characteristic appearance of stained or unstained life cycle stages. Helminth life cycles do *not* include trophozoites, cysts, oocysts, or spores, which are life cycle stages of protozoa (see Chapter 22).

Blood Specimens

Thick and thin blood smears, or blood films, described in Chapter 22, are used to detect **microfilariae** (tiny prelarval stages) of various filarial worms, such as *Wuchereria* spp., *Brugia* spp., *Loa loa*, and occasionally, *Onchocerca* spp. Microfilariae of *Onchocerca* spp. are more commonly observed in skin snips

> Stained blood smears can be used to detect tiny prelarval stages—microfilariae—of filarial worms, such as *Wuchereria* spp., *Brugia* spp., *Loa loa*, and occasionally, *Onchocerca* spp.

(discussed later). Delafield hematoxylin stain is recommended for the staining of microfilariae because it stains their sheaths, if present. Microfilariae are usually not present in large numbers in the bloodstream. Although the entire thin blood smear should be examined, microfilariae are most apt to be found along the edges or the feathered end of the smear.

Stool Specimens

Fresh or preserved stool specimens are processed as described in Chapter 22. The various fixatives available for preserving stool specimens are also discussed in Chapter 22. Most of the fixatives are acceptable for preservation of helminth life cycle stages. The one exception is polyvinyl alcohol (PVA). *Trichuris trichiura* eggs are not concentrated as easily with PVA as with formalin-based fixatives. Also, *Strongyloides stercoralis* microfilarial morphology is poor when PVA is used; it is much better with formalin-based fixatives.

Either sedimentation or flotation concentration techniques can be used to recover helminth life cycle stages from stool specimens. However, operculated eggs and/or very dense eggs, such as unfertilized *Ascaris* eggs, do not concentrate well with the flotation method. Also, thin-shelled eggs are subject to collapse and distortion if the surface film is not removed for examination within 5 minutes of the time the centrifuge stops.

The O&P (ova and parasite) examination, described in Chapter 22, is used to detect helminth life cycle stages—primarily, eggs and larvae—in stool specimens. Microscopes should be equipped with a calibrated ocular micrometer because the size of a helminth egg is often an important identifying characteristic. Ocular micrometers are discussed in Appendix A.

> The O&P examination is used to detect helminth life cycle stages—primarily eggs and larvae—in stool specimens.

Skin Snips

Skin snips are used to diagnose onchocerciasis (river blindness). As the name implies, a skin snip is a small piece of skin collected using either a surgical blade or a needle. Skin snips are placed immediately into a drop of normal saline or distilled water, teased a bit with dissecting needles, and covered with a glass coverslip. If present, microfilariae should emerge from the skin in 30 minutes to 1 hour. The preparation is examined microscopically, using the low-power objective. To enable identification of the microfilariae to species, the skin snip is allowed to dry, methanol fixed, and stained with Giemsa stain.

Culture and Hatching Procedures

Fecal and agar culture methods are available for the culture of *Strongyloides* larvae, but these procedures are not performed

TABLE 23 - 1   Selected Helminth Infections of Humans

Anatomical Location	Infection	Helminth That Causes Infection
Cardiovascular system	Filariasis	*Wuchereria bancrofti* (N) and *Brugia malayi* (N); microfilariae (tiny prelarval stages) of these helminths are found in the bloodstream
	Schistosomiasis (also known as bilharzia or bilharziasis)	Adult worms in the genus *Schistosoma* (T) live in blood vessels
Skin	Onchocerciasis (also known as river blindness)	*Onchocerca volvulus* (N); microfilariae of these helminths are found in the skin
Muscles and subcutaneous tissues	Trichinosis	*Trichinella spiralis* (N)
	Dracunculiasis	*Dracunculus medinensis* (N), also known as the guinea worm
Eyes	Onchocerciasis	*Onchocerca volvulus* (N); microfilariae enter the eyes, causing an intense inflammatory reaction
	Loiasis	*Loa loa* (N), also known as the African eyeworm
Respiratory system	Paragonimiasis	*Paragonimus westermani* (T); the lung fluke
Central nervous system	Cysticercosis	Cysts (the larval stage) of the pork tapeworm, *Taenia solium* (C), are found in various parts of the body, including the brain
	Hydatid cyst disease	*Echinococcus granulosis* (C) or *E. multilocularis* (C); in addition to the brain, hydatid cysts (the larval form of these helminths) can form in many other locations in the body
Gastrointestinal tract, including the liver	Ascariasis	*Ascaris lumbricoides* (N); the large intestinal roundworm of humans
	Hookworm infection	*Ancylostoma duodenale* (N) or *Necator americanus* (N)
	Enterobiasis (pinworm infection)	*Enterobius vermicularis* (N)
	Trichuriasis (whipworm infection)	*Trichuris trichiura* (N)
	Strongyloidiasis	*Strongyloides stercoralis* (N)
	Beef tapeworm infection	*Taenia saginata* (C)
	Dog tapeworm infection	*Dipylidium caninum* (C)
	Dwarf tapeworm infection	*Hymenolepis nana* (C)
	Fish tapeworm infection	*Diphyllobothrium latum* (C)
	Pork tapeworm infection	*Taenia solium* (C)
	Rat tapeworm infection	*Hymenolepis diminuta* (C)
	Fasciolopsiasis	*Fasciolopsis buski* (T), an intestinal fluke
	Fascioliasis	*Fasciola hepatica* (T), a liver fluke
	Clonorchiasis	*Clonorchis sinensis* (T), also known as the Chinese or oriental liver fluke

C, cestode (tapeworm); N, nematode (roundworm); T, trematode (fluke).

TABLE 23 - 2	Clinical Specimens Commonly Used to Diagnose Helminth Infections
Specimen	**Infection**
Blood	Filarial infections (by observation of microfilariae)
Brain tissue biopsy	Cysticercosis, hydatid cyst disease
Eye biopsy	Cysticercosis
Feces, duodenal aspirates, intestinal biopsy specimens	Ascariasis, hookworm infection, schistosomiasis, strongyloidiasis, trichuriasis, various fluke infections, various tapeworm infections
Liver biopsy	Clonorchiasis, hydatid cyst disease
Lung biopsy	Hydatid cyst disease
Muscle biopsy	Cysticercosis, onchocerciasis (nodules), trichinosis
Serum (for antibody detection procedures)	Cysticercosis, echinococcosis, fascioliasis, filariasis, onchocerciasis, paragonimiasis, schistosomiasis, strongyloidiasis, toxocariasis, and trichinellosis
Cellophane (Scotch) tape prep	Pinworm infection
Skin snips	Onchocerciasis (by observation of microfilariae)
Sputum	Paragonimiasis (lung fluke infection); migrating larval stages of *Ascaris lumbricoides*, *Strongyloides stercoralis*, and hookworms
Urine	Schistosomiasis

in CMLs. Likewise, procedures for hatching schistosome eggs are available but not routinely performed in CMLs.

Immunodiagnostic Procedures

Antibody detection tests are available for cysticercosis, echinococcosis, fascioliasis, filariasis, onchocerciasis, paragonimiasis, schistosomiasis, strongyloidiasis, toxocariasis, and trichinellosis, but these procedures are not usually performed in CMLs.

Molecular Diagnostic Procedures

Molecular diagnostic procedures—specifically, polymerase chain reaction procedures—are available for identifying *Brugia*, *Echinococcus*, *Onchocerca*, *Taenia*, and *Wuchereria* spp., but these procedures are not usually performed in CMLs.

SELECTED HELMINTH INFECTIONS

Helminth Infections of the Cardiovascular System

Table 23-3 summarizes the ways in which certain helminth infections are diagnosed by examination of stained blood smears.

Filariasis

Disease. Filariasis is caused by long, threadlike worms known as filarial worms. The adult worms live in lymph nodes, where they can block the flow of lymph. Symptoms include high fever, chills, lymphadenitis, lymphangitis, and eosinophilia. Chronic filariasis leads to an enlargement of legs, breasts, and genitalia—a condition known as **elephantiasis** (Fig. 23-1).

> Filariasis is caused by long, threadlike worms known as filarial worms. Chronic filariasis leads to an enlargement of legs, breasts, and genitalia—a condition known as elephantiasis.

Geographic occurrence. Bancroftian filariasis, caused by *Wuchereria bancrofti*, occurs in Latin America, Africa, Asia, and the Pacific Islands. Brugian filariasis, caused by *Brugia malayi*, is endemic in rural southwest India, Southeast Asia, and the central and northern coastal regions of China and South Korea. Timorean filariasis, caused by *Brugia timori*, occurs on Timor and other southeastern islands of Indonesia. It is estimated that approximately 90 million people are infected with these three filarial worms.

TABLE 23 - 3	Helminth Infections Diagnosed by Examining Stained Blood Smears	
Infection	**Observation Required for Diagnosis**	
Filariasis/elephantiasis	Extracellular microfilariae	
Loiasis (eye worm infection)	Extracellular microfilariae	
Onchocerciasis (river blindness)	Extracellular microfilariae (however, these microfilariae are more commonly observed in skin snips)	

Parasites. Adult male and female worms live in the lymphatic system, where they reach lengths of up to 40 mm. Female worms release tiny, microscopic, prelarval stages called microfilariae, which migrate into the bloodstream (Fig. 23-2). When a mosquito takes a blood meal, it ingests the microfilariae. Within the mosquito, the microfilariae mature into infective larvae. When the mosquito again takes a blood meal, it injects the infective larvae into the human. In the human body, a larva matures into an adult worm. In this parasitic life cycle, the human is the definitive host and the mosquito is the intermediate host. Many mosquito species serve as intermediate hosts, including *Culex*, *Anopheles*, and *Mansonia* spp.

> Filariasis is transmitted by infected mosquitoes. It is diagnosed by observing and recognizing microfilariae in blood.

Laboratory diagnosis. Diagnosis is confirmed by observing and recognizing microfilariae in blood. Microfilariae of *Wuchereria bancrofti* exhibit a nocturnal periodicity,[1] meaning that they appear in greater numbers in peripheral blood during nighttime hours—especially between 10:00 PM and 2:00 AM. Peripheral blood smears are stained with Giemsa stain or Delafield hematoxylin stain. The microfilariae of *W. bancrofti*, *B. malayi*, and *B. timori* retain the egg membrane and are referred to as **sheathed microfilariae.** Delafield hematoxylin stain is better than Giemsa stain for staining microfilarial sheaths. Other characteristics of these three filarial worms are shown in Table 23-4. Sources of information on differentiating these microfilariae from the microfilariae of other filarial worms include the Web sites of the World Health Organization (WHO; http://www.who.int/) and the Division of Parasitic Diseases of the Centers for Disease Control and Prevention (CDC; http://www.dpd.cdc.gov/dpdx/) and parasitology textbooks. Immunodiagnostic and molecular diagnostic procedures are also available for diagnosis of filariasis.

Schistosomiasis

Disease. Schistosomiasis is caused by trematodes in the genus *Schistosoma*—primarily, *S. mansoni*, *S. japonicum*, and *S. haematobium*—which are referred to as blood flukes.

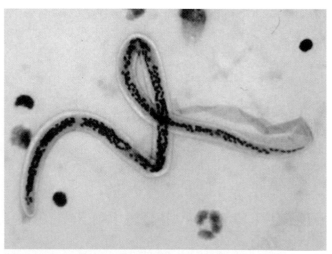

Figure 23-2. Sheathed microfilaria of *Wuchereria bancrofti*. The head is to the left and its tail to the right. Notice that the nuclei do not extend to the tip of the tail. *W. bancrofti* microfilariae range from about 7.5 to 10.0 μm wide by 244 to 296 μm long. (Courtesy of the CDC, Division of Parasitic Diseases.)

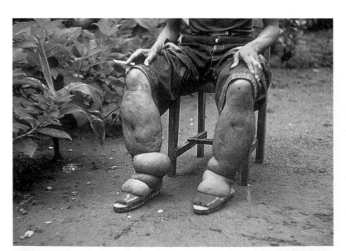

Figure 23-1. Elephantiasis of the legs, resulting from filariasis. (Courtesy of the Centers for Disease Control and Prevention [CDC].)

[1] *The nocturnal periodicity of* W. bancrofti *microfilariae is thought to be related to the nocturnal feeding habits of the mosquito host. Higher concentrations of microfilariae in the bloodstream during the time that a mosquito takes a blood meal increase the chances of the mosquito becoming infected.*

TABLE 23 - 4	Characteristics of Selected Microfilariae	
Species	**Width × Length (μm)**	**Key Features**
Wuchereria bancrofti	7.5 to 10.0 × 244 to 296 (av. 260) in stained blood smears	Found in blood; short, clear headspace; dispersed nuclei; sheath unstained in Giemsa-stained preparation; body in smooth curves; tapered tail; nuclei do not extend to the tip of the tail, resulting in a clear space at tip of the tail
Brugia malayi	5.0 to 6.0 × 177 to 230 (av. 220) in stained blood smears	Found in blood; long, clear headspace; sheath pink in Giemsa-stained preparation; tapered tail; nuclei extend to the tip of the tail; subterminal and terminal nuclei widely separated
Brugia timori	4.4 to 6.8 × 265 to 323 (av. 287) in stained blood smears	Found in blood; long, clear headspace; sheath unstained in Giemsa-stained preparation; tapered tail; nuclei extend to the tip of the tail; subterminal and terminal nuclei are widely separated
Onchocerca volvulus	5.0 to 9.0 × 304 to 315 in skin snips	Found primarily in skin snips and occasionally in blood after treatment; flexed, anucleate tail tapers to a point; microfilariae unsheathed
Loa loa	5.0 to 7.0 × 231 to 250 (av. 238) in stained blood smears	Found in blood; sheath unstained in Giemsa-stained preparations; tapered tail; nuclei irregularly spaced in a single row to the end of the tail

Schistosomiasis is known as bilharzia or bilharziasis in many parts of the world. Female worms produce eggs that are disseminated throughout the body via the bloodstream (hematogenously). The eggs can penetrate tissues, resulting in inflammation, granuloma formation, and scarring. Chronic inflammation in the patient's liver leads to scarification, which causes portal hypertension, or obstructed blood flow through the liver. This, in turn, leads to **ascites,** or buildup of fluid in the abdominal cavity, thus explaining why patients with schistosomiasis frequently have distended or protuberant bellies. Ascites is a common finding in chronic *S. mansoni* and *S. japonicum* infections but is less pronounced in *S. haematobium* infections. Other symptoms of schistosomiasis relate to the number and location of the eggs and include high fever; lymphadenopathy; malaise; eosinophilia; and hepatic, intestinal, and urinary tract complications.

> Schistosomiasis, also known as bilharzia or bilharziasis, is caused by trematodes in the genus *Schistosoma*—primarily, *S. mansoni*, *S. japonicum*, and *S. haematobium*—which are referred to as blood flukes.

Geographic occurrence. *S. mansoni* is found in Africa, the Arabian Peninsula, Brazil, Venezuela, and some Caribbean islands. *S. japonicum* is found in China, Taiwan, the Philippines, and Indonesia. *S. haematobium* is found in Africa and the Middle East. Schistosomiasis occurs only in countries where the appropriate freshwater snail intermediate hosts are found.

Parasites. The adult male and female worms, which are between 1 and 2 cm in length, live in pairs within the human body in blood vessels that surround either the urinary bladder, in the case of *S. haematobium*, or the intestine, in the case of *S. mansoni* and *S. japonicum*. The eggs that are released by the female worms can penetrate blood vessel walls and migrate through tissues, although most eggs are carried via the portal system into the liver.

Eggs of *S. haematobium* gain access to the lumen of the urinary bladder, and eggs of the other two species gain access to the lumen of the intestine. Eggs passed either in urine or feces must reach freshwater. In the water, a ciliated larva called a **miracidium** emerges from the egg. The miracidium penetrates into a snail, where it matures into a mother sporocyst. The mother sporocyst produces daughter sporocysts, each of which matures into a cercaria. The mature cercariae

> In the schistosome life cycle, humans serve as definitive hosts and freshwater snails serve as intermediate hosts. Humans acquire schistosomiasis by penetration of the skin by cercariae present in water in which the people are working, swimming, or wading.

are released from the snail into the water. A person becomes infected by penetration of the skin by a cercaria living in contaminated water in which the person is working, swimming, or wading. Within the human body, the cercaria matures into an adult worm. Adult worms may live throughout the lifetime of the infected human. In this parasitic life cycle, the human is the definitive host and the freshwater snail is the intermediate host.

Laboratory diagnosis. Definitive diagnosis of schistosomiasis requires observation and recognition of characteristic eggs in fecal (*S. mansoni* and *S. japonicum*) or urine (*S. haematobium*) specimens. An *S. mansoni* egg is yellow-brown, elongate, ovoid, and 45 to 73 μm wide by 114 to 180 μm long, with a large, lateral, thornlike spine projecting outward near one end (Fig.

> Definitive diagnosis of schistosomiasis requires observation and recognition of characteristic eggs. The eggs of *Schistosoma haematobium* are primarily found in urine, whereas the eggs of *S. mansoni* and *S. japonicum* are primarily found in feces.

23-3A). An *S. japonicum* egg is yellow-brown and, at 40 to 60 μm wide by 55 to 85 μm long, smaller and more spherical than the *S. mansoni* egg, with a very small lateral spine not seen in all strains (Fig. 23-3B). An *S. haematobium* egg is yellow-brown, elongate, ovoid, and 40 to 70 μm wide by 112 to 170 μm long, with a distinct terminal spine (Fig. 23-3C).

Essentials

Schistosoma **spp.**

- Blood flukes

- Cause of schistosomiasis (bilharzia, bilharziasis)

- Definitive host is human; intermediate hosts are freshwater snails

- Schistosomiasis is acquired by penetration of the skin by cercaria

- Adult worms live in blood vessels

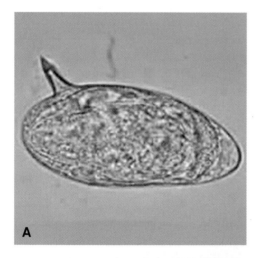
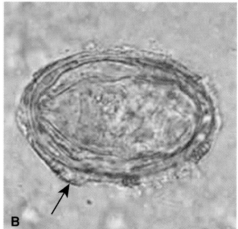
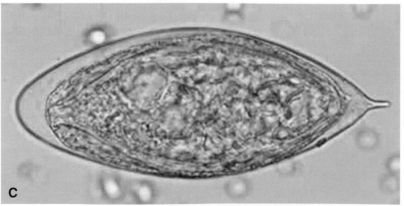

***Figure 23-3. Schistosoma* eggs. A.** *S. mansoni* egg; notice its prominent lateral spine. **B.** *S. japonicum* egg; its small vestigial spine (*arrow*) can be seen here but is often not visible. **C.** *S. haematobium* egg; notice its prominent terminal spine. (Courtesy of the CDC, Division of Parasitic Diseases.)

- Schistosomiasis is diagnosed by observing and recognizing characteristic eggs in urine (*S. haematobium*) or feces (*S. mansoni* and *S. japonicum*)

- Large eggs; the *S. mansoni* egg has a prominent lateral spine; the *S. haematobium* egg has a prominent terminal spine

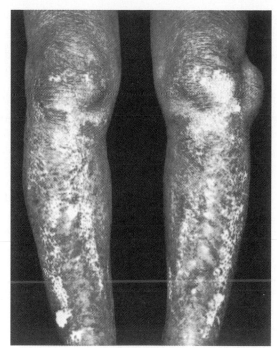

Figure 23-4. **Focal depigmentation, referred to as "leopard skin," in an onchocerciasis patient.** (From Binford CH, Connor DH. Pathology of Tropical and Extraordinary Diseases, vol 1. Washington, DC: Armed Forces Institute of Pathology, 1976.)

Helminth Infections of the Skin

Onchocerciasis

Disease. Onchocerciasis is also known as river blindness for two reasons: it primarily affects people who live near moving bodies of water, such as streams and rivers, and it can lead to blindness. An infected person develops fibrous subcutaneous nodules containing adult worms; a nodule grows near the site where the vector injected infective larvae. The location of the nodules relates to the flying pattern of the arthropod vector. Nodules occur primarily on the head and shoulders in the Western Hemisphere and primarily on the pelvic girdle and lower extremities in Africa. Migrating microfilariae affect the skin and the eyes, causing intense itching of skin, changes in skin pigmentation (leopard skin; Fig. 23-4), skin elasticity, lymphadenitis (Fig. 23-5), and ocular damage. Over the years, continued ocular damage ultimately causes blindness.

Geographic occurrence. In the Western Hemisphere, onchocerciasis is found in Guatemala, southern Mexico, and some countries in South America. In the Eastern Hemisphere, onchocerciasis occurs primarily in sub-Saharan Africa.

Parasite. Adult male and female *Onchocerca volvulus* worms live within fibrous tissue nodules. Female worms

> In the life cycle of *Onchocerca volvulus*, humans serve as definitive hosts and *Simulium* blackflies serve as intermediate hosts. Humans acquire onchocerciasis by the bite of an infected blackfly.

release microscopic prelarval stages called microfilariae, which get into the skin, eyes, and bloodstream (occasionally). When a blackfly (genus *Simulium*) takes a meal of tissue juices, it ingests the microfilariae. Within the blackfly, the microfilariae mature into infective larvae. When the blackfly again takes a blood meal, it injects an infective larva into the human. In the human body, the larva matures into an adult worm. Adult worms may live for 15 years in the human body, producing microfilariae for about 10 years. In this parasitic life cycle, the human is the definitive host and the blackfly is the intermediate host. *Simulium* blackflies live near moving bodies of water because the eggs that the female flies deposit on submerged, aquatic vegetation must be well oxygenated for proper maturation to occur.

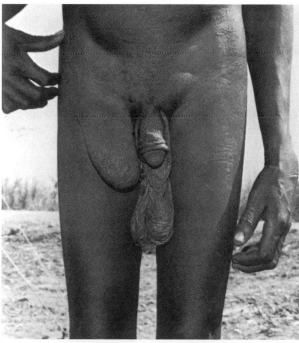

Figure 23-5. **The condition known as "hanging groin," caused by onchocercal lymphadenitis of the underlying femoral lymph nodes.** (From Binford CH, Connor DH. Pathology of Tropical and Extraordinary Diseases, vol 1. Washington, DC: Armed Forces Institute of Pathology, 1976.)

Because the vectors live near streams and rivers, it is the people who also live there that become infected.

Laboratory diagnosis. Diagnosis is most often made by observing and recognizing tiny, unsheathed, *O. volvulus* microfilariae in skin snips (described earlier) that have been incubated in water or saline. Rarely, microfilariae are observed in blood and urine specimens. CML professionals must be able to differentiate *O. volvulus* microfilariae (see Table 23-4) from the microfilariae produced by other filarial worms. Differentiating criteria include whether the microfilaria are sheathed or unsheathed and the distribution of nuclei within their tails. The WHO or CDC web site or a parasitology textbook should be consulted for additional information on differentiating *O. volvulus* microfilariae from the microfilariae of other filarial worms.

> Diagnosis of onchocerciasis is most often made by observing and recognizing tiny, unsheathed *Onchocerca volvulus* microfilariae in skin snips.

Essentials

Onchocerca volvulus

- Filarial nematode

- Cause of onchocerciasis (river blindness), dermatitis, and eye damage

- Definitive host is human; intermediate host is *Simulium* blackfly

- Onchocerciasis is acquired by introduction of larvae during the bite of an infected blackfly

- Adult worms live in onchocercal nodules

- Onchocerciasis is diagnosed by observing and recognizing characteristic microfilariae in skin snips

Helminth Infections of the Muscles and Subcutaneous Tissues

Trichinosis

Disease. Trichinosis, also known as trichiniasis and trichinellosis, is caused by a nematode whose larvae become encapsulated in striated muscles. Muscles having the largest blood supply are most commonly affected, including the diaphragm, tongue, and biceps. Symptoms vary widely depending on the number and location of cysts. They include swelling of the upper eyelids, fever, muscle pain, and eosinophilia. Cardiac and neurologic complications can lead to death.

Geographic occurrence. Trichinosis occurs worldwide.

Parasite. The cause of trichinosis is the nematode *Trichinella spiralis*. Humans become infected by eating raw or undercooked meat (usually pork, products containing pork, and the meat of wild carnivores) that contains encysted *T. spiralis* larvae. Within the epithelium of the human small intestine, the larvae mature into adult male and female worms. Female worms release larvae that penetrate blood vessels and are then hematogenously disseminated throughout the human body. The larvae become encapsulated within striated muscle. Within the cysts, larvae reach lengths of 0.8 to 1 mm. Animals become infected as humans do—by eating the meat of infected animals. Humans are considered accidental hosts and dead-end hosts.

> Trichinosis is caused by the nematode *Trichinella spiralis*, whose larvae become encapsulated in striated muscles. Trichinosis can be diagnosed by observing and recognizing encysted larvae in a muscle biopsy specimen and by immunodiagnostic procedures.

Laboratory diagnosis. Trichinosis can be diagnosed by observing and recognizing encysted larvae in a muscle biopsy specimen (Fig. 23-6) and by immunodiagnostic procedures.

Dracunculiasis

Disease. Dracunculiasis, also known as guinea worm infection, is caused by a long, thin nematode that migrates in the deep connective tissues and subcutaneous tissues of the body. A female worm migrates to a lower extremity—typically, an ankle or foot. There the female discharges larvae into a water source by extending a portion of its posterior end through a blister in the skin. Symptoms include urticaria,

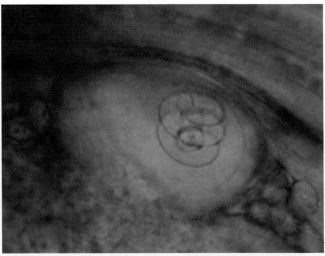

Figure 23-6. **Coiled larva within a *Trichinella spiralis* cyst, in pressed muscle tissue.** (Courtesy of the Division of Parasitic Diseases, CDC.)

eosinophilia, fever, and burning or itching at the site of the blister.

Geographic occurrence. Dracunculiasis occurs in sub-Saharan Africa, India, and Yemen. The WHO and the Carter Center are making excellent progress in their efforts to eliminate dracunculiasis, primarily by educating members of the indigenous population to filter their drinking water. (See the CD-ROM for additional information regarding the dracunculiasis eradication campaign.)

Parasite. The adult *Dracunculus medinensis* (guinea worm) can be up to a meter in length. The female worm usually

> Dracunculiasis, or guinea worm infection, is caused by a long, thin nematode that migrates in the deep connective tissues and subcutaneous tissues of the body. Humans become infected by drinking water that contains a *Cyclops* sp.

migrates to an ankle or foot, where a blister forms. On contact with water, the blister bursts, and a portion of the worm protrudes through the opening. Larvae are discharged into the water. A larva is ingested by a small, freshwater crustacean of the genus *Cyclops*. Within the *Cyclops* sp., it takes about 8 days before the larva becomes infective for humans. Humans become infected by drinking water that contains the infected *Cyclops*. In the human body, the larva matures into an adult worm. In this parasitic life cycle, the human is the definitive host and the *Cyclops* sp. is the intermediate host.

STUDY AID

Cyclops. A genus of freshwater crustaceans, *Cyclops* serves as an intermediate host in both dracunculiasis and fish tapeworm infection (discussed later in the chapter).

Laboratory diagnosis. Diagnosis is made clinically by observing and recognizing a portion of the female worm protruding from the patient's skin—usually, near the ankle. Traditionally, worms were removed by winding them onto a stick (Fig. 23-7), but now removal is done surgically.

> Diagnosis of dracunculiasis is made clinically by observing and recognizing a portion of the female worm protruding from the patient's skin—usually, near the ankle.

Essentials

Dracunculus medinensis

- Guinea worm
- Long, thin nematode
- Cause of dracunculiasis or guinea worm infection

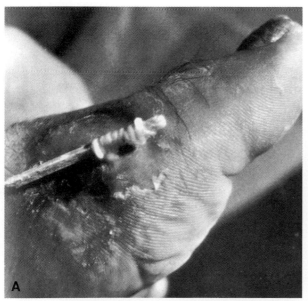

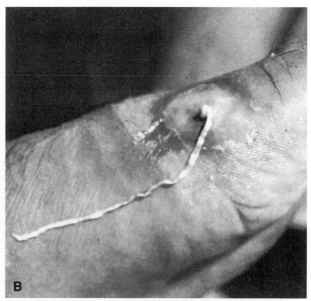

***Figure 23-7.* Guinea worm infection. A.** Adult *Dracunculus medinensis* worm being removed by winding it onto a stick. **B.** Partially removed *D. medinensis* worm. Larvae have been squeezed from the exterior portion, which has caused flattening of that portion of the worm. (From Binford CH, Connor DH. Pathology of Tropical and Extraordinary Diseases, vol 1. Washington, DC: Armed Forces Institute of Pathology, 1976.)

- Definitive host is human; intermediate host is the genus *Cyclops* (a freshwater crustacean)

- Dracunculiasis is acquired by ingestion of a *Cyclops* sp. containing an infective larva

- Adult worms migrate within subcutaneous tissues; the posterior end of a female worm protrudes from a blister in the skin to deposit larvae into freshwater

- Adult worm can be removed by surgery or by winding the worm onto a stick

Helminth Infections of the Eyes

Onchocerciasis

Onchocerciasis, which can cause blindness, was discussed earlier in the section on helminth infections of the skin.

Loiasis

Disease. Loiasis, also known as *Loa loa* or eyeworm infection, is caused by a long, thin filarial worm that migrates through subcutaneous and deeper tissues of the body and sometimes passes beneath the conjunctiva (hence the name eyeworm; Fig. 23-8). Symptoms include localized pain, itching, urticaria, and transient swellings referred to as fugitive swellings or **Calabar swellings.**

Geographic occurrence. Loiasis occurs in Africa, primarily in the rainforests of central Africa.

Parasite. *Loa loa* is a filarial worm. Adult worms are about 0.5 mm wide and up to 7 cm long. Female worms produce microfilariae, which are found in the bloodstream. The microfilariae are ingested by a mango fly (*Chrysops* spp.) when it takes a blood meal and then mature within the fly. Infective larvae are introduced into the skin when the fly takes a blood meal.

> Loiasis is caused by *Loa loa*, a long, thin filarial worm that migrates through subcutaneous and deeper tissues of the body. Because the adult worm sometimes passes beneath the conjunctiva, it is also called the eyeworm. Humans become infected via the bite of an infected *Chrysops* fly.

In this parasitic life cycle, the human is the definitive host and the *Chrysops* fly is the intermediate host.

Laboratory diagnosis. Diagnosis of loiasis is usually made clinically. Laboratory diagnosis is made by observing and recognizing microfilariae in a stained peripheral blood smear. The microfilariae are said to have diurnal[2] periodicity because they are most likely to be present in the bloodstream during the daytime. For this reason, it is recommended that

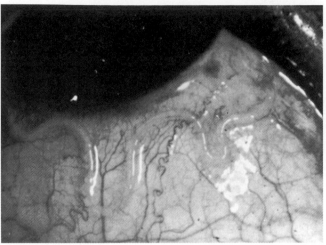

***Figure 23-8.* Adult *Loa loa* worm migrating beneath the conjunctiva.** (From Binford CH, Connor DH. Pathology of Tropical and Extraordinary Diseases, vol 1. Washington, DC: Armed Forces Institute of Pathology, 1976.)

blood specimens be collected between 10:00 AM and 2:00 PM. Like the microfilariae of *Wuchereria* and *Brugia* spp., they are sheathed, but unlike the microfilariae of *Wuchereria* and *Brugia* spp., their nuclei are continuous to the tip of the tail (see Table 23-4).

Essentials

Loa loa

- African eyeworm

- Filarial nematode

- Cause of loiasis

- Definitive host is human; intermediate host is mango fly or deerfly (*Chrysops* sp.)

- Loiasis is acquired by introduction of larvae during the bite of an infected mango fly

- Adult worms migrate within subcutaneous tissues and sometimes pass beneath the conjunctiva

- Migrating worms cause inflammatory responses known as Calabar swellings

- Loiasis is diagnosed clinically or by observing and recognizing characteristic microfilariae in a blood specimen

Helminth Infections of the Respiratory System

Paragonimiasis

Disease. Paragonimiasis, or lung fluke infection, is caused by trematodes in the genus *Paragonimus*, which become

---

[2] *Diurnal pertains to daylight hours. It is the opposite of nocturnal, which pertains to the hours of darkness. The diurnal periodicity of* Loa loa *microfilariae is thought to be associated with the daytime biting habits of the vectors, the* Chrysops *spp.*

encapsulated in the lungs. The most common symptoms of paragonimiasis include cough, hemoptysis (coughing up of blood), and chest pain. The patient's symptoms and chest radiographs can lead to a mistaken diagnosis of pulmonary tuberculosis. Adult worms may invade sites other than the lungs, including the central nervous system, intestinal wall, liver, and lymph nodes.

Geographic occurrence. Paragonimiasis occurs in the Far East, southwestern Asia, India, Africa, Mexico, Central America, and South America.

Parasites. Several species of trematodes in the genus *Paragonimus* cause lung fluke infection. Adult worms are plump, ovoid, and reddish brown. Female worms release eggs,

> Paragonimiasis, or lung fluke infection, is caused by trematodes in the genus *Paragonimus*, which become encapsulated in the lungs. Humans become infected by ingesting raw, pickled, salted, marinated, or partially cooked crabs or crayfish containing larvae called metacercariae.

which are coughed up by the patient and either expelled in sputum or swallowed. Swallowed eggs pass out in the feces, and if they reach freshwater, larvae called miracidia are released into the water. The miracidia infect suitable species of snails, within which cercariae are produced after several intermediate developmental stages. Released cercariae infect crabs and crayfish, within which they encyst, becoming metacercariae. Humans become infected by ingesting raw, pickled, salted, marinated, or partially cooked crabs or crayfish containing metacercariae. The larvae excyst in the intestinal tract, penetrate the intestinal wall, and migrate through various tissues. In this parasitic life cycle, humans are the definitive hosts and snails, crabs, and crayfish serve as intermediate hosts.

Laboratory diagnosis. Diagnosis of paragonimiasis is made by observing and recognizing *Paragonimus* eggs during microscopic examination of a sputum or fecal specimen. Spu-

> Paragonimiasis is diagnosed by observing and recognizing *Paragonimus* eggs during microscopic examination of a sputum or fecal specimen. Sputum specimens are often tinged with orange-brown flecks, called iron filings, that are masses of eggs.

tum specimens are often tinged with orange-brown flecks, referred to as iron filings, that represent masses of eggs. Sputum may also be tinged with blood. The eggs are 45 to 65 μm wide by 80 to 120 μm long, ovoid, brownish yellow, unembryonated, thick shelled, and operculated at one end (Fig. 23-9). The **operculum** is like a trap door, through which the miracidium ultimately emerges. Opercular shoulders are present, and the shell thickens at the abopercular end

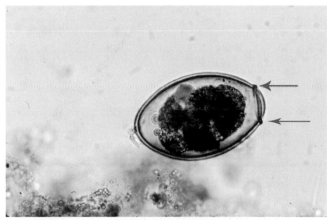

Figure 23-9. Paragonimus westermani egg. Notice the thin, smooth shell and the prominent shouldered operculum (*arrows*). Although similar in appearance to a *Clonorchis sinensis* egg (see Fig. 23-32), it is two to three times larger. It is similar in size to a *Diphyllobothrium latum* egg (see Fig. 23-26), but the latter has a flat rather than raised operculum. (From Winn WC Jr, et al. Koneman's Color Atlas and Textbook of Diagnostic Microbiology. 6th Ed. Philadelphia: Lippincott Williams & Wilkins, 2006.)

(the end of the egg opposite from the operculum). These latter features aid in differentiating *Paragonimus* eggs from the eggs of *Diphyllobothrium latum*, the fish tapeworm, which is described later in the chapter. *Paragonimus* eggs are also larger than *D. latum* eggs, illustrating the importance of using an ocular micrometer to measure the eggs.

Helminth Infections of the Central Nervous System

Cysticercosis

Disease. Cysticercosis, or cysticerciasis, is tissue infection with the larval stage of the pork tapeworm. It usually involves the central nervous system (CNS), although cysts can form in other tissues and organs, such as the eye and heart (Fig. 23-10). Symptoms depend on the number and location of the cysts. Neurocysticercosis (cysts in the CNS) may cause seizures, headache, abnormal behavior, disequilibrium, and visual problems.

Geographic occurrence. Cysticercosis occurs worldwide but is particularly frequent where pork is eaten raw or insufficiently cooked, and where pigs have access to human feces.

Parasite. Cysticercosis is caused by larvae of the pork tapeworm, *Taenia solium*. The adult pork tapeworm (described later in the chapter) lives in the human small intestine, where it produces eggs. Only one tapeworm is necessary for egg production because all tapeworms are **hermaphroditic,** meaning that they contain both male and female reproductive organs. When a human ingests the eggs, the larvae that emerge in the intestinal tract penetrate the intestinal wall, gain access to the lymphatics and

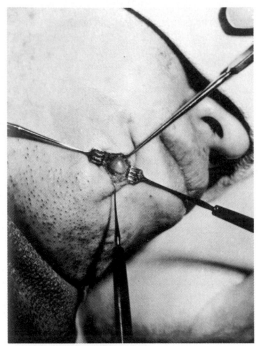

Figure 23-10. **Larval *Taenia solium,* known as a cysticercus, being removed from a patient's face.** (From Binford CH, Connor DH. Pathology of Tropical and Extraordinary Diseases, vol 1. Washington, DC: Armed Forces Institute of Pathology, 1976.)

bloodstream, and are carried to various tissues. An encysted larva is referred to as a cysticercus (pl. *cysticerci*).

Laboratory diagnosis. As described in a later section, infection with an adult pork tapeworm can be diagnosed by a fecal examination. Cysticercosis is diagnosed using immunodiagnostic procedures or by histological examination of an excised cyst.

Hydatid Cyst Disease

Disease. Hydatid cyst disease or echinococcosis is caused by tapeworms in the genus *Echinococcus*. Only infection with one particular species—*E. granulosus*—is described in this section. Cysts may develop in any tissues or organs of the body but are most often found in the liver. Symptoms vary with the number and location of the cysts.

Geographic occurrence. Hydatid cyst disease occurs worldwide, except in Antarctica and Iceland. Infection with *E. granulosus* occurs primarily in sheep-raising regions.

Parasite. In nature, the life cycle of *E. granulosus* usually involves a dog as the definitive host and a sheep as the intermediate host. The adult *E. granulosus* tapeworm lives in the dog's small intestine, where it grows to only about 6 mm in length. Eggs released by the tapeworm are passed in the dog's feces. Each egg contains an embryo called an **oncosphere.** If an egg is eaten by a sheep, the oncosphere develops into a larva, and a fluid-filled cyst called a hydatid cyst grows somewhere in the internal organs of the sheep.

The fluid within the hydatid cyst contains many daughter cysts and scolices (sing. **scolex**), or tapeworm heads, which collectively are referred to as hydatid sand. If the sheep's viscera (internal organs) containing the hydatid cyst are fed to a dog, each scolex can mature into an adult worm. Adult worms can live for up to 20 months in the dog's intestine. If a human ingests an egg, a hydatid cyst develops somewhere in the human body. Developed cysts are usually about 1 to 7 cm in diameter but can exceed 10 cm. Humans are considered accidental hosts and dead-end hosts. Hydatid cysts must be very carefully removed from the human body by surgery. If the cyst is punctured during surgery and the contents of the cyst spill out into a body cavity, a severe allergic reaction (anaphylaxis) can occur, and each daughter cyst can mature into another hydatid cyst.

Laboratory diagnosis. Diagnosis of hydatidosis is usually made by immunodiagnostic procedures or microscopic examination of the hydatid sand following surgical removal of the cyst.

Helminth Infections of the Gastrointestinal Tract, Including the Liver

Table 23-5 summarizes ways in which certain helminth infections are diagnosed by examination of gastrointestinal tract specimens. The helminths are listed in the table in the same order that they are described in this section: nematodes or roundworms first, cestodes or tapeworms second, and trematodes or flukes third.

Ascariasis

Disease. Ascariasis is infection with *Ascaris lumbricoides*, the large intestinal roundworm of humans. It is called the large intestinal roundworm of humans because it is large, not because it lives in the large intestine. In fact, male and female adult worms live in the small intestine. Symptoms depend on the number of worms infecting the patient, referred to as the **worm burden,** and the location(s) of the worm(s). A patient may be infected with one or more worms, sometimes many. Although the adult worms usually remain in the intestinal tract, they can penetrate the intestinal wall and migrate to virtually any part of the body. The worms may be stimulated to migrate by fever or anaesthesia associated with surgery. Problems associated with ascariasis can include nutritional deficiency, bowel obstruction, obstruction of a bile or pancreatic duct, appendicitis, and peritonitis.

Geographic occurrence. Ascariasis is reported worldwide but with greatest frequency in moist tropical countries. Ascariasis is most common in areas where human feces, referred to as night soil, are used to fertilize crops.

Parasite. Adult worms can reach a maximum length of an impressive 35 cm. Female worms release eggs that pass in the feces. The eggs must reach moist, warm soil, where it

TABLE 23 - 5 Diagnosing Intestinal Helminth Infections

Infection	Observation Required for Diagnosis
Nematode infections	
Ascariasis	Whole worms or eggs in feces
Hookworm infection	Eggs in feces
Strongyloidiasis	Larvae in duodenal aspirates or feces
Enterobiasis (pinworm infection)	Eggs in cellophane (Scotch) tape preparations
Trichuriasis (whipworm infection)	Eggs in feces
Cestode infections	
Beef tapeworm infection	Tapeworm segments (proglottids) or eggs in feces
Pork tapeworm infection	Proglottids or eggs in feces
Diphyllobothriasis (fish tapeworm infection)	Proglottids or eggs in feces
Dog tapeworm infection	Proglottids or egg packets in feces
Dwarf tapeworm infection	Proglottids (rarely) or eggs in feces
Rat tapeworm infection	Eggs in feces
Trematode infections	
Fasciolopsiasis (giant intestinal fluke infection)	Eggs in feces
Fascioliasis	Eggs in feces
Clonorchiasis	Eggs in feces

takes about 2 weeks for the larvae within the eggs to become infective. Humans become infected by ingesting infective eggs, often by ingesting unwashed or inadequately washed vegetables. In the human body, the larva then matures into an adult worm. Adult worms can live in the body for one or two years. Humans are the only hosts.

> Ascariasis is infection with *Ascaris lumbricoides*, the large intestinal roundworm of humans. Humans become infected by ingesting infective eggs from soil.

Laboratory diagnosis. Ascariasis is diagnosed by observing and recognizing characteristic eggs during a microscopic examination of a fecal specimen or by identifying an adult worm that has emerged from the patient's anus, mouth, or nose. Adult worms are cylindrical, with a tapering anterior end having three well-developed lips. Female worms are 20 to 35 cm long, and males are 15 to 31 cm long (Fig. 23-11).

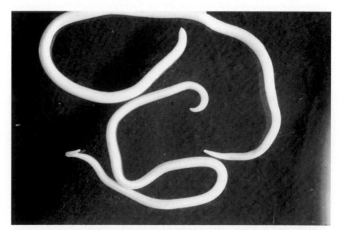

***Figure 23-11.* Adult *Ascaris lumbricoides* worms.** The female worm (*top*) may reach 20 to 35 cm in length. The male worm (*bottom*) is generally shorter (15 to 31 cm) and has a curved tail. (From Winn WC Jr, et al. Koneman's Color Atlas and Textbook of Diagnostic Microbiology. 6th Ed. Philadelphia: Lippincott Williams & Wilkins, 2006.)

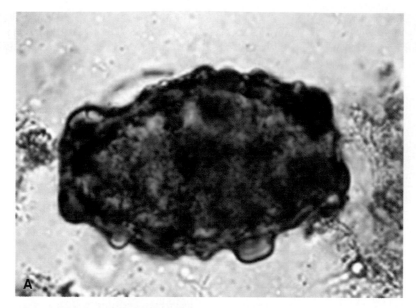

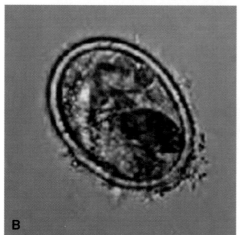 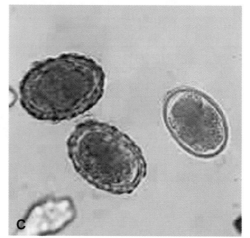

***Figure 23-12. Ascaris lumbricoides* eggs. A.** Unfertilized egg with a mamillated surface. **B.** Decorticated unfertilized egg. **C.** Fertilized eggs; the one on the right is decorticated. (Courtesy of the CDC, Division of Parasitic Diseases.)

Ascaris eggs may be fertilized or unfertilized and may or may not possess a thick, bumpy (**mamillated**) coat. Thus, as shown in Figure 23-12, an *Ascaris* egg may assume any of four possible appearances, any or all of which may be observed in a single fecal specimen:

> Ascariasis is diagnosed by observing and recognizing characteristic eggs during a microscopic examination of a fecal specimen or by identifying an adult worm that has emerged from the patient's anus, mouth, or nose. *Ascaris* eggs may be fertilized or unfertilized and may or may not possess a thick, bumpy coat. Any or all of these forms of eggs may be observed in a single fecal specimen.

- An unfertilized egg with a pronounced mamillated coat; elongated oval; up to 90 μm long (Fig. 23-12A)

- An unfertilized egg with no mamillated coat (the egg is said to be **decorticated**); elongated oval; up to 90 μm long (Fig. 23-12B)

- A fertilized egg with a thin mamillated coat; broadly oval; usually golden brown; up to 50 μm wide and 75 μm long; may or may not possess a motile larva (Fig. 23-12C)

- Decorticated fertilized egg; broadly oval; usually golden brown; up to 50 μm wide and 75 μm long; may or may not possess a motile larva (Fig. 23-12C)

Essentials

Ascaris lumbricoides

- Intestinal nematode

- Cause of ascariasis

- Definitive host is human; no intermediate hosts

- Ascariasis is acquired by ingestion of eggs from contaminated soil (often on inadequately washed vegetables)

- Adult worms live in the small intestine but can migrate to other parts of the body

- Ascariasis is diagnosed by observing and recognizing adult worms or characteristic eggs in feces

- Eggs may be fertilized or unfertilized, and corticated (mamillated) or decorticated

Hookworm Infection

Disease. Human hookworm infection is caused by *Necator americanus*, the New World hookworm, and *Ancylostoma duodenale*, the Old World hookworm. The adult hookworms, which are about 7 to 11 mm in length, live in the small intestine. The worms anchor themselves to the intestinal mucosa by means of well-developed mouthparts: teeth in *A. duodenale* (Fig. 23-13A) and cutting plates in *N. americanus* (Fig. 23-13B). The attachment of the worms causes bleeding. Depending on the worm burden, symptoms may range from none to iron deficiency, anemia, fatigue, abdominal pain, nausea, vomiting, red-to-black diarrheal stools, weakness, and pallor.

Geographic occurrence. Although *N. americanus* is referred to as the New World hookworm and *A. duodenale* is referred to as the Old World hookworm, these terms should not be taken literally. Hookworm infection in the Western Hemisphere, including the United States, is caused primarily, but not exclusively, by *N. americanus*. *A. duodenale* is the cause of hookworm infection in Europe, North Africa, and the Middle East. Hookworm infection in sub-Saharan Africa, southern Asia, and the Far East are caused primarily by *N. americanus*. It has been estimated that more than 1 billion people are infected with hookworm worldwide.

Parasite. Female hookworms release eggs that pass in the feces. The eggs must reach moist, shady, warm soil, where they hatch within 1 to 2 days. In the soil, it takes about 5 to 8 days for immature, noninfective larvae (called rhabditiform larvae) to become mature, infective larvae (called filariform larvae). The infective larvae remain viable in the soil for several weeks. Humans become infected by penetration of the skin—usually, the soles of the feet—by the infective larvae. In the human body, the larvae then mature into adult worms. Adult worms can live in the body for 4 to 20 years. Humans are the only hosts.

> Immature, noninfective hookworm larvae are referred to as rhabditiform larvae. Mature, infective hookworm larvae are referred to as filariform larvae.

Laboratory diagnosis. Diagnosis is confirmed by observing and recognizing characteristic hookworm eggs (Fig. 23-14) during a microscopic examination of a fecal specimen. The eggs of *N. americanus* are identical in appearance to *A. duodenale* eggs. Hookworm eggs are oval and approximately 40 μm wide by 60 μm long, with broadly rounded ends and very thin shells. The eggs are usually in an early stage of cleavage, with a clear space between the

> Humans become infected with hookworms by penetration of the skin by infective larvae from soil. Diagnosis of hookworm infection is confirmed by observing and recognizing characteristic hookworm eggs during a microscopic examination of a fecal specimen.

> It is not possible to differentiate between *Necator americanus* infection and *Ancylostoma duodenale* infection by the appearance of their eggs or larvae.

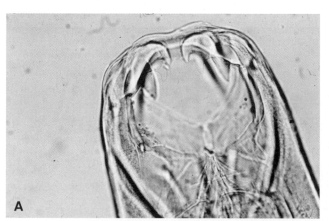
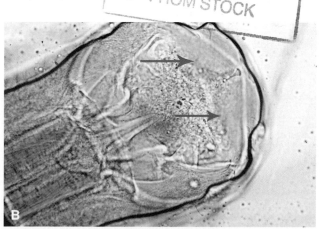

Figure 23-13. **Mouthparts of adult hookworms. A.** Teeth of *Ancylostoma duodenale*. **B.** Cutting plates (*arrows*) of *Necator americanus*. (From Winn WC Jr, et al. Koneman's Color Atlas and Textbook of Diagnostic Microbiology. 6th Ed. Philadelphia: Lippincott Williams & Wilkins, 2006.)

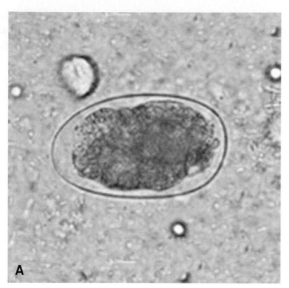
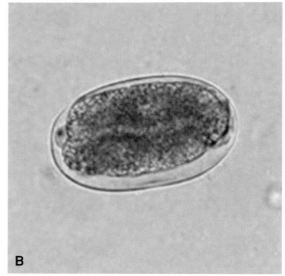

Figure 23-14. **Hookworm eggs. A.** Hookworm eggs usually are either unsegmented or in an early segmentation stage when passed in feces. **B.** When the specimen has been at room temperature for a while, a developing larva may be seen within the eggs. The eggs of *Necator americanus* and *Ancylostoma duodenale* are indistinguishable. Hookworm eggs are also indistinguishable from *Strongyloides stercoralis* eggs, but the latter are rarely seen in fecal specimens. (Courtesy of the CDC, Division of Parasitic Diseases.)

eggshell and the developing embryo. In stool specimens that are more than 24 hours old, eggs containing larvae or free, noninfective (rhabditiform) larvae may be seen. The larvae are very similar in appearance to, and must be differentiated from, *Strongyloides* larvae, because infections of the two different parasites demand different therapies.

Essentials

Hookworms

- *Ancylostoma duodenale* (Old World hookworm) and *Necator americanus* (New World hookworm)

- Intestinal nematodes

- Cause of hookworm infection

- Definitive host is human; no intermediate hosts

- Hookworm infection is acquired by penetration of the skin by infective filariform larvae from contaminated soil

- Adult worms live in the small intestine, where they attach to the intestinal mucosa by teeth (*A. duodenale*) or cutting plates (*N. americanus*) and cause bleeding, which can result in anemia

- Hookworm infection is diagnosed by observing and recognizing characteristic eggs in feces; the eggs of *A. duodenale* cannot be differentiated from those of *N. americanus*

- When passed in the feces, eggs are usually in the 8- to 32-cell stage of development

Strongyloidiasis

Disease. Strongyloidiasis is a roundworm infection of the small intestine. Symptoms depend on the worm burden, ranging from asymptomatic infection to abdominal pain, diarrhea, urticaria, eosinophilia, nausea, weight loss, vomiting, weakness, and constipation. Disseminated strongyloidiasis, including wasting, pulmonary involvement, and death, may occur in immunocompromised patients.

Geographic occurrence. Strongyloidiasis occurs in tropical and temperate areas, most commonly in warm, wet regions.

Parasite. Strongyloidiasis is caused by the roundworm *Strongyloides stercoralis*, sometimes referred to as threadworm. Parthenogenic female worms—able to produce eggs without any assistance from males—live in the mucosa of the human duodenum and upper jejunum. They release eggs that usually hatch in the intestinal tract. Noninfective rhabditiform larvae pass in the feces. In temperate climates, the rhabditiform larvae develop into infective filariform larvae in the soil. In tropical regions, the rhabditiform larvae develop into filariform larvae that then develop into free-living male and female adult worms in the soil. Fertilized female worms produce

> Strongyloidiasis is caused by the roundworm *Strongyloides stercoralis*, sometimes referred to as threadworm. Humans usually become infected by penetration of the skin by filariform larvae in soil.

eggs that develop into rhabditiform larvae that, in turn, develop into filariform larvae. The free-living cycle enables *Strongyloides* to maintain itself in nature without the need to

RHABDITIFORM STAGE

Scale:
0   45   90 μm

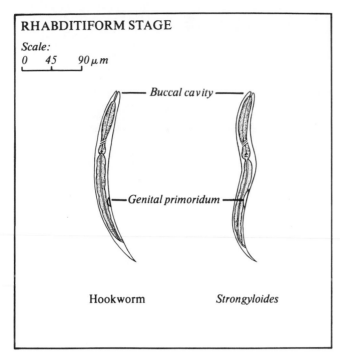

Buccal cavity

Genital primoridum

Hookworm   *Strongyloides*

FILARIFORM STAGE

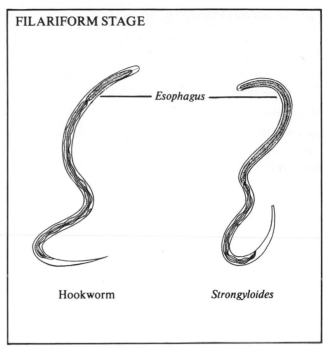

Esophagus

Hookworm   *Strongyloides*

Figure 23-15. **Morphological differences between hookworm and *Strongyloides* larvae.** (From Brooke MM, Melvin DM. Morphology of Diagnostic Stages of Intestinal Parasites of Humans. 2nd Ed. Atlanta, GA: CDC, 1984.)

infect humans. Humans usually become infected by penetration of the skin by filariform larvae in the soil. The larvae enter the bloodstream, pass through the lungs, and ultimately reach the small intestine, where they develop into adult worms. Humans, dogs, and cats can serve as hosts, and morphologically similar worms can infect monkeys.

Autoinfection is also possible with *S. stercoralis.* Sometimes, such as occurs with chronic constipation, rhabditiform larvae produced within the body remain in the intestinal tract long enough to develop into infective filariform larvae. The filariform larvae then penetrate the tissues of the intestinal tract and develop as if they had penetrated the skin, possibly leading to a very high worm burden. Autoinfection, which can also occur in pinworm infection (discussed later), is contrary to the general rule that, once infected with a particular helminth, it does not increase in number within the body.

> *S. stercoralis* is an unusual parasite in that it has both free-living and parasitic life cycles, and autoinfection can occur.

> Diagnosis of strongyloidiasis is usually made by observing and recognizing larvae in a fecal specimen or duodenal aspirate.

Laboratory diagnosis. Diagnosis of strongyloidiasis is usually made by observing and recognizing larvae in a fecal specimen or duodenal aspirate. Specimens may contain rhabditiform larvae and/or filariform larvae. The latter are quite similar to,

and must be distinguished from, hookworm larvae (Fig. 23-15):

- A hookworm rhabditiform larva is 15 to 20 μm wide by 250 to 300 μm long. It has a mouth opening (buccal capsule) approximately three times longer than the buccal capsule of a *Strongyloides* rhabditiform larva. The genital primordium packet of cells, which lies about two-thirds of the way back from the anterior end, is quite small and difficult to see. The tail is stubby.

- A *Strongyloides* rhabditiform larva is 10 to 20 μm wide by 200 to 300 μm long. It has a short buccal capsule and a prominent genital primordium packet of cells that lies about two-thirds of the way back from the anterior end. The tail is sharply pointed.

- A hookworm filariform larva is 10 to 20 μm wide by 300 to 600 μm long. The tail is long and sharply pointed.

- A *Strongyloides* filariform larva is 10 to 20 μm wide by 300 to 600 μm long. The tail is blunt with a small slit.

STUDY AID **Remembering the Differences Between *Strongyloides* and Hookworm Larvae.** It helps some students to remember the differences between *Strongyloides* larvae and hookworm larvae to think of *Strongyloides* larvae as being "short, stubby, and sexy," with a short buccal cavity, stubby tail, and prominent genital primordium.

Enterobiasis (Pinworm Infection)

Disease. Enterobiasis, or pinworm infection, is thought to be the most common helminth infection in the world. Humans—primarily children—are the only hosts. The worms cause perianal itching, disturbed sleep, and irritability.

Geographic occurrence. Enterobiasis occurs worldwide.

Parasite. Enterobiasis is caused by the roundworm *Enterobius vermicularis*. Male and female worms, which reach a maximum length of about 13 mm, live in the cecum, the first part of the colon. Female worms migrate down through the colon, emerge from the anus, and release eggs onto the perianal skin. The eggs are fully embryonated and

> Enterobiasis, or pinworm infection, is caused by a small nematode named *Enterobius vermicularis*. Humans become infected by ingesting infective eggs. Autoinfection is common among children who transfer eggs from their perianal regions to their mouths via fingers.

infective within a few hours. Humans become infected by ingesting the infective eggs. In the human body, the larvae then mature into adult worms. Adult worms can live in the body for several months to several years. Autoinfection is common in pinworm infection. In the process of scratching their perianal regions, children get the eggs on their fingers

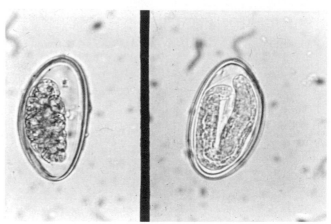

Figure 23-17. Enterobius vermicularis **eggs.** When passed, an egg may contain an embryo (*left*) or a coiled larva (*right*). Notice that one side of the egg is flattened. (From Winn WC Jr, et al. Koneman's Color Atlas and Textbook of Diagnostic Microbiology. 6th Ed. Philadelphia: Lippincott Williams & Wilkins, 2006.)

and beneath their fingernails. The eggs are ingested when they place their fingers into their mouths.

Laboratory diagnosis. Diagnosis is made using a cellophane (Scotch) tape prep. A piece of transparent tape is applied to the patient's perianal region, preferably in the morning before the patient bathes or defecates. The tape is then applied to a glass microscope slide, which is transported to the CML. Commercial collection devices are also available (Fig. 23-16). Diagnosis is confirmed by observing and recognizing characteristic pinworm eggs (Fig. 23-17) during a microscopic examination of the cellophane tape

> Diagnosis of pinworm infection is made using a cellophane (Scotch) tape prep. Thus, it is important to remember to associate the cellophane tape prep with pinworm infection.

prep. The eggs are approximately 20 to 30 μm wide by 50 to 60 μm long. An egg looks like an American-type football with one flattened side.

Adult *E. vermicularis* worms are sometimes present on cellophane tape preps. They are characterized by the presence of cervical alae—winglike flaps on either side of the anterior end (Fig. 23-18). If a worm dries out, these flaps often shrink and are unobservable. Placing the dried out worms into a small amount of water or saline will cause rehydration, and the flaps will pop back out for observation.

Essentials

Enterobius vermicularis

- Pinworm

- Intestinal nematode

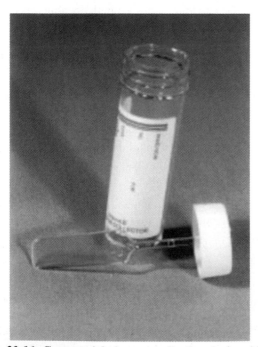

Figure 23-16. **Commercial pinworm collection device.** After the sticky side of the paddle has been pressed firmly against the patient's perianal skin, the paddle is returned to the container. In the parasitology section of the CML, the top of the paddle is snapped off, and the paddle is examined microscopically. (Courtesy of Scientific Device Laboratory Inc., Des Plaines, IL.)

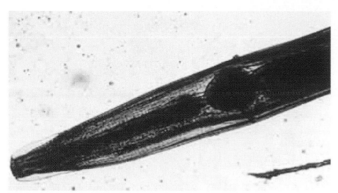

Figure 23-18. **Anterior end of a stained adult pinworm.** Notice the clear winglike flaps (cervical alae) on either side of the tip. (Courtesy of the CDC, Division of Parasitic Diseases.)

- Cause of enterobiasis

- Definitive host is human; no intermediate hosts

- Pinworm infection or enterobiasis is acquired by ingesting eggs

- Enterobiasis is diagnosed by observing characteristic eggs in cellophane (Scotch) tape preparations

- Football-shaped egg, flattened on one side

- Egg contains a larva

Trichuriasis (Whipworm Infection)

Disease. Trichuriasis or whipworm infection is an infection of the large intestine by a roundworm called *Trichuris trichiura,* often referred to by CML professionals as T. trich (pronounced "tee-trick"). Symptoms depend on the worm burden. Many patients are asymptomatic, but heavy infections can result in bloody, mucoid, diarrheal stools; rectal prolapse; anemia; and growth retardation.

Geographic occurrence. Trichuriasis occurs worldwide, especially in warm, moist regions. Cases have been reported in the United States.

Parasite. Adult *T. trichiura* male worms are 30 to 45 mm long, and female worms are 35 to 50 mm long (Fig. 23-19). The whip-shaped adult worms live attached to the mucosa of the colon, with the thin whip end—the anterior end of the worm—embedded in the intestinal mucosa and the thick whip handle end dangling in the intestinal lumen (Fig. 23-20). Female worms produce eggs that pass in the feces. The eggs require a minimum of 10 to 14 days in warm, moist soil to become infective. Humans become infected by ingestion of infective eggs. Humans are the only host.

> Trichuriasis, or whipworm infection, is caused by the roundworm *Trichuris trichiura*. Humans become infected by ingestion of infective eggs.

Laboratory diagnosis. Diagnosis of trichuriasis is made by observation and recognition of characteristic eggs in a fecal specimen or by observation of the worms by sigmoidoscopy. The egg is barrel shaped, with a clear mucoid-appearing plug at each end, and 22 to 23 μm wide by 50 to 54 μm long (Fig. 23-21). Although *T. trichiura* eggs are probably the easiest helminth eggs to recognize, care must be taken not to misidentify them as *Capillaria philippinensis* or *C. hepatica* eggs. *C. philippinensis* causes intestinal capillariasis, and *C. hepatica* causes hepatic capillariasis. Neither disease is endemic in the United States. *Capillaria* eggs (Fig. 23-22) are similar in size (21 by 45 μm) to *Trichuris* eggs, but they have striations on their shells that are not present on *Trichuris* eggs.

> Diagnosis of trichuriasis is made by observation and recognition of characteristic eggs in a fecal specimen or by observation of the adult worms by sigmoidoscopy.

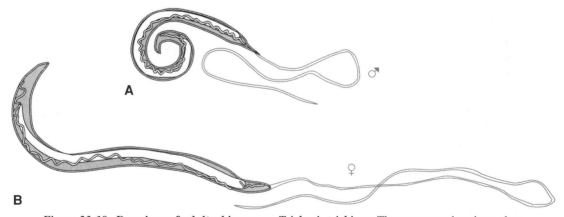

A

B

Figure 23-19. **Drawings of adult whipworms, *Trichuris trichiura*.** The worms anchor themselves within the large intestine by weaving their thin anterior portions into the intestinal mucosa. The male worm (**A**) is shorter than the female (**B**), as is true for most helminths. (Volk WA, et al: Essentials of Medical Microbiology, 5th Ed. Philadelphia, Lippincott-Raven, 1996.)

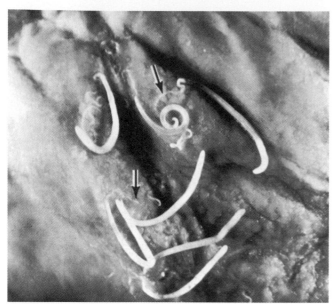

*Figure 23-20. **Adult T. trichiura worms.** Their slender anterior ends (arrows) are threaded beneath the colonic epithelium, and their thicker posterior ends dangle in the lumen of the colon. (From Binford CH, Connor DH. Pathology of Tropical and Extraordinary Diseases, vol 1. Washington, DC: Armed Forces Institute of Pathology, 1976.)*

Essentials

Trichura trichiura

- Whipworm

- Intestinal nematode

- Cause of trichuriasis, or whipworm infection

- Definitive host is human; no intermediate hosts

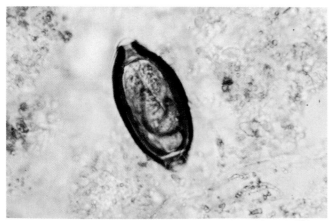

*Figure 23-21. **Typical bile-stained, barrel-shaped T. trichiura egg.** Note the clear (hyaline) plug at each end of the egg. (From Winn WC Jr, et al. Koneman's Color Atlas and Textbook of Diagnostic Microbiology. 6th Ed. Philadelphia: Lippincott Williams & Wilkins, 2006.)*

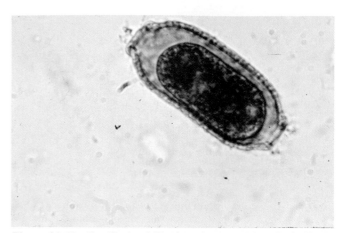

*Figure 23-22. **Capillaria philippinensis egg.** Although similar in appearance to a T. trichiura egg (see Fig. 23-21), the Capillaria egg has a striated shell and broad polar plugs. (From Winn WC Jr, et al. Koneman's Color Atlas and Textbook of Diagnostic Microbiology. 6th Ed. Philadelphia: Lippincott Williams & Wilkins, 2006.)*

- Trichuriasis is acquired by ingestion of infective eggs from contaminated soil

- Adult worms live in the large intestine, where they attach by threading their thin anterior ends through the intestinal mucosa

- Trichuriasis is diagnosed by observing characteristic eggs in feces

- Egg is barrel shaped and has a clear plug at each end (polar plugs)

Beef Tapeworm Infection

Disease. *Taeniasis* is a general term referring to intestinal infection with a *Taenia* sp.—either *T. saginata* (the beef tapeworm) or *T. solium* (the pork tapeworm). Infection with a beef tapeworm may be asymptomatic, or symptoms may include nervousness, insomnia, anorexia, weight loss, abdominal pain, and digestive disturbance. Motile segments of the worm that emerge from the anus can cause itching.

CAUTION **Beware of Similar-Sounding Names.** Do not confuse tinea with *Taenia*. **Tinea** (pronounced "tin-ee-uh") infections are fungal infections (see Chapter 20). Although they are often referred to as ringworm infections, they have nothing to do with worms. *Taenia* (pronounced "teen-ee-uh") is a genus of tapeworm. Both the beef tapeworm and pork tapeworm are members of this genus.

Geographic occurrence. Beef tapeworm infections occur worldwide, particularly where beef is eaten raw or undercooked and where cattle have access to human feces.

Parasite. The adult *Taenia saginata* tapeworm lives in the human small intestine, where it can reach 8 meters in length. Eggs released by the tapeworm are passed in the feces. The egg contains a six-hooked embryo called an oncosphere. When eggs are ingested by cattle, the oncospheres mature into cysticercus larvae in striated muscle of the animals. Humans become infected by ingestion of raw or undercooked beef containing an encysted cysticercus larva. Within the human body, the cysticercus larva matures into an adult worm. Adult worms can live for up to 25 years in the human body. In this parasitic life cycle, the human is the definitive host and cattle are the intermediate hosts.

> Beef tapeworm infection is infection with the cestode *Taenia saginata*. Humans become infected by ingestion of raw or undercooked beef containing an encysted cysticercus larva.

Laboratory diagnosis. Diagnosis of beef tapeworm infection is usually made by observing and recognizing either eggs or segments of the worm called **proglottids**. Less often, the diagnosis is made by finding the head or scolex of the worm. Finding the scolex, usually following specific therapy, would indicate that the worm is no longer present in the small intestine. Figure 23-23 illustrates the general anatomy of a tapeworm.

The eggs of *T. saginata*, which cannot be differentiated from those of *T. solium*, are spheroidal, yellow-brown, thick shelled, and 31 to 43 μm in diameter (Fig. 23-24). The shell is radially striated and contains a six-hooked embryo called an oncosphere.

If a proglottid is seen, it must be distinguished from the proglottid of *T. solium*. Proglottids of both species contain both male and female reproductive systems; tapeworms are hermaphroditic. The uterus of gravid proglottids contains numerous eggs. Table 23-6 contains the criteria by which gravid proglottids and scolices of *T. saginata* and *T. solium* can be differentiated. Figure 23-25 illustrates gravid proglottids and scolices of all of the intestinal cestodes described in this chapter.

> Diagnosis of beef tapeworm infection is usually made by observing and recognizing either eggs or segments of the worm called proglottids. Less often, the diagnosis is made by finding the head or scolex of the worm. Keep in mind that it is not possible to differentiate *Taenia saginata* from *Taenia solium* by the appearance of their eggs.

> The heads or scolices of *Taenia* spp. and some of the other intestinal tapeworms resemble the aliens that are depicted in many science fiction films.

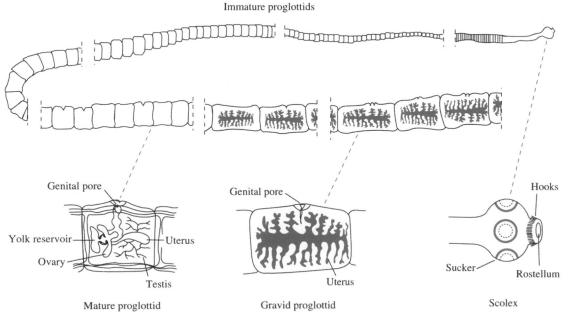

Immature proglottids

Genital pore

Yolk reservoir — Uterus

Ovary

Testis

Mature proglottid

Genital pore

Uterus

Gravid proglottid

Hooks

Sucker — Rostellum

Scolex

Figure 23-23. **Anatomy of a tapeworm.** Tapeworms are generally long and ribbonlike. They consist of a head (scolex) and numerous segments (proglottids). Tapeworms are hermaphroditic, with mature proglottids containing both male and female reproductive organs. Proglottids containing fertilized eggs are referred to as gravid proglottids. (Volk WA et al: Essentials of Medical Microbiology, 5th Ed. Philadelphia, Lippincott-Raven, 1996.)

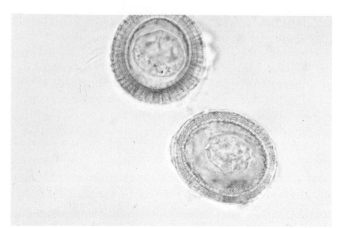

Figure 23-24. **Unstained eggs of a *Taenia* species.** Notice the radial striations in the walls. *T. saginata* eggs are indistinguishable from *T. solium* eggs. (From Winn WC Jr, et al. Koneman's Color Atlas and Textbook of Diagnostic Microbiology. 6th Ed. Philadelphia: Lippincott Williams & Wilkins, 2006.)

STUDY AID **Remembering the Differences Between *T. saginata* and *T. solium* Proglottids.** It helps some students to remember the differences between the gravid proglottids of *T. saginata* and those of *T. solium* by relating the larger number of uterine branches in *T. saginata* proglottids to the fact that the specific epithet *saginata* has more letters than does *solium*. Also, cows are bigger than pigs.

Essentials

Taenia saginata

- Beef tapeworm
- Cause of beef tapeworm infection

- Definitive host is human; intermediate hosts are cattle
- Beef tapeworm infection is acquired by ingestion of encysted larvae present in raw or undercooked beef
- Adult worms live in the small intestine, where they can reach lengths of 25 meters but are usually only about half that length
- Beef tapeworm infection is diagnosed by observing characteristic segments of adult worms (proglottids) or eggs in feces
- Gravid proglottids are longer than they are wide and contain 15 to 20 (average of 18) lateral uterine branches per side
- Egg is round with a thick, striated shell; it contains a six-hooked embryo; *T. saginata* eggs cannot be differentiated from *T. solium* eggs

Pork Tapeworm Infection

Disease. Infection with the pork tapeworm, *Taenia solium*, may be asymptomatic, or symptoms may include nervousness, insomnia, anorexia, weight loss, abdominal pain, and digestive disturbance. Motile segments of the worm that emerge from the anus can cause itching. If humans ingest *T. solium* eggs, cysticercus larvae develop in various tissues within the body. Larvae in the brain can lead to seizures and other CNS problems. This disease—where the larvae of *T. solium* are present in human tissues and organs—is known as cysticercosis (previously described).

Geographic occurrence. Pork tapeworm infection occurs worldwide, particularly where pork is eaten raw or undercooked and where pigs have access to human feces.

Parasite. The adult *T. solium* tapeworm lives in the human small intestine, where it can grow as long as 7 meters. Eggs released by the tapeworm are passed in the feces. The egg

TABLE 23 - 6	Differentiating *Taenia* spp. Gravid Proglottids and Scolices	
Feature	*T. saginata*	*T. solium*
Gravid proglottid	Longer (19 mm) than it is wide (17 mm); contains 15 to 20 lateral branches on each side of the central uterine stem; single lateral pore; usually found singly	Approximately square; contains 7 to 13 lateral branches on each side of the central uterine stem; single lateral pore; occasionally 2 or 3 proglottids seen attached to each other
Scolex	Top of head is roughly square; contains 4 suckers (one at each corner of the square), no rostellum, and no hooklets (referred to as an unarmed scolex)	Top of head is roughly square; contains 4 suckers (one at each corner of the square), contains a raised rostellum surrounded by a double set of hooklets (referred to as an armed scolex)

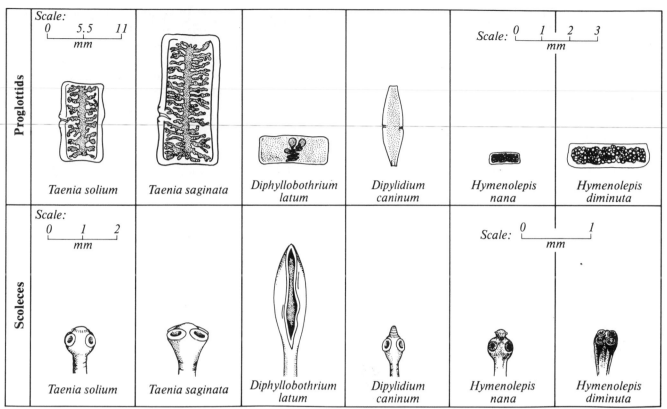

Figure 23-25. **Gravid proglottids and scoleces of the intestinal cestode parasites described in this chapter.** Notice that the scoleces of *T. solium*, *T. saginata*, and *D. caninum* are longer than they are broad, whereas those of *D. latum*, *H. nana*, and *H. diminuta* are broader than they are long. (From Brooke MM, Melvin DM. Morphology of Diagnostic Stages of Intestinal Parasites of Humans. 2nd Ed. Atlanta, GA: CDC, 1984.)

Pork tapeworm infection is infection with the cestode, *Taenia solium*. Humans become infected by ingestion of raw or undercooked pork containing an encysted cysticercus larva. ingestion of raw or undercooked pork containing a cysticercus larva. Within the human body, the cysticercus larva matures into an adult worm. Adult worms can live for up to 25 years in the human body. In this parasitic life cycle, the human is the definitive host and the pig is the intermediate host.

Laboratory diagnosis. Diagnosis of pork tapeworm infection is made by observing and recognizing either eggs (usually), segments of the worm called proglottids, or the head (scolex) of the worm (rarely). Finding the scolex, usually following specific therapy, would indicate that the worm is no longer present in the small intestine. The eggs of *T. solium* cannot be differentiated from those of *T. saginata* (see Fig. 23-24). Ingesting the eggs of *T. solium*, which are infectious, can lead to cysticercosis (previously discussed). The criteria by which gravid proglottids and scolices of *T. solium* and *T. saginata* can be differentiated were presented in Table 23-6.

contains a six-hooked embryo called an oncosphere. If an egg is ingested by a pig, the embryo matures into a cysticercus larva in striated muscle of the animal. Humans become infected by

Diagnosis of pork tapeworm infection is made by observing and recognizing either eggs (usually), segments of the worm called proglottids, or the head (scolex) of the worm (rarely). Remember that the eggs of *Taenia solium* cannot be differentiated from those of *Taenia saginata*. The eggs of *T. solium* are infectious, however, and ingestion of these eggs can lead to cysticercosis.

Essentials

Taenia solium

- Pork tapeworm

- Cause of pork tapeworm infection and cysticercosis

- Definitive host is human; intermediate hosts are pigs

- Pork tapeworm infection is acquired by ingestion of encysted larvae present in raw or undercooked pork

- Adult worms live in the small intestine, where they can reach lengths of 2 to 7 meters

- Pork tapeworm infection is diagnosed by observing characteristic segments of adult worms (proglottids) or eggs in feces

- Gravid proglottids are longer than they are wide and contain 7 to 13 (average of 9) lateral uterine branches per side

- Egg is round with a thick, striated shell and a six-hooked embryo; *T. solium* eggs cannot be differentiated from *T. saginata* eggs

- Cysticercosis is acquired by ingesting eggs of *T. solium*; self-infection is possible when a person is harboring an adult worm

- Encysted larvae of *T. solium* (called cysticerci) can be located anywhere in the body, including the brain

- Cysticerci are observed by radiograph, CT scan, or MRI; they are removed surgically, when possible

Fish Tapeworm Infection

Disease. Fish tapeworm infection, also known as diphyllobothriasis, is infection with the intestinal tapeworm *Diphyllobothrium latum*. Patients harboring one worm may be asymptomatic, but symptoms can include intestinal obstruction, diarrhea, abdominal pain, and vitamin B_{12} deficiency anemia.

Geographic occurrence. Fish tapeworm infection occurs worldwide, primarily in countries where eating raw or partially cooked fish is popular.

Parasite. The adult *D. latum* tapeworm lives in the human small intestine, where it can reach 10 meters in length. Eggs released by the tapeworm are passed in the feces. An egg must reach freshwater, where a ciliated larva called a **coracidium** emerges from the egg. The coracidium is eaten by a *Cyclops* sp. Within the *Cyclops*, the coracidium matures into a procercoid larva. If the *Cyclops* is eaten by a fish, the procercoid larva matures into a plerocercoid larva in the muscle of the fish. (See Fig. 21-1 for a diagram of

> Fish tapeworm infection, also known as diphyllobothriasis, is infection with the intestinal tapeworm *Diphyllobothrium latum*. Humans become infected by eating raw or undercooked fish containing a plerocercoid larva.

the life cycle of the fish tapeworm.) If the raw or undercooked fish is then eaten by a human, the plerocercoid larva matures into an adult worm. Adult worms may live for up to 25 years in the human body. In this parasitic life cycle, the human is the definitive host, the *Cyclops* is the first intermediate host, and the fish is the second intermediate host.

STUDY AID **Coracidium Versus Miracidium.** The ciliated larva that emerges from a *Diphyllobothrium latum* egg is called a **coracidium.** The ciliated larva that emerges from an egg of a *Schistosoma* sp. or other trematode is called a **miracidium.**

Laboratory diagnosis. Diagnosis of fish tapeworm infection requires observation and recognition of eggs and/or proglottids in fecal specimens. The eggs are broadly oval, 40 to 50 μm wide by 58 to 75 μm long, yellow-brown, and operculated (Fig. 23-26). Recall that an operculum is like a trap door—in this

> Diagnosis of fish tapeworm infection requires observation and recognition of eggs and/or proglottids in fecal specimens.

case, allowing the coracidium larva to emerge. Sometimes, eggs are observed with their operculum open or "popped up." Unlike *Paragonimus* eggs, *D. latum* eggs have no prominent shoulders adjacent to the operculum and no thickening of the shell at the abopercular end (the end of the egg opposite from the operculum). A small knob is usually present at the abopercular end of *D. latum* eggs. Compared with *Paragonimus* eggs, *D. latum* eggs are smaller.

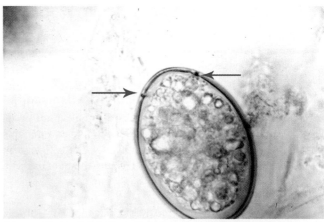

Figure 23-26. Diphyllobothrium latum egg. Although this is an operculated egg, the operculum (*arrows*) is difficult to see because its shoulders are small and inconspicuous. Compare this egg to the egg of *Paragonimus westermani* (see Fig. 23-9). (From Winn WC Jr, et al. Koneman's Color Atlas and Textbook of Diagnostic Microbiology. 6th Ed. Philadelphia: Lippincott Williams & Wilkins, 2006.)

Gravid proglottids of *D. latum* are wider (11 mm) than they are long (3 mm). The reproductive structures, including the genital pore, are located in the center of the proglottid, referred to as a rosette (see Fig. 23-25). Gravid proglottids are often passed in a chain, sometimes up to several feet in length.

Essentials

Diphyllobothrium latum

- Fish tapeworm

- Cause of fish tapeworm infection

- Definitive host is human; intermediate hosts are *Cyclops* (first intermediate host) and freshwater fish (second intermediate host)

- Fish tapeworm infection is acquired by ingestion of encysted plerocercoid larvae present in raw or under-cooked freshwater fish

- Adult worms live in the small intestine, where they can reach lengths of 10 meters or more

- Fish tapeworm infection is diagnosed by observing characteristic segments of adult worms (proglottids) or eggs in feces

- Gravid proglottids are wider than they are long and contain a central rosette-shaped uterine structure

- Eggs are operculated, but the operculum is difficult to see

Dog Tapeworm Infection (Dipylidiasis)

Disease. Dipylidiasis, or infection with the dog tapeworm, *Dipylidium caninum*, usually occurs in children as a result of swallowing an infected flea. The infection is usually asymptomatic, but parents of the child frequently become anxious when they observe the motile proglottids moving in inchworm fashion at the child's anus or on the surface of the child's stool.

> Dipylidiasis, or infection with the dog tapeworm, *Dipylidium caninum*, usually occurs in children as a result of swallowing an infected flea.

Geographic occurrence. *D. caninum* is distributed worldwide in dogs and cats.

Parasite. The adult *D. caninum* tapeworm lives in the dog's small intestine, where it can reach 70 cm in length. Egg packets released by the tapeworm are passed in the feces. If an egg is eaten by a larval flea, a cysticercoid larva develops within the flea. If the flea is then ingested by a dog, cat, or human, the larva matures into an adult worm. Adult worms usually live less than one year in the human body. In this parasitic life cycle, the dog is the usual definitive host and the flea is the intermediate host. Humans are considered accidental hosts, and because fleas are unlikely to ingest human feces, humans are also dead-end hosts.

Laboratory diagnosis. Diagnosis of dog tapeworm infection is made by observing and recognizing either egg packets (usually), single eggs, or proglottids in stool specimens. Individual eggs resemble *Taenia* eggs. The *D. caninum* egg is spherical, 25 to 40 μm in diameter, and thick walled, with a striated eggshell and containing a six-hooked oncosphere. Groups of eggs, referred to as egg packets, are often seen (Fig. 23-27). Individual proglottids resemble cucumber seeds when they are wet and rice grains when they are dry. The *D. caninum* proglottid has two genital pores located on opposite sides of the proglottid.

> Diagnosis of dog tapeworm infection is made by observing and recognizing either egg packets (usually), single eggs, or proglottids in stool specimens.

Essentials

Dipylidium caninum

- Dog tapeworm

- Cause of dog tapeworm infection

- Usual definitive hosts are dogs and cats; intermediate host are fleas from dogs and cats

- Dog tapeworm infection is acquired by ingestion of a cysticercoid larva present in an infected flea

- Adult worms live in the small intestine, where they reach lengths of 10 to 70 cm

- Dog tapeworm infection is diagnosed by observing characteristic segments of adult worms (proglottids) or egg packets in feces

- Gravid proglottids are longer than they are wide, with two lateral pores

- Eggs of *D. caninum* resemble those of *Taenia* spp. but are usually found in packets containing 15 to 25 eggs

Dwarf Tapeworm Infection

Disease. Hymenolepiasis is a general term for intestinal infection with a tapeworm in the genus *Hymenolepis*. *H. nana* is referred to as the dwarf tapeworm because of its small size. *H. diminuta* is referred to as the rat tapeworm, for reasons described in the next section. Dwarf tapeworm infections are usually asymptomatic, but heavy worm

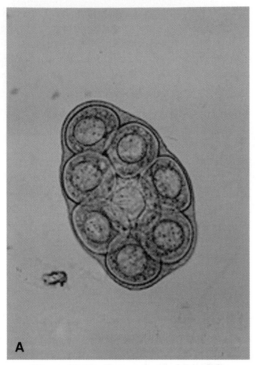 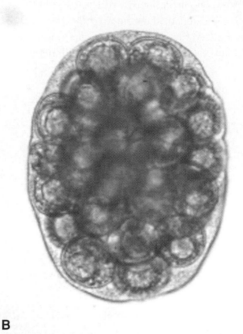

Figure 23-27. **Egg packets of *Dipylidium caninum*. A.** Egg packet containing 8 eggs. **B.** Atypical egg packet containing more than 30 eggs. The usual number of eggs in an egg packet is between 5 and 15. (Courtesy of the CDC, Division of Parasitic Diseases.)

Hymenolepis nana (the dwarf tapeworm) is the smallest tapeworm that infects humans, and *Diphyllobothrium latum* (the fish tapeworm) is the largest.

Geographic occurrence. Dwarf tapeworm infection occurs worldwide but is more common in warm, dry climates than in cold, wet climates. It is the most common human tapeworm infection in the United States.

Parasite. Adult *H. nana* tapeworms live in the human small intestine, where they can reach 4 cm in length (quite small

H. nana is the only human tapeworm that does not require an intermediate host.

for a tapeworm). Eggs released by the tapeworm are passed in the feces. They are infective at the time they are passed. If an egg is ingested by another human, a cysticercoid larva develops within the human. The cysticercoid larva then matures into an adult worm. Usually, humans are the only hosts; an intermediate host is not required. However, it is possible for an insect to ingest an egg, for the cysticercoid larva to develop within the insect, and then for a human to ingest the infected insect.

Laboratory diagnosis. Diagnosis of dwarf tapeworm infection is made by observing and recognizing *H. nana* eggs in a

burdens can cause gastroenteritis with or without diarrhea, abdominal pain, pallor, loss of weight, and weakness.

fecal specimen. The eggs must be differentiated from those of *H. diminuta*. The *H. nana* egg is thin shelled, round to oval, and 30 to 47 μm in diameter (Fig. 23-28). It contains a six-hooked oncosphere that has polar thickenings (one at each end of the egg), from which arise polar filaments that can be seen between the oncosphere and the eggshell. The *H. diminuta* egg does not contain polar filaments.

Diagnosis of dwarf tapeworm infection is made by observing and recognizing *H. nana* eggs in fecal specimens. It is important to remember that the eggs of *Hymenolepis nana* contain polar filaments, whereas those of *Hymenolepis diminuta* do not.

Rat Tapeworm Infection

Disease. Infection with the intestinal tapeworm *Hymenolepis diminuta* is referred to as rat tapeworm infection because rodents are the usual definitive hosts. *H. diminuta* is a very small tapeworm, and infected individuals are rarely symptomatic.

Geographic occurrence. Infection with the rat tapeworm occurs worldwide.

Parasite. In nature, the life cycle of *H. diminuta* typically involves a rodent (the definitive host) and an arthropod, usually a beetle (the intermediate host). The adult *H. diminuta* tapeworm lives in the rodent's small intestine, where it

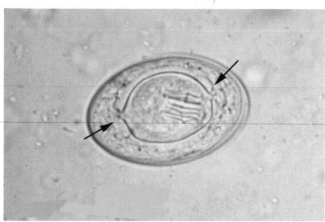

*Figure 23-28. **Hymenolepis nana** egg.* The *H. nana* egg is smaller than that of *H. diminuta* (see Fig. 23-29) and contains polar filaments (*arrows*), which are not present in the *H. diminuta* egg. The *H. nana* egg contains a six hooked oncosphere. (From Winn WC Jr, et al. Koneman's Color Atlas and Textbook of Diagnostic Microbiology. 6th Ed. Philadelphia: Lippincott Williams & Wilkins, 2006.)

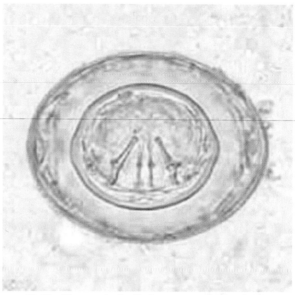

*Figure 23-29. **Hymenolepis diminuta** egg.* *H. diminuta* eggs are larger than *H. nana* eggs (see Fig. 23-28). They do not contain polar filaments but, like *H. nana* eggs, have a six-hooked oncosphere. (Courtesy of the CDC, Division of Parasitic Diseases.)

can reach 60 cm in length. Eggs released by the tapeworm are passed in the feces. If an egg is eaten by a beetle, a cysticercoid larva develops within the beetle. If the beetle is then ingested by a rodent (or a human), the larva matures into an adult worm. Adult worms usually live less than one year in the human body. Humans are considered accidental hosts. Because they are more likely to ingest an infected beetle, children are infected more often than adults. However, infected weevils can invade grains and cereals and thus may be eaten by anyone. Unlike *H. nana* infection, person-to-person transmission of rat tapeworm infection is not possible.

> Infection with the intestinal tapeworm *Hymenolepis diminuta* is referred to as rat tapeworm infection because rodents are the usual definitive hosts. Humans become infected by swallowing an infected beetle containing a cysticercoid larva.

Laboratory diagnosis. Rat tapeworm infection is diagnosed by observing and recognizing *H. diminuta* eggs in a fecal specimen. Proglottids usually dissolve in the intestinal tract and are rarely seen in fecal specimens. The eggs of *H. diminuta* resemble, and must be differentiated from, *H. nana* eggs. *H. diminuta* eggs are round to oval, thin shelled, and 60 to 79 μm in diameter, almost twice as large as *H. nana* eggs (Fig. 23-29). They contain a six-hooked oncosphere, but unlike *H. nana* eggs, the oncosphere has no polar thickenings and no polar filaments.

> Rat tapeworm infection is made by observing and recognizing *H. diminuta* eggs in fecal specimens.

 STUDY AID **The Big *diminuta*.** One has good reason to question why *Hymenolepis diminuta* has the specific epithet *diminuta*, suggesting that it is diminutive, or very small. The adult *H. diminuta* worm is much larger than that of *H. nana* (up to 60 cm long compared with about 4 cm for *H. nana*). Additionally, the egg of *H. diminuta* is twice as large as that of *H. nana*.

Essentials

Hymenolepis spp.

- *H. nana* (the dwarf tapeworm) and *H. diminuta* (the rat tapeworm) are cestodes

- They cause dwarf and rat tapeworm infections, respectively

- Definitive host for *H. nana* is human; no intermediate hosts

- Usual definitive hosts for *H. diminuta* are rodents; intermediate hosts are various arthropods (e.g., beetles)

- Dwarf tapeworm infection is acquired by ingestion of eggs present in feces

- Rat tapeworm infection is acquired by ingestion of a cysticercoid larva present in an infected arthropod

- Adult worms live in the small intestine, where they reach lengths of up to 4 cm (*H. nana*) or 20 to 60 cm (*H. diminuta*)

- Dwarf and rat tapeworm infections are usually diagnosed by observing characteristic eggs in feces

- The eggs of *H. nana* and *H. diminuta* resemble each other, but those of *H. diminuta* (60 to 79 μm in diameter) are much larger than those of *H. nana* (30 to 47 μm in diameter); *H. nana* eggs contain polar filaments, whereas those of *H. diminuta* do not

See Figure 23-30 for a comparison of some of the nematode and cestode eggs that can be found in human fecal specimens.

Fasciolopsiasis

Disease. Fasciolopsiasis, also known as giant intestinal fluke disease, is a trematode infection of the small intestine. Light infections are asymptomatic. Heavier infections may cause diarrhea alternating with constipation, vomiting, anorexia, and eosinophilia. Large worm burdens may cause anemia, intestinal obstruction, and edema of the face, abdominal wall, and legs.

Geographic occurrence. Fasciolopsiasis occurs in rural Southeast Asia, especially Thailand, central and south China, and parts of India. Prevalence is higher in areas where pigs are raised.

Parasite. Adult *Fasciolopsis buski* worms are broad, flat, and 0.8 to 2 cm wide by 2 to 7.5 cm long. The worm has an oral sucker at the anterior end and a ventral sucker nearer to the center of the body. The hermaphroditic worms live attached to the walls of the small intestine: in the duodenum and jejunum in light infections, and throughout the small intestine in heavier infections. Eggs are passed in the feces. If an egg reaches freshwater, larval development occurs, and a motile, ciliated miracidium escapes through the operculum. The miracidium infects an appropriate snail host. After going through several developmental stages, cercariae are released from the snail into the water. Cercariae attach to aquatic vegetation and encyst, becoming metacercariae. Humans, pigs, and some other animals become infected by

> Fasciolopsiasis, also known as giant intestinal fluke disease, is a trematode infection of the small intestine. Humans and animals become infected by ingesting raw or undercooked aquatic vegetation bearing metacercariae.

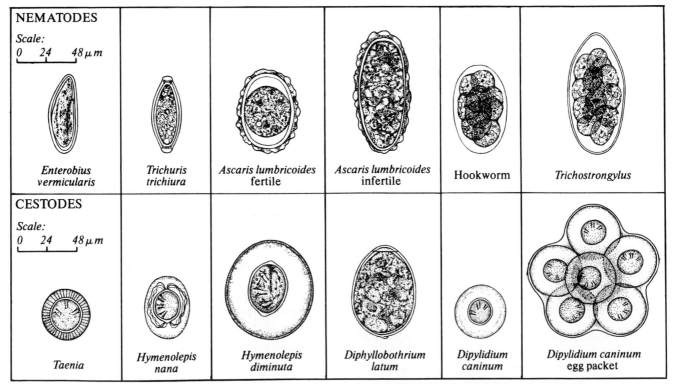

NEMATODES					
Enterobius vermicularis	*Trichuris trichiura*	*Ascaris lumbricoides* fertile	*Ascaris lumbricoides* infertile	Hookworm	*Trichostrongylus*

Scale: 0 24 48 μm

CESTODES					
Taenia	*Hymenolepis nana*	*Hymenolepis diminuta*	*Diphyllobothrium latum*	*Dipylidium caninum*	*Dipylidium caninum* egg packet

Scale: 0 24 48 μm

Figure 23-30. Recap of intestinal nematode and cestode eggs. All these helminths, except *Trichostrongylus*, are described in this chapter. (From Brooke MM, Melvin DM. Morphology of Diagnostic Stages of Intestinal Parasites of Humans. 2nd Ed. Atlanta, GA: CDC, 1984.)

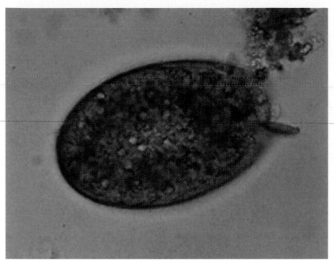

Figure 23-31. Fasciolopsis buski egg. The egg has a small, indistinct operculum, which is open in this photograph. *F. buski* eggs cannot be distinguished from *Fasciola hepatica* eggs. (Courtesy of the Georgia Division of Public Health and the CDC Division of Parasitic Diseases.)

ingesting raw or undercooked aquatic vegetation bearing metacercariae. The metacercariae excyst and attach to the lining of the small intestine, where they develop into hermaphroditic adult worms.

Laboratory diagnosis. Diagnosis of fasciolopsiasis is usually made on clinical grounds and patient history. Adult worms are usually seen in feces only after the patient has received an anthelmintic. Although eggs are observed in fecal specimens, *F. buski* eggs cannot be distinguished from *Fasciola hepatica* eggs. The eggs are ellipsoidal, operculate, yellow-brown, and 80 to 85 μm wide by 130 to 140 μm long (Fig. 23-31). There are no prominent shoulders around the operculum.

> Diagnosis of fasciolopsiasis is usually made on clinical grounds and patient history. Although *Fasciolopsis buski* eggs can be seen in fecal specimens, they cannot be distinguished from *Fasciola hepatica* eggs.

STUDY AID **Beware of Similar-Sounding Names.** Do not confuse fasciolopsiasis with fascioliasis. **Fasciolopsiasis** is an intestinal infection with *Fasciolopsis buski*. **Fascioliasis** is a liver infection usually caused by *Fasciola hepatica*. Both *F. buski* and *F. hepatica* are trematodes.

Fascioliasis

Disease. Fascioliasis is a liver infection, most often caused by the trematode *Fasciola hepatica*. The adult worms live in bile ducts. Medical problems associated with fascioliasis include liver tissue damage, hepatomegaly, liver pain, eosinophilia, and obstruction of bile ducts.

Geographic occurrence. Sheep- and cattle-raising areas of South America, the Caribbean, Europe, Australia, the Middle East, and Asia.

Parasite. Hermaphroditic adult *F. hepatica* worms are about 1.2 cm wide by 2.54 cm long. They can live for up to 9 years in bile ducts. Eggs are passed in the feces. If an egg reaches freshwater, larval development occurs, and a motile, ciliated miracidium escapes through the operculum. The miracidium infects an appropriate snail host. After going through several developmental stages, cercariae are released from the snail into the water. Cercariae attach to aquatic vegetation, such as watercress, and encyst, becoming metacercariae. Humans, sheep, cattle, and some other animals become infected by ingesting raw or undercooked aquatic vegetation bearing metacercariae. The metacercariae excyst in the small intestine, migrate through the intestinal wall, and enter the liver, where they mature into hermaphroditic adult worms. The adult worms then enter the bile ducts.

> Fascioliasis is a liver infection typically caused by the trematode *Fasciola hepatica*. Humans and animals become infected by ingesting raw or undercooked aquatic vegetation bearing metacercariae.

Laboratory diagnosis. Diagnosis is usually made on clinical grounds and patient history. Although *F. hepatica* eggs can be observed in fecal specimens or in bile that has been aspirated from the duodenum, the eggs of *F. hepatica* cannot be differentiated from those of *Fasciolopsis buski*.

> Diagnosis of fascioliasis is usually made on clinical grounds and patient history. Although *Fasciola hepatica* eggs can be observed in fecal specimens or in bile that has been aspirated from the duodenum, the eggs of *F. hepatica* cannot be differentiated from those of *Fasciolopsis buski*.

Clonorchiasis

Disease. Clonorchiasis is a disease of the bile ducts caused by the trematode *Clonorchis sinensis*. *C. sinensis* is referred to as the oriental or Chinese liver fluke. Light infections are usually asymptomatic. Heavier infections may cause loss of appetite, diarrhea, and a sensation of abdominal pressure. Rarely, bile duct obstruction occurs, followed by jaundice, cirrhosis, and enlargement and tenderness of the liver. Clonorchiasis is a chronic disease that can last 30 or more years.

Geographic occurrence. Clonorchiasis occurs in China, Japan, Taiwan, Korea, and Vietnam.

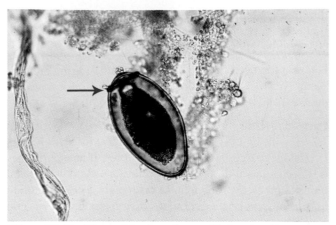

***Figure 23-32. Clonorchis sinensis* egg.** Notice the thin, smooth shell and the prominent shouldered operculum (*arrow*). A tiny knob is sometimes observed at the abopercular end (the end of the egg that is opposite from the operculated end), but it is not visible in this photograph. (From Winn WC Jr, et al. Koneman's Color Atlas and Textbook of Diagnostic Microbiology. 6th Ed. Philadelphia: Lippincott Williams & Wilkins, 2006.)

Parasite. Hermaphroditic adult worms are 0.3 to 0.5 cm wide by 1.0 to 2.5 cm long. Eggs are released in the bile ducts and pass in the feces. Eggs are ingested by freshwater snails, within which miracidia emerge through the operculum. After several developmental stages, cercariae are released from the snail into the water. Cercariae encyst in the skin or flesh of freshwater fish, becoming metacercariae. Humans and other animals become infected by ingesting the metacercariae in raw or undercooked fish. The metacercariae excyst in the duodenum, enter the bile ducts, and develop into hermaphroditic adult worms.

> Clonorchiasis is a disease of the bile ducts caused by the trematode *Clonorchis sinensis*. Humans and other animals become infected by ingesting the metacercariae in raw or undercooked fish.

> Clonorchiasis is diagnosed by observing and recognizing operculated *C. sinensis* eggs in a fecal specimen.

Laboratory diagnosis. Clonorchiasis is diagnosed by observing and recognizing *C. sinensis* eggs in a fecal speci-

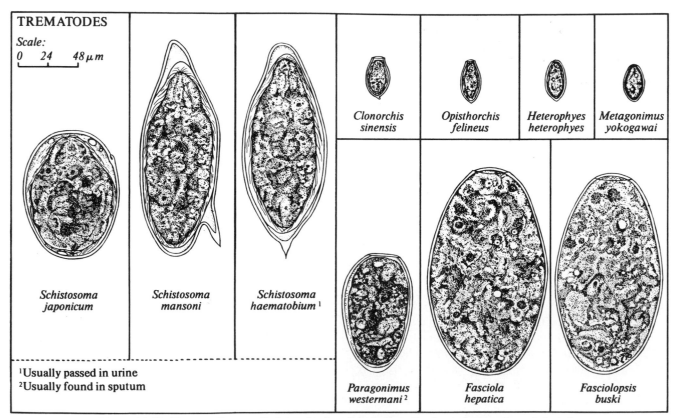

TREMATODES

Scale:
0   24   48 µm

Schistosoma japonicum

Schistosoma mansoni

Schistosoma haematobium [1]

Clonorchis sinensis

Opisthorchis felineus

Heterophyes heterophyes

Metagonimus yokogawai

Paragonimus westermani [2]

Fasciola hepatica

Fasciolopsis buski

[1] Usually passed in urine
[2] Usually found in sputum

Figure 23-33. Trematode eggs that can be found in human fecal specimens. Some helminths shown here are not discussed in this chapter. (From Brooke MM, Melvin DM. Morphology of Diagnostic Stages of Intestinal Parasites of Humans. 2nd Ed. Atlanta, GA: CDC, 1984.)

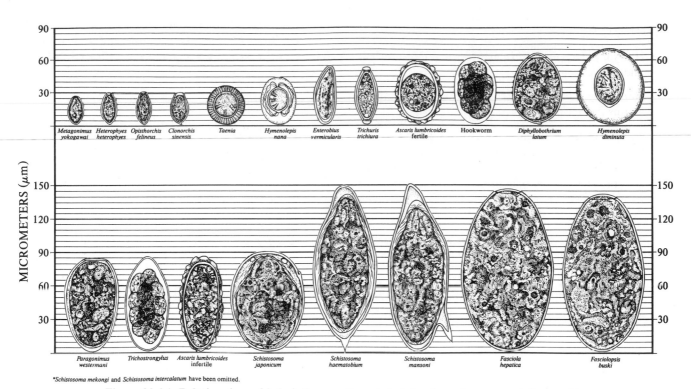

Schistosoma mekongi and *Schistosoma intercalatum* have been omitted.

Figure 23-34. **Relative sizes of helminth eggs.** Some helminths shown here are not discussed in this chapter. (From Brooke MM, Melvin DM. Morphology of Diagnostic Stages of Intestinal Parasites of Humans. 2nd Ed. Atlanta, GA: CDC, 1984.)

men. Eggs are fully embryonated, ovoid, 12 to 19 μm wide by 28 to 35 μm long, and operculated, with a yellow-brown shell (Fig. 23-32). The operculum is surrounded by distinct opercular shoulders. The egg often has a small, comma-shaped knob at the abopercular end. The eggs cannot be differentiated from the eggs of two intestinal flukes: *Heterophyes heterophyes* and *Metagonimus yokogawai*, neither of which is discussed in this book. In heavy *C. sinensis* infections, adult flukes may be observed in fecal specimens.

Figure 23-33 compares trematode eggs that can be found in human fecal specimens, and Figure 23-34 illustrates the relative sizes of helminth eggs.

Chapter Review

- Helminths are multicellular animals. They are *not* microorganisms.

- Nematodes, or roundworms, are long, cylindrical worms that have a complete digestive system.

- Cestodes, or tapeworms, have flat, segmented, ribbonlike bodies and complex life cycles. They vary in length from just a few millimeters to more than 10 meters. They are hermaphroditic, meaning that an individual worm has both male and female reproductive organs.

- Trematodes or flukes are flat, leaf-shaped helminths that have complex life cycles.

- Helminths can cause diseases that affect many anatomical sites, including the cardiovascular system, skin, tissues, eyes, respiratory system, central nervous system, and gastrointestinal tract.

- Specimens used to diagnose helminth infections include blood, biopsy specimens, skin snips, sputum, urine, serum, cellophane tape preps, aspirates, and feces.

- Filariasis is a disease caused by long, threadlike worms known as filarial worms. Chronic filariasis can lead to a condition known as elephantiasis.

- Microfilariae are prelarval stages of filarial worms.

- Trichinosis, caused by the roundworm *Trichinella spiralis*, is acquired by eating raw or undercooked meat (usually pork, products containing pork, or the meat of wild carnivores) that contains encysted *T. spiralis* larvae.

- Dracunculiasis, or guinea worm infection, is acquired by swallowing infected freshwater crustaceans of the genus *Cyclops*.

- Onchocerciasis, also known as river blindness, is caused by the filarial worm *Onchocerca volvulus*.

- The roundworm *Loa loa* is called the eyeworm because the adult worm can migrate beneath the conjunctiva of the eye.

- Paragonimiasis, or lung fluke infection, is caused by trematodes in the genus *Paragonimus*. The adult worms become encapsulated in the lungs.

- Cysticercosis is acquired by ingesting the eggs of the pork tapeworm, *Taenia solium*.

- Hydatid cyst disease is caused by tapeworms in the genus *Echinococcus*. Hydatid sand refers to the many scolices contained within hydatid cysts.

- Intestinal helminth infections are generally diagnosed by observation of whole worms, eggs, or proglottids in feces. Scolices are rarely seen in fecal specimens.

- Ascariasis is infection with the large intestinal roundworm *Ascaris lumbricoides*. *Ascaris* eggs may be fertilized or unfertilized and may or may not possess a thick, bumpy (mamillated) coat.

- Immature, noninfective hookworm and *Strongyloides* larvae are called rhabditiform larvae, whereas the mature, infective larvae are referred to as filariform larvae.

- Humans acquire hookworm infection by penetration of the skin by filariform larvae in the soil.

- Diagnosis of pinworm or *Enterobius vermicularis* infection is made using a cellophane tape preparation and observing characteristic football-shaped *E. vermicularis* eggs.

- Beef and pork tapeworms are in the genus *Taenia*. Humans become infected by eating meat containing encysted larvae.

- The adult fish tapeworm can reach 10 meters or more in length.

- Dog and rat tapeworms are acquired by swallowing infected fleas and beetles, respectively.

- Humans are the only hosts of *Hymenolepis nana*, the dwarf tapeworm.

- Fasciolopsiasis is an intestinal infection, whereas fascioliasis and clonorchiasis are liver infections.

New Terms and Abbreviations

After studying Chapter 23, you should be familiar with the following terms, which are defined within the chapter and in the Glossary at the back of the book:

Ascites

Autoinfection

Calabar swelling

Coracidium

Decorticated

Elephantiasis

Filarial worm

Filariform larva

Hermaphroditic

Mamillated

Microfilariae (sing. microfilaria)

Miracidium

Oncosphere

Operculum

Proglottid

Rhabditiform larva

Scolex (pl. scolices)

Worm burden

References and Suggested Reading

Cox FEG. Taxonomy and classification of human parasites. In: Murray PR, Baron EJ, Jorgensen JH, Pfaller MA, Yolken RH, eds. Manual of Clinical Microbiology. 8th Ed. Washington, DC: ASM Press, 2003.

Garcia LS. Diagnostic medical parasitology. In: Manual of Commercial Methods in Clinical Microbiology. Washington, DC: ASM Press, 2002.

Garcia LS. Practical Guide to Diagnostic Microbiology. Washington, DC: ASM Press, 1999.

Garcia LS, et al. Algorithms for detection and identification of parasites. In: Murray PR, Baron EJ, Jorgensen JH, Pfaller MA, Yolken RH, eds. Manual of Clinical Microbiology. 8th Ed. Washington, DC: ASM Press, 2003.

Garcia LS, et al. Specimen collection, transport, and processing: parasitology. In: Murray PR, Baron EJ, Jorgensen JH, Pfaller MA, Yolken RH, eds. Manual of Clinical Microbiology. 8th Ed. Washington, DC: ASM Press, 2003.

Heymann DL, ed. Control of Communicable Diseases Manual. 18th Ed. Washington, DC: American Public Health Association, 2004 (with 2006 update).

Markell, EK, John DT, Krotoski WA. Markell and Voge's Medical Parasitology. 8th Ed. Philadelphia: WB Saunders, 1999.

Winn WC Jr, et al. Koneman's Color Atlas and Textbook of Diagnostic Microbiology. 6th Ed. Philadelphia: Lippincott Williams & Wilkins, 2006.

 On the CD-ROM

- A Closer Look at the Dracunculiasis Eradication Campaign

- Additional Self-Assessment Exercises

- Case Studies

- Puzzle

Self-Assessment Exercises

Match the parasitic infection or disease in the left column with the appropriate parasite in the right column.

1. _____ Hydatid disease

2. _____ Pinworm

3. _____ Trichinosis

4. _____ Schistosomiasis

5. _____ Loiasis

A. *Enterobius vermicularis*

B. *Schistosoma* spp.

C. *Loa loa*

D. *Echinococcus granulosis*

E. *Trichinella spiralis*

6. List the most appropriate specimen to use for diagnosis of the following parasitic infections:

    A. Pinworm: _____

    B. Hookworm: _____

7. Name two methods by which trichinosis can be diagnosed.

    A. _____

    B. _____

8. A laboratory professional observes several barrel- or football-shaped objects with plugs at each end in a stained fecal specimen.

    A. What is the most likely identification of this parasite? _____

    B. What is the common name of this organism? _____

9. True or false: *Taenia saginata* and *T. solium* can be differentiated based on the appearance of their eggs.

10. True or false: Polyvinyl alcohol is a good fixative for *T. trichiura* eggs.

CHAPTER 24

Introduction to Medical Virology

Chapter Outline

Structure and Classification of Viruses

Viral Replication

Human Diseases Caused by Viruses

Latent Virus Infections

Antiviral Agents

Oncogenic Viruses

Clinical Specimens Required for the Diagnosis of Viral Infections

Laboratory Procedures Used in the Diagnosis of Viral Infections
- Cell Cultures
- Immunodiagnostic Procedures
- Cytology and Histology
- Electron Microscopy

☞ Given a viral disease, state the probable viral pathogen(s) involved

☞ Describe what is meant by a latent viral infection, and cite at least one example of a latent viral infection

☞ Briefly state why antibiotics are not effective against viral infections

☞ Name two examples of oncogenic viruses

☞ Discuss the proper collection and processing of viral specimens, including the temperature, transport medium, and time requirements

☞ Describe and identify the three categories of cell cultures used for propagation of viruses, and give an example of each

☞ Identify the appropriate specimen(s) needed to diagnose a specified disease or clinical manifestation

☞ Describe cytopathic effect and how it is used to identify a viral infection

☞ Name some of the laboratory procedures (e.g., molecular diagnostic procedures) that can be used to diagnose a viral infection

LEARNING OBJECTIVES

After studying this chapter, you should be able to:

☞ Define the terms introduced in this chapter (e.g., *capsid, capsomeres, cell culture*)

☞ Name the five properties of viruses that distinguish them from living cells

☞ Name the six general categories of human viruses based on the type and organization of the viral genome

☞ Given a diagram of the structure of the simplest human virus, correctly label the components

☞ Briefly explain how human viruses replicate, describing each of the six steps

Most scientists do not consider viruses to be living organisms. Thus, they are not included in either the five-kingdom system or three-domain system of classification. Viruses are often referred to as infectious particles or infectious agents rather than microorganisms. The study of viruses is called **virology**, and a person who studies viruses is called a **virologist**. **Medical virology** is the study and use of laboratory methods for the diagnosis of human viral infections. Laboratory procedures described in this chapter are performed in the virology section of the clinical microbiology laboratory (CML). Virology sections are found in the CMLs of large hospitals and medical centers. Specimens collected for the diagnosis of viral infections

> Viruses are not living organisms. They are often referred to as infectious particles or infectious agents.

from patients in small hospitals are usually sent to a reference laboratory.

Viruses are said to have five specific properties that distinguish them from living cells:

- They possess *either* DNA or RNA, unlike living cells, which possess both.

- They are unable to replicate (multiply) on their own; their replication is directed by the viral nucleic acid once it is introduced into a host cell.

- Unlike cells, they do not divide by binary fission, mitosis, or meiosis.

- They lack the genes and enzymes necessary for energy production.

> A virus contains either DNA or RNA, never both.

> Viruses must invade host cells to replicate.

- They depend on the ribosomes, enzymes, and metabolites (building blocks) of the host cell for protein and nucleic acid production.

Complete virus particles, called **virions,** are very small and simple in structure. Most viruses range in size from 10 to 300 nm in diameter (Fig. 24-1), although some, like Ebola virus (Fig. 24-2), can be up to 1 μm in length. The smallest virus is about the size of the large hemoglobin molecule of a red blood cell. Scientists were unable to see viruses until electron microscopes were invented in the 1930s. The first photographs of viruses were obtained in 1940. The negative staining procedure, developed in 1959, revolutionized the study of viruses, making it possible to observe unstained viruses against a dark, electron-dense background. Although electron microscopy was useful in the past to diagnose

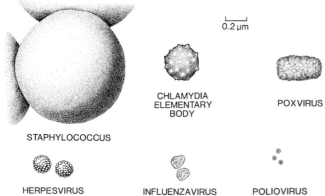

Figure 24-1. Sizes of some viruses compared to the sizes of a *Staphylococcus* cell and a *Chlamydia* elementary body. Poxviruses are among the largest viruses, and poliovirus is among the smallest. (From Winn WC Jr, et al. Koneman's Color Atlas and Textbook of Diagnostic Microbiology. 6th Ed. Philadelphia: Lippincott Williams & Wilkins, 2006.)

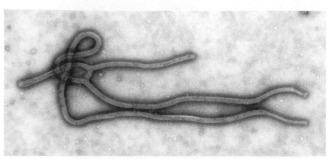

Figure 24-2. Ebola virus. An exceptionally long virus, Ebola virus causes a type of hemorrhagic fever. (Courtesy of Cynthia Goldsmith and the Centers for Disease Control and Prevention [CDC].)

certain human viral infections, it is no longer considered necessary.

STUDY AID **Beware of Similar-Sounding Terms. A virion** is a complete viral particle (i.e., one that has all its parts, including its nucleic acid and a capsid). A **viroid** is an infectious RNA molecule that is *not* surrounded by a protein coat. The suffix *–oid* means "resemble"; thus, viroids are viruslike in the sense that they resemble viruses. Certain plant diseases are caused by viroids.

No type of organism is safe from viral infections; viruses infect humans, animals, plants, fungi, protozoa, algae, and bacterial cells. Many human diseases are caused by viruses. Some viruses, called **oncogenic viruses** or **oncoviruses,** cause specific types of cancer, including human cancers such as lymphomas, carcinomas, and certain types of leukemia.

STRUCTURE AND CLASSIFICATION OF VIRUSES

Although the taxonomy of viruses is controversial and almost constantly in a state of flux, most virologists agree that viruses can be divided into orders, families, subfamilies, genera, and species. The names of orders end in *-virales,* families in *-viridae,* subfamilies in *-virinae,* and genera in *-virus.* For example, one virus family has the name Herpesviridae. Additional information regarding the classification of viruses can be found on the CD-ROM.

There are many ways to classify viruses. The following three criteria are used to differentiate orders, families, and genera of viruses:

- Type and organization of the viral genome

- Manner in which the virus replicates

- Structure of the complete virus particle (virion)

TABLE 24 - 1	Categories of Human Viruses Based on the Type and Organization of the Viral Genome
Category	**Human Viruses**
Single-stranded DNA, linear	Parvovirus B19
Double-stranded DNA, linear	Smallpox virus, human monkeypox virus, cowpox virus, herpesviruses, human adenovirus A to F
Double-stranded DNA, circular	Papillomaviruses (wart viruses), hepatitis B virus
Single-stranded RNA, linear	HIV types 1 and 2, Ebola virus, parainfluenza virus, mumps virus, measles virus, human respiratory syncytial virus, Hendra virus, rabies virus, influenza virus types A to C, California encephalitis virus, La Crosse virus, Hantaan virus, Sin Nombre virus, Crimean-Congo hemorrhagic fever virus, human coronavirus, human enterovirus types A to D, poliovirus, rhinovirus types A and B, hepatitis A virus, Norwalk virus, Sapporo virus, hepatitis E virus, human astrovirus, Ross River virus, Chikungunya virus, O'nyong-nyong virus, rubella virus, tickborne encephalitis virus, dengue virus, Japanese encephalitis virus, Murray Valley virus, St. Louis encephalitis virus, West Nile virus, hepatitis C virus, hepatitis G virus, hepatitis GB virus
Single-stranded RNA, circular	Lassa virus, lymphocytic choriomeningitis virus, Guanarito virus, Junin virus, Machupo virus, Sabia virus, hepatitis D virus
Double-stranded RNA, linear	Reoviruses, rotavirus A and B

Human viruses are divided into six general categories based on the type and organization of the viral genome. (Note: The term *human viruses* is used throughout the chapter in reference to viruses that infect humans.) The six categories of human viruses and examples of viruses in each category are shown in Table 24-1.

Viruses have a simpler structure than do procaryotic and eucaryotic cells. The simplest of human viruses consists of nothing more than nucleic acid surrounded by a protein coat, but most human viruses are somewhat more complex in structure. The protein coat is called a **capsid.** Viral capsids exist in two major geometrical configurations: one is referred to as a helical symmetry, and the other is called an icosahedral symmetry (Fig. 24-3). The capsid of **helical viruses** is composed of multiple copies of a single type of protein subunit known as a **protomer.** The capsid of icosahedral viruses

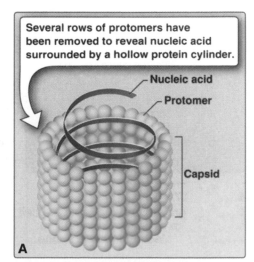
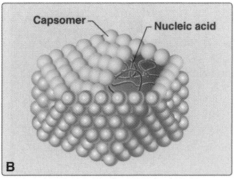

Figure 24-3. **Viral nucleocapsids. A.** Nucleocapsid of a helical virus. **B.** Nucleocapsid of an icosahedral virus. (From Strohl WA, et al. Lippincott's Illustrated Reviews: Microbiology. Philadelphia: Lippincott Williams & Wilkins, 2001.)

is somewhat more complex, comprising protein subunits that consist of several proteins; these subunits are known as **capsomeres** or capsomers. The capsid plus the nucleic acid contained within it is called the **nucleocapsid.**

STUDY AID

Helical Versus Icosahedral Symmetry of Viruses. In helical symmetry, protein subunits called protomers bind to each other in such a way as to surround a helical strand of viral nucleic acid. The connected protomers form a cylinder, within which lies the nucleic acid. In geometry, an icosahedron is described as a solid structure having 20 triangular sides. The capsid of icosahedral viruses is composed of protein subunits called capsomeres, which bind to each other in such a way as to form an icosahedron.

Some viruses, called **enveloped viruses,** have a protective outer envelope composed of lipids and polysaccharides.

> The simplest of human viruses consists of nothing more than nucleic acid surrounded by a protein coat, known as a capsid. The capsid plus the nucleic acid contained within are referred to as the nucleocapsid.

Frequently, the envelope around the capsid makes the virus appear spherical or irregular in shape in electron micrographs. The envelope is acquired by certain viruses as they escape from the nucleus or cytoplasm of the host cell by budding (Figs. 24-4 and 24-5). In other words, the envelope is derived from the host cell's nuclear membrane or cell membrane. Apparently, viruses can then alter these membranes by adding protein fibers, spikes, and knobs that enable the virus to recognize the next host cell to be invaded.

The morphology of selected animal viruses is shown in Figure 24-6.

Thus far, you have learned that viruses can be differentiated on the basis of (1) the type of nucleic acid they possess, (2) their capsid symmetry, and (3) whether or not they are enveloped. Listed here are criteria that can be used to differentiate various species of viruses:

- Relatedness of the genome base pair sequence

- The natural host range—that is, the type of organism the virus infects; for example, some viruses infect humans but not dogs, while others infect dogs but not humans

- Cell and tissue affinity—that is, the type of cell or tissue the virus infects; for example, some viruses can attach to and invade cells that line the respiratory tract but not cells that

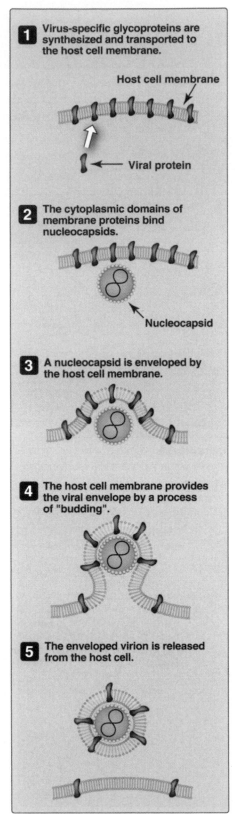

1. Virus-specific glycoproteins are synthesized and transported to the host cell membrane.

Host cell membrane

Viral protein

2. The cytoplasmic domains of membrane proteins bind nucleocapsids.

Nucleocapsid

3. A nucleocapsid is enveloped by the host cell membrane.

4. The host cell membrane provides the viral envelope by a process of "budding".

5. The enveloped virion is released from the host cell.

***Figure 24-4.* Virus particle becoming enveloped in the process of budding.** (From Strohl WA, et al. Lippincott's Illustrated Reviews: Microbiology. Philadelphia: Lippincott Williams & Wilkins, 2001.)

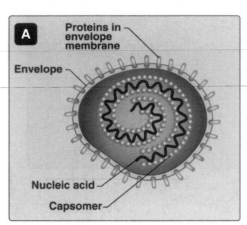
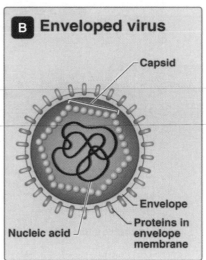

Figure 24-5. **Enveloped viruses. A.** Enveloped helical virus. **B.** Enveloped icosahedral virus. (From Strohl WA, et al. Lippincott's Illustrated Reviews: Microbiology. Philadelphia: Lippincott Williams & Wilkins, 2001.)

line the gastrointestinal tract, while others infect cells of the gastrointestinal tract but not cells of the respiratory tract

• Pathogenicity and cytopathology

• Mode of transmission

• Physicochemical properties of the virions

• Antigenic properties of viral proteins

VIRAL REPLICATION

Because viruses do not contain ribosomes for protein synthesis or mitochondria for energy production, they must invade and take over a functioning cell—referred to as the host cell—to multiply. Some viruses contain enzymes that play a role in viral multiplication within host cells. The steps in the multiplication of animal viruses is shown in Table 24-2.

The first step in the multiplication of human viruses is **attachment,** or adsorption, of the virus to the cell. Human viruses can only attach to cells bearing the appropriate protein or polysaccha-ride receptors on their surface. Why do certain viruses cause infections in dogs but not humans, or vice versa? Why do some viruses cause respiratory infections, while others cause gastrointestinal infections? The answers to these questions boil down to receptors. **A virus can only attach to and invade cells that bear a receptor the virus can recognize.**

> Viruses can only attach to and invade cells bearing appropriate surface receptors.

The second step in the multiplication of human viruses is **penetration.** Usually, the entire virion enters the host cell, sometimes as a result of the host cell phagocytizing the virus. Two types of penetration are shown in Figures 24-7 and 24-8.

In the third step, called **uncoating,** the viral nucleic acid escapes from the capsid. The first three steps in viral replication are shown in Figure 24-9.

From this point on, the viral nucleic acid "dictates" what occurs within the host cell. The fourth step is **biosynthesis,** whereby many viral pieces—viral nucleic acid and viral proteins—are produced. This step can be quite complicated, depending on what type of virus infected the cell (i.e., is it a single-stranded DNA virus? a double-stranded DNA virus? a single-stranded RNA virus? a double-stranded RNA virus?). Some human viruses do not initiate biosynthesis immediately but remain hidden or dormant within the host cell for variable periods. These are referred to as latent viral infections, which are discussed in more detail in a subsequent section.

The fifth step, **assembly,** involves fitting the virus pieces together to produce complete virions. After the virus particles are assembled, they must escape from the cell—the sixth step called **release.** How the virions escape from the cell depends on the type of virus. Some animal viruses escape by destroying the host cell, leading to cell destruction and some of the symptoms associated with infection with that particular virus. Other viruses escape the cell by a process known as budding. Viruses that escape from the host cell cytoplasm by budding become surrounded with pieces of the cell

> Viruses acquire their envelopes by budding from host cells.

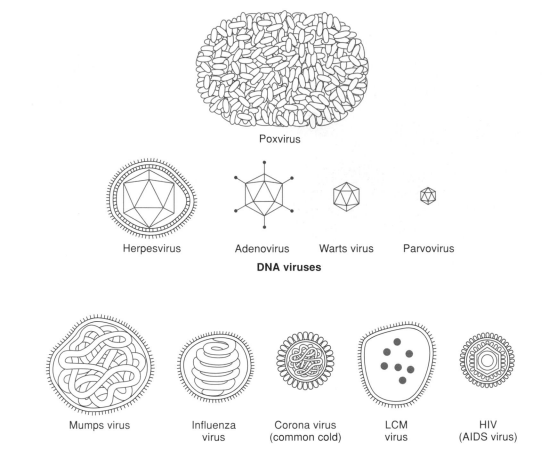

Poxvirus

Herpesvirus   Adenovirus   Warts virus   Parvovirus

DNA viruses

Mumps virus   Influenza virus   Corona virus (common cold)   LCM virus   HIV (AIDS virus)

Rotavirus   Poliovirus   Rabies virus   Eastern equine encephalitis virus

RNA viruses

Figure 24-6. **Morphology of selected animal viruses.** LCM, lymphocytic choriomeningitis virus. (From Schaechter M., et al. eds. Mechanisms of Microbial Disease. 3rd Ed. Philadelphia: Lippincott Williams & Wilkins, 1999.)

TABLE 24 - 2	Steps in the Multiplication of Human Viruses
Step	**Description**
1. Attachment (adsorption)	Virus attaches to a protein or polysaccharide molecule (receptor) on the surface of a host cell
2. Penetration	Entire virus enters the host cell, in some cases because it was phagocytized by the cell
3. Uncoating	Viral nucleic acid escapes from the capsid
4. Biosynthesis	Viral genes are expressed, resulting in the production of many pieces/parts of viruses (i.e., viral DNA and viral proteins)
5. Assembly	Viral pieces/parts are assembled to create complete virions
6. Release	Complete virions escape from the host cell by lysis or budding

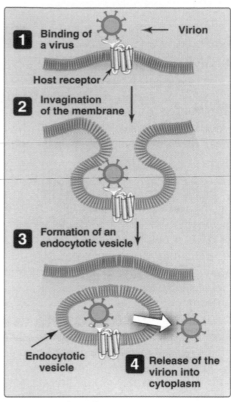

Figure 24-7. **Penetration of a nonenveloped virus by endocytosis.** (From Strohl WA, et al. Lippincott's Illustrated Reviews: Microbiology. Philadelphia: Lippincott Williams & Wilkins, 2001.)

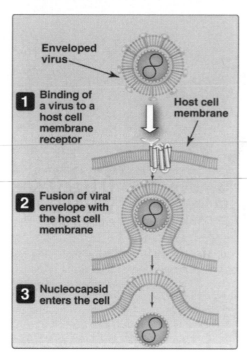

Figure 24-8. **Penetration of a host cell by an enveloped virus.** (From Strohl WA, et al. Lippincott's Illustrated Reviews: Microbiology. Philadelphia: Lippincott Williams & Wilkins, 2001.)

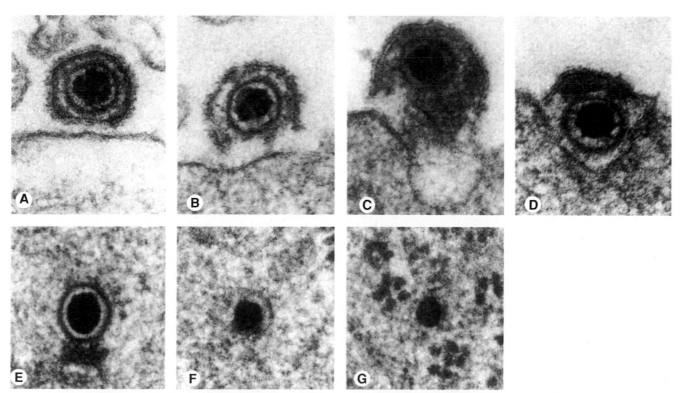

Figure 24-9. **Development of herpes simplex virus on HeLa cells, as deduced from transmission electron micrographs of infected cell sections. A.** Adsorption. **B and C.** Penetration involves local digestion of the viral and cellular membranes. **D.** The result is fusion of the two membranes and release of the nucleocapsid into the cytoplasmic matrix. **E–G.** Uncoating and digestion of the capsid. The naked nucleocapsid is intact in **E**, is partially digested in **F**, and has disappeared in **G**, leaving a core containing DNA and protein. (From Morgan C, et al. Electron microscopy of herpes simplex virus: I. Entry J Virol 1968;2:507.)

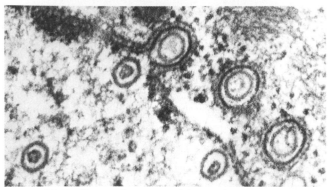

***Figure 24-10.* Herpesviruses acquiring their envelopes as they leave a host cell's nucleus by budding.** From center to right: One virus particle is in the process of leaving the nucleus by budding. Two virus particles have already acquired their envelopes. (From Volk WA, et al. Essentials of Medical Microbiology. 5th Ed. Philadelphia: Lippincott-Raven, 1996.)

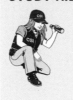

STUDY AID **Understanding Biosynthesis and Assembly.** Picture a jig-saw puzzle in your mind when trying to understand the biosynthesis and assembly steps in viral replication. During the biosynthesis step, the pieces of the puzzle are manufactured. During the assembly step, the pieces are fitted together to create the final picture.

membrane, thus becoming enveloped viruses (Fig. 24-10). **All enveloped viruses escaped from their host cells by budding.**

Remnants or collections of viruses, called **inclusion bodies,** are often seen in infected cells and are used as a diagnostic tool to identify some viral diseases. Depending on the particular disease, inclusion bodies may be found either in the cytoplasm (called cytoplasmic inclusion bodies) or within the nucleus (called intranuclear inclusion bodies). In rabies, the cytoplasmic inclusion bodies in nerve cells are called Negri bodies. The inclusion bodies of AIDS and the Guarnieri bodies of smallpox are also cytoplasmic. Herpes and poliomyelitis viruses produce intranuclear inclusion bodies. In each case, inclusion bodies may represent aggregates or collections of viruses.

HUMAN DISEASES CAUSED BY VIRUSES

Table 24-3 presents an overview of viral infections of humans. Additional information about most of these diseases can be found in Chapter 25.

LATENT VIRUS INFECTIONS

As stated earlier, some human viruses do not initiate biosynthesis immediately after entering the host cell; rather, they remain hidden or dormant within the host cell for some time. These are referred to as latent viral infections. Herpes virus infections, such as cold sores or fever blisters, are good examples of latent virus infections. Infected persons harbor the latent virus in nerve cells. A fever, stress, or excessive sunlight can trigger the viral genes to take over the cells and produce more viruses; in the process, cells are destroyed and a cold sore or fever blister develops. Latent viral infections are usually limited by the defense systems of the human body—phagocytes and antiviral proteins called interferons produced by virus-infected cells. (Interferons are discussed in Chapter 3.) Another example of a latent viral infection is shingles, a painful nerve disease caused by the same herpesvirus that causes chickenpox. Following a chickenpox infection, the virus can remain latent in the human body for many years. Then, when the body's immune defenses become weakened by old age or disease, the latent chickenpox virus resurfaces to cause shingles.

ANTIVIRAL AGENTS

It is very important to understand that antibiotics are not effective against viral infections. Antibiotics function by inhibiting certain metabolic activities within cellular pathogens, and viruses are not cells. However, for certain patients with colds and influenza, antibiotics may be prescribed in an attempt to prevent secondary bacterial infections that might follow the virus infection. In recent years, a relatively small number of chemicals, called antiviral agents, have been developed to interfere with virus-specific enzymes and virus production by either disrupting critical phases in viral cycles or inhibiting the synthesis of viral DNA, RNA, or proteins. Some antiviral agents are discussed in Chapter 7.

> The drugs used to treat viral infections are called antiviral agents. Antibiotics are not effective against viral infections.

Many vaccines are available to protect humans and animals from viral diseases. A good example is the measles-mumps-rubella vaccine, which protects humans from three viral diseases.

ONCOGENIC VIRUSES

Viruses that cause cancer are called oncogenic viruses or oncoviruses. The first evidence that viruses cause cancers came from experiments with chickens. Subsequently, viruses were shown to be the cause of various types of cancers in

TABLE 24 - 3   Overview of Viral Infections of Humans

Anatomical Site	Disease	Viral Pathogens (listed alphabetically)
Central nervous system	Encephalitis	Arboviruses, cytomegalovirus (CMV), Epstein-Barr virus (EBV), hemorrhagic fever viruses, HIV, herpes simplex virus type 1 (HSV-1), measles virus, mumps virus, rabies virus, varicella-zoster virus (VZV)
	Meningitis	Enteroviruses, herpes simplex virus type 2 (HSV-2), lymphocytic choriomeningitis virus
Eyes	Chorioretinitis	CMV, VZV
	Conjunctivitis	Adenoviruses, enteroviruses
	Keratoconjunctivitis	Adenoviruses, HSV-1, HSV-2, VZV
Gastrointestinal tract	Diarrheal diseases	Adenoviruses, astrovirus, CMV, Norwalk virus group, rotavirus
Heart	Myocarditis	Enteroviruses
	Pericarditis	Enteroviruses
Liver	Hepatitis	CMV; EBV; hepatitis A, B, C, D, and E viruses; parvovirus B19
Respiratory system	Bronchiolitis	Influenza viruses, parainfluenza viruses, respiratory syncytial virus (RSV)
	Croup	Parainfluenza viruses, RSV
	Pharyngitis	Adenoviruses, EBV, enteroviruses, HSV-1, HSV-2
	Pneumonia	Adenoviruses, CMV, Hanta virus, influenza viruses, parainfluenza viruses, RSV, VZV
	Rhinitis, coryza	Adenoviruses, coronaviruses, enteroviruses, influenza viruses, parainfluenza viruses, rhinoviruses, RSV
Skin	Maculopapular rash	Adenoviruses, enteroviruses, human herpesvirus 6, measles virus, parvovirus B19, rubella virus
	Vesicular rash	Enteroviruses, HSV-1, HSV-2, poxvirus, VZV

rodents, frogs, and cats. Although the causes of many (perhaps most) types of human cancers remain unknown, it is known that *some* human cancers are caused by viruses. Epstein-Barr virus (a type of herpesvirus), the cause of infectious mononucleosis, also causes three types of human cancers: nasopharyngeal cancer, Burkitt lymphoma, and B-cell lymphoma. Kaposi sarcoma, a type of cancer common in AIDS patients, is caused by human herpesvirus 8. Associations between hepatitis B and C viruses and hepatocellular (liver) carcinoma have been established. Human papillomaviruses (wart viruses) can cause various types of cancer, including cancers of the cervix and other parts of the genital tract. A retrovirus closely related to HIV (the cause of AIDS) called HTLV-1 causes a rare type of adult T-cell leukemia.

CLINICAL SPECIMENS REQUIRED FOR THE DIAGNOSIS OF VIRAL INFECTIONS

The proper selection, collection, transport, and processing of clinical specimens is of the utmost importance in the diagnosis of viral infections. Ideally, clinical specimens should be collected within 3 to 7 days after the onset of symptoms. The type of specimen and its manner of collection depend on the laboratory procedure for which the specimen is collected—that is, whether for virus isolation, viral antigen detection, or some type of molecular diagnostic procedure. Table 24-4 contains information

TABLE 24 - 4	Clinical Specimens Processed in the Virology Section
Clinical Specimen	**Viruses Detected**
Amniotic fluid	Cytomegalovirus (CMV), herpes simplex virus, parvovirus B19, rubella virus
Blood (whole blood, acute-phase serum, convalescent-phase serum)	Arboviruses; arenaviruses; CMV; enterovirus; Epstein-Barr virus; filoviruses, such as Ebola virus; hepatitis A, B, C, D, and E viruses; human herpesvirus 6; measles virus; parvovirus B19; rabies virus; retroviruses (HIV, HTLV); rubella virus; varicella-zoster virus
Bone marrow	CMV, human herpesvirus 6, parvovirus B19, varicella-zoster virus
Cerebrospinal fluid	Adenoviruses, arboviruses, arenaviruses, CMV, enteroviruses, Epstein-Barr virus, herpes simplex virus, human herpesvirus 6, mumps virus, polyomavirus, rabies virus, retroviruses, varicella-zoster virus
Eye specimens (conjunctival swabs, corneal scrapings, aqueous and vitreous fluids)	Adenoviruses, CMV, enteroviruses, herpes simplex virus, rabies virus
Feces	Adenoviruses, astrovirus, calcivirus, coronavirus, CMV, enterovirus, hepatitis A and E viruses, herpes simplex virus, rotaviruses, rubella virus
Genital specimens	CMV, herpes simplex virus, papillomavirus, retroviruses
Pericardial fluid	Enterovirus
Respiratory specimens (throat and nasal swabs, nasal wash, nasopharyngeal aspirate, bronchoalveolar lavage)	Adenoviruses, arenaviruses, coronavirus, CMV, enterovirus, filoviruses, herpes simplex virus, influenza viruses, measles virus, parainfluenza virus, respiratory syncytial virus (RSV), retrovirus, rhinovirus, rubella virus, varicella-zoster virus
Saliva	CMV, mumps virus, rabies virus, retrovirus
Skin	Enterovirus, herpes simplex virus, measles virus, poxviruses, rabies virus, varicella-zoster virus
Tissue	Adenoviruses, arboviruses, coronavirus, CMV, enterovirus, Epstein-Barr virus, hepatitis C virus, herpes simplex virus, human herpesvirus 6, influenza viruses, measles virus, mumps virus, papillomavirus, parainfluenza virus, parvovirus B19, polyomavirus, poxviruses, rabies virus, RSV, retrovirus, rhinovirus, rubella virus, varicella-zoster virus
Urine	Adenoviruses, arenaviruses, CMV, enterovirus, filoviruses, measles virus, mumps virus, polyomavirus, rubella virus

Source: Forman MS, Valsamakis A. Specimen Collection, Transport, and Processing: Virology. In: Murray PR, Baron EJ, Jorgensen JH, Pfaller MA, Yolken RH, eds. Manual of Clinical Microbiology. 8th Ed. Washington, DC: ASM Press, 2003.

about the types of clinical specimens submitted to the virology section of the CML and the viruses that may be detected in each.

After the specimen is collected, it should be transported to the CML as rapidly as possible. In general, all specimens except blood should be kept at 4°C if processing will be delayed by more than 1 hour and frozen (at −60°C) if a delay of 24 hours or longer is anticipated. Specimens for cytomegalovirus (CMV) should not be frozen. Some specimens require the use of viral transport media (VTM), whereas others do not. For example, respiratory specimens such as nasal wash and bronchoalveolar lavage specimens; conjunctival, genital, rectal, and vesicle swabs; and tissue specimens require VTM. Types of specimens that do not require VTM include amniotic fluid, aqueous and vitreous fluids, blood, bone marrow, cerebrospinal fluid, pericardial and pleural fluids, and urine. Various types of VTM are commercially available. The

TABLE 24 - 5	Categories of Cell Lines
Category of Cell Line	**Description**
Primary cell line	Used directly from its tissue of origin or, at most, subcultured only once or twice
Low-passage cell line	Remains viable and sensitive to viral infection through 20 to 50 passages
Continuous culture cell line	Can be subcultured indefinitely without altering its sensitivity to virus infection

primary purposes of VTM are to prevent drying of the specimen and prevent the overgrowth of contaminating microorganisms. VTM contain antimicrobial agents to prevent bacterial and fungal growth, protein to stabilize the virus, and a buffer to control the pH. VTM do not interfere with either immunodiagnostic or molecular diagnostic procedures. The type of VTM supplied or recommended by the manufacturer of the commercial assay should always be used.

LABORATORY PROCEDURES USED TO DIAGNOSE VIRAL INFECTIONS

Cell Cultures

Viruses are obligate intracellular pathogens and as such require live host cells for replication. **Cell cultures** are used for the propagation of viruses. There are three general categories of cell cultures: primary, low-passage, and continuous cell lines (Table 24-5).

As stated earlier, a particular virus can only attach to and infect cells that bear appropriate cell receptors—that is, receptors that the virus can recognize. Thus, it is necessary to maintain several cell lines in the virology section of the CML (see Table 24-6). Cell lines can be purchased from commercial sources.

Cell culture procedures must be performed using biosafety cabinets, not only to protect CML professionals from infection but also to protect the cell cultures from becoming contaminated. Contamination by *Mycoplasma* spp. is an especially common and troublesome problem. Cell cultures can also become contaminated with other viruses present in the specimen.

Processed specimens are inoculated into cell culture vials, each containing a monolayer of the appropriate cells. Inoculated cell cultures are incubated at 35°C to 37°C for most viruses, and the maintenance medium is changed weekly or biweekly. Using either a traditional microscope (Fig. 24-11) or an inverted microscope (Fig. 24-12), the cultures are examined periodically for evidence of morphologic alterations, which is called **cytopathic effect (CPE).** The objective lens of an inverted microscope is *beneath* the stage, enabling examination of the bottom of plates or vials.

Examples of CPE include rounding, swelling, and shrinking of cells, or cells may become granular, glassy, vacuolated, or fused. Fused cells are referred to as multinucleated giant cells or syncytial cells. In some cases, cells become clustered, looking like bunches of grapes, or they detach from the glass vial. Viruses can often be identified by the type of CPE they cause. A particular virus causes a characteristic type of CPE in specific cell lines (Fig. 24-13).

> A particular virus causes a characteristic type of cytopathic effect in specific cell lines.

The use of shell vial cultures, also known as spin-amplified cell cultures, is quite popular in CMLs. Shell vials

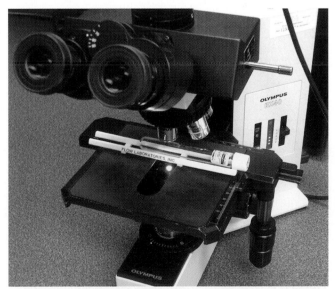

Figure 24-11. **Viral cell culture being examined for cytopathic effect (CPE) using a traditional microscope.** A specially designed plastic tube holder prevents the round tube from rolling off the microscope stage. (Courtesy of Dr. Robert C. Fader.)

TABLE 24 - 6	Examples of Cell Lines Used for Virus Isolation	
Category of Cell Line	**Type of Cell**	**Viruses Most Commonly Isolated Using This Cell Line (listed alphabetically)**
Primary cell lines	African green monkey kidney cells	Herpes simplex virus (HSV), mumps virus, rubella virus, varicella-zoster virus (VZV)
	Human cord blood or peripheral blood mononuclear cells	HIV, human herpesvirus 6, human T-cell lymphotropic virus
	Human neonatal kidney cells	Adenoviruses, HSV, mumps virus, VZV
	Rabbit kidney cells	HSV
	Rhesus or cynomolgus monkey kidney cells	Enteroviruses, influenza viruses, measles virus, mumps virus, parainfluenza viruses, respiratory syncytial virus (RSV)
Low-passage cell lines	Human foreskin fibroblasts	HSV, cytomegalovirus (CMV)
	Human embryonic lung fibroblasts	CMV, HSV, rhinoviruses, VZV
	W1-38 and MRC-5 human fetal lung cells	Adenoviruses, CMV, enteroviruses, HSV, rhinoviruses, RSV, VZV
Continuous cell lines	293 human kidney cells	Adenovirus types 5, 40, 41
	A549 human lung carcinoma cells	Adenoviruses (except types 40 and 41), HSV
	HeLa human cervical carcinoma cells	Enteroviruses, poxviruses, rhinoviruses, RSV
	HEp-2 human larynx carcinoma cells	Adenoviruses, measles virus, RSV
	MDCK canine kidney cells	Influenza viruses, parainfluenza viruses
	Mink lung cells	HSV
	RD human rhabdosarcoma cells	Enteroviruses (coxsackievirus group A)
	RK13 rabbit kidney cells	Poxviruses, rubella virus
	Buffalo, Vero, and CV-1 African green monkey kidney cells	Enteroviruses, HSV, measles virus, parainfluenza viruses, poxviruses, RSV, rubella virus, VZV

Source: Forman MS, Valsamakis A. Specimen Collection, Transport, and Processing: Virology. In: Murray PR, Baron EJ, Jorgensen JH, Pfaller MA, Yolken RH, eds. Manual of Clinical Microbiology. 8th Ed. Washington, DC: ASM Press, 2003.

are small vials containing a coverslip on which a monolayer of cells has grown (Fig. 24-14). With shell vial cultures, the specimen is centrifuged onto the monolayer, which is then stained for viral antigens prior to the development of CPE. The major advantage of the shell vial technique is that viruses that normally take days to weeks to produce CPE can be detected within 1 to 2 days. The shell vial technique has proven especially useful for herpes simplex viruses, CMV, varicella-zoster virus, and influenza viruses.

Immunodiagnostic Procedures

Antigen Detection

Commercial antigen detection procedures such as fluorescence-labeled antibody assays, enzyme immunoassays, and latex agglutination assays are commonly used to detect viral antigen in specimens (Table 24-7). In general, antigen detec-

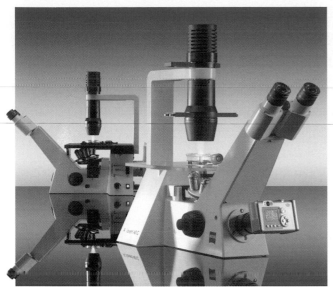

Figure 24-12. **Inverted microscopes used to examine viral cell cultures for CPE.** (Courtesy of Fisher Scientific.)

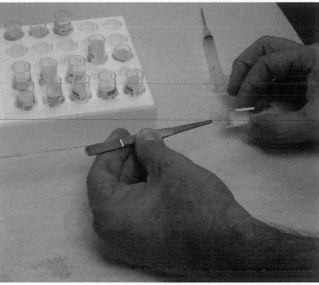

Figure 24-14. **Shell vials used for cell cultures in the virology section of the clinical microbiology laboratory.** The vials contain a round coverslip on which the cells are grown. Following specimen inoculation and incubation of the vial, the coverslip is stained, removed using a needle or forceps, and examined microscopically for CPE. (Courtesy of Dr. Robert C. Fader.)

tion procedures are less sensitive than cell culture or molecular diagnostic techniques.

Antibody Detection

For the most part, cell culture, antigen detection, and molecular diagnostic procedures have replaced serologic detection of antibodies as a means of diagnosing viral infections. However, antibody detection procedures are still used to diagnose diseases caused by viruses that do not replicate in the commonly used cell lines. These viruses include arboviruses, Epstein-Barr virus, hepatitis viruses, HIV, and HTLV-1.

The best methods for diagnosis of current viral disease by antibody detection are (1) assays that specifically detect IgM antibodies in acute-phase specimens, and (2) assays that demonstrate a fourfold rise in antibody titer between acute-phase and convalescent-phase specimens. Both methods are discussed in Chapter 6. For most viral infections, IgM antibodies are detectable within 3 to 5 days of onset of disease and may persist for as long as 6 months.

Molecular Diagnostic Procedures

Many molecular diagnostic procedures for the diagnosis of viral infections are commercially available for detection of

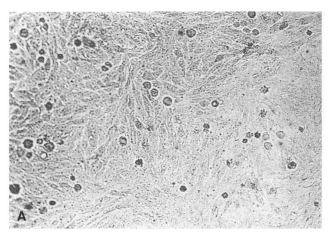

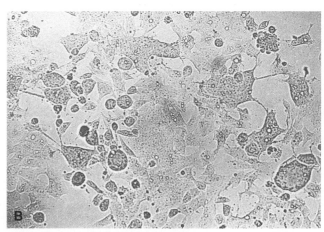

Figure 24-13. **Normal cell line and CPE. A.** Normal appearance of cell culture. **B.** CPE.

| TABLE 24 - 7 | Commercially Available Viral Antigen Detection Assays |

Virus	Antigen Detection Assays
Adenoviruses	Direct fluorescent antibody assay (DFA), enzyme immunoassay (EIA), indirect fluorescent antibody assay (IFA)
Cytomegalovirus	IFA (antigenemia assay)
Herpes simplex viruses (HSV)	DFA, EIA
Influenza viruses, types A and B	DFA, EIA
Rotavirus	EIA, latex agglutination
Respiratory syncytial virus (RSV)	DFA, EIA, IFA

Epstein-Barr virus, CMV, hepatitis B virus, hepatitis C virus, human herpesvirus 6, HIV, herpes simplex viruses, HTLV-1, human papillomaviruses, and varicella-zoster virus. These include nonamplified nucleic acid probe-based assays and nucleic acid amplification techniques (see Chapter 6). Nucleic acid amplification techniques include polymerase chain reaction (PCR) and reverse-transcriptase PCR, among others. Molecular diagnostic procedures are rapid, sensitive, and especially useful for viruses that can-

not be detected either by culture or immunodiagnostic procedures.

Cytology and Histology

Some viral infections can be diagnosed by observing intracytoplasmic or intranuclear inclusions in stained cells. The inclusions represent clusters of viruses or viral macromolecules. Certain of these inclusions have a characteristic morphol-

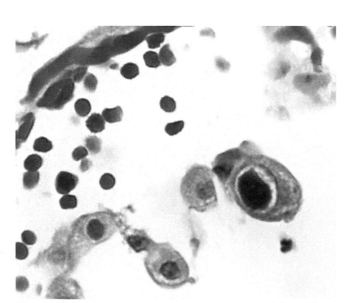

Figure 24-15. **Cytomegalovirus-infected cell containing a characteristic "owl's eye" intranuclear inclusion body.** (Courtesy of Dr. Edwin P. Ewing Jr. and the CDC.)

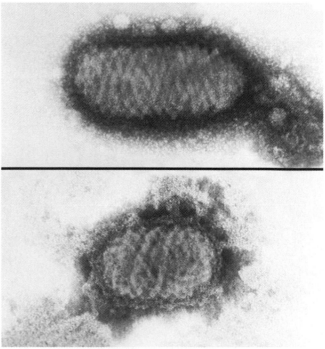

Figure 24-16. **Transmission electron micrographs of an orf virus.** (Courtesy of the CDC.)

ogy, such as the "owl's eye" intranuclear inclusions seen in cells infected with cytomegalovirus (Fig. 24-15). Cytological preparations are usually stained with Papanicolaou, Giemsa, or Wright-Giemsa stains, whereas tissue sections are usually stained with hematoxylin eosin stain. Immunostaining techniques using fluorescent antibodies or horseradish peroxidase–labeled antibodies are also available.

Electron Microscopy

Electron microscopy is not required for the diagnosis of most viral infections. It can be of value for detection of viruses that cannot be cultivated; are highly contagious; or can be identified by their unique morphology, such as the orf virus, a type of poxvirus that causes cutaneous lesions (Fig. 24-16).

Chapter Review

- Because they are not cells, viruses are often referred to as infectious particles or infectious agents, rather than microorganisms.

- Viruses have five properties that distinguish them from living cells: (1) they possess either DNA or RNA, *but not both*; (2) they are unable to replicate on their own; (3) they do not divide by binary fission, mitosis, or meiosis; (4) they lack the genes necessary for energy production; and (5) they depend on the host cell for protein and nucleic acid production.

- Complete virus particles, called virions, are extremely small and simple in structure.

- The three primary criteria used to differentiate viruses are (1) the type and organization of the viral genome, (2) the manner in which the virus replicates, and (3) the structure of the virion.

- The simplest of human viruses consist only of nucleic acid surrounded by a protein coat (capsid). The protein subunits that make up the capsid are called protomers (in helical viruses) or capsomeres (in icosahedral viruses). The capsid plus the nucleic acid within it is called the nucleocapsid.

- Some viruses are surrounded by an envelope, composed of lipids and polysaccharides. Such viruses are called enveloped viruses.

- Viruses must invade and take over a functioning cell, referred to as the host cell, to multiply.

- The six steps in the multiplication of animal viruses are attachment, penetration, uncoating, biosynthesis, assembly, and release.

- Viruses can only attach to and invade cells that bear a receptor they can recognize.

- All enveloped viruses escaped from their host cells by budding. The envelope is derived from either the host cell's nuclear membrane or its cell membrane.

- Remnants or collections of viruses are called inclusion bodies, which may be seen within infected cells. Inclusion bodies are often used as a diagnostic tool to identify some viral diseases.

- Some viruses may remain dormant in the body but reappear later as latent viral infections. Examples include cold sores and shingles. Latent viral infections may be triggered by fever, stress, or excessive sunlight.

- Antibiotics are not effective against viral infections. Some antiviral agents have been developed. These agents work by disrupting viral cycles or by inhibiting the synthesis of viral DNA, RNA, or proteins.

- Viruses that cause cancer are called oncogenic viruses or oncoviruses.

- Many types of samples (e.g., blood, cerebrospinal fluid, feces) may be submitted to the virology section of the CML for processing. Some specimens require the use of viral transport media.

- Samples for viral work-up must be properly collected and transported to the laboratory. Specimens should be processed immediately, but may be kept at 4°C if there is a delay of more than 1 hour. If the delay is 24 hours or more, the sample may be frozen at –60°C.

- Laboratory methods used to diagnose viral infections include cell cultures, antigen detection, antibody detection, molecular diagnostic procedures, and cytology and histology procedures.

- Cell lines used in the identification of viruses include primary, low-passage, and continuous cell lines.

- A particular virus causes a characteristic cytopathic effect (CPE) in a specific cell line or culture. Following inoculation and incubation, a cell culture is examined for a particular type of CPE, such as rounding, swelling, shrinkage, or fused cells.

New Terms and Abbreviations

After studying Chapter 24, you should be familiar with the following terms, which are defined within the chapter and in the Glossary at the back of the book:

Capsid

Capsomere

Cell culture

Cytopathic effect (CPE)

Enveloped virus

Helical virus

Icosahedral virus

Inclusion body

Medical virology

Nucleocapsid

Oncogenic virus

Protomer

Virion

References and Suggested Reading

Büchen-Osmond C. Taxonomy and classification of viruses. In: Murray PR, Baron EJ, Jorgensen JH, Pfaller MA, Yolken RH, eds. Manual of Clinical Microbiology. 8th Ed. Washington, DC: ASM Press, 2003.

Forman MS, Valsamakis A. Specimen collection, transport, and processing: Virology. In: Murray PR, Baron EJ, Jorgensen JH, Pfaller MA, Yolken RH, eds. Manual of Clinical Microbiology. 8th Ed. Washington, DC: ASM Press, 2003.

 ## On the CD-ROM

- Classification of Viruses That Infect Humans
- A Closer Look at HIV
- Additional Self-Assessment Exercises
- Puzzle

Self-Assessment Exercises

1. The viral structure, consisting of nucleic acid surrounded by a protein coat is called a(an)

    A. capsid.

    B. envelope.

    C. capsomere.

    D. nucleocapsid.

2. The best temperature for storage of viral specimens on a short-term basis is

    A. 4°C.

    B. 8°C.

    C. –20°C.

    D. –60°C

3. Methods for identification of viruses include all of the following *except*

    A. antigen detection.

    B. antibody detection.

    C. molecular diagnostic procedures.

    D. biochemical assays.

4. Answer the following as true or false:

    A. _____ Viruses possess both DNA and RNA.

    B. _____ Viruses are unable to replicate on their own.

    C. _____ Viruses lack genes and enzymes necessary for energy production.

    D. _____ Complete virus particles are called viroids.

    E. _____ Viruses can be seen with a compound microscope.

5. An example of a linear, single-stranded DNA virus is

    A. parvovirus.

    B. hepatitis B.

    C. Lassa virus.

    D. HIV.

6. Briefly explain why some viruses cause infections in humans but not in dogs:

_____

_____

7. List the six steps in the replication of human viruses:

A. _____

B. _____

C. _____

D. _____

E. _____

F. _____

8. Name the three general categories of cell cultures, and cite one example of each type of cell.

Category of Cell Line	Type of Cell
A. _____	_____
B. _____	_____
C. _____	_____

9. Name three laboratory methods for detecting viruses.

A. _____

B. _____

C. _____

10. Briefly explain what is meant by *cytopathic effect*.

_____

_____

CHAPTER 25

Laboratory Diagnosis of Selected Viral Infections

LEARNING OBJECTIVES

After studying this chapter, you should be able to:

☛ Define the terms and abbreviations introduced in this chapter (e.g., *arthralgia, Koplik spots, malaise*)

☛ Given a patient's signs and symptoms, identify the most likely viral etiologic agent and whether it is an RNA or DNA virus

☛ Given a particular virus, name any associated diseases, the clinical specimen needed for diagnosis, and the particular requirements for preservation of the specimen

☛ Describe the laboratory tests available for diagnosing the viral infections presented in the chapter

☛ Compare and contrast the hepatitis viruses, citing the name of the virus, mode of transmission, and type of each disease

☛ Given a particular virus, identify which body system it primarily affects (e.g., respiratory, cardiovascular, nervous system, gastrointestinal, genital)

☛ Name three arthropod-borne viral diseases with incidence in the United States, citing the name of the viral pathogen and an example of a reservoir and vector

It would be impossible in a book this size to describe *all* the infectious diseases caused by viruses. Thus, only selected viral diseases are described in this chapter. Readers should keep in mind that, although each disease is described in a particular section of the chapter (e.g., under cardiovascular infections or respiratory infections), many viral diseases have multiple clinical manifestations.

VIRAL INFECTIONS OF THE CARDIOVASCULAR AND IMMUNE SYSTEMS

HIV Infection and AIDS

Disease. The signs and symptoms of acute HIV infection (i.e., infection with "the AIDS virus") usually occur within several weeks to several months after infection with HIV. Initial symptoms include an acute, self-limited mononucleosis-like illness lasting 1 or 2 weeks. Unfortunately, acute HIV infection is often undiagnosed or misdiagnosed because anti-HIV antibodies are usually not present in a high enough concentration to be detected during this early phase of infection. Other signs and symptoms of acute HIV infection include fever, rash, headache, lymphadenopathy, pharyngitis, **myalgia** (muscle pain), **arthralgia** (joint pain), aseptic meningitis, retro-orbital pain, weight loss, depression, gastrointestinal distress, night sweats, and oral or genital ulcers.

Without appropriate anti-HIV treatment, approximately 90% of HIV-infected patients ultimately develop AIDS. AIDS is a severe, life-threatening syndrome that represents the late clinical stage of infection with HIV. Invasion and destruction of helper T cells (see Chapter 3) leads to suppression of the patient's immune system (immunosuppression). Secondary infections caused by viruses (e.g., cytomegalovirus, herpes simplex), protozoa (e.g., *Cryptosporidium, Toxoplasma*), bacteria (e.g., mycobacteria), and/or fungi (e.g., *Candida, Cryptococcus, Pneumocystis*) become systemic and cause death. Persons with AIDS die as a result of overwhelming infections caused by various pathogens, often opportunistic pathogens. Kaposi sarcoma, a previously rare type of cancer, is a frequent complication of AIDS thought to be caused by a type of herpes virus called human herpesvirus 8. Previously considered a universally fatal disease, certain combinations of drugs, referred to as cocktails, are extending the life of some HIV-positive patients. In the absence of effective anti-HIV treatment, the AIDS case fatality rate is very high—approaching 100%.

Pathogens. AIDS is caused by human immunodeficiency virus (Fig. 25-1). Two types have been identified: type 1 (HIV-1), which is the most common type, and type 2 (HIV-2). HIV viruses are RNA viruses in the family Retroviridae (retroviruses). Infected humans serve as reservoirs. Transmission occurs via direct sexual contact (homosexual or heterosexual); sharing of contaminated needles and syringes by

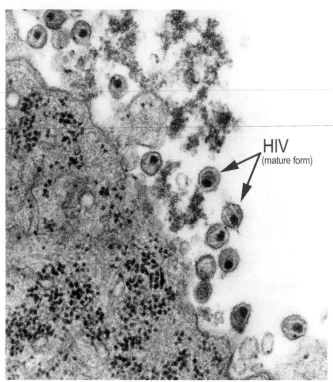

Figure 25-1. **Transmission electron micrograph of enveloped HIV virions that have escaped from experimentally infected tissue by budding.** (Courtesy of the Centers for Disease Control and Prevention [CDC].)

intravenous drug abusers; transfusion of contaminated blood and blood products; transplacental transfer from mother to child; breast-feeding by HIV-infected mothers; transplantation of HIV-infected tissues or organs; and needlestick, scalpel, and broken glass injuries. There is no evidence of HIV transmission via biting insects. Most likely, HIV-1 first invades dendritic cells in the genital and oral mucosa. These cells then fuse with CD4+ lymphocytes (helper T cells) and spread to deeper tissues. HIV-1 can be cultured from plasma about 5 days after infection. A drawing of HIV appears in the Chapter 24 section of the CD-ROM.

Clinical specimens. Serum or plasma are required for immunodiagnostic and molecular diagnostic procedures, depending on the procedure being used; follow manufacturer's instructions. HIV may be cultured from leukocytes (buffy coat) separated from anticoagulated blood.

Specimen preservation. In accordance with current specimen guidelines, serum may be refrigerated for short-term storage and frozen (at less than –20°C) for longer periods. Plasma can be refrigerated for up to 72 hours or frozen (at –70°C) for longer periods. Unfractionated whole blood should be submitted at room temperature and should not be refrigerated.

Laboratory diagnosis. Immunodiagnostic procedures are available for detection of antigen and antibodies. Most HIV-infected patients develop detectable antibodies within

1 to 3 months after infection. However, there may be a more prolonged interval of up to 6 months, or even longer in some cases. The most commonly used screening test is an enzyme-linked immunosorbent assay. If the screening test is positive, a confirmatory test such as the Western blot analysis[1] or indirect fluorescent antibody test is usually performed. Antigen detection procedures detect an HIV antigen known as p24. Molecular diagnostic procedures are also available. Quantitative assessment of viral RNA is used to monitor the effectiveness of antiviral therapy.

STUDY AID   **Viremia.** The presence of viruses in the bloodstream is known as **viremia.** The viruses may be either free in the plasma or attached to or within red blood cells or white blood cells, such as lymphocytes and monocytes. The number of viruses in the bloodstream is referred to as the **viral load,** which may be described as being heavy or light. The degree of viremia varies from one viral disease to another, and often from one stage of a particular viral infection to another.

Infectious Mononucleosis

Disease. Infectious mononucleosis (also called mono or the kissing disease) is an acute viral disease that may be asymptomatic or may be characterized by fever, sore throat, lymphadenopathy (especially posterior cervical lymph nodes), splenomegaly (enlarged spleen), and fatigue. Infectious mononucleosis is usually a self-limited disease of one to several weeks' duration and is rarely fatal.

Pathogen. The etiologic agent of infectious mononucleosis is Epstein-Barr virus (EBV), which is also known as human herpesvirus 4. It is a DNA virus in the family Herpesviridae. EBV infects and transforms B cells, although it also infects other types of cells. EBV is known to be oncogenic (cancer causing), causing or being associated with lymphomas (e.g., Hodgkin disease and Burkitt lymphoma), carcinomas (e.g., nasopharyngeal carcinoma and gastric carcinoma), and sarcomas, among other cancers. Infected humans serve as reservoirs. Transmission occurs from person to person by direct contact with saliva. Kissing facilitates spread among adolescents. EBV can be transmitted via blood transfusion.

Clinical specimens. Serum or plasma should be collected (follow manufacturer's instructions) for immunodiagnostic or molecular diagnostic procedures. Whole anticoagulated blood is needed for culture of virus from buffy coat. Specimens are preserved as described under "HIV Infection and AIDS."

Laboratory diagnosis. Patients with infectious mononucleosis usually present with a lymphocytosis (abnormally

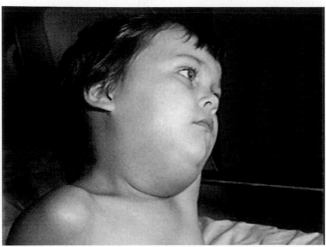

Figure 25-2 **Child with mumps.** (Courtesy of Barbara Rice, the National Immunization Program, and the Centers for Disease Control [CDC].)

high peripheral lymphocyte count), including 10% or more abnormal lymphocyte forms, and abnormalities in liver function tests. Specific diagnosis is usually made by detection of antibodies. Molecular diagnostic procedures are also available. EBV can be cultured from the buffy coat—the layer of white blood cells that appears in centrifuged blood.

Mumps

Disease. Mumps or infectious parotitis is an acute viral infection characterized by fever and swelling and tenderness of the salivary glands (Fig. 25-2). Complications can include orchitis (inflammation of the testes), oophoritis (inflammation of the ovaries), meningitis, encephalitis, deafness, pancreatitis, arthritis, mastitis, nephritis, thyroiditis, and pericarditis.

Pathogen. Mumps is caused by mumps virus, an RNA virus in the genus Rubulavirus, family Paramyxoviridae (Fig. 25-3). Infected humans serve as reservoirs. Transmission occurs via droplet spread and direct contact with the saliva of an infected person.

Clinical specimens. Throat swabs, saliva, urine, or cerebrospinal fluid (CSF) are collected for virus isolation. Serum is required for antibody detection.

Specimen preservation. Throat swabs should be immediately placed into VTM and be kept at 4°C. Urine specimens should be submitted to the laboratory at 4°C.

Laboratory diagnosis. Diagnosis of mumps is made using immunodiagnostic procedures or cell culture.

Viral Hemorrhagic Diseases

Diseases. Viral hemorrhagic diseases are extremely serious, acute viral illnesses. Initial symptoms include sudden onset of fever, malaise (a feeling of general discomfort; feeling

---

[1] *A Western blot analysis is a procedure in which proteins separated by electrophoresis in polyacrylamide gels are transferred (blotted) onto nitrocellulose or nylon membranes and identified by specific complexing with tagged antibodies.*

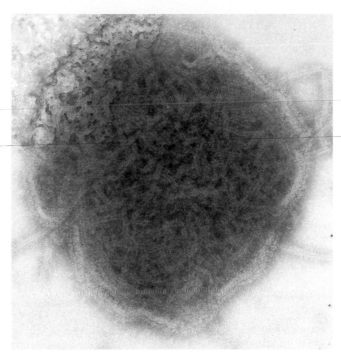

Figure 25-3. **Transmission electron micrograph of mumps virus.** (Courtesy of Dr. F. A. Murphy and the CDC.)

"out of sorts"), myalgia, and headache, followed by pharyngitis, vomiting, diarrhea, rash, and internal hemorrhaging. Case fatality rates for Marburg virus infection and Ebola virus infection have been 25% and 50% to 90%, respectively. All known cases of both diseases occurred in or could be traced back to Africa.

Pathogens. Two of the causes of viral hemorrhagic diseases are Ebola virus and Marburg virus. They are filamentous viruses in the family Filoviridae. Ebola virus is about 80 nm in width and up to 1 μm or longer in length (Fig. 25-4).

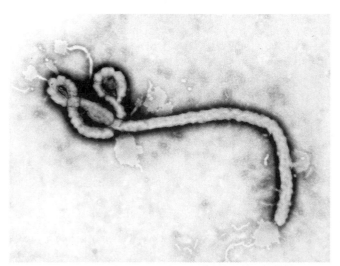

Figure 25-4. **Transmission electron micrograph of Ebola virus.** (Courtesy of Dr. F. A. Murphy and the CDC.)

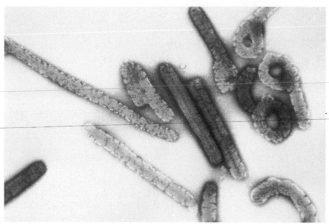

Figure 25-5. **Transmission electron micrograph of Marburg virus.** Several of the virions display the characteristic "shepherd's crook" shape. (Courtesy of Dr. Erskine Palmer, Dr. Russell Regnery, and the CDC.)

Marburg virus is about 80 nm in width and 790 nm in length (Fig. 25-5). Infected humans serve as reservoirs; infected African green monkeys are also reservoirs of Marburg virus. Transmission is from person to person via direct contact with infected blood, secretions, internal organs, or semen, or via needlestick. The risk is highest when the patient is vomiting, having diarrhea, or hemorrhaging.

Clinical specimens. Serum, heparinized plasma, whole blood, throat washings, or urine are required for virus isolation and immunodiagnostic and molecular diagnostic procedures.

Specimen preservation. Specimens must be frozen when shipped.

Laboratory diagnosis. Viral hemorrhagic diseases are diagnosed using immunodiagnostic and molecular diagnostic procedures, cell culture, or electron microscopy. Laboratory studies of viral hemorrhagic fevers represent an extreme biohazard and should be conducted only in biosafety level 4 (BSL-4) containment facilities. Additional hemorrhagic fevers are the arthropod-borne viral hemorrhagic fevers: dengue, yellow fever, and Crimean-Congo hemorrhagic fever. Dengue or dengue hemorrhagic fever and yellow fever are mosquito-borne diseases. Crimean-Congo hemorrhagic fever is tickborne (Fig. 25-6). These diseases are diagnosed either by isolation of the virus from blood, using cell cultures or inoculation of suckling mice, or by immunodiagnostic or molecular diagnostic procedures.

VIRAL INFECTIONS OF THE SKIN

Chickenpox and Shingles

Diseases. Chickenpox, also known as varicella, is an acute, generalized viral infection with fever and a skin rash (Fig. 25-7). Vesicles also form in mucous membranes. It is usually

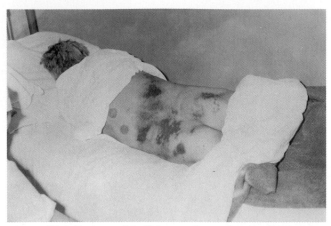

Figure 25-6. **Patient with Crimean-Congo hemorrhagic fever.** This disease, which has been found in Africa, Asia, the Middle East, and Eastern Europe, can be transmitted from person to person and has a 30% fatality rate. (Courtesy of Dr. B. E. Henderson and the CDC.)

a mild, self-limiting disease but can be severely damaging to a fetus. Serious complications include pneumonia, secondary bacterial infections, hemorrhagic complications, and encephalitis. Reye syndrome, a severe encephalomyelitis with liver damage, may follow clinical chickenpox if aspirin is given to children younger than 16 years of age. Chickenpox is the leading cause of vaccine-preventable death in the United States

Shingles, also known as herpes zoster, is a reactivation of the varicella-zoster virus, often the result of immunosuppression. Shingles involves inflammation of sensory ganglia of cutaneous sensory nerves, producing fluid-filled blisters,

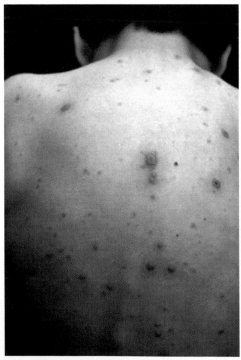

Figure 25-7. **Child with chickenpox.** The pus-filled, blistery lesions usually appear on the face, scalp, and trunk. (Courtesy of the CDC.)

pain, and paresthesia (numbness and tingling). Shingles may occur at any age but is most common after age 50.

Pathogen. Chickenpox and shingles are caused by varicella-zoster virus (Fig. 25-8), a herpesvirus (family Herpesviridae) also known as human herpesvirus 3. Varicella-zoster virus is a DNA virus. Infected humans serve as reservoirs. Person-to-person transmission occurs by direct contact through droplet or airborne spread of vesicle fluid or secretions of the respiratory system of persons with chickenpox.

CAUTION **Beware of Similar-Sounding Names.** It is important not to confuse the terms *varicella*, *variola*, and *vaccinia*. **Varicella-zoster virus,** which is a type of herpesvirus, is the cause of chickenpox. **Variola virus,** a poxvirus, is the cause of smallpox and is often referred to as smallpox virus. **Vaccinia virus,** also a poxvirus, is the cause of cowpox. Vaccinia virus is used to make the vaccine that protects against smallpox. The words *vaccine* and *vaccination* are derived from *vacca*, a Latin word meaning "cow."

Clinical specimens. Swabs of vesicular contents are the appropriate specimens.

Specimen preservation. Swabs should be immediately placed into VTM and be kept at 4°C.

Laboratory diagnosis. Diagnosis is usually made on clinical and epidemiologic grounds. Immunodiagnostic and molecular diagnostic procedures are available, as are cell culture and electron microscopy. Multinucleated giant cells may be seen in Giemsa-stained scrapings from the base of a lesion and in cell cultures (Fig. 25-9).

German Measles (Rubella)

Disease. German measles, or rubella, is a mild, febrile viral disease. A fine, pinkish, flat rash begins 1 or 2 days after the onset of symptoms (Fig. 25-10). The rash starts on the face and neck and spreads to the trunk, arms, and legs. Rubella is a milder disease than hard measles and has fewer complications. If acquired during the first trimester of pregnancy, rubella may cause congenital rubella syndrome in the fetus. This can lead to intrauterine death, spontaneous abortion, or congenital malformations of major organ systems.

Pathogen. Rubella is caused by rubella virus, an RNA virus in the family Togaviridae. Infected humans serve as reservoirs. Transmission occurs via droplet spread or direct contact with nasopharyngeal secretions of infected people.

Clinical specimens. Vesicular swabs or aspirates, throat swabs, or nasopharyngeal secretions are collected for culture, and sometimes cataract tissue or urine is used. Serum is collected for serological procedures.

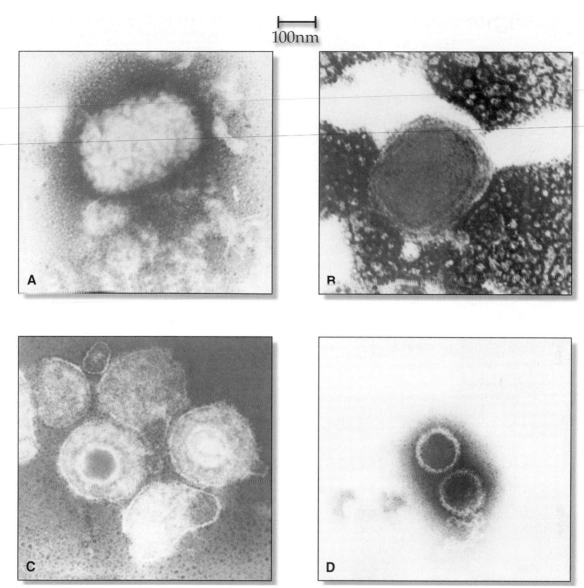

Figure 25-8. **Comparison of smallpox (variola) and varicella-zoster viruses.** Variola is a poxvirus. Surface filaments are seen on the M (mulberry) form (**A**) but not on the C (capsular) form (**B**). Varicella-zoster (**C and D**) is a type of herpesvirus. (Courtesy of Dr. James Nakano and the CDC.)

Specimen preservation. Specimens for culture should be immediately placed into VTM. They can be stored at 4°C for short periods (days) or at −70°C for longer periods (weeks). Serum should be submitted to the laboratory at 4°C.

Laboratory diagnosis. Immunodiagnostic and molecular diagnostic procedures are available for diagnosis of rubella. The virus can be propagated in cell culture.

Measles (Hard Measles, Rubeola)

Disease. Measles, also known as hard measles (to distinguish it from rubella) and rubeola, is an acute, highly communicable viral disease with fever, conjunctivitis, cough, photosensitivity (light sensitivity), Koplik spots in the mouth, and a red blotchy skin rash (Fig. 25-11). Koplik

spots are small red spots, in the center of which can be seen a minute bluish-white speck when observed under a strong light (Fig. 25-12). The red blotchy rash begins on the face between days 3 and 7 and then becomes generalized. Complications include bronchitis, pneumonia, otitis media, and encephalitis. Rarely, autoimmune, subacute, sclerosing panencephalitis (SSPE) may follow a latent period of several years. SSPE is characterized by gradual progressive psychoneurological deterioration, including personality changes, seizures, photosensitivity, ocular abnormalities, and coma.

Pathogen. Measles is caused by measles virus, which is also known as rubeola virus. It is an RNA virus in the family Paramyxoviridae. Infected humans serve as reservoirs. Airborne transmission occurs by droplet spread; direct contact

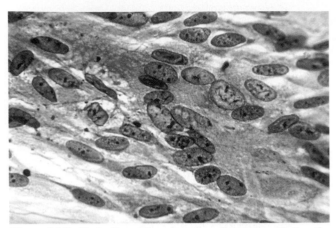

Figure 25-9. **Varicella-zoster virus in cell culture.** Notice the multinucleated giant cells and intranuclear inclusion bodies. (Courtesy of the CDC.)

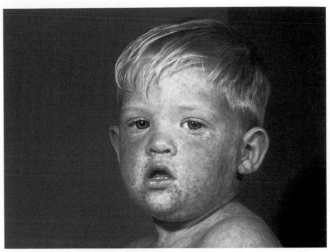

Figure 25-11. **Child with measles.** (Courtesy of the CDC.)

with nasal or throat secretions of infected persons, or with articles freshly soiled with nose and throat secretions.

 CAUTION

Beware of Similar-Sounding Names. Rubella virus is the cause of German measles, whereas **rubeola virus** is the cause of the more common disease known as hard measles.

Clinical specimens. Specimens include vesicular swabs or aspirates, whole blood, serum, throat swabs, nasopharyngeal secretions, urine, and sometimes brain and skin biopsy specimens.

Specimen preservation. Specimens for culture (except blood, serum, and urine) should be immediately placed into VTM and be kept at 4°C.

Laboratory diagnosis. Diagnosis of measles is usually made on clinical and epidemiologic grounds. Immunodiagnostic and molecular diagnostic procedures are available; and the virus can be isolated in cell culture.

Monkeypox

Disease. Monkeypox is a rare viral disease that causes fever, headache, muscle aches, backache, lymphadenitis, malaise, and a rash (Fig. 25-13). A milder disease than smallpox,

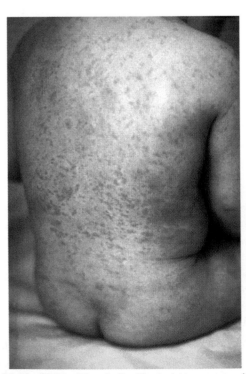

Figure 25-10. **Child with rubella.** The lesions are not as intensely red as those of measles. (Courtesy of the CDC.)

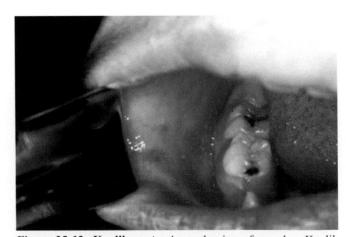

Figure 25-12. **Koplik spots.** An early sign of measles, Koplik spots usually appear before the onset of skin rash. They are irregularly shaped, bright red spots, often having a bluish-white central dot, present on the tongue and check mucosa of this patient. (Courtesy of the CDC.)

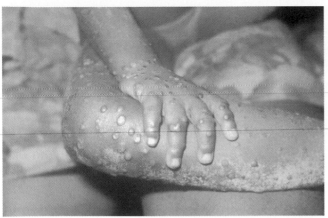

Figure 25-13. **Child with monkeypox.** (Courtesy of the CDC.)

monkeypox occurs primarily in central and western Africa, although several people in the United States became ill in 2003 after handling infected prairie dogs. Unlike smallpox, the disease is rarely fatal.

Pathogen. Monkeypox is caused by monkeypox virus, which is in the same group of viruses (orthopoxviruses) as smallpox virus (variola virus) and the virus that is used in the smallpox vaccine (vaccinia virus; Fig. 25-14). Infected animals serve as reservoirs. Transmission occurs via animal bite or contact with an infected animal's blood, body fluids, or rash. Human-to-human transmission does occur.

Clinical specimens. Swabs of vesicular contents are the appropriate specimens.

Specimen preservation. Swabs should be immediately placed into VTM and be kept at 4°C.

Laboratory diagnosis. Monkeypox can be diagnosed by molecular diagnostic procedures, cell culture, electron microscopy, or immunodiagnostic procedures.

Smallpox
Disease. Smallpox is a systemic viral infection with fever, malaise, headache, prostration, severe backache, a characteristic skin rash (Fig. 25-15), and occasional abdominal

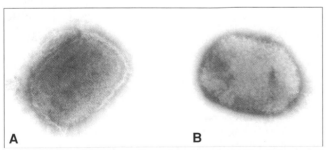

Figure 25-14. **Two forms of monkeypox virus.** The C (capsular) form (**A**) of the virus does not possess the short, whorled filaments that are present on the M (mulberry) form (**B**). (Courtesy of Cynthia S. Goldsmith, Inger K. Damon, Sherif R. Zaki, and the CDC.)

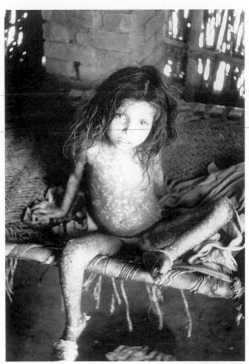

Figure 25-15. **Child with smallpox.** (Courtesy of the CDC.)

pain and vomiting. The rash is similar to, and must be distinguished from, the rash of chickenpox (see Fig. 25-7). Smallpox can become severe, with bleeding into the skin and mucous membranes, followed by death.

Pathogens. Smallpox is caused by two strains of variola virus: variola minor (with a fatality rate of <1%), and variola major (with a fatality rate of 20% to 40% or higher). Variola virus is a double-stranded DNA virus in the genus Orthopoxvirus, family Poxviridae (Fig. 25-16). Before smallpox was eradicated, infected humans were the only source of the virus. Person-to-person transmission is via the respiratory tract (droplet spread) or skin inoculation.. Patients are most contagious before eruption of the rash, by aerosol droplets from oropharyngeal lesions. There are no known animal or environmental reservoirs.

Clinical specimens. Specimens include swabs or aspirates of vesicular contents.

Specimen preservation. Specimens should be immediately placed into VTM and be kept at 4°C.

Laboratory diagnosis. Because of the potential danger of the use of smallpox virus as a bioterrorism agent, physicians must become familiar with the clinical and epidemiologic features of smallpox and how to distinguish smallpox from chickenpox (see Chapter 26). Histopathologic examination of the base of mature smallpox vesicles reveals degenerating cells containing intracytoplasmic inclusion bodies (Fig. 25-17). The inclusion bodies, known as Guarnieri bodies, are of variable

> Associate Guarnieri bodies with smallpox.

Historical Vignette

The World Health Organization (WHO) was able to eradicate smallpox by a combination of isolation of infected persons and vaccination of others in the community. The last known case of naturally acquired smallpox in the world occurred in Somalia in October 1977. In May 1980, the WHO announced the global eradication of smallpox. Smallpox virus is currently stored in several laboratories, including those at the Centers for Disease Control and Prevention and a comparable facility in Russia. Smallpox virus is a potential biological warfare and bioterrorism agent (see Chapter 26).

size, paranuclear,[2] and surrounded by a clear halo. Laboratory diagnosis is by cell culture, virus neutralization tests, molecular diagnostic procedures, or electron microscopy. These procedures are performed only in BSL-4 facilities.

Warts

Diseases. Warts consist of many varieties of skin and mucous membrane lesions, including common warts (verrucae vulgaris), venereal warts, and plantar warts. Most are harmless, but some can become cancerous. Venereal or genital warts are discussed in more detail later in the chapter.

Pathogens. Warts are caused by at least 70 types of human papillomaviruses. Wart viruses are classified in the genus Papillomavirus within the family Papovaviridae. They are DNA viruses. Infected humans serve as reservoirs. Transmission usually occurs by direct contact. Genital warts are sexually transmitted. Warts are easily spread from one area of the body to another, but most are not very contagious from person to person; genital warts are an exception.

Laboratory diagnosis. Diagnosis is made on clinical grounds.

VIRAL INFECTIONS OF THE EYES

Adenoviral Conjunctivitis and Keratoconjunctivitis

Diseases. Adenoviral conjunctivitis and keratoconjunctivitis are acute viral diseases of one or both eyes, associated with inflammation of the conjunctiva, edema of the eyelid and periorbital tissue, pain, photophobia, and blurred vision. The cornea is involved in about 50% of cases, with permanent scarring of the cornea in severe cases.

Pathogens. Adenoviral conjunctivitis and keratoconjunctivitis are caused by various types of adenoviruses. Herpes

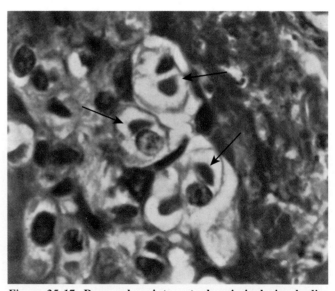

Figure 25-17. **Paranuclear intracytoplasmic inclusion bodies (Guarnieri bodies) of smallpox.** The inclusion bodies (*arrows*) seen here are within skin cells in various stages of ballooning degeneration. (From Binford CH, Connor DH. Pathology of Tropical and Extraordinary Diseases, vol 1. Washington, DC: Armed Forces Institute of Pathology, 1976.)

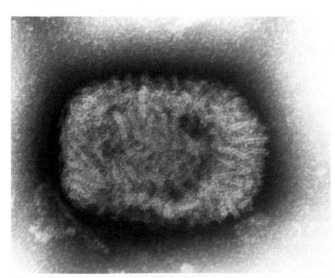

Figure 25-16. **Transmission electron micrograph of a smallpox (variola) virion.** (Courtesy of the CDC.)

---

[2] *The prefix* para- *means "adjacent, alongside, near." Thus,* paranuclear *means "alongside the nucleus."*

simplex and varicella-zoster viruses can also cause keratoconjunctivitis. Infected humans serve as reservoirs. Transmission occurs via direct contact with eye secretions or contact with contaminated surfaces, instruments, or solutions.

Clinical specimens. Eye swabs or conjunctival scrapings are typical specimens.

Specimen preservation. Specimens should be immediately placed into VTM and be kept at 4°C.

Laboratory diagnosis. Diagnosis is made by cell culture or immunodiagnostic or molecular diagnostic procedures.

Hemorrhagic Conjunctivitis

Disease. Hemorrhagic conjunctivitis has a sudden onset, with redness, swelling, and pain in one or both eyes. Small, discrete, subconjunctival hemorrhages may enlarge to form confluent subconjunctival hemorrhages. One adenoviral syndrome, called pharyngoconjunctival fever, is characterized by upper respiratory disease, fever, and minor degrees of corneal epithelial inflammation.

Pathogens. Hemorrhagic conjunctivitis is caused by adenoviruses and enteroviruses. Infected humans serve as reservoirs. Transmission occurs by direct or indirect contact with discharge from infected eyes. Adenovirus transmission may be associated with poorly chlorinated swimming pools; this "swimming pool conjunctivitis" can reach epidemic proportions.

Clinical specimens. Specimens include eye swabs or conjunctival scrapings.

Specimen preservation. Specimens should be immediately placed into VTM and be kept at 4°C.

Laboratory diagnosis. Diagnosis is made by cell culture or immunodiagnostic or molecular diagnostic procedures.

VIRAL INFECTIONS OF THE RESPIRATORY SYSTEM

The Common Cold (Acute Viral Rhinitis, Acute Coryza)

Disease. The common cold is a viral infection of the lining of the nose, sinuses, throat, and large airways. Symptoms include coryza (profuse discharge from nostrils), sneezing, runny eyes, sore throat, chills, and malaise. Additionally, laryngitis, tracheitis, or bronchitis may accompany a cold. Secondary bacterial infections, including sinusitis and otitis media, may follow. The common cold is most common in fall, winter, and spring. On average, most people have one to six colds annually.

Pathogens. Many different viruses cause colds. Rhinoviruses, of which there are more than 100 serotypes, are the major cause in adults. Other cold-causing viruses include coronaviruses, parainfluenza viruses, respiratory

syncytial virus (RSV), influenza viruses, adenoviruses, and enteroviruses. Infected humans serve as reservoirs. Transmission occurs via respiratory secretions by way of hands and fomites, or by direct contact with or inhalation of airborne droplets.

Clinical specimens. The nasopharyngeal swab is the specimen used to identify any of the viruses causing the common cold.

Specimen preservation. Specimens should be immediately placed into VTM and be kept at 4°C.

Laboratory diagnosis. Laboratory diagnosis of the common cold usually is not required, but cell culture techniques can often demonstrate the specific virus.

Acute, Febrile, Viral Respiratory Disease

Disease. Acute, febrile, viral respiratory disease is characterized by fever and one or more of the following systemic reactions: chills, headache, general aching, malaise, anorexia, and sometimes gastrointestinal disturbances in infants. The disease may include rhinitis, pharyngitis, tonsillitis, laryngitis, bronchitis, pneumonia, conjunctivitis, otitis media, and/or sinusitis.

Pathogens. Acute, febrile, viral respiratory disease can be caused by one of many viruses, including parainfluenza viruses, RSV, adenovirus, rhinoviruses, certain coronaviruses, coxsackieviruses, and echoviruses. RSV is the major viral respiratory tract pathogen of early infancy. RSV may cause pneumonia, croup, bronchitis, otitis media, and death. Infected humans serve as reservoirs. Transmission occurs via direct oral contact or by droplets; indirectly via handkerchiefs, eating utensils, other fomites; or for some viruses, via the fecal-oral route.

Clinical specimens. Specimens include nasopharyngeal aspirates, nasal wash, nasopharyngeal swabs, and bronchoalveolar lavage.

Specimen preservation. Specimens should be immediately placed into VTM and be kept at 4°C.

Laboratory diagnosis. Isolation of the etiologic agent from respiratory secretions, using cell cultures, is required. Immunodiagnostic and molecular diagnostic procedures are available.

Influenza (Flu)

Disease. Influenza is an acute, viral respiratory infection with fever, chills, headache, aches and pains throughout the body (most pronounced in the back and legs), sore throat, cough, and nasal drainage. Influenza sometimes causes bronchitis, pneumonia, and death in severe cases. Nausea, vomiting, and diarrhea may occur, particularly in children. Although the term *stomach flu* is often heard, influenza viruses rarely cause gastrointestinal symptoms. Stomach flu, also known as the 24-hour flu, is caused by viruses other than influenza viruses.

Historical Vignette

The 1918–1919 Spanish flu pandemic killed between 20 million and 50 million people worldwide. The 1957–1958 Asian flu and 1968–1969 Hong Kong flu pandemics killed about 70,000 and 34,000 U.S. citizens, respectively. Flu epidemics occur in the United States almost every year, affecting 10% to 20% of the general population.

Pathogens. Influenza is caused by influenza virus types A, B, and C (Fig. 25-18). They are single-stranded RNA viruses in the family Orthomyxoviridae. Influenza A virus causes severe symptoms and is associated with pandemics and widespread epidemics. Influenza B virus causes less severe disease and more localized outbreaks. Influenza C virus usually does not cause epidemics or significant disease. Infected humans are the primary reservoir; pigs and birds also serve as reservoirs. Because pig cells have receptors for both avian and human strains of influenza virus, pigs serve as "mixing bowls," resulting in new strains containing RNA segments from both avian and human strains. Transmission occurs via airborne spread and direct contact.

Clinical specimens. Specimens include nasopharyngeal aspirates, nasal wash, nasopharyngeal swabs, and bronchoalveolar lavage. Serum is required for antibody detection.

Specimen preservation. Specimens should be immediately placed into VTM and be kept at 4°C.

Laboratory diagnosis. Influenza is diagnosed by isolation of an influenza virus from pharyngeal or nasal secretions or washings using cell culture techniques, antigen detection, demonstration of a rise in antibody titer (concentration) between acute and convalescent sera, or molecular diagnostic procedures.

Avian Influenza (Bird Flu)

Disease. Avian influenza, commonly referred to as bird flu, is primarily a disease of birds but can cause human disease. In humans, the virus causes a respiratory infection with manifestations ranging from influenza-like symptoms (fever, cough, sore throat, and muscle aches) to eye infections, pneumonia, acute and severe respiratory distress, and other severe and life-threatening complications.

Pathogens. Bird flu is caused by avian influenza virus type A. The three prominent subtypes of the virus are designated H5, H7, and H9. The strain known as H5N1 is the most virulent strain (Figs. 25-19 and 25-20). Infected wild and domesticated birds serve as reservoirs. Bird-to-human

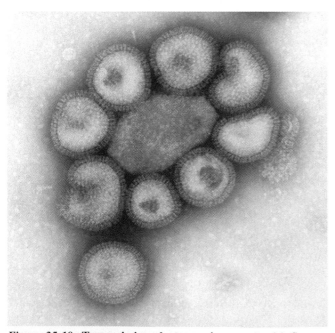

Figure 25-18. **Transmission electron micrograph of influenza virus virions.** (Courtesy of Dr. F. A. Murphy and the CDC.)

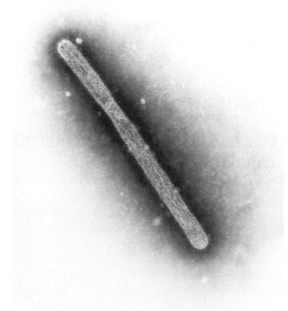

Figure 25-19. **Transmission electron micrograph of an avian influenza A (H5N1) virion.** (Courtesy of Cynthia Goldsmith, Jackie Katz, and the CDC.)

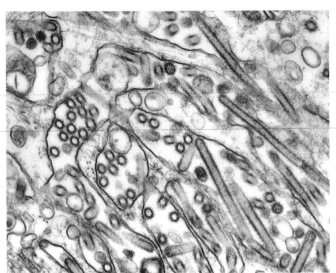

Figure 25-20. **Artificially colorized transmission electron micrograph of avian influenza A (H5N1) virions in cell culture.** The virions are gold and the tissue culture cells are green. (Courtesy of Cynthia Goldsmith, Jacqueline Katz, Sharif R. Zaki, and the CDC.)

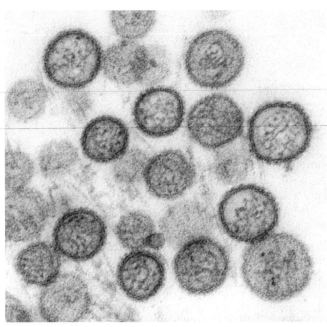

Figure 25-21. **Transmission electron micrograph of the Sin Nombre strain of hantavirus.** (Courtesy of Cynthia Goldsmith, Luanne Elliot, and the CDC.)

transmission occurs via contact with infected poultry or surfaces that have been contaminated with excretions or secretions from infected birds. As of April 2007, approximately 291 human cases had occurred worldwide, with about 172 deaths (a mortality rate exceeding 50%), and the world was preparing for a worldwide pandemic. Most human cases resulted from bird-to-human transmission, and documented human-to-human transmission had occurred in only a small number of cases. However, influenza viruses commonly mutate, and increased instances of human-to-human transmission are likely to occur in the future.

Clinical specimens. Specimens include nasopharyngeal aspirates, nasal wash, nasopharyngeal swabs, and bronchoalveolar lavage.

Specimen preservation. Specimens should be immediately placed into VTM and be kept at 4°C.

Laboratory diagnosis. Molecular diagnostic procedures or cell culture are the means of diagnosis.

Hantavirus Pulmonary Syndrome

Disease. Hantavirus pulmonary syndrome (HPS) is an acute viral disease characterized by fever, myalgias, gastrointestinal complaints, cough, difficulty breathing, and hypotension (decreased blood pressure). The Sin Nombre virus—literally, the "virus with no name"—was the cause of the epidemic that occurred in the Four Corners area of the United States in the spring and summer of 1993. Since then, sporadic cases have been reported in many states as well as in South America.

Pathogens. At least five hantaviruses (Sin Nombre, Bayou, Black Creek Canal, New York 1, and Monongahela) have caused HPS in the United States. The Sin Nombre strain is shown in Figure 25-21. Other strains have caused HPS in South America. Rodents, including the deer mouse, pack rats, and chipmunks, serve as reservoirs. Transmission occurs via inhalation of aerosolized rodent feces, urine, and saliva. Person-to-person transmission is rare.

Clinical specimens. Specimens include nasopharyngeal aspirates, nasal wash, nasopharyngeal swabs, and bronchoalveolar lavage.

Specimen preservation. Specimens should be immediately placed into VTM and be kept at 4°C.

Laboratory diagnosis. HPS can be diagnosed by immunodiagnostic and molecular diagnostic procedures and by cell culture.

Severe Acute Respiratory Syndrome

Disease. Severe acute respiratory syndrome (SARS) is a viral respiratory illness with high fever, chills, headache, a general feeling of discomfort, body aches, and sometimes diarrhea. Most patients develop a dry cough followed by pneumonia. SARS was first reported in southern China in late 2002. In 2002–2003, 8,098 people developed SARS, 774 of whom died. Several cases in China were reported in 2004.

Pathogen. SARS is caused by SARS-associated coronavirus (SARS-CoV; Fig. 25-22). Infected persons serve as reservoirs. Transmission occurs by respiratory droplets or by touching the mouth, nose, or eye after touching a contaminated

viruses, HIV, herpes simplex virus type 1 (HSV-1), measles virus, mumps virus, rabies virus, enteroviruses, and varicella-zoster virus.

Clinical specimens and specimen preservation. See the descriptions under "Arthropod-Borne Viral Encephalitis."

Laboratory diagnosis. Diagnosis is primarily by immunodiagnostic or molecular diagnostic procedures or by cell culture. Differentiation of viruses within this group requires nucleic acid analysis.

Lymphocytic Choriomeningitis

Disease. Lymphocytic choriomeningitis is a rodentborne viral disease that presents as aseptic meningitis, encephalitis, or meningoencephalitis. Asymptomatic or mild febrile disease also occurs. Some patients develop fever, malaise, suppressed appetite, muscle aches, headache, nausea, vomiting, sore throat, coughing, joint pain, chest pain, and salivary gland pain. Possible complications of CNS involvement include deafness and temporary or permanent neurological damage. An association between lymphocytic choriomeningitis virus infection and myocarditis has been suggested.

Pathogen. Lymphocytic choriomeningitis is caused by the lymphocytic choriomeningitis virus, which is a member of the family Arenaviridae. Infected rodents, primarily the common house mouse, serve as reservoirs. Humans become infected following exposure to mouse urine, droppings, saliva, or nesting materials. The virus can enter broken skin; through the nose, eyes, or mouth; or via the bite of an infected rodent. Organ transplantation is a possible means of transmission.

Clinical specimens and specimen preservation. See the descriptions under "Arthropod-Borne Viral Encephalitis."

Laboratory diagnosis. Diagnosis is primarily by immunodiagnostic procedures and cell culture.

Poliomyelitis (Polio, Infantile Paralysis)

Disease. In most patients, poliomyelitis causes a minor illness with fever, malaise, headache, nausea, and vomiting. In about 1% of patients, the disease progresses to severe muscle pain, stiffness of the neck and back, with or without flaccid paralysis. Major illness is more likely to occur in older children and adults. Although once a major health problem in the United States, vaccines became available in the 1950s. The WHO is attempting to eradicate polio worldwide.

Pathogens. Poliomyelitis is caused by polioviruses. They are RNA viruses in the family Picornaviridae (small RNA viruses). Infected humans serve as reservoirs. Transmission is person to person, primarily via the fecal-oral route, or by throat secretions.

Clinical specimens and specimen preservation. See the description under "Arthropod-Borne Viral Encephalitis."

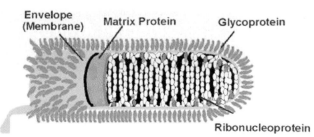

Figure 25-24. **Drawing of a bullet-shaped virion of rabies virus.** (Courtesy of the CDC.)

Laboratory diagnosis. Diagnosis of poliomyelitis is made by isolation of polio virus from stool samples, CSF, or oropharyngeal secretions using cell culture techniques, or by immunodiagnostic or molecular diagnostic procedures.

Rabies

Disease. Rabies is a usually fatal, acute viral encephalomyelitis of mammals, with mental depression, restlessness, headache, fever, malaise, paralysis, salivation, spasms of throat muscles induced by a slight breeze or drinking water, convulsions, and death caused by respiratory failure. Rabies is endemic in every country of the world except Antarctica and in every state except Hawaii. Worldwide an estimated 65,000 to 87,000 people die of rabies annually.

Pathogen. Rabies is caused by the rabies virus—a bullet-shaped, enveloped RNA virus in the family Rhabdoviridae (Fig. 25-24). Reservoirs are various wild and domestic mammals, including dogs, foxes, coyotes, wolves, jackals, skunks, raccoons, mongooses, and bats. Transmission is usually via the bite of a rabid animal, which introduces virus-laden saliva; airborne transmission from bats in caves also occurs. Person-to-person transmission by saliva is theoretically possible but has never been documented.

Clinical specimens. Saliva, serum, CSF, cutaneous nerves, corneal epithelium, and other tissues can be tested for the presence of virions, viral nucleic acid, or viral antigen. All specimens should be considered potentially infectious.

Specimen preservation. If specimens must be shipped, they should be stored frozen at −20°C or below.

Laboratory diagnosis. Diagnosis of rabies is made by cell culture, antibody detection in serum or CSF, antigen detection in tissue samples, molecular diagnostic procedures for brain tissue, or observation of Negri bodies in brain or other tissue. Negri bodies are viral RNA-nucleoprotein complexes found in the cytoplasm of virus-infected cells; that is, they are intracytoplasmic inclusions (Fig. 25-25).

> Associate Negri bodies with rabies.

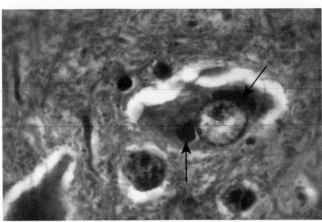

Figure 25-25. Intracytoplasmic inclusion bodies (*arrows*) of rabies virus. The inclusion bodies are called Negri bodies. (Courtesy of Dr. Daniel P. Perl and the CDC.)

VIRAL INFECTIONS OF THE GENITAL TRACT

Anogenital Herpes Viral Infections (Genital Herpes)

Disease. In general, herpes simplex infections are characterized by a localized primary lesion, latency, and a tendency to localized recurrence. In women, the principal sites of primary anogenital herpes virus infection are the cervix and vulva, with recurrent disease affecting the vulva, perineal skin, legs, and buttocks. In men, lesions appear on the penis (Fig. 25-26) and in the anus and rectum of those engaging in anal sex. The initial symptoms are usually itching, tingling, and soreness, followed by a small patch of redness and then a group of small, painful blisters. The blisters break and fuse to form painful, circular sores that become crusted after a few days. The sores heal in about 10 days but may leave scars. The initial outbreak is more painful, prolonged, and widespread than subsequent outbreaks and may be associated with fever.

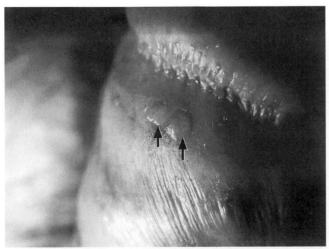

Figure 25-26. Herpes simplex lesions (*arrows*) on a penile shaft. (Courtesy of Susan Lindsley and the CDC.)

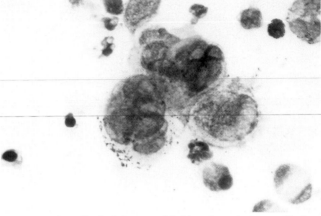

Figure 25-27. Genital herpes. Multinucleated giant cells in a specimen obtained from the base of a penile lesion. (Courtesy of Joe Miller and the CDC.)

Pathogens. Genital herpes is usually caused by herpes simplex virus type 2 (HSV 2) but is occasionally caused by HSV-1. Infected humans serve as reservoirs. Transmission occurs via direct sexual contact or oral-genital, oral-anal, or anal-genital contact during the presence of lesions. Mother-to-fetus or mother-to-neonate transmission occurs during pregnancy and birth.

Clinical specimens. Specimens include swabs of genital lesions or mucus from cervix, vagina, or urethra.

Specimen preservation. Specimens should be immediately placed into VTM and be kept at 4°C.

Laboratory diagnosis. Genital herpes is diagnosed by observation of characteristic cytologic changes in tissue scrapings or biopsy specimens, the presence of multinucleated giant cells with intranuclear inclusions (Fig. 25-27), and confirmation by immunodiagnostic and molecular diagnostic procedures.

Genital Warts (Genital Papillomatosis, *Condyloma acuminatum*)

Disease. Genital warts start as tiny, soft, moist, pink or red swellings that grow rapidly and may develop stalks. Their rough surfaces give them the appearance of small cauliflowers. Multiple warts often grow in the same area, most often on the penis in males and the vulva, vaginal wall, cervix, and skin surrounding the vaginal area in women. Genital warts also develop around the anus and in the rectum in males or females who engage in anal sex. These warts can become malignant.

Pathogens. Genital warts are caused by human papillomaviruses (HPVs) of the Papovaviridae family of DNA viruses (human wart viruses). HPV genotypes 16 and 18 have been associated with cervical cancer. Infected humans serve as reservoirs. Transmission occurs via direct contact, usually sexual; through breaks in skin or mucous membranes; or from mother to neonate during birth.

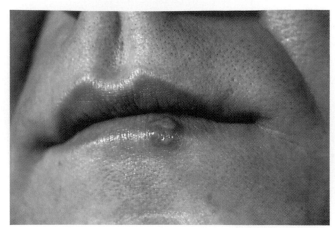

Figure 25-28. **Cold sore caused by herpes simplex.** (Courtesy of Dr. Hermann and the CDC.)

Clinical specimens. Specimens include cervical swabs or excised lesion.

Laboratory diagnosis. Genital warts are usually diagnosed clinically. Molecular diagnostic procedures are available.

VIRAL INFECTIONS OF THE ORAL REGION

Herpes Labialis (Cold Sores, Fever Blisters)

Disease. Cold sores are superficial clear vesicles on an erythematous (red) base occurring on the face or lips (Fig. 25-28). The vesicles crust and heal within a few days. Reactivation can be precipitated by trauma, fever, physiologic changes, or concurrent disease.

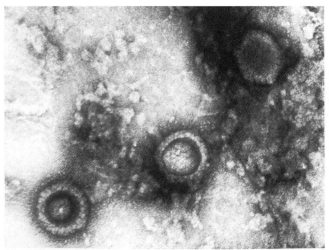

Figure 25-29. **Transmission electron micrograph of three herpes simplex virus particles.** Only the center particle contains a DNA core. Stain has penetrated the other two virus particles, indicating that they lack a DNA core. (Courtesy of Dr. John Hierholzer and the CDC.)

Pathogens. Cold sores are caused by either HSV-1 or HSV-2 (Fig. 25-29). Infected humans serve as reservoirs. Transmission occurs via direct or indirect contact with the saliva of infected persons.

Clinical specimens. Specimens include vesicular swabs, aspirates, or biopsy specimens.

Specimen preservation. Specimens should be immediately placed into VTM and be kept at 4°C.

Laboratory diagnosis. Herpes labialis can be diagnosed by observation of characteristic cytologic changes in tissue scrapings or biopsy specimens in which multinucleated giant cells with intranuclear inclusions are seen. Other means of diagnosis are cell culture, viral antigen detection by immunodiagnostic procedures, and demonstration of HSV DNA in a lesion by polymerase chain reaction.

VIRAL INFECTIONS OF THE GASTROINTESTINAL TRACT

Viral Gastroenteritis (Viral Enteritis, Viral Diarrhea)

Disease. Viral gastroenteritis may be an endemic or epidemic illness in infants, children, and adults. Symptoms include nausea, vomiting, diarrhea, abdominal pain, myalgia, headache, malaise, and low-grade fever. Although most often a self-limiting disease lasting 24 to 48 hours, viral gastroenteritis, especially when caused by a rotavirus, can be fatal in an infant or young child. In developing countries, rotavirus infections are responsible for more than 800,000 diarrheal deaths per year. Although viral gastroenteritis is sometimes referred to as stomach flu or 24-hour flu, keep in mind that *flu* is an abbreviation of *influenza*, which is a respiratory disease.

> The term *stomach flu* is misleading because it implies that the cause is an influenza virus. Influenza viruses cause respiratory diseases. Viral gastroenteritis is caused by other viruses.

Pathogens. The most common viruses infecting children in their first years of life are enteric adenoviruses, astroviruses, caliciviruses (including norovirus-like viruses), and rotaviruses. Those infecting children and adults include norovirus, certain norovirus-like viruses, and rotaviruses. Infected humans are reservoirs of these pathogens; contaminated water and shellfish may also be reservoirs. Transmission is most often via the fecal-oral route. Airborne transmission and contact with contaminated fomites may cause epidemics in hospitals or cruise ships. Foodborne, waterborne, and shellfish transmissions have been reported.

Clinical specimens. Feces or rectal swabs are the specimens used in diagnosing viral gastroenteritis.

TABLE 25 - 2   Common Types of Viral Hepatitis

Name of Disease	Name and Type of Virus	Mode of Transmission	Type of Disease
Type A hepatitis (also known as infectious hepatitis, and epidemic hepatitis)	Hepatitis A virus (HAV), a nonenveloped, linear ssRNA virus in the genus *Hepatovirus,* family Picornaviridae	Fecal-oral transmission; person to person; infected food handlers; fecally contaminated foods and water	Abrupt onset; varies in clinical severity from a mild illness lasting 1 to 2 weeks to a severe, disabling disease lasting several months; no chronic infection
Type B hepatitis (also known as serum hepatitis)	Hepatitis B virus (HBV), an enveloped, circular dsDNA virus in the genus *Orthohepadnavirus,* family Hepadnaviridae; the only DNA virus that causes hepatitis	Sexual or household contact with an infected person; mother to infant before or during birth; intravenous drug abuse; tattooing; needlesticks and other types of nosocomial transmission	Usually has an insidious (gradual) onset; severity ranges from inapparent cases to fulminating, fatal cases; chronic infections occur; may lead to cirrhosis or hepatocellular carcinoma
Type C hepatitis (also known as non-A non-B hepatitis	Hepatitis C virus (HCV), an enveloped, linear ssRNA virus in the genus *Hepacivirus,* family Flaviviridae	Primarily parenterally transmitted (e.g., via blood transfusion); rarely, sexually transmitted	Usually has an insidious onset; 50% to 80% of patients develop a chronic infection; may lead to cirrhosis or hepatocellular carcinoma
Type D hepatitis (also known as delta hepatitis)	Hepatitis D virus (HDV) or delta virus, an enveloped, circular ssRNA viral satellite (a defective RNA virus) in the genus *Deltavirus*	Exposure to infected blood and body fluids; contaminated needles; sexual transmission; coinfection with HBV is necessary	Usually has an abrupt onset; may progress to a chronic and severe disease
Type E hepatitis	Hepatitis E virus (HEV), a spherical, nonenveloped, ssRNA virus in the genus *Calcivirus,* family Calciviridae	Fecal-oral transmission; primarily via fecally contaminated drinking water; also from person to person	Similar to type A hepatitis; no evidence of a chronic form
Type G hepatitis	Hepatitis G virus (HGV); a linear ssRNA virus in the Genus *Hepacivirus,* family Flaviviridae	Parenteral	Can cause chronic hepatitis

ds, double stranded; ss, single-stranded.

Specimen preservation. Specimens should be immediately placed into VTM and be kept at 4°C.

Laboratory diagnosis. Diagnosis is by electron microscopic examination of stool specimens or by immunodiagnostic or molecular procedures.

Viral Hepatitis

Disease. Hepatitis—inflammation of the liver—can be caused by many viruses. Table 25-2 contains information about some of the most common types of viral hepatitis.

Pathogens. See Table 25-2.

TABLE 25 - 3   Methods Used for Diagnosing Viral Infections[a]

Virus	Primary Methods of Diagnosis	Expedited Methods of Diagnosis
Adenovirus	Culture, molecular-amplification test (MAT)	Fluorescent antibody test (FA), enzyme immunoassay (EIA), real-time polymerase chain reaction (RT-PCR)
Adenovirus, enteric	Culture, FA	RT-PCR
Alphaviruses	Culture, MAT	RT-PCR
Arenaviruses	Culture, MAT	EIA, RT-PCR
Astroviruses	MAT	RT-PCR
Bunyaviruses	MAT	RT-PCR
Calciviruses	MAT	RT-PCR
Coronaviruses	Culture, MAT	RT-PCR
Cytomegalovirus	Culture, MAT	Shell vial/spin amplification (SV), FA, quantitative polymerase chain reaction
Enteroviruses	Culture, MAT	RT-PCR
Epstein-Barr virus	Serology,[b] MAT	RT-PCR
Filoviruses	Culture, MAT	RT-PCR
Flaviviruses	Culture, MAT	RT-PCR
Hepatitis A virus	IgM serology	
Hepatitis B virus	Serology	
Hepatitis C virus	Serology, MAT	
Hepatitis D virus	Serology	
Hepatitis E virus	Serology	RT-PCR
Herpes simplex virus	Culture, MAT	SV, FA, EIA, RT-PCR
Human herpesviruses 6 and 7	MAT	RT-PCR
Human herpesvirus 8	MAT	RT-PCR
HIV	Serology, MAT	
Influenza viruses	Culture, MAT	SV, FA, EIA, RT-PCR
Measles virus	Serology	FA, RT-PCR
Metapneumovirus	Culture, MAT	RT-PCR
Mumps virus	Culture, MAT	RT-PCR
Papillomaviruses	MAT	
Parainfluenza viruses	Culture, MAT	SV, FA, EIA, RT-PCR
Parvovirus B19	MAT	RT-PCR

(continued)

TABLE 25 - 3   Continued

Virus	Primary Methods of Diagnosis	Expedited Methods of Diagnosis
Polyomaviruses	MAT	
Poxviruses	Culture, MAT	Electron microscopy, RT-PCR
Rabies virus	Culture, MAT	FA, RT-PCR
Respiratory syncytial virus	Culture, MAT	SV, FA, EIA, RT-PCR
Rhinovirus	Culture, MAT	RT-PCR
Rotavirus	EIA	
Rubella virus	Serology	RT-PCR
Varicella-zoster virus	Culture, MAT	SV, FA, RT-PCR

Source: Winn WC Jr, et al. Koneman's Color Atlas and Textbook of Diagnostic Microbiology. 6th Ed. Philadelphia: Lippincott Williams & Wilkins, 2006.

[a] This table includes some viruses not discussed in this chapter. In addition to the diagnostic methods listed, ancillary, less commonly used methods are also available for diagnosis of most of these viral infections.

[b] Antibody detection.

Clinical specimens. Specimens are usually sera for antibody detection. Liver biopsy specimens may also be taken for immunodiagnostic procedures or electron microscopy.

Specimen preservation. Specimens should be immediately placed into VTM and be kept at 4°C.

Laboratory diagnosis. Diagnosis is by immunodiagnostic or molecular diagnostic procedures or by electron microscopy.

SUMMARY OF VIRAL IDENTIFICATION METHODS

Table 25-3 presents a summary of the methods used for diagnosing viral infections, including some methods not discussed in this chapter.

Chapter Review

- Many infectious diseases are caused by viruses, and viral diseases have various clinical manifestations.

- AIDS is caused by HIV. Both HIV-1 and HIV-2 are RNA viruses. HIV-infected people serve as reservoirs.

- Epstein-Barr virus, the cause of infectious mononucleosis, is a DNA virus and is known to be oncogenic.

- Mumps, an acute viral infection characterized by fever, swelling, and tenderness of the salivary glands, is an RNA virus. It is spread via droplets and direct contact of an infected person.

- Viral hemorrhagic diseases are extremely serious acute viral illnesses caused by Ebola and Marburg viruses.

- Chickenpox, also known as varicella, is an acute viral infection with fever and a skin rash. It is caused by varicella-zoster virus, a DNA virus.

- German measles is a mild, febrile viral disease with a fine, pink rash. It is caused by an RNA virus called rubella virus. When women in the first trimester of pregnancy become infected, the virus may cause congenital rubella syndrome in the fetus.

- Measles is an acute, highly communicable disease with fever, conjunctivitis, cough, light sensitivity, red blotchy skin rash, and Koplik spots. It is caused by an RNA virus called rubeola virus.

- Smallpox is a severe, systemic viral infection that can cause bleeding into the skin and mucous membranes. It is caused by one of two strains of variola virus, variola major and variola minor, which are DNA viruses.

- There are at least 70 types of HPV that cause lesions of the skin and mucous membranes called warts. All these viruses are DNA viruses.

- The common cold can be caused by one of many viruses. Rhinoviruses are the major cause in adults. Other cold-causing viruses include coronaviruses, parainfluenza viruses, influenza viruses, adenoviruses, and enteroviruses.

- The three prominent subtypes of avian influenza (bird flu) viruses are H5, H7, and H9. The strain that has caused the most human cases is H5N1. Wild and domesticated birds serve as reservoirs. Bird-to-human transmission occurs via contact with infected poultry or surfaces that have been contaminated with excretions.

- Hantavirus pulmonary syndrome is caused by one of at least five hantaviruses: Sin Nombre, Bayou, Black Creek Canal, New York 1, and Monongahela.

- Influenza (flu) is caused by influenza viruses types A, B, and C. They are RNA viruses.

- Severe acute respiratory syndrome is a viral respiratory illness that is caused by SARS-associated coronavirus.

- Arthropod-borne viral encephalitides are caused by a variety of RNA viruses and involve a variety of reservoirs and vectors.

- Polio, also known as poliomyelitis and infantile paralysis, is caused by poliovirus, an RNA virus.

- Rabies virus is a bullet-shaped enveloped RNA virus. Reservoirs of the virus include many wild and domestic animals.

- Genital herpes is caused primarily by HSV-2 and occasionally by HSV-1. Cold sores or fever blisters may be caused by either HSV-1 or HSV-2.

- Human papillomaviruses, which are DNA viruses, cause genital warts and may be associated with cervical cancer.

- The most common gastrointestinal viruses infecting children in their first years of life are enteric adenoviruses, astroviruses, caliciviruses (including norovirus), and rotaviruses.

- Hepatitis, or inflammation of the liver, can be caused by one of numerous viruses.

New Terms and Abbreviations

After studying Chapter 25, you should be familiar with the following terms, which are defined within the chapter and in the Glossary at the back of the book:

Arthralgia

Hantavirus pulmonary syndrome (HPS)

Koplik spots

Malaise

Myalgia

Oncogenic

Severe acute respiratory syndrome (SARS)

Viral load

Viremia

References and Suggested Reading

Chin J, ed. Control of Communicable Diseases Manual. 17th Ed. Washington, DC: American Public Health Association, 2000.

Forman MS, Valsamakis A. Specimen collection, transport, and processing: Virology. In: Murray PR, Baron EJ, Jorgensen JH, Pfaller MA, Yolken RH, eds. Manual of Clinical Microbiology. 8th Ed. Washington, DC: ASM Press, 2003.

Protection of Laboratory Workers from Occupationally Acquired Infections: Approved Guideline. 3rd Ed. CLSI Document M29-A3. Wayne, PA: Clinical and Laboratory Standards Institute (CLSI), 2005.

Winn WC Jr, et al. Koneman's Color Atlas and Textbook of Diagnostic Microbiology. 6th Ed. Philadelphia: Lippincott Williams & Wilkins, 2006.

Yolken RH, et al. Algorithms for detection and identification of viruses. In: Murray PR, Baron EJ, Jorgensen JH, Pfaller MA, Yolken RH, eds. Manual of Clinical Microbiology. 8th Ed. Washington, DC: ASM Press, 2003.

 On the CD-ROM

- 2006 Mumps Outbreak
- A Closer Look at Aseptic Meningitis
- Case Study
- Additional Self-Assessment Exercises
- Puzzle

Self-Assessment Exercises

1. Name two viruses considered oncogenic.

A. _____

B. _____

2. Laboratory diagnosis of HIV infection is usually made by which of the following?

A. Biochemical tests

B. Growth of the virus in chicken embryos

C. Immunodiagnostic procedures for detection of antigen and antibodies

D. Light microscopy

3. Name three arthropod-borne viral diseases, a representative vector, and the reservoir.

Disease	**Vector**	**Reservoir**
A. _____	_____	_____
B. _____	_____	_____
C. _____	_____	_____

4. A 4-year-old male presents to his pediatrician with fever and vesicular eruptions of the skin and mucous membranes. A sibling presented with the same signs and symptoms a few weeks previously. What is the most likely cause?

A. Rhinovirus

B. Varicella-zoster virus

C. Rubeola virus

D. Rubella virus

5. Name two general types of laboratory methods or techniques used for diagnosing viral infections.

A. _____

B. _____

6. Which of the following is the cause of smallpox?

A. Varicella-zoster virus

B. Variola virus

C. Vaccinia virus

D. None of the above

7. Identify the following viruses as primarily respiratory (R), gastrointestinal (GI), genital (G), or central nervous system (CNS).

   A. Rabies   _____

   B. HSV-1 and HSV-2   _____

   C. Rotaviruses   _____

   D. Rhinoviruses   _____

   E. Papillomaviruses   _____

8. This hepatitis virus usually has an insidious onset and can lead to chronic infection, cirrhosis, or hepatocellular carcinoma. It is primarily transmitted parenterally and is an enveloped, linear single-stranded RNA virus. What is it?

   A. Hepatitis A virus

   B. Hepatitis B virus

   C. Hepatitis C virus

   D. Hepatitis D virus

9. True or false: Quantitative assessment of viral RNA is used to monitor the effectiveness of antiviral therapy in the case of HIV infection.

10. True or false: Shingles is a reactivation of the varicella-zoster virus.

CHAPTER 26

Health Care Epidemiology and Bioterrorism

Chapter Outline

Role of the Clinical Microbiology Laboratory in Health Care Epidemiology
- Terms and Definitions
- How Clinical Microbiology Professionals Participate in Infection Control

Role of the Clinical Microbiology Laboratory in Bioterrorism
- Category A Biological Warfare and Bioterrorism Agents
- Other Potential Biological Warfare and Bioterrorism Agents
- Bioterrorism Events in the United States
- Bioterrorism and the Clinical Microbiology Laboratory
- Laboratory Response Network

LEARNING OBJECTIVES

After studying this chapter, you should be able to:

- Define the terms and abbreviations introduced in this chapter (e.g., *antibiogram, biological warfare agents, bioterrorism*)

- List four factors that determine the frequency, distribution, and determinants of human diseases

- Differentiate between a nosocomial infection and a community-acquired infection

- List three organisms commonly associated with nosocomial infections

- State three measures taken to control or prevent infections in health care settings

- Name three ways clinical microbiology laboratory professionals participate in infection control

- Briefly explain how clinical microbiology laboratory professionals can determine if a bacterium isolated from an environmental sample is the *same* organism

isolated from patients during a hospital epidemic; describe the two most commonly used methods and general procedures

- List four pathogens most commonly discussed as potential biological weapons

- Briefly describe the Laboratory Response Network, including its purpose, makeup, and structure

ROLE OF THE CLINICAL MICROBIOLOGY LABORATORY IN HEALTH CARE EPIDEMIOLOGY

Terms and Definitions

Epidemiology. *Epidemiology* can be defined as the study of factors determining the frequency, distribution, and determinants of diseases in human populations. With respect to infectious diseases, these factors include the following:

- Characteristics of various pathogens

- Susceptibility of various human populations as a result of overcrowding, lack of immunization, nutritional status, and inadequate sanitation procedures, among others

- Locations (reservoirs) where pathogens lurk

- Various ways infectious diseases are transmitted

It could be said that epidemiologists are concerned with the who, what, where, when, and why of infectious diseases. Who becomes infected? What pathogens are causing the infections? Where do the pathogens come from? What are their modes of transmission? Where do certain diseases occur? Why do they occur in certain places but not elsewhere? When do the diseases occur? Why do some diseases occur only at certain times of the year? Epidemiologists also develop ways to prevent, control, or eradicate diseases in populations. It should be noted that epidemiologists are concerned with *all* types of diseases, not just infectious diseases.

Health care epidemiology. The Society for Healthcare Epidemiology of America (SHEA) defines *health care epidemiology* as "any activity designed to study and/or improve patient care outcomes in any type of health care institution or setting." On its Web site (http://www.shea-online.org), SHEA elaborates on that definition as follows:

Healthcare epidemiology . . . includes a variety of disciplines and activities directed at enhancing the quality of healthcare and preventing and controlling adverse outcomes. Among these activities are epidemiologic and laboratory investigation, surveillance, risk reduction programs focused on device and procedure management, policy development and implementation, education and information dissemination, and cost-benefit assessment of prevention and control programs.

Nosocomial infections. Infectious diseases can be divided into two categories: Those acquired within hospitals or other health care facilities are called **hospital-acquired infections** or **nosocomial infections.** Those acquired outside of health care facilities are called **community-acquired infections.** A hospitalized patient may have either type of infection. According to the Centers for Disease Control and Prevention (CDC), community-acquired infections are those that are present or incubating at the time of hospital admission. All other infections of hospitalized patients are considered to be nosocomial infections, including those erupting within 14 days of hospital discharge. **Iatrogenic infections** are diseases that develop after medical or surgical treatment and are thus caused by surgeons, other physicians, or other health care personnel. Examples of iatrogenic infections are postsurgical wound infections and urinary tract infections resulting from urinary catheterization.

> Infections that people acquire as a result of hospitalization are referred to as hospital-acquired or nosocomial infections. All other infections are referred to as community-acquired infections.

> Infections that result from medical or surgical treatment are known as iatrogenic infections.

Microorganisms commonly associated with nosocomial infections include *Escherichia coli, Staphylococcus aureus, Pseudomonas aeruginosa, Klebsiella pneumoniae, Enterobacter* spp., *Enterococcus* spp., coagulase-negative staphylococci, *Haemophilus influenzae,* and *Candida albicans.* Additional information about nosocomial infections can be found on the CD-ROM.

Hospital outbreaks/epidemics. Outbreaks within a hospital setting do not necessarily involve a large number of patients. An outbreak is defined as an increase in infection rate beyond the expected or usual rate during a defined period.

Infection control. Infection control pertains to the numerous measures taken to prevent infections from occurring in health care settings. These preventive measures include actions taken (1) to eliminate or contain reservoirs of infection, (2) to interrupt the transmission of pathogens, and (3) to protect people (patients, employees, and visitors) from becoming infected. In short, they are ways to break various links in the chain of infection.

Infection control committee. All health care facilities should have some type of formal infection control program. Although its specific functions vary depending on the type of health care facility, any infection control program is responsible for preventing, monitoring, and controlling the spread of infections in that facility. In a hospital setting, the program is often under the jurisdiction of an infection control committee (ICC) or epidemiology service. The ICC is composed of representatives from most of the hospital's departments, including medical and surgical services, the pathology department, nursing, hospital administration, risk management, pharmacy, housekeeping, food services, and central supply. The ICC periodically reviews the hospital's infection control program and the incidence of nosocomial infections. It is a policy-making and review body that may take drastic action, such as instituting quarantine measures, when epidemiologic circumstances warrant. Other ICC responsibilities include patient surveillance, environmental surveillance, investigation of outbreaks and epidemics, and education of the hospital staff regarding infection control.

> A hospital's infection control committee is primarily responsible for preventing, monitoring, and controlling the spread of infections in that facility.

Infection control professionals. The chairperson of the ICC is usually an infection control professional (ICP), such as a physician (e.g., an epidemiologist or infectious disease specialist), an infection control nurse, a microbiologist, or some other person knowledgeable about infection control. Additional information about ICPs can be found on the CD-ROM.

How Clinical Microbiology Professionals Participate in Infection Control

Clinical microbiology laboratory (CML) professionals participate in infection control in three major ways:

- By monitoring the types and numbers of pathogens isolated from hospitalized patients. In most hospitals, this type of monitoring is accomplished using computers and appropriate software programs.

- By promptly notifying the appropriate ICP when an unusual pathogen or an unusually high number of isolates of a common pathogen are detected. The ICP then initiates an investigation of the outbreak. As recommended by Diekema and Pfaller (2003; see "References and Suggested Reading"), "every clinical laboratory, in consultation with the infection control [committee, should] generate a list of epidemiologically important organisms that merit immediate notification of infection control personnel."

- By processing environmental samples collected from within every ward or unit affected by an outbreak. These samples include air and water; environmental surfaces like sink drains, air vents, and bed railings; and samples collected from health care workers, like nasal swabs, open lesions, and hand cultures. Even disinfectants, antiseptics, and soap dispensers can be sources of pathogens. Culturing environmental samples helps to pinpoint the exact source of the pathogen causing the outbreak.

Additional responsibilities of CML professionals in health care epidemiology include strict adherence to guidelines regarding specimen quality, employing accurate methods of identification and susceptibility testing of isolates, and proper storage of all epidemiologically important isolates.

Assume that there is an epidemic of *Klebsiella pneumoniae* infections on the pediatric floor and that *K. pneumoniae* has been isolated from an environmental sample collected on the floor. How do CML personnel determine that the *K. pneumoniae* isolated from the environmental sample is the same strain of *K. pneumoniae* isolated from the infected patients? Traditionally, the two most commonly used methods have been by biotype and antibiogram. If the two strains produce the exact same biochemical test results, they have the same **biotype.** If they produce the exact same susceptibility and resistance patterns when antimicrobial susceptibility testing is performed, they have the same **antibiogram.** Having the same biotype and antibiogram is evidence, but not absolute proof, that two isolates are the same strain.

> When two isolates produce identical biotypes and antibiograms, it is evidence, but not absolute proof, that they are the same strain.

However, because of the limitations of phenotypic methods such as biotypes and antibiograms, most hospitals practice **molecular epidemiology,** which uses genotypic methods to identify strains. Typically, these methods involve genotyping of plasmid and/or chromosomal DNA (see Table 26-1). Genotypic methods provide more accurate data than phenotypic methods. If the two isolates of *K. pneumoniae* in the previously cited example have exactly the same genotype (i.e., possess exactly the same genes), they arc the same strain, and therefore the source of the epidemic has been located.

As pointed out by Soll et al. (see "References and Suggested Reading"), "no dominant [genetic fingerprinting] method has emerged for all of the pathogen categories (bacteria, fungi, and parasites) or even for all species within a category."

TABLE 26 - 1 Examples of Methods Used in Molecular Epidemiology

Method	Substrate	Examples of Pathogens That Can Be Typed Using This Method
Plasmid fingerprinting	Plasmid DNA	Enterobacteriaceae such as *Klebsiella* spp., *Serratia* spp., and *Enterobacter* spp.; *Staphylococcus aureus*; coagulase-negative staphylococci
Polymerase chain reaction	Chromosomal DNA	*Candida* spp., *Clostridium difficile*, Enterobacteriaceae, *S. aureus*
Pulsed-field gel electrophoresis	Chromosomal DNA	*Candida* spp., Enterobacteriaceae, enterococci, *Pseudomonas* spp., staphylococci
Restriction endonuclease analysis of chromosomal DNA with conventional electrophoresis	Chromosomal DNA	*C. difficile*, *Enterococcus faecium*, *S. aureus*
Restriction-fragment length polymorphism analysis with nucleic acid probes	Chromosomal DNA	*Candida albicans*, Enterobacteriaceae, *Mycobacterium tuberculosis*, *S. aureus*

Source: Diekema DJ, Pfaller MA. Role of the clinical microbiology laboratory in hospital epidemiology and infection control. In: McClatchey KD, ed. Clinical Laboratory Medicine. 2nd Ed. Philadelphia: Lippincott Williams & Wilkins, 2002.

ROLE OF THE CLINICAL MICROBIOLOGY LABORATORY IN BIOTERRORISM

Category A Biological Warfare and Bioterrorism Agents

Unfortunately, pathogenic microorganisms sometimes find themselves in the hands of terrorists or extremists who want to use them to cause harm to others. In times of war, the use of microorganisms in this manner is called biological warfare, and the microbes are referred to as **biological warfare (BW) agents.** However, the danger does not exist solely during times of war. The possibility that members of terrorist or radical hate groups might use pathogens to create fear, chaos, illness, and death always exists. These people are referred to as biological terrorists or **bioterrorists,** and the specific microorganisms they use are called **bioterrorism agents.**

Four of the pathogens most often discussed as potential BW or bioterrorism agents are *Bacillus anthracis*, *Clostridium botulinum*, smallpox virus (variola virus), and *Yersinia pestis*, the etiologic agents of anthrax, botulism, smallpox, and plague, respectively. Each of these diseases has been described in previous chapters, but some additional and/or review information is presented here.

> Four of the pathogens most often discussed as potential BW or bioterrorism agents are *Bacillus anthracis, Clostridium botulinum,* smallpox virus (variola virus), and *Yersinia pestis.*

The CDC has classified the etiologic agents of anthrax, botulism, smallpox, and plague as category A bioterrorism agents. Category A agents are those that

- pose the greatest possible threat for a bad effect on public health,

- may spread across a large area or need public awareness, and

- need a great deal of planning to protect the public's health.

Anthrax

Anthrax is caused by *Bacillus anthracis*, a spore-forming Gram-positive bacillus (see Chapters 10 and 18). People can develop anthrax in several ways (Fig. 26-1), resulting in three forms of the disease: cutaneous anthrax, inhalation anthrax, and gastrointestinal anthrax. Anthrax infections involve marked hemorrhaging and serous effusions in various organs and body cavities and are frequently fatal. Of the three forms of anthrax, inhalation anthrax is the most severe, followed by gastrointestinal anthrax and then cutaneous

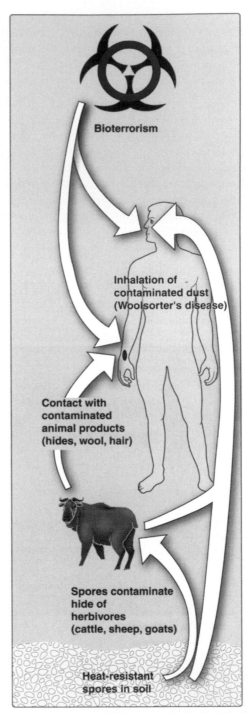

Figure 26-1. **Anthrax transmission.** (From Strohl WA, et al. Lippincott's Illustrated Reviews: Microbiology. Philadelphia: Lippincott Williams & Wilkins, 2001.)

anthrax. Patients with cutaneous anthrax develop lesions like that shown in Figure 26-2 (see also Fig. 18-7). In all three types of anthrax, symptoms can appear within 7 days of coming in contact with the pathogen. Anthrax can be treated using drugs such as ciprofloxacin, levofloxacin, doxycycline, or penicillin. Although a vaccine to prevent

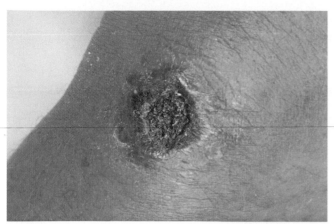

Figure 26-2. Black anthrax lesion (eschar) on a patient's fore-arm. The name of the disease comes from the Greek word *anthrax,* which means "coal," in reference to the black skin lesions of anthrax. (Courtesy of James H. Steele and the CDC.)

anthrax does exist, the vaccine is not yet available for the general public.

Bioterrorists could disseminate *B. anthracis* spores via aerosols or contamination of food supplies. In the fall of 2001, letters containing *B. anthracis* spores were mailed to several politicians and members of the news media. According to the CDC, a total of 22 cases of anthrax resulted: 11 cases of inhalation anthrax with 5 fatalities and 11 cases of cutaneous anthrax with no fatalities. Undoubtedly, many additional cases were prevented as a result of prompt prophylactic antibiotic therapy.

Botulism

Botulism was discussed in Chapter 17. A potentially fatal disease, botulism is caused by botulinal toxin, a neurotoxin produced by *Clostridium botulinum. C. botulinum* is a spore-forming anaerobic Gram-positive bacillus. Bioterrorists could add botulinal toxin to water supplies or food. Botulinal toxin is odorless and tasteless, and only a tiny quantity of the toxin need be ingested to cause a potentially fatal case of botulism. An antitoxin is available for treatment of patients with botulism. If untreated, botulism can result in paralysis of the arms, legs, trunk, and respiratory muscles and death.

Smallpox

Smallpox is a serious, contagious, and sometimes fatal infectious disease (see Chapter 25). Patients with smallpox are shown in Figures 26-3 and 26-4 (see also Fig. 25-15). Smallpox viruses are shown in Figure 26-5. The last case of

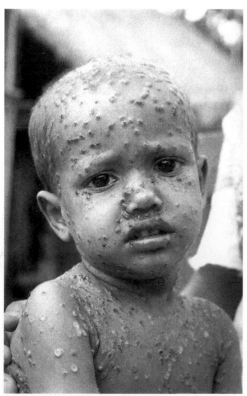

Figure 26-3. Child with smallpox. (Courtesy of Dr. Stan Foster and the CDC.)

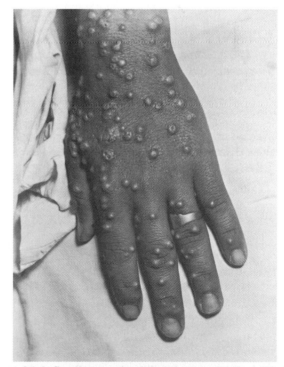

Figure 26-4. Smallpox patient's hand. (From Binford CH, Connor DH. Pathology of Tropical and Extraordinary Diseases, vol 2. Washington, DC: Armed Forces Institute of Pathology, 1976.)

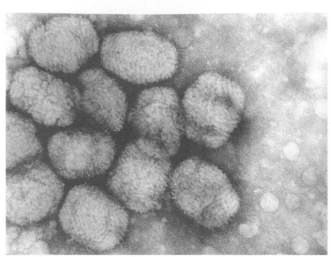

Figure 26-5. **Transmission electron micrograph of smallpox viruses.** (Courtesy of Fred Murphy, Sylvia Whitfield, and the CDC.)

smallpox in the United States was in 1949, and the last naturally occurring case in the world was in Somalia in 1977. Since 1980, when the World Health Organization announced that smallpox had been eradicated, most people no longer receive smallpox vaccinations. Thus, throughout the world, huge numbers of people are highly susceptible to the virus. Although there are no reservoirs for smallpox virus in nature, preserved samples of the virus exist in a few medical research laboratories worldwide. There is always the danger that smallpox virus, or any of the other pathogens mentioned here, could fall into the wrong hands. According to the CDC, the U.S. government has stockpiled enough smallpox vaccine to vaccinate every person in the country in case of a smallpox emergency.

It is important for clinicians to be able to distinguish smallpox from chickenpox, both of which are caused by poxviruses. Information regarding differentiation of these two diseases on clinical grounds is presented in Table 26-2.

Plague

Plague is caused by *Yersinia pestis*, a Gram-negative bacillus in the family Enterobacteriaceae (see Chapters 12 and 18). Plague is predominantly a zoonosis and is usually transmitted to humans by fleas (Fig. 26-6). Plague can manifest itself in several ways: bubonic plague, septicemic plague, pneumonic plague, and plague meningitis. Patients with plague are depicted in Figures 18-4 and 18-5. Bioterrorists could disseminate *Y. pestis* via aerosols, resulting in numerous severe and potentially fatal pulmonary infections. Pneumonic plague can be transmitted from person to person. The incubation period is 1 to 6 days, depending on

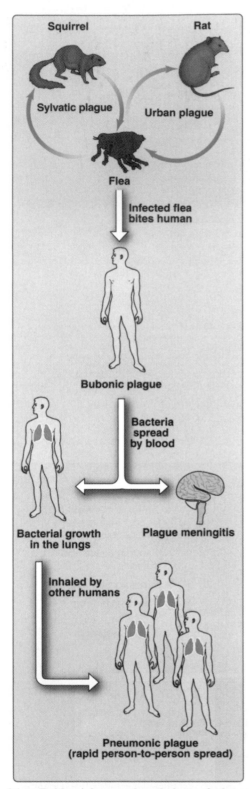

Figure 26-6. **Epidemiology and pathology of plague.** (From Strohl WA, et al. Lippincott's Illustrated Reviews: Microbiology. Philadelphia: Lippincott Williams & Wilkins, 2001.)

TABLE 26 - 2   Clinical Criteria Used to Differentiate Between Chickenpox and Smallpox

Chickenpox	Smallpox
No or mild prodrome	Febrile prodrome occurs 1 to 4 days before rash; fever greater than or equal to 101°F, and at least one of the following: prostration, headache, backache, chills, vomiting, or severe abdominal pain
Lesions are superficial vesicles, described as "dewdrops on a rose petal"	Deep-seated, hard, round, well-circumscribed vesicles or pustules; as they evolve, the lesions may become umbilicated or confluent
Lesions appear in crops; on any one part of the body, lesions may be in different stages (papules, vesicles, crusts)	On any one part of the body, all the lesions are in the same stage of development (i.e., all are vesicles or all are pustules)
Centripetal distribution of lesions, meaning that the greatest concentration of lesions is on the trunk and the fewest on distal extremities; may involve the face or scalp; occasionally, the entire body is equally affected	Centrifugal distribution of lesions, meaning that the greatest concentration of lesions is on the face and distal extremities (not the trunk)
First lesions appear on the face or trunk	First lesions appear on the oral mucosa or palate, face, or forearms
Patients are rarely toxic or moribund (dying)	Patients appear toxic or moribund
Rapid evolution of lesions; lesions evolve from macules to papules to vesicles to crusts quickly (less than 24 hours)	Slow evolution of lesions; lesions evolve from macules to papules to pustules over days; each stage lasts 1 to 2 days
Palms and soles are rarely involved	Lesions occur on palms and soles
Patients lack reliable history of chickenpox or chickenpox vaccination	
50% to 80% of patients recall exposure to chickenpox or shingles 10 to 21 days before onset of rash	

Source: Web site of the Centers for Disease Control and Prevention (http://www.cdc.gov/).

factors such as the number of organisms inhaled. Plague can be treated orally with tetracycline or a fluoroquinolone drug like ciprofloxacin, or intravenously using streptomycin or gentamicin.

Other Potential Biological Warfare and Bioterrorism Agents
Some of the other pathogens viewed as potential BW and bioterrorism agents are the etiologic agents of brucellosis, Q fever, tularemia, viral encephalitis, and viral hemorrhagic fevers. Table 26-3 lists potential bioterrorism agents that,

according to the CDC, pose the greatest threats to civilians—pathogens with which public health agencies must be prepared to cope.

Bioterrorism Events in the United States
In 1996, 45 laboratory employees in a large Texas medical center developed severe, acute diarrheal illness caused by *Shigella dysenteriae* type 2, a rare cause of diarrhea in the United States. An investigation revealed that a portion of the laboratory's stock culture of this organism had been deliberately used to contaminate muffins and doughnuts anonymously

TABLE 26 - 3	Critical Biological Agent Categories for Public Health Preparedness	
Category	**Biological Agent(s)**	**Disease**
Category A: agents having the greatest potential for adverse public health impact; most require broad-based public health preparedness efforts	Variola virus	Smallpox
	Bacillus anthracis	Anthrax
	Yersinia pestis	Plague
	Clostridium botulinum	Botulism (botulinal toxins)
	Francisella tularensis	Tularemia
	Filoviruses and arenaviruses (e.g., Ebola virus, Lassa virus)	Viral hemorrhagic fevers
Category B: agents having a moderate to high potential for large-scale dissemination or a heightened general public health awareness that could cause mass public fear and civil disruption	Coxiella burnetii	Q fever
	Brucella spp.	Brucellosis
	Burkholderia mallei	Glanders
	Burkholderia pseudomallei	Melioidosis
	Alphaviruses (Venezuela equine, eastern equine, and western equine encephalitis viruses)	Encephalitis
	Rickettsia prowazekii	Typhus fever
	Toxins (e.g., ricin [from the castor oil plant], staphylococcal enterotoxin B)	Toxic syndromes
	Chlamydia psittaci	Psittacosis
	Food safety threats (e.g., Salmonella spp., Escherichia coli O157:H7)	
	Water safety threats (e.g., Vibrio cholerae, Cryptosporidium parvum)	
Category C: agents currently not believed to present a high bioterrorism risk to public health but could emerge as future threats	Emerging threat agents (e.g., Nipah virus, hantavirus)	

Source: Rotz LD, et al. Public health assessment of potential biological terrorism agents. Emerging Infectious Diseases 2002;8:225–230 (prepared and published by the National Center for Infectious Diseases, Centers for Disease Control and Prevention, based on unclassified information).

left in the laboratory break room and subsequently eaten by laboratory employees. It is not known whether the culprit was ever apprehended.

An instance of bioterrorism occurred in a small Oregon town in 1984. Members of a religious cult purposely contaminated salad bars at two restaurants with *Salmonella typhimurium* in an attempt to sicken local citizens and thus prevent them from voting in an upcoming election. They also contaminated the drinking water of two county commissioners. More than 750 people became ill, including the two commissioners, but no deaths occurred. The Japanese cult that released nerve gas in the Tokyo subway system in

1995, killing 12 people and injuring about 3,800, has also attempted to develop botulinal toxin and the agents of anthrax, cholera, and Q fever for bioterrorism use.

During the late 1990s, numerous anthrax threats occurred in the United States, but fortunately most turned out to be hoaxes. The events of the fall of 2001, regarding mailing of *Bacillus anthracis* spores, were described earlier in this chapter.

To minimize the danger of potentially deadly microorganisms falling into the wrong hands, the U.S. Antiterrorism and Effective Death Penalty Act of 1996 makes the CDC responsible for controlling shipment of select agents—pathogens and toxins—deemed most likely to be used as BW agents. On its Web site, the American Society for Microbiology (ASM, http://www.asm.org/) offers this definition: "Select agents are microorganisms, biological agents, or biological toxins that have been deemed by the United States Government to be major threats to public safety because they could be used as agents of bioterrorism." The following are some of these select agents:

- *Bacillus anthracis*

- *Brucella abortus*

- *Clostridium botulinum* neurotoxin

- *Coccidioides immitis*

- *Francisella tularensis*

- Hemorrhagic fever viruses

- Reconstructed replication competent forms of the 1918 pandemic influenza H1N1 virus

- Smallpox virus

- *Yersinia pestis*

Authorities must constantly be on the alert for possible theft of these pathogens from biological supply houses and legitimate laboratories. In addition, vaccines, antitoxins, and other antidotes must be available wherever the threat of the use of these biological agents is high, as in various potential war zones.

Bioterrorism and the Clinical Microbiology Laboratory

The ASM has recommended that all CMLs be staffed with persons familiar with the likely agents of bioterrorism and trained to detect, identify, and safely handle these agents. Snyder and Weissfeld (see "References and Suggested Reading") describe the role of CMLs as follows:

Detection and recognition of a possible [bioterrorism] event will be dependent upon several factors, including an active

microbial surveillance and monitoring program, vigilant laboratory staff who are capable of recognizing the unusual or who develop a high index of suspicion, and communication with clinicians (especially emergency medical personnel), infection control personnel, infectious disease specialists, and other local or regional laboratories.

The following excerpt is from a 2001 colloquium report from the American Academy of Microbiology and the American College of Microbiology titled "Bioterrorism Threats to Our Future: The Role of Clinical Microbiology in Detection, Identification, and Confirmation of Biological Agents" (the full report is available at http://www.asm.org/):

In the case of a possible bioterrorism event, the key responsibilities of the hospital-based clinical microbiology laboratory are to be familiar with the likely agents of bioterrorism and to be prepared to use the Level A laboratory algorithms [described later in the chapter] designed for the detection of these agents. Using these algorithms, clinical microbiology laboratories rule out bioterrorism-related microorganisms and identify suspicious isolates.

The clinical microbiology laboratory will have a very significant role in the determination of whether or not a bioterrorism event has taken place and, if an attack is occurring, what kind of agent is being used. In the event of a biological attack, the early recognition and detection of the causative agent will pose a formidable challenge to the microbiologist and the clinical microbiology laboratory staff. Not only will the clinical microbiology laboratory be expected to detect and identify the agent in a timely manner, bit it also will be expected to provide information regarding the selection, collection, safe handling, and transport of specimens to an appropriate laboratory with a level of biosafety capability compatible with the potential threat.

A large-scale bioterrorism attack would place a tremendous burden on CMLs, as illustrated by the following excerpt from a 2006 article by Montoya (see "References and Suggested Reading"):

In the event of an attack and before supplies arrive, physicians and nurses will be faced with massive numbers (hundreds to thousands) of patients presenting with various symptoms, which will require supportive therapy. It is reasonable to expect exposed patients to experience vomiting, diarrhea, dehydration, and numerous other symptoms depending on the toxin [or pathogen] they have been exposed to. Treatment providers will require substantial laboratory work to appropriately treat patients. Tests such as electrolytes, basic chemistries (glucose, renal, and liver function tests), CBCs, and cultures are minimal essentials needed to make objective medical decisions. After treatment supplies arrive from the federal government, and patients are treated, these same basic tests will be required plus other tests necessary to monitor patients.

TABLE 26 - 4 Laboratory Response Network for Bioterrorism

Laboratory Level	Description	Responsibilities
A: Sentinel laboratory	Basic: certified for general laboratory testing; has policies and procedures for referral of diagnostic specimens to an advanced sentinel laboratory; possesses CDC-published algorithms for ruling out suspicious agents Advanced: certified as high-complexity laboratory; must possess a class II or higher certified biological safety cabinet and must comply with BSL-2 practices; possesses CDC-published algorithms for ruling out suspicious agents	Act as sentinels for raising suspicion of a bioterrorism event; capable of making presumptive identifications of some targeted organisms, but must refer suspicious isolates to a reference laboratory; must have personnel who have been trained and certified in packing and shipping of infectious substances
B: Reference laboratory	Local or state public health laboratory or selected academic- or university-based laboratory; follows BSL-3 containment and practice guidelines	Possesses the reagents and technology for definitive confirmation of organisms, including toxin testing, that have been referred by a sentinel laboratory
C: National laboratory	Known as a "hot lab," with BSL-4 containment facilities and practice guidelines; located at the CDC or the U.S. Army Medical Research Institute of Infectious Diseases	Has unique resources to handle highly infectious agents (e.g., Ebola, Marburg, and smallpox viruses) and the ability to identify specific agents; performs specialized tests (such as advanced genetic characterization) and archive isolates

Sources: Web sites of the CDC (http://www.bt.cdc.gov/lrn/factsheet.asp) and the American Society for Microbiology (http://www.asm.org/). BSL, biosafety level; CDC, Centers for Disease Control and Prevention.

Laboratory Response Network

The CDC has established the Laboratory Response Network (LRN), a consortium of laboratories that provides immediate and sustained laboratory testing and communication in support of public health emergencies, particularly in response to acts of bioterrorism. The LRN structure for bioterrorism consists of three levels of laboratories, designated as sentinel, reference, and national laboratories (Table 26-4). The recommended biosafety levels for handling of potential bioterrorism agents are shown in Table 26-5.

Level A laboratories are primarily the microbiology laboratories found in hospitals, clinics, and small public health facilities. These laboratories are capable of handling and processing clinical specimens required for isolation of the most likely potential bacterial agents of bioterrorism, and work with clinical diagnostic cultures for four of these agents; namely, *B. anthracis, Y. pestis, F. tularensis,* and *Brucella* spp. The pathogen identification criteria (algorithms) used by level A laboratories is contained in Table 26-6.

As stated by the previously referenced colloquium report, "Rapid recognition of potential bioterrorism agents by Level A clinical microbiology laboratories will be essential for the public health response to a bioterrorism event."

TABLE 26 - 5	Recommended Biosafety Levels (BSLs) for Handling Potential Bioterrorism Agents	
Agent	**BSL-2 Procedures**	**BSL-3 Procedures**
Alphaviruses (includes various equine encephalitis viruses)	Activities limited to collection and transport of clinical material	Culture handling
Bacillus anthracis	Activities limited to collection of clinical material and handling of diagnostic quantities of infectious cultures	Culture handling; activities with high potential for aerosol or droplet production
Brucella spp. (laboratory-acquired infections have occurred)	Activities limited to collection, transport, and plating of clinical material	All activities involving manipulation of cultures
Burkholderia pseudomallei	Activities limited to collection, transport, and plating of clinical material	All activities involving manipulation of cultures
Burkholderia mallei	Activities limited to collection, transport, and plating of clinical material	All activities involving manipulation of cultures
Coxiella burnetii (laboratory-acquired infections have occurred)	Activities limited to collection and transport of clinical material, including specimens for serological examinations	Culture handling
Clostridium botulinum (toxin is extremely poisonous)	Activities involving materials known to be or potentially containing toxin must be handled in a class II biosafety cabinet, with a lab coat, disposable surgical gloves, and a face shield (as needed)	Culture handling; activities with high potential for aerosol or droplet production
Francisella tularensis (laboratory-acquired infections have occurred)	Activities limited to collection, transport, and plating of clinical material	All activities involving manipulation of cultures
Yersinia pestis	Activities limited to collection of clinical material and handling of diagnostic quantities of infectious cultures; special care should be taken to avoid the generation of aerosols	Culture handling; activities with high potential for aerosol or droplet production
Smallpox virus (laboratory-acquired infections have occurred)	Activities limited to packing and shipping; do not inoculate cell cultures	N/A; culture handling to be performed at BSL-4 facilities
Staphylococcal enterotoxin B	Activities limited to collection of clinical material and handling of diagnostic quantities of infectious cultures	N/A
Hemorrhagic fever viruses (includes Ebola, Marburg, Lassa viruses, etc.); laboratory-acquired infections have occurred	Activities limited to packing and shipping; do not inoculate cell cultures	N/A; culture handling to be performed at BSL-4 facilities

Source: Web site of the American Society for Microbiology (http://www.asm.org/).
N/A, not applicable.

TABLE 26 - 6   Level A Laboratory Criteria for Presumptive Identification of Bioterrorism Agents

Agent	Presumptive Identification Criteria
Bacillus anthracis (see Chapters 10 and 18 for additional information)	Large (1 to 1.5 μm wide by 3 to 5 μm long) aerobic Gram-positive bacilli. In smears of blood or cerebrospinal fluid, short chains of 2 to 4 cells that appear encapsulated. Colonies on sheep blood agar at 15 to 24 hours are 2 to 5 mm in diameter, tenacious, nonhemolytic, flat or slightly convex, irregularly round, with irregular or wavy borders and a ground-glass appearance. Gram stains of colonies reveal that cells contain oval, central-to-subterminal spores that do not cause significant swelling of the cell. Cells are often seen in long chains. Nonmotile, catalase positive. **Perform all subsequent work in a biosafety cabinet.** Report "*Bacillus* sp." and send to a reference laboratory for definitive identification.
Brucella spp.: as soon as *Brucella* is suspected, perform all further work in a biosafety cabinet, BSL-3 (see Chapter 14 for additional information)	Small (0.4 μm wide by 0.8 μm long) Gram-negative coccobacilli. Visible on Gram stain of positive blood culture broth. Poor growth on blood agar and chocolate agar at 24 hours. Does not grow on MAC. Does not satellite around *Staphylococcus aureus* colonies. Oxidase positive, catalase positive, and urea positive. Report "Possible *Brucella* sp." and send to a reference laboratory for definitive identification.
Burkholderia mallei (see Chapter 13 for additional information)	Gram-negative coccobacilli or small bacilli. Poor growth on blood agar at 24 hours. Better growth of gray, translucent colonies at 48 hours. May or may not grow on MAC. No distinctive odor. Resistant to polymyxin B or colistin. No growth on *Burkholderia cepacia* selective agars. Nonmotile, oxidase variable, indole negative, catalase positive. Red slant (no change)/red butt in TSI or KIA. Report "Possible *Burkholderia mallei*" and send to a reference laboratory for definitive identification.
Burkholderia pseudomallei (see Chapter 13 for additional information)	Straight or slightly curved, small Gram-negative bacillus. Poor growth on blood agar at 24 hours but good growth of white colonies at 48 hours. May develop nonpigmented, wrinkled colonies in time. Often has a strong, characteristic musty or earthy odor. On Gram stains of colonies, cells may demonstrate bipolar morphology at 24 hours and peripheral staining when cultures are old. Growth on MAC at 48 hours. Indole negative, oxidase positive. Resistant to polymyxin B or colistin. No growth on *Burkholderia cepacia* selective agars. Red slant (no change)/variable butt in TSI agar or KIA. Report "Possible *Burkholderia pseudomallei*" and send to a reference laboratory for definitive identification.
Francisella tularensis (see Chapters 14 and 18 for additional information)	Aerobic, pleomorphic, tiny (0.2 to 0.5 μm wide by 0.7 to 1.0 μm long), faintly staining Gram-negative coccobacilli. Scant to no growth on blood agar after >48 hours. Produces 1-to-2-mm-diameter, gray-to-grayish-white colonies on chocolate agar after >48 hours. Oxidase negative, weakly catalase positive, β-lactamase positive, urease-negative. Does not satellite around *Staphylococcus aureus* colonies. **Perform all subsequent work in a biosafety cabinet.** Report "Suspect *Francisella tularensis*; could not rule out" and send to a reference laboratory for definitive identification.
Yersinia pestis (see Chapters 12 and 18 for additional information)	Facultative, bipolar-staining, Gram-negative bacilli, 0.5 μm wide by 1.0 to 2.0 μm long. Slow-growing, pinpoint (1-to-2-mm-diameter), gray-white to opaque colonies on blood agar after 24 hours. Non–lactose fermenter. Growth possible on MAC or eosin-methylene blue at 24 hours. Oxidase negative, catalase positive, urease negative, indole negative. Report "Suspect *Yersinia pestis*; could not rule out" and send to a reference laboratory for definitive identification.

Source: Web site of the American Society for Microbiology (http://www.asm.org/).
KIA, Kligler iron agar; MAC, MacConkey agar; TSI, triple-sugar iron.

Chapter Review

- *Epidemiology* is defined as the study of factors that determine the frequency, distribution, and determinants of diseases in human populations. These factors include characteristics of the pathogen, susceptibility of various human populations, lack of immunizations, nutritional status, and sanitation, among others.

- Epidemiologists are concerned with the who, what, where, when, and why of infectious diseases.

- Nosocomial infections are infections acquired within hospitals or other health care facilities, whereas community-acquired infections are acquired elsewhere.

- Patients contract iatrogenic infections following medical or surgical treatment; thus, surgeons, other physicians, or other health care personnel are the cause of these infections.

- Microorganisms commonly associated with nosocomial infections include *Escherichia coli*, *Staphylococcus aureus*, *Pseudomonas aeruginosa*, *Klebsiella pneumoniae*, *Enterobacter* spp., *Enterococcus* spp., coagulase-negative staphylococci, *Haemophilus influenzae*, and *Candida albicans*.

- Measures taken to prevent infections from occurring in health care settings include elimination of reservoirs of infection; interruption of the transmission of pathogens; and protection of patients, employees, and visitors.

- A health care facility's infection control committee is primarily responsible for preventing, monitoring, and controlling the spread of infections in the facility.

- CML professionals participate in infection control by (1) monitoring the types and numbers of pathogens isolated from hospitalized patients; (2) notifying the appropriate infection control practitioner when an unusual pathogen is isolated; and (3) processing environmental samples that have been collected from within the affected ward, floor, or unit.

- The most commonly used methods to determine if a bacterium that has been isolated from an environmental sample is the same as the organisms being isolated from infected patients are comparing their biotypes, comparing their antibiograms, and using molecular epidemiologic techniques.

- Especially virulent microorganisms may be used as biological warfare agents or by bioterrorists. The four most commonly discussed agents are *Bacillus anthracis*, smallpox virus, *Clostridium botulinum*, and *Yersinia pestis*. Other possible agents include those that cause brucellosis, Q fever, tularemia, viral encephalitis, and viral hemorrhagic fevers.

- The Laboratory Response Network of the CDC is a consortium of laboratories that provides immediate and sustained laboratory testing and communication in the response to bioterrorism. The LRN structure for bioterrorism consists of three levels of laboratories designated as sentinel, reference, and national laboratories.

New Terms and Abbreviations

After studying Chapter 26, you should be familiar with the following terms, which are defined within the chapter and in the Glossary at the back of the book:

Antibiogram

Biological warfare (BW) agent

Bioterrorism

Bioterrorism agent

Biotype

Community-acquired infection

Epidemiology

Health care epidemiology

Hospital outbreak

Iatrogenic infection

Infection control

Infection control committee

Infection control professional

Molecular epidemiology

Nosocomial infection

References and Suggested Reading

Diekema DJ, Pfaller MA. Infection control epidemiology and clinical microbiology. In: Murray PR, Baron EJ, Jorgensen JH, Pfaller MA, Yolken RH, eds. Manual of Clinical Microbiology. 8th Ed. Washington, DC: ASM Press, 2003.

Diekema DJ, Pfaller MA. Role of the clinical microbiology laboratory in hospital epidemiology and infection control. In: McClatchey KD, ed. Clinical Laboratory Medicine. 2nd Ed. Philadelphia: Lippincott Williams & Wilkins, 2002.

Montoya ID. Bioterror defense and its impact on the clinical laboratory. Clin Lab Sci 2006;19:68–69.

Snyder JW, Weissfeld AS. Laboratory detection of potential agents of bioterrorism. In: Murray PR, Baron EJ, Jorgensen JH, Pfaller MA, Yolken RH, eds. Manual of Clinical Microbiology. 8th Ed. Washington, DC: ASM Press, 2003.

Soll DR, et al. Laboratory procedures for the epidemiological analysis of microorganisms. In: Murray PR, Baron EJ, Jorgensen JH, Pfaller MA, Yolken RH, eds. Manual of Clinical Microbiology. 8th Ed. Washington, DC: ASM Press, 2003.

Consult the Web sites of the CDC (http://www.bt.cdc.gov/) and the ASM (http://www.asm.org/) for additional information on bioterrorism.

 On the CD-ROM

- A Closer Look at Nosocomial Infections
- Infection Control Professionals
- Additional Self-Assessment Exercises
- Puzzle

Self-Assessment Exercises

1. List four factors that determine the frequency, distribution, and determinants of diseases in human populations.

   A. _____

   B. _____

   C. _____

   D. _____

2. Briefly define *nosocomial*.

   _____

3. List two examples of iatrogenic infections.

   A. _____

   B. _____

4. List three organisms commonly associated with nosocomial infections.

   A. _____

   B. _____

   C. _____

5. List three major ways microbiology laboratory professionals participate in infection control.

   A. _____

   B. _____

   C. _____

6. True or false: If two strains of an organism are found to have the exact same biochemical test results, they are said to have the same antibiogram.

7. Name three bacterial pathogens that could be used by a bioterrorist.

   A. _____

   B. _____

   C. _____

8. What are the three levels of laboratories in the Laboratory Response Network?

A. _____

B. _____

C. _____

9. Based on the following clinical information, identify the most likely bioterrorism agent. The isolate is an aerobic Gram-positive bacillus that is large, nonmotile, and catalase positive. Colonies are flat, have a ground-glass appearance, and are nonhemolytic.

A. *Brucella* sp.

B. *Bacillus anthracis*

C. *Burkholderia mallei*

D. *Yersinia pestis*

10. True or false: If two bacterial isolates, one from a patient and one from the hospital environment, have exactly the same biotype and antibiogram, then the two isolates are the same organism.

Appendix A

Clinical Microbiology Laboratory Procedures

This appendix contains details of laboratory procedures mentioned but not fully described in the text. The procedures, listed in the following table, are presented in a manner conducive to learning but are not in any particular "prescribed" format. As described, the procedures can be performed in a student microbiology laboratory. In an actual clinical microbiology laboratory (CML), all procedures should be performed according to instructions in that laboratory's procedures manual. See "References and Suggested Reading" for a list of the primary sources used to prepare this appendix; these texts should be consulted for additional details.

Procedure	Page
Inoculating and incubating plated culture media	685
Determining a colony count	686
Using a compound light microscope	686
Calibrating an ocular micrometer	687
Wet mount procedure: differentiating between bacterial and yeast colonies	687
Wet mount procedure for diagnosis of vaginal infections	688
Preparing a smear of a clinical specimen for staining	689
Preparing a smear of a bacterial colony for staining	689
Preparing thick and thin blood smears	689
Potassium hydroxide preparation (KOH prep)	690
Direct simple staining	690
India ink preparation	690
Capsule staining	690
Spore staining	691
Gram staining	691
Sputum digestion, decontamination, and concentration	693
Acid-fast staining	693
Ziehl-Neelsen acid-fast stain	693
Kinyoun acid-fast stain	694

(continued)

(Continued)

(Continued)

Procedure	Page
Novobiocin resistance	705
O-F (oxidation-fermentation)	705
ONPG (o-nitrophenyl-β-D-galactopyranoside)	706
Optochin sensitivity (P-disk)	706
Oxidase	707
Modified oxidase	707
PAD (phenylalanine deaminase)	707
PYR (pyrrolidonyl arylamidase)	708
PZA (pyrazinamidase)	708
Rapid hippurate hydrolysis	708
Salt tolerance	709
TCH (thiophene-2-carboxylic acid hydrazide)	709
Urease	709
X and V factors	710

INOCULATING AND INCUBATING PLATED CULTURE MEDIA

Because the ideal growth temperature of most human pathogens is 35°C to 37°C, it is important that clinical specimens be inoculated to appropriate culture media and incubated as soon as possible following collection. Specimens are inoculated to the surface of plated media in a manner conducive to producing isolated colonies. The proper way to inoculate the surface of a plate of solid medium is depicted in Figure A-1, and the results of proper inoculation are shown in Figure A-2. Anyone working with clinical specimens must wear disposable latex gloves.

Procedure

1. Inoculate approximately one-quarter of the surface of the medium by *gently* streaking a swab of the specimen in a zig-zag manner over the surface of the medium.

2. Use a sterile bacteriological inoculating loop to streak the second quarter of the agar surface, being careful not to tear the medium with the loop.

3. Use the inoculating loop to streak the third and fourth quarters of the agar surface.

4. Place the inoculated plate into a incubator at 35°C to 37°C.

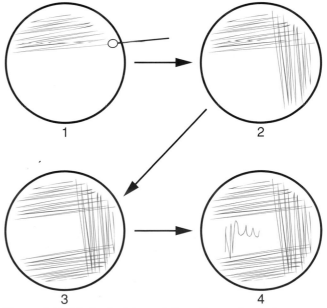

Figure A-1. **Method of inoculating the surface of an agar medium to obtain isolated colonies.** (From Winn WC Jr, et al. Koneman's Color Atlas and Textbook of Diagnostic Microbiology. 6th Ed. Philadelphia: Lippincott Williams & Wilkins, 2006.)

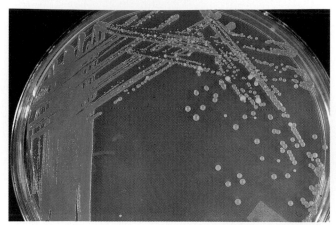

Figure A-2. **Agar medium inoculated to obtain isolated colonies.** (From Winn WC Jr, et al. Koneman's Color Atlas and Textbook of Diagnostic Microbiology. 6th Ed. Philadelphia: Lippincott Williams & Wilkins, 2006.)

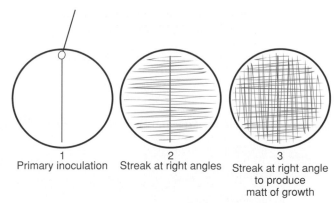

Figure A-3. **Method of inoculating the surface of an agar medium to obtain a colony count.** (From Winn WC Jr, et al. Koneman's Color Atlas and Textbook of Diagnostic Microbiology. 6th Ed. Philadelphia: Lippincott Williams & Wilkins, 2006.)

DETERMINING A COLONY COUNT

Purpose. Although this procedure can be used to determine the number of viable bacteria in any liquid specimen, it is primarily performed on urine specimens. A urine culture has three parts: (1) a colony count, (2) identification of the pathogen, and (3) antimicrobial susceptibility testing. The results of the colony count are reported as the number of colony-forming units (CFUs) per milliliter of urine. Because each colony on the plate theoretically started as a single live bacterial cell, reporting the number of CFUs per milliliter of urine to the clinician informs him or her of the number of live bacteria present in the specimen.

Procedure

1. Dip a sterile 0.01-mL or 0.001-mL calibrated loop into a clean-catch midstream urine specimen. A calibrated loop is a bacteriological loop manufactured to contain a precise quantity of liquid.

2. With the calibrated loop, spread the urine over the entire surface of the plate, using the technique shown in Figure A-3.

3. Incubate the inoculated plate overnight at 35°C to 37°C.

4. Remove the plate from the incubator and count the colonies; experienced CML professionals are able to correctly estimate the number of colonies.

Interpretation of results. To obtain the number of CFUs per milliliter of urine, multiply the number of colonies on the plate by the appropriate dilution factor. With the 0.01-mL calibrated loop, the dilution factor is 100; with the 0.001-mL calibrated loop, the dilution factor is 1,000. For example, a 0.001-mL calibrated loop was used, and 300 colonies grew on the plate. The colony count is $300 \times 1,000 = 300,000$, or 3×10^5 CFU/mL.

What to report. Report the number of CFUs per milliliter.

USING A COMPOUND LIGHT MICROSCOPE
Using the Microscope

1. Remove the microscope from its storage location (if applicable).

2. Remove the dust cover.

3. Plug in the electrical cord.

4. Turn the microscope light on.

5. Make sure that the low-power ($\times$10) objective is in place.

6. Place glass microscope slide on the stage (always make sure that the slide is right side up).

7. Adjust the distance between the oculars (the interocular distance) to match the distance between your eyes.

8. Focus using the coarse-adjustment knob (large inner knob).

9. Make certain that the object to be observed at a higher magnification is centered in the field of view.

10. Swing the high-dry ($\times$40) objective into place.

11. Focus using the fine-adjustment knob (small outer knob).

12. Adjust lighting, if necessary: first, open the iris diaphragm in the condenser; next, open the field diaphragm; finally, turn the rheostat knob to a higher setting.

13. Make certain that the object to be observed at a higher magnification is centered in the field.

14. Swing the $\times$40 objective out of the way.

15. Add one drop of immersion oil to the center of the circle of light coming through the microscope slide.

16. Slowly swing the ×100 objective into place. If it bumps into the microscope slide or coverslip, **something is wrong**—perhaps the microscope slide is upside down—so **seek assistance.**

17. **Caution: Never use the coarse-adjustment knob when the ×100 objective is in place.**

18. Focus using the fine-adjustment knob (small outer knob). Turn the knob very slowly in one direction for only one or two revolutions. If the object does not come into focus, turn the knob very slowly in the other direction for one or two revolutions. If the object still does not come into focus, **seek assistance.**

19. Adjust lighting, if necessary: first, open the iris diaphragm in the condenser; next, open the field diaphragm; finally, turn the rheostat knob to a higher setting.

Putting Away the Microscope

1. Swing the low power (×10) objective into place.

2. Remove the microscope slide from the stage.

3. Turn off the microscope lamp.

4. Check the high-dry (×40) objective for immersion oil. **Check for and remove oil with authorized lens paper only** (if in doubt as to what constitutes **authorized** lens paper, **seek assistance**). If necessary, propanol can be used as a solvent.

5. Remove immersion oil from the oil immersion (×100) lens. **Use authorized lens paper only.**

6. Check the stage for immersion oil; if oil is present, remove it using lens paper.

7. Wrap the electric cord around the base of the microscope.

8. Place dust cover over the microscope.

9. Use two hands to place microscope into its storage cabinet (if applicable).

10. Remove immersion oil from microscope slides that have permanently attached coverslips; do **not** rub oil off stained smears that do not have coverslips.

11. Store slides in their proper locations (if applicable).

CALIBRATING AN OCULAR MICROMETER

Purpose. An ocular micrometer is used to measure the size of objects being examined microscopically. An ocular micrometer is a circular glass wafer that fits into one of the ×10 oculars of a binocular microscope, usually the right ocular. Etched into the wafer is a tiny scale.

Principle. Before it can be used to measure objects, an ocular micrometer must be calibrated for use with the intended microscope and objective lenses. If the ocular micrometer is then transferred to a different microscope, it must be recalibrated.

Procedure

1. Place the ocular micrometer, engraved side down, inside the right-hand ocular, and return the ocular to its usual position. When viewed through both oculars, the ocular micrometer should appear as shown in Figure A-4A.

2. Place the stage micrometer onto the microscope stage. When viewed through the left-hand ocular, it should appear as shown in Figure A-4B.

3. With the high-dry (×40) objective in place and looking through both oculars, move the stage micrometer until the 0 line on the ocular micrometer is exactly superimposed with the 0.0 line, as shown in Figure A-4C.

4. Starting where the left edges of the two scales are superimposed, look to the right until you see two lines that are exactly superimposed. The arrow in Figure A-4D is pointing to that pair of superimposed lines. The lines are 40 on the ocular micrometer scale and 0.09 on the stage micrometer.

Interpretation. Calibration is determined as follows:

1. A reading of 40 units on the ocular scale equals 0.09 mm on the stage micrometer scale.

2. Thus, each division on the ocular scale is equal to 0.09 mm divided by 40, or 0.00225 mm (which is equal to 2.25 μm).

3. Therefore, when measuring an object using the high-dry lens, the size of the object (in μm) is 2.25 times the number of divisions it occupies on the ocular scale.

For example, if the diameter of a spherical object is 20 ocular scale divisions, the object's diameter is 20 × 2.25 μm, or 45 μm.

It is important to understand that a separate calibration must be performed for each of the microscope's objectives, and that the calibration is only good for that particular microscope.

WET MOUNT PROCEDURE: DIFFERENTIATING BETWEEN BACTERIAL AND YEAST COLONIES

Purpose. The wet mount procedure is a very simple method of examining unstained materials (e.g., liquid clinical specimens, broth cultures, bacterial and yeast colonies). Because of the

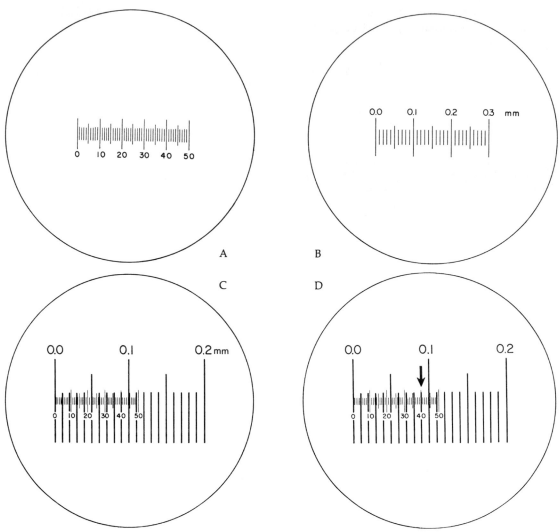

Figure A-4. **Calibration of an ocular micrometer.** (From Winn WC Jr, et al. Koneman's Color Atlas and Textbook of Diagnostic Microbiology. 6th Ed. Philadelphia: Lippincott Williams & Wilkins, 2006.)

similarity in their appearance, it is sometimes impossible to determine if a particular colony is a yeast colony or bacterial colony simply by macroscopic observation. A CML professional can prepare and examine a wet mount of a colony to determine whether the colony comprises yeast cells or bacterial cells.

Procedure

1. Add a drop of sterile water to a clean glass microscope slide.

2. Using a sterile bacteriological inoculating loop, mix a very small portion of the colony into the drop of sterile water.

3. Cover the preparation with a glass coverslip.

4. Examine the preparation under the microscope as described in the section titled "Using a Compound Light Microscope." The oil immersion lens is not used when examining wet mounts.

Interpretation of results. Yeast cells can be distinguished from bacterial cells by size and shape. Yeast cells are larger—up to about 10 times larger than bacteria. Also, yeast cells are usually oval shaped, and some may be observed in the process of budding. Bacteria do not produce buds.

Sometimes, after prolonged examination, nonmotile objects (such as yeast cells) on a wet mount start to "jiggle." This jiggling, technically called **Brownian movement,** is the result of heat generated by the microscope bulb. The heat causes water molecules to move about rapidly, striking the objects, and causing them to jiggle.

WET MOUNT PROCEDURE FOR DIAGNOSIS OF VAGINAL INFECTIONS

Purpose. A wet mount examination of vaginal discharge material can be used in the laboratory diagnosis of vaginal infection. The specimen is examined for the presence of yeasts (*Candida albicans*) or protozoa (*Trichomonas vaginalis*) or evidence of bacterial infection.

Procedure

1. Place a small drop of sterile saline onto a clean glass microscope slide.

2. Obtain some vaginal discharge material using a sterile swab.

3. Gently stir the swab in the drop of saline.

4. Place a glass coverslip over the preparation. Do not allow the specimen to dry.

5. Examine the preparation under the microscope, using reduced lighting. The oil immersion lens is not used when examining wet mounts.

Interpretation of results. The presence of very large quantities of yeast cells is suggestive of yeast vaginitis. A presumptive or tentative diagnosis of trichomoniasis can be made if motile trophozoites of *T. vaginalis* are seen (see Figs. 22-18 and 22-19). The presence of clue cells (squamous epithelial cells densely covered with small coccobacilli; see Fig. 18-23) is suggestive of bacterial vaginosis. If bacterial vaginosis is suspected, a Gram stain of the vaginal fluid should be prepared. Few Gram-positive bacilli (*Lactobacillus* spp.) will be seen in bacterial vaginosis, but large numbers of Gram-negative bacilli (*Bacteroides* spp.), Gram-variable coccobacilli (*Gardnerella vaginalis*), and curved Gram-negative bacilli (*Mobiluncus* spp.) will be seen.

PREPARING A SMEAR OF A CLINICAL SPECIMEN FOR STAINING

Procedure

1. If the specimen is a swab, prepare a smear by rolling the swab over the center portion of a clean glass microscope slide. Check to make sure that you have only one microscope slide; sometimes they stick together. If the specimen is a liquid, dip a sterile swab or sterile bacteriological inoculating loop into the specimen, and then spread a drop of the specimen over the center portion of a glass microscope slide. Always discard used swabs in the appropriate infectious waste container.

2. Allow the smear to air dry.

3. Fix the smear at a staining station by covering it with absolute (100%) methanol. After 30 seconds, tilt the slide to allow the methanol to drain off. If absolute methanol is not available, the smear may be fixed by swiftly passing it two or three times through a Bunsen burner flame.

4. Hold the slide under a stream of gently flowing water to remove the methanol. The smear is now ready for staining.

PREPARING A SMEAR OF A BACTERIAL COLONY FOR STAINING

Procedure

1. Locate the bacterial colony you wish to examine microscopically.

2. Lightly touch the tip of a sterile swab (or sterile loop) to the colony. It is usually not necessary to lift the entire colony from the agar surface.

3. Roll the swab or rub the loop over a 1-inch area in the center of a glass microscope slide. Discard the swab or loop in the appropriate infectious waste container. (If using a nondisposable wire loop, sterilize it before setting it aside.)

4. Allow the smear to air dry.

5. Fix the smear as described in the section titled "Preparing a Smear of a Clinical Specimen for Staining." The fixed smear is now ready for staining.

PREPARING THICK AND THIN BLOOD SMEARS

Thick and thin blood smears are prepared in the parasitology section. After staining, they are examined microscopically for the presence of parasites. The following sections summarize the methods recommended by the Centers for Disease Control and Prevention.

Preparing a Thick Blood Smear

1. Place a small drop of blood in the center of a precleaned, labeled slide.

2. Using the corner of another clean slide or an applicator stick, spread the drop in a circular pattern until it is the size of a dime (1.5 cm in diameter). A thick smear of proper density is one that, if placed over newsprint while wet, allows you to barely read the words.

3. Lay the slide flat, and allow the smear to dry thoroughly. Protect it from dust and insects. At room temperature, drying can take several hours; 30 minutes is the strict minimum. Drying can be accelerated by using a fan, hair drier, incubator, or slide warmer. Use only moderate heat, if any, to avoid heat-fixing the smear. Do not fix the smear.

Preparing a Thin Blood Smear

1. Place a small drop of blood on a precleaned, labeled slide, near its frosted end.

2. Bring another clean slide at a 30- to 45-degree angle up to the drop, allowing the drop to spread along the entire width of the second slide.

3. While holding the upper slide at the same angle, quickly push it smoothly along the lower slide toward the unfrosted end.

4. Make sure the smears have a feathered edge. This is achieved by using the proper amount of blood and correct spreading technique. In the feathered edge, the red blood cells should be in a monolayer, or even more distant from one another.

5. Allow the thin smears to dry. They dry much faster than the thick smears.

6. Fix the smears by dipping them in absolute methanol. Fixing makes thin blood smears less subject to detachment than thick blood smears.

POTASSIUM HYDROXIDE PREPARATION (KOH PREP)

Purpose. A KOH prep is often used to determine if fungi are present in a clinical specimen. The most common specimen types on which KOH preps are performed are skin scrapings, hair clippings, and fingernail and toenail clippings.

Principle. The function of the potassium hydroxide is to dissolve keratin in the specimen, making it easier to see any fungal elements (yeasts or hyphae) that might be present. Thus, the KOH acts as a clearing agent.

Reagent. 10% potassium hydroxide.

Procedure

1. Place the specimen (pus, exudate, tissue, skin, hair, nail clipping) into a drop of 10% potassium hydroxide on a clean glass microscope slide. Mix and then wait for 5 to 30 minutes before proceeding. (Gentle warming may be required to clear the specimen.) A drop of lactophenol cotton blue stain can then be added to enhance the visibility of fungal elements, but this is optional.

2. Cover the preparation with a glass coverslip.

3. Examine the preparation under the microscope, with reduced lighting, looking for fungal elements (hyphae, yeast cells, pseudohyphae).

DIRECT SIMPLE STAINING

Purpose. In nature, bacteria are usually colorless, transparent, and quite difficult to see. The primary purpose of the direct simple staining procedure is to stain bacteria to determine their size, basic cell shape, and morphological arrangement.

Reagent. Methylene blue.

Procedure

1. Prepare a fixed smear as described in the section titled "Preparing a Smear of a Clinical Specimen for Staining."

2. Place the fixed smear onto a staining rack.

3. Flood the smear with methylene blue. After one minute, wash off the methylene blue, using a stream of gently flowing water.

4. Allow the stained smear to air dry, or gently blot the smear with bibulous paper or a paper towel. **Blot, do not rub.**

5. Examine the stained smear under the microscope, following the instructions in the section titled "Using a Compound Light Microscope."

Interpretation of results. One use for the direct simple staining procedure is to distinguish between bacteria and yeasts. Although both bacteria and yeasts stain blue with methylene blue, yeast cells can be distinguished from bacterial cells by size and shape. Yeast cells are larger than bacteria—up to about 10 times larger—and usually oval shaped, and some may be observed in the process of budding.

INDIA INK PREPARATION

Purpose. The India ink preparation is an example of a negative staining procedure. In a negative staining procedure, the background becomes stained but all objects of interest remain unstained. Most often, the India ink preparation (India ink prep) is performed on cerebrospinal fluid (CSF) to presumptively diagnose a type of yeast meningitis called cryptococcosis. Cryptococcosis is caused by an encapsulated yeast named *Cryptococcus neoformans*. The test can also be performed on sputum, blood, or urine. CSF is used as an example in the procedure steps that follow.

Reagent. India ink or nigrosin dye (a black dye).

Procedure

1. Place a drop of CSF on a sterile glass microscope slide.

2. Add a glass coverslip.

3. Place a drop of India ink or nigrosin on the glass slide next to the coverslip.

4. Allow the India ink to diffuse under the slide, creating an ink gradient.

5. Examine the preparation microscopically, starting with the $\times 10$ objective. Then switch to the $\times 40$ objective. Examine the region where the ink particle density is neither too light nor too heavy.

Interpretation of results. The presence of budding encapsulated yeasts is interpreted as a presumptive or tentative diagnosis of cryptococcal meningitis (see Fig. 20-48). Culture and identification by biochemical tests are necessary for definitive diagnosis.

CAPSULE STAINING

Purpose. The capsule-staining procedure is used to determine if a particular bacterium does or does not possess a capsule. The procedure is rarely used in CMLs. The capsule-staining procedure is an example of a negative staining procedure. In such procedures, the background becomes stained and the objects of interest are seen as unstained objects against a dark background.

Principle. Because of their chemical composition, bacterial capsules do not stain with most biological dyes. In the capsule-staining procedure, the bacterial cells take up one dye, and the background stains with the other dye. Because the capsules do not stain, they appear as colorless "halos" against the stained background (see Fig. 2-6).

Reagents. Congo red stain and Maneval stain.

Procedure

1. Add a drop of Congo red stain to one end of a clean glass microscope slide.

2. Add a drop of serum to the stain, and then, using a bacteriological inoculating loop, mix in a small amount of the organism to be stained.

3. Using a second glass microscope slide, spread the mixture over the entire length of the first slide.

4. Air dry. Do not heat fix.

5. Flood the slide with Maneval stain and let stand for 1 minute.

6. Rinse the slide with water and blot dry using bibulous paper. Do not rub.

7. Observe the preparation using the oil immersion lens.

Interpretation of results. If capsules are present, they appear as colorless halos against the stained background.

SPORE STAINING

Purpose. The spore-staining procedure is used to determine if a bacterial isolate produces spores and, if so, where the spores are produced within the cells.

Principle. The Wirtz-Conklin spore stain causes the bacterial cells to stain one color, and the spores to stain a different color.

Reagents. Malachite green and safranin.

Procedure

1. Flood the air-dried fixed smear with 5% to 10% aqueous malachite green. Allow the stain to remain on the smear for 45 minutes, or gently heat to steaming for 3 to 6 minutes. Heating is the preferred technique because it enhances the uptake of the stain into the spores.

2. Rinse with tap water.

3. Flood the smear with 0.5% aqueous safranin.

4. After 30 seconds, rinse with tap water, blot dry, and examine at ×400 or ×1,000.

Interpretation of results. Cells stain red and spores stain green. Also note the location of the spores. Are they produced at the tips of the cells (terminal spores), or are they produced elsewhere in the cells (subterminal spores)? Do the spores cause the cells to swell?

GRAM STAINING

Purpose. The Gram staining procedure is the most important staining procedure used in the bacteriology section of the CML. It is used to determine if a bacterial isolate is Gram positive or Gram negative.

Principle. The structure of the organism's cell wall determines the color the organism will stain using the Gram staining procedure. Because of the thicker layer of peptidoglycan in their cell walls, organisms possessing Gram-positive-type cell walls are more difficult to decolorize during the staining procedure than are organisms having Gram-negative-type cell walls. The thicker the layer of peptidoglycan in the cell wall, the more difficult it is to remove the crystal violet from the cell. Also, the decolorization step of the staining procedure dissolves the lipid in the cell walls of Gram-negative bacteria, causing the crystal violet to flow out of the cell. A more complete explanation can be found in Chapter 8.

Reagents. Two dyes are used in the Gram staining procedure: crystal violet and safranin. Other reagents are Gram's iodine and a decolorizing agent—either 95% ethanol or a mixture of acetone and ethanol (400 mL of acetone in 1,200 mL of 95% ethanol).

Procedure

1. **Use latex gloves to avoid getting stains on your fingers.**

2. Place the fixed smear on a staining rack over a sink. Be careful not to turn the slide upside down at any time during the staining procedure.

3. Cover the fixed smear with crystal violet (the primary stain). Allow the crystal violet to remain in contact with the smear for 30 seconds. It is during this step that all bacteria become blue.

4. Wash off the excess crystal violet using a stream of gently flowing water. Too strong a stream will wash the smear off the slide.

5. Cover the smear with Gram's iodine (the mordant). Allow the Gram's iodine to remain in contact with the smear for 30 seconds. The Gram's iodine becomes chemically bonded to the crystal violet, making it more difficult to remove the blue color in step 7. All bacteria remain blue.

6. Wash off the excess Gram's iodine using a stream of gently flowing water.

7. **This is the most critical step in the gram staining procedure.** Using a forceps or spring-type

clothespin, hold the slide at an angle over the sink. Drip the decolorizing agent over the smear until no further blue color washes off the smear. This usually takes only a few drops and a few seconds. If performed correctly, Gram-negative bacteria become decolorized (go back to being colorless), and Gram-positive bacteria remain blue.

8. **Immediately** stop the decolorization process when the drops coming off the end of the slide are no longer blue. The decolorization process is stopped by holding the slide under a stream of gently flowing water. Allowing the alcohol to remain on the smear too long will cause decolorization of Gram-positive bacteria.

9. Place the slide back on the staining rack. Cover the smear with safranin (the counterstain or secondary stain). Allow the safranin to remain in contact with the smear for 1 minute. Safranin is a bright red dye. It is during this step that Gram-negative bacteria become pink to red—pink if they only take up a little of the safranin, red if they take up a lot.

10. Wash off the excess safranin with a stream of gently flowing water.

11. Allow the stained smear to air dry. To speed up the drying process, clean bibulous paper or a clean paper towel may be used to gently blot the smear. **Blot. Do not rub.** Stain can be partially removed from fingers using 95% ethanol, stain remover, or an acid-alcohol solution.

12. Examine the Gram-stained slide as described in the section titled "Using a Compound Light Microscope."

Interpretation of results. When the Gram staining procedure is performed correctly, Gram-positive bacteria are blue to purple, and Gram-negative bacteria are pink to red.

The following table illustrates what happens to the bacteria during each step of the Gram staining procedure. Assume that all bacteria are colorless at the start of the staining procedure.

Step	Purpose	Resulting Color of Gram-Positive Bacteria	Resulting Color of Gram-Negative Bacteria
1. Apply the primary stain (crystal violet)	Stains all bacteria blue	Blue	Blue
2. Rinse with water	Removes excess crystal violet	Blue	Blue
3. Apply the mordant (Gram's iodine)	Iodine forms a chemical complex with the crystal violet, making it more difficult to remove the crystal violet from the cells	Blue	Blue
4. Rinse with water	Removes excess iodine	Blue	Blue
5. Decolorize (using 95% ethanol)	Removes the blue color from Gram-negative bacteria	Blue	Colorless
6. Rinse with water	Removes the decolorizing agent and stops the decolorizing process	Blue	Colorless
7. Apply the counterstain (safranin)	Stains the Gram-negative bacteria	Blue to purple	Pink to red (pink if the cells take up only a small amount of safranin; red if they take up a lot of safranin)
8. Rinse with water	Removes excess safranin	Blue to purple	Pink to red

Quality control information. Quality control (QC) organisms are used to test each newly received lot of Gram stain reagents, and the reagents are checked weekly. Any Gram-positive organism (e.g., *Staphylococcus aureus* subsp. *aureus* ATCC 25923) can be used as the positive control, and any Gram-negative organism (e.g., *Escherichia coli* ATCC 25922) can be used as the negative control. Commercially prepared Gram stain QC slides are available.

SPUTUM DIGESTION, DECONTAMINATION, AND CONCENTRATION

The recovery of mycobacteria from sputum is greatly enhanced when steps are taken to release the organisms from mucus, reduce the number of contaminant organisms, and concentrate the number of mycobacteria present in the specimen. The following procedure can be used to accomplish these goals. Be sure to perform all work in the mycobacteriology section (TB lab) and adhere to all appropriate safety procedures.

Procedure

1. Add 1.5 mL of N-acetyl-L-cysteine (NALC) to 50 mL TB base digestant (containing sodium hydroxide [NaOH]). NALC is a mucolytic agent. NaOH is used as a decontaminating agent.

2. Add the specimen to a sterile 50-mL conical polypropylene screw-capped centrifuge tube. Then add an amount of the NALC-NaOH mixture equal to the volume of the specimen. Avoid using excessive NaOH, which would kill any mycobacteria present.

3. With the cap tightly secured, agitate the tube on a vortex mixture for not more than 30 seconds. Excessive agitation should be avoided, because NALC is unstable in the presence of oxygen.

4. Let stand for 15 minutes at room temperature.

5. Add sterile distilled water or sterile 0.067 M phosphate buffer (pH 6.8) to the 50-mL mark on the tube. Recap the tube and invert several times.

6. Centrifuge the tube at 300 g for 15 to 20 minutes. Be sure to use an aerosol-free sealed centrifuge cup.

7. Pour the supernatant into a splash-proof discard container filled with disinfectant.

8. Remove some of the sediment with a bacteriological loop and prepare a smear on a clean glass microscope slide. This smear will be used for acid-fast staining.

9. Suspend the remaining sediment in 1 to 2 mL of TB buffer or sterile distilled water and inoculate appropriate media (e.g., 7H11 agar slant and/or BACTEC vial) immediately. Never use tap water, which could contain environmental *Mycobacterium* spp.

ACID-FAST STAINING

Acid-fast staining procedures are differential staining procedures. They are used primarily for the tentative or presumptive diagnosis of tuberculosis and are therefore routinely performed in the TB lab. There are several acid-fast staining methods, four of which are described here.

The cell walls of certain organisms contain fatty substances (e.g., waxes) that cause the cell walls to be impervious to certain dyes. Heat or a detergent must be used to enable penetration of the primary dye into the bacterial cell. Once the dye has entered the cell, it is difficult to remove, and once mycobacteria take up the bright red primary dye (carbolfuchsin), they resist decolorization with a mixture of acid and alcohol. Because they resist decolorization, the bacteria are said to be acid fast.

All *Mycobacterium* spp. are acid fast, as are *Nocardia* spp. and a few other bacteria. Certain parasites (e.g., *Cryptosporidium*, *Isospora*, and *Cyclospora* spp.) are also acid fast; thus, acid-fast staining is also used in the parasitology laboratory.

Ziehl-Neelsen Acid-Fast Stain

Purpose. The Ziehl-Neelsen acid-fast staining procedure is used to differentiate between acid-fast and non-acid-fast bacteria. It is used primarily for the tentative or presumptive diagnosis of tuberculosis.

Principle. In the Ziehl-Neelsen acid-fast staining procedure, heat is used to force the carbolfuchsin into the bacterial cells. (In the Kinyoun modification, described next, phenol is used in place of heat.)

Reagents. Two dyes are used: Ziehl-Neelsen carbolfuchsin and either malachite green or methylene blue. The decolorizing agent is a mixture of acid and alcohol (97 mL of 95% ethanol and 3 mL of hydrochloric acid).

Procedure

1. Place the fixed smear on a staining rack. Cover the smear with the bright red primary dye (carbolfuchsin).

2. Heat the slide slowly to steaming and continue steaming for 3 to 5 minutes. Heating is usually accomplished using an electric staining rack or by holding a Bunsen burner flame under the slide. Do not overheat.

3. After cooling, wash off the carbolfuchsin using a stream of gently flowing water.

4. Decolorize for 2 minutes using acid-alcohol.

5. Wash using a stream of gently flowing water, and counterstain with methylene blue or malachite green.

6. After 1 minute, wash off the counterstain using a stream of gently flowing water.

7. Allow the stained smear to air dry. Blotting is not recommended because of the possibility of transferring

acid-fast organisms from one stained smear to another when the same piece of bibulous paper is used to blot more than one smear.

8. Examine the acid-fast stained slide as described in the section titled "Using a Compound Light Microscope."

Interpretation of results. At the conclusion of the acid-fast staining procedure, acid-fast organisms are red. Non-acid-fast organisms are either blue or green, depending on which counterstain was used.

Quality control information. QC organisms are used to test each newly received lot of acid-fast stain reagents, and the reagents are checked weekly. Any acid-fast organism (e.g., a *Mycobacterium* sp.) can be used as the positive control, and any non-acid-fast organism (e.g., *Escherichia coli*) can be used as the negative control. *Nocardia asteroides*, which is acid fast with the Kinyoun method but non–acid fast with the Ziehl-Neelsen method, can be used as a negative control.

Kinyoun Acid-Fast Stain
Purpose. As stated for the Ziehl-Neelsen method.

Principle. As stated for the Ziehl-Neelsen method, except that heat is not used in the Kinyoun method. The high concentration of phenol in the carbolfuchsin reagent dissolves lipids in the bacterial cell walls, allowing penetration of the stain.

Reagents. Two dyes are used: Kinyoun carbolfuchsin and either malachite green or methylene blue. The decolorizing agent is a mixture of acid and alcohol (97 mL of 95% ethanol and 3 mL of hydrochloric acid).

Procedure

1. Place the fixed smear on a staining rack. Cover the smear with the bright red primary dye (Kinyoun carbolfuchsin).

2. Allow the stain to remain on the smear for 5 minutes. Do not heat.

3. Wash off the carbolfuchsin using a stream of gently flowing water.

4. Decolorize for 3 minutes using acid-alcohol.

5. Wash using a stream of gently flowing water, and counterstain with methylene blue or malachite green.

6. After 3 to 4 minutes, wash off the counterstain using a stream of gently flowing water.

7. Allow the stained smear to air dry. Do not blot.

8. Examine the acid-fast stained slide as described in the section titled "Using a Compound Light Microscope."

Interpretation of results. At the conclusion of the acid-fast staining procedure, acid-fast organisms are red. Non-acid-fast organisms are either blue or green, depending on which counterstain was used.

Quality control information. As stated for the Ziehl-Neelsen method.

Modified Kinyoun Acid-Fast Stain
Purpose. As stated for the Ziehl-Neelsen method.

Principle. The modified Kinyoun procedure is useful when staining weakly acid-fast organisms, such as *Nocardia* spp., which become decolorized when either the Ziehl-Neelsen or Kinyoun method is used.

Procedure. The modified Kinyoun acid-fast staining procedure is performed in the same manner as the Kinyoun method, except that a weaker decolorizing agent (0.5% to 1.0% sulfuric acid) is used in place of 3% acid-alcohol.

Quality control information. *Nocardia asteroides* can be used as a positive control. Any non-acid-fast organism can be used as a negative control.

Auramine-Rhodamine Fluorescent Acid-Fast Stain
Purpose. As stated for the Ziehl-Neelsen method.

Principle. Using this procedure, acid-fast organisms emit a bright yellow fluorescence when observed using short-wave ultraviolet light. The potassium permanganate counterstain causes the background debris to fluoresce pale yellow.

Reagents. Three reagents are used: auramine-rhodamine stain, 0.5% potassium permanganate counterstain (0.5 g potassium permanganate in 100 mL distilled water), and 0.5% acid-alcohol decolorizer (0.5 mL concentrated hydrochloric acid plus 100 mL 70% ethanol).

Procedure

1. Flood heat-fixed smear with auramine-rhodamine stain. Let stand for 15 minutes.

2. Rinse with tap water. Drain.

3. Decolorize with 0.5% acid-alcohol for 2 minutes.

4. Rinse with tap water. Drain.

5. Flood smear with 0.5% potassium permanganate counterstain. Let stand for 2 minutes.

6. Rinse with tap water. Drain.

7. Air dry. Do not blot.

8. Examine immediately, using a fluorescence microscope fitted with a BG-12 or 52112 primary filter and an OG-1 barrier filter.

Interpretation of results. Acid-fast organisms emit a bright yellow fluorescence against a pale yellow background. Stained smears can be restained using any of the carbolfuchsin staining procedures.

Quality control information. As stated for the Ziehl-Neelsen method.

MOTILITY: HANGING DROP

Purpose. The hanging drop method is one way to determine whether a bacterial isolate is motile or nonmotile.

Principle. If motile, organisms will be seen "swimming" around in a suspended drop of broth culture.

Procedure

1. Obtain a clean glass depression slide, and place a narrow, thin film of petroleum jelly around the outer edge of the well. Be careful not to get any of the petroleum jelly in the well.

2. Obtain a broth culture of the organism to be tested. Gently invert the tightly capped tube several times to obtain a homogeneous suspension of the organism.

3. Using aseptic (sterile) techniques, transfer a loopful of the broth culture to a clean glass coverslip, using a sterile, plastic inoculating loop. Dispose of the used inoculating loop in the appropriate infectious waste container.

4. Turn the depression slide upside down, and then lower the slide over the coverslip, so that the drop is within the well.

5. Quickly, but gently, turn the depression slide right side up. The drop should now be hanging down into the well. (The petroleum jelly will keep the coverslip from slipping, and the seal will prevent the drop from drying out; see Fig. 8-19).

6. Examine the preparation under the microscope, in the manner described in the section titled "Using a Compound Light Microscope." It should not be necessary to use the oil immersion objective. Lower the light intensity, if necessary.

Interpretation of results. Motile bacteria can be seen darting around within the drop, whereas nonmotile bacteria are stationary. If the slide is left in place too long, however, nonmotile organisms start to "jiggle." Why is that? (If you don't recall, see the section titled "Wet Mount Procedure: Differentiating Between Bacterial and Yeast Colonies.")

MOTILITY: SEMISOLID AGAR

Purpose. The semisolid agar method is one way of determining whether a bacterial isolate is motile or nonmotile.

Principle. If nonmotile, organisms can be observed only where they are inoculated into the semisolid agar. If they are motile, they can also be seen in the surrounding medium.

Procedure

1. Obtain a sterile bacteriological inoculating wire (not a loop) and a tube of semisolid agar.

2. Using aseptic (sterile) techniques, dip the inoculating wire into a broth culture of the organism to be tested.

3. Using aseptic (sterile) techniques, stab the wire into the semisolid agar. Use one straight stab; do not wiggle the inoculating loop in the medium. It is not necessary for the tip to reach the bottom of the tube.

4. Recap the tube, and place it into the incubator at 35°C to 37°C. Incubate overnight.

5. Examine the tube the next day for evidence of motility.

Interpretation of results. If the organism is nonmotile, growth occurs only along the stab line. If the organism is motile, evidence of growth (turbidity) can be seen away from the stab line into the surrounding medium (see Fig. 8-18).

GERM TUBE

Purpose. The germ tube test is used in the identification of the yeast *Candida albicans*.

Principle. In the presence of serum, *Candida albicans* blastoconidia (yeast cells) produce hyphal elements (germ tubes) more rapidly than do most other species of yeast. Unlike some other yeast species, no constriction exists between the *C. albicans* mother cell and the germ tube.

Reagent. It is best to use fetal or newborn calf serum, but outdated human blood bank serum can be used if it has been shown to produce correct test results with positive and negative control organisms.

Procedure

1. Inoculate a small amount of the yeast colony into 0.5 mL of serum.

2. Incubate at 35°C.

3. After at least 30 minutes of incubation, examine a wet preparation of the yeast suspension at ×400 magnification. Look for characteristic hyphal elements (see Fig. 19-8).

4. Continue to incubate and periodically examine the contents for up to 3 hours.

Interpretation of results. The presence of germ tubes having no constriction at the site of origin is considered a positive test result, consistent with *C. albicans*. However, the absence of germ tubes does not rule out *C. albicans*.

Quality control information. Use a known germ-tube-producing strain of *C. albicans* as a positive control and a non-germ-tube-producing yeast, such as *C. glabrata*, as a negative control.

TEASE MOUNT

Purpose. The tease mount is used for the microscopic examination of mould colonies. Microscopic features are important clues in the identification (speciation) of moulds.

Procedure

1. Place a drop of lactophenol cotton blue (LPCB) stain on a glass microscope slide.

2. Using a pair of dissecting needles (often referred to as teasing needles), dig out a small section of the mould colony to be examined. Include both surface and subsurface portions of the colony.

3. Place the section of the mould colony into the drop of LPCB stain.

4. Use the dissecting needles to **gently** tease apart the section of mould colony. Excessive or vigorous teasing sometimes damages the microscopic features that are valuable clues in the identification of moulds.

5. Place a coverslip over the preparation, and gently exert pressure on the coverslip surface using an eraser at the end of a pencil.

6. Examine the preparation microscopically, first using the ×10 objective and then increasing magnification.

7. Examine the hyphae, fruiting bodies, and conidia. Notice whether the hyphae are septate or aseptate, branched or not branched, and pigmented or not pigmented. Are arthroconidia present? Notice the appearance of fruiting bodies and the manner in which conidia are produced. Notice also the size, shape, and arrangement of conidia. Are both macroconidia and microconidia present?

CELLOPHANE TAPE PREPARATION

Purpose. A cellophane (Scotch) tape preparation can be used as a substitute for the tease mount. The technique is inexpensive, rapid, and simple to perform and often preserves microscopic features better than a tease mount. Perform all steps in a biosafety cabinet while wearing gloves.

Procedure

1. Using a piece of unfrosted, clear cellophane tape that is about 6 cm (2½ inches) long, press the sticky side gently but firmly to the surface of the mould colony to be examined.

2. Keeping the tape outstretched, place it over the drop of LPCB stain, anchoring the ends of the tape to the slide on either side of the drop. With practice, you can overcome the problem of the tape sticking to your gloved fingers. Try to avoid trapping air bubbles beneath the tape.

3. Examine the preparation microscopically, first using the ×10 objective and then increasing magnification. The tape may interfere with examination under oil immersion. Examine for the structures mentioned in the section titled "Tease Mount."

MICROSLIDE CULTURE

Purpose. Microslide cultures are used for the microscopic examination of mould colonies. They are more tedious and time consuming to perform than are either tease mounts or cellophane tape preparations, but they provide a better view of aerial and vegetative hyphae. Microslide cultures can be used to prepare permanent slide mounts.

Procedure

1. Place a round piece of sterile filter paper or a piece of sterile gauze in the bottom of a sterile Petri dish.

2. Place a pair of thin glass rods or wooden applicator sticks on the filter paper or gauze. These will serve as supports for a glass microscope slide.

3. Place a 3-inch-by-1-inch glass microscope slide onto the supports.

4. Place a square block of cornmeal or potato dextrose agar on top of the slide (Fig. A-5).

5. Using a straight inoculating wire or the tip of a dissecting needle, inoculate the margins of the agar block in several places with material obtained from the mould colony to be studied.

6. Gently heat a glass coverslip by passing it through a Bunsen burner flame, and immediately place it onto the surface of the agar block. Heating the coverslip causes it to adhere tightly to the surface of the agar block.

7. Using a pipette, saturate the filter paper or gauze with sterile water.

8. Place the lid on the Petri dish and incubate at room temperature or in a 30°C incubator for 3 to 5 days.

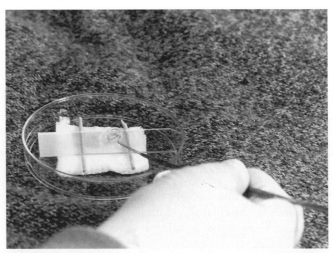

***Figure A-5.* Microslide culture setup.** The setup includes a Petri dish, gauze pad, two slide supports, a glass microscope slide, and an agar block being placed on the slide. (From Winn WC Jr, et al. Koneman's Color Atlas and Textbook of Diagnostic Microbiology. 6th Ed. Philadelphia: Lippincott Williams & Wilkins, 2006.)

9. When the growth appears to be mature, place a drop of LPCB stain on a glass microscope slide.

10. Very gently remove the coverslip and place it on top of the drop of LPCB stain.

11. If a permanent preparation is desired, either mounting fluid or clear fingernail polish can be added around the entire perimeter of the coverslip.

12. Examine the preparation microscopically, first using the ×10 objective and then increasing magnification. Examine for the structures mentioned in the section titled "Tease Mount."

13. If desired, examine material on the original microscope slide after the agar block is removed and properly discarded. Add a drop of LPCB stain and a coverslip, and examine microscopically. A permanent preparation can be prepared by adding either mounting fluid or clear fingernail polish around the perimeter of the coverslip.

ACETAMIDE UTILIZATION

Purpose. The acetamide utilization test is used to determine if a bacterial isolate can use acetamide as the sole source of carbon.

Principle. Bacteria capable of growing on an acetamide slant cause the deamination of acetamide and the release of ammonia. The presence of ammonia increases the pH of the medium, causing the medium to change from green to royal blue.

Reagent. An acetamide agar slant.

Procedure

1. Lightly inoculate an acetamide agar slant, using growth from an 18-to-24-hour-old culture. Do not use a broth culture as inoculum.

2. Incubate the slant at 35°C for up to 7 days.

Interpretation of results. A change in the color of the medium from green to royal blue constitutes a positive test result. No color change in the medium constitutes a negative test result.

Quality control information. Use *Pseudomonas aeruginosa* as a positive control and *Stenotrophomonas maltophilia* as a negative control.

ARYLSULFATASE

Purpose. The arylsulfatase test is of value in the identification of some *Mycobacterium* and *Nocardia* spp. Rapidly growing members of the *Mycobacterium fortuitum* complex are usually arylsulfatase positive within 3 days. Most *Nocardia* spp. are arylsulfatase negative, but *N. africana* and *N. nova* are exceptions.

Principle. The enzyme arylsulfatase splits free phenolphthalein from the tripotassium salt of phenolphthalein. If free phenolphthalein is present, the medium turns pink to red following addition of sodium carbonate.

Reagents. Arylsulfatase broth (the broth contains phenolphthalein disulfate tripotassium salt, but the exact composition of the broth varies depending on whether the 3-day or 14-day arylsulfatase test is being performed) and 2N sodium carbonate solution.

Procedure

1. Inoculate a tube of arylsulfatase broth with a slightly turbid suspension of the test organism in sterile water. Thoroughly emulsify the culture in the broth.

2. Incubate the tube for 3 days or 14 days at 35°C in a non-CO_2 incubator.

3. Remove from the incubator and add 1 mL of the 2N sodium carbonate reagent, mix, and observe for a color change.

Interpretation of results. A color change to pink to red constitutes a positive test result. No color change constitutes a negative test result.

Quality control information. *Mycobacterium fortuitum* is used as a positive control, and *M. intracellulare* is used as a negative control. Specific American Type Culture Collection (ATCC) strains are required, depending on whether the 3-day or 14-day test is being performed. Fresh, actively growing cultures must be used.

BACITRACIN SENSITIVITY (A-DISK)

Purpose. The A-disk or bacitracin sensitivity test was the traditional method of differentiating *Streptococcus pyogenes* from other β-hemolytic *Streptococcus* spp. of human origin. Thus, the A-disk test was used whenever a β-hemolytic *Streptococcus* sp. was isolated from a clinical specimen. It is called the A-disk test because *S. pyogenes* is also known as group A strep. The A-disk test has largely been replaced by other, more reliable methods.

Principle. The A-disk is a small circular piece of filter paper that is saturated with bacitracin, an antibiotic produced by *Bacillus subtilis*. The test determines whether an organism is susceptible or resistant to the concentration of bacitracin used in the test.

Reagent. Bacitracin.

Procedure

1. Heavily inoculate a section of a blood agar plate with the β-hemolytic *Streptococcus* sp. to be tested.

2. Gently press an A-disk (a 0.04-U bacitracin disk) to the inoculated surface.

3. Incubate the plate overnight in a CO_2 incubator at 37°C.

Interpretation of results. The organism is either susceptible to (killed by) the bacitracin or it is not. If the organism is susceptible to the bacitracin, a zone of no growth forms around the disk (see Fig. 9-18). Any zone of inhibition of growth is considered a positive test result. A zone of no growth is referred to as a positive A-disk result. Absence of a zone of no growth is considered a negative A-disk result.

What to report. *S. pyogenes* is bacitracin sensitive. However, some β-hemolytic, group B, C, and G streptococci are also bacitracin sensitive; thus, they cause false-positive test results. Therefore, if the organism is killed by the bacitracin, it may or may not be *S. pyogenes*; report "Bacitracin-sensitive β-hemolytic *Streptococcus* sp." If the organism is not killed by the bacitracin, report "Bacitracin-resistant β-hemolytic *Streptococcus* sp."

Quality control information. QC organisms are used to test each newly received lot of A-disks, and the disks are checked at least weekly. A strain of *S. pyogenes* is used as the positive control (e.g., ATCC 19615) and a bacitracin-resistant β-hemolytic *Streptococcus* sp. is used as the negative control (e.g., ATCC 12386).

β-LACTAMASE

Purpose. The β-lactamase test is used to detect the production of a β-lactamase enzyme by a bacterial isolate. Several methods are available for detecting β-lactamase production. The method described here is known as the chromogenic cephalosporin or nitrocefin test.

Principle. Nitrocefin changes from yellow to red when the amide bond in the β-lactam ring is hydrolyzed by a β-lactamase.

Reagent. A commercial disk saturated with nitrocefin (the cefinase disk) is available from BD Biosciences.

Procedure

1. Place a cefinase disk onto the surface of a clean glass microscope slide.

2. Moisten the disk with 1 drop of sterile water.

3. Smear some colonial growth onto the surface of the moistened disk.

4. Observe for the development of a red color.

Interpretation of results. Development of a red color is interpreted as a positive test result. The color change occurs only where the test organism was applied to the disk. A positive result usually occurs within 5 minutes, although some strains take up to 1 hour.

Quality control information. Use a known β-lactamase producer, such as a β-lactamase-positive strain of *Staphylococcus aureus*, as a positive control. Use a non-β-lactamase producer, such as a β-lactamase-negative strain of *Haemophilus influenzae*, as a negative control. Alternatively,

β-lactamase-positive and β-lactamase-negative strains of *Neisseria gonorrhoeae* can be used as controls (e.g., ATCC 31426 and ATCC 43069, respectively).

BILE-ESCULIN HYDROLYSIS

Purpose. The bile-esculin hydrolysis test is of value in the identification of group D streptococci and *Enterococcus* spp.

Principle. Some bacteria are capable of hydrolyzing esculin in the presence of bile (either 4% bile salts or 40% bile). Bile-esculin-positive bacteria are able to grow on the medium (in the presence of bile) and hydrolyze esculin. One of the products of esculin hydrolysis, esculetin, reacts with ferric ions in the medium, causing the formation of a black diffusible complex.

Reagent. Bile-esculin agar slants or plates.

Procedure

1. Using an inoculating loop, inoculate the slant with two or three colonies of the test organism, using an S-shaped motion, or inoculate the surface of a plate to obtain isolated colonies.

2. Incubate the inoculated slant or plate at 35°C for 24 to 48 hours in a non-CO_2 incubator.

Interpretation of results. Diffuse blackening of more than half of the slant is interpreted as a positive test result (see Fig. 9-24). On plates, black halos around isolated colonies or any blackening of the medium is considered a positive test result.

Quality control information. Use an *Enterococcus* sp. as a positive control and one of the non–group D viridans streptococci as a negative control.

BILE SOLUBILITY

Purpose. The bile solubility test is of value in the identification of *Streptococcus pneumoniae*.

Principle. *S. pneumoniae* produces autolytic enzymes (autolysins) that cause lysis of older cells. These autolysins are responsible for the sunken centers that are observed in older *S. pneumoniae* colonies on agar media. The bile solubility test uses bile salts to accelerate the lytic process.

Reagents. 10% sodium deoxycholate, 1% aqueous phenol red solution, and 0.10N sodium hydroxide (NaOH) solution.

Procedure

1. Transfer approximately 0.5 mL of an 18-to-24-hour broth culture to two clean test tubes. Label one tube "test" and the other tube "control." Alternatively, a suspension of the test organism can be prepared by transferring colonial growth to tubes containing phosphate-buffered saline (pH 7.0).

2. Add one drop of phenol red solution to each tube.

3. Add NaOH solution to the suspensions to adjust the pH to 7.0; at pH 7.0, the liquid is light pink. This pH adjustment is not necessary if the suspension was prepared from colonial growth.

4. Add 0.5 mL of 10% sodium deoxycholate to the "test" tube.

5. Add 0.5 mL sterile normal saline to the control tube.

6. Gently agitate both tubes, and then place them in an incubator or water bath at 35°C for 3 hours, checking hourly for clearing of the suspension in the "test" tube.

The bile solubility test can also be performed by adding a drop of 2% sodium deoxycholate to a few well-isolated colonies on sheep blood agar. *S. pneumoniae* colonies disappear, leaving an α hemolytic spot where the colony had been.

Interpretation of results. Visible clearing of the suspension in the "test" tube and no change in the turbidity of the suspension in the control tube constitute a positive test result. No change in the turbidity of the suspension in the "test" tube relative to the turbidity in the control tube constitutes a negative test result. Most strains of *S. pneumoniae* are bile solubility positive.

Quality control information. Use *Streptococcus pneumoniae* (e.g., ATCC 6305) as a positive control and one of the α-hemolytic viridans group streptococci (e.g., *S. gallolyticus* ATCC 49147) as a negative control.

CAMP

Purpose. The CAMP test is used in the identification of *Streptococcus agalactiae* (group B strep). The CAMP test is named for the scientists who first described the test: Christie, Atkins, and Munich-Petersen.

Principle. The hemolytic activity of the β-hemolysin (β-lysin) produced by most strains of *Staphylococcus aureus* is enhanced by an extracellular protein (called CAMP factor) produced by *S. agalactiae*. This synergistic hemolysis is seen with both hemolytic and nonhemolytic strains of *S. agalactiae*.

Reagents. A sheep blood agar plate and a β-hemolysin-producing strain of *S. aureus*.

Procedure

1. Make a single straight-line streak of the *S. aureus* down the center of a blood agar plate.

2. Perpendicular to the staph streak, make one 3-to-4-cm-long straight-line streak of the test organism, making sure that the staph and test organism streaks do not touch.

3. Inoculate the streptococcal control strains on the same plate.

4. Incubate the plate at 35°C for 18 to 24 hours in a non-CO$_2$ incubator. Do not incubate in a candle jar, in a CO$_2$ incubator, or under anaerobic conditions.

Interpretation of results. An area of increased hemolysis at the juncture of the test organism streak and the staph streak, often in the shape of an arrowhead, is interpreted as a positive test result (see Fig. 9-19). A bacitracin-resistant, trimethoprim-sulfamethoxazole-resistant, CAMP test–positive, β-hemolytic *Streptococcus* sp. can be reported as "β-Hemolytic group B *Streptococcus* sp. by CAMP test."

Quality control information. Use *S. agalactiae* as a positive control and *S. pyogenes* as a negative control.

CATALASE: SLIDE

Purpose. Catalase is an enzyme that enables some bacteria (and other cells) to remove the potentially harmful hydrogen peroxide (H$_2$O$_2$) that accumulates in their environment as a result of the reduction of oxygen. Bacteria that produce catalase are catalase positive, whereas those that do not produce catalase are catalase negative. The most common use for the catalase test is to differentiate between *Staphylococcus* spp. (catalase positive) and *Streptococcus* spp. (catalase negative). Thus, the catalase test can be used whenever a Gram-positive coccus is isolated from a clinical specimen. Many bacteria other than *Staphylococcus* spp. also produce catalase. Likewise, many bacteria other than *Streptococcus* spp. do not produce catalase. Thus, the catalase test can be used as a clue to the identification (speciation) of organisms in addition to *Staphylococcus* and *Streptococcus* spp. For example, all *Bacillus* spp. are catalase positive, whereas all *Clostridium* spp. are catalase negative.

Principle. Catalase catalyzes the conversion of H$_2$O$_2$ to water (H$_2$O) and oxygen (O$_2$), as shown in the following reaction:

$$2\ H_2O_2 + Catalase \rightarrow 2\ H_2O + O_2$$

Reagent. 3% hydrogen peroxide; use 15% hydrogen peroxide when testing anaerobes.

Procedure

1. Using a sterile inoculating loop, transfer a colony to a glass microscope slide and prepare a smear.

2. Add one drop of the 3% H$_2$O$_2$.

3. Observe for the immediate formation of bubbles.

Interpretation of results. The immediate formation of bubbles constitutes a positive test result (see Fig. 9-2). If no bubbles are produced, the test is negative. The bubbles are bubbles of oxygen (O$_2$).

What to report. Report that the organism is either catalase positive or catalase negative. If the organism is a Gram-positive coccus, keep in mind that all *Staphylococcus* spp. are catalase positive, whereas all *Streptococcus* spp. are catalase negative.

Quality control information. QC organisms are used to test each newly received lot of catalase, and the disks are checked on each day of use. Any strain of *Staphylococcus* (e.g., *S. aureus* subsp. *aureus* ATCC 25923) can be used as a positive control, and any strain of *Streptococcus* (e.g., *S. pyogenes* ATCC 19615) can be used as a negative control.

68°C CATALASE

Purpose. The 68°C catalase test is useful for identifying some *Mycobacterium* spp. For example, members of the *M. tuberculosis* complex are 68°C catalase negative.

Principle. As discussed in the section titled "Catalase: Slide," catalase is an enzyme that splits hydrogen peroxide into water and oxygen. Oxygen is detected by the presence of bubbles. Some forms of catalase are inactivated by heating at 68°C for 20 minutes.

Reagents. 30% hydrogen peroxide (also known as Superoxol; this is not the same hydrogen peroxide used in the slide catalase test) in a solution of 10% Tween 80, and sterile 0.067 M phosphate buffer. Tween 80 is a strong detergent that helps to disperse the tightly clumped mycobacteria, maximizing the detection of catalase.

Procedure

1. Add 0.5 mL of phosphate buffer to a test tube.

2. Inoculate the buffer with growth from a 2-to-4-week-old, actively growing subculture of the test organism. Thoroughly emulsify the culture in the buffer.

3. Incubate the tube in a 68°C water bath for exactly 20 minutes.

4. Remove the tube from the water bath and cool to room temperature.

5. Add 0.5 mL of freshly prepared Tween 80 hydrogen peroxide reagent. Avoid contact of the reagent with skin.

6. Allow the tube to remain at room temperature for 20 minutes. Do not shake the tube.

7. Observe for bubbles.

Interpretation of results. The presence of bubbles constitutes a positive test result. The absence of bubbles constitutes a negative test result. Heating to 68°C causes *M. tuberculosis* and some other mycobacteria to lose their catalase activity.

Quality control information. Use *M. tuberculosis* ATCC 15177 as a negative control (bubbles at 22°C to 25°C, but no bubbles at 68°C) and *M. fortuitum* ATCC 6841 as a positive control (bubbles at 22°C to 25°C and at 68°C).

COAGULASE: SLIDE

Purpose. Both the slide coagulase test and the tube coagulase test (described next) are used to differentiate *Staphylococcus aureus* from other species of *Staphylococcus*. Thus, the coagulase test is performed whenever a *Staphylococcus* sp. has been isolated from a clinical specimen. The slide test, which detects bound coagulase (or clumping factor) is quicker and easier to perform than the tube test. The tube test, which detects free coagulase, is the more sensitive of the two tests, meaning that the tube test can detect smaller quantities of coagulase than the slide test. The slide coagulase test is performed first. Only if the slide test is negative will the more sensitive tube coagulase test be performed.

Principle. Coagulase causes the formation of clots. Specifically, it catalyzes the conversion of fibrinogen (a plasma protein) to a sticky substance called fibrin.

Reagent. Rabbit plasma with ethylenediamine tetraacetic acid. Rabbit serum cannot be used in this test because serum lacks the clotting factors found in plasma.

Procedure

1. Using a wax pencil, draw two circles on a glass microscope slide.

2. Place a drop of sterile water into each circle.

3. Using a sterile inoculating loop, mix a colony of the organism to be tested into each of the drops of water, making a suspension of the bacteria.

4. Stir a drop of rabbit plasma into the bacterial suspension.

5. Gently rock the slide back and forth while observing for agglutination (clumping of the bacteria).

Interpretation of results. The formation of clumps within 10 to 15 seconds is a positive test result (see Fig. 9-10). The bacteria are being held together by sticky fibrin. If no clumps are formed, the test is considered negative.

What to report. *S. aureus* is the most likely coagulase-positive, Gram-positive coccus to be encountered in human clinical specimens. Thus, if clumping occurs, report the identity of the organism as *Staphylococcus aureus*. Alternatively, it can be reported as a "Coagulase-positive *Staphylococcus* sp." If clumping does not occur, perform the more sensitive tube coagulase test.

Quality control information. QC organisms are used to test each newly received lot of rabbit plasma, and the rabbit plasma is checked on each day of use. A strain of *S. aureus* (e.g., *S. aureus* subsp. *aureus* ATCC 25923) is used as the positive control, and a coagulase-negative *Staphylococcus* sp. (e.g., *S. epidermidis* ATCC 12228) is used as the negative control. The rabbit plasma can also be tested by adding one drop of 5% calcium chloride to 0.5 mL of the plasma. A clot should form within 10 to 15 seconds.

COAGULASE: TUBE

Purpose. The more sensitive tube coagulase test is used to differentiate *Staphylococcus aureus* from other species of *Staphylococcus*, when the less sensitive slide coagulase test result is negative.

Principle. See "Coagulase: Slide."

Reagent. Rabbit plasma with ethylenediamine tetraacetic acid. Rabbit serum cannot be used in this test because serum lacks the clotting factors found in plasma.

Procedure

1. Add 0.5 mL of rabbit plasma to a small test tube.

2. Add 2 drops of a broth culture of the organism to be tested to the rabbit plasma, or emulsify a small amount of a colony in the rabbit plasma.

3. Place the tube into a 35°C water bath.

4. Check the tube every 30 minutes for up to 4 hours to see if a clot has formed. The tube is checked every 30 minutes because some strains of *S. aureus* also produce an enzyme that dissolves clots. A tube left unchecked until 4 hours of incubation and showing no clot formation does not necessarily represent a negative result because a clot may have formed and subsequently dissolved.

5. If no clot is observed at 4 hours, incubate the tube at room temperature for 18 hours, and then check again for clot formation.

Interpretation of results. Formation of a clot represents a positive test result (see Fig. 9-11). If no clot has formed by the end of 18 hours, the test is considered negative.

What to report. Of all the *Staphylococcus* spp. likely to be encountered in clinical specimens, only *S. aureus* is tube coagulase positive. Thus, if a clot is formed, the report would identify the organism as *Staphylococcus aureus*. If a clot does not form, the organism is some other species of *Staphylococcus*, and the report would state "*Staphylococcus* sp. other than *Staphylococcus aureus*" or "Coagulase-negative *Staphylococcus*." The most commonly isolated coagulase-negative staphylococci are *S. epidermidis* and *S. saprophyticus*. In general, coagulase-negative staphylococci are less virulent than *S. aureus*.

Quality control information. QC organisms are used to test each newly received lot of rabbit plasma, and the rabbit plasma is checked on each day of use. A strain of *S. aureus* is used as the positive control, and any coagulase-negative *Staphylococcus* sp. is used as the negative control. (See "Coagulase: Slide" for suggestions.)

DECARBOXYLASE

Purpose. Decarboxylase tests are performed to determine which decarboxylase enzymes a bacterial isolate is producing. As stated in Chapter 12, decarboxylase enzymes cause the removal of the acid end of amino acid molecules—a process known as decarboxylation. The three most commonly tested substrates are lysine, ornithine, and arginine. Each decarboxylase enzyme is specific for a particular amino acid. For example, lysine decarboxylase is the enzyme that causes decarboxylation of lysine.

Principle. Möeller decarboxylase broth, containing glucose and a particular amino acid, is inoculated with the test organism. During the initial stages of incubation, the medium turns yellow as a result of glucose fermentation and the formation of acid. (Keep in mind that all members of the family Enterobacteriaceae ferment glucose.) Once the broth has become acidic, decarboxylation can take place. If the organism produces the appropriate decarboxylase, an alkaline product is formed, causing the medium to return to its original purple color.

Reagent. Möeller decarboxylase medium containing glucose and the amino acid being tested.

Procedure

1. Inoculate two tubes of Möeller decarboxylase broth. One tube contains the amino acid being tested. The other tube lacks the amino acid and serves as a negative control.

2. Overlay the medium in both tubes with sterile mineral oil.

3. Incubate the tubes at 35°C for 18 to 24 hours.

Interpretation of results. If the control tube is yellow and the amino acid–containing tube is purple, the test result is positive. If both tubes are yellow, the test result is negative (see Fig. 12-12).

What to report. If the amino acid being tested is ornithine and the test result is positive, the organism is reported as being ornithine decarboxylase positive. However, if the organism produces a negative result, it is reported as being ornithine decarboxylase negative.

Quality control information. The organisms shown in the following table can be used as controls.

Amino Acid	Positive Control	Negative Control
Lysine	*Enterobacter aerogenes*	*Enterobacter cloacae*
Ornithine	*Enterobacter cloacae*	*Klebsiella pneumoniae*
Arginine	*Enterobacter cloacae*	*Enterobacter aerogenes*

ESCULIN HYDROLYSIS

Purpose. The esculin hydrolysis test is of value in the identification of some nonfermenters. This is not the bile-esculin test.

Principle. Some bacteria are capable of hydrolyzing esculin to yield glucose and esculetin. Although esculin fluoresces under long-wave (360-nm) ultraviolet light, the end products of esculin hydrolysis do not. Thus, a loss of fluorescence indicates that esculin was hydrolyzed. Also, the medium turns black as a result of the reaction of esculetin and ferric ions in the medium.

Reagent. Esculin agar slant or esculin broth.

Procedure

1. Inoculate the surface of an esculin agar slant or esculin broth with one well-isolated colony of the test organism.

2. Incubate at 35°C for 18 to 24 hours.

Interpretation of results. Loss of fluorescence or the development of a black color is interpreted as a positive test result. Fluorescence or lack of a black color is interpreted as a negative test result.

Quality control information. Use *Aeromonas hydrophila* as a positive control, and *Pseudomonas aeruginosa* as a negative control.

FURAZOLIDONE SENSITIVITY

Purpose. Furazolidone sensitivity can be used to differentiate between staphylococci and micrococci.

Principle. Growth of staphylococci is inhibited by furazolidone, whereas growth of micrococci is not.

Reagent. Furazolidone, also known as Furoxone or FX.

Procedure

1. Prepare a suspension of the organism to be tested in sterile distilled water or broth. The suspension should be equivalent to a 0.5 McFarland turbidity standard.

2. Using a sterile swab, spread some of the suspension over one-half of the surface of a blood agar plate.

3. Aseptically place a 100-μg furazolidone disk in the center of the inoculated area. Gently press the disk until it is flush with the agar surface.

4. Incubate the plate at 35°C in a non-CO_2 incubator for 18 to 24 hours.

5. Check for a zone of no growth and if present, measure its diameter.

Interpretation of results. *Micrococcus* spp. are FX resistant, with zone diameters up to 9 mm. *Staphylococcus* spp. are FX susceptible, with zone diameters of 15 mm or larger (see Figs. 9-4 and 9-5).

Quality control information. Controls should be run weekly and with each new lot of disks. Use a *Staphylococcus* sp. as a positive (susceptible) control and a *Micrococcus* sp. as a negative (resistant) control.

IMViC

The IMViC test is a combination of four tests. In the acronym IMViC, *I* stands for indole, the *M* stands for methyl red, *V* stands for Voges-Proskauer, and *C* stands for citrate (the lowercase *i* in the abbreviation has no meaning). IMViC reactions can be used to differentiate *Escherichia coli* from other lactose-fermenting members of the family Enterobacteriaceae (e.g., *Enterobacter aerogenes*, *Enterobacter cloacae*, and *Klebsiella pneumoniae*). All these organisms look alike on primary culture media.

Three or four tubes can be used for IMViC testing: one tube of tryptophan broth for the indole test, one or two tubes of MRVP broth for the methyl red and Voges-Proskauer tests, and one Simmons citrate agar slant for the citrate utilization test (see Fig. 12-17).

Indole Production

Purpose. As the name implies, the indole production test is used to determine if the organism is capable of producing indole. Indole production is a useful test for differentiating *E. coli* (indole positive) from Enterobacteriaceae in the *Klebsiella-Enterobacter-Hafnia-Serratia* group of bacteria, most of which are indole negative.

Principle. The indole test is actually a test to determine if the organism possesses several enzymes collectively referred to as tryptophanase. In the presence of tryptophanase, the amino acid tryptophan is broken down (hydrolyzed and deaminated) into indole, pyruvic acid, ammonia, and energy. Thus, following incubation of the organism with tryptophan, the presence of indole in the tube is evidence that the organism possesses tryptophanase.

Reagents. The medium to be used must contain tryptophan. A 1% tryptophan broth is prepared using trypticase, sodium chloride, and water. Either Kovac or Ehrlich reagent can be used; both reagents contain para-dimethylaminobenzaldehyde.

Procedure. The procedure varies slightly, depending on whether Kovac or Ehrlich reagent is being used.

1. Inoculate tryptophan broth (or another suitable medium) with the test organism.

2. Incubate at 35°C for 18 to 24 hours.

3. If Ehrlich reagent is used, add 1 mL xylene to the tube. This step is not necessary if Kovac reagent is used.

4. Add 15 drops of either Ehrlich or Kovac reagent, letting the reagent flow down the inner wall of the tube.

5. Observe for the immediate formation of a bright red color at the interface of the reagent and the broth (or

the xylene layer). A red complex is produced when indole reacts with the aldehyde group of para-dimethylaminobenzaldehyde.

Commercial filter paper strips saturated with para-dimethylaminobenzaldehyde are available for screening bacteria that are prompt indole producers.

Interpretation of results. A bright red color indicates the presence of indole and is interpreted as a positive test result. The absence of a bright red color is interpreted as a negative test result.

What to report. The organism is either indole positive or indole negative.

Quality control information. Use *E. coli* as a positive control and *Klebsiella pneumoniae* as a negative control.

Methyl Red

Purpose. The methyl red (MR) test is used to detect the production of large amounts of acid by a test organism. Like the indole test, the MR test is useful for differentiating between *E. coli* (MR positive) and the *Klebsiella-Enterobacter-Hafnia-Serratia* group (MR negative).

Principle. Methyl red is a pH indicator. Only organisms that produce large amounts of strong acids (e.g., lactic, acetic, and/or formic acids) and maintain a very low pH (pH 4.4 and below) after prolonged incubation will produce a positive test result.

Reagents. The most commonly used medium is methyl red Voges-Proskauer (MRVP) broth, which is used for both the MR and Voges-Proskauer tests. Methyl red pH indicator is also used.

Procedure

1. Inoculate a tube of MRVP broth with a pure culture of the organism to be tested.

2. Incubate the broth at 35°C for 48 to 72 hours (a minimum of 48 hours).

3. Add 5 drops of the methyl red reagent to the broth.

Interpretation of results. The immediate formation of a stable, bright red color at the surface of the broth indicates a pH of 4.4 or lower and is a positive test result. Neither a red-orange color (a weakly positive test result) nor a yellow color (a negative test result) should be reported as MR positive.

Quality control information. Use *E. coli* as a positive control and *Enterobacter aerogenes* as a negative control.

Voges-Proskauer

Purpose. Like the indole and methyl red tests, the Voges-Proskauer (V-P) test is useful for differentiating between *E. coli* (V-P negative) and the *Klebsiella-Enterobacter-Hafnia-Serratia* group (V-P positive).

Principle. Organisms in the *Klebsiella-Enterobacter-Hafnia-Serratia* group produce acetoin as the major end product of glucose metabolism. In the presence of atmospheric oxygen and 40% potassium hydroxide (KOH), acetoin is converted to diacetyl. When α-naphthol is added to diacetyl, a pink-to-red complex is formed.

Reagents. MRVP broth, 5% α-naphthol, and 40% KOH.

Procedure

1. Inoculate a tube of MRVP broth with a pure culture of the organism to be tested.

2. Incubate the broth at 35°C for 24 hours.

3. Transfer 1 mL of the broth to a clean test tube.

4. Add 0.6 mL of 5% α-naphthol and then 0.2 mL of 40% KOH to the tube. Do not reverse the order of the reagents added to the tube.

5. Shake the tube gently to expose the mixture to atmospheric oxygen.

6. Allow the tube to remain undisturbed for 10 to 15 minutes.

Interpretation of results. The development of a pink-to-red color 15 minutes or more (up to 1 hour) after the addition of the reagents indicates the presence of diacetyl; this is interpreted as a positive test result. A yellow color indicates a negative test result.

Quality control information. Use *Enterobacter aerogenes* as a positive control and *E. coli* as a negative control.

Citrate Utilization

Purpose. The citrate utilization test is used to determine if a bacterial isolate can utilize citrate as the sole carbon source.

Principle. The test medium contains sodium citrate (a salt of citric acid) as the only source of carbon. It also contains ammonium phosphate as a nitrogen source. Any organism capable of using citrate as a sole carbon source can also extract nitrogen from the inorganic ammonium salt, leading to the production of ammonia and alkalization of the medium.

Reagent. The most commonly used test medium is Simmons citrate medium, which is green.

Procedure

1. Inoculate the slant surface of a tube of Simmons medium, using a single streak line.

2. Incubate the tube at 35°C for 24 to 48 hours.

Interpretation of results. Growth on the medium with or without the development of a deep blue color (indicative of the production of alkaline products) is interpreted as a positive test result. No growth is interpreted as a negative test result.

Quality control information. Use *Enterobacter aerogenes* as a positive control and *E. coli* as a negative control.

LAP (LEUCINE AMINOPEPTIDASE)

Purpose. The LAP test is useful in the identification of streptococci, enterococci, and some *Streptococcus*-like organisms. The test identifies the presence of the enzyme leucine aminopeptidase; aminopeptidase is also called arylamidase.

Principle. Leucine aminopeptidase hydrolyzes the substrate leucine-α-naphthylamide to leucine and free α-naphthylamine. α-Naphthylamine reacts with para-dimethylaminocinnamaldehyde (DMACA) to produce a red color.

Reagents. Commercial disk containing leucine-α-naphthylamide and DMACA reagent.

Procedure

1. Moisten a disk with sterile water.

2. Heavily inoculate the moistened disk with colonial growth.

3. After 10 minutes, add a drop of the DMACA reagent.

4. Observe for a red color after 3 minutes.

Interpretation of results. Development of a red color on the disk constitutes a positive test result. A pink color is a weakly positive result. A yellow color is a negative result. All *Streptococcus* and *Enterococcus* spp. are LAP positive. Some less frequently isolated *Streptococcus*-like Gram-positive cocci are LAP positive, whereas others are LAP negative.

Quality control information. Use a known LAP-positive organism, such as *S. pyogenes*, as a positive control. Use a known LAP-negative organism, such as a *Leuconostoc* sp., as a negative control.

LYSOSTAPHIN SUSCEPTIBILITY

Purpose. The lysostaphin susceptibility test helps to differentiate between *Staphylococcus* (lysostaphin susceptible) and *Micrococcus* (lysostaphin resistant) spp. Some *Staphylococcus* spp. are more susceptible to the enzyme than others.

Principle. Lysostaphin is an endopeptidase that cleaves peptidoglycan cross bridges in the cell walls of staphylococci, rendering the bacterial cells susceptible to osmotic lysis.

Reagent. Commercial lysostaphin tube test. A filter paper disk diffusion test is also commercially available.

Procedure

1. Using growth on a beef peptone-based culture medium, prepare a heavy suspension of the test organism in 0.2 mL sterile saline.

2. Add 0.2 mL of lysostaphin solution.

3. Incubate at 35°C for 2 hours.

4. Observe for clearing of the suspension.

Interpretation of results. Clearing of the suspension indicates that the organism is susceptible to lysostaphin; this constitutes a positive test result. *Staphylococcus* spp. are susceptible to lysostaphin, whereas *Micrococcus* spp. are not.

Quality control information. Use a *Staphylococcus* sp. as a positive control and a *Micrococcus* sp. as a negative control.

MUG (4-METHYLUMBELLIFERYL-β-D-GLUCURONIDE)

Purpose. The MUG test is used to determine if a bacterial isolate can produce the enzyme β-D-glucuronidase.

Principle. In the presence of β-D-glucuronidase, the substrate 4-methylumbelliferyl-β-D-glucuronide is hydrolyzed to yield the 4-methylumbelliferyl moiety, which fluoresces blue under long-wave (360-nm) ultraviolet light.

Reagent. Commercial MUG disk.

Procedure

1. Wet a MUG disk with a drop of water.

2. Using a wooden applicator stick or a bacteriological loop, roll a portion of a colony onto the disk.

3. Incubate at 35°C in a closed container for up to 2 hours.

4. Observe the disk using a long-wave ultraviolet light.

Interpretation of results. An electric-blue fluorescence constitutes a positive test result. Lack of fluorescence constitutes a negative test result.

Quality control information. Use *Escherichia coli* as a positive control and a *Proteus* sp. as a negative control.

NIACIN ACCUMULATION

Purpose. The niacin accumulation test is used to differentiate between certain *Mycobacterium* spp. For example, *M. tuberculosis* is niacin accumulation positive, whereas *M. bovis* is niacin accumulation negative.

Principle. Although all *Mycobacterium* spp. can produce niacin ribonucleotide from niacin, some strains cannot further convert niacin ribonucleotide to nicotinamide adenine dinucleotide (NAD). Niacin accumulates in the culture medium of *Mycobacterium* spp. unable to convert niacin ribonucleotide to NAD.

Reagent. A niacin filter paper strip.

Procedure

1. Add 1 mL of sterile distilled water to a tube of Löwenstein-Jensen culture medium containing heavy growth of the organism to be tested. Stab the medium with the pipette tip to allow the water to access the underlying medium.

2. Tilt the tube so that the water covers the surface of the slant. Let stand 20 to 30 minutes at room temperature to allow extraction of niacin from the medium.

3. Carefully remove 0.5 mL of the extract liquid without touching the medium, and transfer to a small screw-capped test tube.

4. Using forceps, drop a niacin filter paper test strip into the tube, with the arrow on the strip pointing downward. Screw the cap on tightly.

5. Gently shake the tube. Shake again after 5 and 10 minutes.

6. After 12 to 15 minutes, observe for a yellow color.

Interpretation of results. Development of a yellow color in the fluid (not on the strip) indicates the presence of niacin. Thus, a yellow color in the fluid represents a positive test result (see Fig. 10-15). Virtually all strains of *M. tuberculosis* and *M. simiae* and some strains of *M. chelonae* are niacin accumulation test positive.

Quality control information. Use *M. tuberculosis* as a positive control and *M. intracellulare* as a negative control.

NITRATE REDUCTION

Purpose. The nitrate reduction test is used to determine if a bacterial isolate is capable of reducing nitrates. Some organisms reduce nitrates to nitrites, while others reduce nitrates beyond nitrites—sometimes all the way to nitrogen gas.

Principle. Following incubation of the test organism in nitrate broth or on a nitrate agar slant, reagents are added to determine if nitrite is present in the medium. The presence of nitrites indicates that the organism is capable of reducing nitrates. The absence of nitrites shows that either the organism was unable to reduce nitrates or the nitrates were reduced beyond nitrites. The nitrate reduction test is designed to determine which of these possibilities occurred (see Fig. 12-15).

Reagents. Nitrate broth or a nitrate agar slant, α-naphthylamine in acetic acid (referred to as reagent A), and sulfanilic acid in acetic acid (referred to as reagent B).

Procedure

1. Inoculate the nitrate medium with one loopful of the test organism.

2. Incubate at 35°C for 18 to 24 hours.

3. Add 1 mL of reagent A and then 1 mL of reagent B to the test medium. **Do not reverse the order of the reagents added to the tube.**

Interpretation of results. Development of a red color within 30 seconds of addition of reagents indicates the presence of nitrites and represents a positive test result. The organism can be reported as nitrate positive (see Fig. 12-16).

No red color at this point represents the absence of nitrites. Either the organism was unable to reduce nitrates or it reduced the nitrates beyond nitrites. Add a small amount of zinc dust to the tube. If nitrates are present, they are reduced to nitrites, and a red color develops. At this point, a red color is interpreted as a negative test result—that the organism was unable to reduce nitrates. If no red color develops following the addition of zinc dust, there are no nitrates present in the tube because they were reduced beyond nitrites. Thus, no red color following the addition of zinc dust constitutes a positive test result; the organism is nitrate positive.

Quality control information. Use *Escherichia coli* as a positive control and *Acinetobacter baumannii* as a negative control.

NOVOBIOCIN RESISTANCE

Purpose. Novobiocin resistance is a useful test in the speciation of coagulase-negative staphylococci.

Principle. Growth of some species of coagulase-negative staphylococci (e.g., *S. epidermidis*) will be inhibited by novobiocin, whereas growth of other species (e.g., *S. saprophyticus*) will not.

Reagent. Novobiocin, which is an antibiotic produced by some *Streptomyces* spp.

Procedure

1. Prepare a suspension of the organism to be tested in sterile distilled water or broth. The suspension should be equivalent to a 0.5 McFarland turbidity standard.

2. Using a sterile swab, spread some of the suspension over one-half of the surface of a blood agar plate.

3. Aseptically place a 5-μg novobiocin disk in the center of the inoculated area. Gently press the disk so that it is flush with the agar surface. (Furazolidone sensitivity can be assessed on the same plate. Place the disks about 4 cm apart.)

4. Incubate the plate at 35°C in a non-CO_2 incubator for 18 to 24 hours.

5. Check for a zone of no growth and, if present, measure its diameter.

Interpretation of results. *S. saprophyticus* is novobiocin resistant, with zone diameters up to 12 mm. A novobiocin-resistant, coagulase-negative *Staphylococcus* sp. isolated from a positive urine culture can be presumptively identified as *S. saprophyticus* (see Fig. 9-13). Other coagulase-negative staphylococci and *S. aureus* are novobiocin susceptible, with zone diameters of 16 mm or larger.

Quality control information. Controls should be run weekly and with each new lot of disks. Use *S. saprophyticus* ATCC 49453 as a novobiocin-resistant control and *S. epidermidis* ATCC 12228 as a novobiocin-susceptible control.

O-F (OXIDATION-FERMENTATION)

Purpose. The O-F test is used to determine if a bacterial isolate is capable of catabolizing a particular carbohydrate and, if so, whether the organism does so via an oxidative pathway, a fermentative pathway, or both.

Principle. The test organism is inoculated into two tubes of medium containing a particular carbohydrate. The medium in one tube is overlaid with mineral oil; whatever happens in this tube, happens in the absence of oxygen (anaerobically). The other tube remains open (no mineral oil overlay); whatever happens in this tube happens in the presence of oxygen (aerobically).

Reagents. Tubes of O-F carbohydrate media, each tube containing a single carbohydrate and phenol red indicator, and sterile mineral oil or melted paraffin.

Procedure

1. Inoculate two tubes of O-F medium containing the same carbohydrate. Inoculate each tube by stabbing the semisolid medium 3 or 4 times halfway to the bottom of the tube. Inoculate two tubes for each carbohydrate to be tested.

2. Overlay the medium in one of the tubes with 1 cm of sterile mineral oil or melted paraffin. This tube is referred to as the closed tube. The other tube is the open tube.

3. Incubate both tubes at 35°C and examine daily for several days.

Interpretation of results. A change in the color of the medium from green to yellow indicates the production of acid and constitutes a positive test result. No color change constitutes a negative test result. Results are interpreted as shown in the following table.

Open Tube	Closed Tube	Interpretation
Yellow	Green	Organism is an oxidizer of this particular carbohydrate (Fig. 13-3)
Yellow	Yellow	Organism is a fermenter of this particular carbohydrate (Fig. 13-4)
Green	Green	Organism is unable to catabolize this particular carbohydrate; sometimes referred to as a nonoxidizer

Quality control information. For glucose, use *Escherichia coli* as a fermenter control, *Pseudomonas aeruginosa* as an oxidizer control, and a *Moraxella* sp. as a nonoxidizer control. Other QC organisms are used as controls for other carbohydrates.

ONPG (O-NITROPHENYL-β-D-GALACTOPYRANOSIDE)

Purpose. The ONPG test detects the ability of a bacterial isolate to ferment lactose. A positive ONPG test is especially useful in identifying late lactose fermenters (e.g., *Citrobacter* and *Serratia* spp.).

Principle. The abbreviation ONPG stands for o-nitrophenyl-β-D-galactopyranoside, a molecule that is structurally similar to lactose. If a bacterial isolate produces the enzyme β-galactosidase, ONPG is hydrolyzed to produce galactose and o-nitrophenyl (which is yellow).

Reagents. Physiologic saline, toluene, and buffered ONPG solution.

Procedure

1. Remove a loopful of growth from a medium containing lactose. Kligler iron agar or triple-sugar iron agar give the best results.

2. Emulsify the growth in 0.5 mL of physiologic saline to produce a heavy suspension.

3. Add 1 drop of toluene to the suspension, and mix vigorously for a few seconds to release the β-galactosidase from the cells.

4. Add an equal quantity of buffered ONPG solution, and place the mixture in a 37°C water bath.

5. If using a commercial ONPG tablet, place the tablet into a small test tube. Add 1 mL of distilled water. Mix in a loopful of growth. Mix vigorously, and place the tube in a 37°C water bath for up to 24 hours.

Interpretation of results. Production of a yellow color constitutes a positive test result (see Fig. 12-22). The reaction may occur rapidly (within 5 to 10 minutes) or may take longer. The test should not be interpreted as negative before 24 hours of incubation.

Quality control information. Use *Escherichia coli* as a positive control and a *Proteus* sp. as a negative control.

OPTOCHIN SENSITIVITY (P-DISK)

Purpose. The P-disk test is used whenever an α-hemolytic *Streptococcus* sp. is isolated from a clinical specimen. It is used to differentiate *S. pneumoniae* from other α-hemolytic streptococci. The *P* in *P*-disk test stands for *pneumoniae*.

Principle. The P-disk is a small circular piece of filter paper saturated with a chemical called optochin. The test determines whether an organism is susceptible or resistant to optochin.

Reagent. Optochin.

Procedure

1. Heavily inoculate a section of a blood agar plate with the α-hemolytic *Streptococcus* sp. to be tested.

2. Gently press a P-disk to the inoculated surface.

3. Incubate the plate overnight in a CO_2 incubator at 37°C.

Interpretation of results. Either the organism is killed by optochin or it is not. If the organism is killed by optochin, a zone of no growth forms around the disk; this constitutes a positive P-disk result (see Fig. 9-22). If the organism is not killed by optochin, a zone of no growth does not form, and the P-disk result is negative.

What to report. The only α-hemolytic *Streptococcus* sp. killed by optochin is *S. pneumoniae*. Thus, if the P-disk test indicates that the organism has been killed by optochin, the organism has been identified and should be reported as *S. pneumoniae*. If the organism was not killed by optochin, the report should read, "α-Hemolytic *Streptococcus* sp. other than *Streptococcus pneumoniae*."

Quality control information. QC organisms are used to test each newly received lot of P-disks, and the disks are checked at least weekly. A strain of *S. pneumoniae* (e.g., ATCC 6305) is used as the positive control, and any other α-hemolytic *Streptococcus* sp. (e.g., *S. gallolyticus* ATCC 49147) is used as the negative control.

OXIDASE

Purpose. The oxidase test is useful in identifying Gram-negative bacilli (GNB). Some GNB produce the enzyme oxidase (e.g., *Neisseria* spp. and *Pseudomonas aeruginosa*), but other GNB do not (e.g., *Escherichia coli* and other members of the family Enterobacteriaceae). Organisms that produce oxidase are said to be oxidase positive, while those that do not produce oxidase are said to be oxidase negative. The oxidase test is performed whenever a GNB is isolated from a clinical specimen.

Principle. *Oxidase* is an abbreviation for the enzyme cytochrome oxidase. This enzyme plays an important role in the electron transport chain. Specifically, it is responsible for transferring electrons to oxygen (the terminal electron acceptor), thus enabling the oxygen to combine with hydrogen ions to form molecules of water.

Reagent. Tetramethyl-para-phenylenediamine dihydrochloride. Because of its lengthy name, this reagent is usually simply referred to as the oxidase reagent.

Procedure

1. Saturate a piece of filter paper with the oxidase reagent.

2. Using a sterile bacteriological inoculating loop, rub a colony of the organism to be tested onto the saturated filter paper.

3. Observe for the formation of a deep blue-to-purple color.

Interpretation of test results. The appearance of deep blue-purple within 10 seconds is interpreted as a positive test,

meaning that the organism is producing oxidase (see Fig. 11-5). The oxidase reagent has been oxidized, leading to the formation of the end product called indophenol blue. If no deep blue-purple color appears, the test is interpreted as negative, meaning that the organism is not producing oxidase.

What to report. An organism cannot be identified solely on the basis of an oxidase test. If a report is needed at this point, the organism is reported as being either an oxidase-positive or oxidase-negative GNB.

Quality control information. QC organisms are used to test each newly received lot of oxidase reagent, and the reagent is checked on each day of use. A strain of *P. aeruginosa* is used as the positive control, and a strain of *E. coli* is used as the negative control.

MODIFIED OXIDASE

Purpose. The modified oxidase test is primarily used to differentiate *Staphylococcus* spp. from *Micrococcus* spp.

Principle. See "Oxidase" for a discussion of the principle. Dimethyl sulfoxide (DMSO) is used in the modified procedure to render the bacterial cells permeable to the oxidase reagent.

Reagent. Commercial filter paper disk containing the oxidase reagent (tetramethyl-para-phenylenediamine dihydrochloride) and DMSO. The disks, called Microdase Test Disks, are available from Remel (http://www.remelinc.com/).

Procedure

1. Using an applicator stick, remove a colony from the growth medium and rub it into a Microdase Test Disk.

2. Observe for the development of a blue-purple color within 30 seconds.

Interpretation of results. Development of a blue-purple color within 30 seconds is considered a positive test result (see Fig. 9-6). No color development within this time frame is considered a negative test result. *Micrococcus* spp., *Macrococcus* spp., and some other Gram-positive cocci are modified oxidase positive, whereas most *Staphylococcus* spp. and some other Gram-positive cocci are modified oxidase negative.

Quality control information. Use any *Micrococcus* sp. as a positive control and *Staphylococcus epidermidis* as a negative control.

PAD (PHENYLALANINE DEAMINASE)

Purpose. The only members of the Enterobacteriaceae family that produce phenylalanine deaminase are *Proteus*, *Morganella*, and *Providencia* spp. Thus, the PAD test is useful in the identification of members of these genera.

Principle. The enzyme phenylalanine deaminase causes deamination of the amino acid, phenylalanine. Deamination involves the removal of the amino end of phenylalanine.

The resulting products are phenylpyruvic acid and ammonia. A ferric chloride solution is added to detect the presence of phenylpyruvic acid. Phenylpyruvic acid and the ferric ion (Fe^{+++}) combine to produce a green complex.

Reagents. Phenylalanine agar and 10% ferric chloride solution.

Procedure

1. Inoculate a phenylalanine agar slant with the organism to be tested.

2. Incubate at 35°C for 18 to 24 hours.

3. Add 4 or 5 drops of ferric chloride reagent to the surface of the agar slant, while rotating the tube to dislodge the surface colonies.

Interpretation of results. The immediate appearance of an intense green color indicates the presence of phenylpyruvic acid, which is interpreted as a positive test result (see Fig. 12-24). The absence of a green color is interpreted as a negative test result.

Quality control information. Use a *Proteus* sp. as a positive control and *Escherichia coli* as a negative control.

PYR (PYRROLIDONYL ARYLAMIDASE)

Purpose. The PYR test is used in the rapid identification of *Streptococcus pyogenes* (β-hemolytic) and most strains of *Enterococcus* (which may be α- or β-hemolytic or nonhemolytic), all of which are PYR positive. The test can also be used to differentiate *Staphylococcus lugdunensis* (PYR positive) from *Staphylococcus epidermidis* (PYR negative).

Principle. The substrate in the PYR test is L-pyrrolidonyl-β.-naphthylamide. If present, the enzyme pyrrolidonyl arylamide (pyrrolidonase) hydrolyzes that substrate to free β-naphthylamide and L-pyrrolidone. The reagent para-dimethylaminocinnamaldehyde (DMACA) couples with naphthylamide to produce a red product.

Reagents. PYR broth containing L-pyrrolidonyl-β-naphthylamide and PYR reagent containing DMACA.

Procedure

1. Emulsify two or three colonies of the organism to be tested in 0.20 mL of PYR broth.

2. Incubate the tube at 35°C for 4 hours.

3. Add 1 drop of the PYR reagent, wait 1 minute, and then observe for a color change.

The PYR test can also be performed using commercial filter paper disks or strips.

Interpretation of results. The development of a deep cherry red color is interpreted as a positive test result. A yellow or orange color is interpreted as a negative reaction.

Quality control information. Use *Enterococcus faecalis* or *Streptococcus pyogenes* as a positive control and *Streptococcus agalactiae* as a negative control.

PZA (PYRAZINAMIDASE)

Purpose. The PZA test is used to determine the presence of the enzyme pyrazinamidase and thus to differentiate between certain *Mycobacterium* spp.

Principle. Pyrazinamidase deaminates pyrazidamide to ammonia and pyrazinoic acid. The test determines whether pyrazinoic acid has been produced.

Reagents. Pyrazinamidase substrate medium and 1% ferrous ammonium sulfate.

Procedure

1. Heavily inoculate the surface of two tubes of pyrazinamidase substrate medium.

2. Incubate with caps loose at 37°C for 4 days. Also incubate two uninoculated control tubes.

3. Remove one inoculated tube and one control tube from the incubator, and add 1.0 mL of freshly prepared 1% ferrous ammonium sulfate to each tube.

4. After 30 minutes at room temperature, examine the tubes for a pink band in the reagent layer on the surface of the agar. Use incident room light against a white background. Refrigerate negative tubes for 4 hours, and reexamine for the presence of a pink band.

5. If negative, repeat the procedure with the remaining two tubes after 7 days of incubation.

Interpretation of results. Development of a pink band indicates the presence of pyrazinoic acid. Thus, the presence of a pink band constitutes a positive test result (see Fig. 10-18). *M. tuberculosis* is pyrazinamidase positive, whereas *M. bovis* is pyrazinamidase negative. *M. marinum* is pyrazinamidase positive, whereas *M. kansasii* is pyrazinamidase negative.

Quality control information. Use *M. intracellulare* as a positive control and *M. kansasii* as a negative control.

RAPID HIPPURATE HYDROLYSIS

Purpose. The rapid hippurate hydrolysis test is used to differentiate *Streptococcus agalactiae* (group B strep) from other β-hemolytic streptococci.

Principle. Hydrolysis of sodium hippurate produces benzoic acid and the amino acid glycine. When ninhydrin (a protein detector) is added, it reacts with glycine to produce a deep blue color.

Reagents. 1% sodium hippurate and ninhydrin solution.

Procedure

1. From a fresh subculture on blood agar, add a heavy inoculum of the test organism to a tube containing 0.4 mL of 1% sodium hippurate. Be careful not to transfer any of the agar medium during inoculation; the protein present in the agar would cause a weak positive test result.

2. Emulsify the test organism in the sodium hippurate substrate.

3. Incubate the tube for 2 hours in a 37°C heating block or water bath.

4. Add 0.2 mL of ninhydrin solution and mix gently. Do not shake or vigorously agitate the tube.

5. Return the tube to the heating block or water bath and wait 10 minutes. Incubation longer than 30 minutes may cause a false-positive result.

6. Observe the color of the tube contents.

Interpretation of results. A deep blue color is indicative of a positive test result. Virtually all strains of *S. agalactiae* produce positive test results. If the liquid is colorless or has a faint tinge of purple, the test result is negative.

Quality control information. Use fresh subcultures of *S. agalactiae* ATCC 12386 as a positive control and *S. pyogenes* ATCC 19615 as a negative control. The control organisms should be growing on soybean casein digest agar with 5% sheep blood.

SALT TOLERANCE

Purpose. The salt tolerance test is primarily used to differentiate between certain Gram-positive cocci. *Enterococcus* spp. are salt tolerant, whereas the group D streptococci *S. bovis* and *S. equinus* are not salt tolerant. (Both *Enterococcus* spp. and group D streptococci are bile-esculin positive.)

Principle. The salt tolerance test determines the ability of a bacterial isolate to grow in 6.5% sodium chloride (NaCl) broth.

Reagent. 6.5% NaCl broth, with or without bromcresol purple indicator.

Procedure

1. Inoculate two or three colonies into a tube of 6.5% NaCl broth.

2. Incubate overnight at 35°C in a non-CO_2 incubator.

3. Observe for growth.

A different salt tolerance test is used to test mycobacteria.

Interpretation of results. Growth in the 6.5% NaCl broth, with or without a color change in the pH indicator (if present), constitutes a positive test result (see Fig. 9-24). No evidence of growth constitutes a negative test result.

Quality control information. Use *Enterococcus faecalis* ATCC 29212 as a positive control and *Streptococcus gallolyticus* ATCC 9809 as a negative control.

TCH (THIOPHENE-2-CARBOXYLIC ACID HYDRAZIDE)

Purpose. The TCH test is useful for differentiating between *Mycobacterium tuberculosis* and *M. bovis*.

Principle. Growth of *M. bovis* is inhibited by thiophene-2-carboxylic acid hydrazide (TCH or T2H), whereas growth of *M. tuberculosis* is not.

Reagents. Quadrant plates containing TCH susceptibility medium: quadrants I and III contain Middlebrook 7H10 medium without TCH (referred to as control quadrants), and quadrants II and IV contain Middlebrook 7H10 medium with TCH (referred to as TCH quadrants).

Procedure

1. Prepare a suspension of the unknown mycobacterium in sterile deionized water. Use a 3-to-4-week-old culture on Löwenstein-Jensen or Middlebrook 7H10 medium. The suspension should be equivalent to a 1 McFarland turbidity standard.

2. Prepare two dilutions (10^{-3} and 10^{-4}) in sterile deionized water.

3. Inoculate 3 drops of each dilution onto a control quadrant and 3 drops of each dilution onto a TCH quadrant.

4. Cover the plate with brown paper and leave it at room temperature for several minutes to allow adsorption of the inoculum.

5. Place the plate into a CO_2-permeable zipper bag, invert the plate, and incubate it at 37°C in 8% to 10% CO_2 for 3 weeks.

6. Remove the plate from the incubator, and count the colonies on each quadrant.

Interpretation of results. The organism is considered resistant to TCH if the number of colonies on the TCH medium is greater than 1% of the growth on the control medium (see Fig. 10-17).

Quality control information. Use *M. bovis* ATCC 35734 as a positive (susceptible) control and *M. tuberculosis* ATCC 25177 as a negative (resistant) control.

UREASE

Purpose. The urease test is performed to determine if a bacterial isolate is producing the enzyme urease.

Principle. Urease hydrolyzes urea to ammonia and carbon dioxide. The presence of ammonia causes an increase in the pH of the test medium.

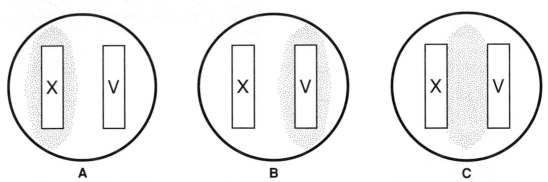

Figure A-6. **X and V factor test results (stippling represents growth of the test organism). A.** Results obtained with an organism that requires X factor but not V factor. **B.** Results obtained with an organism that requires V factor but not X factor. **C.** Results obtained with an organism that requires both X and V factors. (From Winn WC Jr, et al. Koneman's Color Atlas and Textbook of Diagnostic Microbiology. 6th Ed. Philadelphia: Lippincott Williams & Wilkins, 2006.)

Reagents. The two media most commonly used to detect urease activity are Stuart urea broth and Christensen urea agar. Both contain phenol red as a pH indicator.

Procedure

1. Inoculate either the broth or the agar slant with the organism to be tested.

2. Incubate at 35°C for 18 to 24 hours.

A different urease test is used to test mycobacteria.

Interpretation of results. A red color throughout the Stuart broth indicates alkalization and is interpreted as a positive test result. The test is negative if the broth remains yellow. With Christensen agar, a red color throughout the medium is indicative of a rapid urea splitter, such as a *Proteus* sp. Slow urea splitters, such as *Klebsiella* spp., produce a red slant that gradually converts the entire tube to red. The test is negative if the medium remains yellow (see Figs. 12-14 and 12-24).

Quality control information. Use a *Proteus* sp. as a positive control, a *Klebsiella* sp. as a weak positive control, and *Escherichia coli* as a negative control.

X AND V FACTORS

Purpose. Determining a requirement for X and V factors is useful for identifying *Haemophilus* spp.

Principle. This test determines a bacterial isolate's requirement for X factor (hemin or hematin) and/or V factor (nicotinamide adenine dinucleotide).

Reagents. Filter paper strips saturated with X and V factors and an agar medium lacking these factors (e.g., trypticase soy or brain-heart infusion agar).

Procedure

1. Prepare a light suspension of the organism to be tested in brain-heart infusion broth. Be careful not to transfer any of the culture medium during inoculation of the broth.

2. Using this suspension, inoculate the entire surface of an appropriate agar medium (one that is lacking X and V factors).

3. Place one X-factor strip and one V-factor strip on the plate. The strips should be flush with the agar surface and placed about 1 cm apart.

4. Incubate the plate at 35°C in 3% to 5% CO_2 for 18 to 24 hours.

Interpretation of results. Examine the plates for visible growth (Fig. A-6). If the organism is growing only around the X-factor strip, it has a requirement for X factor. If it is growing only around the V-factor strip, it has a requirement for V factor. If it is growing only between the X- and V-factor strips, it has a requirement for both X and V factors.

Quality control information. Use *H. parainfluenzae* (requires only V factor) and *H. influenzae* (requires both X and V factors) as controls.

References and Suggested Reading

Abbreviated Identification of Bacteria and Yeast: Approved Guideline. CLSI Document M35-A. Wayne, PA: Clinical and Laboratory Standards Institute (CLSI), 2002.

American Type Culture Collection (ATCC). http://www.atcc.org/.

Murray PR, Baron EJ, Jorgensen JH, Pfaller MA, Yolken RH, eds. Manual of Clinical Microbiology. 8th Ed. Washington, DC: ASM Press, 2003.

Winn WC Jr, et al. Koneman's Color Atlas and Textbook of Diagnostic Microbiology. 6th Ed. Philadelphia: Lippincott Williams & Wilkins, 2006.

Appendix B

Useful Conversions

LENGTH CONVERSIONS

- To convert inches into centimeters, multiply by 2.54.

- To convert centimeters into inches, multiply by 0.39.

- To convert yards into meters, multiply by 0.91.

- To convert meters into yards, multiply by 1.09.

1 mile (mi) = 1.609 kilometers
1 yard (yd) = 0.914 meter
1 foot (ft) = 30.48 centimeters
1 inch (in) = 2.54 centimeters
1 kilometer (km) = 0.62 mile
1 meter (m) = 39.37 inches
1 centimeter (cm) = 0.39 inch
1 millimeter (mm) = 0.039 inch

Note: Information about micrometers and nanometers can be found in Figure 6-1.

VOLUME CONVERSIONS

- To convert gallons into liters, multiply by 3.78.

- To convert liters into gallons, multiply by 0.26.

- To convert fluid ounces into milliliters, multiply by 29.6.

- To convert milliliters into fluid ounces, multiply by 0.034.

1 gallon (gal) = 3.785 liters
1 quart (qt) = 0.946 liter
1 pint (pt) = 0.473 liter
1 fluid ounce (fl oz) = 29.573 milliliters
1 liter (L) = 1.057 quarts
1 milliliter (mL) = 0.0338 fluid ounce

WEIGHT CONVERSIONS

- To convert ounces into grams, multiply by 28.4.

- To convert grams into ounces, multiply by 0.035.

- To convert pounds into kilograms, multiply by 0.45.

- To convert kilograms into pounds, multiply by 2.2.

1 pound (lb) = 0.454 kilogram
1 ounce (oz) = 28.35 grams
1 kilogram (kg) = 2.2 pounds
1 gram (gm) = 0.035 ounce
1 gram = 1,000 milligrams (mg)
1 gram = 1,000,000 micrograms (μg)

TEMPERATURE CONVERSIONS

- To convert Celsius (°C) into Fahrenheit (°F), use °F = (°C × 1.8) + 32.

- To convert Fahrenheit (°F) into Celsius (°C), use °C = (°F − 32) × 0.556.

Appendix C

Answers to Self-Assessment Exercises

CHAPTER 1

1. c
2. b
3. b
4. c
5. b
6. c
7. d
8. c
9. c
10. c

CHAPTER 2

1. d
2. c
3. d
4. d
5. c
6. c
7. c
8. a
9. c
10. d

CHAPTER 3

1. b
2. c
3. a
4. c

5. a
6. d
7. b
8. c
9. d
10. d

CHAPTER 4

1. c
2. a
3. c
4. c
5. d
6. b
7. c
8. d
9. a
10. b

CHAPTER 5

1. c
2. d
3. b
4. c
5. a
6. d
7. a
8. b
9. b
10. d

CHAPTER 6

1. d
2. d
3. d
4. c
5. c
6. a
7. c
8. c
9. d
10. b

CHAPTER 7

1. d
2. c
3. c
4. a
5. c
6. a
7. a
8. a
9. c
10. b

CHAPTER 8

1. b
2. a
3. a
4. b
5. c
6. b
7. b
8. d
9. a
10. d

CHAPTER 9

1. e
2. c
3. b
4. a
5. d
6. a
7. b
8. True
9. False
10. True

CHAPTER 10

1. a. *Corynebacterium*; b. *Nocardia*; c. *Mycobacterium*
2. Lungs
3. c
4. a
5. d
6. c
7. d
8. a
9. b
10. d

CHAPTER 11

1. a
2. b
3. d
4. c
5. True
6. False
7. True
8. a
9. d
10. c

CHAPTER 12

1. b
2. a
3. d
4. c
5. e
6. False
7. a
8. b
9. c
10. a. Glucose fermentation; b. Gas production; c. H_2S production

CHAPTER 13

1. b
2. d
3. c
4. a
5. a
6. True
7. True
8. True
9. d
10. b

CHAPTER 14

1. c
2. a
3. c
4. c
5. d
6. a
7. b
8. e
9. d

10. *Satelliting* refers to the fact that an organism can only grow in the vicinity of an organism that is producing an essential nutrient that is not present in the culture medium (e.g., on a blood agar plate, *Haemophilus influenzae* can only grow in the vicinity of a V factor-producing organism, such as *Staphylococcus aureus* or an *Enterococcus* sp.)

CHAPTER 15

1. a
2. e
3. d
4. b
5. c
6. True
7. False
8. d
9. c
10. a. Growth on Campy agar at 42°C; b. Curved GNB; c. Motile; d. Oxidase positive and catalase positive

CHAPTER 16

1. c
2. d
3. e
4. a
5. b
6. c
7. Following entry into a host cell, the elementary body (EB) reorganizes into a reticulate body (RB); the RB then divides repeatedly; the RBs then reorganize into EBs; the host cell ruptures, releasing the infectious EBs, which then infect neighboring cells
8. False
9. True
10. False

CHAPTER 17

1. a. An organism that can multiply in the presence of some oxygen but grows best in an anaerobic environment

b. An organism that can survive in either the presence or absence of oxygen

c. An organism that can survive only in an anaerobic environment

2. a. Electrons that would normally participate in metabolic reactions are used to reduce oxygen; cellular activity ceases, but the organisms remain alive.

b. Organisms are destroyed by the byproducts of oxygen reduction.

3. a. Gram-negative; bacilli

b. Gram-positive; spore-forming bacilli

c. Gram-negative; spindle-shaped bacilli

d. Gram-positive; cocci

e. Gram-negative; cocci

f. Gram-negative; pitting bacilli

g. Gram-positive; branching bacilli

h. Gram-positive, but stain Gram-negative; curved bacilli

i. Gram-positive; bifurcated bacilli

4. True

5. False

6. a. *B. fragilis*; b. *B. ovatus*; c. *B. stercoris*; d. *B. thetaiotaomicron*; e. *B. vulgatus*

7. True

8. a. U; b. A; c. A; d. U; e. U; f. A; g. U; h. U; i. A; j. A

9. a. Brucella blood agar; b. bacteroides bile esculin (BBE) agar; c. laked blood-kanamycin-vancomycin (LBKV) agar; d. phenylethyl alcohol (PEA) agar

10. a. Catalase; b. Spot indole; c. Fluorescence; d. Oxidase; e. Urease

CHAPTER 18

1. c

2. d

3. b

4. a

5. a. Enterobacteriaceae; b. Staphylococci; c. Streptococci

6. b

7. False

8. c

9. a. Thayer-Martin agar; b. Löwenstein-Jensen medium; c. Cycloserine-cefoxitin-fructose agar

10. True

CHAPTER 19

1. A dimorphic fungus is a fungus that can exist either as a yeast and a mould, depending upon growth conditions; demonstrate dimorphism in the laboratory by converting the mould phase to the yeast phase

2. c

3. True

4. False

5. a

6. a

7. d

8. Yeasts are larger than bacteria, are usually oval-shaped, and are often seen in the process of budding

9. Aerial hyphae (also known as reproductive hyphae)

10. a. Rate of growth; b. Macroscopic appearance; c. Microscopic appearance

CHAPTER 20

1. b

2. a

3. d

4. c

5. Black piedra, *Piedraia hortae*

6. Tinea versicolor, *Malassezia furfur*

7. Cryptococcosis, *Cryptococcus neoformans*

8. a. *Cladophialophora*; b. *Phialophora*

9. a. *Coccidioides immitis*; b. *Histoplasma capsulatum*

10. a. *Epidermophyton*; b. *Microsporum*; c. *Trichophyton*

CHAPTER 21

1. Parasites are organisms that live on or in other living organisms (hosts), at whose expense they gain some advantage

2. A definitive host is a host that harbors the adult or sexual stage of the parasite or the sexual phase of the life cycle

3. A facultative parasite is an organism that can be parasitic, but is also capable of a free-living existence

4. a. Amebae, pseudopodia; b. Flagellates, flagella; c. Ciliates, cilia

5. A cyst is a dormant stage in a protozoan's life cycle

6. a. *Giardia lamblia*; b. *Trichomonas vaginalis*

7. a. Egg; b. Larva; c. Adult worm

8. True

9. False

10. d

CHAPTER 22

1. b

2. d

3. c

4. c

5. a

6. Blood

7. Stool

8. Stool

9. False

10. True

CHAPTER 23

1. d

2. a

3. e

4. b

5. c

6. a. Cellophane tape preparation; b. Stool

7. a. By observing encysted larvae in muscle biopsy specimens; b. Immunodiagnostic procedures

8. a. *Trichuris trichiura*; b. Whipworm

9. False

10. False

CHAPTER 24

1. d

2. a

3. d

4. a. False; b. True; c. True; d. False; e. False

5. a

6. Viruses can only attach to and invade cells that bear a receptor that they can recognize; in this specific example, human cells bear the appropriate receptor, but dog cells do not

7. a. Attachment; b. Penetration; c. Uncoating; d. Biosynthesis; e. Assembly; f. Release

8. a. Primary cell line/African green monkey kidney cells; b. Low-passage cell line/human embryonic lung fibroblasts; c. Continuous culture cell line/HeLa human cervical carcinoma cells

9. a. Antigen detection; b. Antibody detection; c. Molecular diagnostic procedures

10. Cytopathic effect (CPE) refers to morphologic alterations in cell cultures that are caused by viruses; a particular virus causes a characteristic type of CPE in specific cell lines

CHAPTER 25

1. a. Epstein-Barr virus; b. HPV

2. c

3. a. Eastern equine encephalitis/birds, horses/mosquitoes; b. St. Louis encephalitis/birds/mosquitoes; c. West Nile virus encephalitis/birds/mosquitoes

4. b

5. a. Immunodiagnostic procedures; b. Molecular diagnostic procedures

6. b

7. a. CNS; b. G; c. GI; d. R; e. G

8. c

9. True

10. True

CHAPTER 26

1. a. Characteristics of the pathogens; b. Susceptibility of human populations; c. Reservoirs; d. Modes of transmission

2. Nosocomial infections are infections that are acquired within a hospital or other healthcare setting

3. a. A urinary tract infection following urinary catheterization; b. A postsurgical wound infection

4. a. *Escherichia coli*; b. *Staphylococcus aureus*; c. *Pseudomonas aeruginosa*

5. a. Monitor pathogens that are isolated from hospitalized patients; b. Notify the appropriate infection control professional if an unusual pathogen is isolated or if an unusually large number of isolates of a common pathogen is detected; c. Process environmental samples that are collected during a hospital outbreak

6. False

7. a. Smallpox virus; b. *Bacillus anthracis*; c. *Yersinia pestis*

8. a. Basic sentinel laboratories; b. Reference laboratories; c. National laboratories

9. b

10. False

Glossary

Accidental host. A living organism that can serve as a host in a particular parasite's life cycle but is not a usual host in that life cycle; some accidental hosts are dead-end hosts.

Acellular microbe. A microbe that is not composed of cells, is smaller than a cell, and has structures far less complex than those of a cell; e.g., virus, prion; also known as an *infectious agent* or *infectious particle*.

Acid-fast bacterium. A bacterium that retains the red color of carbolfuchsin dye following the decolorization step of the acid-fast staining procedure.

Acquired immunity. Immunity or resistance acquired at some point in a person's lifetime.

Acquired resistance. As the term applies to bacteria, the resistance that bacteria develop to a drug to which they were once susceptible.

***Actinomyces*-like.** Having the branched appearance of *Actinomyces* spp.

Actinomycetoma. A mycetoma caused by an actinomycete, such as a *Streptomyces* or *Nocardia* sp.

Active acquired immunity. Immunity or resistance acquired as a result of the active production of antibodies.

Acute disease. A disease having a sudden onset and short duration.

Adhesin. A molecule on the surface of a pathogen that enables the pathogen to recognize and bind to a particular receptor on the surface of a host cell; also known as a *ligand*.

Aerial hypha. A hypha that rises above the surface on which a fungal mycelium is growing; also known as a *reproductive hypha* because spores are produced on it.

Aerotolerant anaerobe. An organism that can live in the presence of oxygen but grows best in an anaerobic environment—an environment containing no oxygen.

Agammaglobulinemia. The absence of, or extremely low levels of, the γ-fraction of serum globulin; the absence of immunoglobulins in the bloodstream.

Algicidal agent. A disinfectant or chemical that specifically kills algae.

α-Hemolysis. Greenish discoloration of the blood agar medium surrounding a bacterial colony; an organism that produces α-hemolysis is *α-hemolytic*.

Amastigote. A small, round-to-oval-shaped, intracellular life cycle stage of *Leishmania* spp. and *Trypanosoma cruzi*; it has no external flagellum; called a *Leishman-Donovan (LD) body* in visceral leishmaniasis; observation of amastigotes within macrophages is the primary method of diagnosing leishmaniasis.

Ameboflagellate. A protozoan parasite that can exist as either an ameba or a flagellate in its free-living state but only as an ameba in its parasitic state; e.g., *Naegleria fowleri*.

Ameboma. A nodular, tumorlike focus of proliferative inflammation that develops in chronic amebiasis.

Amphitrichous bacterium. A bacterium that possesses one flagellum or more than one flagellum at each end (pole) of the cell.

Anabolic reaction. A metabolic reaction that requires energy for the creation of chemical bonds; also known as a *biosynthetic reaction*.

Anabolism. Refers to all the anabolic reactions that occur within a cell.

Anaerobe. An organism that does not require oxygen for survival; one that can exist in the absence of oxygen.

Anorexia. Loss of appetite.

Antagonism. The use of two drugs that work against each other.

Antibacterial agent. Technically, any physical or chemical agent that kills or inhibits the growth of bacteria; in this book, the term is reserved for a drug used to treat bacterial diseases.

Antibiogram. The pattern of antimicrobial susceptibility test results obtained when such tests are performed on a bacterial isolate; whenever two strains of the same species produce exactly the same antimicrobial susceptibility test results, they are said to have the same antibiogram.

Antibody. A glycoprotein produced by lymphocytes in response to an antigen; if it protects the host in some manner, it is called a *protective antibody*.

Antifungal agent. Technically, any physical or chemical agent that kills or inhibits the growth of fungi; in this book, the term is reserved for a drug used to treat fungal diseases.

Antigen. A substance, usually foreign, that stimulates the production of antibodies; an *anti*body-*gen*erating substance; also known as an *immunogen*.

Antigenic. Refers to a molecule that stimulates the immune system to produce antibodies.

Antigenic determinant. The smallest part of an antigen capable of stimulating the production of antibodies; an antigenic molecule; also known as an *epitope*.

Antigen-presenting cell (APC). A macrophage that is displaying antigenic determinants on its surface.

Antimicrobial agent. Technically, any physical or chemical agent that kills or inhibits the growth of microorganisms; in this book, the term is reserved for a drug used to treat infectious diseases.

Antimicrobial susceptibility testing. The laboratory procedure used to determine the antimicrobial agents to which a microorganism is susceptible and resistant.

Antiprotozoal agent. Technically, any physical or chemical agent that kills or inhibits the growth of protozoa; in this book, the term is reserved for a drug used to treat protozoal diseases.

Antisepsis. Prevention of infection by inhibiting the growth of pathogens.

Antiseptic technique. Procedures taken to effect antisepsis; the use of antiseptics.

Antiserum. A serum containing specific antibodies; also known as an *immune serum*.

Antitoxin. An antibody produced in response to a toxin; often can neutralize the toxin that stimulated its production.

Antiviral agent. Technically, any physical or chemical agent that inactivates viruses; in this book, the term is reserved for a drug used to treat viral diseases.

Arthralgia. Pain in a joint.

Arthropod-borne disease. A disease transmitted by an arthropod (usually an insect or an arachnid).

Artificial active acquired immunity. Active acquired immunity induced artificially (e.g., by a vaccine injection).

Artificial medium. A culture medium prepared in the laboratory; it does not occur naturally; also known as a *synthetic medium*.

Artificial passive acquired immunity. Passive acquired immunity induced artificially (e.g., by an antibody injection).

Ascites. Buildup of fluid in the abdominal cavity, leading to a distended or protuberant abdomen; common in chronic schistosomiasis caused by either *Schistosoma mansoni* or *S. japonicum*.

Asepsis. Literally, "without infection"; a condition in which living pathogens are absent.

Aseptate hypha. Hypha that possesses few or no cross walls (septa); if present, septa are irregularly produced; the cytoplasm within an aseptate hypha is multinucleated; also known as a *coenocytic hypha*.

Aseptic techniques. Measures taken to ensure that living pathogens are absent; see also *sterile techniques*.

Asymptomatic disease. A disease having no symptoms; also known as a *subclinical disease*.

Attenuated vaccine. A vaccine prepared from an attenuated (weakened) microbe.

Autoclave. An apparatus used for sterilization by steam under pressure.

Autogenous vaccine. A vaccine prepared from microorganisms or cells obtained from the person's own body.

Autoinfection. Self-infection with a particular pathogen, such as frequently occurs in children with pinworm infection and sometimes occurs in patients with strongyloidiasis.

Autolysis. Self-destruction of cells caused by enzymes produced within the cells.

Avirulent strain. A strain of an organism that is not virulent, not pathogenic, or not capable of causing disease.

B cell (B lymphocyte). The leukocyte that produces antibodies.

Bacillus (pl. *bacilli*). A rod-shaped bacterium; also, the bacterial genus *Bacillus*, which is composed of aerobic, Gram-positive, spore-forming bacilli.

Bacteremia. The presence of bacteria in the bloodstream.

Bactericidal agent. A chemical agent or drug that kills bacteria; also known as a *bactericide*.

Bacteriology. The study of bacteria.

Bacteriophage. A bacterial virus—that is, a virus that infects bacteria.

Bacteriostatic agent. A chemical agent or drug that inhibits the growth of bacteria.

Bacteriuria. The presence of bacteria in the urine.

Bartholinitis. Inflammation of the Bartholin ducts in females.

β-Hemolysis. Complete clearing of the blood agar medium surrounding a bacterial colony as a result of destruction of red blood cells in the medium; an organism that produces β-hemolysis is described as being *β-hemolytic*.

β-Lactam antibiotic. An antibiotic containing a β-lactam ring in its structure; also known as a *β-lactam*.

β-Lactam ring. One of the double-ringed structures found in penicillin and cephalosporin molecules.

β-Lactamase. An enzyme that destroys the β-lactam ring in β-lactam antibiotics; e.g., penicillinase, cephalosporinase.

Binary fission. A method of reproduction whereby one cell divides to become two cells; the method by which bacteria reproduce.

Biofilm. A complex and tenacious community of assorted bacteria; e.g., dental plaque, the slippery coating on a rock in a stream, the slime that accumulates on the inner walls of various types of pipes and tubing.

Biological vector. An arthropod, such as a flea or tick, capable of transmitting a pathogen and within which the pathogen multiplies and/or matures.

Biological warfare agent. A microorganism used specifically to harm people during wartime; also known as a *BW agent*.

Biosafety cabinet (BSC). An apparatus designed to protect people and the environment from pathogens; also used to protect specimens, cultures of microorganisms, or cell cultures from contamination.

Biosafety level (BSL or BL). There are four biosafety levels (BSL-1, BSL-2, BSL-3, BSL-4), based on the degree of hazard associated with particular pathogens.

Bioterrorism. The use of microorganisms to harm people during times other than wartime; also known as *biological terrorism*.

Bioterrorism agent. A microorganism used specifically to harm people during times other than wartime; a person using such an agent is called a *bioterrorist*.

Biotype. The pattern of biochemical test results obtained when such tests are performed on a bacterial isolate; whenever two strains of the same species produce the exact same biochemical test results, they are said to have the same biotype.

Biphasic system. A culture system consisting of both a liquid medium and a solid medium.

Blastoconidium or blastospore. Alternative terms for a yeast cell.

Blepharoplast. A small, darkly staining body located near the base of a flagellum; also known as a *basal body*.

Botulinal toxin. The neurotoxin produced by *Clostridium botulinum*; causes botulism.

Brightfield microscope. Alternative name for a compound light microscope; *brightfield* refers to the bright background or field against which objects are observed.

Broad-spectrum antibiotic. An antibiotic that is effective against a wide range of bacteria; it is effective against both Gram-positive and Gram-negative bacteria.

Bronchitis. Inflammation of the mucous membrane lining of the bronchial tubes.

Bronchopneumonia. The combination of bronchitis and pneumonia.

Brownian movement. The vibration of nonmotile objects that sometimes occurs during examination of a wet mount; heat from the microscope bulb causes water molecules to move about rapidly, striking the objects and causing them to vibrate.

Calabar swelling. The transient swelling associated with loiasis; also known as *fugitive swelling*.

Capnophile. An organism that grows best in the presence of increased concentrations of carbon dioxide; such an organism is said to be *capnophilic*.

Capsid. Part of the structure of a virion; the protein coat that surrounds the viral nucleic acid.

Capsomeres. The protein subunits that make up the capsid of an icosahedral virus.

Capsule. An organized layer of glycocalyx, firmly attached to the outer surface of a bacterial cell wall; some yeasts are also encapsulated.

Carbuncle. A deep-seated pyogenic (pus-producing) infection of the skin, usually arising from a coalescence of furuncles.

Carrier. A person having an asymptomatic infection that can be transmitted to other susceptible persons.

Catabolic reaction. A metabolic reaction that involves the breaking of chemical bonds and the release of energy; also known as a *degradative reaction*.

Catabolism. Refers to all the catabolic reactions that occur within a cell.

Catalase. An enzyme that causes the breakdown of hydrogen peroxide into water and oxygen; bacteria that produce catalase are said to be catalase positive, and those that do not are said to be catalase negative.

Cell culture. An in vitro culture technique using live cells in place of an artificial culture medium.

Cell-mediated immunity. A type of immunity in which many cell types (e.g., macrophages, various types of lymphocytes) are involved but antibodies play only a minor role, if any; also known as *delayed hypersensitivity*.

Cell membrane. The structure that forms the protoplasmic boundary of all cells, providing selective permeability and other important functions.

Cell wall. The outermost layer of many types of cells (e.g., algal, bacterial, fungal, and plant cells); it serves to protect the cell.

Cellulitis. Inflammation of subcutaneous, loose connective tissue.

Centers for Disease Control and Prevention (CDC). The federal public health agency within the Department of Health and Human Services with a mission to help prevent and control infectious diseases and environmental health threats, among other things; conduct research; work with states and other partners to provide a system for monitoring and preventing disease outbreaks (including bioterrorism); implement disease prevention strategies; maintain national health statistics; and guard against international disease transmission.

Cephalosporinase. An enzyme that destroys the β-lactam ring of cephalosporin antibiotics.

Cerebrospinal fluid (CSF). Fluid that fills cavities in the brain and spinal cord.

Cervicitis. Inflammation of the cervix (the part of the uterus that opens into the vagina).

Cestode. A type of parasitic flatworm in the class Cestoidea or Cestoda; also known as a *tapeworm*.

Chancre. A painless ulcerated lesion seen in primary syphilis.

Chemically defined medium. A type of culture medium in which the exact chemical composition is known.

Chemokine. A chemotactic agent produced by one of several types of cells in the body.

Chemotactic agent. A chemical substance that attracts leukocytes; also known as a *chemotactic factor*, *chemotactic substance*, or *chemoattractant*.

Chemotaxis. The movement of cells in response to a chemical (e.g., the attraction of phagocytes to an area of injury).

Chemotherapeutic agent. Any chemical used to treat any disease or medical condition.

Chemotherapy. The use of a chemical substance or drug to treat a disease, including an infectious disease.

"Chinese letter" arrangement. Clusters of bacteria that resemble Chinese letters.

Chitin. A complex polysaccharide found in the cell walls of fungi but not in the cell walls of other microorganisms; chitin is found in the exoskeleton of beetles and crabs.

Chromatin. The darkly staining, DNA-containing portion of the protozoan nucleus; a single, compact mass in some protozoa but fragmented in others.

Chromatoidal bar. A darkly staining inclusion found within the cytoplasm of some amebae; may be bar shaped, round, or splinter shaped; contains chromatin; also known as a *chromatoid body* or *chromatoid*.

Chromosomes. Cellular structures where most (sometimes all) of the cell's genes are located; eucaryotic chromosomes consist of linear double-stranded DNA molecules and proteins (histones and nonhistone proteins); a procaryotic chromosome usually consists of a single, long, supercoiled, circular, double-stranded DNA molecule.

Chronic disease. A disease having an insidious (slow) onset and a long duration.

Ciliates. Ciliated protozoa (i.e., protozoa that move by means of cilia); in the phylum Ciliophora.

Cilium (pl. *cilia*). A thin, usually short, hairlike organelle of motility; possessed by some eucaryotic cells.

Clean-catch midstream (CCMS) urine. The type of specimen appropriate for urine culture; *clean-catch* means that the area around the external opening of the urethra is cleansed prior to collection of urine; *midstream* means that urine is collected after the initial portion of the urine stream is directed into a toilet or bedpan.

CLIA '88. A U.S. federal regulation that mandates quality standards for laboratory testing, to include quality control, personnel, and proficiency testing standards for clinical laboratories; CLIA guidelines are based on test complexity; the more complicated the test, the more stringent the requirements.

Clinical and Laboratory Standards Institute (CLSI). Formerly the National Committee for Clinical Laboratory Standards (NCCLS). Organization that enhances the value of medical testing within the healthcare community through the development and dissemination of standards, guidelines, and best practices.

Clinical laboratory scientist (CLS). A laboratory professional possessing a bachelor's degree in clinical laboratory science (medical technology); also known as a *medical technologist (MT)*.

Clinical laboratory technician (CLT). Laboratory professional possessing an associate's degree in clinical laboratory technology (medical laboratory technology); also known as a *medical laboratory technician (MLT)*.

Clinically relevant results. Laboratory test results that provide useful information about a patient's infectious disease.

Clinical microbiology. The subdiscipline of microbiology associated with the diagnosis of human infectious diseases; also known as *diagnostic microbiology*.

Clinical microbiology laboratory (CML). A laboratory within a hospital, clinic, or other health care facility where microbiological procedures are performed on human clinical specimens to assist clinicians in the diagnoses of infectious diseases; procedures include isolation of pathogens from human clinical specimens, tests to identify or speciate pathogens, and tests to determine the susceptibility or resistance of pathogens; also known as the *diagnostic microbiology laboratory*.

Clinical specimens. The various types of specimens collected from patients and used to diagnose or follow the progress of infectious diseases, as well as other types of diseases.

Clinician. In this book, refers to a physician, physician's assistant, nurse practitioner, or any other health care professional who is authorized and licensed to make diagnoses, write prescriptions, and initiate appropriate therapy.

Clumping factor. A protein located on the surface of *Staphylococcus aureus* cells; it is capable of binding to fibrinogen but does not convert fibrinogen to fibrin; it is also known as *bound coagulase*.

Coagglutination. Technical term for the clumping that results from the combination of either red blood cells and bacteria or latex particles and bacteria.

Coagulase. A bacterial enzyme that causes plasma to clot; converts fibrinogen (a plasma protein) into fibrin; bacteria that produce coagulase are said to be coagulase-positive; those that are said to be coagulase-negative.

Coagulase-negative staphylococci (coagNS). *Staphylococcus* spp. that do not produce coagulase.

Coccobacillus (pl. *coccobacilli*). A very short bacillus.

Coccus (pl. *cocci*). A spherical bacterium.

Coliforms. Refers to lactose-fermenting members of the family Enterobacteriaceae, including *Escherichia coli*, *Enterobacter* spp., and *Klebsiella* spp.

Colitis. Inflammation of the colon (large intestine).

Collagenase. A bacterial enzyme that causes the breakdown of collagen.

Colonization. When a microbe has landed on or in the human body and has taken up residence there; the person is said to be *colonized* with that organism.

Colony. In terms of bacteria, a mound or pile of millions of bacterial cells.

Colostrum. The first milk secreted at the termination of pregnancy.

Communicable disease. A disease capable of being transmitted from person to person.

Community-acquired infection. An infection acquired outside a health care facility.

Complement. A protein complex of 25 to 30 components (including proteins designated C1 through C9) found in blood; involved in inflammation, chemotaxis, phagocytosis, and lysis of bacteria.

Complement cascade. The stepwise manner in which proteins of the complement system (complement components) interact with each other.

Complex medium. A culture medium, the exact chemical composition of which is unknown; often contains ground animal organs (e.g., brain, heart, liver) and/or yeast extract.

Compound light microscope. A compound microscope that uses visible light as its source of illumination.

Compound microscope. A microscope containing more than one magnifying lens.

Conjugate vaccine. A vaccine prepared by linking a weakly antigenic molecule (e.g., bacterial capsule material) to a powerful antigen.

Conjunctiva. The thin, tough lining that covers the inner wall of the eyelid and the sclera (the white of the eye).

Conjunctivitis. Inflammation of the conjunctiva.

Contagious disease. A disease easily transmitted from one person to another; a type of communicable disease.

Contaminant. An undesirable or accidentally introduced microorganism.

Convalescent period. The period in the course of an infectious disease cycle in which the patient is getting better (convalescing).

Coracidium. Microscopic, ciliated life cycle stage that emerges from a *Diphyllobothrium latum* egg.

Coryneform bacteria. Club-shaped bacteria.

Culture medium (pl. *culture media*). One of various types of nutrient-containing liquid and solid mixtures used in clinical microbiology laboratories to culture (grow) microorganisms.

Cyst. As the term applies to parasitology, the dormant, survival stage in the protozoal life cycle; its tough wall enables it to resist desiccation and temperature extremes; called an *oocyst* in some species of parasitic protozoa.

Cystitis. Inflammation of the urinary bladder.

Cytopathic effect (CPE). A particular type of morphologic alteration of, or damage to, cells in a cell culture, caused by the presence of a virus.

Cytoplasm. A type of protoplasm found in both procaryotic and eucaryotic cells.

Cytostome. A primitive mouth possessed by some protozoa through which they ingest "food" particles.

Cytotoxic T cells. T cells that kill other types of cells (e.g., foreign cells, virus-infected cells, cancer cells).

Darkfield microscope. A compound light microscope fitted with a darkfield condenser; *darkfield* refers to the dark background or field against which objects are observed.

Dead-end host. A host from which a parasite cannot continue its life cycle.

Deamination. Enzymatic removal of the amino end of an amino acid molecule.

Decarboxylation. Enzymatic removal of the carboxyl (acid) end of an amino acid molecule.

Decorticated. Refers to an *Ascaris* egg that has lost its mamillated outer coat.

Definitive host. In a parasitic relationship, the host that harbors the adult or sexual stage of a parasite, or the sexual phase of the parasite's life cycle.

Dematiaceous fungus. A fungus with dark hyphae, resulting in a dark or black mycelium.

Dental caries. Tooth decay or cavities.

Dermatitis. Inflammation of the skin.

Dermatophyte. One of a group of moulds that cause tinea (ringworm) infections; e.g., *Epidermophyton, Microsporum, Trichophyton* sp.

Dermis. The layer of skin containing blood and lymphatic vessels, nerves, and nerve endings, glands, and hair follicles.

Diarrhea. An abnormally frequent discharge of semisolid or fluid fecal matter.

Differential medium. A culture medium that enables microbiologists to readily differentiate between groups of organisms growing on the medium.

Differential staining procedure. A bacterial staining procedure that enables microbiologists to differentiate between two groups of stained bacteria; e.g., Gram staining, acid-fast staining.

Dimorphic fungus. A fungus capable of living as both a yeast and a mould.

Dimorphism. The ability to exist in two forms.

Diphtheria toxin. The exotoxin produced by *Corynebacterium diphtheriae* that causes diphtheria.

Diphtheroid. Bacteria that resemble *Corynebacterium diphtheriae* in appearance.

Diphtheroid-like. Having the appearance of *Corynebacterium diphtheriae* or diphtheroids; alternative terms are *diphtheroidal* or a *diphtheroid appearance*.

Diplobacilli. Bacilli arranged in pairs.

Diplococci. Cocci arranged in pairs.

Disinfectant. A chemical agent used to destroy pathogens or inhibit their growth and vital activity; usually refers to a chemical agent used on nonliving materials.

DNA vaccine. An experimental type of vaccine that stimulates host cells to produce numerous copies of a harmless microbial protein (antigen); the host's immune system then produces antibodies directed against the protein, and these antibodies protect the person from infection with the pathogen that possesses the protein; also known as a *gene vaccine*.

Drug binding site. A specific molecule on the surface of a cell to which a particular drug attaches.

Dysentery. Frequent watery stools accompanied by abdominal pain, fever, and dehydration; the stool specimens may contain blood and/or mucus.

Dysphagia. Difficulty swallowing.

Ectoparasite. A parasite that lives on the external surface of its host.

Ectothrix infection. A fungal infection of hair shafts in which fungal spores are located on the outside of the shafts.

Edema. Swelling caused by an accumulation of watery fluid in cells, tissues, or body cavities; the swollen areas are described as being *edematous*.

Electron micrograph. A photograph taken through the lens system of an electron microscope; e.g., transmission electron micrograph, scanning electron micrograph.

Electron microscope. A type of microscope that uses electrons as a source of illumination.

Elementary body (EB). One of the two stages in the developmental cycle of chlamydiae; an EB is metabolically inactive, infectious, and capable of surviving in an extracellular environment.

Elephantiasis. Enlargement of a lower limb or the genitalia, usually caused by long-standing obstruction of lymphatic vessels; most commonly the result of many years of infection with a filarial worm.

Empirical therapy. Treatment or therapy initiated by a clinician before receipt of test results.

Empty magnification. An increase in magnification without any concurrent increase in resolving power.

Encephalitis. Inflammation of the brain.

Encephalomyelitis. Inflammation of the brain and spinal cord.

Endemic disease. A disease that is always present in a particular community or geographic area.

Endocarditis. Inflammation of the endocardium—the endothelial membrane that lines the cavities of the heart.

Endocytosis. A general term for ingestion of material from outside the cell; phagocytosis is a type of endocytosis.

Endoenzyme. An enzyme produced by a cell that remains within the cell; an intracellular enzyme.

Endoflagella. Flagella that lie between the cell membrane and an outer membrane of the cell; endoflagella connect to both ends of the cell, resulting in both corkscrew and oscillating movements of the cell.

Endogenous anaerobe. An anaerobe that originates from within the body.

Endogenous microbe. A microbe that originates from within the body.

Endometritis. Inflammation of the endometrium (the inner layer of the uterine wall).

Endoparasite. A parasite that lives within the body of its host.

Endoplasmic reticulum (ER). A network of membranous tubules and flattened sacs in the cytoplasm of a eucaryotic cell; ER with attached ribosomes is called rough ER (RER) or granular ER; ER having no attached ribosomes is called smooth ER (SER).

Endospore. Thick-walled, resistant body formed within a bacterial cell for the purpose of survival; a bacterial cell produces only one endospore, and from that endospore emerges (by a process known as germination) one bacterial cell; also known as a *bacterial spore*.

Endothrix infection. A fungal infection of hair shafts, in which fungal spores are located on the inside of the shafts; there is no conspicuous external sheath of spores.

Endotoxin. The lipid portion of the lipopolysaccharide found in the cell walls of Gram-negative bacteria; an intracellular toxin.

Enriched medium. A culture medium that enable microbiologists to isolate fastidious organisms from samples or specimens and grow them in the laboratory.

Enrichment medium. A liquid medium (broth) containing specific nutrients that encourage growth of a particular organism.

Enteritis. Inflammation of the intestines, usually referring to the small intestine.

Enterotoxin. A bacterial exotoxin specific for cells of the intestinal mucosa.

Enterovirulent *E. coli*. Certain serotypes of *Escherichia coli* that are always pathogenic.

Enveloped virus. A virion having an outer covering called an envelope, which is derived from either the nuclear membrane or cell membrane of the host cell.

Enzyme. A biological catalyst; a protein molecule that causes a biochemical reaction to occur or speeds it up; the enzyme itself remains unchanged in the process.

Epidemic disease. A disease occurring in a higher-than-usual number of cases in a particular population during a given time interval.

Epidemiology. The study of factors that determine the frequency, distribution, and determinants of diseases in human populations.

Epidermis. The superficial epithelial portion of the skin.

Epididymitis. Inflammation of the epididymis (an elongated structure connected to the testis).

Epiglottitis. Inflammation of the epiglottis (the mouth of the windpipe).

Erysipelas. A disease characterized by hot, red, edematous, cutaneous eruptions, usually accompanied by severe constitutional symptoms; caused by *Streptococcus pyogenes*.

Erysipeloid. A cutaneous infection with purplish red bumps (usually located on the hands and fingers) and less commonly, septicemia, endocarditis, and arthritis; caused by *Erysipelothrix rhusiopathiae*.

Erythema. Redness of the skin; a reddened area of skin is described as being *erythematous*.

Erythema migrans. A raised red ring with advancing firm borders and central clearing; in Lyme disease, the characteristic skin lesion that radiates from the site of a tick bite; also known as *erythema chronicum migrans*.

Erythrocyte. A red blood cell.

Erythrogenic toxin. The exotoxin produced by *Streptococcus pyogenes* that causes scarlet fever; *erythrogenic* means "produces redness," referring to the red rash of scarlet fever.

Etiologic agent. The pathogen that causes a particular infectious disease; the causative agent.

Eucaryote. An organism that is eucaryotic, meaning that its cells contain a true nucleus; can also be spelled *eukaryote*.

Eumycetoma. A mycetoma caused by a true fungus.

Exfoliatin. An exotoxin produced by some strains of *Staphylococcus aureus*; causes a serious skin condition known as staphylococcal scalded skin syndrome (SSSS); also known as *exfoliative toxin*.

Exoenzyme. An enzyme produced by a cell that is released from the cell; an extracellular enzyme.

Exogenous anaerobe. An anaerobe that originates from outside the body (i.e., from the external environment).

Exogenous microbe. A microbe that originates from outside the body (i.e., from the external environment).

Exotoxin. A toxin that is released from the cell that produced it; an extracellular toxin.

Facultative anaerobe. An organism that can live in either the presence or absence of oxygen.

Facultative intracellular pathogen. A pathogen that can live either intracellularly or extracellularly.

Facultative parasite. An organism that can be a parasite but is also capable of a free-living existence.

Fasciae (sing. *fascia***).** The fibrous tissue that envelops the body beneath the skin and encloses muscles or groups of muscles.

Fasciitis. Inflammation of the fasciae.

Fastidious pathogen. A microorganism difficult to isolate from a specimen and grow in the laboratory because of complex nutritional requirements or other factors.

Favic infection. A fungal infection of hair shafts, in which hyphae, air bubbles, tunnels, and fat droplets occur within the shafts.

Fermentative pathway. A biochemical pathway that does not involve oxygen.

Fermenter. In the oxidation-fermentation (O-F) test, an organism that uses a particular substrate via a fermentative pathway.

Filarial worms. Long, thin roundworms that cause diseases such as filariasis, loiasis, and onchocerciasis.

Filariform larva. The mature, infective larva of hookworms and *Strongyloides* spp.

Final report. The last report furnished by the laboratory, pertaining to a particular specimen.

Fixed macrophage. A macrophage that remains localized within certain organs and tissues; also known as a *histocyte* or *histiocyte*.

Flagellate. A flagellated protozoan (i.e., a protozoan that moves by means of flagella).

Flagellum (pl. *flagella***).** Whiplike organelle of motility; procaryotic and eucaryotic flagella differ in structure; the procaryotic flagellum is composed of a protein called *flagellin*; the eucaryotic flagellum is composed of nine doublet microtubules arranged around two central microtubules (called a 9 + 2 arrangement).

Fleshy fungus. A large fungus that grows outdoors; e.g., mushroom, toadstool, puffball, bracket fungus.

Fluorescence microscope. A type of compound light microscope that employs an ultraviolet light source.

Folliculitis. Inflammation of a hair follicle, the sac that contains a hair shaft.

Fomite. Any inanimate object capable of transmitting a pathogen; e.g., patients' clothing, bed linen, towel, eating utensil.

"Fried egg" colony. A colony that resembles a sunny-side-up fried egg; it has an opaque granular center surrounded by a flat translucent zone.

Fungemia. The presence of fungi in the bloodstream.

Fungicidal agent. A chemical agent or drug that kills fungi; also known as a *fungicide* or *mycocide*.

Furuncle. A localized pyogenic infection of the skin, usually resulting from folliculitis; also known as a *boil*.

Fusiform. An adjective that refers to a shape that is long, thin, and tapered at the ends; sometimes called spindle shape; fusiform bacteria include *Fusobacterium* spp., *Bacteroides gracilis, B. forsythus,* and microaerophilic *Capnocytophaga* spp.

Gametocyte. A sexual stage in the malarial parasite's life cycle; within an *Anopheles* mosquito's stomach, macrogametocytes (female gametocytes) develop into a female gamete, and microgametocytes (male gametocytes) produce male gametes.

γ-Hemolysis. No observable effect on the blood agar surrounding a bacterial colony; a synonym for nonhemolytic; an organism that produces γ-hemolysis is described as being *γ-hemolytic*.

Gangrene. Tissue necrosis (death) resulting from local anemia (ischemia).

Gas gangrene. A type of gangrene that is always caused by *Clostridium* spp.; *gas* refers to gaseous byproducts—primarily hydrogen and nitrogen—of the clostridial metabolism that accumulate in necrotic tissues.

Gastritis. Inflammation of the mucosal lining of the stomach.

Gastroenteritis. Inflammation of the mucosal linings of the stomach and intestines.

Gene. A functional unit of heredity that occupies a specific space (locus) on a chromosome; contains the genetic information that enables a cell to produce a protein (usually), an rRNA molecule, or a tRNA molecule.

Gene product. The molecule (usually a protein) coded for by a gene.

Generation time. The time required for a cell to split into two cells; also known as the *doubling time*.

Genotype. The complete genetic constitution of an organism (i.e., all of that organism's genes); also known as the *genome*.

Genus (pl. *genera*). The first part in the name of a species; e.g., *Escherichia* in *Escherichia coli*.

Gingivitis. Inflammation of the gingiva (gums).

Glycocalyx. Extracellular polysaccharide material that may or may not be firmly attached to the outer surface of the cell wall; e.g., capsule, slime layer.

Golgi apparatus. A membranous system located within the cytoplasm of a eucaryotic cell; associated with the transport and packaging of secretory proteins; also known as the *Golgi complex* or *Golgi body*.

Gonococcemia. The presence of *Neisseria gonorrhoeae* in the bloodstream.

Gonococci (GC; sing. *gonococcus*). Slang term referring to *Neisseria gonorrhoeae*.

Granulocyte. A type of leukocyte with prominent cytoplasmic granules; e.g., neutrophil, eosinophil, basophil.

Granuloma. A nodular, inflammatory lesion, containing various types of phagocytic cells.

HACEK group. Fastidious Gram-negative bacteria grouped together because they can all be found as indigenous microflora of the oral cavity and can cause a particular type of endocarditis; HACEK stands for *Haemophilus*, *Actinobacillus*, *Cardiobacterium*, *Eikenella*, and *Kingella*.

Hantavirus pulmonary syndrome (HPS). A respiratory disease caused by several hantaviruses.

Hapten. A small, nonantigenic molecule that becomes antigenic when combined with a larger molecule (e.g., a carrier protein).

Health care epidemiology. Activities designed to study and/or improve patient care outcomes in any type of health care institution or setting.

Helical virus. A virus having a helical capsid (a capsid having a helical symmetry).

Helminth. A parasitic worm.

Helper T cell. A type of T cell that, among other things, assists B cells in the production of antibodies.

Hemagglutination. The agglutination or clumping together of red blood cells.

Hematogenous dissemination. Dissemination of something by way of the bloodstream; a term often used when discussing how pathogens are distributed throughout the body.

Hemoflagellate. A flagellated protozoan found in the blood; e.g., *Trypanosoma* sp.

Hemolysin. A bacterial enzyme capable of lysing erythrocytes.

Hemolysis. Usually refers to the destruction of red blood cells; an organism that produces hemolysis is said to be *hemolytic*.

Hemoptysis. Spitting of blood.

Hepatitis. Inflammation of the liver.

Hermaphroditic. Refers to an organism possessing both male and female reproductive organs and capable of self-fertilization.

High-efficiency particulate (HEPA) filter. A filter that very efficiently removes particles from the air.

Hospital outbreak or epidemic. An outbreak of infection occurring within a hospital setting; an outbreak is defined as an increase in the infection rate beyond the expected or usual rate during a defined period.

Host. In a parasitic relationship, the organism on or in which a parasite lives.

Host defense mechanism. A mechanism that serves to protect the body from pathogens and the infections they cause.

Humoral immunity. A type of immunity in which antibodies play a major role; also known as *antibody-mediated immunity (AMI)*.

Hyaline fungus. A fungus that produces colorless or transparent hyphae.

Hyalohyphomycosis. An infection caused by a hyaline fungus.

Hyaluronidase. A bacterial enzyme that breaks down hyaluronic acid; sometimes called *diffusing* or *spreading factor* because it enables bacteria to invade deeper into tissue.

Hybridoma. A tumor produced in vitro by fusion of mouse tumor cells and specific antibody-producing cells; used in the production of monoclonal antibodies.

Hypha (pl. *hyphae*). A long, thin, intertwined, cytoplasmic filament, many of which make up a fungal mycelium.

Hypogammaglobulinemia. Decreased quantity of the γ-fraction of serum globulin, including a decreased quantity of immunoglobulins.

Iatrogenic infection. An infection that results from medical or surgical treatment; therefore, an infection caused by a surgeon, other physician, or other health care worker.

Icosahedral virus. A virus with an icosahedral capsid (a capsid with an icosahedral symmetry).

Immune. Free from the possibility of acquiring a particular infectious disease; to be resistant to an infectious disease.

Immunity. The status of being immune or resistant to an infectious disease.

Immunocompetent. Refers to a person who is able to mount a normal immune response; a person whose immune system is functioning properly.

Immunodiagnostic procedure (IDP). A laboratory procedure used to diagnose an infectious disease by using the principles of immunology; IDPs are used to detect either antigen or antibody in patients' specimens.

Immunoglobulin. A class of glycoproteins containing antibodies.

Immunology. The study of immunity and the immune system.

Immunosuppressed. Refers to a person whose immune system is not functioning properly; such persons are also said to be *immunodepressed* or *immunocompromised*.

IMViC reactions. The reactions from four tests represented by the letters in the acronym: the *I* stands for indole, *M* for methyl red, *V* for Voges-Proskauer, and *C* for citrate; the lowercase *i* has no meaning; used to differentiate *Escherichia coli* from other lactose-fermenting members of the family Enterobacteriaceae.

In vitro. In an artificial environment, such as a laboratory setting; used in reference to what occurs *outside* an organism.

In vivo. Used in reference to what occurs *within* a living organism.

Inactivated vaccine. A vaccine prepared from inactivated (killed) microorganisms.

Inclusion body. A cluster of viruses or viral remnants within a host cell; an inclusion body may either be within the host cell's nucleus (a nuclear or intranuclear inclusion body) or within its cytoplasm (a cytoplasmic or intracytoplasmic inclusion body).

Incubation. In microbiology, refers to holding a culture at a particular temperature for a certain length of time.

Incubation period. The period in the course of an infectious disease between time of entry of the pathogen into the body and the time the patient first experiences symptoms.

Incubator. In microbiology, the chamber within which cultures are held at a particular temperature for a certain length of time.

Indigenous microflora. Microorganisms that live on and in the healthy body; also known as *indigenous microbiota* or *normal flora*.

Infection control. The numerous measures taken to prevent infections from occurring in health care settings.

Infection control committee. A hospital committee primarily responsible for preventing, monitoring, and controlling the spread of infections in the facility.

Infection control professional. Person who is knowledgeable about infection control and responsible for enforcing the hospital's infection control policy; may be an epidemiologist, infectious disease specialist, infection control nurse, or microbiologist.

Infectious disease. Any disease that is caused by a microorganism and follows colonization of the body by that microorganism.

Inflammation. A nonspecific pathologic process consisting of a dynamic complex of cytologic and histologic reactions that occur in response to an injury or abnormal stimulation by a physical, chemical, or biological agent.

Inflammatory exudate. An accumulation of fluid, cells, and cellular debris at a site of inflammation.

Inoculation. In microbiology, refers to adding a specimen to some type of culture medium.

Interferon. A small antiviral glycoprotein produced by a cell infected with an animal virus; an interferon is cell and species specific but not virus specific.

Intermediate host. In a parasitic relationship, the host that harbors the larval or asexual stage of a parasite, or the asexual phase of the parasite's life cycle.

Intraerythrocytic pathogen. A pathogen that lives within erythrocytes; e.g., *Plasmodium* sp., *Babesia* sp.

Intraleukocytic pathogen. A pathogen that lives within leukocytes, e.g., *Ehrlichia* sp.

Intrinsic resistance. As the term applies to bacteria, the resistance to a particular drug that is the result of some naturally occurring property of the bacterial cell.

Ischemia. Local anemia that results from an obstruction, loss, or reduction of blood supply and leads to a lack of oxygen.

Jaundice. Yellowish pigmenting of the skin, eyes, deeper tissues, and excretions resulting from the presence of bile pigments.

Karyosome. A mass of chromatin found within protozoal nuclei; the nucleus of a given protozoan may contain one or more karyosomes.

Keratitis. Inflammation of the cornea of the eye.

Keratoconjunctivitis. Inflammation of both the cornea and the conjunctiva.

Kinase. A bacterial enzyme capable of dissolving clots; also known as *fibrinolysin*.

Kinetoplast. The darkly staining part of a large DNA-containing mitochondrion found in the cytoplasm of certain protozoa (e.g., *Leishmania* sp., *Trypanosoma* sp.); located adjacent to the basal body or blepharoplast at the base of a flagellum.

Koplik spot. A small red spot that may appear in the mouth of a measles patient; under a strong light, a minute bluish-white speck can be seen in the center of the spot.

Laboratory diagnosis of infectious diseases. In this book, refers to the various laboratory test results that, when received and evaluated by clinicians, help them to correctly diagnose infectious diseases and initiate appropriate therapy.

Lactose fermenter (LF). An organism that ferments lactose.

Laryngitis. Inflammation of the mucous membrane of the larynx (voice box).

Latent infection. An asymptomatic infection capable of manifesting symptoms under particular circumstances or if activated.

Lawn of growth. Refers to a microorganism that is growing over the entire surface of the agar.

Lecithinase. A bacterial enzyme capable of breaking down lecithin (a name given to several types of phospholipids that are essential constituents of animal and plant cells).

Leishman-Donovan body. An intracellular amastigote observed in a stained smear from the bone marrow, spleen, liver, lymph node, or blood of a patient with visceral leishmaniasis.

Leukemia. A type of cancer characterized by the proliferation of abnormal leukocytes in the blood.

Leukocidin. A bacterial exotoxin capable of destroying leukocytes.

Leukocytes. White blood cells.

Localized infection. An infection that remains localized (i.e., does not spread); also known as a *local infection* or *focal infection*.

Lophotrichous bacterium. A bacterium that possesses two or more flagella at one end (pole) of the cell.

Lymphadenitis. Inflamed and swollen lymph nodes.

Lymphadenopathy. Diseased lymph nodes.

Lymphangitis. Inflamed lymphatic vessels.

Lysosome. A membrane-bound vesicle in the cytoplasm of a eucaryotic cell; contains a variety of digestive enzymes, including lysozyme.

Macroconidium (pl. *macroconidia*). In fungi, the larger of two distinctly different-sized types of conidia in a particular species; may be thick or thin walled and composed of anywhere from 2 to 10 cells.

Macrophage. A large phagocytic leukocyte that arises from a monocyte.

Malaise. A feeling of general discomfort, uneasiness, or extreme fatigue; feeling "out of sorts."

Mamillated. Refers to the thick, bumpy, nipple-like projections on the outer surface of an *Ascaris* egg.

Material safety data sheet (MSDS). A form required by the Occupational Safety and Health Administration (OSHA) containing important safety information about a particular chemical.

Mechanical vector. An arthropod, such as a housefly, capable of transmitting a pathogen by merely transporting it from point A to point B. The pathogen neither multiplies nor matures in the process.

Medical bacteriology. The study of bacteria that cause human diseases.

Medical mycology. The study of fungi that cause human diseases.

Medical parasitology. The study of parasites that cause human diseases.

Medical virology. The study of viruses that cause human diseases.

Meninges. The membranes that surround the brain and spinal cord.

Meningitis. Inflammation of the meninges.

Meningococcal meningitis. Meningitis caused by *Neisseria meningitidis*.

Meningococcemia. A type of septicemia in which the bloodstream contains meningococci (*Neisseria meningitidis*).

Meningococcus (pl. *meningococci*). Slang term for *Neisseria meningitidis*.

Meningoencephalitis. Inflammation of the brain and meninges.

Merozoite. A stage in the malarial parasite's life cycle; merozoites are produced within intraerythrocytic schizonts and schizonts located within liver cells (hepatocytes); within red blood cells, merozoites develop into trophozoites.

Metabolic reaction. Chemical reaction that occurs within cells; may be either catabolic or anabolic.

Metabolism. The sum of all the chemical reactions occurring in a cell; consists of anabolism and catabolism.

Methicillin-resistant *Staphylococcus aureus* (MRSA). A strain of *S. aureus* that is resistant to the usually prescribed dosages of methicillin and other penicillinase-resistant penicillins.

Methicillin-resistant *Staphylococcus epidermidis* (MRSE). A strain of *S. epidermidis* that is resistant to the usually prescribed dosages of methicillin and other penicillinase-resistant penicillins.

Microaerophile. An organism that requires an environment with only about 5% oxygen, roughly one-fourth the oxygen found in air; such an organism is said to be *microaerophilic*.

Microbial intoxication. A disease that results from ingestion of a toxin produced by a pathogen in vitro (outside the body).

Microbiology. The study of microbes (acellular microbes and microorganisms).

Microconidium (pl. *microconidia*). In fungi, the smaller of two distinctly different-sized conidia in a particular species; usually single celled and spherical, ovoid, pyriform (pear shaped), or clavate (club shaped).

Microfilaria (pl. *microfilariae*). The tiny, prelarval stage of filarial worms; if it has retained the egg membrane, it is called a *sheathed microfilaria*; if it has not retained the egg membrane, it is called an *unsheathed microfilaria*.

Micrometer. A metric unit of length equal to one-millionth of a meter and one-thousandth of a millimeter.

Microorganism. A microbe composed of cells; e.g., bacterium, archaean, microscopic alga, protozoan, microscopic fungus (yeast, mould); also known as a *cellular microbe*.

Minimum bactericidal concentration (MBC). The lowest concentration of a drug that kills 99.9% of the organisms tested.

Minimum inhibitory concentration (MIC). The lowest concentration of a drug that inhibits visible growth of the organism tested.

Minisystem. A miniaturized biochemical test system; often used to speciate microorganisms isolated from clinical specimens.

Miracidium. Microscopic, ciliated life cycle stage that emerges from the eggs of *Schistosoma* spp. and other trematodes.

Mitochondrion (pl. *mitochondria*). The eucaryotic organelle involved in cellular respiration for the production of energy; the "energy factory" of the cell.

Molecular diagnostic procedure (MDP). A method of diagnosing an infectious disease using genotypic methods; by discovering a particular pathogen's DNA or RNA in the patient's specimen.

Molecular epidemiology. The use of genotypic typing methods, such as genotyping of plasmid and/or chromosomal DNA, to characterize a bacterial isolate and prove that two isolates are the same strain; e.g., if two isolates of *Escherichia coli* have exactly the same genotype (i.e., possess exactly the same genes), they are the same strain.

Monoclonal antibodies. Antibodies produced by a clone of genetically identical hybrid cells; often used in immunodiagnostic procedures.

Monotrichous bacterium. A bacterium with only one flagellum.

Morula (pl. *morulae*). As used in this chapter, refers to a microscopic colony of a few to more than 40 *Ehrlichia* cells within a vacuole in the cytoplasm of a host cell.

Myalgia. Muscular pain.

Mycelium (pl. *mycelia*). A mould colony.

Mycetoma. A chronic infection involving subcutaneous tissue, skin, and contiguous bone; characterized by the formation of localized lesions with tumefactions (swellings) and multiple draining sinuses; the exudate contains granules, the color of which depends on the causative agent.

Mycology. The study of fungi.

Mycosis (pl. *mycoses*). A fungal infection.

Mycotoxicosis (pl. *mycotoxicoses*). A disease caused by a mycotoxin.

Mycotoxin. A toxin produced by a fungus.

Myelitis. Inflammation of the spinal cord.

Myocarditis. Inflammation of the myocardium—the muscular walls of the heart.

Nanometer. A metric unit of length, equal to one-billionth of a meter and one-thousandth of a micrometer.

Narrow-spectrum antibiotic. An antibiotic that is only effective against a narrow range of bacteria; e.g., it is effective only against certain Gram-positive bacteria or against certain Gram-negative bacteria.

National Fire Protection Association (NFPA). Organization whose mission is to reduce the worldwide burden of fire and other hazards on the quality of life by providing and advocating consensus codes and standards, research, training, and education.

Natural active acquired immunity. Active acquired immunity that is acquired naturally (e.g., by being infected with a particular pathogen).

Natural passive acquired immunity. Passive acquired immunity that is acquired in a natural manner (e.g., when a fetus receives the mother's antibodies in utero).

Necrotizing enzyme. An enzyme that destroys tissue.

Nemathelminthes. Phylum of roundworms containing the parasitic roundworms of humans; also known as the phylum *Nematoda* or *nematodes*.

Nephritis. Inflammation of the kidneys.

Neuritis. Inflammation of a nerve.

Neurotoxin. A bacterial exotoxin that attacks the nervous system.

Neutrophil. A type of granulocyte found in blood; its granules contain neutral substances that attract neither acidic nor basic dyes; also known as a *polymorphonuclear cell*, *poly*, or *PMN*.

Non-acid-fast bacterium. A bacterium that loses the red color of carbolfuchsin dye during the decolorization step of the acid-fast staining procedure; i.e., it becomes decolorized.

Noncommunicable disease. A disease that is not transmitted from person to person; e.g., tetanus, botulism, gas gangrene.

Nonfermenter. An organism lacking the ability to ferment any sugars.

Non–lactose fermenter (NLF). An organism that does not ferment lactose; also known as a *lactose nonfermenter*.

Nonoxidizer. In the oxidation-fermentation (O-F) test, an organism that cannot utilize a particular substrate.

Nonpathogen. A microorganism that does not cause disease; the organism is said to be *nonpathogenic*.

Nonphotochromogen. A *Mycobacterium* sp. that produces nonpigmented colonies whether grown in the presence or absence of light.

Nonspecific host defense mechanisms. Host defense mechanisms directed against all types of invading pathogens and other foreign substances.

Nonsterile site. An anatomical site inhabited by indigenous microflora.

Nonsterile specimen. A clinical specimen collected from a nonsterile site.

Nontuberculous mycobacteria (NTM). *Mycobacterium* spp. that are not part of the *Mycobacterium tuberculosis* complex; they can cause diseases other than tuberculosis; also known as *mycobacteria other than tuberculosis (MOTT)*.

Nosocomial infection. Any infection a patient acquires while in the hospital or some other health care facility; also known as a *hospital-acquired infection*.

Nuclear membrane. The membrane that surrounds the nucleus of a eucaryotic cell.

Nucleocapsid. Viral nucleic acid plus the protein coat (capsid) that surrounds it.

Nucleolus. A dense portion of the nucleus of a eucaryotic cell; where ribosomal RNA (rRNA) is produced.

Nucleoplasm. The gelatinous matrix or base material of the nucleus in which chromosomes arc cmbcddcd or suspended; like cytoplasm, nucleoplasm is a type of protoplasm.

Nucleus, pl., *nuclei*. An organelle containing nucleoplasm and chromosomes; found in eucaryotic cells but not in procaryotic cells.

Obligate aerobe. An organism that requires 20% to 21% oxygen (the concentration of oxygen found in air) to survive.

Obligate anaerobe. An organism that cannot survive in an atmosphere containing oxygen.

Obligate intracellular pathogen. A pathogen that must reside within another living cell; e.g., virus, *Chlamydia* sp., *Rickettsia* sp.

Obligate parasite. An organism that can only exist as a parasite; incapable of a free-living existence.

Occupational Safety and Health Administration (OSHA). Federal agency whose mission is to assure the safety and health of Amcrica's workers by setting and enforcing standards; providing training, outreach, and education; establishing partnerships; and encouraging continual improvement in workplace safety and health.

Octad. A packet of eight cocci.

Ocular micrometer. A tiny ruler located within the eyepiece (ocular) of the compound light microscope.

Oncogenic. Cancer causing; synonym for *oncogenous*.

Oncogenic virus. A cancer-causing virus; also known as an *oncovirus*.

Oncosphere. A spherical embryo that can be seen in certain cestode eggs (e.g., *Echinococcus* sp., *Hymenolepis* sp., *Taenia* sp.)

Oocyst. A life cycle stage of certain sporozoan parasites (e.g., *Cryptosporidium* sp., *Cyclospora* sp.), within which sporozoites are produced.

Oophoritis. Inflammation of an ovary.

Operculum. The cover, similar to a lid or cap, that a cestode or trematode egg might have and through which the larva escapes from the egg.

Ophthalmia neonatorum. Gonococcal conjunctivitis in a neonate (newborn).

Opportunistic pathogen. A microbe that could cause disease but does not do so under ordinary circumstances; e.g., may cause disease in susceptible persons with lowered resistance; also known as an *opportunist*.

Opsonin. A substance (such as an antibody or complement fragment) that enhances phagocytosis.

Opsonization. The process by which bacteria (or other particles) are altered to enable phagocytes to engulf them more readily and efficiently; often involves coating the bacteria with antibodies and/or complement fragments.

Orchitis. Inflammation of the testis.

Organelle. General term for any of the various and diverse structures contained within a eucaryotic cell (e.g., mitochondrion, Golgi apparatus, nucleus, endoplasmic reticulum, lysosome).

Oropharyngitis. Inflammation of the oral portion of the throat.

Otitis externa. Infection of the outer ear canal.

Otitis media. Infection of the middle ear.

Oxidase. An abbreviation of *cytochrome oxidase*, an enzyme that participates in the electron transport chain; a bacterium that produces oxidase is termed *oxidase positive*, and one that does not is *oxidase negative*.

Oxidative pathway. A biochemical pathway in which oxygen participates.

Oxidizer. In the oxidation-fermentation (O-F) test, an organism that uses a particular substrate via an oxidative pathway.

Palisade arrangement. Bacteria lined up side by side; also known as a *picket fence arrangement*.

Pandemic disease. A disease occurring in epidemic proportions in several to many countries, sometimes worldwide.

Parasite. An organism that lives on or in another living organism (called the host) and derives benefit from the host (usually in the form of nutrients).

Parasitemia. The presence of parasites in the bloodstream.

Parasitism. A symbiotic relationship that is beneficial to one party (the parasite) and detrimental to the other party (the host).

Parasitologist. A person specializing in the science of parasitology.

Parasitology. The study of parasites.

Paroxysm. A sudden onset of symptoms (e.g., chills and fever in malaria).

Passive acquired immunity. Immunity or resistance acquired as a result of receipt of antibodies produced by another person or by an animal.

Pathogen. Disease-causing microbe; such a microbe is said to be *pathogenic*.

Pathogenesis. The steps or mechanisms involved in the development of a disease.

Pathogenicity. The ability to cause disease.

Pathologist. A physician with extensive, specialized training in pathology.

Pathology. The study of disease, especially structural and functional changes that result from disease processes.

Pelvic inflammatory disease (PID). Inflammation of female pelvic structures (e.g., endometrium, uterine tube, pelvic peritoneum).

Penicillinase. An enzyme that destroys the β-lactam ring in penicillin antibiotics.

Perfect fungus. A fungus with both a sexual form (referred to either as the perfect state or the teleomorph) and an asexual form (known as the imperfect state or the anamorph).

Pericarditis. Inflammation of the pericardium—the fibrous sac within which the heart is encased.

Periodontitis. Inflammation of the periodontium—tissues that surround and support the teeth, including the gingiva and supporting bone.

Peritrichous bacterium. A bacterium that possesses flagella over its entire surface.

Personal protective equipment (PPE). Items for personal protection; e.g., gloves, gowns, lab coats, face shields, goggles, respirators.

Phaeohyphomycosis. An infection caused by a dematiaceous fungus.

Phagocyte. A cell capable of ingesting bacteria, yeasts, and other particulate matter; e.g., ameba, certain white blood cells.

Phagocytosis. Ingestion of particulate matter involving the use of pseudopodia to surround the particle.

Phagolysosome. A membrane-bound vesicle formed by the fusion of a phagosome and a lysosome; found in phagocytic cells.

Phagosome. A membrane-bound vesicle containing an ingested particle (e.g., a bacterial cell); found in phagocytic cells.

Pharyngitis. Inflammation of the mucous membrane and underlying tissue of the pharynx; commonly called a *sore throat*.

Phase contrast microscope. A type of compound light microscope that can be used to observe unstained living microorganisms.

Phenotype. Manifestation of a genotype; all of the traits, attributes, or characteristics of an organism.

Phialide (pl. *phialides*). In fungi, a conidia-producing cell; conidia are extruded out to form chains.

Photochromogen. A *Mycobacterium* sp. that produces pigmented colonies only in the presence of light.

Photomicrograph. A photograph taken through the lens system of a compound light microscope.

Phycology. The study of algae; also known as *algology*.

Pilus (pl. *pili*). A hairlike surface projection possessed by some bacteria (called *piliated bacteria*); most pili are organelles of attachment; also known as a *fimbria* (pl. *fimbriae*).

Plasma cell. A differentiated B cell capable of secreting antibodies.

Plasmid. An extrachromosomal genetic element; a molecule of DNA that can function and replicate while physically separate from the bacterial chromosome.

Plastid. A membrane-bound organelle containing photosynthetic pigment; the site of photosynthesis; a *chloroplast* is a plastid containing chlorophyll.

Platyhelminthes. Phylum of flatworms containing the parasitic cestodes and trematodes.

Pleomorphism. Existing in more than one form; also known as *polymorphism*; an organism that exhibits pleomorphism is said to be *pleomorphic*.

PMN. Acronym for *polymorphonuclear leukocyte*, a type of granulocyte; one of the two major phagocytic cells in the body; also known as a *neutrophil* or *poly*.

Pneumococcal pneumonia. Pneumonia caused by *Streptococcus pneumoniae*.

Pneumococcus (pl. *pneumococci*). Slang term for *Streptococcus pneumoniae*.

Pneumonia. Inflammation of one or both lungs.

Polymerase chain reaction (PCR). An amplification procedure that uses the enzyme DNA polymerase to make many copies of existing segments of DNA.

Polymicrobial infection. An infection caused by the combined actions of two or more microorganisms; e.g., trench mouth, bacterial vaginosis; also known as a *synergistic infection*.

PRAS medium. A prereduced, anaerobically sterilized culture medium.

Preliminary report. Any report furnished by the laboratory before publication of the final report.

Primary disease. The initial disease; often creates the conditions that lead to a secondary disease; if the primary disease is an infection, it is called the *primary infection*.

Primary response. The immune response that occurs the first time an antigen enters a person's body.

Primary setup. The various media inoculated with a particular type of clinical specimen.

Prions. Infectious protein molecules; i.e., proteins capable of causing certain diseases of animals and humans.

Probiotics. The use of live microorganisms, such as various *Lactobacillus* spp., in the treatment of certain diseases.

Procaryote. An organism with cells that do not contain a true nucleus; can also be spelled *prokaryotic*; such an organism is said to be *procaryotic*.

Proctitis. Inflammation of the mucous lining of the rectum.

Prodromal period. The period in the course of an infectious disease just before the period of illness; during the prodromal period, the patient feels "out of sorts," as if "coming down with something."

Professional phagocytes. Refers to the two most important phagocytic cells in the body: neutrophils and macrophages.

Proglottid. A tapeworm segment; proglottids containing eggs are called *gravid proglottids*.

Prostatitis. Inflammation of the prostate.

Protective antibodies. Antibodies that protect a person from infection or reinfection.

Protists. Members of the Kingdom Protista; includes algae and protozoa.

Protomers. The identical protein subunits that make up the capsid of a helical virus.

Protoplasm. The semifluid matter within living cells; *cytoplasm* and *nucleoplasm* are two types of protoplasm.

Protozoology. The study of protozoa.

Pseudohypha (pl. *pseudohyphae*). A chain of elongated buds; resembles and is sometimes mistaken for a hypha.

Pseudomonicidal agent. A drug or disinfectant that kills *Pseudomonas* spp. (pseudomonads).

Pure culture. When an organism has been isolated/separated from other organisms and is growing alone.

Purulent exudate. A thick, greenish-yellow exudate that contains many live and dead leukocytes; also known as *pus*.

Pyelonephritis. Inflammation of the renal parenchyma (the basic cellular tissue of the kidney).

Pyocyanin. A blue, water-soluble, diffusible pigment produced by *Pseudomonas aeruginosa*; when pyocyanin combines with pyoverdin, the characteristic greenish or blue-green color of *P. aeruginosa* is produced.

Pyogenic. Pus producing; causing the production of pus.

Pyogenic microorganisms. Pathogens that cause pus-containing infectious processes.

Pyoverdin. A fluorescent, yellow-green or yellow-brown pigment produced by some *Pseudomonas* spp., which are called the *fluorescent group of pseudomonads.*

Quality assurance (QA) program. A program within a health care facility that attempts to continuously identify, monitor, evaluate, and improve the reliability and efficiency of every aspect of patient care in the institution; also known as a *quality assessment program.*

Quality control (QC) organism. An organism maintained in a laboratory for use in quality control procedures; usually an organism known to give positive or negative test results.

Quality control (QC) program. A laboratory program designed to monitor the accuracy, reliability, and reproducibility of all tests performed and to identify and correct any problems that exist; it is an integral part of a health care facility's QA program.

Reaginic antibody. An antibody produced in response to lipoidal material released from damaged host cells and possibly also in response to lipoprotein-like material and cardiolipin released from treponemes; produced in response to a treponemal infection, autoimmune disease, pregnancy, or other condition causing tissue damage; also known as a *reagin.*

Receptor. A molecule on the surface of a host cell that a particular pathogen is able to recognize and attach to; also known as an *integrin.*

Reservoir of infection. A place where a pathogen lives and from which it can be transmitted to humans; a reservoir of infection may be living or nonliving; also known as simply a *reservoir.*

Resistance factor (R factor). A plasmid containing more than one drug resistance gene; a bacterium that possesses an R factor is multidrug resistant; it is a "superbug."

Resolving power. The ability of the eye or any other optical instrument to distinguish detail, such as the separation of closely adjacent objects; also known as *resolution.*

Reticulate body (RB). One of the two stages in the developmental cycle of chlamydiae; reticulate bodies are metabolically active, noninfectious, and incapable of surviving in extracellular environments.

Reticuloendothelial system (RES). A collection of phagocytic cells that includes macrophages and cells that line the sinusoids of the spleen, lymph nodes, and bone marrow.

Rhabditiform larva. The immature, noninfective larva of hookworms and *Strongyloides* spp.

Ribosome. An organelle that is the site of protein synthesis in both procaryotic and eucaryotic cells.

Ringworm. A tinea infection; caused by a dermatophyte.

Salpingitis. Inflammation of the uterine tube.

Scanning electron micrograph. A photograph taken through the lens system of a scanning electron microscope.

Scanning electron microscope. A type of electron microscope that enables the operator to observe the outer surface of a specimen (i.e., to observe surface detail).

Schizont. A stage in the malaria parasite's life cycle, within which merozoites are produced; schizonts are produced within liver cells and red blood cells.

Scolex (pl. *scolices*). The head or anterior end of a tapeworm; if it possesses hooks, it is called an *armed scolex*; an *unarmed scolex* has no hooks.

Scotochromogen. A *Mycobacterium* sp. that produces pigment in either the presence or absence of light.

Sebaceous glands. Glands in the dermis that usually open into hair follicles and secrete an oily substance known as *sebum.*

Sebum. See *sebaceous glands.*

Secondary disease. A disease that follows an initial disease; if the secondary disease is an infection, it is called a *secondary infection.*

Secondary response. The immune response that occurs the second time an antigen enters a person's body; also known as a *memory response* or *anamnestic response.*

Selective medium. A culture medium that allows a certain organism or group of organisms to grow while inhibiting growth of all other organisms.

Semisynthetic antibiotic. An antibiotic that has been chemically altered, usually to increase its spectrum of activity.

Sepsis. The presence of pathogens and/or their toxins in the bloodstream; often used as a synonym for *septicemia.*

Septate hypha. A hypha that possesses cross walls (septa); the cytoplasm within a septate hypha is divided into cells.

Septic shock. A type of shock resulting from sepsis or septicemia.

Septicemia. A systemic disease characterized by chills, fever, prostration (extreme fatigue), and the presence of bacteria and/or their toxins in the bloodstream.

Sequela (pl. *sequelae*). A complication that develops in the course of, or as a result of, a disease.

Serovars. Serovars of a particular species differ from each other primarily as a result of differences in surface antigens; sometimes, as in the case of *Chlamydia trachomatis* and *Escherichia coli*, different serovars of a particular species cause different diseases; the terms *serotypes* and *serovars* are synonyms.

Severe acute respiratory syndrome (SARS). A disease caused by the SARS-associated coronavirus (SARS-CoV).

Shock. A sudden, often severe, physical and/or mental disturbance, usually resulting from low blood pressure and a lack of oxygen in organs.

Signs of a disease. Abnormalities indicative of disease that are discovered on examination of a patient; objective findings; e.g., abnormal lab results; abnormal heart or breath sounds; lumps; abnormalities revealed by radiograph, computerized tomography, magnetic resonance imaging, electrocardiogram, ultrasound.

Simple microscope. A microscope containing only one magnifying lens.

Simple staining procedure. The use of a single dye to stain objects (e.g., bacterial cells), enabling scientists to gain information about the objects (e.g., size, shape, morphological arrangement).

Sinusitis. Inflammation of the lining of one or more of the paranasal sinuses.

Slime layer. An unorganized, loosely attached layer of glycocalyx surrounding a bacterial cell.

Species (pl. *species*). A member of a genus; e.g., *Escherichia coli* is a species in the genus *Escherichia*; the name of a species consists of two parts: the generic name and the specific epithet; singular *species* is abbreviated *sp.*, and plural *species* is abbreviated *spp.*

Specific epithet. The second part of the name of a species; e.g., *coli* in *Escherichia coli*; the specific epithet cannot be used alone.

Specific host defense mechanisms. Defense mechanisms that the host directs against a specific invading pathogen; synonym for the *immune system* or the *third line of defense*.

Sporadic disease. A disease that occurs occasionally, usually affecting only one person; neither endemic nor epidemic.

Sporangiospore. An asexual spore produced within a saclike structure known as a *sporangium* (pl. *sporangia*).

Spore. A thick-walled, resistant body formed by bacteria (for survival) and fungi (for reproduction).

Sporicidal agent. A chemical agent that kills bacterial spores (endospores); also known as a *sporicide*.

Sporozoan. Parasitic protozoan that does not possess pseudopodia, flagella, or cilia; classified in the phylum Sporozoa.

Sporozoite. The stage in the malaria parasite's life cycle that is introduced into humans when an infected *Anopheles* mosquito takes a blood meal; sporozoites are produced within oocysts attached to the outer wall of the mosquito's stomach; having nothing to do with malaria, sporozoites are also produced within the oocysts of *Cryptosporidium* and *Cyclospora* spp.

Sporulation. Production of spores.

Sputum. The pus that accumulates deep within the lungs of a patient with pneumonia, tuberculosis, or other lower respiratory tract infection.

Standard precautions. Safety measures taken by health care workers to protect themselves and their patients from infection; these precautions are taken for *all* patients and *all* patient specimens (body substances); includes precautions previously termed *universal precautions* or *universal body substance precautions*.

Staphylocoagulase. Coagulase enzyme produced by *Staphylococcus aureus* that is not bound to the surface of the cells; also known as *free coagulase*.

Staphylococci. Cocci arranged in clusters, as in the genus *Staphylococcus.*

Staphylokinase. An enzyme produced by some strains of *Staphylococcus aureus* that dissolves fibrin clots.

Sterile. Free of all living microorganisms, including spores.

Sterile site. An anatomic site that does not harbor indigenous microflora; e.g., blood, cerebrospinal fluid.

Sterile techniques. Techniques used in an attempt to create an environment that is sterile (devoid of microorganisms).

Sterilization. The destruction of *all* microorganisms in or on something (e.g., on surgical instruments).

Streptobacilli. Bacilli arranged in chains of varying lengths.

Streptococci. Cocci arranged in chains, as in the genus *Streptococcus.*

Structural staining procedure. A staining procedure used to stain a particular bacterial structure, such as capsules, flagella, and endospores.

Sty (or **stye**). Inflammation of a sebaceous gland that opens into a follicle of an eyelash.

Subacute disease. A disease that comes on more suddenly than a chronic disease but less suddenly than an acute disease; subacute diseases are usually of moderate duration.

Substrate. The chemical substance that an enzyme acts on or alters.

Subunit vaccine. A vaccine that uses antigenic (antibody-stimulating) portions of a pathogen, rather than using the whole pathogen; also known as an *acellular vaccine*.

Superbug. A multidrug-resistant microorganism; the term is usually used in reference to multidrug-resistant bacteria.

Superinfection. An overgrowth or "population explosion" of one or more pathogens, often pathogens that are resistant to an antimicrobial agent that a patient is receiving.

Symptomatic disease. A disease in which the patient experiences symptoms; also known as a clinical disease.

Symptoms of a disease. Indications of disease that are experienced by the patient; subjective; e.g., aches, pains, chills, blurred vision, nausea.

Synergism. When two or more drugs work together to accomplish a cure rate that is greater than either drug could accomplish by itself; also known as *synergy*.

Systemic infection. An infection that has spread throughout the body; also known as a *generalized infection*.

Taxon (pl. *taxa*). A group in taxonomy; the usual taxa are kingdom, phylum (or division), class, order, family, genus, species, and subspecies.

Taxonomy. The systematic classification of living organisms.

T cell (T lymphocyte). A type of leukocyte that plays several important roles in the immune system.

T-dependent antigen. An antigen that requires T helper cells for its processing in the body.

Tetanospasmin. The neurotoxin produced by *Clostridium tetani*; causes tetanus.

Tetrad. A packet of four cocci.

Thermophilic. Literally "heat-loving"; an organism that prefers to live at high temperatures is said to be *thermophilic*.

Thrush. An oral infection caused by the yeast *Candida albicans*.

T-independent antigen. An antigen that does not require T helper cells for its processing in the body.

Toxemia. The presence of toxins in the bloodstream.

Toxin. In this book, refers to a poisonous substance produced by a microorganism.

Toxoid. A toxin altered in such a way as to destroy its toxicity but retain its antigenicity; certain toxoids are used as vaccines.

Toxoid vaccine. A vaccine prepared from a toxoid.

Transferrin. A glycoprotein synthesized in the liver and used to store iron and deliver it to host cells.

Transmission electron micrograph. A photograph taken through the lens system of a transmission electron microscope.

Transmission electron microscope. A type of electron microscope in which electrons are transmitted through very thin sections of specimens; enables the operator to observe internal detail.

Trematode. A type of parasitic flatworm in the class Digenea or Trematoda; also known as a *fluke*.

Trophozoite. The motile, feeding, dividing stage in the protozoal life cycle.

Trypomastigote. A flagellated form of hemoflagellates such as *Trypanosoma brucei* and *Trypanosoma cruzi*.

Tuberculocidal agent. A chemical or drug that kills the bacterium that causes tuberculosis (*Mycobacterium tuberculosis*); also known as a *tuberculocide*.

Twitching motility. The ability of some nonflagellated bacteria to "crawl" over a solid surface because of the presence of pili or fimbriae, which apparently act like grappling hooks.

Ureteritis. Inflammation of the ureter.

Urethritis. Inflammation of the urethra.

Urinary tract infection (UTI). An infection of any of the organs that comprise the urinary tract.

Vaccine. Any preparation that, following injection (or ingestion, in some cases), produces active acquired immunity.

Vaginitis. Inflammation of the vagina.

Vaginosis. A noninflammatory infection of the vagina; bacterial vaginosis (usually referred to as BV) is a synergistic infection, caused by a mixture of different bacteria.

Vancomycin-intermediate *Staphylococcus aureus* (VISA). A strain of *S. aureus* that is resistant to the usually prescribed dosages of vancomycin.

Vancomycin-resistant enterococcus (VRE). An *Enterococcus* sp. that is resistant to the usually prescribed dosages of vancomycin.

Vancomycin-resistant *Staphylococcus aureus* (VRSA). A strain of *S. aureus* that is resistant to higher than usually prescribed dosages of vancomycin.

Vasodilation. An increase in the diameter of blood vessels.

Vectors. In this book, refers to invertebrate animals (e.g., ticks, mites, mosquitoes, fleas) capable of transmitting pathogens among vertebrates.

Vegetative hypha. A hypha that lies beneath the surface that a fungal mycelium is growing on.

V factor. Nicotinamide adenine dinucleotide (NAD), a coenzyme.

Viral load. The quantity of a virus in the bloodstream.

Viremia. The presence of viruses in the bloodstream.

Viricidal agent. A chemical or drug that inactivates a virus, rendering it noninfectious; can also be spelled *virucidal agent*; also known as a *viricide* or *virucide*.

Viridans group streptococci (VGS). α-Hemolytic streptococci other than *S. pneumoniae*; members of the indigenous microflora; occasionally involved in serious infections; also known as *oral streptococci*.

Virion. A complete viral particle; i.e., one that has all its components.

Virology. The branch of science concerned with the study of viruses.

Virulence. A measure of pathogenicity (i.e., some pathogens are more or less *virulent* than others).

Virulence factors. Attributes or properties of a microorganism that contribute to its virulence or pathogenicity (e.g., certain exoenzymes and toxins produced by pathogenic bacteria).

Virulent strain. A strain that is pathogenic (i.e., capable of causing disease).

Vulvovaginitis. Inflammation of the vulva (the external genitalia of females) and the vagina.

Wandering macrophage. A macrophage that migrates in the bloodstream and tissues; also known as a *free macrophage*.

Wet mount. A method of observing microorganisms in which an unstained liquid suspension of a clinical specimen or organism removed from a colony is examined under the microscope.

World Health Organization (WHO). The United Nations' specialized agency for health whose mission is the attainment by all peoples of the highest possible level of health (complete physical, mental, and social well-being).

Worm burden. Refers to the number of worms that are infecting the patient; symptoms associated with a particular helminth infection often depend upon the worm burden.

X factor. Another name for hemin, a chloride of heme (the oxygen-carrying group of hemoglobin).

Xenodiagnosis. A method of diagnosing American trypanosomiasis (Chagas disease) in which noninfected triatomic bugs are allowed to take blood meals from a patient suspected of having the disease.

Zone of no growth. In disk diffusion antimicrobial susceptibility testing, the area around an antimicrobial agent–containing disk where the organism tested is not growing; also known as a *zone of inhibition* or *zone of inhibition of growth*.

Zoonosis (pl. *zoonoses*). An infectious disease that is transmissible from an animal to a human; also known as a *zoonotic disease*.

Zygomycosis. A disease caused by one of the many fungi in the class Zygomycetes (e.g., bread moulds); older terms for this disease are *mucormycosis* and *phycomycosis*.

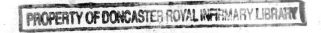

Index

Page numbers in *italics* denote figures; those followed by a t denote tables.